Streptococcus pneumoniae

Molecular Biology & Mechanisms of Disease

Streptococcus pneumoniae

Molecular Biology & Mechanisms of Disease

Editor

Alexander Tomasz, Ph.D.
Laboratory of Microbiology
The Rockefeller University
New York, New York

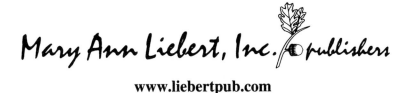

www.liebertpub.com

Library of Congress Cataloging-in-Publication Data

Streptococcus pneumoniae: molecular biology & mechanisms of disease/editor, Alexander Tomasz.
    p. cm.
    Based on a workshop held Sept. 23–29, 1996, in Portugal.
    Includes bibliographical references and index.
    ISBN 0–91311–385–9
    1. Streptococcus pneumoniae—Congresses. 2. Pneumonia—Congresses. I. Tomasz, Alexander.
    [DNLM: 1. Streptococcus pneumoniae—genetics—Congresses. 2. Streptococcus pneumoniae—
pathogenicity—Congresses. 3. Drug Resistance, Microbial—Congresses. 4. Pneumococcal
Infections—drug therapy—Congresses. 5. Pneumococcal Infections—physiopathology—Congresses.
QW 142.5.C6 S9153 1999]
QR201.S7 S77 1999
616′.01455 21—dc21
                                                99-043059

Background and Purpose of this Book

Concern over pneumococcal disease, particularly in the forms caused by antibiotic-resistant and multidrug-resistant strains, has been frequently expressed in recent medical literature and in the public media. *Streptococcus pneumoniae* has remained a major human pathogen with an estimated annual worldwide mortality of several million, in the same range as that of tuberculosis. Antibiotic-resistant strains of this bacterium have recently achieved worldwide spread, posing serious challenges to chemotherapy.

Streptococcus pneumoniae has also remained a major model organism for studies on the mechanism of pathogenesis and on the molecular and cell biology of a gram-positive bacterium.

It was last in 1981 that a Workshop of Pneumococcal Disease was held, in Santa Inez, California, sponsored by the Kroc Foundation. That Workshop, the contributions of which were published in an issue of *Reviews of Infectious Diseases* in 1981, is still considered by many colleagues in the field as a watershed meeting, remaining an important resource of information.

Since that time an enormous amount of information on all aspects of pneumococcal microbiology and disease has accumulated. In order to provide an updated overview of this large body of new information and also to exchange views on new strategies for intervention with pneumococcal disease, an International Workshop was held from September 23–29, 1996 in Portugal ("*Streptococcus pneumoniae*: Molecular Biology and Mechanisms of Disease—Update for the 1990s"). The Workshop brought together key experts—50 scientists from over 12 countries—in the molecular biology of this bacterium, and also experts on various aspects of pneumococcal disease.

It was the general consensus of the participants that reproduction in book form of the contributions to the meeting will provide a timely update and useful resource for information. Contributors to the book were encouraged to follow a free format, providing either a technically-detailed documentation of their topic or a more general overview of their field.

Alexander Tomasz, Ph.D.
Editor

Contents

Contributors

Piet C. Aerts
Eijkman-Winkler Institute for Microbiology,
  Infectious Diseases & Inflammation
Utrecht University Medical Center
Utrecht University Hospital
Room G04.614
Heidelberglaan 100
3584 CX Utrecht
The Netherlands

Peter William Andrew
Professor
Department of Microbiology & Immunology
University of Leicester
P.O. Box 138
University Road
Leicester LE1 9HN
United Kingdom

Carlos Arrecubieta
Research Scientist
Departamento de Microbiologia Molecular
Consejo Superior de Investigaciones
  Científicas (CSIC)
Velázquez 144
28006 Madrid
Spain

Robert Austrian
Professor and Chairman Emeritus
Department of Molecular & Cellular
  Engineering
University of Pennsylvania
School of Medicine
552 Johnson Pavilion
Philadelphia, PA 19104-6088

Richard H. Baltz
Consultant
Dow AgroSciences
9330 Zionsville Road
Indianapolis, IN 46268

Kimberly A. Benton
ORISE Fellow
Center for Biologics Evaluation and Research
U.S. Food and Drug Administration
1401 Rockville Pike
HFM 521
Rockville, MD 20852

Anne Marie Berry
Senior Research Officer
Women's and Children's Hospital
72 King William Road
North Adelaide, SA 5006
Australia

Helmut Brade
Professor
Research Center Borstel
Center for Medicine and Biosciences
Parkallee 37
D-23845 Borstel
Germany

Lara E. Braverman
Research Associate
Eli Lilly and Company
Lilly Corporate Center
D.C. 3322
Indianapolis, IN 46285

Robert F. Breiman
Centers for Disease Control and Prevention
Atlanta, GA 30333

David E. Briles
Professor of Microbiology
Department of Microbiology
University of Alabama at Birmingham
845 19th Street South
Room 658
Birmingham, AL 35294

Alexis Brooks-Walter
University of Alabama at Birmingham
845 19th Street South
BBRB 670, Box 10
Birmingham, AL 35294

Stanley Burgett
Associate Scientist
Eli Lilly and Company
Lilly Corporate Center
Indianapolis, IN 46285

Jay C. Butler
Director, Arctic Investigations Program
Centers for Disease Control and Prevention
4055 Tudor Centre Drive
Anchorage, AK 99508

Carmen Cabellos
Attending Physician
Infectious Diseases Department
Ciutat Sanitària i Universitària de Bellvitge
Feixa Llarga s/n
08907 L'Hospitalet de Llobregat
Barcelona
Spain

Melissa J. Caimano
Postdoctoral Fellow
University of Connecticut Health Center
Center for Microbial Pathogenesis
263 Farmington Avenue
Farmington, CT 06030-3710

Jean-Pierre Claverys
Directeur de Recherche
Centre National de la Recherche Scientifique
   (CNRS)
Laboratoire de Microbiologie et Génétique
   Moléculaire CNRS-UPR 9007
Université Paul Sabatier
118, route de Narbonne
31062 Toulouse Cedex 04
France

Marilyn J. Crain
Associate Professor of Pediatrics
Department of Pediatrics
Division of Infectious Diseases
University of Alabama at Birmingham
School of Medicine
1616 Sixth Avenue South
Suite 204
Birmingham, AL 35294-0011

Ronald de Groot
Professor of Pediatrics
Chief of the Division of Pediatric Infectious
   Diseases and Immunology
Sophia Children's Hospital
Dr. Molewaterplein 60
3015 GJ Rotterdam
The Netherlands

Adela Gonzalez De La Campa
Cientifico Titular del CSIC Consejo Superior
   de Investigaciones Científicas (CSIC)
Unidad de Genética Bacteriana
Centro Nacional de Biología Fundamental
Instituto de Salud Carlos III
28220 Majadahonda, Madrid
Spain

Herminia de Lencastre
Unidade de Genética Molecular
Instituto de Tecnologia Química e
Biológica da Universidade Nova de Lisboa
   (ITQB/UNL)
Oeiras
Portugal

Bradley S. DeHoff
Associate Senior Microbiologist
Eli Lilly and Company
Lilly Corporate Center
Indianapolis, IN 46285

M. Angeles Domínguez
Microbiologist
Department of Microbiology
Ciutat Sanitària i Universitària de Bellvitge
Feixa Llarga s/n
08907 L'Hospitalet de Llobregat
Barcelona
Spain

Christopher G. Dowson
Reader in Microbiology
Department of Biological Sciences
University of Warwick
Coventry CV4 7AL
United Kingdom

Roman Dziarski
Northwest Center for Medical Education
Indiana University
3400 Broadway
Gary, IN 46408

Volker El-Samalouti
Laboratorium für Klinische Forschung GmbH
Lise-Meitner-Strasse 25-29
24223 Raisdorf
Germany

Mark C. Enright
Research Fellow
Department of Zoology
The Wellcome Trust Centre for the
*   Epidemiology of Infectious Disease*
University of Oxford
South Parks Road
Oxford, Oxfordshire OX1 3FY
United Kingdom

Asunción Fenoll
Chief, Pneumococcal Reference Laboratory
Centro Nacional de Microbiología
Instituto de Salud Carlos III
28220 Majadahonda, Madrid
Spain

Werner Fischer
Professor of Biochemistry
Institute of Biochemistry
Medical Faculty
University Erlangen-Nürnberg
Fahrstrasse 17
D-91054 Erlangen
Germany

Hans-Dieter Flad
Professor
Research Center Borstel
Center for Medicine and Biosciences
Parkallee 22
D-23845 Borstel
Germany

Ernesto García
Professor
Departamento de Microbiologia Molecular
Consejo Superior de Investigaciones Científicas
*   (CSIC)*
Velázquez 144
28006 Madrid
Spain

José L. García
Senior Researcher
Department of Molecular Microbiology
Centro de Investigaciones Biológicas
Consejo Superior de Investigaciones Científicas
*   (CSIC)*
Velázquez 144
28006 Madrid
Spain

Pedro García
Assistant Professor
Centro de Investigaciones Biológicas
Consejo Superior de Investigaciones Científicas
*   (CSIC)*
Velázquez 144
28006 Madrid
Spain

Anne-Marie Gasc
Ingenieur de Recherche
Centre National de la Recherche Scientifique
*   (CNRS)*
Laboratoire de Microbiologie et Génétique
*   Moléculaire*
118, route de Narbonne
31062 Toulouse Cedex 04
France

Pierre Geslin
Centre National de Références des
*   Pneumocoques*
CHU
40, avenue de Créteil
94010 Créteil
France

Philippe Giammarinaro
Laboratoire de Microbiologie et Génétique
*   Moléculaire*
Centre National de la Recherche Scientifique
*   (CNRS)*
Université Paul Sabatier
118, route de Narbonne
31062 Toulouse Cedex 04
France

G. Scott Giebink
Professor
Departments of Pediatrics & Otolaryngology
University of Minnesota
School of Medicine
Box 296
420 Delaware Street SE
Minneapolis, MN 55455

Robert J.C. Gilbert
Division of Structural Biology
University of Oxford
Wellcome Trust Centre for Human Genetics
Roosevelt Drive
Headington, Oxford OX3 7BN
United Kingdom

Francesc Gudiol
Professor of Medicine, Head of Infectious
  Diseases
Hospital de Bellvitge
University of Barcelona
Feixa Llarga s/n
08907 L'Hospitalet de Llobregat
Barcelona
Spain

Dipika Gupta
Assistant Professor of Biochemistry and
  Molecular Biology
Northwest Center for Medical Education
Indiana University
3400 Broadway
Gary, IN 46408

Regine Hakenbeck
Professor of Microbiology
Department of Microbiology
University of Kaiserslautern
Paul Ehrlichstrasse 23
D-67663 Kaiserslautern
Germany

Gail G. Hardy
Postdoctoral Research Associate
Department of Molecular Microbiology
Washington University School of Medicine
Room 864, Box 8230
4566 Scott Avenue
St. Louis, MO 63110

Jørgen Henrichsen
Head of Department
Statens Serum Institut
Artillerivej 5
DK 2300 Copenhagen S
Denmark

Peter W.M. Hermans
Laboratory of Pediatrics
Erasmus University Rotterdam
P.O. Box 1738, Room EE 15-02
3000 DR Rotterdam
The Netherlands

Ann Hermansson
Associate Professor
Department of ENT
University Hospital of Lund
SE-221 85 Lund
Sweden

Susan K. Hollingshead
Research Associate Professor
Department of Microbiology
University of Alabama at Birmingham
845 19th Street South
BBRB 654
Birmingham, AL 35294

J. Hoskins
Eli Lilly and Company
Lilly Corporate Center
Indianapolis, IN 46285

Margaret K. Hostetter
Professor of Pediatrics
Yale University
School of Medicine
464 Congress Ave.
New Haven, CT 06519-1313

Odile Humbert
Postdoctoral Researcher
Institut de Pharmacologie et Biologie
  Structurale
Centre National de la Recherche Scientifique
  (CNRS)
205, route de Narbonne
31077 Toulouse Cedex
France

Edward N. Janoff
Professor of Medicine
Minneapolis VA Medical Center
University of Minnesota
School of Medicine
One Veterans Drive
Minneapolis, MN 55417

I. Jenkins
Eli Lilly and Company
Lilly Corporate Center
Indianapolis, IN 46285

Johannis P. Kamerling
Professor of Organic Chemistry of Natural
  Products
Department of Bio-Organic Chemistry
Bijvoet Center
Utrecht University
P.O. Box 80.075
3508 TB Utrecht
The Netherlands

Kristina Kaminski
Max Planck Institut für Molekulare Genetik
Ihnestrasse 73
14195 Berlin
Germany

David L. Klein
Bacterial Respiratory Disease Program Officer
National Institutes of Health/National Institute
  of Allergy and Infectious Diseases
6700-B Rockledge Drive
Room 3130
Bethesda, MD 20892

Keith P. Klugman
Professor and Chairman
School of Pathology
Director
South African Institute for Medical Research
Hospital Street
Hillbrow
Johannesburg 2000
South Africa

Andrea König
Max Planck Institut für Molekulare Genetik
Ihnestrasse 73
14135 Berlin
Germany

Karl G. Kristinsson
Department of Microbiology
National University Hospital
V/Baronstig
121 Reykjavik
Iceland

Shoichi Kusumoto
Faculty of Science
Department of Chemistry
Osaka University
Toyonaka 560, Osaka
Japan

Sanford A. Lacks
Senior Geneticist
Biology Department
Brookhaven National Laboratory
Upton, NY 11973-5000

Josefina Liñares
Head of Antibiotic Laboratory
Department of Microbiology
Ciutat Sanitària i Universitària de Bellvitge
Feixa Llarga s/n
08907 L'Hospitalet de Llobregat
Barcelona
Spain

Robert Arthur Lock
Royal Perth Hospital Medical Research
  Foundation
Perth, Western Australia 6000
Australia

Rubens López
Professor
Centro de Investigaciones Biológicas
Consejo Superior de Investigaciones Científicas
  (CSIC)
Velázquez 144
28006 Madrid
Spain

Ana C. Martín
Research Scientist
Departamento de Microbiologia Molecular
Consejo Superior de Investigaciones Científicas
  (CSIC)
Velázquez 144
28006 Madrid
Spain

Bernard Martin
Maître de Conférences
Centre National de la Recherche Scientifique
  (CNRS)
Laboratoire de Microbiologie et Génétique
  Moléculaire CNRS-UPR 9007
Université Paul Sabatier
118, route de Narbonne
31062 Toulouse Cedex 04
France

H. Robert Masure
Director of Research and Development
JESE, Genomic Search Engines
12617 Juniper Circle
Leawood, KS 66209

Patti J. Matsushima
Associate Senior Microbiologist
Eli Lilly and Company
Lilly Corporate Center
D.C. 0428
Indianapolis, IN 46285

Taila Mattern
Assistant Professor for Immunology
Universitätsklinikum Essen
Forschergruppe Shock and Multiple Organ
  Failure
Hufelandstrasse 55
D-45122 Essen
Germany

Larry S. McDaniel
Associate Professor of Microbiology and
  Surgery
University of Mississippi
Medical Center
2500 North State Street
Jackson, MS 39216

Lesley McGee
MRC/WITS/Pneumococcal Diseases Research
  Unit
Department of Clinical Microbiology and
  Infectious Diseases
South African Institute for Medical Research
P.O. Box 1038
Johannesburg 2000
South Africa

M.A. McHenney
Eli Lilly and Company
Lilly Corporate Center
Indianapolis, IN 46285

Francisco Javier Medrano
Research Assistant
Centro de Investigaciones Biológicas
Consejo Superior de Investigaciones Científicas
  (CSIC)
Velázquez 144
28006 Madrid
Spain

Åsa Melhus
Department of Medical Microbiology
Malmö University Hospital
Malmö S-205 02
Sweden

Timothy J. Mitchell
Professor
Division of Infection and Immunity
Institute of Biomedical and Life Sciences
Joseph Black Building
University of Glasgow
Glasgow G12 8QQ
United Kingdom

Marta Mollerach
Research Scientist
Departamento de Microbiologia
Facultad de Farmacia y Bioquímica
Universidad de Buenos Aires
Junin 956
1113 Buenos Aires
Argentina

Pete Morgan
Group Leader, Protein Purification and
  Characterization
Murex Biotech Limited
Central Road
Dartford, Kent DA1 5LR
United Kingdom

Judy K. Morona
Research Officer
Molecular Microbiology Unit
Women's and Children's Hospital
72 King William Road
North Adelaide, SA 5006
Australia

Renato Morona
Department of Microbiology and Immunology
The University of Adelaide
Adelaide, South Australia 5005
Australia

Donald A. Morrison
Professor
Laboratory for Molecular Biology
Department of Biological Sciences
University of Illinois at Chicago
900 South Ashland Avenue
Chicago, IL 60607

Isabelle Mortier-Barriere
Ph.D. Student
Centre National de la Recherche Scientifique
  (CNRS)
Laboratoire de Microbiologie et Génétique
  Moléculaire CNRS-UPR 9007
Université Paul Sabatier
118, route de Narbonne
31062 Toulouse Cedex 04
France

Rosarío Muñoz
Research Scientist
Departamento de Microbiologia Molecular
Consejo Superior de Investigaciones
  Científicas (CSIC)
Velázquez 144
28006 Madrid
Spain

Daniel M. Musher
Head of Infectious Diseases
Professor of Medicine
Professor of Microbiology & Immunology
Baylor College of Medicine
VA Hospital
2002 Holcombe Blvd.
Houston, TX 77030

Susanne Vinther Nielsen
Statens Serum Institut
Artillerivej 5
DK 2300 Copenhagen S
Denmark

Fred H. Norris
Eli Lilly and Company
Lilly Corporate Center
Indianapolis, IN 46285

Karin Overweg
Department of Pediatrics
Erasmus Medical Center Rotterdam
P.O. Box 1738
3000 DR Rotterdam
The Netherlands

Johanna Paik
Postdoctoral Research Fellow
Imperial Cancer Research Fund
Clare Hall Laboratories
Blanche Lane
South Mimms, Potters Bar
Hertfordshire EN6 3LD
United Kingdom

Roman Pallares
Professor, Consultant Physician
Hospital Bellvitge and
University of Barcelona
08907 L'Hospitalet de Llobregat
Barcelona
Spain

James C. Paton
Associate Professor
Molecular Microbiology Unit
Women's and Children's Hospital
72 King William Road
North Adelaide, SA 5006
Australia

R. Peery
Eli Lilly and Company
Lilly Corporate Center
Indianapolis, IN 46285

Andrew Paul Pickerill
Experimentalist
Zeneca Agrochemicals
Jealotts Hill Research Station
Bracknell RG42 6ET
United Kingdom

Gina Porter
Senior Technician
Eli Lilly and Company
Lilly Corporate Center
D.C. 0424
Indianapolis, IN 46285

Karin Prellner
Medical Director
Department of Otorhinolaryngology, Head and
 Neck Surgery
University Hospital of Lund
SE-221 85 Lund
Sweden

Marc Prudhomme
Maître de Conférences
Centre National de la Recherche Scientifique
 (CNRS)
Laboratoire de Microbiologie et Génétique
 Moléculaire CNRS-UPR 9007
Université Paul Sabatier
118, route de Narbonne
31062 Toulouse Cedex 04
France

Peter Reichmann
Scientist
Department of Microbiology
University of Kaiserslautern
Paul Ehrlichstrasse 23
D-67663 Kaiserslautern
Germany

Ernst Theodor Rietschel
Director
Research Center Borstel
Center for Medicine and Biosciences
Parkallee 22
D-23845 Borstel
Germany

Pamela Rockey
Associate Scientist
Eli Lilly and Company
Lilly Corporate Center
Indianapolis, IN 46285

Paul R. Rosteck, Jr.
Senior Research Scientist
Eli Lilly and Company
Lilly Corporate Center
Indianapolis, IN 46285

Jeffrey B. Rubins
Staff Pulmonary Physician
Associate Professor of Medicine
Minneapolis VA Medical Center
University of Minnesota
Pulmonary (111N)
One Veterans Drive
Minneapolis, MN 55417

Ilda Santos Sanches
Faculdade de Ciências e Tecnologia
Universidade Nova de Lisboa (FCT/UNL)
Monte da Caparica
Portugal

Ana R. Sánchez-Beato
Research Scientist
Departamento de Microbiologia Molecular
Consejo Superior de Investigaciones Científicas
 (CSIC)
Velázquez 144
28006 Madrid
Spain

Merle A. Sande
Professor and Chairman
Department of Internal Medicine
University of Utah
50 North Medical Drive
4C104 SOM
Salt Lake City, UT 84132

Jens Schletter
Cardiogene AG
Max-Planck-Strasse 15a
40699 Erkrath
Germany

Anatoly Severin
Infectious Diseases Unit
Wyeth Ayerst Research
401 North Middletown Road
Pearl River, NY 10965

Ulrich Seydel
Professor
Head of Division, Biophysics
Research Center Borstel
Center for Medicine and Biosciences
Parkallee 10
D-23845 Borstel
Germany

Michel Sicard
Centre National de la Recherche Scientifique
 (CNRS)
Laboratoire de Microbiologie et Génétique
 Moléculaire
Université Paul Sabatier
118, route de Narbonne
31062 Toulouse Cedex 04
France

Paul L. Skatrud
Research Scientist
Eli Lilly and Company
Lilly Corporate Center
Indianapolis, IN 46285

Marcel Sluijter
Department of Pediatrics
Erasmus Medical Center Rotterdam
P.O. Box 1738
3000 DR Rotterdam
The Netherlands

Patricia Solenberg
Associate Senior Biologist
Eli Lilly and Company
Lilly Corporate Center
Indianapolis, IN 46285

Edwin Swiatlo
Assistant Professor of Medicine
University of Mississippi
Medical Center
2500 North State Street
Jackson, MS 39216

Alexander J. Szalai
Assistant Professor
Department of Medicine
Division of Clinical Immunology and
  Rheumatology
University of Alabama at Birmingham
THT 437
1900 University Boulevard
Birmingham, AL 35294-0006

Martin G. Täuber
Professor of Medicine, Chief of Infectious
  Diseases, and Co-Director
Institute for Medical Microbiology
University of Berne
Friedbühlstrasse 51
CH-3010 Berne
Switzerland

Alexander Tomasz
The Rockefeller University
Laboratory of Microbiology
1230 York Avenue
New York, NY 10021-6399

Bao Ton-Hoang
INRA
Laboratoire de Biologie Moléculaire des
Relations Plantes-Micro-organismes
Chemin de Borde Rouge
Auzeville, BP 27
31326 Castanet-Tolosan Cedex
France

Marie-Claude Trombe
Maître de Conférences
Université Paul Sabatier
Bactériologie
CHU Rangueil/Bat L1
Avenue J. Poulhès
31403 Toulouse
France

Fe Tubau
Microbiologist
Department of Microbiology
Ciutat Sanitària i Universitària de Bellvitge
Feixa Llarga s/n
08907 L'Hospitalet de Llobregat
Barcelona
Spain

Elaine I. Tuomanen
Chair, Infectious Diseases
St. Jude Children's Research Hospital
332 North Lauderdale
Memphis, TN 38105

Artur J. Ulmer
Professor
Research Center Borstel
Center for Medicine and Biosciences
Parkallee 22
D-23845 Borstel
Germany

Mark van der Giezen
EMBO Research Fellow
Department of Zoology
The Natural History Museum
Cromwell Road
London SW7 5BD
United Kingdom

Mark Van Der Linden
Scientist
Department of Microbiology
University of Kaiserslautern
Paul Ehrlichstrasse 23
D-67663 Kaiserslautern
Germany

Hans van Dijk
Professor
Eijkman-Winkler Institute for Microbiology,
  Infectious Diseases & Inflammation
Utrecht University Medical Center
Utrecht University Hospital
Room G04.614
Heidelberglaan 100
3584 CX Utrecht
The Netherlands

Pedro F. Viladrich
Infectious Disease Specialist
Associate Professor of Medicine
Ciutat Sanitària i Universitària de Bellvitge
Hospital de Bellvitge
Feixa Llarga s/n
08907 L'Hospitalet de Llobregat
Barcelona
Spain

Anni Virolainen
Assistant Professor
Haartman Institute
Department of Bacteriology and Immunology
P.O. Box 21 (Haartmaninkatu 3)
00014 University of Helsinki
Finland

Jeffrey N. Weiser
Assistant Professor of Pediatrics and
  Microbiology
University of Pennsylvania
301 B Johnson Pavilion
Philadelphia, PA 19104-6076

Peter White
Physician
Department of Otorhinolaryngology, Head and
  Neck Surgery
University Hospital of Lund
SE-221 85 Lund
Sweden

Carol Ann Widdowson
Doctoral Student
South African Institute for Medical Research
P.O. Box 1038
Johannesburg 2000
South Africa

Birgit Weidemann
Research Center Borstel
Center for Medicine and Biosciences
Parkallee 22
D-23845 Borstel
Germany

Janet Yother
Associate Professor of Microbiology
Department of Microbiology
BBRB 661/12
University of Alabama at Birmingham
845 19th Street South
Birmingham, AL 35294

M. Young
Eli Lilly and Company
Lilly Corporate Center
Indianapolis, IN 46285

Dorothea Zähner
Scientist
Department of Microbiology
University of Kaiserslautern
Paul Ehrlichstrasse 23
D-67663 Kaiserslautern
Germany

Ulrich Zähringer
Chemist
Research Center Borstel
Center for Medicine and Biosciences
Parkallee 22
D-23845 Borstel
Germany

Piotr Zawadski
Procter & Gamble
Sulzbacher Strasse 40
65824 Schwabach/Ts
Germany

Acknowledgments

Contributions to this book originate from the International Workshop on "*Streptococcus pneumoniae*: Molecular Biology and Mechanisms of Disease—Update for the 1990s," which was held from September 23–29, 1996 in Oeiras, Portugal, and was hosted by Herminia de Lencastre, Professor and Head of the Molecular Genetics Unit at the Instituto de Tecnologia Química e Biológica (ITQB) of the Universidade Nova de Lisboa (UNL).

Alexander Tomasz, Professor and Head, Laboratory of Microbiology, The Rockefeller University, New York, NY was responsible for convening the Workshop.

We would like to express gratitude to the members of the Organizing Committee: Robert Breiman (CDC, Atlanta), David Briles (University of Alabama at Birmingham), G. Scott Giebink (University of Minnesota, Minneapolis), Regine Hakenbeck (Max Planck Institut for Molekulare Genetik, Berlin), Rubens López (CSIC, Madrid), and James C. Paton (Women's and Children's Hospital, North Adelaide, S. Australia).

We would like to thank Professors António Xavier (Director of ITQB), Manuel Carrondo (Director of IBET), and Herminia de Lencastre (Professor and Head of the Molecular Genetics Unit, ITQB) for hosting the Workshop, and acknowledge the indispensable assistance of Ms. Margaret Geller (The Rockefeller University) and Mrs. Manuela Nogueira (ITQB) with virtually every aspect of the meeting. We express our gratitude to organizations that provided funding for the Workshop: Fundação Luso-Americana, Junta Nacional de Investigação Científica e Technológica (JNICT), and the following pharmaceutical companies: Abbott, Bayer, Eli Lilly, Merck, Pfizer, Smith-Kline Beecham, Roche, and Roussel Uclaf.

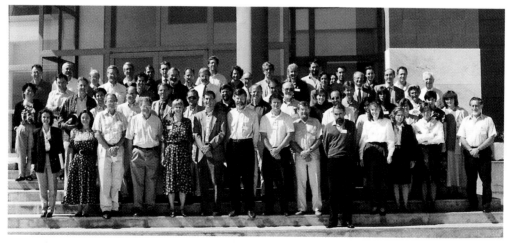

Attendees of the Streptococcus pneumoniae: *Molecular Biology and Mechanisms of Disease Conference, Oeiras, Portugal.*

Part 1

Introduction

The Enduring Pneumococcus:
Unfinished Business and Opportunities for the Future

ROBERT AUSTRIAN

MORE THAN A CENTURY HAS ELAPSED since George Miller Sternberg injected a rabbit with his own saliva and recovered pneumococci from the stricken animal.[41] Since that eventful experiment was performed, it is doubtful that the study of any other organism has contributed more to the understanding of bacterial infection than has the pneumococcus. Despite the large store of knowledge that has accumulated, many questions in the realms of bacteriology, immunology, and vaccinology remain to be answered; with the ever-increasing sophistication of modern technology, their solutions may provide new insights into the relationships between man and his microflora and into the pathogenesis and prevention of disease. Accordingly, knowing that many of you have been traveling many hours, rather than presenting an array of data, I have assembled a number of problems for which I have no answers, with the thought that some might seem worth exploring by one or another of the persons in this talented group.

Morphologic variation in pneumococcus is a phenomenon that seems worthy of further investigation. As noted by Sternberg in 1889: "I object to the name 'diplococcus pneumoniae' because this micrococcus in certain culture media forms longer or shorter chains and it is in fact a streptococcus,"[41] an observation of which American taxonomists have taken cognizance only in recent years. As isolated from man, pneumococci grow diffusely in liquid medium as single cells, diplococci, and in short chains, morphologies favoring access to nutrients. In contrast, when widely spaced inocula on blood agar plates are incubated for 5 to 10 days, rough excrescences appear at colonial margins composed of chains of pneumococci of 100 or more cells that fail to separate after division. These filamentous variants have greater access to nutrients by virtue of the pseudomotility imparted by buckling of the chains or filaments. Both filamentous and nonfilamentous variants autolyze in the presence of detergents, can produce Cs and conventional capsules, are comparably sensitive to penicillin; each can be transformed to the other.[2,3,8] The mechanism or enzyme responsible for cellular separation after division remains undefined. Phenocopies of the filamentous variant can be obtained by growing nonfilamentous variants in a medium in which the concentration of divalent cations has been markedly reduced or in a synthetic medium in which choline has been replaced by an amino alcohol such as ethanolamine.[47] Phenocopies of the former kind revert promptly to the nonfilamentous form when ions such as magnesium are restored to the medium. It would be of interest to discover the molecular basis of these phenomena and their potential applicability to other members of the genus *Streptococcus*.

Under normal circumstances, pneumococcus enjoys a commensal relationship with its principle host: man. Colonization of man with pneumococci may occur on the day of birth, and as many as four capsular types may be carried simultaneously in childhood.[13,14] Seemingly essential to its successful survival in the human nasopharynx is the ability to produce a significant quantity of one or another of 90 or more extracellular capsular polysaccharides which diffuse away from the surface of the bacterium and render it significantly less susceptible to phagocytosis. When viewed microscopically in preparations fixed in a variety of ways, the polysaccharide appears in the form of a capsule. Although isolation of noncapsulated pneumococci from the human nasopharynx has been reported from time to time in the past, their certain identification is open to question; one attempt to study their survival after instillation of a culture into the nose was followed by inability to detect them by colonial morphology or immunologic means after more than several weeks.[6] Colonization with capsulated pneumococci is influenced by the presence or absence of homotypic anticapsular antibody.[27] If an individual has antibody to a given pneumococcal type, the likelihood of his/her becoming colonized with organisms of that type is reduced by approximately half. In contrast, if an individual is already colonized with a given type of pneumococcus and subsequently develops antibody to that type, the antibody will not eliminate the carrier state. The foregoing observations indicate that its capsule is an attribute important to the survival in nature of pneumococcus and similar observations have been made with regard to a number of other bacterial species.

Pneumococcus produces capsules of a great variety of chemical compositions. How did such capsules arise? The organism is surrounded by a cell wall including a polysaccharide composed of glucose, 2-acetamido-4-amino-2,4,6 trideoxygalactose, N-acetyl galactosamine, galactosamine, ribitol-5-phosphate, and phosphocholine.[20] When noncapsulated pneumococci derived from capsulated variants of several types are grown in liquid medium containing antibodies to surface con-

Department of Molecular and Cellular Engineering, University of Pennsylvania, School of Medicine, Philadelphia, PA 19104–6088.
Reprinted from *Microbial Drug Resistance*, Vol. 3, No. 2, 1997.

stituents other than cell wall or C polysaccharide, capsulated mutants, selected because of their nutritional advantage of growing diffusely in the menstruum, can be recovered.[8] Examination of the capsule, designated Cs, shows it to be composed of the same constituents as the cell wall, prompting the question: is the mutation giving rise to this capsule the forerunner of the other previously characterized capsules? Each component of pneumococcal C polysaccharide can be found as a constituent of one or more of the pneumococcal capsular polysaccharides. The trideoxygalactose is a component of type 1 capsular polysaccharide;[25] phosphocholine is found in the capsular polysaccharides of types 24A, 27, 28F, 28A, 32F, and 32A,[40] and galactosamine and/or ribitol in a number of others.[50] Did the latter arise from translocation and mutations of genes concerned with synthesis of the cell wall? With the increasingly sophisticated techniques of genetic analysis now available, it would be of interest to determine the relation in the pneumococcal genome of the genes controlling cell wall synthesis to those controlling capsular synthesis and also to discover, if possible, the mutation leading to the production of the Cs pneumococcal capsule.

Pneumococcal capsular types differ significantly in their virulence for man and for other mammalian species for reasons that are not well understood. Type 3 bacteremic pneumococcal pneumonia treated with penicillin has a case fatality rate of 50%, attributed in part to the large size of the capsule of this type, and one colony forming unit may cause lethal infection in a mouse or rat. By contrast, pneumococcus type 37, which has a capsule of a size comparable to that of type 3, composed solely of glucose, is rarely carried by or a cause of illness in man, and 10^7 organisms are required to cause a lethal infection in rodents.[23] When organisms of each type were grown in human plasma, three times as much capsular polysaccharide was found in the supernatant fluid of a culture of pneumococcus type 37 as that associated with the cells whereas with a similar culture of pneumococcus type 3, a significantly greater portion of the polysaccharide remained cell-associated. What factors other than the chemistry and quantity of polysaccharide produced by individual capsular types affect their behavior in man seems worthy of further investigation.

Two pairs of capsular polysaccharides, that of types 6A and 6B[22] and that of types 19F and 19A[21] are each composed of the same constituents, the differences in the members of each pair resulting from a difference in a single linkage between two components of the polymer. How similar are the genomes and enzymes controlling the synthesis of the individual members of each cross-reacting pair? Also noteworthy are the limited data suggesting differences in human responses to vaccination with the individual polysaccharides of each pair. Whereas the capsular polysaccharide of type 6A or 6B each stimulates antibodies cross reactive with the other,[36] those of types 19F and 19A seemingly fail to do so.[34] More data are needed.

Pneumococcal infections of species other than man are uncommon but do occur, having been reported in primates, horses, goats, sheep, and feral rats. One of the more interesting of such relationships is the fulminant infections in guinea pigs caused almost exclusively by pneumococcus type 19F. The latter will wreak havoc, for reasons unclear, in a guinea pig colony, causing septicemic disease.[11,32] Here again is a model that may be fruitful to study.

The normal mammalian respiratory tract is relatively impervious to pneumococcal infection and the latter seems to occur most commonly after injury not always apparent to the upper or lower respiratory tract. Harford et al.[15] showed that normal mice exposed to an aerosol of type 1 pneumococci in particles of a sufficiently small size to reach the pulmonary alveoli rapidly cleared the bacteria from the lungs. Similarly, mice infected with the virus of influenza A cleared pneumococci at a time when viral titer in the lung was maximal, yet histologic evidence of viral infection was absent. Only when histologic evidence of epithelial injury in the lung was apparent did pneumonia evolve following exposure. Pulmonary edema, whether caused by a rodenticide or by instillation of serum into the lung increased susceptibility to infection with inhaled pneumococci and the evolution of pneumonia.[16]

Pneumococcal bacteremia is observed not uncommonly in infants and less often in adults in the absence of any clinically detectable lesion in the upper or lower respiratory tract, though involvement of the former seems perhaps more likely as it is the site of colonization. Animal experiments suggest strongly that the organisms are taken up in the lymphatic vessels draining the upper respiratory tract and pass to the cervical lymph nodes.[38] If not checked in the sinuses of these glands, they pass through the efferent lymphatics to the venous circulation, giving rise to bacteremia and, at times, to local metastatic infection, such as inappropriately named "primary" pneumococcal arthritis. That experimental infection followed this route from the nasopharynx was confirmed by canulating cervical lymphatic vessels and the finding that the presence of pneumococci in the lymph antedated that in the blood. Similar findings have followed injection of pneumococci into the footpads of rodents.[49]

Until recently, spontaneous recovery from pneumococcal bacteremia in the adult had not been recognized although it had been observed in infants. In 1938 White wrote:

> From time to time, bacteriologists have alleged that virulent pneumococci as well as streptococci are to be found in the blood of healthy persons as well as those ill with afflictions to which these organisms are not related. The validity of these claims is always highly questionable, and it is problematical if pneumococcus invades the circulatory system unless a specific focus of infection exists at some point in the body.[48]

In the course of trials in South Africa designed to quantify the efficacy of pneumococcal vaccine, 16 adult patients with headache, malaise, and fever of varying degree but lacking symptoms of respiratory infection were hospitalized for 1 to 3 days and treated symptomatically prior to discharge with a diagnosis of "other disease, medical".[5] Because of requirements of the trial's protocol, each had had a blood culture on admission which was found to contain pneumococci of one of the prevailing types in the population, including the highly virulent type 12, after the patient's discharge. Two of the 16 relapsed but the other 14 remained well and returned to work. Twelve of these illnesses occurred during the first 3 months of employment during which time it is possible that some type specific antibody might have developed as a sequel to nasopharyngeal colonization although such is problematical. What led to the recovery of these patients? In his Harvey lecture delivered in December 1951, W. Barry Wood, Jr. described the intravascular activation of polymorphonuclear leukocytes and their phagocytosis of Friedländer's bacilli following IV injection of the latter and in the absence of antibody, a finding attributed to the phenomenon he designated *surface phagocytosis*.[49] Did such a phenomenon play a role in the recoveries of 14 of the 16 patients described? Unfortunately, no immunologic data are available to correlate with these illnesses. The phenomena in man just described have their counterparts in other species, bacteremia having been observed in mice, rats, rabbits, and rhesus monkeys following inoculation of the nasopharynx with pneumococci or *Haemophilus influenzae* type b. These models offer opportunities to explore further the relative roles of humoral and cellular defenses in protecting the presumably nonimmune host against pneumococcal infection and that caused by some other capsulated bacterial species.

Turning back to man, there are notable deficiencies in our knowledge of the pneumococcal carrier state in adults. Because of the importance of the turnover of pneumococcal types to the understanding of the efficacy of polyvalent pneumococcal vaccines, it would be highly desirable to supplement the information now available suggesting that two to four new pneumococcal types may be acquired annually.[7] In certain settings, such as those in military barracks, individual soldiers have been shown to be colonized with as many as eight different capsular types in a period of 10 weeks.[19] The issue of turnover is important because the observed aggregate efficacy of polyvalent pneumococcal vaccines over time will be influenced by the individual's exposure to one or more of the several pneumococcal types represented in the vaccine. Previous studies of the pneumococcal carrier state dictate that, if they are to be meaningful, mouse inoculation with material from nasopharyngeal swabbings must be included as part of the protocol for isolating pneumococci.[4,19] The studies of Hodges et al. show quite clearly that half the pneumococcal isolates recovered from over 2000 nasopharyngeal swabbings in their study of adult carriers would not have been recognized had mice not been employed. Because of expense and lay opposition to the use of animals, mice have been rarely employed in recent studies of the pneumococcal carrier state, but it should be recognized clearly that studies excluding mice provide only minimal data on pneumococcal carriage and underestimate significantly its true extent.

Pneumococcal infections continue to be endemic in all societies in which their recognition has been sought and are responsible for significant mortality. After a period of the successful management of most over a period of four decades, the rapid rise in the last decade in the resistance of pneumococci to beta lactams and to other antimicrobial drugs has posed an increasing problem in their treatment. The situation is not without its ironic aspects. One of the first, if not the first, observation of the emergence of drug-resistant bacteria *in vivo* was reported by Morgenroth and Kaufmann in 1912 when Optochin-resistant pneumococci were recovered from infected mice treated with this drug.[31] Five and 6 years later, similar resistant isolates were recovered from man treated with Optochin.[29,30] In less than 5 years after the introduction of sulfonamide therapy of pneumococcal infection, sulfapyridine-resistant pneumococci were identified without reference to the earlier observations cited.[25] In 1943, the year before the strik-

ing efficacy of benzyl penicillin in the treatment of both bacteremic and nonbacteremic pneumococcal pneumonia was reported, pneumococci showing an incremental increase in resistance to penicillin were isolated by Schmidt and Sesler from infected mice treated with this drug.[37] The latter observation created little, if any, alarm and two decades were to elapse before reports of similar isolates from man were described. Why did it take so long? Heidelberger et al. showed that 10 billion pneumococci of types 1 or 2 yielded 30 to 40 micrograms of capsular polysaccharide,[18] and Frisch et al. reported isolating a gram or more of capsular polysaccharide from the consolidated lobes of patients succumbing to pneumococcal pneumonia,[12] suggesting populations of 10^{14} pneumococcal cells might be present in the infected respiratory tract if one makes some allowance for a greater production of polysaccharide *in vivo*. Perhaps the fact that high levels of resistance to penicillin in pneumococci are the result of multiple mutational events may be responsible in part for the long hiatus between the laboratory and clinical observations. Although most pneumococcal infections can be treated successfully today with large doses of penicillin because of its minimal toxicity, management of pneumococcal meningitis remains a serious problem and the need to discover new anti-pneumococcal drugs remains acute. Whether or not pneumococcal sensitivity to vancomycin like that of group A streptococci to penicillin will persist, is uncertain but even if it does, vancomycin is less than an ideal drug.

The problem posed by pneumococcal resistance to most antimicrobial drugs gives added impetus to prophylaxis. Much still remains to be learned about the currently available 23-valent vaccine of type specific capsular polysaccharides. To begin, there is a paucity of information regarding the optimal age at which to vaccinate otherwise healthy adults. Relatively few data are available regarding levels of antibody to a given antigen throughout the human life span. Studies of Thompsen and Kettel in the 1920s of the A,B,O blood group isoagglutinins from birth to age 100 show them to rise from infancy to age 30 after which they begin a gradual but steady decline.[44] Is it wise to delay vaccination of otherwise healthy adults until the age of 65 as is currently recommended? There is a growing body of experimental evidence suggesting that more antibody forming cells may be recruited at an earlier age and that the antibody formed has greater protective value than that resulting from immunization at a later age.[28,33] More studies of age-related responses to the vaccine are needed. In addition, especially in light of current recommendations by some that vaccine be re-administered after 5 to 7 years, studies of the kinetics of antibody decay after re-vaccination at different stages of life are needed, ones encompassing a time period of a minimum of 1 or more years. Data from the large case control study of Shapiro et al.[39] strongly suggest that the degree of protection after vaccination wanes with increasing rapidity with advancing years.

An additional phenomenon of potential interest is the failure of some recipients of polyvalent pneumococcal vaccine to respond to one or more antigens in the vaccine. It would seem worthwhile to select several such individuals as propositi and to examine the responsiveness to the same antigens in members of their kindreds to determine whether or not genetic factors play a role in determining failure to respond to specific antigens.

There also needs to be more widespread recognition of the impact on pneumococcal vaccine's efficacy of its high degree of polyvalency. What is loosely called the *polyvalent formulation's efficacy* is, in fact, its *aggregate efficacy*. If the average efficacy of each of the vaccine's antigens is 90% and one is exposed to four of the pneumococcal types represented in the vaccine, the likelihood of being infected by none would be 0.9^4 or 64%, a value of a magnitude quite similar to that of several studies. It has been known for many years that purified polysaccharides are poor antigens in infancy but that antibodies to them will be generated if the polysaccharide is injected after chemical conjugation to a protein. Such conjugate vaccines are currently under development,[24] and the question has arisen whether or not such conjugate vaccines will be more immunogenic also in adults. Few data relating to this issue are yet available, but those that are do not suggest that conjugates will be significantly superior in the adult to the polysaccharides alone.[35] More information, however, is clearly needed and doubtless will forthcoming.

Finally, there is the issue of the role of other components of the pneumococcal surface and cell as potentially useful immunogens for the prevention of pneumococcal infection. Some protection against infection with pneumococcus type 1 of rabbits immunized with a noncapsulated variant of pneumococcus type 2 was demonstrated by Tillett in 1928.[45] Although protection could be transferred passively to other rabbits, such was not the case with mice.[46] A somewhat similar degree of protection in a different rabbit model was reported by Street in 1942.[43] More recently, a participatory role in stimulating host defense of several better defined pneumococcal components, among them the surface protein(s) PspA,[10] C polysaccharide,[9] and pneumolysin,[1] has been described, antibodies to each of which may modify the outcome of pneumococcal infection in the mouse. Were antibodies to one or more of them to prove comparably effective to antibodies to capsular polysaccharide, the problem of the prophylaxis of pneumococcal infection would be simplified greatly. As knowledge of noncapsular antigens advances, however, it seems relevant that their efficacy be contrasted with that of capsular polysaccharides in a variety of ways. Such studies should include challenge at lengthening times after vaccination, determination of the number of lethal doses against which protection is afforded by antibodies to each, the inclusion of species other than the mouse, measurement of opsonic activity in tests of phagocytosis *in vitro*, the protective effect of passively acquired immunity and ultimately, if feasible, tests in small numbers of primates. Until such data are available, it seems questionable that other than small scale tests of immunogenicity in man should be carried out, with examination of the protective effect of passively transferred vaccinee's serum in animal models. It may be worth recalling that the unit of therapeutic antiserum in the era of serum therapy was defined as "that amount of antibody which will protect at least 50 percent of a series of inoculated standard white mice against 1,000,000 fatal doses of a standardized pneumococcus culture of the same type."[17] The potency of therapeutic antisera of several types ranged from 150 to 900 units per cubic cm. Although the amount of antibody required for prophylaxis is significantly smaller than that required for therapy, one would like to stimulate an amount well in excess of the minimal requirement.

The foregoing list of topics is by no means exhaustive and we can look forward in the days ahead to presentation and discussion of additional important issues. It does suggest strongly, however, that, even after more than a century of study, the pneumococcus and the diseases it causes remain worthy objects of scrutiny.

REFERENCES

1. **Alexander, J.E., R.A. Lock, C.C.A.M. Peeters, J.T. Poolman, P.W. Andrew, I.J. Mitchell, D. Hansman, and J.C. Paton.** 1994. Immunization of mice with pneumolysin toxoid confers a significant degree of protection against at least nine serotypes of *Streptococcus pneumoniae*. Infect. Immun. **62:**5683–5688.
2. **Austrian R.** 1953. Morphologic variation in pneumococcus. I. an analysis of the bases for morphologic variation in pneumococcus and description of a hitherto undefined morphologie variant. J. Exp. Med. **98:**21–34.
3. **Austrian, R.** 1953. Morphologic variation in pneumococcus. II. control of pneumococcal morphology through transformation reactions. J. Exp. Med. **98:**35–40.
4. **Austrian, R.** 1986. Some aspects of the pneumococcal carrier state. J. Antimicrob. Chemother. **18 suppl A:**35–45.
5. **Austrian, R.** 1986. Untreated pneumococcal bacteremia of cryptic origin in the human adult with spontaneous recovery. S. African Med. J. **70 suppl** 11 Oct: 46–49.
6. **Austrian, R.** Unpublished observations.
7. **Bliss, E.A., W.D. McClasky, and P.H. Long.** 1934. A study of pneumococcus carriers. J. Immunol. **27:**95–103.
8. **Bornstein, D.L., G. Schiffman, H.P. Bernheimer, and R. Austrian.** 1968. Capsulation of pneumococcus with soluble C-like (Cs) polysaccharide. I. biological and genetic properties of Cs pneumococcal strains. J. Exp. Med. **128:**1385–1400.
9. **Briles, D.E., C. Forman, J.C. Horowitz, J.E. Volanakis, W.H. Benjamin Jr., L.S. McDaniel, J. Eldridge, and J. Brooks.** 1989. Antipneumococcal effects of C-reactive protein and monoclonal antibodies to pneumococcal cell wall and capsular antigens. Infect. Immun. **57:** 1457–1464.
10. **Briles, D.E., J.D. King, M.A. Gray, L.S. McDaniel, E. Swiatlo, and K.A. Benton.** 1996. PspA, a protection-eliciting pneumococcal protein: Immunogenicity of isolated native PspA in mice. Vaccine **14:**858–867.
11. **Finland, M.** 1942. Recent advances in the epidemiology of pneumococcal infections. Medicine **21:**307–344.
12. **Frisch, A.W., J.W. Tripp, C.D. Barrett, and B.E. Pidgeon.** 1942. The specific polysaccharide content of pneumonic lungs. J. Exp. Med. **76:**505–510.
13. **Gundel, M., and G. Okura.** 1933. Untersuchungen über das gleichzeitige Vorkommen mehrer Pneumokokkentypen bei Gesunden und ihrer Bedeutung für Epidemiologie. Zeitschr f. Hyg u Infektionskr **114:**678–704.
14. **Gundel, M., and F.K.T. Schwartz.** 1932. Studien über die Bakterienflora der obern Atmungswege Neugeborner (im Vergleich mit der Mundhöhlen flora der Mutter und des Pflegepersonals) unter besonderer Berucksichtigung ihrer Bedeutung für das Pneumonieproblem. Zeitschr f Hyg u Infektionskr. **113:**411–436.
15. **Harford, C.G., V. Leidler, and M. Hara.** 1949. Effect of the lesion due to influenza virus in the resistance of mice to inhaled pneumococci. J. Exp. Med. **89:**53–68.
16. **Harford, C.G., and M. Hara.** 1950. Pulmonary edema in influenzal pneumonia of the mouse and the relation of fluid in the lung to the inception of pneumococcal pneumonia. J. Exp. Med. **91:**245–260.
17. **Heffron, R.** 1979. Pneumonia with special reference to pneumococcus lobar pneumonia. 2nd printing. Harvard University Press, Cambridge, MA, pp. 826–828.

18. **Heidelberger, M., C.M. MacLeod, S.J. Kaiser, and B. Robinson.** 1946. Antibody formation in volunteers following injection of pneumococci or their type-specific polysaccharides. J. Exp. Med. **83**:303–320.

19. **Hodges, R.G., C.M. MacLeod, and W.G. Bernhard.** 1946. Epidemic pneumococcal pneumonia. III, carrier studies. Am. J. Hyg. **44**:207–230.

20. **Jennings, H.J., C. Lugowski, and N.M. Young.** 1980. Structure of the complex polysaccharide C-substance from *Streptococcus pneumoniae* type I. Biochemistry **19**:4712–4719.

21. **Katzenellenbogen, E., and H.J. Jennings.** 1983. Structural determination of the capsular polysaccharide of *Streptococcus pneumoniae* type 19A (57). Cbhy Rsrch **124**:235–245.

22. **Kenne, L., B. Lindberg, and J.K. Madden.** 1979. Structural studies of the capsular antigen from *Streptococcus pneumoniae* type 26. Cbhy. Rsrch. **73**:175–182.

23. **Knecht, J., G. Schiffman, and R. Austrian.** 1970. Some biological properties of pneumococcus type 37 and the chemistry of its capsular polysaccharide. J. Exp. Med. **132**:475–487.

24. **Leach, A., S.J. Ceesay, W.A.S. Banya, and B. Greenwood.** 1996. Pilot trial of a pentavalent pneumococcal protein/conjugate vaccine in Gambian infants. Pediatr. J. Infect. Dis. **15**:333–339.

25. **Lindberg, B., B. Lindqvist, J. Lönngren, and D.A. Powell.** 1980. Structural studies of the capsular polysaccharide from *Streptococcus pneumaniae* type I. Cbhy. Rsrch. **78**:111–117.

26. **MacLean, I.H., K.B. Rogers, and A. Fleming.** 1939. M & B693 and pneumococci. Lancet **1**:562–568.

27. **MacLeod, C.M., R.G. Hodges, M. Heidelberger, and W.G. Bernhard.** 1945. Prevention of pneumococcal pneumonia by immunization with specific capsular polysaccharides. J. Exp. Med. **82**:445–465.

28. **Miller, R.A.** 1996. The aging immune system: Primer and prospectus. Science **273**:70–74.

29. **Moore, H.F., and A.M. Chesney.** 1917. A study of ethylhydrocuprein (optochin) in the treatment of acute lobar pneumonia. Arch. Int. Med. **19**:611–682.

30. **Moore, H.F., and A.M. Chesney.** 1918. A further study of ethylhydrocuprein (optochin) in the treatment of acute lobar pneumonia. Arch. Int. Med. **21**:659–681.

31. **Morgenroth, J., and M. Kaufmann.** 1912. Arzneifestigkeit bei Bakterien (Pneumokokken). Zeitschr f Immunitätsforsch (I) **15**:610–614.

32. **Neufeld, F., and R. Etinger-Tulczynska.** 1932. Untersuchungen über die Pneumokokkenseuche des Meerschweinchens. Zeitschr f Hyg u Infektionskr **114**:324–346.

33. **Nicoletti, C., X. Yang, and J. Cermy.** 1993. Repertoire diversity of antibody response to bacterial antigens in aged mice. III. phosphorylcholine antibody from young and aged mice differ in structure and protective activity against infection with *Streptococcus pneumoniae.* J. Immunol. **150**:543–549.

34. **Penn, R.L., E.B. Lewin, R.G. Jr. Douglas, G. Schiffman, C-J. Lee, and J.B. Robbins.** 1982. Antibody responses in adult volunteers to pneumococcal polysaccharide types 19F and 19A administered singly and in combination. Infect. Immun. **36**:1261–1262.

35. **Powers, D.C., E.L. Anderson, K. Lottenbach, and C.A.M. Mink.** 1996. Reactogenicity and immunogenicity of protein-conjugated pneumococcal oligosaccharide vaccine in older adults. J. Infect. Dis. **173**:1014–1018.

36. **Robbins, J.B., C.-J. Lee, S.C. Rastogi, G. Schiffman, and J. Henrichsen.** 1979. Comparative immunogenicity of group 6 pneumococcal type 6A (6) and type 6 B(26) capsular polysacchrides. Infect. Immun. **26**:1116–1122.

37. **Schmidt, L.H., and C.L. Sesler.** 1943. Development of resistance to penicillin by pneumococci. Proc. Soc. Exp. Biol. Med. **52**:353–357.

38. **Schultz, R.Z., M.F. Warren, and C.K. Drinker.** 1938. The passage of rabbit virulent type III pneumococci from the respiratory tract of rabbits into the lymphatics and blood. J. Exp. Med. **68**:251–261.

39. **Shapiro, E.D., A.T. Berg, R. Austrian, D. Schroeder, V. Parcells, A. Margolis, R.K. Adair, and J.D. Clemens.** 1991. The protective efficacy of pneumococcal polysaccharide vaccine. N. Engl. J. Med. **325**:1453–1460.

40. **Sørensen, U.B.S., R. Agger, J. Bennedsen, and J. Henrichsen.** 1984. Phosphocholine determinants in six pneumococcal capsular polysaccharides detected by monoclonal antibody. Infect. Immun. **43**:876–878.

41. **Sternberg, G.M.** 1881. A fatal form of septicemia in the rabbit produced by subcutaneous injection of human saliva: An experimental research. Natl. Bd. Health Bull. **2**:781–783.

42. **Sternberg, G.M.** 1897. The etiology of croupous pneumonia. Natl. Med. Rev. **7**:175–177.

43. **Street, J.A.** 1942. Studies of the mechanism of species-specific immunity against pneumococcal infection. J. Immunol. **44**:53–68.

44. **Thomsen, O., and K. Kettel.** 1929. Die Stärke der menschichen Isogglutine und entsprechender Blutkörperchenrezeptoren in verschieden Lebensaltern. Zeitschr Immunitätsforsch u Exp Therapie **63**:67–93.

45. **Tillett, W.S.** 1928. Active and passive immunity to pneumococcus infection induced in rabbits by immunization with R pneumococci. J. Exp. Med. **48**:791–804.

46. **Tillett, W.S.** 1927. Studies on immunity to pneumococcus mucosus (type III) III: Increased resistance to type III infection induced in rabbits by immunization with R and S forms of pneumococcus. J. Exp. Med. **46**:343–356.

47. **Tomasz, A.** 1968. Biological consequences of the replacement of choline by ethanolamine in the cell wall of peumococcus: Chain formation, loss of transformability and loss of autolysis. Proc. Natl. Acad. Sci. **59**:86–93.

48. **White, B.** 1979. The biology of pneumococcus, 2nd printing. Harvard University Press, Cambridge, MA, p. 227.

49. **Wood, W.B., Jr.** 1953. Studies on the cellular immunology of acute bacterial infections. Harvey Lectures **47**:72–98.

50. **Van Dam, J.E.G., A. Fleer, and H. Snippe.** 1990. Immunogenicity and immunochemistry of *Streptococcus pneumoniae* capsular polysaccharides. Antonie van Leeuwenhoek **58**:1–47.

Address reprint requests to:
Robert Austrian
Dept. of Molecular and Cellular Engineering
The University of Pennsylvania
School of Medicine
Philadelphia, PA 19104–6088

Streptococcus pneumoniae: Functional Anatomy

ALEXANDER TOMASZ

THE PURPOSE OF THIS BRIEF CHAPTER on the functional anatomy of *Streptococcus pneumoniae* is to provide a kind of "visual framework" for the topics of the other chapters in this book. It is also hoped that some of the intriguing morphological observations reproduced here will stimulate new approaches to explore the cell biology of this interesting microbe.

THE FINE STRUCTURE OF *S. pneumoniae*

A high-resolution electron microscopic study of laboratory strain R6 (a derivative of R36A) has identified the basic morphological feature of *S. pneumoniae*.[22] This strain represents a prototype of the Pneumococcus: most laboratory studies conducted over the past decades on the physiology, biochemistry, and genetics of *S. pneumoniae* have used strain R36A or its laboratory derivatives and these studies included the characterization of the complete genome of *S. pneumoniae*.[1] The parent strain of R36A was a serotype 2 clinical isolate D39 from which serial passage in anti-capsular 2 antibody selected the nonencapsulated strain R36A in which the type 2 capsular locus is inactivated by a 7,504-bp deletion in 9 capsular genes.[9]

Pneumococci were grown in synthetic or semisynthetic media, harvested in the exponential phase of growth, fixed and stained according to the procedure of Ryter and Kellenberger,[15] and embedded in crosslinked methacrylate; thin sections with the interference color of silver to silver-gray were examined with the electron microscope (Fig. 1).

Several of the basic morphological features of *S. pneumoniae* may be identified in Fig. 1.

NUCLEAR REGION

The central region of the cell with relatively low electron density is filled with more or less packed fibrils of uniform 25–30 angstroms (Å) width, representing the appearance of the bacterial chromosome after the electron microscopic procedure. In dividing bacteria sectioned in the appropriate plane, a bipolar distribution of the nuclear region and nuclear fibrils is apparent, suggesting the progressive physical separation of the duplicated bacterial chromosome into the emerging daughter cells during cell division (Fig. 2).

CYTOPLASM

The cytoplasm of pneumococci contains a large number of electron dense particles with the diameter of approximately 150 Å, representing, presumably, ribosomes and polysomes which are distributed homogeneously throughout the cytoplasm.

MEMBRANOUS "ORGANELLES"

A striking feature of the thin sections of strain R36A is the frequent presence of intracellular membranous organelles, often referred to in the cytological literature as "mesosomes"[24] or "chondrioids."[22] Because the functions of these organelles are unknown, we shall simply refer to them as intracellular membranes, or *icm-s*.

In an examination of over 100 pneumococcal cells in electron microscopic serial sections (which enabled us to examine two-thirds to three-quarters of the complete width of the bacteria), no bacterial cells could be identified without any *icm-s* (unpublished observations). The most frequent location of the *icm-s* was at developing septa and/or at the pointed poles of the bacterial cells. No septa were seen without an *icm* attached. The *icm-s* were also frequently shown in apparent "contact" with a nuclear region, and the majority of *icm-s* examined in detail (49 out of a total of 64) were shown to have a common boundary with the plasma membrane in a few section planes. The number and geometry of *icm-s* as determined in serial sections of 13 *S. pneumoniae* cells is shown in Table 1.

The lumenal space of *icm-s* seems to be of two kinds: membrane-limited islands with the electron density of cytoplasm alternate with low-density, empty-looking areas. We interpret this as a regular alteration of cytoplasmic-and "extracellular" space (*i.e.,* space between the plasma membrane and the cell wall) originating from consecutive invaginations (*i.e.,* first-, second-, *etc.* order infoldings of the plasma membrane) so that the lumen of every odd-numbered infolding is extracellular space, while the lumen of even-numbered infoldings is essentially cytoplasm. Cross sections of the *icm-s* strongly suggest that their structural subunit is the complete plasma membrane. The identification of both plasma membrane surfaces in the *icm-s* is facilitated by the asymmetric staining of the plasma membrane (*i.e.,* the outer layer providing a stronger osmiophylic staining than the inner layer) (Fig. 3).

The Rockefeller University, New York, NY 10021.

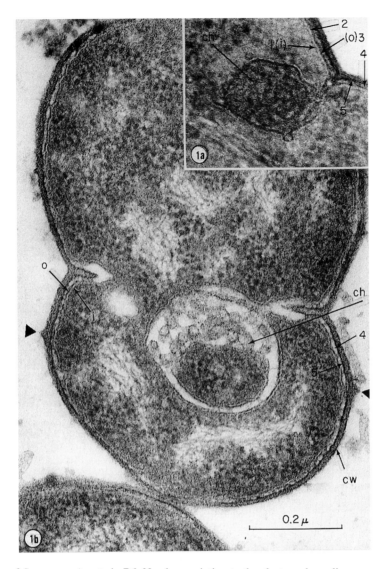

FIG. 1. Fine structure of *S. pneumoniae* strain R6. Numbers pointing to the electron-dense lines represent parts of the plasma membrane and cell wall (i) and (o) refer to the inner and outer layer of the plasma membrane; ch, chondrioid or intracellular membrane (*icm*); cw, cell wall. Black arrowheads refer to the equatorial ring structure. (Reproduced with permission from *Journal of Cell Biology.*[22])

The peculiar geometry of *icm-s, i.e.,* their frequent association with septa and the frequent alignment of pairs of *icm-s* with the dividing chromosome, suggests that they may be involved with the equatorial biosynthesis of cell wall or separation of the chromosomes during cell division.

PLASMA MEMBRANE

Inside the cell wall, five osmiophylic bands of different staining intensity can be identified in thin sections (see Fig. 1). We interpret bands number 1, 2, and 3 as representing the plasma membrane of pneumococci, specifically, number 1 representing the inner leaflet (i in Fig. 1) and number 3 the outer leaflet (o in Fig. 1) of a unit membrane. Of the rest of the five bands,

the number 5 represents the inner surface of the cell wall, and the low-density "band" number 4 appears to represent something morphologically and/or functionally analogous to the "periplasmic space" of Gram-negative bacteria (Fig. 1). The two electron-dense bands, each 25–30 Å wide, of the plasma membrane of pneumococci enclose a less dense band of approximately the same width. These dimensions correspond to that of the "unit membrane" identified in many cellular membrane systems.[13] A degree of asymmetry is observable in the pneumococcal plasma membrane in thin sections of intact cells, in which the "outer" electron-dense band appears to be wider (35–40 Å) than the inner one. Numerous "bridges" or invaginations connect the plasma membrane and the cell wall and in thin sections of pneumococci exposed briefly to hypertonic sucrose prior to fixation; these bridges appear to penetrate the en-

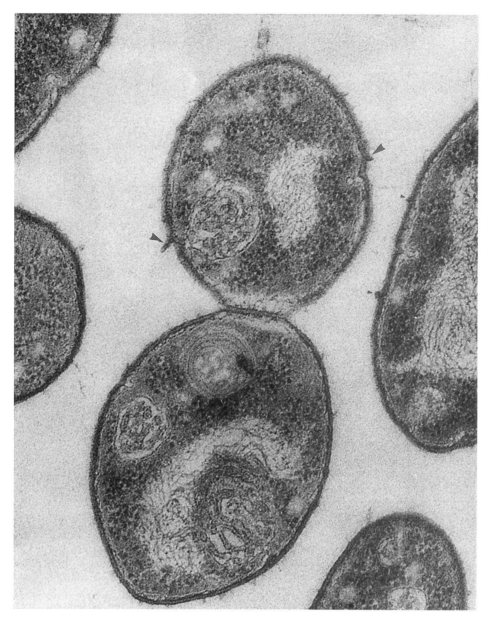

FIG. 2. Alignment of the membranous organelles (*icm-s*) with the dividing chromosome. Large arrowhead, residual equatorial ring after its division; small arrowhead, equatorial ring.

tire width of the cell wall (Fig. 4). These images suggest a close anatomical and/or functional interdigitation of the plasma membrane and the cell wall in pneumococci, perhaps similar to the cell membrane-wall junctions described in Gram-negative bacteria.[2]

CELL WALL

The outermost structure on the surface of the nonencapsulated pneumococcus, composed of an electron-dense outer and inner band, each of about 30–40 Å wide and enclosing a less electron-dense band of about 60–80 Å, represents the bacterial cell wall. In encapsulated pneumococci, this trilaminated struc-

ture is covered from the outside with a less structured layer of the polysaccharide capsule, which may have very different appearances depending on the details of the cytological procedure used (Fig. 5). The chemical composition of the cell wall peptidoglycan and teichoic acid are described in two accompanying contributions to this book.

MORPHOLOGICAL ALTERATIONS DURING CELL DIVISION

Electron microscopy of thin sections of pneumococci in different stages of cell division allows one to identify tentatively and put in chronological order what appears to be a sequel of

TABLE 1. NUMBERS AND GEOMETRIC ARRANGEMENTS OF *ICM-S* IN 13 *S. PNEUMONIAE* CELLS OBSERVED IN ELECTRON MICROSCOPIC SERIAL SECTIONS

Cell	Division Stage	Number of Nuclei	Number of *icm*-s	Number of *icm*-s classified as			Arrangement
				Septal	Polar	Extra	
1	$\frac{1}{4} < \ < \frac{1}{2}$	1	3	1	2(1)	0	
2	$\frac{1}{4} >$	1	7	3(3)	2	2	
3	$\frac{1}{4} < \ < \frac{1}{2}$	1	4	4(2)	0	0	
4	$\frac{1}{4} >$	1	11	6(2)	4(1)	1(1)	
5	$\frac{1}{4} >$	1	4	2(2)	0	2(1)	
6	$\frac{1}{4} >$	1	2	1(1)	1(1)	0	
7	$\frac{1}{4} >$	1	4	4(4)	0	0	
8	$\frac{1}{4} >$	1	3	2(1)	1(1)	0	
9	$\frac{1}{4}$	1	3	2(1)	1(1)	0	
10	$\frac{1}{4}$	1	6	4(2)	2(2)	0	
11	$\frac{1}{4}$	1	4	3(3)	1	0	
12	$\frac{1}{4} >$	1	3	3(2)	0	0	
13	$\frac{1}{4} >$	1	2	1(1)	1	0	

carefully regulated and symmetrical morphological events involving the cell wall and plasma membrane of pneumococci. Similar to other streptococci, pneumococci divide in a single plane in the central equatorial region of the cell, and the site of incipient septum is marked by a morphological alteration at the cell wall, which appears as a "hump" of the cell wall located at the precise middle of the cell surface.[7] This structure is, in fact, the cross section of an equatorial ring: an enlargement of

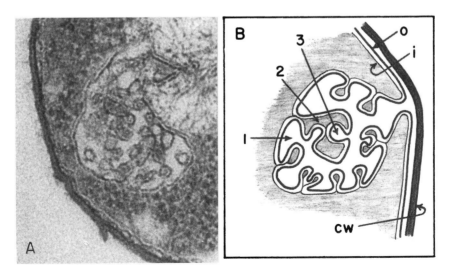

FIG. 3. Interpretation of the lumenal structure of *icm-s*. cw, cell wall; (o) and (i), outer and inner layer of the plasma membrane; numbers indicate the extracellular (1 and 3) and cytoplasmic (2) space.

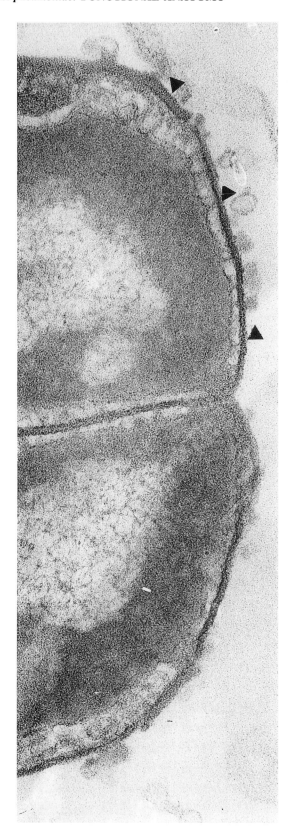

FIG. 4. Cell wall–plasma membrane junctions observed in *S. pneumoniae* exposed to hypertonic medium. (Reproduced with permission from *Journal of Bacteriology.*[16a])

the cell wall which divides the bacterial surface into two equal-size hemispheres, and which may be related to the morphological marker of cell division in *Escherichia coli.*[14]

The morphological and staining properties of the equatorial ring indicate that it is made up of cell wall material and the "next" observable morphological event involves the division of the equatorial ring into two, presumably by the localized action of an autolysin. This splitting event coincides with the first signs of a centripetally growing cell wall or septum. As the inward growth of the septum progresses, the addition of new material at the leading tip also seems to feed into the peripheral wall, pushing the "old" hemispheres symmetrically to the left and to the right. The two equatorial rings move along and become recognizable age markers of the cell surface: The cell wall enveloping the dividing bacterium between the equatorial ring and the septal tip is one generation "younger" in biosynthetic age than the cell wall between the equatorial rings and the left or right poles of the bacterium. Experimental evidence for this interpretation comes from experiments in which the inheritance of pneumococcal cell wall was examined.

INHERITANCE AND CONSERVATIVE SEGREGATION OF CELL WALL

The nutritional requirement of pneumococci for the amino alcohol choline[12] and the unique localization of most of this compound as a component of the cell wall teichoic acid[18] has allowed examination of the inheritance of pneumococcal cell walls during cell division. Bacteria grown in the presence of radiolabeled choline were transferred into a growth medium in which the choline component was replaced by ethanolamine. One of the consequences of the nutritional shift from the use of choline to the use of ethanolamine is an inhibition in the separation of daughter cells at the end of cell division. Pneumococci growing in ethanolamine-containing medium form infinite chains, which represent linear clones of this bacteria. Examination of the localization of radioactively labeled cells in such an ethanolamine-induced chain or linear clone by autoradiography has shown that the "old" choline-labeled surface of the pneumococcus is inherited intact and passed on during cell division from one daughter cell to the other in the form of choline-labeled hemispheres.[4] In this experimental system, cells labeled with radioactive choline appear preferentially as the terminal cells in the pneumococcal chains (Fig. 6). A model providing the interpretation of this autoradiographic assay is shown in Fig. 7. A similar conservation of the cell surface was demonstrated earlier by immunological techniques in group A streptococci, whereas a more diffuse intercalation of new into old cell wall material and a consequent lack of conservation of cell wall was shown in *E. coli* and other bacilli.

EQUATORIAL GROWTH ZONE

Inherent in the results of a segregation experiment(s) is the notion of a single, equatorially located growth zone in which new cell wall material enters the pneumococcal surface. Direct experimental demonstration of this was made possible by exploiting yet another feature of the pleiomorphy that is associ-

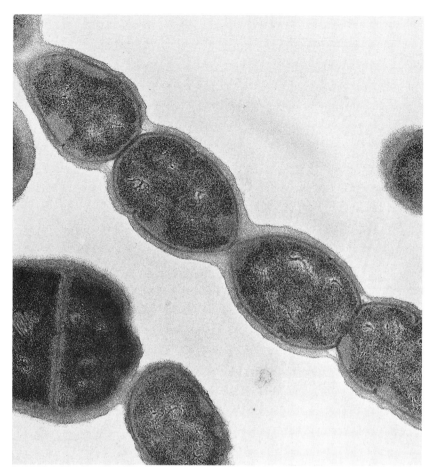

FIG. 5. Chain of an encapsulated strain of *S. pneumoniae.* Outermost low-density layer enveloping the bacterial cell represents capsular material.

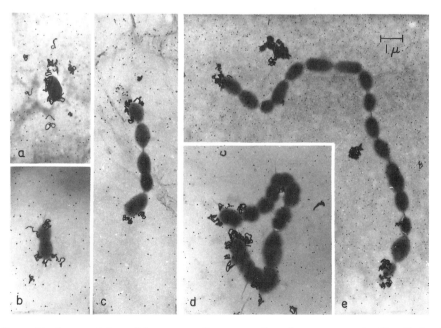

FIG. 6. Autoradiographic documentation of the conservative segregation of pneumococcal cell wall. Sections (a) through (e) represent bacterial cells grown for increasing numbers of cell divisions in the presence of ethanolamine-containing medium. Bacterial cells carrying the original radioactive choline-labeled surface are represented by the radioautographic markers (see "root-like" tracks of tritium decay in the nuclear emulsion). (Reproduced with permission from *Journal of Cell Biology.*[4])

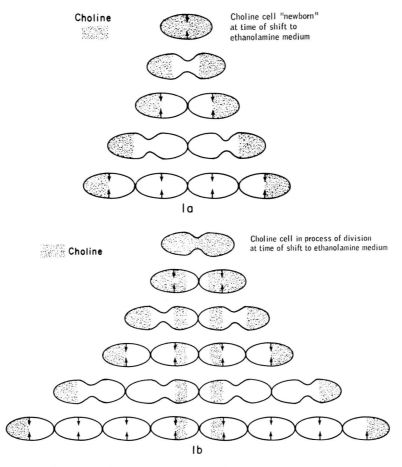

Choline

Choline cell "newborn" at time of shift to ethanolamine medium

Ia

Choline

Choline cell in process of division at time of shift to ethanolamine medium

Ib

FIG. 7. Model for the conservative segregation of pneumococcal cell wall. (Reproduced with permission from *Journal of Cell Biology.*[4])

CELL WALL PREPARATION	TOTAL CPM	TOTAL CPM RELEASED BY AUTOLYSIN
$[^{14}C]$-ETHANOLAMINE (choline pulse)	85,590	1,700 (2%)
ETHANOLAMINE ($[^{3}H]$-choline pulse)	106,252	101,200 (95%)

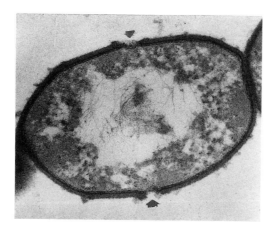

FIG. 8. Selective removal of the choline-containing nascent cell wall from an ethanolamine-grown bacterium pulse-labeled with choline. The missing piece of cell wall from the middle of the bacterium (arrowheads) was removed by exposure of the cells to the pneumococcal autolysin, resulting in the release of 95% of the radioactive choline label but only 2% of radioactive ethanolamine label, which represented the biosynthetically "old" cell wall material. (Reproduced with permission from *Journal of Biological Chemistry.*[22a])

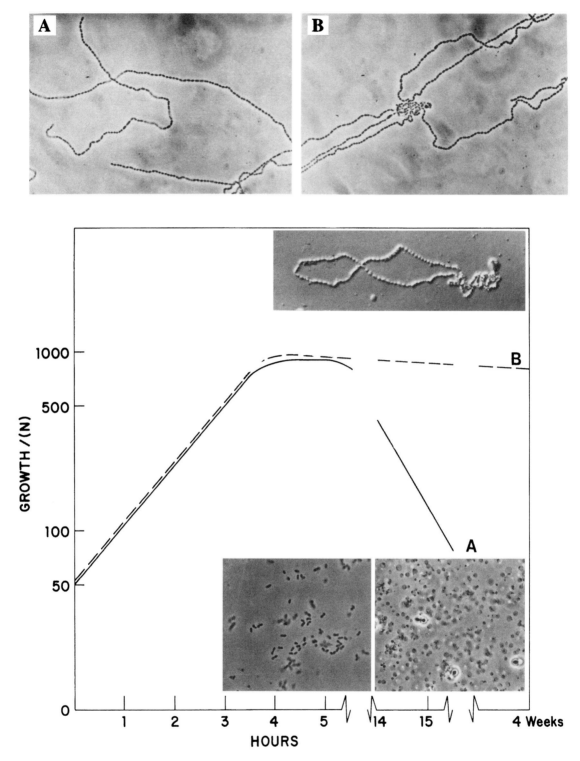

FIG. 9. Effect of interference with choline metabolism on the separation of daughter cells and autolysis. (**A**): Pneumococci growing in the presence of high concentrations of choline (5 mg/ml). (**B**) Choline-independent pneumococcal mutant Cho⁻ growing in choline-free growth medium. Lower panel: Pneumococci growing in a medium containing choline (**A**) or ethanolamine instead of choline (**B**). Spontaneous autolysis of culture A and lack of autolysis in culture B are indicated. Also shown (top of panel), the appearance of bacteria from culture B (extensive formation of chains) and the appearance of bacteria from culture A from the exponential growing culture (left panel) and after extensive autolysis (right panel).

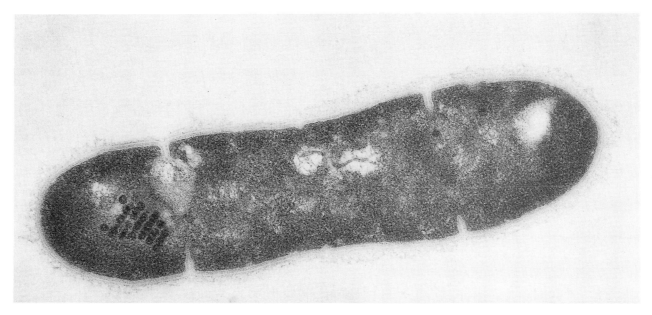

FIG. 10. Inhibition of cell division and septation by mitomycin C. On the left side of the bacterium, assembly of phage particles induced by the mitomycin treatment is apparent. (Reproduced with permission from *Journal of Bacteriology.*[11])

ated with replacing choline residues with the structural analog ethanolamine in the cell wall teichoic acid. A series of experiments has demonstrated that the physical attachment and subsequent degradation of the pneumococcal cell wall by the pneumococcal autolytic amidase has an absolute requirement for the presence of choline residues in the wall teichoic acid.[5,8] Cell walls of pneumococci grown on ethanolamine-containing medium produce a cell wall in which the choline residues are replaced by ethanolamine, and such cell walls are totally resistant to the amidase. When pneumococci growing in ethanolamine-containing medium were exposed to choline in the growth medium for a short time (up to 1 min, corresponding to 1–2% of the culture's mass doubling time), the bacteria immediately shifted to the use of this nutrient and the production of choline-containing cell wall teichoic acids which, along with the peptidoglycan, incorporated into the pneumococcal surface. The site of this incorporation was identified by exposing such bacteria containing a "hybrid" of ethanolamine-containing ("old") and choline-containing ("nascent") cell walls to exogenous autolysin, which resulted in the selective removal of the choline-containing portion of the cell wall. Electron microscopic observation of thin sections showed that the "missing" cell wall piece was located in the precise geometric center of the cell, *i.e.*, the site of cell wall incorporation was located at the equatorial zone of the bacterium (Fig. 8).[21] A simple modification of this experimental system has been used for the direct biochemical analysis of nascent and biosynthetically old bacterial cell wall.[10]

DAUGHTER CELL SEPARATION AT THE END OF CELL DIVISION

The appearance of daughter cells as independent "viable units" physically separated from one another occurs in a process

that is not carefully synchronized with cell division, *i.e.*, a pneumococcus may engage in a new cycle of cell division before physical separation from the daughter cell is accomplished. This situation leads to the appearance of "chains" of cells in pneumococcal cultures, the length of which varies with growth conditions. There are a number of experimental interventions that specifically block the cell separation event, and these are associated with the choline metabolism of pneumococci. Conditions that cause inhibition of cell separation and formation of long bacterial chains include (i) growing pneumococci in a medium in which choline is replaced by the structural analog ethanolamine,[19] and (ii) increasing the concentration of choline from the nutritional level of a few micrograms to several milligrams per milliliter.[3] (iii) The recently isolated mutant Cho⁻,[17] which lost its nutritional requirement for an amino alcohol, and another mutant with a preference for the utilization of ethanolamine over choline,[25] both form long chains (Fig. 9). All these conditions cause complete inhibition of autolysis as well. Nevertheless, a deletion mutant of *lytA* (the genetic determinant of the pneumococcal autolysin) forms only short[16] or virtually no chains,[23] indicating that the activity responsible for the ultimate physical separation of daughter cells may involve the activity of a choline-dependent enzyme yet to be identified.

INHIBITION OF CELL DIVISION AND ABNORMAL SEPTUM FORMATION

Addition of the DNA inhibitor mitomycin C at appropriate concentrations to the growth medium of pneumococci causes rapid reduction in the viable titer of bacteria without inhibition of the mass increase and growth of the cells. During this residual growth, which may continue for a considerable length of time, pneumococci undergo morphological change which involves an abnormal elongation of bacteria caused by an appar-

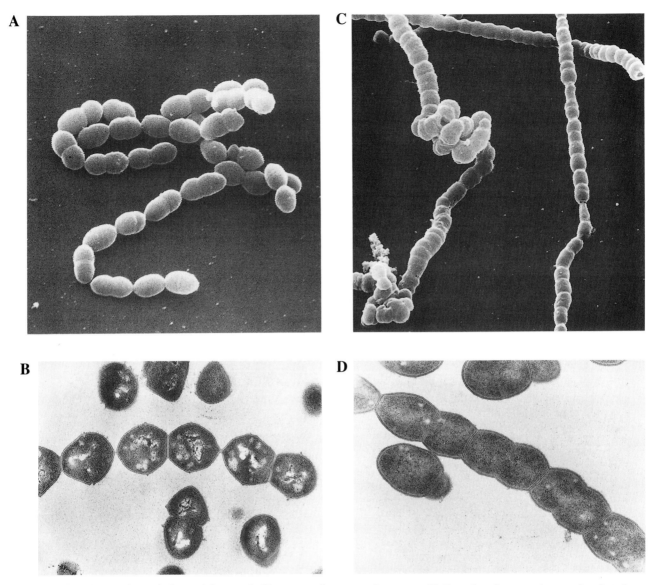

FIG. 11. Abnormal morphology of the pseudo-filamentous *S. pneumoniae* mutant *fil*. Scanning electron micrographs of strain R6 (**A**) and mutant *fil* (**C**). Thin sections of strain R6 showing normal septation and cell separation (**B**) and the abnormal cell septation in mutant *fil* (**D**).

ent block of cell division and inhibition of the formation and progress of septal growth (Fig. 10).[11]

A different type of interference with septum formation was identified in a morphological mutant "*fil*" of pneumococcus isolated in the laboratory. The characteristic phenotype of this mutant is shown by Fig. 11, A–D, which compares the scanning electron micrographs and thin-section electron micrographs of normal and mutant bacteria. Individual cells of the mutant no longer have the characteristic pointed "football" shape of pneumococci. Characteristics of this pseudofilamentous mutant is the formation of extremely long multiseptate chains. However, in contrast to the chains formed in bacteria with inhibited choline metabolism, the chains of the *fil* mutant are extremely resistant to mechanical shear. Cell walls of these mutants can be isolated as long tubular structures representing multiples of

covalently interlinked units of hundreds of individual cells, and such structures prevail even after extraction with hot sodium dodecyl sulfate. The genetic defect in *fil* appears to be some abnormality of the structure and/or physical separation of the crosswall laid down at the septum.

GENETIC TRANSFORMATION

The chain formation of ethanolamine-grown pneumococci was exploited to demonstrate the strikingly high frequency with which individual cells in a pneumococcal culture can internalize exogenous DNA molecules after "activation" with the pneumococcal competence-inducing factor.[6] A culture of pneumo-

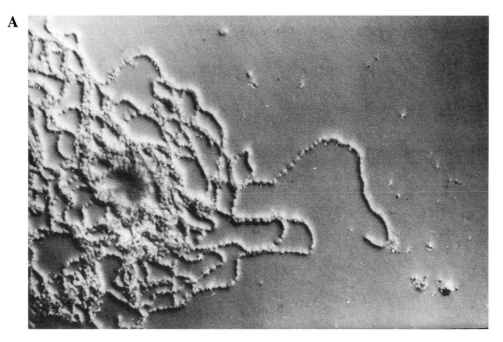

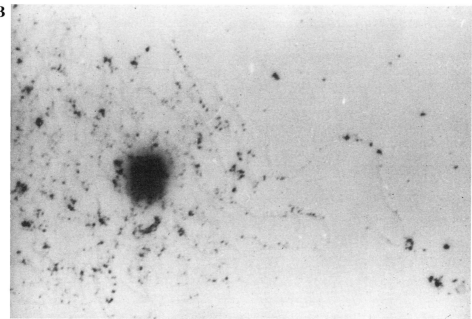

FIG. 12. Radioautographic demonstration of the frequency of DNA uptake in *S. pneumoniae*. An ethanolamine-induced chain of pneumococcus treated with choline, the competence activating factor and tritiated thymidine-labeled DNA was assayed for cells that absorbed radioactive DNA, using autoradiography. (**A**) Nomarsky optics was focused on the cells. (**B**) Nomarsky optics was focused on the autoradiographic grains.

cocci grown in ethanolamine was exposed to a brief, few-minute pulse of choline in the growth medium, accompanied by purified competence factor and DNA labeled with radioactive thymidine at very high specific radioactivity. After a short 10- to 15-min incubation with these reagents, the culture was treated with DNase, washed briefly to remove exogenous DNA, and deposited on microscope slides that were covered with nuclear emulsion capable of detecting cells that have taken up DNA. Figure 12, A and B, demonstrates the very high frequency with which these bacteria can participate in genetic transformation events. In a second experiment, pneumococci made competent by treatment with the competence activator were mixed with a low concentration of transforming DNA and were delivered onto the surface of a colloidal balance containing a monolayer of a basic protein. Sampling of the surface with electron microscope grids followed by uranium shadow casting of the specimen and observation under the electron microscope has allowed the detection of images shown in Fig. 13, suggesting that

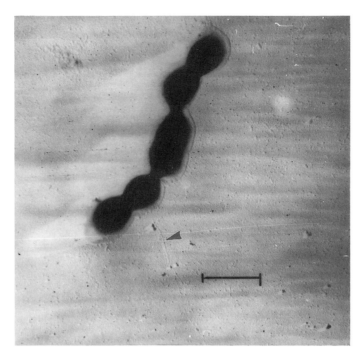

FIG. 13. Chain of *S. pneumoniae* with a strand of DNA attached to one of the cells seen by electron microscopy. Arrowhead points to DNA strand. Size marker, 1 μm.

they represented the morphological documentation of a stage in the uptake of DNA molecules in genetic transformation.[20]

REFERENCES

1. **Baltz, R.H., F.H. Norris, P. Matsushima, B.S. DeHoff, P. Rockey, G. Porter, S. Burgett, R. Peery, J. Hoskins, L. Braverman, I. Jenkins, P. Solenberg, M. Young, M.A. McHenney, P.L. Skatrud, and P.R. Rosteck, Jr.** 1998. DNA sequence sampling of the *Streptococcus pneumoniae* genome to identify novel targets for antibiotic development. Microb. Drug Resist. **4:**1–9.

2. **Bayer, M.E.** 1968. Areas of adhesion between wall and membrane of *Escherichia coli.* J. Gen. Microbiol. **53:**395–404.

3. **Briese, T., and R. Hakenbeck.** 1985. Interaction of the pneumococcal amidase with lipoteichoic acid and choline. Eur. J. Biochem. **146:**417–427.

4. **Briles, E.B., and A. Tomasz.** 1970. Radioautographic evidence for equatorial wall growth in a gram positive bacterium: segregation of choline ^{3}H-labeled teichoic acid. J. Cell Biol. **47:**786–790.

5. **Giudicelli, S., and A. Tomasz.** 1984. Attachment of pneumococcal autolysin to wall teichoic acids, an essential step in enzymatic wall degradation. J. Bacteriol. **158:**1188–1190.

6. **Havarstein, L.S., G. Coomaraswamy, and D.A. Morrison.** 1995. An unmodified heptadecapeptide pheromone induces competence for genetic transformation in *Streptococcus pneumoniae.* Proc. Natl. Acad. Sci. USA **92:**11140–11144.

7. **Higgins, M.L., and G.D. Shockman.** 1970. Model for cell wall growth of *Streptococcus faecalis.* J. Bacteriol. **101:**643–648.

8. **Holtje, J.-V., and A. Tomasz.** 1975. Specific recognition of choline residues in the cell wall teichoic acid by the N-acetylmuramyl-L-alanine amidase of pneumococcus. J. Biol. Chem. **250:**6072–6076.

9. **Iannelli, F., B.J. Pearce, and G. Pozzi.** 1999. The type 2 capsule locus of *Streptococcus pneumoniae.* J. Bacteriol. **181:**2652–2654.

10. **Laitinen, H., and A. Tomasz.** 1990. Changes in composition of peptidoglycan during maturation of the cell wall in pneumococci. J. Bacteriol. **172:**5961–5967.

11. **Ramirez, M., E. Severina, and A. Tomasz.** 1999. A high incidence of prophage carriage among natural isolates of *Streptococcus pneumoniae.* J. Bacteriol. **181:**3618–3625.

12. **Rane, L., and Y. Subbarow.** 1940. Nutritional requirements of the pneumococcus. 1. Growth factors for types I, II, V, VII, VIII. J. Bacteriol. **40:**695–704.

13. **Robertson, J.D.** 1959. The ultrastructure of cell membranes and their derivatives, p. 3. In The Structure and Function of Subcellular Components. Biochem. Soc. Symp. 16. Cambridge University Press, Cambridge, UK.

14. **Rothfield, L.I., and S.S. Justice.** 1997. Bacterial cell division: the cycle of the ring. Cell **88:**581–584.

15. **Ryter, A., and D. Kellenberger.** 1958. Étude au microscope electronique de plasmas contenant de l'acide désoxyribonucleique. A. Naturforsch. **13b:**597.

16. **Sanchez-Puelles, J.M., C. Ronda, J.L. Garcia, P. Garcia, R. Lopez, and E. Garcia.** 1986. Searching for autolysin functions. Characterization of a pneumococcal mutant deleted in the *lytA* gene. Eur. J. Biochem. **158:**289–293.

16a. **Seto, H., R. Lopez, and A. Tomasz.** 1975. Cell surface-located DNA receptors in transformable pneumococci. J. Bacteriol. **122:**1339–1350.

17. **Severin, A., D. Horne, and A. Tomasz.** 1997. Autolysis and cell wall degradation in a choline-independent strain of *Streptococcus pneumoniae.* Microb. Drug Resist. **3:**391–400.

18. **Tomasz, A.** 1967. Choline in the cell wall of a bacterium: novel type of polymer-linked choline in pneumococcus. Science **157:**694–697.

19. **Tomasz, A.** 1968. Biological consequences of the replacement of

choline by ethanolamine in the cell wall of pneumococcus: chain formation, loss of transformability, and loss of autolysis. Proc. Natl. Acad. Sci. USA **59**:86–93.

20. **Tomasz, A., and W. Stoeckenius.** 1963. Electronmicroscopic studies of cells and DNA molecules during the genetic transformation of bacteria. XIth International Congress Genetics, The Hague.

21. **Tomasz, A., E. Zanati, and R. Ziegler.** 1971. DNA uptake during genetic transformation and the growing zone of the cell envelope. Proc. Natl. Acad. Sci USA **68**:1848–1852.

22. **Tomasz, A., J.D. Jamieson, and E. Ottolenghi.** 1964. The fine structure of *Diplococcus pneumoniae.* J. Cell. Biol. **22**:453–467.

22a. **Tomasz, A., M. McDonnell, M. Westphal, and E. Zanati.** 1975. Coordinated incorporation of nascent peptidoglycan and teichoic acid into pneumococcal cell walls and conservation of peptidoglycan during growth. J. Biol. Chem. **250**:337–341.

23. **Tomasz, A., P. Moreillon, and G. Pozzi.** 1988. Insertional inactivation of the major autolysin gene of *Streptococcus pneumoniae.* J. Bacteriol. **170**:5931–5934.

24. **Van Interson, W., and W. Leene.** 1964. A cytochemical localization of reductive sites in a gram-positive bacterium. Tellurite reduction in *Bacillus subtilis.* J. Cell Biol. **20**:361.

25. **Yother, J., Leopold, K., White, J. and Fischer, W.** 1998. Generation and properties of a *Streptococcus pneumoniae* mutant which does not require choline or analogs for growth. J. Bacteriol. **180**:2093–2101.

Address reprint requests to:
Dr. Alexander Tomasz
Laboratory of Microbiology
The Rockefeller University
1230 York Avenue
New York, NY 10021

Part 2

Chromosome Structure, Recombination, and Cloning

Structural Organization of the *Streptococcus pneumoniae* Chromosome and Relatedness of Penicillin-Sensitive and -Resistant Strains in Type 9V

ANNE-MARIE GASC,[1] PHILIPPE GIAMMARINARO,[1] BAO TON-HOANG,[1] PIERRE GESLIN,[2] MARK van der GIEZEN,[3] and MICHEL SICARD[1]

ABSTRACT

Fragmentation of *Streptococcus pneumoniae* genomic DNA with low-frequency-cleavage restriction endonucleases and separation of the fragments by field-inversion gel electrophoresis (FIGE) provides a DNA-fingerprint of a strain. This method enables us to construct a physical and genetic map of the R6 laboratory strain what will be presented. The origin of replication containing several Dna boxes was located in the dnaA region. It was of interest to compare the profiles of subclones. Two clones of strain R36A (R6 and Cl3) were cultivated separately for more than 15,000 generations in two laboratories. FIGE profiles differed by only one band. Another R36A descendant, isolated in 1958 by Ravin, strain Rx was of interest since it was deficient in Dpn restriction enzymes and methylases and in the hex B function. Its origin was questionable; its profile is identical to others R6 descendants, demonstrating that Rx is derived from R36A. FIGE analysis was carried out on several penicillin-resistant strains of type 9V because penicillin-resistance in this type increased recently. The profiles of a collection of a number of these resistant isolates were very similar, showing that they result from a clone. The profiles of penicllin sensitive isolates of the same type are very similar to the resistant isolates. This suggests that the 9V type has spread recently from a clone, and the resistance genes have mutated and were selected when penicillin was extensively used.

INTRODUCTION

STREPTOCOCCUS PNEUMONIAE IS A COMMON MICROORGANISM of the human respiratory flora and a major cause of morbidity and mortality worldwide. Moreover the spread of penicillin resistance is a major concern for antimicrobial therapy. Although the pneumococcal transformation system has been extensively investigated and used for genetic studies, the mechanisms of this important health problem are very poorly understood. The absence of a genetic map has been a major impediment to the investigation of the molecular genetics of *S. pneumoniae*. The ability to separate large fragments of DNA by pulsed-field gel electrophoresis (FIGE) has provided the technology to map bacterial chromosomes. We will present the map of chromosome of *S. pneumoniae*. Genetic markers are located on this map. We have also utilized the FIGE method to compare the profiles of several strains. As this method is an effective tool for typing *S. pneumoniae* strains with a very good discrimination,[24] we used it to answer several questions: what will be the divergeance of strains that were cultivated separately in different laboratories for many generations? When the origin of a strain is questionable can we determine its genealogy? In the spread of penicillin resistance of a given serotype (9V), is there a clonal origin and is it due to penicillin treatment or does it pre-exist this treatment?

[1]Laboratoire de Microbiologie et Génétique Moléculaire du CNRS and Université Paul Sabatier, 118 route de Narbonne 31062 Toulouse Cedex, France.
[2]Centre National de Références des Pneumocoques, CHU 40 avenue de Créteil 94010 Créteil, France.
[3]Department of Microbiology, University of Groningen, P.O. Box 14, NL-9750 AA Haren, The Netherlands.
Reprinted from *Microbial Drug Resistance*, Vol. 3, No. 1, 1997.

TABLE 1. CHARACTERISTICS OF *S. PNEUMONIAE* CLINICAL ISOLATES SEROTYPE 9V STRAINS[a]

Strain	Origin	Serotype	Antibiotic resistance markers	MIC of Pe (mg ml^{-1})
19590	Le Mans	9V	PeTp	0.5
17700	Paris (Debré)	9V	PeTp	4
17365	Tours	9V	Pe Tp	1
17534	Paris (Bichat)	9V	Pe Tp	4
17316	Paris (St. Antoine)	9V	Pe Tp	2
17114	Créteil	9V	Pe Tp	1
17438	Brive	9V	Pe Tp	2
18044	Brive	9V	Pe Tp	0.5
18997	Paris (St Joseph)	9V	Pe Tp Em Cm	2
16415	Aulnay sous Bois	9V	Pe Tp Em	0.5
665	Spain	9V	Pe Tp	1
676	Spain	9	Pe Tp	1
4491	Le Mans	9V	—	0.016
5349	Clermont-Ferrand	9V	Tp	0.016
10197	Reims	9V	Tp Em	0.032
14893	Brive	9V	—	0.016
14609	Arras	9V	Tp	0.032
30298	Bordeaux	9V	Em	0.032

[a]The French isolates were kindly donated by P. Geslin (Centre National de Référence des Pneumocoques, Créteil (France). The two spanish strains 665 and 676 were a generous gift of R. Hakenbeck (Max Planck Institut, Berlin, Germany). Resistance makers: Pe, penicillin; Tp, trimethoprim; Em, erythromycine; Cm, chloramphenicol.

MATERIALS AND METHODS

Bacterial strains and growth conditions

All bacteria used to construct the map described in the text are derived from pneumococcus strain R6. A subculture of *S. pneumoniae* 800 or 801 was used in this study[23] along with a multiply marked strain (strain 119) resistant to 200 µg of streptomycin (*str-4l*) per ml, 75 µg of fusidic acid (*fus-*rA) per ml, 4 µg of novobiocin (*nov-rl*) per ml, 2 µg of optochin (*opt-r2*) per ml, 1 µg of rifampin (*rif-rF*) per ml, and 5 µg of streptolydigin (*stg-rF*) per ml.[47] The *uvr* resistance gene[48] was located with the use of the cloned gene.[44] To map the *amiA* gene, strain 801 bearing *amiA3* was used.[13] The methotrexate-sensitive bacteria in the resistant population were selected in synthetic medium containing an excess of isoleucine.[45] Bacterial 9V strains and their relevant properties are listed in Table 1. Ten French clinical isolates of penicillin-resistant *S. pneumoniae* were studied and compared with two Spanish strains.[11] The culture media and transformation procedures have been described elsewhere.[8] For several experiments, pneumococci were grown in brain heart infusion broth (Difco Laboratories Inc.) supplemented with 40 µg of thymidine per ml and 150 µg of glutamine per ml. Cultures were incubated at 37°C without aeration and were maintained during growth at pH 7.8 with the addition of 1N NaOH.

DNA preparation and digestion with restriction enzymes

S. pneumoniae DNA embedded in agarose beads was prepared by the method described previously for *Haemophilus influenzae*,[21] with the exception that lysozyme was omitted in the lysis buffer. A number of *S. pneumoniae* genes have been cloned in plasmids[46] and used for genome mapping. Restriction enzymes were obtained from New England Biolabs, Pharmacia (Uppsala, Sweden), and Bethesda Research Laboratories (Cergy Pontoise, France). The reaction conditions were those recommended by Bethesda Research Laboratories.

Electrophoresis and hybridization

Southern blot hybridization and nick translation were performed essentially as described by Sambrook et al.[40] The field inversion gel electrophoresis (FIGE) has been described in detail elsewhere.[20]

Gene mapping

In order to correlate genetic markers with the physical map, two procedures were utilized: Southern blot hybridization of cloned genes and transformation of fragments separated by FIGE. The cloned genes were labeled with ^{32}P by nick translation and were hybridized to fragments of restriction digests transferred to nylon membranes. To test for transforming activity, the restriction digests were separated by FIGE in 1% low-melting-point agarose (FMC Corp., Rockland, ME). Following electrophoresis, a portion of the gel was stained with ethidium bromide and DNA bands were detected with the UV transilluminator. The gel was sliced, individual bands were melted at 68°C for 10 min and equilibrated at 37°C with 5 mM EDTA-100 mM NaCl (pH 8.0), and agarase (Calbiochem) was added to 40 U/ml. After overnight digestion, the DNAs were ethanol precipitated and dissolved in 35 µl of 30 mM sodium citrate (pH 7.0). An aliquot of 5 µl from each sample was used to transform competent pneumococcal cultures, which were selected for donor markers. In some experiments, the individual bands were extracted by electroelution. For equivalent amounts of DNA in the gels, electroeluted DNA gave gels of lower biological activity than agarase-digested DNA did.

RESULTS AND DISCUSSION

Evolution of the chromosome of S. pneumoniae

The original transformable pneumococcus used by Avery and coworkers was the strain R36A, a rough spontaneous mutant derived from the type II smooth strain, D39.[4] A subclone of R36A, strain R6 was used later on in the Rockefeller Institute by Rollin Hotchkiss and coworkers. In 1947 Harriett Ephrussi-Taylor moved from this laboratory to the Faculté des Sciences de Paris carrying the R36A strain. In order to obtain more efficient competent cultures, she isolated a subclone (clone 3 or Cl3) that was transformable in this laboratory. Thus the two clones (R6 and Cl3) derived from a unique strain R36A were geographically separated and cultured for many generations. This situation is an excellent opportunity to study the evolution of these strains by FIGE analysis of their chromosome.

In the routine protocol of strains maintenance in the Paris laboratory, strain Cl3 was subcultured every month from cultures stored in the refrigerator. Cell death was very high. Often cultures were re-established from several colonies at the surface of Petri dishes. As competence was difficult to obtain routinely, strains were often subcultured every day from a 1 to 20 dilution. Under such conditions genetic drift was necessarily important. Thus Cl3 has been cultured for more than 15,000 generations. The Rockefeller strain, R6, a sister strain of Cl3 was also continuously, but less frequently, subcultured by a passage every 3 months.[18] In any case more than 15,000 generations separated these two strains. The DNA of these two strains were analyzed by the FIGE method using *Sma*I and *Apa*I restriction enzyme treatments and two different migration programs. Only one band was changed out of the 30 well defined bands obtained

TABLE 2. *S. PNEUMONIAE* GENES AND THEIR LOCALIZATION ON FIGE SEPARATED DNA FRAGMENTS PREVIOUSLY DIGESTED WITH *Sma*I, *Apa*I, OR *Sac*II RESTRICTION ENZYMES

| Genes | Restriction fragments | | | Reference |
	*Sma*I	*Apa*I	*Sac*II	
hexA	5	4	13–17	28
malM	5	4	12	46
dnaA	5	4	—	unpublished
aspS	5	4	—	27
polA	13–14	14	24–26	30
comAB	7–8	14	3	7
pspA	7–8	3	3–4	31
hexB	11	3	3–4	36
str-41	13	3	6	47
fus-rA	15–16	3	6	47
hya	3	3	6–7	35
sul abcd	3	3	6	25
pbp x	3	12–13	6–7	22
ponA	3	13	13–17	26
cap3A	3	13	13–17	3
aliA	3	13	13–17	1
ply	9–10	8–9	8–9	5
rif23	8–10	8–10	9–12	47
stg rF	8–10	8–10	9–12	47
lytA	8–10	8–9	9	10
penA	7–9	9	2	9
mms	8	9	2	29
nanA	8	9	2	6
ami	6	16–18	2	2
recP	12	11	13–17	39
ciaR/ciaH	1	2	4–5	16
dacA	1	2	4–5	41–42
nov-rl	1	2	4–5	47
ung	2	1	1	32
mutX	2	1	1	33
uvs 402	2	1	1	44
Target region for Ω BM6001	2	1	1	49
Target region for Ω BM4200	2	10	18–20	17
opt-r2	—	5	8	47

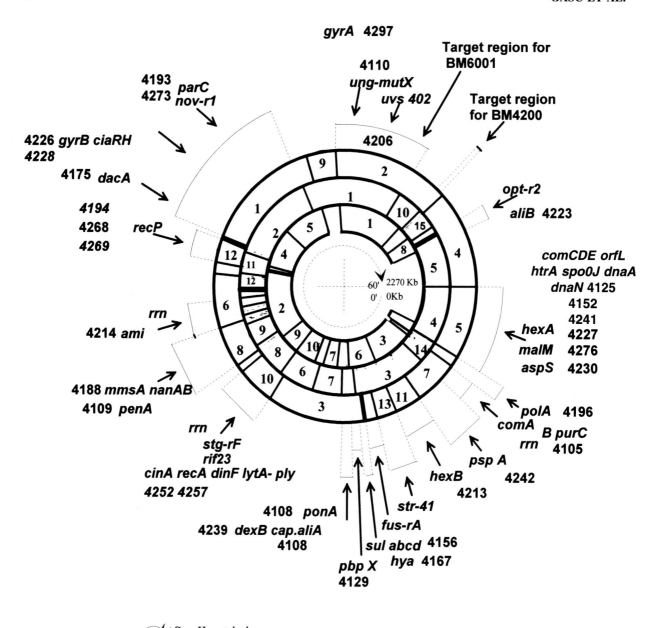

FIG. 1. Physical and genetic map of *Streptococcus pneumoniae* R6 made by using *Sma*I, *Apa*I and *Sac*II restriction enzymes. The sequences of genes listed in Table 2 were localized on *Streptococcus pneumoniae* TIGR Microbial Database. The numbers near the genes refer to TIGR Microbiol Database.contigs. Sequences data were obtained from The Institute for Genomic Research Website at http:www.tigr.org.

by these analysis. This shows that FIGE patterns are quite stable and evolution is fairly slow. This genomic drift is also exemplified by genetic divergence. When in the early sixties a synthetic medium was devised to grow *S. pneumoniae*, it was found that Cl3 requires uracil (ura) while the strains from which it arose do not (R36A, D39).[45] Cl3 appears to have become uracil⁻ during 1960 since most (24/25) of the aminopterin-resistant mutants selected in that year and there after are also ura⁻ whereas

mutants selected within Cl3 prior to this date proved all to be ura⁺. Other differences of unknown determinants such as transformability and growth in complete medium were observed when these two sister strains were cultured in our laboratory.

Strain R_x is another rough pneumococcal strain routinely used in several microbial genetic laboratories. When used as recipient, all markers yield equal transformation frequencies whereas in R6 or Cl3 recipients these markers differed in their transformation frequencies by a factor of 10. This observation first reported by D. MacDonald Green in A. Ravin laboratory[15] was eventually explained at the molecular level by the discovery of the mismatch-repair system requiring the *hex A*[28] and *hex B* genes.[36,37] Strain Rx is mutated in the *hexB* gene.[36] Moreover Rx has lost the *Dpn*I pneumococcal restriction system acting on methylated adenine at the GATC sequence.[34] Furthermore it has been observed that the release of the competence peptide in the culture medium is more efficient than in strain R6. Arnold Ravin reports its isolation[38] from the following experiments. In 1950, strain R36A was transformed by DNA from Smooth type III-1. A Smooth type III-1-T50 transformant was selected and in 1954 it was used as recipient to be transformed by DNA from Smooth type III-2. A Smooth type III-N-T54 transformant containing the normal amount of capsule was recovered and cultured. This strain, treated by DNA from smooth type III-1-str, yielded some rough colonies that were unexpected. One of them was the strain R$_x$. It might be a spontaneous rough mutant present in the last recipient culture or from an unknown origin. As pointed out by A. Ravin[38] (in the experiments lacking adequate control of the spontaneous R mutation), the R36A genetic background of strain R$_x$ is questionable. To define its origin, we have analyzed the DNA from strain Rx by FIGE methodology. The FIGE profiles were identical to the R6 profiles showing that indeed it is a rough mutant of strains derived from R36A. Other mutations such as *Dpn*0 should have accumulated during subculturing at an undefined date.

Physical and genetic map of strain R6

The basic strategy for chromosomal mapping consists of immobilizing cells in a solid matrix, such as in low-melting-temperature agarose, and subsequently removing cellular components by treatment with agents that dissolve the outer surface and proteins. The intact chromosome(s) embedded in agarose can then be directly cut with restriction enzymes, producing fragments separable in an agarose gel. The restriction enzymes are chosen on the basis of the number of fragments produced per chromosome. *Apa*I (GGGCCC), *Sma*I (CCCGGG), and *Sac*II (CCGCGG) each gave less than 30 fragments that could be conveniently separated by FIGE, and they were chosen for this study. DNA fragment sizes were determined from agarose gels and the estimated genome sizes was 2,200 kbp. The approach used was to separate individual fragments label them with ^{32}P deoxyribonucleoside triphosphate, and hybridize them to separated, restriction enzyme-digested chromosomal DNA fragments. A single DNA fragment should produce a single band of hybridization to DNA digested with the same enzyme, but it may produce one or several bands hybridizing with the DNA fragments from other restriction enzyme digests. Hybridization with two or more fragments of another restriction enzyme digest was evidence for an overlap and was used to construct the map. By this procedure, almost all *Sma*I and *Apa*I fragments could be located unambiguously on the *S. pneumoniae* map. However, *Apa*I fragments 20 and 22 hybridized to the same *Sma*I fragment (fragment 4), and their positions relative to each other are assigned arbitrarily. In a like manner, *Apa*I fragments 16,17,18,19, and 21 and *Sma*I fragments 16 and 19 could not be precisely ordered within the physical map.[12]

Assignment of genetic markers

The ability to transform chromosomal markers is a unique property of naturally competent bacteria such as *S. pneumoniae*. We have used this property to map genetic markers to specific restriction fragments. DNA from multiply marked strain 119 was digested by the three restriction enzymes *Apa*I, *Sac*II and *Sma*I, separated by FIGE, and used for mapping. Whenever possible, the DNA from each individual band was extracted and used to transform competent recipient cells. Biological activity was often found in a single band only when this band could be isolated without contamination from adjacent or similar-size fragments. Cloned genes obtained from various sources were labeled and hybridized to separated *Sma*I, *Apa*I, and *Sac*II restriction digest fragments. All these genes and the hybridization or transformations results are listed in Table 2. The physical and genetic map of strain R6, resulting from these studies is shown in Fig. 1.

Replication origin of strain R6

To determine where is the origin of replication of the pneumococcal chromosome, we have located the genes and sequences that are usually near the origin in several bacteria. The dnA protein plays an important role in initiation of chromosomal replication. Richter and Messer have characterized a fragment carrying a part of *dnaA* gene of *S. pneumoniae*. Fig. 2 gives FIGE separation of *Sma*I, *Sma*I and *Apa*I, *Apa*I and *Sac*II restriction fragments of *S. pneumoniae* strain R6. The program used yields maximal separation of the largest fragments. Near every profile we have the corresponding hybridization with a

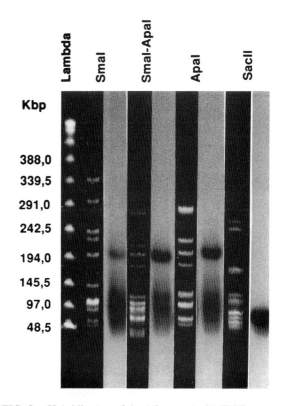

FIG. 2. Hybridization of *dnaA* fragment with FIGE separated restriction enzyme digests of strain R6.

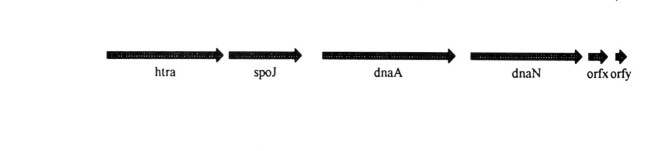

FIG. 3. Genetic map of *Streptococcus pneumoniae dnaA* region.

part of dnaA gene labelled with [32]P. By this procedure this gene was localized on the physical map (Fig. 1). In order to study the neighboring genes and sequences, we have selected a lambda Zap phage[43] which hybridizes with the labeled dnaA fragment. This phage came from the phage-bank of *S. pneumoniae* DNA, constructed by B. Martin. It carries a 6-kb insert that was sequenced. Downstream of *dnaA* we have found a gene homologous to *dnaN* and upstream a gene homologous to *SpoOJ*. There is another open reading frame and the deduced amino acid sequence of the putative product is similar to a serine protease. Genes at the right or at the left of dnaA are transcribed in the same direction. The order of these genes is shown in Fig. 3. We also found several dnaA box sequences in this region suggesting a putative origin of replication.

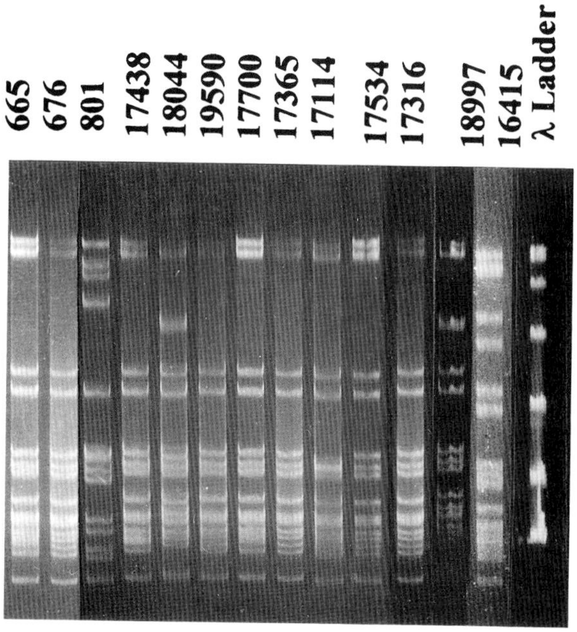

Relatedness of penicillin-resistant and -sensitive strains of type 9

Although more than 80 types are known in *S. pneumoniae*, most of the penicillin-resistant clinical isolates belongs to only

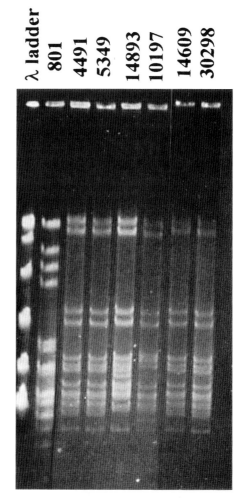

FIG. 4. FIGE separation of SmaI restriction fragments of *S. pneumoniae* penicillin resistant type 9V strains.

FIG. 5. FIGE separation of SmaI restriction fragments of *S. pneumoniae* sensitive type 9V strains.

a few groups. The first type 9V strain resistant to penicillin was isolated in Spain in 1987.[19] In France, after the emergence of the first strain in 1988, the frequency of penicillin resistance in type 9V rose to 15% in 1993.[14] To test if these strains emerged independently or resulted from the spreading of one or few clones, we compared the FIGE profiles of fragments of their genomic DNA. Similar analysis was performed for penicillin-sensitive strain of the same type.

Ten penicillin-resistant 9V strains isolated in French Hospital and two strains isolated in Spain were submitted to the FIGE analysis after a *Sma*I treatment of their DNA. In Fig. 4 we can see that all of the French 9V strains are genetically related and share a similar profile to strains first isolated in Spain. This suggests that the 10 French and the Spanish isolates originated from a clone. However within this group of 12 related strains, penicillin resistance varied by up to 8-fold. This might mean that resistance genes had accumulated in a parental clone or that the population of penicillin-sensitive strains from type 9V was already genetically homogeneous prior to mutations to resistance to varied concentrations of penicillin.

We have analyzed six penicillin sensitive strains from type 9V by FIGE after digestion of genomic DNA by *Sma*I or *Apa*I. Their FIGE profiles were similar (Fig. 5) and similar to the pattern of the resistant isolates. A more extensive study of twenty six sensitive strains yield the same results (Ramuz, pers. com.). This suggests that generation of a clone of type 9V have occured first in sensitive strains, accounting for the homogeneity of the group followed by further selection of resistant strains. It is noteworthy that clonal origin of strains is not restricted to antibiotic usage, but can be found in sensitive strains of type 9V. It would be interesting to investigate the reason for the selective advantage of 9V.

ACKNOWLEDGMENTS

The authors thank the Institute for Genomic Research (Website at http:www.tigr.org.) where *Streptococcus pneumoniae* sequences were available. This work was partly supported by an INSERM BECHAM grant.

REFERENCES

1. **Alloing, G., P. de Philip, and J.P. Claverys.** 1994. Three highly homologous membrane-bound lipoproteins participate on oligopeptide transport by the Ami system of the Gram-positive *Streptococcus pneumoniae*. J. Molec. Biol. **241**:44–58.

2. **Alloing, G., M.C. Trombe, and J.P. Claverys.** 1990. The ami locus of the Gram- positive bacterium *Streptococcus pneumoniae* is similar to binding protein-dependent transport operons of Gram-negative bacteria. Mol. Microbiol. **4**:633–644.

3. **Arrecubieta, C., R. Lopez, and E. Garcia.** 1994. Molecular characterization of *cap*3A, a gene from the operon required for the synthesis of the capsule of *Streptococcus pneumoniae* type 3: Sequencing of mutations responsible for the unencapsulated phenotype and localization of the capsular cluster on the pneumococcal chromosome. J. Bacteriol. **176**:6375–83.

4. **Avery, O.T., C.M. MacLeod, and M. McCarty.** 1944. Studies on the chemical nature of the substance inducing transformation of pneumococcal types. J. Exp. Med. **79**:137–58.

5. **Boulnois, G.L., J.C. Paton, T.J. Mitchell, and P.W. Andrew.** 1991. Structure and function of pneumolysin, the multifunctional, thiol activated toxin of *Streptococcus pneumoniae*. Mol. Microbiology. **5**:2611–2616.

6. **Camara, M., T.J. Mitchell, P.W. Andrew, and G.L. Boulnois.** 1991. *Streptococcus pneumoniae* produces at least two distinct enzymes with neuraminidase activity: Cloning and expression of a second neuraminidase gene in *Escherichia coli*. Infection and Immunity. **59**:2856–2858.

7. **Chandler, M.S., and D.A. Morrison.** 1987. Competence for genetic transformation in *Streptococcus pneumoniae*: Molecular cloning of *com*, a competence control locus. J. Bacteriol. **169**:2005–2011.

8. **Claverys, J.P., M. Roger, and A.M. Sicard.** 1980. Excision and repair of mismatched base pairs in transformation of *Streptococcus pneumoniae*. Mol. Gen. Genet. **178**:191–201.

9. **Dowson, C.G., A. Hutchison, and B.G. Spratt.** 1989. Nucleotide sequence of the penicillin-binding protein 2B gene of *Streptococcus pneumoniae* strain R6. Nucleic Acids Res. **17**:7518.

10. **Garcia, P., J.L. Garcia, and R. Lopez.** 1986. Nucleotide sequence and expression of the pneumococcal autolysin gene from its own promoter in *Escherichia coli*. Gene. **43**:265–72.

11. **Gasc, A.M., P. Geslin, and A.M. Sicard.** 1995. Relatedness of penicillin-resistant *Streptococcus pneumoniae* serogroup 9 strains from France and Spain. Microbiology. **141**:623–627.

12. **Gasc, A.M., L. Kauc, P. Barraillé, A.M. Sicard, and S. Goodgal.** 1991. Gene localization, size, and physical map of the chromosome of *Streptococcus pneumoniae*. J. Bacteriol. **173**:7361–7367.

13. **Gasc, A.M., A.M. Sicard, and J.P. Claverys.** 1989. Repair of single and multiple substitution mismatches during recombination in *Streptococcus pneumoniae*. Genetics. **120**:29–36.

14. **Geslin, P., A. Fremaux, and G. Sissia.** 1993. Infections à pneumocoques de sensibilité diminuée aux bêta-lactamines. pp. 55–71. C. Carbon, C. Chastang and J.M. Decazes (eds.), *In* Epidémiologie de la Résistance de *Streptococcus pneumoniae* aux Bêta-lactamines, en France et dans le Monde. Springer-Verlag, Paris.

15. **Green, D.M.** 1959. A host-specific variation affecting relative frequency of transformation of two markers in pneumococcus. Exp. Cell. Research. **18**:466–480.

16. **Guenzi, E., A.M. Gasc, A.M. Sicard, and R. Hakenbeck.** 1994. A two-component signal-transducing system is involved in competence and penicillin susceptibility in laboratory mutants of *Streptococcus pneumoniae*. Mol. Microbiol. **12**:505–515.

17. **Guild, W.R., S. Hazum, and M.D. Smith.** 1981. Chromosomal location of conjugative R determinants in strain BM4200 of *Streptococcus pneumoniae*. p. 610. S.B. Levy, R.C. Clowes and E.L. Koenig (eds.) *In* Molecular Biology, Pathogenicity, and Ecology of Bacterial Plasmids. Plenum, New York.

18. **Hotchkiss, R.D.** Personal communication.

19. **Hakenbeck, R., T. Briese, L. Chalkley, H. Ellerbrok, R. Kallioloski, C. Latorre, m. Leinonen, and C. Martin.** 1991. Antigenic variation of penicillin-binding proteins from penicillin-resistant clinical strains of *Streptococcus pneumoniae*. J. Infect. Dis. **164**:313–319.

20. **Kauc, L., and S.H. Goodgal.** 1989. The size and physical map of the chromosome of *Haemophilus parainfluenzae*. Gene. **83**:377–380.

21. **Kauc, L., M. Mitchell, and S.H. Goodgal.** 1989. Size and physical map of the chromosome of *Haemophilus influenzae*. J. Bacteriol. **171**:2474–2479.

22. **Laible, G., R. Hakenbeck, A.M. Sicard, B. Joris, and J.M. Ghuysen.** 1989. Nucleotide sequences of the pbp X genes encoding the penicillin-binding proteins 2X from *Streptococcus pneumoniae* R6 and a cefotaxime-resistant mutant C506. Mol. Microbiol. **3**:1337–1348.

23. **Lefèvre, J.C., J.P. Claverys, and A.M. Sicard.** 1979. Donor deoxyribonucleic acid length and marker effect in pneumococcal transformation. J. Bacteriol. **138**:80–86.

24. **Lefèvre, J.C., G. Faucon, A.M. Sicard, and A.M. Gasc.** 1993.

DNA finger printing of *Streptococcus pneumoniae* strains by pulsed field electrophoresis. J. Clin. Microbiol. **31:**2724–2728.

25. **Lopez, P., M. Espinoza, and S.A. Lacks.** 1984. Physical structure and genetic expression of sulfonamide-resistance plasmid pLS80 and its derivatives in *Streptococcus pneumoniae* and *Bacillus subtilis.* Mol. Gen. Genet. **195:**402–410.

26. **Martin, C., T. Briese, and R. Hakenbeck.** 1992. Nucleotide sequences of genes encoding penicillin-binding proteins from *Streptococcus pneumoniae* and *Streptococcus oralis* with high homology to *Escherichia coli* penicillin-binding proteins 1A and 1B. J. Bacteriol. **174:** 4517–4523.

27. **Martin, B., O. Humbert, M. Camara, E. Guenzi, J. Walker, T. Mitchell, P. Andrew, M. Prudhomme, G. Alloing, R. Hakenbeck, D.A. Morrison, G.J. Boulnois, and J.P. Claverys.** 1992. A highly conserved repeated DNA element located in the chromosome of *Streptococcus pneumoniae.* Nucleic Acids Research. **20:**3479–3483.

28. **Martin, B., H. Prats, and J.P. Claverys.** 1985. Cloning of the *hex*A mismatch repair gene of *Streptococcus pneumoniae* and identification of the product. Gene **34:**293–303.

29. **Martin, B., G.J. Sharples, O. Humbert, R.G. Lloyd, and J.P. Claverys.** 1996. The mms A locus of *Streptococcus pneumoniae* encodes a RecG-like protein involved in DNA repair and in three-strand recombination. Mol. Microbiol. **19:**1035–1045.

30. **Martinez, S., P. Lopez, M. Espinoza, and S.A. Lacks.** 1986. Cloning of a gene encoding a DNA polymerase exonuclease of *Streptococcus pneumoniae.* Gene **44:**79–88.

31. **McDaniel, L., S.J. Yother, M.N. Vijamakumar et al.** 1987. Use of insertional inactivation to facilitate studies of biological properties of pneumococcal surface protein A (PspA). J. Exp. Med. **165:**381–394.

32. **Méjean, V., J. Rives, and J.P. Claverys.** 1990. Nucleotide sequence of *Streptococcus pneumoniae ung* gene encoding uracil-DNA glycosylase. Nucleic Acids Res. **18:**6693.

33. **Méjean, V., C. Salles, L.C. Bullions, M.J. Bessman, and J.P. Claverys.** 1994. Characterization of the *mutX* gene of *Streptococcus pneumoniae* as a homologous of *Escherichia coli* mutT, and tentative definition of a catalytic domain of the dGTP pyrophosphohydrolases. Mol. Microbiol. **11:**323–330.

34. **Muckerman, C.C., S.S. Springhorn, B. Greenberg, and S.A. Lacks.** 1982. Transformation of restriction endonuclease phenotype in *Streptococcus pneumoniae.* J. Bacteriol. **152:**183–190.

35. **Paton, J.C., P.W. Andrew, G.J. Boulnois, and T.J. Mitchell.** 1993. Molecular analysis of the pathogenicity of *Streptococcus pneumoniae*: The role of pneumococcal proteins. Ann. Rev. Microbiol. **47:**89–115.

36. **Prats, H., B. Martin, and J.P. Claverys.** 1985. The *Hex*B mismatch repair gene of *Streptococcus pneumoniae.* Characterization, cloning and identification of the product. Mol. Gen. Genet. **200:** 482–489.

37. **Prudhomme, M., B. Martin, V. Méjean, and J.P. Claverys.** 1989. Nucleotide sequence of the *Streptococcus pneumoniae hex*B mismatch repair gene: Homology of HexB to mutL of *Salmonella typhimurium* and to PMS1 of *Saccharomyces cerevisiae.* J. Bacteriol. **171:**5332–5338.

38. **Ravin, A.** 1959. Reciprocal capsular transformation of pneumococci. J. Bacteriol. **77:**296–309.

39. **Rhee, D.K., and D.A. Morrison.** 1988. Genetic transformation in *Streptococcus pneumoniae*: Molecular cloning and characterization of *rec*P, a gene required for genetic recombination. J. Bacteriol. **170:**630–637.

40. **Sambrook, J., E.F. Fritsch, and T. Maniatis.** 1989. Molecular cloning, a laboratory manual. Cold Spring Harbor Laboratory Press, New York.

41. **Schuster, C., B. Dobrinski, and R. Hakenbeck.** 1990. Unusual septum formation in *Streptococcus pneumoniae* mutants with an alteration in the D,D-carboxypeptidase penicillin-binding protein 3. J. Bacteriol. **172:**6499–6505.

42. **Selakovitch-Chenu, L., L. Seroude, and A.M. Sicard.** 1993. The role of penicillin-binding protein 3 (PBP 3) in cefotaxime resistance in *Streptococcus pneumoniae.* Mol. Gen. Genet. **239:**77–80.

43. **Short, J.M., J.M. Fernandez, J.A. Sorge, and W.B. Huse.** 1988. λ Zap: A bacteriophage λ expression vector with *in vivo* excision properties. Nucl. Acids Res. **16:**7583–7600.

44. **Sicard, N., and A.M. Estevenon.** 1990. Excision-repair in *S. pneumoniae*: Cloning and expression of an uvr-like gene. Mutat. Res. **235:**195–201.

45. **Sicard, A.M.** 1964. A new synthetic medium for *Diplococcus pneumoniae* and its use for the study of reciprocal transformations at the *ami*A locus. Genetics. **50:**31–44.

46. **Stassi, D.L., P. Lopez, M. Espinosa, and S.A. Lacks.** 1981. Cloning of chromosomal genes in *Streptococcus pneumoniae.* Proc. Natl. Acad. Sci. USA **78:**7028–7032.

47. **Tiraby, G., and M. Fox.** 1973. Marker discrimination in transformation and mutation of pneumococcus. Proc. Natl. Acad. Sci. USA **70:**3541–3545.

48. **Tiraby, G., and A.M. Sicard.** 1973. Integration efficiency in DNA-induced transformation of pneumococcus. II. Genetic studies of mutant integrating all the markers with a higher efficiency. Genetics **75:**35–48.

49. **Vijayakumar, M.N., S.D. Priebe, and W.R. Guild.** 1986. Structure of a conjugative element in *Streptococcus pneumoniae.* J. Bacteriol. **166:**978–984.

Address reprint requests to:
Anne-Marie Gasc
Laboratoire de Microbiologie et de Génétique Moléculaire
du CNRS
118 route de Narbonne
31062 Toulouse Cedex, France

DNA Sequence Sampling and Gene Disruption for Identification of New Antibacterial Targets in *Streptococcus pneumoniae*

RICHARD H. BALTZ, FRED H. NORRIS, PATTI MATSUSHIMA, BRADLEY S. DEHOFF,
PAMELA ROCKEY, GINA PORTER, STANLEY BURGETT, R. PEERY, J. HOSKINS,
LARA BRAVERMAN, I. JENKINS, PATRICIA SOLENBERG, M. YOUNG, M.A. McHENNEY,
PAUL R. ROSTECK, Jr. and PAUL L. SKATRUD

ABSTRACT

We initiated a survey of the *Streptococcus pneumoniae* genome by DNA sequence sampling. More than 9,500 random DNA sequences of approximately 500 bases average length were determined. Partial sequences sufficient to identify approximately 95% of the aminoacyl tRNA synthetase genes and ribosomal protein (*rps*) genes were found by comparing the database of partial sequences to known sequences from other organisms. Many genes involved in DNA replication, repair, and mutagenesis are present in *Streptococcus pneumoniae*. Genes for the major subunits of RNA polymerase are also present, as are genes for two alternative sigma factors, *rpoD* and *rpoN*. Many genes necessary for amino acid or cofactor biosynthesis and aerobic energy metabolism in other bacteria appear to be absent from the *Streptococcus pneumoniae* genome. A number of genes involved in cell wall biosynthesis and septation were identified, including six homologs to different penicillin binding proteins. Interestingly, four genes involved in the addition of D-alanine to lipoteichoic acid in other gram positive bacteria were found, even though the lipoteichoic acid in *Streptococcus pneumoniae* has not been shown to contain D-alanine. The *Streptococcus pneumoniae* genome contains a number of chaperonin genes similar to those found in other bacteria, but apparently does not contain genes involved in the type III secretion commonly observed in gram negative pathogens. The G + C content of *Streptococcus pneumoniae* genomic DNA is approximately 43 mole percent and the size of the genome is approximately 2.0 Mb as determined by pulsed-field gel electrophoresis. Many of the genes identified by sequence sampling have been physically mapped to the 19 different *Sma*I fragments derived from the *Streptococcus pneumoniae* genome. We developed a gene disruption system for *Streptococcus pneumoniae* that is mediated by conjugation from *Escherichia coli*. Partial genomic sequences were used as probes to clone internal segments of open reading frames which were in turn used to carry out gene disruption in *Streptococcus pneumoniae*. By this procedure, we have identified several potential lethal targets for antibiotic intervention.

INTRODUCTION

GENOME SEQUENCING is a powerful method to generate fundamental information on the genetics, biochemistry, and physiology of bacteria. Nearly every kb of sequence yields a gene and approximately 60% of open reading frames encode proteins of known function based on gene sequences already in the databases.[5,7,11,12,18] Therefore, genome sequencing can be particularly valuable for the analysis of poorly characterized bacteria. As the number of gene sequences known to researchers expands, the probability of identifying genes from homology relationships will also increase. Comparative analysis of multiple genomes should also provide a wealth of information on the basic processes of mutation, recombination, and genome evolution.[4,11,24] In addition, bacterial genomics should help identify many basic functions that, at present, are not understood and functions that are unique to certain groups of bacteria.

From the practical view of drug development, genomics can be used to identify genes of known function common to many microorganisms, genes unique to a single pathogen, and genes of unknown function that may be potential targets for anti-

---

Lilly Research Laboratories, A Division of Eli Lilly and Company, Indianapolis, Indiana.

biotic development, based on specific criteria for target development. For example, if the strategy is to pick novel lethal targets present in all pathogenic bacteria, then genomics can be used to initiate a series of steps as follows: (i) identify all genes in *S. pneumoniae* that are of unknown function and that are present in other gram positive and gram negative bacteria; (ii) clone an internal segment from each of these genes and carry out gene disruption to identify potentially lethal targets; (iii) obtain a complete sequence for the genes with indispensable function(s); (iv) clone and express the genes in *Escherichia coli* or in some other expression host; (v) purify the protein and develop an assay; (vi) screen for inhibitors of the protein using natural product, combinational chemical, and other chemical libraries; (vii) optimize lead inhibitors using traditional or combinatorial chemical approaches; and (viii) proceed to clinical evaluation. Obviously, this scenario has the difficult proviso that assays be developed for proteins of unknown function. Different sets of criteria can be put in place to simplify assay development (e.g., pick targets of known function), to develop narrow spectrum antibacterials, or to develop drugs directed at virulence factors. In this chapter, we focus on the identification of genes in *S. pneumoniae* by DNA sequence sampling and on gene disruption to identify potential lethal targets for antibiotic development. The data on DNA sequence sampling is from Baltz *et al.*[2a]

STRATEGIES FOR GENOMIC DNA SEQUENCE ANALYSIS

There are at least two additional DNA sequencing strategies for extracting the basic genetic information from a bacterium beyond the traditional approach of identifying, cloning, and sequencing individual genes. The first is random, whole genome sequencing.[1,11,12] This approach identifies the complete nucleotide sequence of a bacterial genome and, thus, provides extensive information on gene organization, potential transcriptional and translational units, potential regulatory sequences for specific genes, and other features such as repeat elements. Coupled with data from other bacteria, it can also provide insights into genome evolution. A current limitation of this approach is that it requires either DNA sequencing capacity and bioinformatics available only at a small number of institutions or a concerted, highly coordinated effort by many institutions. As DNA sequencing techniques and DNA sequence assembly and analysis methods are improved and made generally available to the scientific community, this approach should become the method of choice.

A second approach is genome sequence sampling or sequence scanning.[3,4,17,29] This approach can provide much information about the genetic makeup of a bacterium without determining the complete sequence. Since the function of approximately 60% of bacterial genes can be identified by DNA sequence alone, a partial sequence of one strand is often sufficient to identify the presence of the gene in a bacterium. In addition, the isolated clones and the partial sequences obtained from them (genome sequence tags or GSTs) are valuable reagents for additional molecular biology and bioinformatics applications.[29] Sequence sampling at a multiplicity of one, or one-fold coverage of all bases in a genome,[11] should give ac-

tual sequence for approximately 63% of all bases ($P = 1 - e^{-1}$, from the Poisson Distribution at a multiplicity of 1). Since a gene of known sequence can be identified by a partial sequence of either DNA strand, the actual multiplicity for identifying known genes is higher than 63%. For example, if each individual sequence determined is approximately 500 b, then the probability for identifying known genes is closer to 2 at a multiplicity of 1 for identifying all bases. If the sequence sampling is truly random, then twofold sequence coverage should be sufficient to identify over 95% of all known genes (i.e., $P = 1 - e^{-4}$), based on partial DNA sequence homology to other genes in the databases. This is substantially less than the approximately sixfold random coverage required to initiate the assembly of the complete genomic sequence of *Haemophilus influenzae*. Sequence sampling can be coupled with focused sequencing of individual genes or chromosomal segments to facilitate the analysis and exploitation of specific genes or specific clustered biosynthetic pathways. This approach can be particularly fruitful in poorly studied pathogenic bacteria to quickly identify, clone, and express genes that encode functions suitable for antibiotic development. In such cases, the complete genomic sequence may not be needed since only a fraction of the genes identified are likely to encode functions that present attractive targets for antibiotic intervention. Sequence sampling also provides a platform for complete sequence analysis if that is desirable as assembly and annotation techniques become more routine.

RANDOM DNA SEQUENCE SAMPLING

We calculated the probability of missing particular genes by sequence sampling as a function of fractional sequence coverage, assuming a genome size of 2×10^6 bp containing approximately 2,000 genes of approximately 1 kb average size, and individual, random sequences of approximately 500 b using the Poisson equation, $P = m^x e^{-m}/x!$, where P is the probability of x sequencing hits occurring per one 1 kb gene at a given multiplicity (m) of sequencing runs per gene. We generated over 9,500 random nucleotide sequences from libraries constructed by cloning *S. pneumoniae* genomic DNA partially digested with various restriction enzymes in the bacteriophage vector M13mp19.[29] This amount of sequence data is equivalent to a coverage of approximately 2.3-fold and a multiplicity (of partially sequencing an average gene of 1 kb) of over fourfold. At this coverage, random sequence sampling should identify approximately 98% of 1 kb-sized genes ($P = 1 - e^{-4}$).

Initially, we assessed the randomness of sequence sampling by surveying amino-acyl tRNA synthetase and ribosomal protein genes, both of which are highly conserved in bacteria. In *E. coli* and *H. influenzae*, individual tRNA synthetases are responsible for the charging of the individual 20 natural amino acids to their respective tRNAs. In *B. subtilis*, 19 tRNA synthetases charge the 20 amino acids to their respective tRNAs.[15] *B. subtilis*, *B. megaterium*, *Lactococcus acidophilus*, and *Mycoplasma genitalium* lack a glutamine tRNA synthetase. In these gram-positive bacteria, tRNA Gln is first charged with Glu by the cognate tRNA synthetase and Glu is converted to Gln by an amidotransferase.[15] Table 1 shows the results of *S. pneumoniae* sequence sampling and searches for tRNA synthetase genes using the sequence comparison algorithm BLAST.[1] We identified 18 tRNA synthetase genes, but a glutamine tRNA synthetase gene (gluS) was not found, consistent with the lack of this gene in other gram positive bacteria. We found a homolog to the *B. subtilis* glutamyl-tRNA transamidase, also consistent with the mechanism described above. The tRNA Trp gene (trpS) was also not found by DNA sequence sampling. If we assume that this gene is present in the *S. pneumoniae* genome, then we identify about 95% of the aminoacyl tRNA synthetase genes by a sequence sampling. Since the aminoacyl tRNA synthetase genes are essential for all bacteria,[24] their gene products are potential targets for antibiotic development.

We surveyed ribosomal protein (rps) genes to determine the efficiency of identifying relatively small genes (20 of the rps genes are smaller than 1 kb). For these, we have summed the number of sampling hits for each of the genes. Table 2 shows that all of the genes except rpsF and rpsT were identified at least twice by sampling. A possible rpsF homolog was found once, but it had relatively poor homology to rpsF genes from other organisms (Table 2); we therefore assume, for the sampling analysis, that this is not a legitimate match. Of the 21 rps genes present in *E. coli*, only rpsT has not been found in *H. influenzae*, *M. genitalium*, and *Methanococcus jannaschii*.[5,11,12] Therefore, the inability to find the rpsT gene in *S. pneumoniae* suggests that it may not be present in the genome. With these assumptions, it appears that we have identified 19 of 20 (95%) of the rps genes in *S. pneumoniae*.

The average number of matches to the individual rps genes was seven, higher than the predicted multiplicity of 4–5 for 1 kb-sized genes. This is probably due to the identification of more than one physically linked rps gene in a number of individual random sequences. These data may also indicate that the sequence sampling was not completely random because of the unusually high number of matches observed with rpsB and rpsG and the apparent lack of sequences similar to rpsF. Nonetheless, these data, coupled with the data on tRNA synthetase genes, support the notion that approximately twofold coverage may be sufficient to identify up to 95% of genes. At this level of sampling the method should be useful for determining the presence or absence of genes with some precision, particularly genes involved in multistep pathways. We have begun to survey different sets of genes and discuss the results in the following sections.

Amino acid biosynthesis

The defined medium for *S. pneumoniae* contains the following amino acids: Arg, Asp, Cys, Glu, Gly, His, Ile, Leu, Lys, Met, Thr, and Val.[31] In early studies on the development of a synthetic medium for *S. pneumoniae*, Sicard[31] noted that the addition of Ser or Gly was needed for growth, suggesting that *S. pneumoniae* expressed serine hydroxymethyl transferase activity. We identified a partial sequence with a very high deduced amino acid sequence similarity to that encoded by the glyA gene of *E. coli* ($P(n) = 1.5e − 119$), confirming the prediction made 32 years ago. We surveyed many other genes in-

TABLE 1. AMINOACYL-tRNA SYNTHETASE
GENES IDENTIFIED IN *S. pneumoniae*

Gene	Homolog[a]	Blast p value[b]
alaS	H. influenzae	3.5e–41
argS	S. cerevisiae (mito)	1.2e–50
asnS	B. subtilis	6.0e–53
aspS	E. coli	6.7e–71
cysS	B. subtilis	2.6e–81
gltX	B. subtilis	7.8e–20
glnS[c]	—	—
glyS	E. coli	1.4e–36
hisS	S. equissimilis	3.1e–118
ileS	S. aureus	1.6e–97
leuS	B. subtilis	4.9e–79
lysS	S. aureus	7.9e–219
metG	B. subtilis	1.1e–53
pheS	B. subtilis	1.1e–72
proS	E. coli	4.3e–38
serS	B. subtilis	2.7e–55
thrS	B. sutbilis	3.4e–99
trpS	—	—
tyrS	B. subilitis	4.7e–57
valS	L. casei	7.7e–62

[a]Organism with gene giving best P(n), the smallest Poisson probability.

[b]The p value calculated from the probability of two random sequences showing similarity. The lower the p value, the higher the probability of significance of the match.

[c]Absent in *B. subtilis*, *B. megaterium*, and *Lactobacillus acidophilus*. *S. pneumoniae* has Glu amidotransferase homolog of that found in *B. subtilis*.

TABLE 2. DISTRIBUTION OF DNA SEQUENCE MATCHES
WITHIN RIBOSOMAL PROTEIN GENES

Gene	Protein	Mol wt[a]	Sampling hits[b]
rpsA	S1	61,159	4
rpsB	S2	26,613	28
rpsC	S3	25,852	5
rpsD	S4	23,137	4
rpsE	S5	17,151	5
rpsF	S6	15,704	1[c]
rpsG	S7	19,732	17
rpsH	S8	13,996	9
rpsI	S9	14,569	2
rpsJ	S10	11,736	14
rpsK	S11	13,726	2
rpsL	S12	13,606	5
rpsM	S13	12,968	9
rpsN	S14	11,063	6
rpsO	S15	10,001	3
rpsP	S16	9,191	12
rpsQ	S17	9,573	12
rpsR	S18	8,896	6
rpsS	S19	10,299	9
rpsT	S20	9,553	0
rpsU	S21	8,369	4

[a]*E. coli* proteins[28] in daltons.

[b]Based on sampling of 10,500 sequences.

[c]This hit had a $P(n)$ of $1.7e^{−6}$.

volved in amino acid biosynthesis by sequence sampling. In some cases, there was a good correlation between our inability to identify specific amino acid biosynthetic genes and the growth requirements for specific amino acids. The most prominent examples were Arg, His, Ile, Lys, Met, and Val. In each of these cases, three or more genes involved in biosynthesis were not found by sequence sampling. On the other hand, most of the genes involved in the biosynthesis of amino acids not added to the defined medium were identified by sequence sampling (Table 3). The exception was Ala, where neither of the two genes searched for was found. The results suggest that the biochemical pathways for amino acid biosynthesis in S. pneumoniae are generally similar to those in other bacteria and that a relatively large number of genes required for the biosynthesis of Arg, His, Ile, Lys, Met, and Val may be missing.

Cofactor biosynthesis

The synthetic medium for S. pneumoniae is supplemented by biotin, choline, nicotinamide, pantothenate, pyridoxal, riboflavin, and thiamine.[31] We found significant DNA sequence homologies to only three of 34 genes involved in the biosynthesis of biotin, nicotinamide, pantothenate, pyridoxal, and thiamine. In contrast, we found significant sequence homologies

TABLE 3. AMINO ACID AND COFACTOR BIOSYNTHETIC GENES IDENTIFIED IN S. pneumoniae

Amino acid or cofactor	Added to synthetic medium[a]	Genes identified
ala	−	0/2
arg	+	5/8
asn	+	1/2
asp	−	2/2
cys	+	3/3
glu	−	1/2
gln	+	1/1
gly	+	1/1
his	+	2/8
ile	+	8/11
leu	+	3/4
lys	+	2/7
met	+	3/6
phe	−	6/7
pro	−	1/3
ser	−	2/3
thr	+	2/3
trp	−	7/8
val	−	8/11
biotin	+	1/7
choline	+	—
folic acid	−	5/6
molybdopterin	−	0/8
nicotinamide	+	2/7
pantothenate	+	0/5
pyridoxal	+	0/4
riboflavin	+	5/7
thiamine	+	0/11

[a]From Sicard.[31]

to five of seven genes involved in riboflavin biosynthesis. Although riboflavin is added to the synthetic medium, Sicard[31] pointed out that it improved growth, but was dispensable, consistent with our results suggesting that the riboflavin biosynthetic pathway is present in S. pneumoniae. We also found genes homologous to five of seven genes involved in folic acid biosynthesis, a cofactor not required for S. pneumoniae growth. Furthermore, we found no homologs to the eight molybdopterin genes surveyed, even though this cofactor is not required for S. pneumoniae growth. This finding suggests that nitrate reductase activity, which requires molybdopterin, is not required for normal growth of S. pneumoniae. The inability to find many other cofactor genes by sequence sampling strongly suggests that these genes are not present on the S. pneumoniae genome.

DNA and RNA metabolism

We surveyed the S. pneumoniae data base for DNA replication genes encoding well-characterized functions in E. coli.[21] Five of the eight genes searched for identified matches with significant amino acid sequence homologies. These were dnaA, dnaB, dnaE, dnaG, and dnaN. Of the three genes not identified in S. pneumoniae, the dnaC gene also was not identified in M. genitalium[12] and the dnaX gene was not found in H. influenzae.[11] It is possible, therefore, that one or both of these functions also may be missing in S. pneumoniae. We identified gyrA and gyrB genes encoding DNA gyrase subunits; uvrA, uvrB, uvrC, and uvrD genes, involved in repair of damage to DNA; mutS (hexA), and mutL (hexB) involved in mismatch repair;[20,26] and mutT, mutM, and mutY, involved in repair of oxidative damage to DNA.[22] We surveyed genes involved in transcription and found rpoA, rpoB and rpoC, which encode RNA polymerase subunits; and rpoD and rpoN, which encode sigma subunits of the RNA polymerase. The rpoD gene encodes the major sigma factor in bacteria and is needed for the transcription of the major highly conserved promoter sequence associated with many housekeeping genes.[9] S. pneumoniae is known to contain an abundance of homologs of these sequences that function as promoters in E. coli.[23] The rpoN homologue is interesting in that it represents a possible sigma factor that has not been identified previously in S. pneumoniae. The rpoN gene product sigma[54] is involved in a variety of cellular functions in other bacteria that generally require positive regulatory proteins for transcriptional activation.[30] Sigma[54] recognizes promoter sequence distinct from those recognized by the rpoD gene product.[21] A number of these genes involved in DNA or RNA metabolism are known or potential targets for therapeutic intervention.

Energy metabolism

S. pneumoniae is an anaerobe and, as such, may not express complete pathways associated with robust aerobic growth. We surveyed the S. pneumoniae partial sequence database for twenty-nine genes involved in aerobic respiration in E. coli (cyoA-cyoE, ddl, hyaA-F, lctD, lctR, ndh, and nuoA-N) and found no partial sequences with significant homologies to any of the genes. Similarly, we found none of eighteen genes encoding functions in the TCA cycle (acnAB; citD-F; fumA, fumB; gltA; icdC, E; mdh, sdhA, B D; and sucA-D) and none of five genes encoding functions in gluconeogenesis. However, we found partial sequences with significant homologies to seven of seventeen genes involved in glycolysis. These data are consistent with the notion that the relatively small genome of *S. pneumoniae* simply lacks many genes associated with aerobic growth.

Cell wall biosynthesis and septation

The enzymes involved in cell wall biosynthesis and septation are potential and, in some cases, well-documented targets for antibiotic intervention. We searched our *S. pneumoniae* random sequence library for homologs to *fts* genes, stem peptide biosynthetic genes, and penicillin binding proteins. We identified homologs to *murA*, *murB*, *murC*, *murD*, *murE*, *murG*, *ddl*, and *murI* (Table 4). We also identified homologs to nine *fts* genes and possibly six *pbp* genes (Table 4).

Chaperonins and heat shock proteins

We surveyed the *S. pneumoniae* database of partial sequences for heat shock and chaperonin genes known to be expressed in other organisms.[16,34] *S. pneumoniae* contains linked *groEL* and *groES* homologs with very high amino acid similarities to those of the *Lactococcus lactis* gene products. *S. pneumoniae* also contains ORFs that potentially encode proteins with high amino acid similarities to those of the *dnaJ*, *dnaK*, *grpE*, *clpA*, *clpP*, *clpX*, and *clpY*. Interestingly, two of the putative genes showed high amino acid similarities to genes from *Saccharomyces cerevisiae* and *Arabidopsis thaliana*. Additional work is needed to determine if these define genes other than those discussed above.

Type III secretion systems and pathogenicity islands

A number of animal and plant pathogens secrete antihost proteins by a mechanism that does not involve cleavage of a signal peptide. In *Yersenia*, the type III secretion system delivers Yop proteins into eukaryotic cells upon contact and the secretion of Yop proteins is assisted by apparently dedicated chaperone proteins called Syc.[33] These chaperones have homologs in other bacteria with type III secretion systems. In *Salmonella*, a number of genes involved in export of virulence determinants have been identified. These genes also have homologs in other gram negative bacteria.[13] We searched the *S. pneumoniae* partial genome library for 15 of the genes involved in type III secretion and found a potential homolog to only one gene, *invA* from *Salmonella*. These data indicate that type III secretion probably is not a mechanism used by *S. pneumoniae*. This search demonstrates that genomic sequence sampling is an efficient means of assessing quickly the presence or absence of specific pathways associated with processes such as virulence and pathogenicity.

TABLE 4. GENES INVOLVED IN CELL WALL BIOSYNTHESIS OR SEPTATION IDENTIFIED IN *S. pneumoniae*

Gene	Homolog[a]	p(n)[b]
murA	*B. subtilis*	1.1e–62
murB	*S. typhimurium*	6.8e–17
murC	*B. subtilis*	8.4e–08
murD	*B. subtilis*	6.3e–44
murE	*B. subtilis*	2.1e–10
murF	none found	—
murG	*B. subtilis*	9.9e–11
ddl	*H. influenzae*	9.7e–35
murI	*P. pentosaceus*	9.9e–78
ponA	*S. pneumoniae*	5.5e–192
pbp1A	*B. subtilis*	4.2e–24
pbpX	*S. pneumoniae*	2.8e–221
pbpB	*B. subtilis*	2.2e–42
pbp2B	*S. pneumoniae*	1.6e–218
pbp4	*S. aureus*	8.2e–18
ftsA	*B. subtilis*	1.3e–41
ftsE	*E. coli*	1.3e–35
ftsH	*L. lactis*	1.2–57
ftsQ	*S. coelicolor*	1.0e–16
ftsW	*C. paradoxa*	5.8e–15
ftsX	*E. coli*	4.1e–06
ftsY	*H. influenzae*	8.7e–41
ftsZ	*B. subtilis*	3.7e–62

[a]Organism with gene giving best score.
[b]The *p* value calculated from the probability of two random sequences showing similarity. The lower the *p* value, the higher the probability of significance of the match.

FOCUSED DNA SEQUENCING

An advantage of DNA sequence sampling is that specific genes can be identified rapidly and targeted for complete sequence analysis. In some cases, obtaining a complete sequence can be as simple as extending an initial random sequence, or genome sequence tag (GST), on an M13 clone by additional oligonucleotide primer directed sequencing, In other cases, the complete gene sequence can be obtained by identifying the gene in a large fragment library, then obtaining the complete sequence from the clone by any of several techniques. Furthermore, because of the known functional linkage relationships identified in the well-studied bacteria (e.g., *E. coli*, *B. subtilis*, *H. influenzae*, and others), the clone from a large fragment library often can provide information on other genes in the same pathway, some of which may be additional potential targets for antibiotic development.

We pursued two approaches to developing large fragment libraries of *S. pneumoniae* DNA. The first, cosmid cloning, was not successful. We prepared libraries in the cosmid vectors, SuperCos1 (Stratagene) and pOJ434,[2] and only incomplete libraries not representative of the complete genome were obtained. These results suggested a biological bias introduced by the cloned DNA. This is consistent with observations of others suggesting that *S. pneumoniae* DNA is difficult to clone in *E. coli*, possibly because of the abundance of *E. coli* consensus promoter sequences and other reasons. Since bacteriophage lambda libraries do not require continued propagation of viable *E. coli* cells and, therefore, should be less sensitive to the effects of unregulated transcription of foreign DNA inserts, and since lambda libraries have been prepared successfully from *Streptococcus sobrinus* DNA, we prepared a sheared DNA library of *S. pneumoniae* R6 *hex* DNA in the vector Lambda DASHII (Stratagene). We analyzed a number of different clones and the average insert size was 18 kb, similar to the mean size for allowable inserts. We also examined three different clones that hybridized to the "trigger factor" gene homolog of *S. pneumoniae* by long fragment PCR using primers to the lambda vector and the trigger factor gene. Each of the clones contained inserts of different sizes and different positioning of the trigger factor gene. This was as expected for a sheared DNA library designed to contain random, overlapping fragments. These preliminary experiments suggest that cosmid libraries may not be feasible for *S. pneumoniae* DNA, but that lambda libraries may provide a source for sequencing linked segments of the *S. pneumoniae* genome.

Lipoteichoic acid

One interesting example of sequence sampling coupled with focused sequencing is the identification of a *dlt* operon of *S. pneumoniae*. We identified a primary random sequence that contained an ORF that predicted an amino acid sequence that showed high similarity to the *dltA* gene. This is interesting since *dltA* encodes a D-alanine activating enzyme involved in adding D-ala to lipoteichoic acid (LTA) in *B. subtilis* and in *Lactococcus casei*.[25] *S. pneumoniae* LTA has not been shown to contain D-ala.[10] Additional DNA sequence was obtained from the primary M13 clone and three other ORFs apparently encoding other genes in the *dlt* operon, *dltB*, *dltC*, and *dltD*, were identified and their organization is similar to that of the *dlt* operon observed in *L. casei* and *B. subtilis*.[25] The *dlt* operon of *S. pneumoniae* may represent a silent or defective set of genes. Alternatively, D-ala may be present on LTA only under specific physiological conditions that have not yet been identified. This intriguing possibility merits further work.

GENERAL FEATURES OF THE *S. pneumoniae* R6 *hex* GENOME

The *S. pneumoniae* genome has been estimated to be approximately 2.3 Mb in size by FIGE analysis.[7,14] We estimated the *S. pneumoniae* genome to be approximately 2.0 Mb by CHEF analysis (Table 5). In our analysis, we did not observe the *Sma*I fragment labeled 16 in the *S. pneumoniae* genome. Also, CHEF analysis is generally more accurate since conditions can be modified readily to focus in different molecular weight ranges. We therefore think that 2.0 Mb is probably closer to the actual size. The *S. pneumoniae* genome is approximately three times the size of the *Mycoplasma genitalium* genome,[12] approximately one-half the size of the genomes of *E. coli* and *Bacillus subtilis*,[7] and one-quarter the size of the genome of *Streptomyces coelicolor*.[27]

The G+C content of the *S. pneumoniae* genome, based on analysis of over 2 Mb of random sequence, is 43%. The codon usage based on analysis of 1,469 partial ORFs is shown in Table 6. Codons containing A or T in the third position are generally preferred, with some exceptions [e.g., TTG (Leu) is more abundant than TTA (Leu) and ATC (Ile) is substantially more abun-

TABLE 5. SIZES OF *Sma*I FRAGMENTS
OF THE *S. pneumoniae* GENOME

| Fragment | Fragment size | |
	FIGE[a]	CHEF
1	380	325
2	340	292
3	290	244
4	260	231
5	235	206
6	150	142
7	110	108
8	104	104
9	95	97
10	90	91
11	60	63
12	52	50
13	26	30
14	25	21
15	19	12
16	19	—
17	7.6	8.0
18	5.8	5.9
19	3.2	3.7
Total	2,271.6	2,033.6

[a]Data from Gasc *et al.*[14]

dant than ATA (Ile)]. We also searched the first 700 random sequences using the GCG program FIND[8] and identified at least 14 sequences similar to *E. coli* consensus promoters (Table 7). This high density of *E. coli*-like promoters is consistent with the observation that sigma 70 promoter consensus sequences are readily cloned from *S. pneumoniae* and contain promoter activity in *E. coli*.[9,23] This feature of *S. pneumoniae* DNA is relevant in choosing methods to prepare large fragment libraries as discussed above.

PHYSICAL MAPPING OF *S. pneumoniae* GENES

To gain a better understanding of the genetic organization of the *S. pneumoniae* genome, we initiated physical mapping of many partial DNA sequences (GSTs) based on the current physical map of *S. pneumoniae*.[14] The published *S. pneumoniae* physical map has approximately 25 genes assigned to *Sma*I and *Apa*I fragments. We isolated individual *Sma*I fragments from digestions of total chromosomal DNA and used them as hybridization probes against 1500 M13 clones containing *S. pneumoniae* DNA. Using this procedure, we mapped individual partial DNA sequences to the specific *Sma*I fragments. Figure 1 shows a summary of approximate map locations of a representative group of *S. pneumoniae* genes of known or predicted function based on homology to genes from other bacteria. This strategy of using hybridization of GSTs and larger genomic DNA fragments rapidly generates information regarding the physical location and linkage of individual genes and is applicable in the study of other bacterial genomes.

TABLE 6. CODON USAGE FOR *S. pneumoniae*[a]

	T			C			A			G		
T	Phe	0.651	Ser	0.259	Tyr	0.613	Cys	0.597	T
T	Phe	0.349	Ser	0.103	Tyr	0.387	Cys	0.403	C
T	Leu	0.166	Ser	0.221	STOP	0.357	STOP	0.404	A
T	Leu	0.281	Ser	0.066	STOP	0.239	Trp	1.000	G
C	Leu	0.210	Pro	0.327	His	0.585	Arg	0.395	T
C	Leu	0.138	Pro	0.135	His	0.415	Arg	0.161	C
C	Leu	0.104	Pro	0.446	Gln	0.649	Arg	0.109	A
C	Leu	0.102	Pro	0.091	Gln	0.351	Arg	0.062	G
A	Ile	0.515	Thr	0.319	Asn	0.629	Ser	0.205	T
A	Ile	0.377	Thr	0.242	Asn	0.371	Ser	0.146	C
A	Ile	0.109	Thr	0.314	Lys	0.608	Arg	0.182	A
A	Met	1.000	Thr	0.125	Lys	0.392	Arg	0.091	G
G	Val	0.389	Ala	0.408	Asp	0.646	Gly	0.419	T
G	Val	0.232	Ala	0.233	Asp	0.354	Gly	0.153	C
G	Val	0.196	Ala	0.254	Glu	0.698	Gly	0.292	A
G	Val	0.184	Ala	0.105	Glu	0.302	Gly	0.137	G

[a]Unique open reading frames were predicted in the sequence data and used to tally the codon usage.

CONJUGAL TRANSFER OF DNA FROM *E. coli* TO *S. pneumoniae* AND GENE DISRUPTION ANALYSIS

We developed a procedure to introduce plasmid DNA into *S. pneumoniae* by conjugation from *E. coli* (P. Matsushima *et al.*, manuscript in preparation). Plasmid pCZA342 (Fig. 2) containing a ~0.5 kb internal segment of the *S. pneumoniae nanA* gene which is not required for viability was utilized as the test plasmid for conjugation. This plasmid has replication functions for *E. coli*, *oriT* for conjugal transfer and the *Enterococcus faecalis* erythromycin resistance gene (EmR) for selection of transconjugants in *S. pneumoniae*. Since this plasmid has no replication functions for *S. pneumoniae*, transconjugants can be formed only by the insertion of the plasmid into the chromosome by homologous recombination at the *nanA* locus or by illegitimate recombination elsewhere in the chromosome. Under conditions optimized for conjugation, the integration frequencies at the *nanA* locus typically range from about 10^{-4} to 2×10^{-3} per recipient cell. Figure 3 shows the frequency of transconjugants per *S. pneumoniae* recipient as a function of DNA insert size, using internal fragments of *ponA*, another nonessential gene. Optimum transconjugant frequencies were obtained with inserts of 0.7–1.1 kb. The transconjugant frequency was about 100-fold lower with an insert of 0.4 kb.

Internal segments of ORFs identified by random DNA sequence sampling were cloned into plasmid pCZA342 in *E. coli* S17-1, then introduced into *S. pneumoniae* R6 *hex* by conjugation. Viable transconjugants can be formed only if the disrupted gene still retains function, or if the gene is not required

TABLE 7. HYPOTHETICAL *S. pneumoniae* PROMOTERS[a]

Contig	200	agcgc**TTGACA**aaggaaacggtttcattg.**TATAAT**
Contig	243	gatgc**TTGtCA**aagcctag..ctttcttgt**TATAAT**
Contig	246	gaaaa**TaGACA**caaaagaaa.agtttttgg**TATAAT**
Contig	356	agtag**TTGACA**aaacata..aaaaggctg.**TATAAT**
Contig	420	ataat**TTGACA**aaaactgt.actttggtt.**TATAAT**
Contig	422	agagc**TTGcCA**gcattctt.gaaaagtag.**TATAAT**
Contig	466	atggt**TTGAaA**aat.tactctctttcgtt.**TATAAT**
Contig	470	ttctg**TTGACA**actttctg.aaaagagtc.**TATAAT**
Contig	586	agacc**TTGACA**aataaaaa..taaaatggt**TATtAT**
Contig	642	atgtt**TTGACA**aatgaacac.aaataatga**TATAAT**
Contig	694	atctg**TTGACA**tattntgaa.attaagtac**TATAAT**
Contig	919	gacta**TTGACA**agtagtt...taaaaatga**TATAAT**
Contig	929	agtag**TTGACA**aaacata..nanaggctg.**TATAAT**
Contig	960	cagac**TTGcCA**gcattctt.gaaaagtag.**TATAAT**
Consensus		.....**TTGACA**aa .. n{16–19} tg.**TATAAT**

[a]The *S. pneumoniae* random sequence database was searched for *E. coli* –35 (TTGACA) and –10 (TATAAT) consensus promoter sequences allowing up to one mismatched nucleotide in each putative promoter element and a range of spacing between the elements of 16–19 nucleotides.

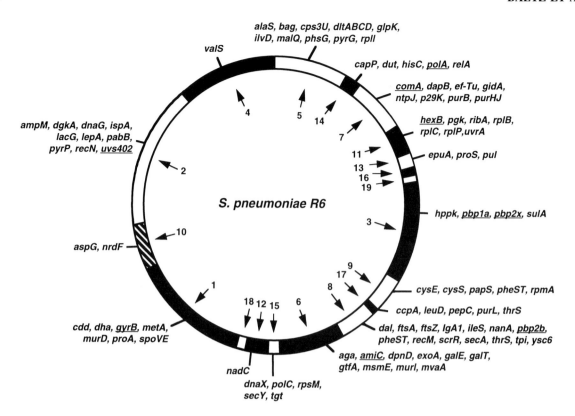

FIG. 1. Genetic map of *Streptococcus pneumoniae* R6 *hex*. The map is based on the *Sma*I linkage relationships established by Gasc *et al.*[11] Gene locations were established by Southern blot hybridizations of isolated *Sma*I fragments with individual M13mp19 clones containing inserts of *S. pneumoniae* DNA. Numbers with arrows refer to the individual *Sma*I fragments. The genes listed on the map refer to the BLAST hits with the highest probability of significance (the lowest *p* value). The underlined genes were mapped previously[14] and confirmed in this study. *aga* (EC 3.2.1.22), *S. mutans*; *alaS, H. influenzae*; *amiC, S. pneumoniae*; *ampM* (EC 3.4.11.18), *B. subtilis*; *aspG* (EC 3.5.1.1), *B. licheniformis*; *bag, S. agalactiae*; *capP, C. glutamicum*; *ccpA, L. casei*; *cdd* (EC 3.5.4.5), *B. subtilis*; *comA, S. pneumoniae*; *cps3U, S. pneumoniae*; *cysE* (EC 2.3.1.30), *B. subtilis*; *cysS, B. subtilis*; *dacA* (EC 3.4.16.4), *Bacillus* sp.; *dal, B. subtilis*; *dapB, Synechocystis* sp.; *dgkA* (EC 2.7.1.107), *S. mutans*; *dha* (EC 1.4.1.1), *Bacillus* sp; *dltABCD, L. casei*; *dnaG* (EC 2.7.7.—); *L. lactis*; *dnaX* (EC 2.7.7.7), *B. subtilis*; *dpnD, S. pneumoniae*; *dut* (EC 3.6.1.23), bacteriophage rit; *ef-Tu, S. oralis*; *epuA, S. pneumoniae*; *exoA* (EC 3.1.11.2), *S. pneumoniae*; *ftsA, B. subtilis*; *ftsZ, Streptomyces griseus*; *galE* (EC 5.1.3.2). *B. subtilis*; *galT* (EC 2.7.7.10), *Butyrivibrio fibrisolvens*; *gidA, B. subtilis*; *glpK* (EC 2.7.1.30), *B. subtilis*; *glfA* (EC 2.4.1.5), *S. mutans*; *gyrB, S. pneumoniae*; *hexB, S. pneumoniae*; *hisC, B. subtilis*; *hppk* (EC 2.7.6.3), *S. pneumoniae*; *Igal, S. pneumoniae*; *ileS, S. aureus*; *ilvD* (EC 4.2.1.9), *Synechocystis* sp.; *ispA* (EC 2.5.1.10), *B. stearothermophilus*; *lacG* (EC 3.2.1.85), *L. lactis*; *lepA, B. subtilis*; *leuD* (EC 4.2.1.33), *L. lactis*; *malQ, S. pneumoniae*; *metA* (EC 2.3.1.46), *E. coli*; *msmE, S. mutans*; *murD, B. subtilis*; *murI, B. subtilis*; *mvaA* (EC 1.1.1.88), *P. mevalorii*; *nadC* (EC 2.4.2.19), *Rhodospirillum rubrum*; *nanA, S. pneumoniae*; *nrdF* (EC 1.17.4.1), *M. tuberculosis*; *ntpJ* (EC 3.6.1.34), *E. hirae*; *p29K, S. pneumoniae*; *pabB* (EC 4.1.3.—), *B. subtilis*; *papS* (EC 2.7.7.19), *B. subtilis*; *pbp1a, S. pneumoniae*; *pbp2b, S. pneumoniae*; *pbp2x, S. pneumoniae*; *pepC, S. thermophilus*; *pgk, Arabidopsis thaliana*; *pheS,T, B. subtilis*; *phsG* (EC 2.4.1.1), *B. subtilis*; *polA, S. pneumoniae*; *polC, S. aureus*; *proA* (EC 1.2.1.41), *H. influenzae*; *proS, E. coli*; *pul, Bacillus* sp.; *purB* (EC 4.3.2.2), *B. subtilis*; *purHJ* (EC 2.1.2.3/3.5.4. 10), *B. subtilis*; *purL* (EC 6.3.5.3), *Synechocystis* sp.; *pyrG* (EC 6.3.4.2), *B. subtilis*; *pyrP, Bacillus* sp.; *recM, S. thermophilus*; *recN, B. subtilis*; *relA* (EC 2.7.6.5), *S. equisimilis*; *ribA* (EC 3.5.4.25), *B. subtilis*; *rplB, B. stearothermophilus*; *rp1C, B. subtilis*; *rpff, B. subtilis*; *rplP, B. subtilis*; *rpmA, B. stearothermophilus*; *rpsM, B. subtilis*; *scrR, S. mutans*; *secA, B. subtilis*; *secY, L. lactis*; *spoVE, B. subtilis*; *sulA, S. pneumoniae*; *tgt* (EC 2.4.2.29), *E. coli*; *thrS, B. subtilis*; *tpi* (EC 5.3.1.1), *L. lactis*; *uvrA, S. mutans*; *uvs402, S. pneumoniae*; *valS, L. casei*; *ysc6* (EC 3.4.24.—), *S. gordonii*.

for viability. Alernatively, viable recombinants might be formed if an internal segment of an essential gene inserts illegitimately into some other site on the chromosome. To explore the conjugation system as a method to obtain homologous insertions into *S. pneumoniae* genes, we have examined the frequencies of recombinants obtained with pCZA342 containing internal segments of genes known to be required for viability in other bacteria, genes known not to be required for viability, and other genes. For genes apparently required for viability, conjugations

were repeated at least five times. Both *ponA* and *nanA* are not essential for viability, and can be disrupted without affecting viability. In both cases, homologous recombination was confirmed by Southern hybridization analysis. Also, the neuraminidase activity of a *nanA*-disrupted mutant was reduced to background (~2% of the control; T. Nicas, unpublished data). These results confirmed that homologous insertions do occur in *S. pneumoniae* following conjugation of plasmid DNA from *E. coli* S17-1. Several genes required for cell wall biosynthesis

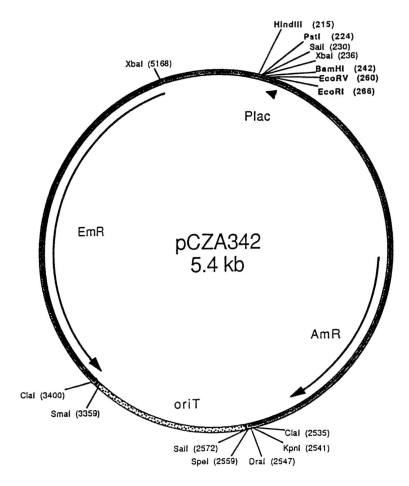

FIG. 2. Cloning vector for conjugation and insertional mutagenesis in *S. pneumoniae*. pCZA342 is derived from pOJ260[2] and contains EmR (erythromycin resistance) from *E. faecalis* for selection in *S. pneumoniae*, *oriT* for conjugal transfer from *E. coli* to *S. pneumoniae*, and a multiple cloning site for the insertion of *S. pneumoniae* DNA. (Data from Matsushima *et al.*, manuscript in preparation.)

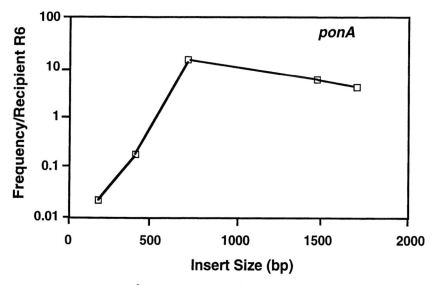

FIG. 3. Transconjugation frequency ($\times 10^{-5}$) as a function of DNA insert size during conjugation from *E. coli* S17-1 to *S. pneumoniae* R6 hex.

TABLE 8.   SUMMARY OF GENE DISRUPTION ANALYSIS[a]

Gene homologue	Predicted function	Transconjugants obtained
amiC	ABC transporter	+
amiE		+
amiF		+
dltA	D-alanyl-lipoteichoic biosynthesis	+
dltB	D-alanyl-lipoteichoic biosynthesis	+
dltC	D-alanyl-lipoteichoic biosynthesis	+
dltD	D-alanyl-lipoteichoic biosynthesis	+
ftsE	Cell division; membrane protein	+
glpF	Glycerol facilitator	+
murA1	Cell wall: UDP-GlcNAc-enolpyruvoyltransferase	+
murA2	Cell wall: UDP-GlcNAc-enolpyruvoyltransferase	+
nanA	Neuraminidase	+
ponA	Penicillin-binding protein (PBP1a)	+
pyrG	CTP synthetase	+
tig	Trigger factor; chaperone in cell division	+
ddl	Cell wall; D-ala-D-ala ligase	−
divIB	Cell division	−
era	GTP-binding protein	−
ftsW	Cell division	−
ftsY	Cell division	−
ftsZ	Cell division	−
lig	DNA ligase	−
mraY	Cell wall; UDP-acetylmuramoyl-pentapeptide: undecarprenyl-PO_4 phosphatase	−
murB	Cell wall; UDP-N-acetylglucosaminyl-3-enolpyruvate reductase	−
murD	Cell wall; UDP-N-acetylmuramoyl-L-ala; D-glu ligase	−
murE	Cell wall; lysine-adding enzyme	−
murI	Cell wall; glutamate reacemase	−
pbp2B	Cell wall; transpeptidase/transglycosylase	−
pbp2X	Cell wall; transpeptidase/transglycosylase	−
secY	Secretion; membrane scanning translocator	−

[a]Internal segments of genes of about 0.5 kb were PCR amplified from M13 clones and inserted into the BamHI site of pCZA342. Conjugations were repeated at least five times for genes that yielded no recombinants. Positive control (nanA) were included in each conjugation experiment. (Data from Matsushima et al., manuscript in preparation.)

or septation, including ddl, ftsW, mraY, murB, murD, murE, murI, and pbp2X did not produce viable transconjugants containing homologous integration events (Table 8). This result is generally consistent with data obtained in other bacteria. However, further analysis is needed to rule out potential polar effects on genes downstream in operons.

Interestingly, an internal fragment of the murA gene inserted into two different loci in the S. pneumoniae chromosome resulted in viable transconjugants. Since the loss of murA function in E. coli is lethal, our data suggest that S. pneumoniae has two functional copies of murA, tentatively designated murA1 and murA2. Other apparently essential genes based upon the lack of viable insertion mutants include dnaG, lig and secY. Genes identified as nonessential by this method included dltABCD, an operon homologous to the dlt operons of Bacillus subtilis and Lactococcus casei that encode enzymes associated with the addition of D-alanine to lipoteichoic acid.[10,25] Since S. pneumoniae lacks D-alanine in its lipoteichoic acid, and since the dlt genes are not essential in Bacillus subtilis, it was not surprising that these genes were nonessential in S. Pneumoniae. Other genes that are apparently not essential for viability are listed in Table 8. This conjugation approach to gene disruption can be used to screen a large number of genes, including those of unknown function, for their effects on viability.

PROSPECTS FOR ANTIBIOTIC DEVELOPMENT

DNA sequence sampling and whole genome sequencing will provide many potential new targets for antibiotic screen development. Some of the most novel targets may be proteins of unknown function. Gene disruption analysis can begin to identify candidate genes, but a daunting challenge is posed by the large number of genes of unknown function.[5,11,12] Many of these genes could be potential targets for drug development. A corollary challenge is how to develop assays for compounds that inhibit proteins of undefined function, albeit ones required for viability or virulence as defined by gene disruption tests. This latter problem may be addressed best by collaborative efforts between academic and industrial scientists and, if pursued successfully, should offer novel approaches to attacking the problem of antibiotic resistant pathogens, including β-lactam resistant S. pneumoniae.

REFERENCES

1. **Altschul, S.F., W. Gish, W. Miller, E.W. Myers, and D.J. Lipman.** 1990. Basic local alignment search tool. J. Mol. Biol. **215:**403–410.

2a. **Baltz, R.H., F.H. Norris, P. Matsushima, B.S. DeHoff, P. Rockey, G. Porter, S. Burgett, R. Peery, J. Hoskins, L. Breaverman, I. Jenkins, P. Solenberg, M. Young, M.A. McHenney, P.L. Skatrud, and P.R. Rosteck, Jr.** 1998. DNA sequence sampling of the *Streptococcus pneumoniae* genome to identify novel targets for antibiotic development. Microbiol. Drug Resist. **4:**1–9.

2. **Bierman, M., R. Logan, K. O'Brien, E.T. Seno, R.N. Rao, and B.E. Schoner.** 1991. Plasmid cloning vectors for the conjugal transfer of DNA from *Escherichia coli* to *Streptomyces spp.* Gene **116:**43–49.

3. **Borges, K.M., S.R. Brummet, A. Bogert, M.C. Davis, K.M. Hujer, S.T. Domke, J. Szasz, J. Ravel, J. DiRuggiero, C. Fuller, J.W. Chase, and F.T. Robb.** 1996. A survey of the genome of the hyperthermophilic archaeon, *Pyrococcus furiosus.* Genome Sci. Tech. **1:**37–46.

4. **Bork, P., C. Ouzounis, G. Casari, R. Schneider, C. Sander, M. Dolan, W. Gilbert, and P.M. Gillevet.** 1995. Exploring the *Mycoplasma capriolum* genome: a minimal cell reveals its physiology. Mol. Microbiol. **16:**955–967.

5. **Bult, C.J., O. White, G.J. Olsen, L. Zhou, R.D. Fleischmann, G.G. Sutton, J.A. Blake, L.M. FitzGerald, R.A. Clayton, J.D. Gocayne, A.R. Kerlavage, B.A. Dougherty, J.-F. Tomb, M.D. Adams, C.I. Reich, R. Overbeek, E.F. Kirkness, K.G. Weinstock, J.M. Merrick, A. Glodek, J.L. Scott, N.S.M. Geoghagen, J.F. Weidman, J.L. Fuhrmann, D. Nguyen, T.R. Utterback, J.M. Kelley, J.D. Peterson, P.W. Sadow, M.C. Hanna, M.D. Cotton, K.M. Roberts, M.A. Hurst, B.P. Kaine, M. Borodovsky, H.-P. Klenk, C.M. Fraser, H.O. Smith, C.R. Woese, and J.C. Venter.** 1996. Complete genome sequence of the methanogenic archaeon. *Methanococcus jannaschii.* Science **273:**1058–1072.

6. **Chen, Y.-Y.M., and D.J. LeBlanc.** 1992. Genetic analysis of *scrA* and *scrB* from *Streptococcus sobrinus* 6715. Infect. Immunol. **60:**3739–3746.

7. **Cole, S.T., and I. Saint Girons.** 1994. Bacterial genomics. F.E.M.S. Microbiol. Rev. **14:**139–160.

8. **Devereux, J., P. Haeberli, and O. Smithies.** 1984. A comprehensive set of sequence analysis programs for the VAX. Nucleic Acids Res. **12:**387–395.

9. **Dillard, J.P., and J.L. Yother.** 1991. Analysis of *Streptococcus pneumoniae* sequences cloned into *Escherichia coli*: effect of promoter strength and transcription terminators. J. Bacteriol. **173:**5105–5109.

10. **Fischer, W.** 1988. Physiology of lipoteichoic acids in bacteria. Adv. Microb. Physiol. **29:**233–302.

11. **Fleischmann, R.D., M.D. Adams, O. White, R.A. Clayton, E.F. Kirkness, A.R. Kerlavage, C.J. Bult, J.-F. Tomb, B.A. Dougherty, J.M. Merrick, K. McKenney, G. Sutton, W. FitzHugh, C. Fields, J.D. Gocayne, J. Scott, R. Shirley, L.-I. Liu, A. Glodek, J.M. Kelley, J.F. Weidman, C.A. Phillips, T. Spriggs, E. Hedblom, M.D. Cotton, T.R. Utterback, M.C. Hanna, D.T. Nguyen, D.M. Saudek, R.C. Brandon, L.D. Fine, J.L. Fritchman, J.L. Fuhrmann, N.S.M. Geoghagen, C.L. Gnehm, L.A. McDonald, K.V. Small, C.M. Fraser, H.O. Smith, and J.C. Venter.** 1995. Whole-genome random sequencing and assembly of *Haemophilus influenzae* Rd. Science **269:**496–512.

12. **Fraser, M., J.D. Gocayne, O. White, M.D. Adams, R.A. Clayton, R.D. Fleischmann, C.J. Bult, A.R. Kerlavage, G. Sutton, J.M. Kelley, J.L. Fritchman, J.F. Weidman, K.V. Small, M. Sandusky, J. Fuhrmann, D. Nguyen, T.R. Utterback, D.M. Saudek, C.A. Phillips, J.M. Merrick, J.-F. Tomb, B.A. Dougherty, K.F. Bott, P.-C.-Hu, T.S. Lucier, S.N. Peterson,

H.O. Smith, C.A. Hutchison III, and J.C. Venter.** 1996. The minimal gene complement of *Mycoplasma genitalium.* Science **270:**397–403.

13. **Galen, J.E.** 1996. Molecular genetic basis of *Salmonella* entry into host cells. Mol. Microbiol. **20:**263–271.

14. **Gasc, A.M., L. Kane, P. Barraille, M. Sicard, and S. Goodgal.** 1991. Gene localization, size, and physical map of the chromosome of *Streptococcus pneumoniae.* J. Bacteriol. **173:**7361–7367.

15. **Green, C.J., and B.S. Vold.** 1993. tRNA, tRNA processing, and aminoacyl-tRNA synthetases. *In* A.L. Sonenshein, J.A. Hock, and R. Losick (eds.), *Bacillus subtilis* and other gram-positive bacteria. American Society for Microbiology, Washington, DC, pp. 683–698.

16. **Hendrick, J.P., and F.-U. Harti.** 1993. Molecular chaperone functions of heat-shock proteins. Annu. Rev. Biochem. **62:**349–384.

17. **Kamb, A., C. Wang, A. Thomas, B.S. DeHoff, F.H. Norris, K. Richardson, J. Rine, M. Skolnick, and P.R. Rosteck, Jr.** 1995. Software trapping: a strategy for finding genes in large genomic regions. Comput. Biomed. Res. **28:**140–153.

18. **Koonin, E.V., A.R. Mushegian, and K.E. Rudd.** 1996. Sequencing and analysis of bacterial genomes. Curr. Biol. **6:**404–416.

19. **Loretto, M., M. Gribskov, and C.A. Gross.** 1991. The sigma^{70} family: sequence conservation and evolutionary relationships. J. Bacteriol. **174:**3843–3844.

20. **Matic, I., C. Rayssiguier, and M. Radman.** 1995. Interspecies gene exchange in bacteria: the role of SOS and mismatch repair systems in evolution of species. Cell **80:**507–515.

21. **Merrick, M.J.** 1993. In a class of its own—the RNA polymerase sigma factor 54. Mol. Microbiol. **10:**903–909.

22. **Michaels, M.L., and J.H. Miller.** 1992. The GO system protects organisms from the mutagenic effect of the spontaneous lesion 8-hydroxyguanine (7,8-dihydro-8-oxoguanine). J. Bacteriol. **174:**6321–6325.

23. **Morrison, D.A., and B. Jaurin.** 1990. *Streptococcus pneumoniae* possesses canonical *Escherichia coli* (sigma 70) promoters. Mol. Microbiol. **4:**1143–1152.

24. **Mushegian, A.R., and E.V. Koonin.** 1996. A minimal set for cellular life derived by comparison of complete bacterial genomes. Proc. Natl. Acad. Sci. U.S.A. **93:**10268–10273.

25. **Neuhaus, F.C., M.P. Heaton, D.V. Debabov, and Q. Zhang.** 1996. The *dlt* operon in the biosynthesis of D-alanyl-lipoteichoic acid in *Lactobacillus casei.* Microbiol. Drug Resist. **2:**77–84.

26. **Prudhomme, M., V. Mejeas, B. Martin, and J.-P. Claverys.** 1991. Mismatch repair genes of *Streptococcus pneumoniae: HexA* confers a mutator phenotype in *Escherichia coli* by negative complementation. J. Bacteriol. **173:**7196–7203.

27. **Redenback, M., H.M. Kieser, D. Denapaite, A. Eichner, J. Cullum, H. Kinashi, and D.A. Hopwood.** 1996. A set of ordered cosmids and a detailed genetic and physical map for the 8 Mb Strep*tomyces coelicolor* A3(2) chromosome. Mol. Microbiol. **21:**77–96.

28. **Riley, M., and B. Labedan.** 1996. *Escherichia coli* gene products: physiological functions and common ancestries. *In* F.C. Neidhardt, R. Curtiss III, J.L. Ingraham, E.C.C. Lin, K.B. Low, B. Magasanik, W.S. Reznikoff, M. Riley, M. Schaechter, and H.E. Umbarger (eds.), *Escherichia coli* and *Salmonella.* Cellular and molecular biology. American Society for Microbiology, Washington, DC, pp. 2118–2202.

29. **Rosteck, P.R., Jr., F.H. Norris, P.M. Rockey, and B.H. DeHoff.** Bacterial genomics and genome informatics. *In* A.L. Demain and J. Davies (eds.), Manual of industrial microbiology and biotechnology, 2nd ed. American Society for Microbiology, Washington, DC, pp. 493–500.

30. **Schingler, V.** 1996. Signal sensing by sigma^{54}-dependent regulators: Derepression as a control mechanism. Mol. Microbiol. **19:**409–416.

31. **Sicard, A.M.** 1964. A new synthetic medium for *Diplococcus pneumoniae*, and its use for the study of reciprocal transformations at the *amiA locus*. Genetics. **50:**31–44.

32. **Sutton, G.G., O. White, M.D. Adams, and A.R. Kerlavage.** 1995. TIGR Assembler: a new tool for assembling large shotgun sequencing projects. Genome Sci. Technol. **1:**9–19.

33. **Wattiau, P., S. Woestyn, and G.R. Cornelis.** 1996. Customized secretion chaperones in pathogenic bacteria. Mol. Microbiol. **20:**255–262.

34. **Wawrzynow, A., B. Banecki, and M. Zylicz.** 1996. The Clp ATPases define a novel class of molecular chaperones. Mol. Microbiol. **21:**895–899.

Address reprint requests to:
R.H. Baltz
Dow Agrosciences LLC
9330 Zionsville Rd.
Indianapolis, IN 46268

Streptococcal Competence for Genetic Transformation: Regulation by Peptide Pheromones

DONALD A. MORRISON

ABSTRACT

Although the capacity for genetic transformation is perhaps the most famous attribute of pneumococcus, use of this genetic phenomenon as a tool for study of the biology of the organism and of its pathogenicity has been largely restricted to a few favored unencapsulated strains, both by the delicacy of the conditions required for development of competence, and by experience that encapsulated strains transformed poorly. We discuss here the recent discovery of a small stable inexpensive peptide pheromone that acts as a quorum-sensing signal and that induces competence under a wide variety of conditions and in encapsulated strains. Its use circumvents some if not all limitations to the expression of transformability in pneumococcus and therefore expands opportunities for application of tools of molecular genetics to many strains of pneumococcus without prior genetic manipulation.

INTRODUCTION: STREPTOCOCCAL COMPETENCE

TWO STREPTOCOCCAL SPECIES POSSESS natural transformation systems that are efficient and have been studied in some detail. For both of them, *Streptococcus gordonii* and *Streptococcus pneumoniae*, genetic transformation depends on a special physiological state, termed competence. Entry into this state depends, in an ill-defined way, on the genetic background, growth medium, and regimen employed,[3,66] and, in a better-defined way, on cell number.[58,78] Streptococcal competence is coordinated between cells by a quorum-sensing mechanism that operates in such a way that most cells of a culture become competent for DNA uptake simultaneously at some point in the exponential phase of growth as a critical cell density is achieved. The broad phenomena of competence regulation in pneumococcus and *S. gordonii* are quite similar,[28,58,77,78] although in pneumococcus there is a sharper peak of competence, with a rapid rise and fall, while in *S. gordonii* the regulation is more relaxed.

Pneumococcal competence has gradually become more amenable to laboratory investigation and application since the demonstration of the transformation reaction in vitro,[14] which brought the phenomenon observed in vivo by Griffith[23] into the laboratory. Succeeding innovations included the use of drug-resistance markers,[28] a defined medium supporting competence,[80] the discovery that competent cells could be frozen and recovered with good competence,[18] and description of the interaction of cells and DNA in terms of the kinetics of a simple two-component reaction.[18] Endogenous competence in pneumococcus may appear at cell densities varying from 10^5/ml to 5×10^8/ml.[8,66] Both the coordination of competence and its density dependence were found to depend on a protease-sensitive intercellular signal, termed activator or competence factor (CF),[74,78] which was thus one of the first bacterial pheromones and quorum-sensing signals to be described. Tomasz and Mosser[79] characterized an activator that had properties of a small basic protein and was obtained from competent pneumococcal cells of strain R6 by heat treatments, but was not found in culture supernatants. Although in early reports CF was obtained from streptococcal cell surfaces by heat treatments at pH 2,[16] in many *S. gordonii* isolates including the Challis strain[19,57,59] and in the pneumococcal strain Rx,[51] significant levels of CF activity were also obtained in simple culture supernatants; yet in the pneumococcal strain R6, the bulk of recoverable activity was bound to the cell surface, although it could pass from cell to cell without intimate cell contact.[78] As discussed on page 33, the stable CF activity found in culture supernatants of strain Rx has been useful for obtaining competence in many strains of pneumococcus;[84] yet, a reproducible, convenient source of pure activator remained elusive.

An interesting strain specificity was discovered by P. Gaus-

University of Illinois at Chicago, Chicago, Illinois 60607
Reprinted from *Microbial Drug Resistance*, Vol. 3, No. 1, 1997.

tad, at the National Hospital in Oslo, using inter-strain competence activation surveys among strains of *S. gordonii*.[20,21] Within one specificity group, all strains respond to CF preparations from members of the same group, though not all members of the group are CF-producers, and none respond to naturally produced pheromone from other groups. No such CF specificity distinctions have been reported for pneumococcus, nor have similarly extensive surveys been reported for this species.

Although the conditions required for development of competence are not well defined, several influential variables have been noted frequently. One aspect of the pneumococcal cell's metabolism with a strong influence on transformability is its capsule state: encapsulated strains are usually incompetent, in contrast to their rough derivatives. Other parameters that have long been observed to influence competence are external, including the presence of calcium ions and albumin and the pH of the culture medium.[8,66,71,78] Although the basis of a strong dependence on pH is still unknown, much of the effect must be at the level of CF production, since high doses of synthetic activator can overcome it.[30] Transformation is usually studied in liquid suspension, but it also occurs within a colony of cells growing in semi-solid media;[39,46,56,66,73] this has proven valuable in screening for mutants with altered transformability, and it may reflect the natural context of transformation more closely than do uniform suspension cultures.

The nature of the competent state is also not well defined, although competent cells are distinguishable from noncompetent ones in several ways beyond the sudden display of a highly efficient DNA uptake capacity. However, it is known that protein and RNA synthesis are required for its induction,[77] and that it is accompanied by a major but brief switch of protein synthesis pattern.[52,65] Among proteins induced at competence, other than CF (discussed below), are the products of the *cinA* locus including *RecA*, and a competence-specific DNA-binding protein that coats the DNA strands formed upon uptake.[53]

Although many features of the regulatory circuit controlling competence have been defined by investigations using crude culture supernatants or more highly enriched cell extracts, and the existence of secreted signals for streptococcal competence induction was known for many years, the precise molecular nature of the signals eluded identification until recently. In the past 12 months, four streptococcal competence activators have been identified by a collaborative effort involving six laboratories in three countries. As described below, each activator was identified as a small unmodified peptide: two from pneumococcus are 17 residues long; two from *S. gordonii* are 19 residues long. The recent progress rested, in the first instance, on genetic indications that the active molecule might be not a protein but a peptide, with subsequent application of fractionation strategies suitable for peptide purification, and, in the remaining cases, on recognition of the circumstance that the structural genes for the peptides are flanked by highly conserved stretches of DNA. This chapter discusses results of the first year of investigations on the nature and role of these streptococcal competence pheromone peptides.

A PNEUMOCOCCAL COMPETENCE STIMULATING PEPTIDE

The first streptococcal competence pheromone to be identified was purified directly from competent cultures of *S. pneumoniae*.[30] Beginning with a 1.5-liter competent culture of strain Rx, L. S. Håvarstein, at the Agricultural University of Norway, purified approximately 2 micrograms of CF after five steps, which included ammonium sulfate precipitation, Amberlite XAD-16 adsorption, ion exchange chromatography in 7*M* urea, reverse-phase HPLC, and SDS PAGE. Assays of activity used Rx cells in a standard transformation reaction. Two fractions of the final column chromatography step were sufficiently pure to give identical sequences upon Edman degradation and visible 2-kd bands in a silver-stained SDS gel. The sequence of the product, shown in Figure 1, describes a short basic peptide with a pI of 11.5 and molecular weight 2243. To ask whether there might be any undetected modification of the peptide important for biological activity, the sequence was prepared by solid phase synthesis and assayed for competence-stimulating activity. As the synthetic peptide is active at a level matching that seen in vivo, it appears that the unmodified product itself is the active signal.

Although the peptide was isolated by virtue of its activating effects on a genetically transformable strain of Rx, it was soon shown that is also complemented the competence deficiency caused by mutation of the gene, *comA* (Fig. 2). This reproduced the effect of crude CF preparations on *comA* mutants and is consistent with a direct role of ComA in production of the peptide (see discussion of information suggesting a specific role

---

```
           * *        *              * .**       *   * .*.   . **..*                    .           .*
Challis    M K K K N K Q N L L P K E L Q Q F E I L T E R K L E Q V T G G D V R S N K I R L W W E N I F F N K K
7865       M K K K N K Q N L L P K E L Q Q F E I L T E R K L E Q V T G G D I R H R I N N S I W R D I F L K R R
Rx         M K N T V K - - - - - - L E Q F V A L K E K D L Q K I K G G E M R L S K - - - F F R D F I L Q R K K
A66        M K N T V K - - - - - - L E Q F V A L K E K D L Q K I K G G E M R I S R - - - I I L D F L F L R K K
           Double-glycine motif:        F     L S     E L     I   G G|
```

FIG. 1. Streptococcal peptide pheromones. Alignment of deduced precursors of four competence signalling peptides. *S. gordonii* pheromones CSP-1 and CSP-2 are encoded by strains Challis and 7865, respectively. *S. pneumoniae* pheromones CSP-1 and CSP-2 are encoded by strains Rx and A66, respectively. The mature peptide sequences form the C-terminal moiety of each precursor, following the GlyGly cleavage site (|). *, residues identical in all four cases; ., conservative substitutions.

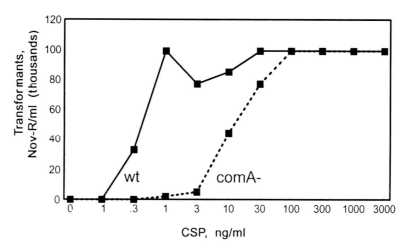

FIG. 2. Pheromone dose-response. Competence of *S. pneumoniae* Rx strains CP1200 (ComA$^+$) and CP1415 (ComA$^-$) induced by exposure to synthetic CSP at the indicated levels. 10^7 cells/ml were treated with peptide and Nov^R DNA (100 ng/ml) for 120 min at 37C in CTM (8). Induction of competence by the lower levels of synthetic pheromone depends on function of the pheromone secretion gene *comA*, described in the text.

below). Antibody prepared against a conjugated preparation of the synthetic peptide was found to abolish both endogenous and peptide-induced competence unless overwhelmed by synthetic peptide.[13] Thus, for strain Rx, the described competence-stimulating peptide (CSP) is both necessary and sufficient for induction of competence. In the discussion below, we attempt to use nomenclature distinguishing the hypothetical active component of unpurified preparations (CF or activator) from the identified active peptide (CSP).

Under 'optimal' conditions, strain Rx derivatives respond to CSP in a reproducible manner.[30] In a noncompetent growing culture, addition of CSP causes a strong but brief induction of competence which reaches a maximal level by about 15–20 min and then decays at a similar rate (Fig. 3). Parameters known to be crucial for endogenous induction of competence also affect the response to CSP. For three factors we have examined (pH, Ca^{++}, BSA), the effect of suboptimal values of the parameter was to reduce somewhat (2–5x) the sensitivity to CSP, but there was less effect, or none at all, on the response at high doses of CSP. This pattern suggests that many of these 'environmental' factors modulate the sensitivity to CSP (readily confused with effects on CSP production because of its autoinducing character, discussed below) or the basal production of CSP, with less effect, if any, on the capacity of cells to respond to high doses of the signal. In Rx strains, 0.2 ng/ml can be sufficient to induce a significant level of competence (Fig. 2). Although the recovery was not measured, the 2000 ng obtained from 1.5 L of Rx culture[30] implies that competent cultures contain at least 2 ng/ml CSP, more than that minimum effective amount. Indirect evidence suggests that while an intact competence quorum-sensing system can be activated by 0.2–1 ng/ml CSP, a pheromone-defective strain requires 20–100 ng/ml for full induction and that the typical competent Rx cultures used for production of CF contain 100 ng CSP/ml or more. Finally, the stability of the biological activity of synthetic pheromone should be noted. In contrast to the activator obtained from the surface of strain R6 cells, which has a half-life of 2 h at 0°C,[79] syn-

thetic CSP proved to be quite stable, with a half-life of 15 days at 20°C.[13]

MULTIPLE PHEROMONE STRUCTURAL GENES AND PHEROTYPES

The CSP described above is one in a family of closely related streptococcal quorum-sensing signals important in regulation of competence. The second pneumococcal competence pheromone described activates strain A66, known as the source of type III capsule genes in the experiments of Avery, MacLeod, and McCarty.[3] It was discovered in a survey of CSP genes among encapsulated pneumococcal strains and defines a second 'pherotype' in this species, apparently following a pheromone-specificity pattern like that previously described for *S. gordonii*.[62] The two competence pheromones described to date in *S. gordonii*[32] represent two of the specificity groups previously described in that species.[20,21] In each of these four cases, the active peptide is encoded within a larger open reading frame, which encodes a putative precursor peptide containing a few dozen extra N-terminal residues. The structures of the three additional pheromones were predicted from nucleotide sequences and were verified by synthesis; in all three cases, the unmodified synthetic peptide is biologically active and strain-specific. Amplification of the gene for pneumococcal CSP-1 was accomplished by PCR using degenerate oligonucleotide primers designed from the peptide sequence; PCR walking recovered its larger context.[30] PCR using primers targeted to conserved flanking sequences retrieved homologues from the three additional strains.[32,62]

As shown in Figure 1, there are several levels of sequence similarity between these peptides. The N-terminal extensions are identical within conspecific pairs, share eleven fully conserved residues between the species, and all contain a conserved double-glycine motif, discussed below. The mature peptides diverge more than the leader moieties, both within a species and

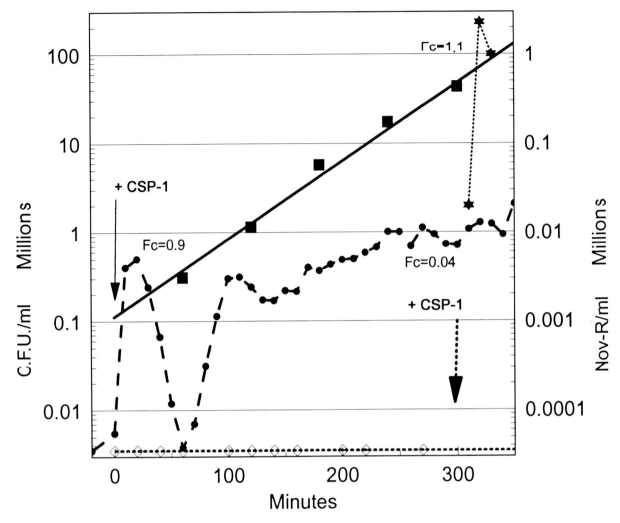

FIG. 3. Acute and chronic responses to peptide pheromone. Early and late responses to continuous exposure to CSP were compared in the Rx strain CP1200. After CSP (400 ng/ml) was added to a dilute culture growing in CTM (8), viable cell titer (squares) and competence of this (circles) and a parallel untreated control culture (diamonds) was monitored at intervals by exposing samples to 100 ng/ml Nov[R] DNA for 20 min at 37°C, terminating the reaction with DNase I (0.01 mg/ml), and challenging with Novobiocin. To verify responsiveness of non-competent cells at higher cell densities, a portion of the untreated control culture was treated with CSP at 300 min (dashed arrow; stars). Fc, fraction of cells competent, was estimated for the acute and chronic responses at the indicated points of this regimen in a separate culture by the congression method of Porter and Guild,[61] but after allowing segregation of individual recipient DNA strands.

between species, but are all rich in basic and hydrophobic residues and share other features.

PHEROMONE PROCESSING AND SECRETION

The four streptococcal competence pheromones identified to date are thought, on the basis of their gene sequences, to be produced by post-translational removal of an N-terminal extension ending in two glycine residues. Furthermore, these extensions match (6 of 8 sites) a motif characteristic of the "double-glycine" class of leader peptides[33] (Fig. 1). The GlyGly consensus is shared with a family of precursors of secreted bacterial peptides including those for many so-called nonlantibiotic bacteriocins, certain lantibiotics, and several Gram-posi-

tive intercellular signals not known to be bacteriocins.[33,36] The genes for members of the double-glycine family of peptide precursors are usually linked to members of a subfamily of ABC-transporters required for their production. As one of these membrane proteins has been shown to carry a protease domain capable of making the proteolytic cut following the GlyGly motif, and, as this domain is uniquely conserved in this subfamily,[31] it is thought that in the usual mode of release of these products, both transport and processing depend on the associated ABC-transporter.

Although CF-responsive competence-defective mutants were mentioned as early as 1965,[75] specific genetic causes of defects in CF production were not identified until recently.[7,86] In the case of the pneumococcal competence pheromone peptide CSP-1, no ABC transporter gene is closely linked to the peptide gene; however, there is an unlinked ABC-transporter gene known which carries the conserved protease domain, and which is required for CF production.[29] It is therefore reasonable to think that production of CSP follows the same path as for other member of the double-glycine peptide class, with proteolytic processing and transport both dependent on a single membrane protein. However there is as yet no direct evidence that streptococcal pheromones are made as larger precursors, or that a ComA-like protein processes them, beyond the CF-deficient phenotype of *comA* mutants. Evidence for the processing of the three more recently identified peptide signals is less complete than for CSP-1 of pneumococcus, since, for example, the mature molecules have not been isolated. However, the strong conservation of the GlyGly motif suggests that they are produced in the same way as the pneumococcal peptide, CSP-1.

The nature and mode of synthesis of competence pheromone in pneumococcal strain R6 is not yet clear. R6 derivatives are induced by CSP-1 and by Rx supernatant preparations,[2] but they do not release much soluble CF.[79,85] It is not known whether the activator in R6 extracts is different from CSP-1, or is like CSP-1 but is bound to some other molecule. Although activator is found mainly on the R6 surface, this could represent either a slower release step or a more rapid high-affinity capture step than occurs in Rx.

Pheromone self-regulation

A remarkable feature of pneumococcal competence is the suddenness with which it appears in most or all cells of a population. If the pheromone accumulates in proportion to cell number due to basal synthesis, doubling once per generation, this abrupt induction suggests the existence of either a steep dose-response curve for signal perception or a mechanism to accelerate the accumulation of the signal. Measurement of activator levels before and during competence induction[51,76] has suggested a competence-associated increase consistent with the hypothesis of an autoinducing signal. The prototype quorum-sensing system of Gram-negative bacteria, the LuxIR system of *Vibrio fischeri*,[72] which employs an acyl homoserine lactone signal to regulate luminescence, also exhibits such a self-inducing signal,[9] as does an autoregulating circuit controlling production of the lantibiotic nisin.[37]

By joining a *lacZ* reporter to *comC*, it was possible to demonstrate that transcription of the gene for CSP-1 is in fact regulated in a manner consistent with the autoinduction hypothesis.[60] A basal level of expression (12 Miller units) occurs in non-competent cultures, and induction with the synthetic peptide causes accumulation of much higher levels of LacZ (550 Miller units). Thus, the expression of *comC* itself responds to its product, in a fashion that would allow an abrupt transition to high levels of the pheromone once an inducing threshold had been crossed. Extrapolating to events in natural competence induction it may be expected that: 1) trace levels of CSP provoke *comC* expression but a delayed competence response, 2) trace levels of CSP cause release of higher amounts of CSP, and 3) CSP levels rise sharply at the point of endogenous competence development. The effectiveness of this autoinduction is reflected by the reduced (20-fold) sensitivity of a *comA* mutant to CSP (Fig. 2).

PHEROMONE RECEPTORS

Two classes of surface proteins which have been implicated in perception of Gram-positive peptide signals are oligopeptide permeases[17,43,70] and members of two-component signal transduction systems.[15,24,69] Examples of both classes of protein are known in *S. pneumoniae*, and are involved in unknown ways in competence regulation.

S. pneumoniae possesses a complex oligopeptide uptake system, Ami, which includes a four-protein ABC-transporter, AmiCDEF, and three homologous substrate-binding lipoproteins, AmiA, AliA, and AliB, located on the cell surface. Each of the three lipoproteins contributes to metabolic utilization of oligopeptides.[1] The pneumococcal oligopeptide permease is implicated in competence regulation by several mutations which alter the pattern of endogenous competence induction. However, as neither single-gene nor multigene mutations in this system block response to CSP,[2] it is unlikely that it acts as an essential part of the pheromone receptor.

Two genes, names *ciaHR*, encode a two-component response regulator system originally identified via *ciaH* mutations recovered at a step in the accumulation of cefotaxime resistance mutations at which there was no alteration of a penicillin binding protein and at which competence was also lost.[25] Isolated CiaH transfers phosphate to CiaR.[85] Point mutations (A203V and T230P) near the active site His226, hypothesized to cause elevated phosphotransfer, suppress competence and CF production and are not activated to competence by crude CF culture supernatant preparations. This phenotype, combined with regulator/receptor homologies, suggested that CiaH might act in CF recognition; yet, disruptions of *ciaH* or *ciaR* are fully competent. Assuming that competence in these mutants depends on CSP, this two-component regulator must not act as the CSP receptor, but appears to modulate the sensitivity to the signal, since its action reduces sensitivity to CSP, but its absence does not. Clearly, we are only starting to learn what signals are integrated with the quorum-sensing signal to regulate competence.

In a third category is a protein, defined biochemically, that was isolated by Horne, Plotch and Tomasz[27] from the cell membrane and has a capacity to inactivate (bind) CF in a reversible (by heating) fashion. Named AIP (for activator inhibiting protein) to represent the latter property, its location at the cell surface and the reversible binding to CF suggested a possible role as CF receptor. However, neither the cognate gene nor relevant mutations have yet been identified, and no further characterization or genetic analysis has been reported. The reported size (68,000 MW) and pI (4.2) of AIP are substantially different from those predicted for ComD, described below (pI 6.2, MW 51,350).

More recently, two additional candidate genes in the two-component regulator class were found near *comC* itself. These were implicated initially by virtue of their close linkage to *comC* and by homology to two-component regulatory gene families. They possess especially high similarity to genes regulating operons for secretion of peptides of the GlyGly type. The genes are found immediately downstream of the CSP gene both in pneumococcus and *S. gordonii*, are named *comD* and *comE*, and encode a histidine protein kinase homologue and a response

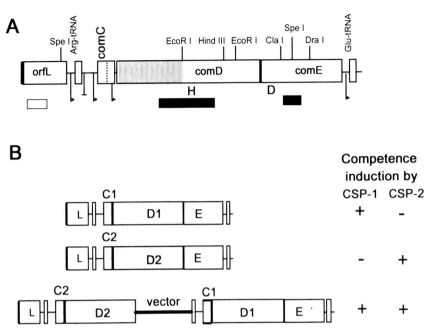

FIG. 4. Map and genetic analysis of pheromone and receptor locus, comCDE. A. Elements of the *S. pneumoniae* pheromone and pheromone receptor locus.[30] tRNA[Arg] and tRNA[Glu] genes and an unidentified gene, *orfL*, flank the locus. The locus encodes ComC, the pheromone precursor peptide containing a double-glycine protease processing site (:), ComD, a histidine protein kinase homologue with an N-terminal set of membrane-spanning helices (striped), and ComE, a response regulator homologue. Conserved histidine and aspartate residues in ComD and ComE involved in phosphotransfer by two-component regulatory systems,[71] are indicated (H, D). Below the map are shown the segments of three genes used to target gene disruption by insertion-duplication (open, Com[+]; filled, Com[−]). Locations of putative promoter sequences are indicated by descending flags. B. Identification of ComD as the pheromone receptor in *S. gordonii* by construction of a hybrid locus, as described by Havarstein *et al.*[32] Gene organization in two strains of *Streptococcus gordonii* responding to two different pheromone peptides, and in a strain constructed with portion of both loci to determine whether the peptide specificity of competence induction was conferred by ComD. The strains are Wicky (NTCT9124, CSP-1 pherotype), 7865 (NTCT7865, CSP-2 pherotype), and STG1 (*comC2comD2*::[pLPV-SKII]::*comC1comD1comE*). The hybrid strain was constructed by insertion-duplication with plasmid pLPV-SKII(Em-R) containing tRNA[Arg], *comC2*, and *comD2* from 7865. Peptides inducing competence in the strains are indicated at right. Experimental details are presented in Håvarstein *et al.*[32]

regulator homologue, respectively. Two lines of genetic evidence link these genes directly to CSP perception. In *S. pneumoniae*, disruption of either gene produces a CSP-blind phenotype.[60] Although this shows that the signal transduction pair is important for CSP response, the linkage could still be indirect. Evidence for a direct linkage was obtained from two homologous *S. gordonii* competence regulation systems. For one of the *S. gordonii* phenotypes, the ComD homologue was shown directly to be the receptor by showing that its gene determines the peptide specificity of the competence response (Fig. 4).[32] Assuming the same to be true for pneumococcus, the non-responsive phenotype of *comE* mutants strongly suggests that ComE acts as a downstream link in the pathway.

Homologous sensing systems, found in a variety of Gram-positive species, participate in regulation of secreted polypeptide products such as plantaricin A, sakacin P, and carnobacteriocin B2, as well as virulence determinants. In some of these cases, the quorum-sensing signal has also been identified as a small peptide. Genes for production of and response to the much smaller and modified peptide pheromones regulating *B. subtilis* competence are more distantly related to the CSP circuit genes.[45,69] It appears that while Gram-negative bacteria rely principally on acyl homoserine lactone signals for quorum-sens-

ing,[9] in Gram-positive species peptides or modified peptides often play that role; streptococcal competence may now be seen as conforming to this pattern.

PNEUMOCOCCAL COMPETENCE IS SELF-LIMITING

When the response to a signal entails a strong switch in protein synthesis pattern, as in streptococcal competence regulation, a corresponding mechanism of attenuation may be required to allow resumption of normal cell growth, especially if there is no arrangement to remove the signal from the milieu. Indeed, a frequently observed hallmark of pneumococcal competence is a rapid decay of competence following induction. A competence inhibitor was found in late-log-phase and post-competent cultures of both *S. gordonii* and *S. pneumoniae* during early studies of competence regulation and, although inhibitory activity was not restricted to competent cultures and it was never directly or intimately linked to the decay of competence, it was suggested that this activity could be responsible for the brevity of competence.[78]

Identification of CSP enabled us to reinvestigate the causes of competence decay, by allowing induction both at very low cell densities and without supplementation by culture supernatant fluids, and allowed a direct test of the importance of extracellular inhibitors in pneumococcal competence shutdown.[13] In Rx strains, competence reaches a maximum approximately 20 min after exposure of cells to CSP, but largely disappears by 40 min; thereafter, cells remain refractory to CSP for about one generation.[13] In these CSP-induced cultures, the kinetics of shutoff were independent of cell density over the range of 10^4–10^7 cells/ml, and culture supernatants taken immediately after competence shut-down supported full competence induction among added log-phase tester cells. Thus, it appears that an internal timing mechanism brings about a competence shut-off as the final act in a chain of CSP-stimulated events, without a requirement for any further cell-to-cell communication.

What then happens during chronic exposure to CSP? It appears that the internal timer leads to a cycling of competence in cells grown in a high constant level of CSP, a cycling that mimics the competence cycling often seen in endogenously induced cultures. Indeed, chronic CSP exposure (Fig. 3) reproduces rather closely a pattern of successive cycles of competence described, for example, by R. Hotchkiss[28] and later by Chen and Morrison.[8] Hotchkiss attributed the waves to experimental phasing of the cell cycle; the present data suggest that the synchrony instead reflects phasing of the competence attenuation timer. The cycling of competent cohorts within a culture also inferred by Hotchkiss is consistent with the finding that a short period of synchronized competence is followed by a longer refractory period. Since the cycling occurs even at low cell densities with high levels of CSP, it seems likely that it reflects repeated activation and loss of the signal attenuation mechanism switch. As the refractory period is longer than the competence period, it is not surprising that some synchrony to persists through several cycles, or that continued exposure to CSP generates a population that maintains a low proportion of competent cells.

PHEROMONE GENES AND PHEROMONE RESPONSIVENESS ARE WIDESPREAD IN PNEUMOCOCCUS

Although it was long known that some *S. gordonii* strains are CF producers while others are not, the first indication that CF was sometimes the competence-limiting element for encapsulated pneumococcal strains was the finding by Yother, McDaniel, and Briles[84] that CF-containing supenatants from strain Rx could provoke competence in some encapsulated strains which were not themselves endogenously competent. They showed that capsule itself is not a barrier to full activation by CF, that some strains require CF even after removal of their capsule, but also that others are not activated by CF, even without capsule. Since the initial report, the CF supernatant preparation from strain Rx has been applied for transformation of encapsulated strains of serotypes 2,[4] 3,[4,34] 5 and 6b,[35] 7,[83] 10,[5] and 19f.[26] Nonetheless, competence failed despite addition of CF in some cases. The specific causes of failure were not identified.

A new perspective on the matter is provided by a study conducted by G. Pozzi and colleagues at the Universities of Siena and Cagliari and at Glaxo-Wellcome in Verona. By sequencing the *comC* gene and assaying response to both synthetic peptides CSP-1 and CSP-2 in a panel of encapsulated strains of *S pneumoniae*, they showed that a large fraction of 42 isolates examined was activated to some degree of competence by at least one of the two synthetic CSP molecules available (Fig. 5). Also, every strain was found to carry either of two allelic forms of the CSP gene, *comC*1 or *comC*2.[62] Thus, some strains, including A66, apparently fail to respond to the Rx CF preparations because they belong to the second pherotype, carrying a different allele of *comC* and a correspondingly specific receptor. Responsive strains included serotypes 2, 3, 6, 9, 17, 18, and 19, and two or three additional types not specifically identified. Bearing in mind that only one culture medium was used for the survey studies, the clear impression is that encapsulated strains, usually characterized as 'nontransformable,' may fail to transform for any of several different reasons, some, but not all, of which can be overcome by exogenous CSP of the appropriate specificity. (Although induced competence levels were high for

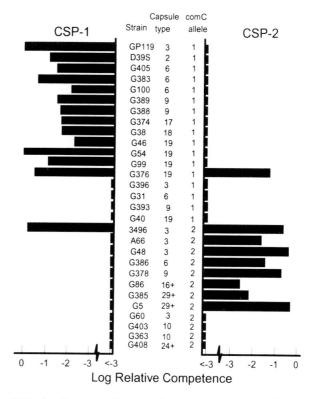

FIG. 5. Response of encapsulated pneumococcal strains to synthetic pheromones. Response to competence pheromone peptides of representative strains *from* survey described in detail in.[62] In summary, approximately 10^7 cfu/ml in Tryptic Soy Broth (Difco) supplemented with BSA, CaCl₂, synthetic peptide pheromone, and Str^R donor DNA (1000 ng/ml) were held for 2.5 hrs at 37°C, then were plated for Str-R transformants. None of these strains transformed above the minimal levels of detection (0.1%) without pheromone. Level of transformation is presented relative to that of a control culture of strain GP119. Capsule types were determined using Statens Seruminstitut typing sera; *comC* alleles were determined by sequencing PCR amplification products. Capsule serotype groups indicated as: 16+, 16/36/37; 24+, 24/31/40; 29+, 29/34/35/42/47.

some strains of both pheretypes, there is as yet no characterization of an 'intact' CSP-2 regulatory system, with high levels of endogenous induction). If the pattern seen in this survey is typical, one must conclude that 'highly transformable' isolates are not rare, even if not universal. Although Rx CF preparations have been applied to induce competence in a variety of encapsulated strains, synthetic CSP allows higher and more reproducible doses. Since commercial peptide synthesis is inexpensive and the activity of the synthetic pheromone is stable, synthetic pheromone should probably be considered as the tool of choice for much routine genetic work.

OPEN QUESTIONS

Although the nature of the competence-regulating signal now seems clear, and some aspects of its functional context have come into view, much more of this context remains to be described. For example, with definition of the signaling molecule, the lack of definition of the targets of this quorum-sensing circuit is highlighted. Only a very few genes regulated for transformation have been defined; we do not know whether other aspects of cell function are also regulated by the same sensor of population density; and the steps linking the receptor to these 'competence-induced' genes are still undefined.

Although several genes important for CSP production have been identified, the sources of the signal are still uncertain. It is unknown whether or how basal synthesis is regulated, or what the influence of capsule or capsule synthesis on CSP production may be. The mode(s) of presentation of CSP are not clear, including whether there is a complex form of CSP which might explain the properties of strain R6. Finally, the nature and significance of pheretype specificity is totally unknown.

One should note that while the role of the competence signalling mechanism in streptococci might be simply to turn on a DNA uptake system when there is a good chance of encountering DNA from the same species, it could be regulating other 'group activities' as well. The circumstance that the CSP quorum-sensing circuit was recognized via its role in competence regulation should not be taken to imply that this is its only, or even its principal, role in the biology of these organisms. For example, the prevalence of bacteriocins among the streptococci raises the possibility that the 'competence' quorum-sensing circuit also may regulate bacteriocin synthesis. A concerted activation of bacteriocin synthesis and competence would provide an interesting source of DNA for natural transformation.

GENETIC APPLICATIONS

Such open questions notwithstanding, the observation that conditions required for competence development are relaxed when induction is accomplished with synthetic peptides, and the high frequency of responsive strains found in an exploratory survey suggests that there already is a broad opportunity for application of gene transfer methods to encapsulated strains of pneumococcus. While the principal outcome of the streptococcal transformation process is allele replacement, varied opportunities for genetic manipulations are also offered by the known fates of chimeric DNA after uptake by the natural transformation pathway, including targeted gene disruption, allele exchange during facilitated plasmid transformation, and simple plasmid transfer. Conjugation systems are also available to complement the transformation route.[63,64]

During several decades of research into the mechanism of natural transformation, only one pathway of DNA uptake has been demonstrated. So far as is known, all DNA taken up by competent streptococci suffers at least one obligatory endonucleolytic scission[54,55] and reduction to single-strand form.[38] A cut end enters first, with uptake proceeding processively in the 3-5′ direction.[49] Despite the disruption of the genetic continuity of the donor molecule attendant on this mode of uptake, the subsequent fate of donor DNA is orderly, with outcomes that depend on the presence and organization of resident base sequences homologous to the donor molecule. Recombination is rapid, being largely completed within 5–10 min at 37°C.[22] However, expression of new characters and segregation of new alleles from old typically require several additional generations. The classes of recombinants recovered depend on the selection employed and the location of the selected element among homologous and heterologous (if any) sequences in the donor molecule. For an integrated view of these processes, the essay by S. Lacks[40] may be consulted. Four principal cases can usefully be distinguished. 1) For small allelic differences between donor and recipient, the donor replaces the recipient allele with a high efficiency (~50%),[6,47] albeit with possible loss by mismatch repair.[11,48] 2) Larger allelic differences are incorporated as well, though with some loss of efficiency, if substantial amounts of flanking homology are present on both sides of a heterologous marker. However, if the homology flanks the selected gene on only one side, integration is much less frequent[12] and is associated with adjacent deletions. 3) Circular chimeras that include a segment of pneumococcal DNA yield either of two different products, depending on whether they carry a replicon active in pneumococcus: closed replicative circles[44] or chromosomal inserts surrounded by duplications of the homologous targeting sequence;[50,81,82] the yield of such products depends on the length of the homologous segment. Finally, 4) heterologous plasmids, bearing no homology to recipient DNA, are reassembled from separate donor molecules.[68]

Each of these pathways has a characteristic efficiency, which varies with the length of homology available for recombination.[6,41,42] However, the overall efficiency of natural transformation in a population of 100% competent cells is so high that events with low relative efficiencies still yield practicable numbers of transformants. The most efficient event in natural transformation is simple homologous allele replacement; for chromosomal donor DNA carrying a point marker, 10^6 transformants are readily obtained among 10^8 competent cells, while a cloned donor copy of such a marker can transform 50% of the cells. Thus events with relative efficiencies as low as 10^{-5} can be used in practice without difficulty. For example, while the efficiency of insertion-duplication events is lower than that of homologous allele replacement and is also length-dependent, its gene targeting is quite reliable: fragments as small as 180 bp have been found to target homologous insertion with high specificity.[60,67] It is, however, important to recognize that the environment for gene expression in pneumococcus is significantly different from those in *E. coli* or *B. subtilis*, though the nature of all differences is not understood, so that the suitability of a selective marker should be verified for each application. For example, some markers with effective expression when carried on plasmid vectors appear to be expressed in single copy form only if joined to an active promoter.[10]

ACKNOWLEDGMENTS

Parts of the recent work discussed in this chapter carried out in Chicago were supported by the National Science Foundation (MCB-9506785). D. Mehan provided excellent technical assistance. Other recent results discussed are the work of collaborators at the Agricultural University of Norway, Ås (L. S. Håvarstein), the Universita di Cagliari (F. Iannelli and L. Masala), the Universita di Siena (R. Manganelli and G. Pozzi), the Institute of Microbiology, National Hospital, Oslo (P. Gaustad), Glaxo Wellcome S. P. A., Verona (L. Piccoli and D. Simon), and the Universite Paul Sabatier, Toulouse (G. Alloing, J. Claverys, and C. Granadel).

REFERENCES

1. **Alloing, G., P. de Philip, and J.P. Claverys.** 1994. Three highly homologous membrane-bound lipoproteins participate in oligopeptide transport by the Ami system of the Gram-positive *Streptococcus pneumoniae*. J. Mol. Biol. **241**:44–58.

2. **Alloing, G., C. Granadel, D.A. Morrison, and J.-P. Claverys,** 1996. Competence pheromone, oligopeptide permease, and induction of competence in *Streptococcus pneumoniae*. Mol. Microbiol. **21**:471–478.

3. **Avery, O.T., C.M. MacLeod, and M. McCarty.** 1944. Studies on the chemical nature of the substance inducing transformation of pneumococcal types. Induction of transformation by a desoxyribonucleic acid fraction isolated from pneumococcus type III. J. Exp. Med. **79**:137–157.

4. **Berry, A.M., R.A. Lock, D. Hansman, and J.C. Paton.** 1989. Contribution of autolysin to virulence of *Streptococcus pneumoniae*. Infect. Immun. **57**:2324–2330.

5. **Berry, A.M., J.C. Paton, and D. Hansman.** 1992. Effect of insertional inactivation of the genes encoding pneumolysin and autolysin on the virulence of *Streptococcus pneumoniae* type-3. Microbial Pathogenesis **12**:87–93.

6. **Cato, A., and W.R. Guild.** 1968. Transformation and DNA size: I. Activity of fragments of defined size and a fit to a random double-crossover model. J. Mol. Biol. **37**:157–178.

7. **Chandler, M.S., and D.A. Morrison.** 1988. Identification of two proteins encoded by *com*, a competence control locus of *Streptococcus pneumoniae*. J. Bacteriol. **170**:3136–3141.

8. **Chen, J.D., and D.A. Morrison.** 1987. Modulation of competence for genetic transformation in *Streptococcus pneumoniae*. J. Gen. Microbiol. **133**:1959–1967.

9. **Choi, S.H., and E.P. Greenberg.** 1992. Genetic dissection of DNA binding and luminescence gene activation by the *Vibrio fischeri* LuxR protein. J. Bacteriol. **174**:4064–4069.

10. **Claverys, J.P., A. Dintilhac, E.V. Pestova, B. Martin, and D.A. Morrison.** 1995. Construction and evaluation of new drug-resistance cassettes for gene disruption mutagenesis in *Streptococcus pneumoniae*, using an ami test platform. Gene **164**:123–128.

11. **Claverys, J.P., and S.A. Lacks.** 1986. Heteroduplex deoxyribonucleic acid base mismatch repair in bacteria. Microbiol. Rev. **50**:133–165.

12. **Claverys, J.P., J.C. Lefevre, and A.M. Sicard.** 1980. Induction of genetic transformation in *Streptococcus pneumoniae* by a *S. pneumoniae*-lambda phage hybrid DNA: Induction of deletions. Proc. Natl. Acad. Sci. U.S.A. **77**:3534–3538.

13. **Coomaraswamy, G.** 1996. PhD Thesis: Induction of competence for genetic transformation in *Streptococcus pneumoniae* by a pheromone peptide and its synthetic analogues. University of Illinois at Chicago, Chicago, Il.

14. **Dawson, M.H., and R.H. Sia.** 1931. In vitro transformation of pneumococcal types. I. A technique for inducing transformation of pneumococcal types in vitro. J. Exp. Med. **54**:681–699.

15. **Diep, D.B., L.S. Håvarstein, and I.F. Nes.** 1995. A bacteriocin-like peptide induces bacteriocin synthesis in *Lactobacillus plantarum* C11. Mol. Microbiol. **18**:631–639.

16. **Dobrzanski, W.T., and H. Osowiecki.** 1967. Isolation and some properties of the competence factor from Group H Streptococcus strain Challis. J. Gen. Microbiol. **48**:299–304.

17. **Dunny, G.M., B.A. Leonard, and P.J. Hedberg.** 1995. Pheromone inducible conjugation in *Enterococcus faecalis*: Interbacterial and host-parasite chemical communication. J. Bacteriol. **177**:871–876.

18. **Fox, M., and R.D. Hotchkiss.** 1957. Initiation of bacterial transformation. Nature **179**:1322–1325.

19. **Gaustad, P.** 1983. Genetic transformation in *Streptococcus sanguis*. Kinetics of production in different media and specific interaction of competence factor and competence inactivator. Acta Pathol. Microbiol. Immunol. Scand. Sect. B **91**:193–200.

20. **Gaustad, P.** 1985. Genetic transformation in *Streptococcus sanguis*: Effects on genetic transformation by culture filtrates of *Streptococcus sanguis* (serogroups H and W) and *Streptococcus mitits* (mitior) with reference to identification. Acta Pathol. Microbiol. Immunol Scand. Sect. B **93**:283–287.

21. **Gaustad, P.** 1993. Genetic transformation and competence factors in the identification of *Streptococcus sanguis*, p 51–54. *In* E. Balla (ed.), DNA transfer and gene expression in microorganisms. Intercept, Andover.

22. **Ghei, O.K., and S.A. Lacks.** 1967. Recovery of donor deoxyribonucleic acid marker activity from eclipse in pneumococcal transformation. J. Bacteriol. **93**:816–829.

23. **Griffith, F.** 1928. The significance of pneumococcal types. J. Hyg. **27**:108–159.

24. **Guangyong, J., R.C. Beavis, and R.P. Novick.** 1995. Cell density control of staphylococcal virulence mediated by an octapeptide pheromone. Proc. Natl. Acad. Sci. U.S.A. **92**:12055–12059.

25. **Guenzi, E., A.-M. Gasc, M.A. Sicard, and R. Hakenbeck.** 1994. A two-component signal-transducing system is involved in competence and penicillin susceptibility in laboratory mutants of *Streptococcus pneumoniae*. Mol. Microbiol. **12**:505–515.

26. **Guidolin, A., J.K. Morona, R. Morona, D. Hansman, and J.C. Paton.** 1994. Nucleotide-sequence analysis of genes essential for capsular polysaccharide biosynthesis in *Streptococcus pneumoniae* type 19F. Infect. Immun. **62**:5384–5396.

27. **Horne, D., S. Plotch, and A. Tomasz.** 1977. Cell surface components implicated as attachment sites for the pneumococcal competence activator, pp. 11–34. *In* A. Portoles (ed.), Bacterial Transformation and transfection. Proceedings of the Third European Meeting on Genetic Transformation. Amsterdam, North Holland.

28. **Hotchkiss, R.D.** 1954. Cyclical behaviour in pneumococcal growth and transformability occasioned by environmental changes. Proc. Natl. Acad. Sci. U.S.A. **40**:49–55.

29. **Hui, F., and D.A. Morrison.** 1991. Competence for transformation in *Streptococcus pneumoniae*: Nucleotide sequence analysis shows comA, a gene required for competence induction, to be a member of the bacterial ATP-dependent transport protein family. J. Bacteriol. **173**:372–381.

30. **Håvarstein, L.S., G. Coomaraswamy, and D.A. Morrison.** 1995. An unmodified heptadecapeptide pheromone induces competence

for genetic transformation in *Streptococcus pneumoniae*. Proc. Natl. Acad. Sci. U.S.A. **92:**11140–11144.

31. **Håvarstein, L.S., D. Diep, and I.F. Nes.** 1995. A family of bacteriocin ABC transporters carry out proteolytic processing of their substrates concomitant with export. Mol. Microbiol. **16:**229–240.

32. **Håvarstein, L.S., P. Gaustad, I.F. Nes, and D.A. Morrison.** 1996. Identification of the streptococcal competence pheromone receptor. Mol. Microbiol. **21:**863–869.

33. **Håverstein, L.S., H. Holo, and I.F. Nes.** 1994. The leader peptide of colicin V shares consensus sequences with leader peptides that are common among peptide bacteriocins produced by Grampositive bacteria. Microbiol. **140:**2383–2389.

34. **Johnson, M.K., J.A. Hobden, R.J. O'Callaghan, and J.M. Hill.** 1992. Confirmation of the role of pneumolysin in ocular infections with *Streptococcus pneumoniae*. Curr. Eye Res. **11:**1221–1225.

35. **Kelly, T., J.P. Dillard, and J. Yother.** 1994. Effect of genetic switching of capsular type on virulence of *Streptococcus pneumoniae*. Infect. Immun. **62:**1813–1819.

36. **Klaenhammer, T.R.** 1993. Genetics of bacteriocins produced by lactic acid bacteria. pp 39–85. *In* FEMS Microbiol. Rev. September, 1993, W.M. De Vos, J.H.J. Huisin't Veld and B. Poolman (eds.), Amsterdam, Elsevier.

37. **Kuipers, O.P., M.M. Beerthuyzen, P.G. De Ruter, E.J. Luesink, and W.M. De Vos.** 1995. Autoregulation of nisin biosynthesis in *Lactococcus lactis* by signal transduction. J. Biol. Chem. **270:**27299–27304.

38. **Lacks, S.** 1962. Molecular fate of DNA in genetic transformation of pneumococcus. J. Mol. Biol. **5:**119–131.

39. **Lacks, S.A.** 1970. Mutants of *Diplococcus pneumoniae* that lack deoxyribonucleases and other activities possibly pertinent to genetic transformation. J. Bacteriol. **101:**373–383.

40. **Lacks, S.A.** 1988. Mechanisms of genetic recombination in Grampositive bacteria. pp. 43–86. *In* R. Kucherlapati and G.R. Smith, (eds.), Genetic recombination. Amer. Soc. Microbiol. Press, Wash DC.

41. **Lataste, H., J.P. Claverys, and A.M. Sicard.** 1981. Relation between the transforming activity of a marker and its proximity to the end of the DNA particle. Mol. Gen. Genet. **183:**199–201.

42. **Lefevre, J.C., J.P. Claverys, and A.M. Sicard.** 1979. Donor deoxyribonucleic acid length and marker effect in pneumococcal transformation. J. Bacteriol. **138:**80–86.

43. **Leonard, B.A., A. Podbielski, P.J. Hedberg, and G.M. Dunny.** 1996. *Enterococcus faecalis* pheromone binding protein, PrgZ, recruits a chromosomal oligopeptide permease system to import sex pheromone cCF10 for induction of conjugation. Proc. Natl. Acad. Sci. U.S.A. **93:**260–264.

44. **Lopez, P., M. Espinosa, D.L. Stassi, and S.A. Lacks.** 1982. Facilitation of plasmid transfer in *Streptococcus pneumoniae* by chromosomal homology. J. Bacteriol. **150:**692–701.

45. **Magnuson, R., Solomon, J., and Grossman, A.D.** 1994. Biochemical and genetic characterization of a competence pheromone from *B. subtilis*. Cell **77:**207–216.

46. **McCarty, M., H.E. Taylor, and O.T. Avery.** 1946. Biochemical studies of environmental factors essential in transformation of pneumococcal types. Cold Spring Harbor Symp. Quant. Biol. **11:** 177–183.

47. **Mejean, V., and J.P. Claverys.** 1984. Use of a cloned DNA fragment to analyze the fate of donor DNA in transformation of *Streptococcus pneumoniae*. J. Bacteriol. **158:**1175–1178.

48. **Mejean, V., and J.P. Claverys.** 1984. Effect of mismatched base pairs on the fate of donor DNA in transformation of *Streptococcus pneumoniae*. Mol. Gen. Genet. **197:**467–471.

49. **Mejean, V., and J.P. Claverys.** 1993. DNA processing during entry in transformation of *Streptococcus pneumoniae*. J. Biol. Chem. **268:**5594–5599.

50. **Mejean, V., J.P. Claverys, H. Vasseghi, and A.M. Sicard.** 1981. Rapid cloning of specific DNA fragments of *Streptococcus pneumoniae* by vector integration into the chromosome followed by endonucleolytic excision. Gene **15:**289–293.

51. **Morrison, D.A.** 1981. Competence-specific protein synthesis in *Streptococcus pneumoniae*. pp. 39–53. *In* M. Polsinelli and G. Mazza (eds.), Transformation 1980: Proceedings of Fifth European Meeting on Bacterial Transformation and Transfection. Cotswold Press, Oxford.

52. **Morrison, D.A., and M. Baker.** 1979. Competence for genetic transformation in pneumococcus depends on the synthesis of a small set of proteins. Nature (London) **282:**215–217.

53. **Morrison, D.A., M. Baker, and B. Mannarelli.** 1979. A protein component of the pneumococcal eclipse complex, pp. 43–52 *In* S.W. Glover and L.O. Butler (eds.), Transformation—1978. Cotswold Press, Oxford.

54. **Morrison, D.A., and W.R. Guild.** 1972. Transformation and DNA size: Extent of degradation on entry varies with size. J. Bacteriol. **112:**1157–1168.

55. **Morrison, D.A., and W.R. Guild.** 1973. Breakage prior to entry of donor DNA in pneumococcus transformation. Biochem. Biophys. Acta. **299,** 545–556.

56. **Morrison, D.A., S.A. Lacks, W.R. Guild, and J.M. Hageman.** 1983. Isolation and characterization of three new classes of transformation-deficient mutants of *S. pneumoniae* that are defective in DNA transport and genetic recombination. J. Bacteriol. **156:**281–290.

57. **Osowiecki, H., J. Nalecz, and Dobrzanski, W.T.** 1969. The mechanism of competence in the transformation of Streptococcus of serological group H. Purification and some properties of the competence factor. Mol. Gen. Genet. **105:**16–20.

58. **Pakula, R., M. Piechowska, E. Bankowska, and W. Walczak.** 1962. A characteristic of DNA mediated transformation systems of two streptococcal strains. *Acta Microbiol. Polonica* **11:**205–222.

59. **Pakula, R., and W. Walczak.** 1963. On the nature of competence of transformable streptococci. J. Gen. Microbiol. **31:**125–133.

60. **Pestova, E.V., L.S. Håvarstein, and D.A. Morrison.** 1996. Regulation of competence for genetic transformation in *Streptococcus pneumoniae* by an autoinduced peptide pheromone and a two-component regulatory system. Mol. Microbiol. **21:**853–862.

61. **Porter, R.D., and W.R. Guild.** Number of transformable units per cell in *Diplococcus pneumoniae*. J. Bacteriol. **97:**1033–1035.

62. **Pozzi, G., L. Masala, F. Iannelli, R. Manganelli, L. Håvarstein, L. Piccoli, D. Simon and D. Morrison.** 1996. Competence for genetic transformation in encapsulated strains of *Streptococcus pneumoniae*: two allelic variants of the peptide pheromone. J. Bacteriol. **178:**6087–6090.

63. **Pozzi, G., R.A. Musmanno, E.A. Renzoni, M.R. Oggioni, and M.G. Cusi.** 1988. Host-vector system for integration of recombinant DNA into chromosomes of transformable and non-transformable streptococci. J. Bacteriol. **170:**1969–1972.

64. **Priebe, S.D., and S.A. Lacks.** 1989. Region of the streptococcal plasmid pMV158 required for conjugative mobilization. J. Bacteriol. **171:**4778–4784.

65. **Raina, J.L., and A.W. Ravin.** 1980. Switches in macromolecular synthesis during induction of competence for transformation of *Streptococcus sanguis*. Proc. Natl. Acad. Sci. U.S.A. **77:**6062–6066.

66. **Ravin, A.W.** 1954. A quantitative study of autogenic and allogenic transformations in pneumococcus. Exp. Cell Res. **7:**58–82.

67. **Rhee, D.K., and D.A. Morrison.** 1988. Genetic transformation in *Streptococcus pneumoniae*: molecular cloning and characterization of *recP*, a gene required for genetic recombination. J. Bacteriol. **170:**630–637.

68. **Saunders, C.W., and W.R. Guild.** 1981. Monomer plasmid DNA transforms *Streptococcus pneumoniae*. Mol. Gen. Genet. **181:**57–62.

69. **Solomon, J.M., and Grossman, A.D.** 1996. Who's competent and when? Regulation of natural genetic competence in bacteria. Trends Genet. **12**:150–155.

70. **Solomon, J.M., Magnuson, R., Srivastava, A., and Grossman, A.D.** 1995. Convergent sensing pathways mediate response to two extracellular competence factors in *Bacillus subtilis*. Genes Dev. **9**:547–558.

71. **Stock, J.B., M.G. Surette, M. Levit, and P. Park.** 1995. Two-component signal transduction systems: Structure-function relationships and mechanism of catalysis. *In* J.A. Hoch and T.J. Silhavy (eds.), Two-component signal transduction. Amer. Soc. Microbiol., Washington.

72. **Swift, S., M.K. Winson, P.F. Chan, N.J. Nainton, M. Birdsall, P.J. Reeves, C.E. Rees, S.R. Chhabra, P.J. Hill, J.P. Throup, B.W. Bycroft, G.P. Salmond, P. Williams, and G.S. Stewart.** 1993. A novel strategy for the isolation of luxI homologues: evidence for the widespread distribution of a LuxR:LuxI superfamily in enteric bacteria. Mol. Microbiol. **10**:511–520.

73. **Tiraby, G., J.P. Claverys, and A.M. Sicard.** 1973. Integration efficiency in DNA-induced transformation of pneumococcus. I. A method of transformation in solid medium and its use for isolation of transformation-deficient and recombination-modified mutants. Genetics **75**:23–33.

74. **Tomasz, A.** 1965. Control of the competent state in Pneumococcus by a hormone-like cell product: an example for a new type of regulatory mechanism in bacteria. Nature **208**:155–159.

75. **Tomasz, A.** 1965. The activation of pneumococcus to competence (Abstract). Genetics **52**:480.

76. **Tomasz, A.** 1966. Model for the mechanism controlling the expression of competent state in Pneumococcus cultures. J. Bacteriol. **91**:1050–1061.

77. **Tomasz, A.** 1970. Cellular metabolism in genetic transformation of pneumococci: requirement for protein synthesis during induction of competence. J. Bacteriol. **101**:860–871.

78. **Tomasz, A., and R. Hotchkiss.** 1964. Regulation of the transformability of pneumococcal cultures by macromolecular cell products. Proc. Natl. Acad. Sci. U.S.A. **51**:480–487.

79. **Tomasz, A., and J.L. Mosser.** 1966. On the nature of the pneumococcal activator substance. Proc. Natl. Acad. Sci. U.S.A. **55**:58–66.

80. **Tomasz, A., E. Zanati, and R. Ziegler.** 1971. DNA uptake during genetic transformation and the growing zone of the cell envelope. Proc. Natl. Acad. Sci. U.S.A. **68**:1848–1852.

81. **Vasseghi, H., and J.P. Claverys.** 1983. Amplification of a chimeric plasmid carrying an erythromycin-resistance determinant introduced into the genome of *Streptococcus pneumoniae*. Gene **21**:285–292.

82. **Vasseghi, H., J.P. Claverys, and A.M. Sicard.** 1981. Mechanism of integrating foreign DNA during transformation of *Streptococcus pneumoniae*, pp. 137–153. *In* M. Polsinelli and G. Mazza (eds.), Transformation 1980: Proceedings of Fifth European Meeting on Bacterial Transformation and Transfection. Cotswold Press, Oxford.

83. **Watson, D.A., and D.M. Musher.** 1990. Interruption of capsule production in *Streptococcus pneumoniae* serotype-3 by insertion of transposon TN916. Infect. Immun. **58**:3135–3138.

84. **Yother, J., L.S. McDaniel, and D.E. Briles.** 1986. Transformation of encapsulated *Streptococcus pneumoniae*. J. Bacteriol. **168**:1463–1465.

85. **Zahner, D., T. Grebe, E. Guenzi, J. Krauss, M. Linden, K. Terhunen, J. Stock, and R. Hakenbeck.** 1996. Resistance determinants for beta-lactam antibiotics in laboratory mutants of *Streptococcus pneumoniae* that are involved in genetic competence. Microbial Drug Res. **2**:187–191.

86. **Zhou, L., F.M. Hui, and D.A. Morrison.** 1995. Competence for genetic transformation in *Streptococcus pneumoniae*: Organization of a regulatory locus with homology to two lactococcin A secretion genes. Gene **153**:25–31.

Address reprint requests to:
Donald A. Morrison
Laboratory for Molecular Biology
University of Illinois
900 South Ashland Ave.
Chicago, Illinois 60607

Control of Recombination Rate During Transformation of *Streptococcus pneumoniae*: An Overview

ISABELLE MORTIER-BARRIERE,[1] ODILE HUMBERT,[2] BERNARD MARTIN,[1]
MARC PRUDHOMME,[1] and JEAN-PIERRE CLAVERYS[1]

ABSTRACT

Despite the fact that natural transformation was described long ago in *Streptococcus pneumoniae*, only a limited number of recombination genes have been identified. Two of them have recently been characterized at the molecular level, *recA* which encodes a protein essential for homologous recombination and *mmsA* which encodes the homologue of the *Escherichia coli* RecG protein. After a survey of the available information regarding the function of RecA, RecG, and other proteins such as the mismatch repair proteins HexA and HexB that can affect the outcome of recombinants, the different levels at which horizontal genetic exchange can be controlled are discussed. It is shown that the specific induction of the *recA* gene which occurs in competent cells is required for full recombination proficiency. Results regarding the ability of the Hex generalized mismatch repair system to prevent recombination between partially divergent sequences during transformation are also summarized. A structural analysis of homeologous recombinants which suggests that formation of mosaic recombinants can occur independently of mismatch repair in a single-step transformation is also reported. Finally, arguments in favor of an evolutionary origin of transformation as a means of genome evolution are discussed and the different types of recombination events observed which could potentially contribute to *S. pneumoniae* genome evolution are listed.

INTRODUCTION

GENETIC TRANSFORMATION, DEFINED AS THE ABILITY OF BACTERIA to take up high molecular weight exogenous DNA, was first discovered in *Streptococcus pneumoniae*.[20] Several observations suggest that competence for genetic transformation in *S. pneumoniae* is a global response to changes in environmental conditions (for a review see[4]). Many hypotheses have been advanced to explain the evolutionary origin of competence mechanisms. The model proposing evolution of transformational recombination as a means of increasing fitness of a bacterial population[14] is particularly attractive, at least for *S. pneumoniae* and naturally transformable oral streptococci. Horizontal transfer of genetic material by transformation has been proposed to account for the alteration of *pbp* genes in penicillin-resistant clinical isolates of *S. pneumoniae*.[12]

Despite the fact that natural transformation was described long ago, only a limited number of recombination genes have been identified. We first summarize the available information

regarding the function of some recombination proteins. The different levels at which horizontal genetic exchange can be controlled are discussed, particularly the role of the specific induction of the *recA* gene which has been observed in competent cells.[26,35] Also, we address the ability of the Hex generalized mismatch repair system to prevent recombination between partially divergent (homeologous) sequences during transformation.[23] Results of a structural analysis of homeologous recombinants which suggest that formation of mosaic recombinants can occur independently of mismatch repair in a single-step transformation are summarized. Finally, the biological significance of transformation is discussed and the different types of recombination events observed in *S. pneumoniae* are listed. This article is not intended to be an exhaustive review of recombination in *S. pneumoniae*. We hope to give an overview including the most recent advances in the field. The mechanisms of recombination in *S. pneumoniae* have been the subject of a more extensive review by Lacks[24] to which the interested reader is referred.

---

[1]Laboratoire de Microbiologie et Génétique Moléculaire CNRS–UPR 9007, Université Paul Sabatier, 118 Route de Narbonne, 31062 Toulouse Cedex, France.

[2]Present address: Imperial Cancer Research Fund, Clare Hall Laboratories, South Mimms, Herts - EN6 3LD, UK.

Reprinted from *Microbial Drug Resistance*, Vol. 3, No. 3, 1997.

GENETICS AND BIOCHEMISTRY
OF RECOMBINATION

The rec genes

The approach to understanding recombination mechanisms based on the isolation of mutants blocked in the process has led to the identification of mutants in *S. pneumoniae*. With one exception (see below) the corresponding genes have not been characterized. Several mutants reducing the frequency of transformation have been isolated. These include strains 405 and 500 (3- to 5-fold reduction),[48] a mutant for an ATP-dependent deoxyribonuclease (6-fold reduction),[52] and mutants decreasing either chromosomal and plasmid transformation (100-fold) or only chromosomal recombination (20-fold).[34] The mutated gene has been identified only in the case of *recP*, belonging to the last group.[42] Although the *recP* gene has been sequenced,[40] the puzzling observation that it belongs to a family of transketolases[41] sheds no light on its role in recombination (Table 1).

Apart from these, only two recombination genes, *recA* and *mmsA*, have been characterized at the molecular level (Table 1). The *recA* gene was identified by immunoscreening a pneumococcal genomic library cloned in lambda with antibodies raised against the *Escherichia coli* RecA protein.[28] Inactivation of the gene resulted in a $>10^5$-fold recombination defect indicating that the RecA protein is essential for transformational recombination.[26]

The *mmsA* gene was identified in a recent re-investigation of strain 500,[48] a mutant previously isolated on the basis of its sensitivity to MMS. The mutant strain also exhibited increased sensitivity to UV light and to X-rays, together with a reduced capacity in recombination and in Hex-mediated generalized mismatch repair (see below). The original mutant strain turned out to contain mutations in two unlinked genes, *mmsA* and *pms* (for phenotype of <u>m</u>ms<u>A</u> <u>s</u>uppressed, see below). The primary structure predicted for MmsA suggested that it could be a homologue of the RecG protein of *E. coli*, a helicase promoting branch migration of Holliday junctions. In agreement with this hypothesis, a plasmid carrying the intact *mmsA* gene complemented *recG* mutants of *E. coli* with respect to resistance to UV light and to mitomycin C.[29] An *mmsA*-null mutant constructed by insertion of a chloramphenicol resistance gene exhibited a 25-fold reduction in recombination during transformation. We suggested that MmsA recognizes and branch migrates three-strand transformation intermediates to extend donor–recipient heteroduplex regions.[29] The *mmsA*-null mutant also exhibited other phenotypes of the original (double) mutant, with the exception of mismatch repair deficiency. In addition, an alteration in colony-forming ability was recorded. In the *pms* mutant background, all phenotypes caused by the *mmsA* mutation were attenuated. Therefore, the *pms* mutation, although it affected mismatch repair and, to some extent, DNA repair and recombination, acted as a suppressor of the *mmsA* mutation.

The hex genes

Genetic evidence for the presence of a generalized mismatch repair system in *S. pneumoniae* (Hex) acting on recombination intermediates first came from investigation of variations in marker transformation efficiencies (for a review see[5]). *Transition* mutations exhibit a low efficiency of transformation (LE markers). The Hex system is very efficient in repairing both types of transition mismatches (i.e., G/T and A/C) at the donor–recipient heteroduplex stage during the transformation process. *Transversion* mutations, on the other hand, generally exhibit a 10- to 20-fold higher efficiency of transformation (HE markers), because either one or both transversion mismatches are not corrected by Hex. The Hex system is a DNA replication editor correcting potentially mutagenic mismatches. It was found to repair different base–base mismatches with various degrees of efficiency.[18]

A strategy based on the inactivation of genes by homology-directed integration of recombinant molecules, the so-called insertion–duplication (ID) mutagenesis (see p. 240), was devel-

TABLE 1. GENES INVOLVED IN RECOMBINATION AND REPAIR IN *S. PNEUMONIAE*

Gene/ operon	Map location[a] (min)	Protein size	Function	Mutant phenotype		Competence- induced expression
				Recombination	Repair	
cinA[26,35]	21–24	418 aa	Recombination accessory protein?	Rec⁻ (90% deficient)[35]	?	+[26,35]
recA[28]	21–24	388 aa	single-strand transfer into duplex DNA	Rec⁻ ($>10^5$ fold)[26] Plasmid transf. Deficient[26]	UV[S26]	+[26,35]
hexA[36]	1–6.5	844 aa	mismatch recognition[37]	Hyperrec (20-fold) for transitions-frameshifts	Mutator	−[23]
hexB[38]	10–11	649 aa	mismatch-repair accessory protein	Hyperrec (20-fold) for transitions-frameshifts	Mutator	−[23]
mmsA[29]	24–26	671 aa	heteroduplex extension	Rec⁻ (25-fold) Decreased viability	MMS[S] UV[S] X-rays[S]	?
pms[29]	44–50	?	?	Rec⁻ (2.5-fold)	Mismatch-repair part. def.	?
recP[40]	31–33	656 aa	transketolase?[41]	Rec⁻ (35- to 100-fold)[40] Plasmid transf. proficient	?	?

[a]The map location in minutes (min) is defined as previously.[27] The circular chromosomal map of *S. pneumoniae*[27] has been divided in 60 min, with the 0/60 position at the top and a clockwise increase.

oped to identify *hex* genes.[7,19] Using this approach, two genes, *hexA* and *hexB*, were characterized. Inactivation of either gene confers a mutator phenotype and abolishes mismatch repair in transformation. Similarities are detected with the *E. coli* proteins involved in mismatch repair. Homologies between HexA and MutS,[36] and between HexB and MutL,[38] support the hypothesis that the Hex system and its *E. coli* counterpart, the Mut system (for a review see[33]), are evolutionarily related.[5] The HexA protein has been shown to bind mismatches *in vitro*[37] as does its homologue MutS. The role of HexB as yet remains obscure, although this protein is essential for mismatch repair.

A third gene possibly involved in mismatch repair is defined by the *pms* mutation. As mentioned, the *pms* mutation by itself affected DNA repair, recombination, and Hex-mediated mismatch repair. The characterization of the *pms* gene may help explain the basis for the suppression of *mmsA* mutations and advance our understanding of the relationship between mismatch repair and recombination.

Role of MmsA, RecA, and Hex in transformation

A diagrammatic representation of the process of recombination during transformation in *S. pneumoniae* is shown in Fig. 1. The *S. pneumoniae* RecA protein is likely to play a role similar to that demonstrated for *E. coli* RecA (for a review see[43]) in the initiation of recombination (Fig. 1, I). The RecG-like protein MmsA is also required in recombination. It was suggested that MmsA could extend heteroduplex regions (Fig. 1, II), at a lower ATP cost than RecA.[29] Finally, a specific resolvase could be required to incise both donor and recipient strands (Fig. 1, III), followed by ligation to create the novel joint.

The antirecombinogenic action of the Hex system could result from inhibition of the RecA-catalyzed process of donor single-strand assimilation (invasion) in the recipient duplex (Steps I–II in Fig. 1). This has been suggested in the case of the Mut system of *E. coli* on the basis of *in vitro* experiments.[53] Alternatively, Hex could destroy potential recombinants at the heteroduplex stage in transformation, after formation of the donor–recipient heteroduplex as shown in Fig. 1 (IV). The kinetics data of Guild and Shoemaker[45] support the latter hypothesis (at least in the case of point mismatches). Although genetic and biochemical data are consistent with destruction of the entire donor strand,[5,39] the mechanism of donor strand rejection remains unknown. It may involve displacement by a DNA helicase and subsequent exonucleolytic degradation. Finally, although the displaced recipient strand (R in Fig. 1) is drawn intact in Fig. 1 (IV), it is not known whether this strand has already been degraded at the time of Hex action. Depending on whether removal of this strand occurs, restoration of the duplex may or may not require repair synthesis.

REGULATION OF RECOMBINATION AND MISMATCH REPAIR GENE EXPRESSION

The recA gene is part of a competence-induced operon

Previous studies from our group[26] have demonstrated that the *recA* gene is part of an operon that is inducible by the competence-stimulating peptide, CSP. This operon was shown to be composed of at least three genes: *cinA* (<u>c</u>ompetence <u>in</u>ducible

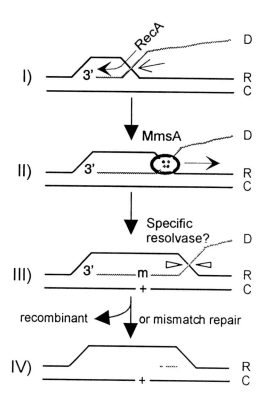

FIG. 1. Processing of recombination intermediates during transformation. (I) The RecA protein initiates the process of donor single-strand assimilation leading to the formation of a donor–recipient heteroduplex region. The structure formed (light arrow) differs from classical Holliday junctions by the lack of a fourth strand. Following 3′ end invasion, extension of the heteroduplex would require a 3′ → 5′ polarity which is opposite to the direction of RecA filament assembly and strand exchange (indicated by a curved arrow). (II) It is proposed that the RecG-like MmsA protein of *S. pneumoniae* specifically recognizes and binds the three-stranded structure, and branch migrates the junction (heavy arrow) to extend the heteroduplex region. (III) Simultaneous incision (indicated by triangles) of the recipient and donor may require the intervention of a putative specific resolvase. Ligation would then generate the final recombinant product (not shown). (IV) Alternatively, in the presence of a mismatch (m/+), the Hex system aborts recombination. D, donor single-strand; R, recipient strand of same polarity; C, recipient, complementary strand. Neither RecA nor an SSB-like protein which covers the incoming donor DNA[51] are represented.

<u>A</u>) which has been suggested to encode a recombination-accessory protein,[35] *recA* which encodes a protein essential for homologous recombination, and *dinF*.[26] Two polycistronic transcripts were identified: a basal transcript (4.3 kb) and a competence-specific transcript (5.7 kb). Both transcripts differed at their 5′ ends, the competence-specific transcript including the additional *cinA* gene.[26] More recently, Northern blot experiments with a *lytA* probe demonstrated that the *lytA* gene which encodes the pneumococcal autolysin[16] was present both on the *recA* 5.7 kb competence-specific transcript as well as on the 4.3 kb basal transcript (A. de Saizieu, personnal communication). This is consistent with our unpublished observations that *recA* was localized on the same *Sac*II generated fragment (n°9; Table

1) as *lytA* and that a tight genetic linkage could be detected between two markers, *recA::cat*[26] (chloramphenicol resistance) and *lytA::ermAM*[49] (erythromycin resistance).

Western blotting experiments revealed that competence-specific induction resulted in a three-fold[26] to five-fold[35] increase in the concentration of RecA.

The hex genes are not competence-induced

Western blotting experiments with antibodies raised against HexA or HexB were used to compare extracts from competent and noncompetent cultures. No change in the amount of HexA and HexB proteins was detected suggesting that *hexA* and *hexB* genes were not induced at competence.[23] In addition, no increase in the amount of the two *hex* transcripts was detected in competent cells exhibiting strong competence-specific induction of the *recA* mRNA.[23] Thus, unlike *recA*, the two *hex* genes did not appear to be induced at competence.

RecA CONCENTRATION-DEPENDENT CONTROL OF RECOMBINATION RATE

In their independent identification of the *rec* locus, Pearce et al.[35] isolated a *cinA-phoA* fusion (called *exp10-phoA* by these authors) which resulted in the synthesis of a truncated CinA protein. The fusion protein had alkaline phosphatase activity, which suggested that CinA was a membrane protein. This mutant exhibited a 70-fold decrease in transformation efficiency, leading to the suggestion that CinA could be required for recombination of donor DNA.[35] However, because *cinA* is the first gene in an operon including *recA*, the hypothesis that the transformation-deficient phenotype conferred by the *cinA-phoA* fusion resulted from a polar effect on the expression of downstream genes was not ruled out.

To check this hypothesis, we took advantage of strain R214 (Fig. 2). This strain generated by ID (see p. 240) of a recombinant plasmid, pR322, which carried a fragment overlapping the 3' extremity of the *cinA* gene and the 5' extremity of the *recA* gene is *cinA*[+] and *recA*[+].[26] Northern-blot analysis confirmed that plasmid insertion in this strain was polar;[26] it prevented the competence-specific induction of *recA* and downstream genes (I. M.-B., B.M., and J.-P.C., in preparation). The recombination rate in strain R214 was compared to that in wild-type cells by using radioactively labelled DNA as donor in transformation. R214 exhibited a 20-fold reduction in recombination (Fig. 2). As expected, inactivation of *recA* in strain R209[26] resulted in an absolute chromosomal recombination deficiency. A similar plasmid ID strategy was used to inhibit the competence-specific induction of only *dinF* and *lytA*. The resulting strain exhibited a normal recombination rate (I. M.-B., B.M., and J.-P.C., in preparation).

Therefore, we conclude that the specific induction of *recA* expression that occurs in *S. pneumoniae* competent cells is required for full recombination proficiency. As prevention of *recA* induction by a polar construct alone leads to a 20-fold reduction in recombinants, a reappraisal of the role of CinA in transformation would require the construction of a nonpolar *cinA*-null mutation.

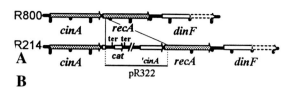

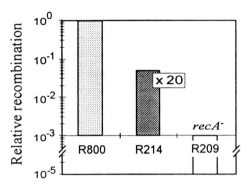

FIG. 2. RecA concentration-dependent control of recombination rate in *S. pneumoniae* transformation: Effect of prevention of the competence-specific induction of *recA*. *Top*: Genetic map of the *S. pneumoniae cinA–recA* chromosomal region in the wild type strain (R800) and in strain R214. Genes identified in the region are indicated by shaded arrows except for the *dinF* homologue the putative 5' extremity of which has not been sequenced. Hairpin structures that flank the chloramphenicol resistance *cat* gene in pR322 and have been shown to function as efficient transcription terminators[26] are indicated by ter. The structure of the *recA*[−] strain R209 has been described previously.[26] *Bottom*: Uptake and transformation were measured in aliquots of the same batch of cells activated with 25 ng/ml synthetic CSP. Radioactive M13mp19 DNA prepared as described[26] corresponding to 10[5] dpm (for 150 to 400 μl of competent cells) was used for DNA uptake measurements. Counts taken up after 15-min contact between cells and DNA were measured in washed cells after DNase I treatment as described previously.[31] Competent cells were transformed with R119 chromosomal DNA, which contains the *str41* marker conferring resistance to 200 μg/ml streptomycin. Recombination proficiencies of the different strains were compared by measuring uptake of [32P] uniformly labelled donor DNA in parallel with scoring of transformants for the *str41* reference marker. After calculation of Sm[R] dpm[−1] ratios, recombination values were expressed relative to the wild type R800 recipient.

HOMOLOGY-DEPENDENT CONTROL OF RECOMBINATION RATE

Because DNA uptake in *S. pneumoniae* is not sequence-specific,[31] any native DNA present in the environment could be taken up as single strands. It is known that restriction systems are not a barrier to gene exchange by transformation in this organism as single strands are refractory to digestion.[3] The major limitation to gene transfer would then be genomic sequence divergence. In *E. coli*, a minimal length segment of sequence identity is required by the recombination enzymes at the initial stage of the strand exchange process.[44] Once initiated, strand exchange can proceed despite a large number of mismatches. However, mismatch-repair systems can be potent inhibitors of recombination between related species. Thus, the frequency of recombination between *E. coli* and *Salmonella ty-phimurium* is reduced as much as a 1000-fold in mismatch-repair proficient cells (for a review see[30]).

In *S. pneumoniae*, mismatch repair reduces transformation frequencies for point mutations in homologous DNA (see above) but appears essentially unable to prevent interspecies transformation.[23] The ability of the Hex generalized mismatch repair system to prevent recombination between partially divergent (also called *homeologous*) sequences was investigated using well-defined cloned *pbp2b* and *pbp2x* DNA fragments as donor in transformation. These fragments which conferred resistance to penicillin (PenR) varied in size (from 1.5 to 3.2 kb) and were from 1.7% to 17.5% divergent in DNA sequence from the recipient. It was observed that the Hex system prevented chromosomal integration of the least and the most divergent fragments but frequently failed to do so for other fragments. In the latter case, the Hex system became saturated (inhibited) due to an excess of mismatches. It was unable to repair a single mismatch located elsewhere on the chromosome. Further investigation with chromosomal donor DNA, carrying only one genetically marked divergent region, revealed that a single divergent fragment can lead to saturation of the Hex system.[23] Heterospecific transformation by chromosomal DNA from two related streptococcal species, *Streptococcus oralis* and *Streptococcus mitis*, also led to complete saturation of the Hex system.

Finally, an increase in cellular concentration of either HexA or HexB was shown to restore repair ability in previously saturating conditions.[23] Together with the observation that, unlike *recA*, the *hex* genes are not induced at competence (see above), this suggested that the Hex system has not evolved to cope with excess mismatches and to abort interspecies recombination.

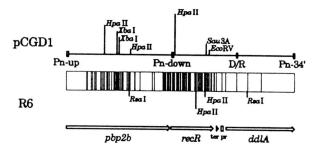

FIG. 3. Restriction polymorphism and base mismatches between donor (pCGD1) and recipient (R6) sequences in the region of the *pbp2b* gene. Construction of plasmid pCGD1 which carries a 3205 bp (*Mbo*I partial digest) fragment of chromosomal DNA from strain 64147, a penicillin-resistant clinical isolate of *S. pneumoniae*, has been described.[13] This fragment contains part of the *pbp2b* gene (coding region for the 486 carboxy-terminal residues) and two downstream genes. With the exception of the downstream sequences of the wild type and 64147 *pbp2b* genes (C.G.D., in preparation), sequence data have appeared in the EMBL/Genbank databases under the accession numbers X13137 (*pbp2b*-wild type) and X13136 (*pbp2b*-64147). Sequences were aligned using the MULTALIN program;[9] each potential mismatch between the Pen[r] donor fragment and the corresponding chromosomal region in the Pen[s] recipient strain is indicated by a vertical bar. Only restriction sites that differ between the two sequences and have been used in the analysis of recombinant structures are indicated. Five oligonucleotide primers used to amplify or to distinguish between donor and recipient sequences are also indicated by Pn-up, Pn-down, D,R, and Pn-34'.

FORMATION OF MOSAIC RECOMBINANTS BY TRANSFORMATION

To investigate the structure of recombinants formed between partially divergent sequences, a strain carrying only one genetically marked divergent region was first obtained by transformation of a wild-type recipient with plasmid pCGD1 DNA. This plasmid[13] carries a 3205 bp fragment from the PenR, clinical isolate strain 64147, containing part of the *pbp2b* gene and downstream sequences (Fig. 3). This fragment is 4.6% divergent from the recipient (149 potential mismatches). A combination of restriction digests, hybridization with specific oligonucleotides, and DNA sequencing was used to confirm the integration of an intact donor fragment[22] (Fig. 3; O.H., C.G. Dowson, and J.P.C., in preparation). This chromosomal DNA with only one divergent region was used to transform Hex[+] and Hex[−] recipient strains. 38 Hex[−] and 43 Hex[+] PenR recombinants were then isolated and their molecular structure was established as just described. Recombinants with alternating blocks of donor and recipient sequences were obtained in both recipients (recombinant types 5 to 9 in Table 2). These structures are reminiscent of the mosaic *pbp* genes found in clinical isolates of *S. pneumoniae* resistant to penicillin.[12] We conclude that, at least under laboratory conditions, formation of mosaic recombinants can occur during transformation with divergent DNA. This is a single-step recombination event and independent of the Hex genetic background of the recipient strain.

TABLE 2. STRUCTURE OF PenR RECOMBINANTS IN HEX[−] AND HEX[+] RECIPIENTS

Type of recombinants	Number of recombinants	
	Hex[−] (38)	Hex+ (43)
1	18	12
2	7	20
3	4	3
4	0	4
5	6	1
6	0	1
7	2	0
8	0	1
9	1	1

BIOLOGICAL SIGNIFICANCE OF TRANSFORMATION: GENOME EVOLUTION?

Several hypotheses have been advanced to explain the evolutionary origin of competence mechanism, including a role in nutrient acquisition, in repair of chromosome damage, and in genome evolution.[14] Nutrient acquisition is obviously unlikely in the case of transformable gram-negative bacteria that exhibit sequence-specific uptake. This hypothesis is not particularly attractive for gram-positive bacteria either. As pointed out for *Bacillus subtilis*,[14] secretion of a nuclease together with the existence of high-affinity transport mechanisms would provide the basis for an effective feeding on exogenous DNA. It is also difficult to understand why the *recA* gene in *S. pneumoniae* and *B. subtilis* or the *B. subtilis addAB* genes (the homologues of the *E. coli recBC* genes)[21] should be induced at competence for this purpose.

On the other hand, induction of *rec* genes would be consistent with both the genome repair and evolution hypotheses. The observation of a coordination of competence development, particularly in *S. pneumoniae* cultures is, however, difficult to accommodate in the repair hypothesis. Synchronization of competence would be most consistent with the idea that transformational recombination has evolved as a means of increasing fitness of a bacterial population by facilitating the acquisition of new genetic traits. Whereas mutations are frequently neutral or deleterious, transformation is expected to replace genes or gene fragments by sequences that were functional in the original species. In this view, transformation would be an extremely powerful mechanism for rapid evolution because each individual cell in a culture can experiment with new combinations of genes. Each cell may randomly take up several independent fragments (up to 1%–5% of the genome). The probability of integrating these fragments varies from close to 1 for homologous DNA to 0.1–0.5 for 2%–10% divergent DNA.[23] As only a few new combinations of genes are expected to be beneficial, coordination of competence development through CSP could be essential to ensure that a sufficient number of cells of the species is present to engage in the process.

The finding that the Hex genes are not induced at competence, whereas an increase in cellular concentration of either HexA or HexB would increase repair ability and prevent saturation by excess mismatches, is also consistent with the genome evolution hypothesis. It strongly suggests that the Hex system has not been tuned to cope with excess mismatches and therefore to abort interspecies recombination. This is unlike the situation in non transformable bacteria.[30] Thus, uptake of DNA from related species present in the same ecological niche (e.g., *S. mitis, S. oralis, S. gordonii,* or *Streptococcus viridans*) followed by recombination into the chromosome can provide the *S. pneumoniae* genome with enhanced plasticity. Moreover, sequences that are only distantly related to *S. pneumoniae* and could not be directly recombined in this organism, could be first integrated in another transformable streptococcus, as there is accumulating evidence that several oral streptococci are transformable (Havarstein and Gaustad, 1996, Evidence for natural genetic transformation within the *Streptococcus milleri* group, Proc. 12th European Mtg. Bacterial Gene Transfer and Expression, Abstr. no. P40). Hybrid sequences could then be donated from the transformable streptococcus to *S. pneumoniae,* se-

quences from the intermediate host providing homology for efficient recombination in *S. pneumoniae.*

Mosaic *pbp* genes found in clinical isolates of *S. pneumoniae* resistant to penicillin are possible examples of replacement of parts of sensitive genes by sequences from related species; *S. oralis* and *S. mitis* are likely donors of some of these sequences.[11,46] Transformation of *S. pneumoniae* from optochin-sensitivity (a characteristic trait of the species) to optochin-resistance has also been observed under laboratory conditions using *S. oralis* chromosomal DNA as donor.[15] It is tempting to speculate that transformation has also played a role in the evolution of the more than 90 different capsular types that have been reported for *S. pneumoniae.* Some of these capsular types may yet prove to result from expression of capsular synthesis genes originating from other streptococci. The same possibility applies to the evolution of other determinants of pathogenicity of this species.

A WIDE VARIETY OF RECOMBINATION EVENTS POTENTIALLY CONTRIBUTING TO GENOME EVOLUTION IN *S. PNEUMONIAE*

Substitutive recombination

Recombination during transformation in bacteria is generally substitutive, leading to replacement of recipient sequences by homologous or homeologous donor sequences. Homologous recombination events can lead to exchange of point mutations thus altering gene expression. Homeologous recombination events that integrate partially divergent sequences (DNA from related species) can have more profound effects on genome expression. They can result in exchange of gene fragments but also in the formation of mosaic recombinants (i.e., new combination of sequences) in a single-step transformation (see above). The latter process can lead to shuffling of protein domains and is, therefore, of significant evolutionary potential. Homologous recombination can also result in exchange of individual genes or combination of linked (or even unlinked) genes. The latter can potentially result in modification or acquisition of multiproteic complexes in a single step.

In addition, integration of completely heterologous DNA has been reported in several instances. The corresponding recombination events can be classified into three categories, ID, cassette insertion, and insertion–deletion.

Insertion–duplication

ID was first observed in *S. pneumoniae* following transformation with nonreplicative recombinant plasmids[32] and is now widely used for insertional inactivation of chromosomal genes. The term ID refers to the structure of the recombinant product, a tandem duplication of the homologous fragment bracketing the heterologous DNA. As the donor DNA is frequently a circle, the mechanism of ID is often diagrammed as the product of a single crossover between a circular molecule and the recipient chromosome (Fig. 4, I) and is referred to as *Campbell-type recombination* (see comment in[24]). However, models of integration must take into account the breakage of donor DNA that occurs upon binding and the subsequent uptake of single strands.[31] In view of the higher absolute efficiency of integra-

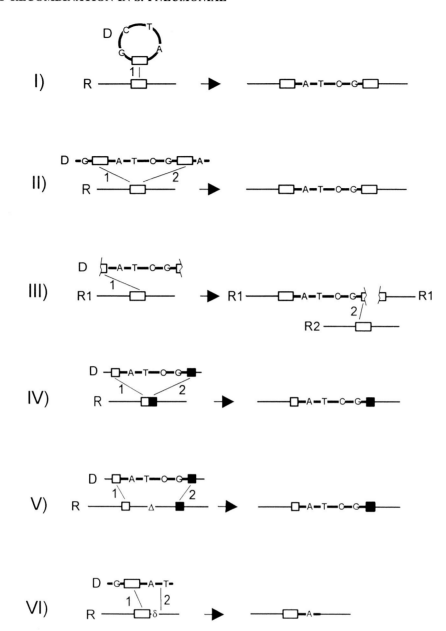

FIG. 4. Models for insertion–duplication, cassette insertion, and insertion–deletion events during transformation in *S. pneumoniae*. Heterologous donor sequences are represented by a thick line with the sequence ATCG. White and black rectangles represent homologous fragments present on both donor (D) and recipient (R). The recipient molecule is shown as a single line although it is double stranded. In any case, replication is required following integration of the donor single strand to restore doublestrandedness. I, Diagrammatic representation of an insertion–duplication event, with a single-cross-over (1) leading to integration of a circular donor molecule. II, Linear synapsis model for integration of a dimeric donor molecule. The donor molecule is represented as cut within the heterologous region upon binding and uptake. Integration of a monomer in the final recombinant involves pairing between each homologous fragment from the donor with a unique copy in the chromosome. Two cross-overs (1 and 2) are required for integration.[50] III, Linear synapsis model for integration of a monomer. The donor molecule is shown as cut within the homologous fragment; cutting upon entry within the heterologous region prohibits subsequent integration. Integration requires independent pairing (synapsis) between each extremity of the interrupted homologous donor fragment and the homologous region in two different recipient chromosomes (R1 and R2). Ligation of each extremity of the donor molecule with a different chromosome generates a dimeric chromosome which should then be resolved by homologous recombination or by a site-specific recombination mechanism as described in *E. coli*.[8] IV and V, Integration of a heterologous fragment by a cassette mechanism, in a recipient containing no material at the particular point of insertion (IV) or in a recipient containing a different cassette (△) which is therefore lost in the process (V). The donor molecule is represented as cut within homologous flanking sequences. VI, Insertion–deletion involving illegitimate recombination (2) leading to the integration of some heterologous sequences and the simultaneous loss of some recipient sequences (δ). The donor molecule is drawn as cut within heterologous DNA upon binding and uptake.

tion of dimeric molecules*,[50] Lacks[24] favored a linear synapsis model in the case of transformation with dimeric forms (Fig. 4, II) and a circular synapsis model for monomeric forms. A previously proposed linear model[50] could as well account for monomeric integration. We present a modified version of this model in Fig. 4 (III). Neither of these models has been supported or ruled out by experimental data.

Transformation can also constitute a means for entry of mobile DNA elements. Insertion sequences and transposons are generally thought to contribute to genome plasticity by promoting illegitimate recombination events,[2] but they can also provide flanking homology for additive homology-dependent recombination events. Thus, a linear donor fragment of heterologous DNA bordered by direct repeats of an element (e.g., an IS) also present in the recipient chromosome could be efficiently processed by the recombination machinery (through a mechanism formally identical to that in Fig. 4, II). Heterologous DNA would be readily integrated and the final recombinant would resemble a classical ID product. Such an additive mechanism may explain the appearance of transformants expressing both the donor and recipient capsular types, a phenomenon called *binary encapsulation*.[1]

The *S. pneumoniae* chromosome contains conserved repeated elements called BOX.[27] These elements are highly conserved (less than 10% divergence) and have a modular structure. Each subunit, *boxA, boxB,* and *boxC* is close to 50 nucleotide long. Therefore, BOX elements are long enough to provide homology for recombination and could be involved in genomic rearrangements following transformation, although no such event has been reported yet.

Cassette insertion

Transfer of gene cassettes represents another example of flanking-homology directed addition of heterologous genetic material. However, unlike ID recombinants, homologous sequences located on both sides of the heterologous cassette differ from each other (Fig. 4, IV and V). Therefore, cassette integrants are stable whereas ID recombinants always show some degree of instability, as recombination between the duplicated regions can lead to spontaneous excision. A cassette mechanism was first demonstrated in the case of the complementary *Dpn*I and *Dpn*II restriction systems of *S. pneumoniae*.[25] Although a cassette mechanism has been suspected long ago to account for the exchange of genes for capsular polysaccharide biosynthesis,[47] convincing evidence has only been obtained recently.[10] Cassette insertion could be simply additive if the recipient chromosome contained no material at the particular point of insertion (Fig. 4, IV), but in general, as in the two examples just mentioned, cassettes are mutually exclusive (Fig. 4, V).

Insertion–deletion

Illegitimate recombination events called insertion–deletions have been first observed during transformation with hybrid

DNA molecules.[6] The name insertion–deletion was introduced because insertion of heterologous DNA and deletion of chromosomal sequences occurred simultaneously. This type of event has been shown to represent about 0.5% of total recombination events during transformation with hybrid DNA[6] whereas ID generated by integration of an entire recombinant plasmid molecule should be about 20-fold more frequent (our unpublished observations). The homologous region in the hybrid molecule is absolutely required for production of insertion–deletions. Therefore, we propose to call the underlying recombination mechanism homology-directed illegitimate (HDI) recombination. A schematic model for HDI recombination is shown in Fig. 4 (VI). Our hypothesis was that pairing between homologous donor and recipient sequences could favor transient pairing between heterologous flanking donor and recipient sequences.[6] Resolution of the heteroduplex would then occur within very short stretches of nucleotide identity. Recent analysis of several junctions suggested that this hypothesis was essentially correct (M.P. and J.P.C., in preparation).

Such a mechanism is of great potential in terms of genome evolution because depending on the point of exchange between donor and recipient, it can lead to the acquisition of completely heterologous genes or to the production of new chimeras. Note that, as in the case of ID, IS, or transposons when present on both donor and recipient DNA can also promote the acquisition of immediately adjacent heterologous sequences, by HDI recombination.

In conclusion, analysis of the recombination potential of *S. pneumoniae* strongly suggests that transformation is a very powerful means of genome evolution. Altogether, coordination of competence development, induction of *recA* expression, inhibition of mismatch repair, and a wide variety of recombination events combine to provide a great deal of genome plasticity to this important human pathogen.

ACKNOWLEDGMENTS

This work was supported in part by a contrat de recherche externe (n° 920102) from the Institut National de la Santé et de la Recherche Médicale and by a Subvention (n° RECH/ 9407531) from the Région Midi Pyrénées. I.M.B. was the recipient of a fellowship from the Ministère de l'Enseignement Supérieur et de la Recherche. O.H. was the recipient of a fellowship from the Association pour la Recherche Contre le Cancer.

REFERENCES

1. **Austrian, R., H.P. Bernheimer, E.E.B. Smith, and G.T. Mills.** 1959. Simultaneous production of two capsular polysaccharides by pneumococcus. II. The genetic and biochemical basis of binary encapsulation. J. Exp. Med. **110:**585–602.

2. **Berg, D.E., and Howe, M.M.** 1989. Mobile DNA. Washington, DC: American Society for Microbiology.

3. **Cerritelli, S., S.S. Springhorn, and S.A. Lacks.** 1989. DpnA, a methylase for single-strand DNA in the *Dpn* II restriction system, and its biological function. Proc. Natl. Acad. Sci. USA **86:** 9223–9227.

---

*Dimeric forms of a recombinant molecule have been shown to yield at least 75-fold more transformants than monomeric forms.[50] As ID mutagenesis is widely used in *S. pneumoniae*, note that concatemeric recombinant molecules should therefore be used as donor to improve the probability of integration for mutagenic purposes, particularly in the case of short homologous inserts.

4. **Claverys, J.P., A. Dintilhac, I. Mortier-Barrière, B. Martin, and G. Alloing.** 1997. Regulation of competence for genetic transformation in *Streptococcus pneumoniae*. J. Appl. Bacteriol. Symposium Series (in press).

5. **Claverys, J.P., and S.A. Lacks.** 1986. Heteroduplex deoxyribonucleic acid base mismatch repair in bacteria. Microbiol. Rev. **50**:133–165.

6. **Claverys, J.P., J.C. Lefèvre, and A.M. Sicard.** 1980. Transformation of *Streptococcus pneumoniae* with *Streptococcus pneumoniae*-lambda phage hybrid DNA: Induction of deletions. Proc. Natl. Acad. Sci. USA **77**:3534–3538.

7. **Claverys, J.P., H. Prats, H. Vasseghi, and M. Gherardi.** 1984. Identification of *Streptococcus pneumoniae* mismatch repair genes by an additive transformation approach. Mol. Gen. Genet. **196**:91–96.

8. **Cornet, F., J. Louarn, J. Patte, and J.M. Louarn.** 1996. Restriction of the activity of the recombination site *dif* to a small zone of the *Escherichia coli* chromosome. Genes Dev. **10**:1152–1161.

9. **Corpet, F.** 1988. Multiple sequence alignment with hierarchical clustering. Nucl. Acids Res. **16**:10881–10890.

10. **Dillard, J.P., and J. Yother.** 1994. Genetic and molecular characterization of capsular polysaccharide biosynthesis in *Streptococcus pneumoniae* type 3. Mol. Microbiol. **12**:959–972.

11. **Dowson, C.G., T.J. Coffey, C. Kell, and R.A. Whiley.** 1993. Evolution of penicillin resistance in *Streptococcus pneumoniae*: The role of *Streptococcus mitis* in the formation of a low affinity PBP2B in *S. pneumoniae*. Mol. Microbiol. **9**:635–643.

12. **Dowson, C.G., A. Hutchison, J.A. Brannigan, R.C. George, D. Hansman, J. Liñares, A. Tomasz, J.M. Smith, and B.G. Spratt.** 1989. Horizontal transfer of penicillin-binding protein genes in penicillin-resistant clinical isolates of *Streptococcus pneumoniae*. Proc. Natl. Acad. Sci. USA **86**:8842–8846.

13. **Dowson, C.G., A. Hutchison, and B.G. Spratt.** 1989. Extensive re-modelling of the transpeptidase domain of penicillin-binding protein 2B of a penicillin-resistant South Africa isolate of *Streptococcus pneumoniae*. Mol. Microbiol. **3**:95–102.

14. **Dubnau, D.** 1991. Genetic competence in *Bacillus subtilis*. Microbiol. Rev. **55**:395–424.

15. **Fenoll, A., R. Muñoz, E. García, and A.G. de la Campa.** 1994. Molecular basis of the optochin-sensitive phenotype of pneumococcus: Characterization of the genes encoding the F_0 complex of the *Streptococcus pneumoniae* and *Streptococcus oralis* H^+-ATPases. Mol. Microbiol. **12**:587–598.

16. **Garcia, E., J.L. Garcia, C. Ronda, P. Garcia, and R. Lopez.** 1985. Cloning and expression of the pneumococcal autolysin gene in *Escherichia coli*. Mol. Gen. Genet. **201**:225–230.

17. **Gasc, A.M., L. Kauc, P. Baraillé, M. Sicard, and S. Goodgal.** 1991. Gene localization, size, and physical map of the chromosome of *Streptococcus pneumoniae*. J. Bacteriol. **173**:7361–7367.

18. **Gasc, A.M., A.M. Sicard, and J.P. Claverys.** 1989. Repair of single- and multiple-substitution mismatches during recombination in *Streptococcus pneumoniae*. Genetics **121**:29–36.

19. **Gherardi, M., and J.P. Claverys.** 1982. Molecular characterization of gene(s) involved in mismatch repair in *Streptococcus pneumoniae*. Proc. 6th European Mtg. Bacterial Transformation and Transfection. **Abstr. n°. 14**:35.

20. **Griffith, F.** 1928. The significance of pneumococcal types. J. Hyg. **27**:113–159.

21. **Haijema, B.J., L.W. Hamoen, J. Kooistra, G. Venema, and D. van Sinderen.** 1995. Expression of the ATP-dependent deoxyribonuclease of *Bacillus subtilis* is under competence-mediated control. Mol. Microbiol. **15**:203–211.

22. **Humbert, O.** 1994. Recombinaison entre séquences partiellement divergentes et réparation des mésappariements chez *Streptococcus pneumoniae*. Ph.D. Dissertation, Univ. P. Sabatier, Toulouse, France.

23. **Humbert, O., M. Prudhomme, R. Hakenbeck, C.G. Dowson, and J.P. Claverys.** 1995. Homeologous recombination and mismatch repair during transformation in *Streptococcus pneumoniae*: Saturation of the Hex mismatch repair system. Proc. Natl. Acad. Sci. USA **92**:9052–9056.

24. **Lacks, S.A.** 1988. Mechanisms of genetic recombination in gram-positive bacteria. *In* R. Kucherlapati and G. R. Smith (eds.) Genetic recombination. American Society for Microbiology, Washington, DC, pp. 43–86.

25. **Lacks, S.A., B.M. Mannarelli, S.S. Springhorn, and B. Greenberg.** 1986. Genetic basis of the complementary *DpnI* and *DpnII* restriction systems of *S. pneumoniae*: An intercellular cassette mechanism. Cell **46**:993–1000.

26. **Martin, B., P. Garcia, M.P. Castanié, and J.P. Claverys.** 1995. The *recA* gene of *Streptococcus pneumoniae* is part of a competence-induced operon and controls lysogenic induction. Mol. Microbiol. **15**:367–379.

27. **Martin, B., O. Humbert, M. Camara, E. Guenzi, J. Walker, T. Mitchell, P. Andrew, M. Prudhomme, G. Alloing, R. Hakenbeck, D.A. Morrison, G.J. Boulnois, and J.P. Claverys.** 1992. A highly conserved repeated DNA element located in the chromosome of *Streptococcus pneumoniae*. Nucl. Acids. Res. **20**:3479–3483.

28. **Martin, B., J.M. Ruellan, J.F. Angulo, R. Devoret, and J.P. Claverys.** 1992. Identification of the *recA* gene of *Streptococcus pneumoniae*. Nucl. Acids. Res. **20**:6412.

29. **Martin, B., G.J. Sharples, O. Humbert, R.G. Lloyd, and J.P. Claverys.** 1996. The *mmsA* locus of *Streptococcus pneumoniae* encodes a RecG-like protein involved in DNA repair and in three-strand recombination. Mol. Microbiol. **19**:1035–1045.

30. **Matic, I., F. Taddei, and M. Radman.** 1996. Genetic barriers among bacteria. Trends Microbiol. **4**:69–73.

31. **Méjean, V., and J.P. Claverys.** 1993. DNA processing during entry in transformation of *Streptococcus pneumoniae*. J. Biol. Chem. **268**:5594–5599.

32. **Méjean, V., J.P. Claverys, H. Vasseghi, and A.M. Sicard.** 1981. Rapid cloning of specific DNA fragments of *Streptococcus pneumoniae* by vector integration into the chromosome followed by endonucleolytic excision. Gene **15**:289–293.

33. **Modrich, P.** 1991. Mechanisms and biological effects of mismatch repair. Annu. Rev. Genet. **25**:229–253.

34. **Morrison, D.A., S.A. Lacks, W.R. Guild, and J.M. Hageman.** 1983. Isolation and characterization of three new classes of transformation deficient mutants of *Streptococcus pneumoniae* that are defective in DNA transport and genetic recombination. J. Bacteriol. **156**:281–290.

35. **Pearce, B.J., A.M. Naughton, E.A. Campbell, and H.R. Masure.** 1995. The *rec* locus, a competence-induced operon in *Streptococcus pneumoniae*. J. Bacteriol. **177**:86–93.

36. **Priebe, S., S. Hadi, B. Greenberg, and S.A. Lacks.** 1988. Nucleotide sequence of the *hexA* gene for DNA mismatch repair in *Streptococcus pneumoniae* and homology of HexA to MutS of *Escherichia coli* and *Salmonella typhimurium*. J. Bacteriol. **170**:190–196.

37. **Prudhomme, M.** 1991. Caractérisation du gène *hexB* et étude du rôle des protéines HexA et HexB dans la réparation des mésappariements de l'ADN chez la bactérie *Streptococcus pneumoniae*. Ph.D. Dissertation, Univ. P. Sabatier, Toulouse, France.

38. **Prudhomme, M., B. Martin, V. Méjean, and J.P. Claverys.** 1989. Nucleotide sequence of the *Streptococcus pneumoniae hexB* mismatch repair gene: Homology of HexB to MutL of *Salmonella typhimurium* and to PMS1 of *Saccharomyces cerevisiae*. J. Bacteriol. **171**:5332–5338.

39. **Prudhomme, M., V. Méjean, B. Martin, O. Humbert, and J.P. Claverys.** 1991. Generalized mismatch repair in *Streptococcus pneumoniae*. *In* G.M. Dunny, P.P. Cleary, and L.L. McKay (eds.)

Genetics and Molecular Biology of Streptococci, Lactococci, and Enterococci. American Society for Microbiology, Washington, DC, pp. 67–70.

40. **Radnis, B.A., D.-K. Rhee, and D.A. Morrison.** 1990. Genetic transformation in *Streptococcus pneumoniae*: Nucleotide sequence and predicted amino acid sequence of *recP*. J. Bacteriol. **172:** 3669–3674.

41. **Reizer, J., A. Reizer, A. Bairoch, and M.H. Saier, Jr.** 1993. A diverse transketolase family that includes the RecP protein of *Streptococcus pneumoniae*, a protein implicated in genetic recombination. Res. Microbiol. **144:**341–347.

42. **Rhee, D.-K., and D.A. Morrison.** 1988. Genetic transformation in *Streptococcus pneumoniae*: Molecular cloning and characterization of *recP*, a gene required for genetic recombination. J. Bacteriol. **170:**630–637.

43. **Roca, A.I., and M.M. Cox.** 1990. The RecA protein: Structure and function. CRC Crit. Rev. Biochem. Mol. Biol. **25:**415–456.

44. **Shen, P., and H.V. Huang.** 1986. Homologous recombination in *Escherichia coli*: Dependence on substrate length and homology. Genetics **112:**441–457.

45. **Shoemaker, N.B., and W.R. Guild.** 1974. Destruction of low efficiency markers is a slow process occurring at a heteroduplex stage of transformation. Mol. Gen. Genet. **128:**283–290.

46. **Sibold, C., J. Henrichsen, A. König, C. Martin, L. Chalkley, and R. Hakenbeck.** 1994. Mosaic *pbpX* genes of major clones of penicillin-resistant *Streptococcus pneumoniae* have evolved from *pbpX* genes of a penicillin-sensitive *Streptococcus oralis*. Mol. Microbiol. **12:**1013–1023.

47. **Taylor, H.E.** 1949. Additive effects of certain transforming agents from some variants of pneumococcus. J. Exp. Med. **89:**399–424.

48. **Tiraby, G., J.P. Claverys, and A.M. Sicard.** 1973. Integration efficiency in DNA-induced transformation of pneumococcus. I. A method of transformation in solid medium and its use for isolation of transformation-deficient and recombination-modified mutants. Genetics **75:**23–33.

49. **Tomasz, A., P. Moreillon, and G. Pozzi.** 1988. Insertional inactivation of the major autolysin gene of *Streptococcus pneumoniae*. J. Bacteriol. **170:**5931–5934.

50. **Vasseghi, H., J.P. Claverys, and A.M. Sicard.** 1981. Mechanism of integrating foreign DNA during transformation of *Streptococcus pneumoniae*. *In* M. Polsinelli and G. Mazza (eds.) Transformation-1980. Cotswold Press, Oxford, pp. 137–154.

51. **Vijayakumar, M.N., and D.A. Morrison.** 1983. Fate of DNA in eclipse complex during genetic recombination in *Streptococcus pneumoniae*. J. Bacteriol. **156:**644–648.

52. **Vovis, G.F.** 1973. Adenosine triphosphate-dependent deoxyribonuclease from *Diplococcus pneumoniae*: Fate of transforming deoxyribonucleic acid in a strain deficient in the enzymatic activity. J. Bacteriol. **113:**718–723.

53. **Worth, L., Jr., S. Clark, M. Radman, and P. Modrich.** 1994. Mismatch repair proteins MutS and MutL inhibit RecA-catalyzed strand transfer between diverged DNAs. Proc. Natl. Acad. Sci. USA **91:**3238–3241.

Address reprint requests to:
Jean-Pierre Claverys
Laboratoire de Microbiologie et
Génétique Moléculaire CNRS–UPR 9007
Université Paul Sabatier
118 Route de Narbonne
31062 Toulouse Cedex, France

Cloning and Expression of Pneumococcal Genes in *Streptococcus pneumoniae*

SANFORD A. LACKS

ABSTRACT

An overview of gene cloning in *Streptococcus pneumoniae* is presented. The advantages of such cloning, especially for pneumococcal genes, are enumerated. The molecular fate of DNA in transformation of *S. pneumoniae*, in particular, the conversion of DNA to single-strand segments on entry, determines the mechanisms for plasmid establishment and interaction with the chromosome. One of these mechanisms, the chromosomal facilitation of plasmid establishment, is useful for obtaining recombinant plasmids and for introducing an allele from the chromosome into a plasmid. The difference between linear and circular synapsis of donor DNA strands with the chromosome is illustrated. Circular synapsis can give rise to circular integration, which is useful for insertional mutagenesis of chromosomal genes, for coupled cloning in *Escherichia coli*, and for sequential cloning of DNA along the pneumococcal chromosome. Cloning in *S. pneumoniae* is not notably affected by DNA mismatch repair or restriction systems in the host cell. Unusual features of gene expression in *S. pneumoniae* are discussed. Transcription begins most often at promoters with extended −10 sequences, and in a small but significant number of cases, translation does not require a ribosome-binding site with a Shine–Dalgarno sequence.

PURPOSE

MOLECULAR MANIPULATION OF PNEUMOCOCCAL GENES— their cloning and mutational alteration—can be accomplished within cells of *Streptococcus pneumoniae*, itself.[83] One motivation for cloning in *S. pneumoniae* derives from the toxicity of some pneumococcal DNA segments, for example those containing *malXMP*[82] and *hexA*,[55] in the commonly used *Escherichia coli* systems. Another motivation is to examine the expression of a pneumococcal gene or regulatory signal in its normal setting. A third reason for manipulation in *S. pneumoniae* is to alter genes within the chromosome. There are certain peculiarities in the use of *S. pneumoniae* as a genetic system, in which it differs from other bacterial systems, notably that of *E. coli*. These differences result from the use of the natural process of transformation in *S. pneumoniae* for purposes of genetic transfer. Exploitation of this process for genetic manipulation requires an understanding of the various mechanisms underlying DNA-mediated transformation in this species.

MECHANISM OF TRANSFORMATION

S. pneumoniae cells are competent to take up DNA only at a late stage in the culture cycle, when the cells have achieved a certain density.[86] The cells can sense the accumulated concentration of a competence factor that is released into the medium. This factor, known for some time to be a protein, was recently shown to be a specific polypeptide of 17 amino acid residues.[25] Action of the competence factor on the cell results in the synthesis of a special class of proteins, including one that binds to the single strands of DNA that enter the cell.[62]

Fate of transforming DNA on uptake

To be taken up efficiently, DNA must be double-stranded. Uptake occurs in two stages:[36,76] (a) binding of DNA to the outside of the cell and (b) its entry into the cell. Bound DNA is still susceptible to external agents, but it is irreversibly adsorbed and has undergone single-strand breaks ~3 kb apart on

Biology Department, Brookhaven National Laboratory, Upton, NY 11973.
Reprinted from *Microbial Drug Resistance*, Vol. 3, No. 4, 1997.

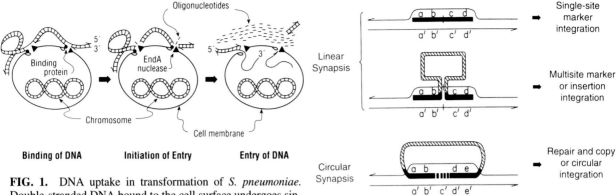

FIG. 1. DNA uptake in transformation of *S. pneumoniae*. Double-stranded DNA bound to the cell surface undergoes single-strand cleavage at random sites, presumably by action of a hypothetical binding protein. The membrane-located EndA nuclease initiates entry of the bound strand by endonucleolytic cleavage of the complementary strand to give a double-strand break. Processive action of the DNase degrades the complementary strand to oligonucleotides which remain outside the cell and allows donor strands to enter in a 3′ to 5′ direction. Segments from either strand may enter.

FIG. 3. Linear and circular synapsis. Depending on the manner of attachment of homologous (solid bar) and heterologous (hatched bar) donor DNA, entering donor strands can interact with recipient double-stranded DNA (thin lines) by either linear or circular synapsis. Circular synapsis can lead to either plasmid establishment or circular integration into the chromosome. Vertical marks indicate mutated sites. Broken bars indicates repair synthesis.

either strand of the duplex DNA.[34] Entry of DNA requires action of a membrane nuclease encoded by the *endA* gene,[70] that degrades one strand to oligonucleotides[33,62] and allows the complementary strand to enter the cell,[27,35] which it does in a 3′ to 5′ direction[57] (Fig. 1). Foreign DNA is taken up as efficiently as pneumococcal DNA.[35] The conversion of DNA to single-stranded segments on entry determines its modes of interaction within the cell and the mechanisms of chromosomal transformation and plasmid establishment.

Chromosomal integration by linear synapsis

If the incoming strands are homologous to DNA in the chromosome, they presumably interact with the chromosome to give a three-stranded intermediate, which was proposed to have either a triple-helical[28] or displaced D-loop structure[37] (Fig. 2). The recipient strand segment corresponding to the donor strand in this intermediate is then eliminated by an unknown mechanism, possibly involving helicases or nucleases, to give a heteroduplex intermediate[21] with strand breaks bracketing the donor DNA segment. Subsequently, the donor DNA is ligated into the chromosomal DNA, which on replication, gives rise to a homoduplex product.

Ordinary chromosomal transformation with point markers (corresponding to single-site mutations) is mediated by linear synapsis in which the linear donor segment is matched point-for-point with its complement in the chromosome, except for the point of mismatch at the marker (Fig. 3, upper). An insertion of nonhomologous DNA within such a segment, for example, the DNA segment missing in a mutant recipient harboring a deletion, or a drug-resistance marker inserted to disrupt a gene, would also give linear synapsis on both sides of a loopout of foreign DNA in the donor strand (Fig. 3, middle). However, if the foreign DNA is attached to the ends of the homologous region, as in a recombinant plasmid, its interaction with the chromosome is by circular synapsis, as shown in Fig. 3, lower. The strand break required for DNA uptake must occur in the homologous region. Any missing donor DNA in this region will be resynthesized on the recipient template to complete the circle. The several possible fates of the circularly synapsed DNA are discussed next.

MECHANISMS OF PLASMID ESTABLISHMENT

Interaction of monomer plasmid strands

Plasmids that contain no homology with the chromosome require two independent entry events for establishment.[75] This follows from the fate of DNA on uptake—any donor DNA must suffer at least one single-strand break and conversion to a single strand.[32] With a monomeric plasmid, the largest structure that can enter is a single, linear plasmid strand. This structure cannot circularize, and it must interact with a complementary strand from another entry event to circularize and replicate, as

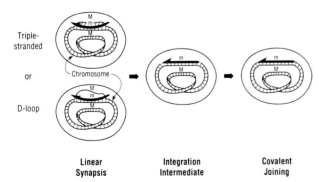

FIG. 2. Chromosomal transformation. It is not known whether synapsis is mediated by a triple-stranded or D-loop structure. Heavy line, donor DNA strand segment. Thin line, chromosomal DNA. Cross hatches indicate hydrogen bonding. M and m, marker difference between donor and recipient.

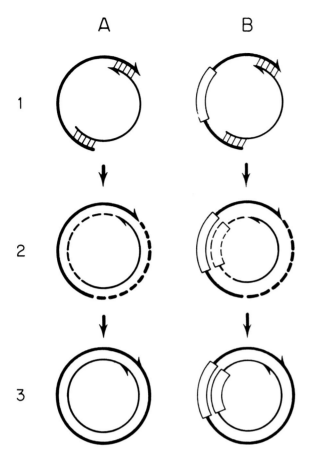

FIG. 4. Plasmid establishment via the transformation pathway. (A) Reconstitution from separately entering monomeric plasmid strand fragments: 1, annealing of complementary fragments; 2, repair synthesis; 3, completed replicon. (B) Reconstitution of recombinant plasmid from separately entering recombinant (rare) and vector (common) plasmid fragments: 1, annealing of complementary fragments; 2, repair synthesis of vector and recombinant portions; 3, completed recombinant plasmid replicon. Heavy line, plasmid. (+)-strand. Thin line, plasmid (−)-strand. Open bar, cloned chromosomal DNA insert. Broken line, newly synthesized DNA. Hatchmarks, hydrogen-bonded regions.

shown in Fig. 4A. Proof of this requirement is the quadratic dependence on monomer plasmid DNA concentration of plasmid establishment.[52,75] Dimeric plasmids that contain redundant information can circularize to a monomer after linearization and require only a single entry event for establishment.[75]

Chromosomal facilitation of plasmid transfer

If an entering plasmid carries homology to the chromosome, the linear single strand derived from it can interact with the chromosome by circular synapsis. As long as the break made during uptake falls in the homologous segment, the chromosomal interaction will circularize the plasmid replicon[52] (Fig. 5). Even if a segment is missing, it will be restored by repair replication and the circular strand will be sealed by DNA ligase. Inasmuch as the vectors usually used in *S. pneumoniae* replicate by a rolling-circle mechanism, they carry a minus-strand

origin of replication[16] that allows conversion of the synapsed plasmid strand to a duplex form, at the same time releasing it from synapse with the chromosome. During repair of the original strand template and its replication, markers from the chromosome can substitute for markers originally on the plasmid.[52] Depending on the length of the homologous segment (and hence, the likelihood of its central portion being absent in the introduced plasmid strand) and the position of the marker within it, as much as 90% of the established plasmids will carry a recipient cell marker.[52] However, the frequency of plasmid establishment is greatly increased by the homology, by a factor of 10 to 100, again depending on the length of the homologous segment. Furthermore, such facilitated transfer is linearly dependent on plasmid concentration.[52]

Establishment of recombinant plasmids

A recombinant plasmid is formed in the usual way by ligating a segment of DNA from *S. pneumoniae*, or another source, into a pneumococcal vector plasmid.[83] The mode of establishment of this plasmid, however, will depend on whether or not the introduced segment carries homology to the recipient cell chromosome.

In the absence of chromosomal homology. If the DNA to be cloned is of foreign origin or if it is not present in all strains of *S. pneumoniae* (like a restriction system gene[48]), or if the recipient chromosome is deleted for that particular DNA (as in the cloning of *mal* genes[83]), there will be no interaction between the recombinant plasmid and the chromosome. The recombinant plasmid must be established by the interaction of two separately entering fragments. However, establishment need not depend on the simultaneous entry of two copies of a particular recombinant, which could be an exceedingly rare event. It can result from interaction of a recombinant strand fragment in which the insert DNA is bordered by vector DNA, with a complementary strand fragment from the vector portion alone, which could come from any plasmid in the mixture, as shown in Fig. 4B.

Effect of chromosomal facilitation. If the recombinant plasmid carries a gene homologous to the chromosome, establishment of the plasmid will be facilitated, but in many cases, the allele present in the chromosome will be cloned in the plasmid. In as many as 90% of the cells in which the plasmid is established, the plasmids could carry the recipient allele.[52] If the original donor allele is desired, the cell carrying it must be selected, either by a bulk screening mechanism depending on properties conferred to the cell (e.g., drug resistance in the case of *sul* cloning[83]) or by individually examining the plasmid size, restriction pattern, or even sequence of the plasmids from as many as 20 different cells. Although this facilitation makes isolation of the donor allele a little more laborious, it makes it very easy to purposely introduce particular alleles, which may include the wild-type as well as different mutants, into the cloned gene.[40] This opportunity to readily clone various forms of the gene far outweighs the complication of identifying individual types among the transformants.

A cloned gene that is itself absent from the chromosome but carries homologous DNA on both sides of it will also be subject to removal by chromosomal facilitation. This was observed in cloning the *Dpn*II restriction system, where the *Dpn*I system

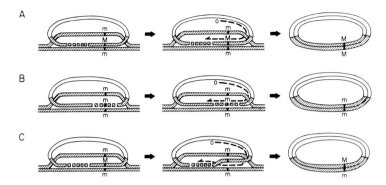

FIG. 5. Mechanism of chromosomal facilitation of plasmid establishment. (A) Formation of plasmid with homoduplex plasmid marker. Circular synapsis with the donor strand break distant from the marker is followed by repair synthesis and ligation to close the plasmid strand. Synthesis of the complementary strand from the plasmid origin replicates the plasmid marker. The plasmid is established with the plasmid marker present in both strands. (B) Formation of plasmid with homoduplex chromosomal marker. Circular synapsis with the donor strand gap covering the marker is followed by repair synthesis that replicates the chromosomal marker. Complementary strand synthesis again replicates the chromosomal marker. The chromosomal marker is present in both strands of established plasmid. (C) Formation of plasmid with heteroduplex marker configuration. Circular synapsis occurs with the break distant from the marker. Complementary strand synthesis shifts to the chromosomal template in the region of the marker before it returns to the plasmid strand. A heteroduplex plasmid is established; upon replication it gives rise to a mixed plasmid pool in the host cell. In each case, the chromosome is released unchanged (not shown) after establishment of the plasmid. Linear bar, segment of double-strand chromosomal DNA. Curvilinear bar, introduced fragment of plasmid DNA. Hatched portion, homologous DNA. Open portion, heterologous (vector) DNA. Broken bar, repair synthesis of introduced plasmid strand. Broken line, synthesis of complementary plasmid strand. M and m, marker alleles; o, origin of plasmid replication. Reproduced from Lacks.[38]

from the chromosome replaced it in the plasmid.[45] However, if homology exists only on one side of the cloned gene, as was the case for a segment of the *Dpn*II system carrying only the *dpnM* gene,[48] the cloned gene is not subject to removal.

Technical pitfall of phosphate removal. When cloning in *E. coli*, a convenient method for preventing religation of the vector is removal of terminal 5′-phosphate from the vector but not the cloned fragment. This method is effective in *E. coli* because the DNA enters in a double-stranded form and a single phosphodiester bond at each junction suffices. However, in the case of *S. pneumoniae*, entering single strands containing the cloned segment would be joined to a vector segment only at one end. Especially in "shotgun" cloning of random chromosomal fragments, it would be unlikely for this strand to encounter a complementary cloned fragment joined at the other end to reconstitute the recombinant replicon. Thus, it was experimentally shown that "shotgun" cloning of heterogeneous DNA is blocked by phosphatase treatment of the vector, although cloning of homogeneous DNA can successfully use this procedure even in *S. pneumoniae*.[4]

Examples of gene cloning in S. pneumoniae

A listing that includes most of the pneumococcal chromosomal genes that have been cloned so far in *S. pneumoniae* is give in Table 1. The vectors shown are all derivatives of pMV158, which was originally isolated from *Streptococcus agalactiae*.[7] In a majority of cases, the pneumococcal genes were cloned *de novo* in *S. pneumoniae*; in some cases, the genes were first cloned in *E. coli* and then transferred to the streptococcal vector. Depending on the genes cloned, various selective and screening procedures were used.

CHROMOSOMAL INTEGRATION BY CIRCULAR SYNAPSIS

Ectopic insertion

Early experiments on cloning of the *malXMP* segment in *S. pneumoniae*, using as a recipient strain a mutant with a large deletion in the *mal* region, revealed the appearance of Mal⁺ transformants at a low frequency, even when no vector was present in a ligated mixture of chromosomal fragments used as donor DNA.[83] It was surmised that ligation of *mal* fragments with other, random restriction fragments of the pneumococcal DNA resulted in integration of the *mal* marker at the locus of the fragment(s) to which it was ligated. As a result, *mal* was not in its normal position but was present as an ectopic insertion. Later, it was shown that ligation of the *mal* fragment to another single fragment to give a circular structure sufficed to give ectopic integration, presumably via circular synapsis.[54]

Ectopic insertion also occurs during cloning experiments in the presence of vector, but such clones contain no plasmid and, therefore, can be readily distinguished from recombinant plasmid clones. Ectopic insertion is of great practical use to introduce new genes or disrupt existing genes in the chromosome of *S. pneumoniae*. Homologous fragments as small as 0.5 kb can direct a foreign segment as large as 10 kb into a specific location in the chromosome.

Additive transformation

After cloning an *amiA* gene segment of *S. pneumoniae* in the *E. coli* plasmid pBR325 (which cannot replicate in *S. pneumoniae*), it was observed that the recombinant plasmid could be

TABLE 1. CLONING OF CHROMOSOMAL GENES IN *S. PNEUMONIAE*

Cloned gene	Function	Recombinant plasmid	Vector	Selection or screening	Reference
Primary cloning					
dpnCD	*Dpn*I restriction	pLS207	pLS101	Chromosomal facilitation; size	45
dpnM	DNA methylation	pMP10	pMP5	Plasmid resistance to *Dpn*II	48
dpnMAB	*Dpn*II restriction	pLS201	pLS101	Plasmid resistance to *Dpn*II	45
endA	Membrane nuclease	pLS10	pAPC30	Nuclease colony assay	70
exoA	DNA exonuclease	pLS10	pLS301	Nuclease colony assay	69
hexA	Mismatch repair	pLS120	pLS101	Enrichment of Hex- cells	5
malXMP	Amylomaltase	pLS70	pMV158	Maltose utilization	83
polA	DNA polymerase I	pSM22	pLS1	Nuclease colony assay	53
recP	Genetic recombination	p561	pSP21	Plate transformation screen	71
sulABCD	Folate biosynthesis	pLS80	pLS1	Sulfonamide resistance	42, 51
ung	DNA uracil glycosylase	pSP61	pSP2	Restriction fragment enrichment	59
uvrB	UV damage repair	pSP2800	pSP2	Mitomycin resistance	80
Secondary cloning[a]					
cap3B	Capsule formation	pLSE3B	pLSE1	Size screening in *E. coli*	2
hexA	Mismatch repair	pSP11	pSP2	Probed with *E. coli* clone	55
hexB	Mismatch repair	pSP41	pSP2	Artificially linked EM[r]	65
lytA	Cell wall amidase	pRG2	pLS1	Lysin colony screen	72

[a]Substantial portions of the gene were initially cloned in *E. coli*.

integrated into the *S. pneumoniae* chromosome in its entirety when it was used as donor DNA for pneumococcal transformation.[87] Inasmuch as the product was duplicated in the segment of *amiA* cloned and the duplicated segments bracketed the pBR325 vector, it was evident that the entire recombinant plasmid had been added to the *ami* locus.[87] This additive transformation could result from linear synapsis with a strand derived from dimeric plasmid DNA, but it also resulted from monomeric plasmid DNA, apparently via circular synapsis.[87]

Insertional mutagenesis

Homology-directed insertion of foreign DNA, particularly easily selectible drug-resistance markers, has been a useful method for disrupting genes and producing mutations.[24,58,63] If a cloned gene is available or the gene sequence is known, a construct consisting of a marker gene bracketed by proximal and distal parts the gene can be introduced by linear synapsis to give a stable mutation. However, in other circumstances, it may only be possible to use circular synapsis, where only a single fragment of the gene is required. The homologous fragment must be small enough to fall entirely within the host gene to prevent translation of a normal product. Due to the presence of repeated DNA segments, such an insertion mutation can be reversed by recombination, so the mutants are not stable,[87] but the reversion rates are low enough to be tolerable for most purposes. Because an entire *E. coli* vector plasmid, such as pBR325, can be inserted, a convenient method for cloning genes in *E. coli* depends on the removal of the insert together with adjacent DNA on the chromosome by treating the chromosomal DNA with an appropriate restriction enzyme.[58] This fragment when circularized by ligation gives a recombinant plasmid that may contain much or all of the mutated gene. The *E. coli* plasmid may be tailored to prevent possible harmful transcription out of the insert, as in the vector pJDC9,[11] and libraries of such inserts can be maintained in *E. coli*. Cultures of

S. pneumoniae transformed by such a library can be used, in turn, as a library source of clonable mutants.[70]

Circular integration

The various interactions in which DNA originally circular in structure interacts with and integrates into the chromosome after uptake via the transformation pathway of *S. pneumoniae* share a common mechanism based on circular synapsis.[37] Such chromosomal integration was first observed in *Bacillus subtilis*,[19] which has a transformation system that processes DNA similarly to *S. pneumoniae*.[18] In addition to ectopic insertion,[83] additive transformation,[87] ectopic integration,[54] and insertion-duplication mutagenesis,[63] the interaction has been called Campbell-like[1] integration after the discoverer of the mode of phage lambda integration (a double-stranded circular interaction) in *E. coli*.[8] Because of its generality, simplicity, and descriptive accuracy, as well as its basis on circular synapsis, I propose the term *circular integration*, to be a most appropriate name for the process.

CASE STUDY OF INSERTIONAL MUTAGENESIS AND CLONING

An example of the cloning of a pneumococcal gene that made use of insertional mutagenesis, a gel enzyme renaturation assay to confirm the "knockout" mutation, cloning in *S. pneumoniae*, and chromosomal facilitation to convert the cloned allele to wild-type is illustrated for the case of *endA*, the gene encoding the membrane nuclease (EndA) implicated in DNA entry[70] (Fig. 6). *Alu*I fragments (mean size 0.25 kb) of *S. pneumoniae* wild-type DNA were ligated into the *Sma*I blunt-cut pJDC9 *E. coli* plasmid. After transformation of *E. coli* and selecting for *erm*, which confers resistance to erythromycin in both species, the library was used to transform an *S. pneumo-*

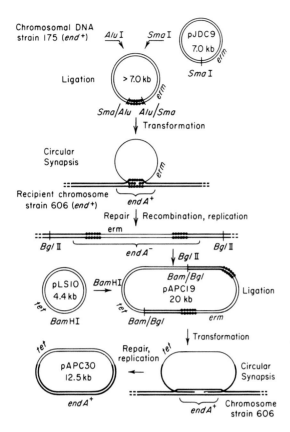

FIG. 6. Procedure used to clone *endA*. *Alu*I fragments of pneumococcal DNA were cloned in the *E. coli* plasmid pJDC9. A recombinant plasmid library transformed *S. pneumoniae* to give insertion mutants in the *endA* gene. A mutant gene was cloned by ligation of a *Bgl*II chromosomal fragment to the streptococcal plasmid pLS10. The wild-type allele of *endA* was recovered after chromosomal facilitation of plasmid establishment. Single and double lines represent single- and double-stranded DNA. Heavy lines correspond to chromosomal DNA; thin lines to vector DNA. The beaded segment indicates an internal *Alu*I fragment of *endA*. (Reproduced from Puyet *et al.*[70] with permission from Academic Press.)

niae strain that produced EndA. Erythromycin-resistant transformants were conveniently screened for absence of the nuclease by an agar plate colony assay for nucleases, and the *endA* mutation was confirmed by a gel renaturation assay employing crude cell extracts.[73] The mutant chromosomal DNA was cut with *Bgl*II and cloned in the *Bam*HI site of the streptococcal vector pLS10. Selection for *erm* gave the chromosomal segment containing *endA* with the pJDC9 insert in the recombinant plasmid pAPC19. Transformation of *S. pneumoniae* with pAPC19 and selection for *tet*, the pLS10 vector gene conferring tetracycline resistance, gave rise by chromosomal facilitation to pAPC30, which carries wild-type *endA*.

SEQUENTIAL CLONING

A procedure was developed for extending the cloning of DNA along the chromosome of *S. pneumoniae* in both direc-

tions, starting from a small cloned segment, such as might result from insertional mutagenesis.[41] The method is based on alternate cycles of circular integration in *S. pneumoniae* of the *E. coli* vector containing small segments, as the vector walks along the chromosome, and cloning in the *E. coli* host of large segments coupled to the vector. The design of the vector is critical in terms of the restriction sites it contains.[41] An example of a vector and two cycles of sequential cloning are illustrated in Fig. 7. Three cycles of this procedure, using the vector pWG5, were successful in extending cloning from the originally cloned *mal* segment which only contained part of the *malP* gene for an additional 8 kb.[41] The newly cloned region included the entire *malP* gene and extended out of the *malMP* operon.

DNA MISMATCH REPAIR

At the stage of transformation when the donor segment is in a heteroduplex structure but not yet ligated into the chromosome (Fig. 2, center), the donor segment is subject to elimination by the Hex mismatch repair system of *S. pneumoniae* (see ref. 13 for a detailed review). This system, which also acts to avoid mutations after DNA replication,[40,84,85] is homologous to the Mut system of *Salmonella typhimurium* and *E. coli*.[39,67,68] In fact, mismatch repair systems homologous to Hex appear to be present in all cells; in humans, defects in these genes lead to cancer.[22] In transformation, up to 95% of the potential transformants are eliminated, depending on the specific mismatch (only mismatches corresponding to base changes or deletion/insertions <5 nt in length are at all recognized).[14,23,40] Mismatch repair does not usually interfere with genetic manipulation in *S. pneumoniae*, but if it does, *hex* mutants lacking the system are readily obtainable and can be used as recipient strains.

RESTRICTION SYSTEM EFFECTS

The only restriction systems that have been reported in *S. pneumoniae* are the complementary *Dpn*I and *Dpn*II systems, one or the other of which is found in wild strains.[45] The *Dpn*I endonuclease is unusual in that it cleaves only *methylated* DNA at GATC sequences where adenine is methylated. Conversely, *Dpn*II, an ordinary restriction endonuclease cleaves only at unmethylated GATC. Neither endonuclease can act on single-stranded DNA or on hemimethylated DNA,[88] so chromosomal transformation is not affected in either type of recipient by the methylation status of donor DNA. With respect to plasmid transfer, *Dpn*I strains do not discriminate strongly against methylated donor plasmids because most of the reconstituted plasmid DNA has undergone repair synthesis and would be hemimethylated at GATC sites.[49] The *Dpn*II system is unusual in that it contains two methyltransferases that act on GATC, DpnM and DpnA.[15] DpnM methylates only double-stranded DNA, but DpnA methylates single-stranded DNA very well, so that entering DNA strands in a *Dpn*II recipient are methylated prior to reconstitution.[9] This protects unmethylated plasmids from destruction; only in *dpnA* mutants is plasmid transfer drastically affected.[9] Thus, restriction system effects can be ignored, for the most part, in the genetic manipulation of *S. pneumoniae*.

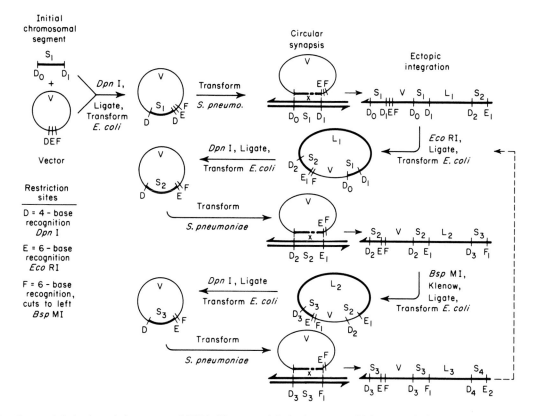

FIG. 7. Sequential cloning of chromosomal DNA. V, sequential cloning vector. Unique restriction sites in vector: D, *Dpn*I (or *Dpn*II); E, *Eco*RI; F, *Bsp*MI. D_0, D_1, etc., successive *Dpn*II sites demarcating short cloned segments: S_1, S_2, etc., successive short cloned segments; L_1, L_2, etc., successive long cloned segments. The small chromosomal segment (S_1) directs the vector insertion in the chromosome and the circular mode of integration results in a duplication of the segment bracketing the vector. The chromosomal DNA is then cut with *Eco*RI, which cleaves at one end of the vector and at another point down the chromosome, to give a fragment that when ligated can transform *E. coli* to give a recombinant plasmid in which a substantial segment of the chromosome is cloned. To walk further down the chromosome, the previous plasmid is cut with *Dpn*I and ligated. In general, there are multiple *Dpn*I sites in the cloned *Eco*RI fragment. Such cutting will, therefore, remove most of the insert and leave only a distal segment between the closest *Dpn*I site to the end of the insert at the *Eco*RI site. Ligation produces a reduced plasmid carrying the fragment S_2. Transformation of *S. pneumoniae* again inserts the vector into the chromosome but further downstream at the site of homology with S_2. This time *Bsp*MI is used to cut out a large fragment of the chromosome containing the vector. This enzyme cleaves upstream of its recognition sequence in the vector so that the adjacent *Eco*RI site is retained. The enzyme produces a 4-nt 5'-overhang which is filled in by Klenow fragment. Circularization of this DNA fragment by ligation and transformation of *E. coli* gives a plasmid containing the second large chromosomal segment (including L_2 and S_3). This plasmid is again reduced by treatment with *Dpn*I (so that it contains only S_3) and is once again integrated into the *S. pneumoniae* chromosome. Cutting with *Eco*RI is repeated, followed by the other steps, and, after the next integration, cutting with *Bsp*MI and subsequent steps are repeated. In this manner, alternate segments down the chromosome are cloned as *Eco*RI and *Bsp*MI fragments. (Reproduced from Lacks and Greenberg[41] with permission from Elsevier.)

GENE EXPRESSION

Transcription: Promoters in S. pneumoniae

Most genes in *S. pneumoniae* are transcribed from promoters having the same consensus sequence as the sigma[70] promoters of *E. coli*, that is a −35 site of TTGACA, an interval of 15 to 20 nt, and a −10 site of TATAAT. However, more than 60% of pneumococcal promoters have an extended −10 site, TNTGNTATAAT, and one promoter (P_1 in the *Dpn*II system) consisted only of an extended −10 site.[74] Although the extended site is found in *E. coli* and does enhance promoter activity, it is much less frequent in that species. However, the frequent occurrence of the extended sites may not be confined to *S. pneumoniae* but be characteristic of streptococcal species in

general. In any event, the extended sequence helps considerably in the identification of functional promoters and operons in uncharted sequences of *S. pneumoniae* DNA. Note that not all promoters in *S. pneumoniae* have the sigma[70] consensus. No such sequence is present at P_2 in the *Dpn*II system (Ayalew and Lacks, unpublished), for which promoter activity has been demonstrated.[43]

Translation: Ribosome binding sites

Shine–Dalgarno sequences. Most structural genes of *S. pneumoniae* are accompanied by an upstream ribosome-binding site (RBS) similar to the Shine–Dalgarno sequence in *E. coli*. However, on account of the slight difference in the 3'-terminus of the pneumococcal 16S rRNA,[3] the corresponding site in *S.*

pneumoniae is a subset of 5'-AAAGGAGGTGA, where the central A is a mean distance of 10 nt from the translation start codon.

Downstream binding sites. Three instances have been observed, for *polA*,[53] *dpnM*,[74] and *rnhB*,[90] where transcription of a structural gene begins right at the translation start site. It is likely that, in these cases, ribosome binding is mediated by a downstream binding site within the coding region of the mRNA,[74,90] as has been proposed for lambda *cI*[78] and, as a contributing factor, for genes of *E. coli*.[81]

Atypical binding sites. In addition to the instances just mentioned, when the absence of a 5'-leader in the mRNA precludes the presence of an upstream RBS, three cases were found where a leader is present but without a discernible Shine–Dalgarno sequence.[79] However, in all three cases, a different consensus sequence was present, that is, 5'-ATTTCT-N_{4-5}-TATANT-N_{7-8} ATG, where the last 3 nt represent the translation start codon. These cases are the *dpnM* (when transcription begins at the putative P_0 promoter) and *dpnA* genes of the *DpnII* system,[15] and the *repB* gene of plasmid pLS1.[44] The consensus sequence may represent an atypical RBS,[15,46] but no experimental evidence has so far supported (or excluded) this possibility.

These findings suggest caution in identifying translation start sites for structural genes in new sequence information; they may not always be associated with Shine–Dalgarno sequences.

MATERIALS AND TECHNIQUES

Transformation procedures

Protocols for transformation can be found in published articles.[28,52,89] Competent cultures, at least of strain R36A derivatives, are regularly obtained by growth in a semisynthetic medium,[28] although more complex media have also been successfully employed.[10,89] Serum albumin must be added to all the media[26] and various conditions of pH and ionic composition must be maintained.[10,31,77] The discovery of the composition of the competence signalling peptides and their synthetic production promise to facilitate the use of transformation for genetic analysis in *S. pneumoniae*.[60] Because these oligopeptides can render poorly competent cultures transformable, in particular cultures of encapsulated cells, their use should make more strains from the wild accessible to analysis by transformation.[60]

Plasmid vectors

As seen in Table 1, virtually all cloning in *S. pneumoniae* has been performed with pMV158 or derivatives thereof, like pLS1. However, there is no reason to think that unrelated plasmids that can replicate in *S. pneumoniae*,[6] such as pAM77 or pSA5700 (which originated in *Streptococcus sanguis* and *Staphylococcus aureus*, respectively) could not also be used as vectors. One derivative of pMV158, pSP2, has an inverted, repeated sequence positioned to allow positive selection of recombinant products.[66] Alternatively, chromosomal facilitation may be used to enrich the recombinant products in a plasmid population.[4]

Another type of plasmid vector of interest, here, is one that cannot replicate in *S. pneumoniae* but can enter by circular integration into the chromosome and then be excised, along with adjacent chromosomal DNA, and propagated in *E. coli*. First used in this way was a pBR325 clone of *amiA*.[58] The sequential cloning plasmids,[41] pWG5 and pWG6 (like pWG5 but contains *Eco*RI instead of *Sph*I) which contain *cat* markers, are examples of such vectors. Plasmid pJDC9, with an *erm* marker, was constructed to place transcription terminators on each side of a cloned segment,[11] and pEVP3 contains a *cat* marker and a *lacZ* reporter for transcriptional fusions.[12] Plasmid pFL10, based on pLS1, makes use of a *tet* marker and a *cat* reporter gene for transcriptional fusions in a pneumococcal plasmid setting.[50] A reporter plasmid based on *lytA* was also made.[17]

Markers and mutants available

Markers from other species have been expressed on both plasmids and chromosome of *S. pneumoniae*; they include *tet*, *erm*, *cat*, and *kan*, which confer resistance to tetracycline, erythromycin, chloramphenicol, and kanamycin, respectively. Pneumococcal genes that have been useful as markers both in plasmids and ectopically in the chromosome are *malM*, *amiA*, and *sulA*-d, which confer the ability to use maltose, aminopterin resistance, and sulfonamide resistance, respectively. The *str* and *nov* markers conferring streptomycin and novobiocin resistance have been widely used in chromosomal transformation.

Many genes of *S. pneumoniae* have been intensively studied and mutants are available in most of them. In some loci, such as *malM*,[28] *amiA*,[20] and *malR*[29] (a repressor of *malM*), numerous spontaneous mutations were isolated. Thymidine-requiring[33] and pyrimidine-requiring[64] mutants are useful for labeling of nucleic acids. Mutants defective in the major cellular DNases, *endA* and *exoA*, have been useful in detecting other less prominent DNases and RNases.[36,56,90]

Renaturation gel electrophoresis

A technique that was developed to detect and analyze nucleases in crude cell extracts may prove particularly useful in examining the effects of "knockout" mutations on gene function. Dr. Allan Rosenthal discovered that it is possible to subject enzymes to denaturing polyacrylamide gel electrophoresis in the presence of sodium dodecyl sulfate, so that the enzyme proteins are separated by molecular weight, and then to renature the enzymes and detect their activities.[73] It was shown that this technique can be used for various types of enzyme as long as the active protein is a monomer or an oligomer of identical subunits.[47] Using this technique, it is relatively easy to test a putative knockout mutant for loss of the corresponding function by subjecting a crude extract to electrophoresis and determining whether the activity band at the expected position is absent.

ACKNOWLEDGMENTS

I thank my various coworkers and colleagues in the field whose research findings formed the basis for this overview. This work was performed under the auspices of the U.S. Department of Energy Office of Health and Environmental Research and supported by U.S. Public Health Service Grant AI14885.

REFERENCES

1. **Albano, M., R. Breitling, and D.A. Dubnau.** 1982. Nucleotide sequence and genetic organization of the *Bacillus subtilis comG* operon. J. Bacteriol. **171:**5386–5404.

2. **Arrecubieta, C., R. Lopez, and E. Garcia.** 1996. Type 3-specific synthase of *Streptococcus pneumoniae* (Cap3B) directs type 3 polysaccharide biosynthesis in *Escherichia coli* and in pneumococcal strains of different serotypes. J. Exp. Med. **184:**449–455.

3. **Bacot, C.M., and R.H. Reeves.** 1991. Novel tRNA gene organization in the 16S–23S intergenic spacer of the *Streptococcus pneumoniae* rRNA gene cluster. J. Bacteriol. **173:**4234–4236.

4. **Balganesh, T.S., and S.A. Lacks.** 1984. Plasmid vector for cloning in *Streptococcus pneumoniae* and strategies for enrichment for recombinant plasmids. Gene **29:**221–230.

5. **Balganesh, T.S., and S.A. Lacks.** 1985. Heteroduplex DNA mismatch repair system of *Streptococcus pneumoniae:* Cloning and expression of the *hexA* gene. J. Bacteriol. **162:**979–984.

6. **Barany, F., and A. Tomasz.** 1980. Genetic transformation of *Streptococcus pneumoniae* by heterologous plasmid deoxyribonucleic acid. J. Bacteriol. **144:**698–709.

7. **Burdett, V.** 1980. Identification of tetracycline resistant R-plasmids in *Streptococcus agalactiae* (group B). Antimicrob. Agents Chemother. **18:**753–760.

8. **Campbell, A.** 1962. Episomes. Advanc. Genet. **11:**101–145.

9. **Cerritelli, S., S.S. Springhorn, and S.A. Lacks.** 1989. DpnA, a methylase for single-strand DNA in the *Dpn*II restriction system, and its biological function. Proc. Nat. Acad. Sci. USA **86:**9223–9227.

10. **Chen, J.-D. and D. Morrison.** 1987. Modulation of competence for genetic transformation in *Streptococcus pneumoniae.* **133:**1959–1967.

11. **Chen, J.-D., and D. Morrison.** 1988. Construction and properties of a new insertion vector, pJDC9, that is protected by transcriptional terminators and useful for cloning of DNA from *Streptococcus pneumoniae.* Gene **64:**155–164.

12. **Claverys, J.P., A. Dintilhac, E.V. Pestova, B. Martin, and D.A. Morrison.** 1995. Construction and evaluation of new drug-resistance cassettes for gene disruption mutagenesis in *Streptococcus pneumoniae*, using an *ami* test platform. Gene **164:**123–128.

13. **Claverys, J.P., and S.A. Lacks.** 1986. Heteroduplex deoxyribonucleic acid base mismatch repair in bacteria. Microbiol. Rev. **50:**133–165.

14. **Claverys, J.P., V. Mejean, A.M. Gasc, and A.M. Sicard.** 1983. Mismatch repair in *Streptococcus pneumoniae:* Relationship between base mismatches and transformation efficiencies. Proc. Natl. Acad. Sci. USA **80:**5956–5960.

15. **de la Campa, A.G., P. Kale, S.S. Springhorn, and S.A. Lacks.** 1987. Proteins encoded by the *Dpn*II restriction gene cassette: Two methylases and an endonclease. J. Mol. Biol. **196:**457–469.

16. **del Solar, G.H., A. Puyet, and M. Espinosa.** 1987. Initiation signals for the conversion of single stranded to double stranded DNA forms in the streptococcal plasmid pLS1. Nucl. Acids Res. **15:**5561–5580.

17. **Diaz, E., and J.L. Garcia.** 1990. Construction of a broad-host range pneumococcal promoter-probe plasmid. Gene **90:**163–167.

18. **Dubnau, D.** 1991. Genetic competence in *Bacillus subtilis.* Microbiol. Rev. **55:**395–424.

19. **Duncan, C.H., G.A. Wilson, and F.E. Young.** 1978. Mechanism of integrating foreign DNA during transformation of *Bacillus subtilis.* Proc. Natl. Acad. Sci. USA **75:**3664–3668.

20. **Ephrussi-Taylor, H., A.M. Sicard, and R. Kamen.** 1965. Genetic recombination in DNA-induced transformation of pneumococcus. I. The problem of relative efficiency of transforming factors. Genetics **51:**455–475.

21. **Fox, M.S., and M.K. Allen.** 1964. On the mechanism of deoxyribonucleate integration in pneumococcal transformation. Proc. Natl. Acad. Sci. USA **52:**412–419.

22. **Friedberg, E.C., G.C. Walker, and W. Siede.** 1995. DNA repair and mutagenesis. American Society for Microbiology, Washington, DC.

23. **Gasc, A.M., P. Garcia, D. Batz, and A.M. Sicard.** 1987. Mismatch repair during pneumococcal transformation of small deletions produced by site-directed mutagenesis. Mol. Gen. Genet. **210:**369–372.

24. **Haldenwang, W., C. Banner, J. Ollington, R. Losick, J. Hoch, M. O'Connor, and A. Sonenshein.** 1980. Mapping a cloned gene under sporulation control by insertion of a drug resistance marker into the *Bacillus subtilis* chromosome. J. Bacteriol. **142:**90–98.

25. **Haverstein, L.S., G. Coomaraswamy, and D.A. Morrison.** 1995. An unmodified hepadecapeptide induces competence for genetic transformation in *Streptococcus pneumoniae.* Proc. Natl. Acad. Sci. USA **92:**11140–11144.

26. **Hotchkiss, R.D., and H. Ephrussi-Taylor.** 1951. Use of serum albumin as source of serum factor in pneumococcal transformation. Fed. Proc. **10:**200.

27. **Lacks, S.** 1962. Molecular fate of DNA in genetic transformation of pneumococcus. J. Mol. Biol. **5:**119–131.

28. **Lacks, S.** 1966. Integration efficiency and genetic recombination in pneumococcal transformation. Genetics **53:**207–235.

29. **Lacks, S.** 1968. Genetic regulation of maltosaccharide utilization in pneumococcus. Genetics **60:**685–706.

30. **Lacks, S.** 1970. Mutants of *Diplococcus pneumoniae* that lack deoxyribonucleases and other activities possibly pertinent to genetic transformation. J. Bacteriol. **101:**373–383.

31. **Lacks, S.** 1977. Binding and entry of DNA in pneumococcal transformation, pp. 35–44. *In* A. Portoles, R. Lopez, and M. Espinosa (eds.), Modern trends in bacterial transformation and transfection, Elsevier/North-Holland, Amsterdam.

32. **Lacks, S.** 1979. Uptake of circular deoxyribonucleic acid and mechanism of deoxyribonucleic acid transport in genetic transformation of *Streptococcus pneumoniae.* J. Bacteriol. **138:**404–409.

33. **Lacks, S., and B. Greenberg.** 1973. Competence for deoxyribonucleic acid uptake and deoxyribonuclease action external to cells in the genetic transformation of *Diplococcus pneumoniae.* J. Bacteriol. **114:**152–163.

34. **Lacks, S., and B. Greenberg.** 1976. Single-strand breakage on binding of DNA to cells in the genetic transformation of *Diplococcus pneumoniae.* J. Mol. Biol. **101:**255–275.

35. **Lacks, S., B. Greenberg, and K. Carlson.** 1967. Fate of donor DNA in pneumococcal transformation. J. Mol. Biol. **29:**327–347.

36. **Lacks, S., B. Greenberg, and M. Neuberger.** 1974. Role of a deoxyribonuclease in the genetic transformation of *Diplococcus pneumoniae.* Proc. Natl. Acad. Sci. USA **71:**2305–2309.

37. **Lacks, S.A.** 1984. Modes of DNA interaction in bacterial transformation, pp. 149–158. *In* V.L. Chopra, B.C. Joshi, R.P. Sharma, and H.C. Bansal (eds.), Genetics: New frontiers, vol. 1, Oxford and IBH, New Delhi.

38. **Lacks, S.A.** 1988. Mechanisms of genetic recombination in grampositive bacteria. *In* R. Kucherlapati, and G. Smith (eds.), Genetic recombination, pp. 43–85, American Society for Microbiology, Washington, DC.

39. **Lacks, S.A.** 1989. Generalized DNA mismatch repair—Its molecular basis in *Streptococcus pneumoniae* and other organisms, pp. 325–339. *In* L.O. Butler, C. Harwood, and B.E.B. Moseley (eds.), Genetic transformation and expression, Intercept, Wimbourne, England.

40. **Lacks, S.A., J.J. Dunn, and B. Greenberg.** 1982. Identification of base mismatches recognized by the heteroduplex-DNA-repair system of *Streptococcus pneumoniae.* Cell **31:**327–336.

41. **Lacks, S.A. and B. Greenberg.** 1991. Sequential cloning by a vector walking along the chromosome. Gene **104:**11–17.

42. **Lacks, S.A., B. Greenberg, and P. Lopez.** 1995. A cluster of four genes encoding enzymes for five steps in the folate biosynthetic pathway of *Streptococcus pneumoniae*. J. Bacteriol. **177:**66–74.

43. **Lacks, S.A., B. Greenberg, and A.G. Sabelnikov.** 1995. Possible regulation of DNA methyltransferase expression by RNA processing in *Streptococcus pneumoniae*. Gene **157:**209–212.

44. **Lacks, S.A., P. Lopez, B. Greenberg, and M. Espinosa.** 1986. Identification and analysis of genes for tetracycline resistance and replication functions in the broad-host-range plasmid pLS1. J. Mol. Biol. **192:**753–765.

45. **Lacks, S.A., B.M. Mannarelli, S.S. Springhorn, and B. Greenberg.** 1986. Genetic basis of the complementary *Dpn*I and *Dpn*II restriction systems of *S. pneumoniae:* An intercellular cassette mechanism. Cell **46:**993–1000.

46. **Lacks, S.A., A.G. Sabelnikov, J.-D. Chen, and B. Greenberg.** 1993. Gene expression in the *Dpn*I and *Dpn*II restriction enzyme systems of *Streptococcus pneumoniae*, pp. 169–178. *In* E. Balla, G. Berencsi, and A. Szentirmai (eds.), Genetic transformation: DNA transfer and gene expression in microorganisms, Intercept. Ltd., Andover, England.

47. **Lacks, S.A., and S.S. Springhorn.** 1980. Renaturation of enzymes after polyacrylamide gel electrophoresis in the presence of sodium dodecyl sulfate. J. Biol. Chem. **255:**7467–7473.

48. **Lacks, S.A., and S.S. Springhorn.** 1984. Cloning in *Streptococcus pneumoniae* of the gene for *Dpn*II DNA methylase. J. Bacteriol. **157:**934–936.

49. **Lacks, S.A., and S.S. Springhorn.** 1984. Transfer of recombinant plasmids containing the gene for *Dpn*II DNA methylase into strains of *Streptococcus pneumoniae* that produce *Dpn*I or *Dpn*II restriction endonucleases. J. Bacteriol. **158:**905–909.

50. **Lopez de Felipe, F., M.A. Corrales, and P. Lopez.** 1994. Comparative analysis of gene expression in *Streptococcus pneumoniae* and *Lactococcus lactis*. FEMS Microbiol. Lett. **122:**289–296.

51. **Lopez, P., M. Espinosa, B. Greenberg, and S.A. Lacks.** 1987. Sulfonamide resistance in *Streptococcus pneumoniae:* DNA sequence of the gene encoding dihydropteroate synthase and characterization of the enzyme. J. Bacteriol. **169:**4320–4326.

52. **Lopez, P., M. Espinosa, D.L. Stassi, and S.A. Lacks.** 1982. Facilitation of plasmid transfer in *Streptococcus pneumoniae* by chromosomal homology. J. Bacteriol. **150:**692–701.

53. **Lopez, P., S. Martinez, A. Diaz, M. Espinosa, and S.A. Lacks.** 1989. Characterization of the *polA* gene of *Streptococcus pneumoniae* and comparison of the DNA polymerase I it encodes to homologous enzymes from *Escherichia coli* and phage T7. J. Biol. Chem. **264:**4255–4263.

54. **Mannarelli, B.M., and S.A. Lacks.** 1984. Ectopic integration of chromosomal genes in *Streptococcus pneumoniae*. J. Bacteriol. **160:**867–873.

55. **Martin, B., H. Prats, and J.P. Claverys.** 1985. Cloning of the *hexA* mismatch repair gene of *Streptococcus pneumoniae* and identification of the product. Gene **34:**293–303.

56. **Martinez, S., P. Lopez, M. Espinosa, and S.A. Lacks.** 1986. Cloning of a gene encoding a DNA polymerase-exonuclease of *Streptococcus pneumoniae*. Gene **44:**79–88.

57. **Mejean, V., and J.P. Claverys.** 1988. Polarity of DNA entry in transformation of *Streptococcus pneumoniae*. Mol. Gen. Genet. **213:**444–448.

58. **Mejean, V., J.P. Claverys, H. Vasseghi, and A.M. Sicard.** 1981. Rapid cloning of specific DNA fragments of *Streptococcus pneumoniae* by vector integration into the chromosome followed by endonucleolytic excision. Gene **15:**289–293.

59. **Mejean, V., J.C. Devedjian, I. Rives, G. Alloing, and J.P. Claverys.** 1991. Uracil-DNA glycosylase affects mismatch repair efficiency in transformation and bisulphite-induced mutagenesis in *Streptococcus pneumoniae*. Nucl. Acids Res. **19:**5525–5531.

60. **Morrison, D.A.** 1997. Streptococcal competence for genetic transformation: Regulation by peptide pheromones. Microb. Drug. Resist. **3:**27–37.

61. **Morrison, D.A., and W.R. Guild.** 1973. Breakage prior to entry of donor DNA in *pneumococcus* transformation. Biochim. Biophys. Acta **299:**545–556.

62. **Morrison, D.A., and B. Mannarelli.** 1979. Transformation in pneumococcus: Nuclease resistance of deoxyribonucleic acid in the eclipse complex. J. Bacteriol. **140:**655–665.

63. **Morrison, D.A., M-C. Trombe, M.K. Hayden, G.A. Waszak, and J.-D. Chen.** 1984. Isolation of transformation-deficient *Streptococcus pneumoniae* mutants defective in control of competence, using insertion-duplication mutagenesis with the erythromycin resistance determinant of pAMβ1. J. Bacteriol. **159:**870–876.

64. **Morse, H.G., and L.S. Lerman.** 1969. A genetic analysis by transformation of a group of uracil-requiring mutants of *Diplococcus pneumoniae*. Genetics **61:**41–60.

65. **Prats, H., B. Martin, and J.P. Claverys.** 1985. The *hexB* mismatch repair gene of *Streptococcus pneumoniae:* Characterization, cloning and identification of the product. Mol. Gen. Genet. **200:**482–489.

66. **Prats, H., B. Martin, P. Pognonec, A.-C. Burger, and J.P. Claverys.** 1985. A plasmid vector allowing positive selection in *Streptococcus pneumoniae*. Gene **39:**41–48.

67. **Priebe, S.D., S.M. Hadi, B. Greenberg, and S.A. Lacks.** 1988. Nucleotide sequence of the *hexA* gene for DNA mismatch repair in *Streptococcus pneumoniae* and homology of *hexA* to *mutS* of *Escherichia coli* and *Salmonella typhimurium*. J. Bacteriol. **170:**190–196.

68. **Prudhomme, M., B. Martin, V. Mejean, and J.P. Claverys.** 1989. Nucleotide sequence of the *Streptococcus pneumoniae hexB* mismatch repair gene: Homology of HexB to MutL of *Salmonella typhimurium* and to PMS1 of *Saccharomyces cerevisiae*. J. Bacteriol. **171:**5332–5338.

69. **Puyet, A., B. Greenberg, and S.A. Lacks.** 1989. The *exoA* gene of *Streptococcus pneumoniae* and its product, a DNA exonuclease with apurinic endonuclease activity. J. Bacteriol. **171:**2278–2286.

70. **Puyet, A., B. Greenberg, and S.A. Lacks.** 1990. Genetic and structural characterization of EndA, a membrane-bound nuclease required for transformation of *Streptococcus pneumoniae*. J. Mol. Biol. **171:**727–738.

71. **Rhee, D.K., and D.A. Morrison.** 1988. Genetic transformation in *Streptococcus pneumoniae:* Molecular cloning and characterization of *recP*, a gene required for genetic recombination. J. Bacteriol. **170:**630–637.

72. **Ronda, C., J.L. Garcia, E. Garcia, J.M. Sanchez-Puelles, and R. Lopez.** 1987. Biological role of the pneumococcal amidase: Cloning of the *lytA* gene in *Streptococcus pneumoniae*. Eur. J. Biochem. **164:**621–624.

73. **Rosenthal, A.L., and S.A. Lacks.** 1977. Nuclease detection in SDS-polyacrylamide gel electrophoresis. Anal. Biochem. **80:**76–90.

74. **Sabelnikov, A.G., B. Greenberg, and S.A. Lacks.** 1995. An extended −10 promoter alone directs transcription of the *Dpn*II operon of *Streptococcus pneumoniae*. J. Mol. Biol. **250:**144–155.

75. **Saunders, C.W., and W.R. Guild.** 1981. Monomer plasmid DNA transforms *Streptococcus pneumoniae*. Mol. Gen. Genet. **181:**57–62.

76. **Seto, H., and A. Tomasz.** 1974. Early stages in DNA binding and uptake during genetic transformation of pneumococci. Proc. Natl. Acad. Sci. USA **71:**1493–1498.

77. **Seto, H., and A. Tomasz.** 1976. Calcium-requiring step in the uptake of deoxyribonucleic acid through the surface of competent pneumococci. J. Bacteriol. **126:**1113–1118.

78. **Shean, C.S., and M.E. Gottesman.** 1992. Translation of the prophage λ *cI* transcript. Cell **70:**513–522.

79. **Shine, J., and L. Dalgarno.** 1975. Determinant of cistron specificity in bacterial ribosomes. Nature (London) **254:**34–38.

80. **Sicard, N., and A.M. Estevenon.** 1990. Excision-repair capacity in *Streptococcus pneumoniae:* Cloning and expressin of a uvr-like gene. Mutat. Res. **235:**195–201.

81. **Sprengart, M.L., H.P. Fatscher, and E. Fuchs.** 1990. The initiation of translation in *E. coli:* Apparent base pairing between the 16s rRNA and downstream sequences of the mRNA. *Nucl. Acids Res. 18:*1719–1723.

82. **Stassi, D.L., and S.A. Lacks.** 1982. Effect of strong promoters on the cloning in *Escherichia coli* of DNA fragments from *Streptococcus pneumoniae.* Gene **18:**319–328.

83. **Stassi, D.L., P. Lopez, M. Espinosa, and S. A. Lacks.** 1981. Cloning of chromosomal genes in *Streptococcus pneumoniae.* Proc. Natl. Acad. Sci. USA **78:**7028–7032.

84. **Tiraby, G., and M.S. Fox.** 1973. Marker discrimination in transformation and mutation of pneumococcus. Proc. Natl. Acad. Sci. USA **70:**3541–3545.

85. **Tiraby, G., and M.A. Sicard.** 1973. Integration efficiencies of spontaneous mutant alleles of *amiA* locus in pneumococcal transformation. J. Bacteriol. **116:**1130–1135.

86. **Tomasz, A.** 1966. Model for the mechanism controlling the expression of competent state in pneumococcus cultures. J. Bacteriol. **91:**1050–1061.

87. **Vasseghi, H., J.P. Claverys, and A.M. Sicard.** 1981. Mechanism of integrating foreign DNA during transformation in *Streptococcus pneumoniae*, pp. 137–154. *In* M. Polsinelli, and G. Mazza (eds.), Transformation 1980, Cotswold Press, Oxford.

88. **Vovis, G.F., and S. Lacks.** 1977. Complementary action of restriction enzymes Endo R.*Dpn*I and Endo R.*Dpn*II on bacteriophage fl DNA. J. Mol. Biol. **115:**525–538.

89. **Yother, J., L.S. McDaniel, and D.E. Briles.** 1986. Transformation of encapsulated *Streptococcus pneumoniae.* J. Bacteriol. **168:**1463–1465.

90. **Zhang, Y.-B., S. Ayalew, and S.A. Lacks.** 1997. The *rnhB* gene encoding ribonuclease HII of *Streptococcus pneumoniae* and evidence of conserved motifs in eucaryotic genes. J. Bacteriol. **179:**3828–3836.

Address reprint requests to:
Sanford A. Lacks
Biology Department
Brookhaven National Laboratory
Upton, NY 11973

Part 3

*Capsule, Cell Wall, and
Virulence Factors*

Pneumococcal Polysaccharides: A Chemical View

JOHANNIS P. KAMERLING

It is hoped that further work in this field will eventually give us more thorough understanding of the chemical basis underlying the specificity of the many types of pneumococci

Report on the analysis of the CPS of serotype 3
(Reeves and Goebel[255])

INTRODUCTION

SINCE ITS FIRST ISOLATION, independently by Sternberg[302] and Pasteur[299] in 1881, the Gram-positive encapsulated[92,302] bacterium *Streptococcus pneumoniae* (pneumococcus) has been one of the most widely studied microorganisms in medicine, biology and chemistry. Early reviews, mainly focusing on the bacteriology of the pneumococcus and the infections it causes, have been published by White[332] and Heffron,[105] and reviews by Austrian updating the newer insights concerning the pneumococcus, the diseases it causes, and the potential for their prevention, appeared in 1981.[16,17]

In the twenties, Avery and coworkers made a number of observations that formed the basis for the scientific bridge between the pathogenic bacterium and the carbohydrate world. At first instance, the presence was reported of a type-specific soluble substance in filtrates of pneumococcal cultures and in the sera and urine of infected humans and rabbits.[82] The specific soluble substances turned out to be type-specific capsular polysaccharides (CPSs).[20,107] Of high importance was the antigenicity of these polysaccharides, a finding that paved the way for the use of pneumococcal polysaccharides as vaccines. It has to be said that the capsules of the pneumococcus were the first nonprotein substances shown to be antigenic in humans.

S. pneumoniae, formerly known as *Diplococcus pneumoniae*, forms part of the normal microflora, and most humans carry pneumococci in the upper respiratory tract. Children may be colonized with pneumococci on the day of birth, usually with a serotype also found in the mother. The organism is an oval or spherical coccus of 0.5–1.25 μm in diameter, surrounded by the polysaccharide capsule. The capsules, highly hydrated shells around the bacterium, are almost invariably polyanionic, and they modulate the passage of molecules and ions to the bacterial cell envelope, the adherence of the bacterium to biological and inorganic surfaces, and the formation of biofilms and microcolonies.[142]

The epidemiology of *S. pneumoniae* is highly complex. Infections with this bacterium is still one of the leading causes of death. Disease occurs when the host is invaded and infection established. The most common infections caused by pneumococci are otitis media, pneumonia, meningitis, bacteremia, and septicemia. The nontoxic CPSs are mainly responsible for the virulence of the bacterium,[216] and during infection they inhibit phagocytosis by polymorphonuclear neutrophils. The defense mechanism of *S. pneumoniae* is based on humoral immunity, whereby antibodies directed to the CPS will protect humans to infections with viable pneumococci.

Nowadays, a total of 90 serotypes have been described.[111,153,201] They are distinguished by chemical differences in their CPSs, and, in turn, on the ability of the immune system of rabbits to recognize these structural differences and to respond with specific antibodies against the antigens of each different type.[286] Two different systems of nomenclature exist for the pneumococcal serotypes, namely, the Danish system and the American system.[110,111,153,200,201] The Danish system is based on cross-reactions between different types, so that serologically cross-reactive types are assigned to a common serogroup, with individual serotypes within each group distinguished by the trailing letter. In the American system, serotypes are numbered sequentially (connected with the order of their discovery); it does not recognize antigenic cross-reactivity among types. In Table 1, a survey of the *S. pneumoniae* serotypes, as updated in 1995 by Henrichsen in the generally used Danish system, is presented,[111] together with the antigenic formulas that represent arbitrary designations of cross-reactions as observed by the capsular reaction.[110,111,153,200,201] For completeness, in Table 2, depicting the primary structures (repeating units) of the CPSs analyzed so far, both the Danish and the American nomenclature system are included.

Early vaccines that were used were crude, whole-cell preparations.[335] The progress in the subsequent application of pneumococcal CPSs as vaccines against *S. pneumoniae* was highly influenced by the discovery of antibiotics. It meant a decreased interest in the capsules after the initial discoveries.[107] It should be noted that although the efficacy of a four-valent polysaccharide vaccine was demonstrated convincingly in 1945,[202] the introduction of commercial six-valent polysaccharide vaccines

---

Bijvoet Center, Department of Bio-Organic Chemistry, Utrecht University, 3508 TB Utrecht, The Netherlands.

TABLE 1.   TYPE DESIGNATIONS (DANISH NOMENCLATURE) AND ANTIGENIC FORMULAS OF
90 TYPES OF *Streptococcus pneumoniae*, AS UPDATED IN 1995 BY HENRICHSEN[111]

Type	Antigenic formula	Type	Antigenic formula
1[@]	1a	19C	19a, 19c, 19f, 7h
2[@]	2a	20[@]	20a, 20b, 7g
3[@]	3a	21	21a
4[@]	4a	22F[@]	22a, 22b
5[@]	5a	22A	22a, 22c
6A	6a, 6b	23F[@]	23a, 23b, 18b
6B[@]	6a, 6c	23A	23a, 23c, 15a
7F[@]	7a, 7b	23B	23a, 23b, 23d
7A	7a, 7b, 7c	24F	24a, 24b, 24d, 7h
7B	7a, 7d, 7e, 7h	24A	24a, 24c, 24d
7C	7a, 7d, 7f, 7g, 7h	24B	24a, 24b, 24e, 7h
8[@]	8a	25F	25a, 25b
9A	9a, 9c, 9d	25A	25a, 25c, 38a
9L	9a, 9b, 9c, 9f	27	27a, 27b
9N[@]	9a, 9b, 9e	28F	28a, 28b, 16b, 23d
9V[@]	9a, 9c, 9d, 9g	28A	28a, 28c, 23d
10F	10a, 10b	29	29a, 29b, 13b
10A[@]	10a, 10c, 10d	31	31a, 20b
10B	10a, 10b, 10c, 10d, 10e	32F	32a, 27b
10C	10a, 10b, 10c, 10f	32A	32a, 32b, 27b
11F	11a, 11b, 11e, 11g	33F[@]	33a, 33b, 33d
11A[@]	11a, 11c, 11d, 11e	33A	33a, 33b, 33d, 20b
11B	11a, 11b, 11f, 11g	33B	33a, 33c, 33d, 33f
11C	11a, 11b, 11c, 11d, 11f	33C	33a, 33c, 33e
11D	11a, 11b, 11c, 11e	33D	33a, 33c, 33d, 33f, 6a
12F[@]	12a, 12b, 12d	34	34a, 34b
12A	12a, 12c, 12d	35F	35a, 35b, 34b
12B	12a, 12b, 12c, 12e	35A	35a, 35c, 20b
13	13a, 13b	35B	35a, 35c, 29b
14[@]	14a	35C	35a, 35c, 20b, 42a
15F	15a, 15b, 15c, 15f	36	36a, 9e
15A	15a, 15c, 15d, 15g	37	37a
15B[@]	15a, 15b, 15d, 15e, 15h	38	38a, 25b
15C	15a, 15d, 15e	39	39a, 10d
16F	16a, 16b, 11d	40	40a, 7g, 7h
16A	16a, 16c	41F	41a, 41b
17F[@]	17a, 17b	41A	41a
17A	17a, 17c	42	42a, 20b, 35c
18F	18a, 18b, 18c, 18f	43	43a, 43b
18A	18a, 18b, 18d	44	44a, 44b, 12b, 12d
18B	18a, 18b, 18e, 18g	45	45a
18C[@]	18a, 18b, 18c, 18e	46	46a, 12c, 44b
19F[@]	19a, 19b, 19d	47F	47a, 35a, 35b
19A[@]	19a, 19c, 19d	47A	47a, 43b
19B	19a, 19c, 19e, 7h	48	48a

[@], serotypes of which the CPSs are present in the commercial 23-valent vaccine.[267]
The antigenic formulas represent arbitrary designations of cross-reactions as observed by the capsular reaction.

was not met with great enthusiasm. The climate changed in the 1960s, because then it turned out that the mortality from systemic pneumococcal infections remained high despite the early institution of appropriate antimicrobial treatment. In 1977 a commercial 14-valent polysaccharide vaccine was introduced,[17,267] followed in 1983 by a commercial 23-valent vaccine (Pneumovax II; Pnu-Immune 23) that covers almost 90% of the infections caused by *S. pneumoniae* in the United States.[267] The addition "in the USA" is essential, because it has

been shown that large variations can exist in the occurrence of serotypes of *S. pneumoniae* in different geographic areas and, in a specific region, also in time. The serotypes that furnish the components for the 23-valent vaccine have been indicated in Table 1. The vaccine contains 25 μg of purified CPS from each serotype.

Indications for immunization with the 23-valent CPS vaccine have been formulated elsewhere[286] as follows: "(1) Adults with chronic illnesses or conditions that are associated with increased frequency and/or severity of serious pneumococcal infections. These include chronic pulmonary or chronic cardiovascular disease, chronic renal failure, alcoholism, diabetes mellitus, splenic dysfunction or anatomic asplenia, Hodgkin's disease, multiple myeloma, cirrhosis, CSF leaks, and conditions associated with immunosuppression; (2) Elderly adults, especially those over 65 years of age, who otherwise are healthy; (3) Children 2 years of age or older with chronic illnesses or conditions such as anatomic or functional asplenia, nephrotic syndrome, CSF leak, and conditions associated with immunosuppression."

Infections with *S. pneumoniae* continue to cause significant morbidity and mortality in humans, despite the availability of effective antibiotic therapy (although the presence of drug-resistant pneumococci is growing) and of a multispecific capsular polysaccharide vaccine. Focusing on vaccination, a number of disadvantages still remain with the commercial 23-valent polysaccharide vaccine (serotypes 1, 2, 3, 4, 5, 6B, 7F, 8, 9N, 9V, 10A, 11A, 12F, 14, 15B, 17F, 18C, 19F, 19A, 20, 22F, 23F, 33F). The immune response in infants less than two years old is poor. The latter situation is highly undesirable, as the children experience one of the highest incidence of disease caused by pneumococci. Unfortunately, CPSs form the classical example of T-cell–independent immunogens (thymus-independent type 2 antigens). Typically the antibody response drops rapidly in children, and a poor immunological memory exists; there is no response in neonates. However, a switch from thymus-independent to thymus-dependent immunogens can be realized by coupling the polysaccharides to proteins (proteins are predominantly thymus-dependent immunogens). Although early studies appeared already around 1930,[21,22] recently, much attention is paid to the clinical value of these polysaccharide-protein conjugates as vaccines.[84,154,161,266,268,280,300] The finding of a thymus-independent → thymus-dependent switch for fragments of CPSs coupled to proteins, has also initiated the testing of oligosaccharide-protein conjugates.[84,154] Some pneumococcal conjugate vaccines are already the subject of clinical phase-III trials. Typical multivalent preparations tested are Pn-CRM (CPSs or CPS fragments of serotypes 4, 6B, 9V, 14, 18C, 19F, 23F; carrier CRM$_{197}$, a non-toxic variant of diphtheria toxin), Pn-D (CPSs of serotypes 3, 4, 6B, 9V, 14, 18C, 19F, 23F; carrier diphtheria toxoid), Pn-T (CPSs of serotypes 3, 4, 6B, 9V, 14, 18C, 19F, 23F; carrier tetanus toxoid), and Pn-OMPC (CPSs of serotypes 4, 6B, 9V, 14, 18C, 19F, 23F; carrier meningococcal outer membrane protein complex).[154,161] For information on spontaneous capsular transformation events occurring among pneumococcal strains, which may have implications for the construction of effective conjugate vaccines, see other sources[15,23,31,101,220] and references cited therein.

In addition to the CPSs, the pneumococci produce two common antigenic polysaccharides: A teichoic acid (C-polysaccharide or C-substance) and a lipoteichoic acid (Forssman antigen; F-antigen).[294] The C-polysaccharide of the pneumococcus was first described by Tillett and Francis[309] in 1930, and the F-antigen by Goebel and coworkers[99] in 1943. The structure of the teichoic acid part of the F-antigen is identical to that of the C-polysaccharide.[91] In pneumococcal infections, both compounds may have a pathophysiological role. For the interaction with the autolytic enzyme, *N*-acetylmuramyl-L-alanine amidase, the phosphocholine residues of both polymers are essential.

Studies on the attachment of the CPSs to the bacterial cells demonstrated for the examined serotypes 2, 4, 6A, 6B, 7F, 8, 14, 19F, and 23F a so far unknown linkage to the peptidoglycan present in the cell wall.[293,298] Only the outer surface of the walls is decorated with CPSs.[295] For serotype 3, such a linkage was not indicated.[298] Also the C-polysaccharide is linked by an unknown linkage region to the peptidoglycan layer,[310] whereby it is uniformly distributed on both the inside and the outside of the cell walls.[295,297] Combining these data, it has been suggested that the CPS and the C-polysaccharide of the pneumococcus have different attachment sites on the peptidoglycan, which means that they are connected indirectly to each other.[293,298] The F-antigen is hydrophobically anchored in the cytoplasmic membrane by its ester-linked fatty acids.[118,297,310]

Over the years the "pneumococcal area" has been extensively reviewed, and only a selection of reviews is included in the present chapter. For reviews mainly dealing with biological, immunological, and pathogenetic aspects, see other sources.[6,17,22,54,70,90,98,106,138,155,219,230,246,286,310,312,316] For reviews especially focused on vaccines, see these sources.[17–19,22,51,53,55,89,90,132–135,161,180,182,209,211,265–268,278,286,287] Information with respect to clinical resistance to antibiotics is found elsewhere[12,31,49,122,163,187,217,311] and references cited therein.

In this chapter, specific attention is paid to the structural chemistry and biochemistry of pneumococcal polysaccharides. Furthermore, chemical aspects related to pneumococcal carbohydrate conjugates are discussed.

STRUCTURAL ANALYSIS OF BACTERIAL POLYSACCHARIDES

The primary structure of carbohydrate chains is defined by several parameters: (i) nature and number of the constituent monosaccharides; (ii) sequence and ring size of the monosaccharides; (iii) type and anomeric configuration of the glycosidic linkages; and (iv) nonsugar substituents (Fig. 1).

Over the years protocols for the structure determination of bacterial polysaccharides have changed rapidly, and especially the introduction of combined gas-liquid chromatography/electron impact mass spectrometry (GLC-EIMS) and nuclear magnetic resonance (NMR) spectroscopy in the period 1965–1975 were real landmarks. In parallel with these analytical improvements and the possibilities to scale down the amounts of material necessary for structural analysis, useful degradation protocols were improved or developed. The more recent fascinating developments in mass spectrometry (MS) contribute in another way to the enhancement of the reliability of followed analysis strategies. Several comprehensive reviews on GLC, MS, and NMR of carbohydrates related to bacterial polysaccharide analysis have already appeared and a series of relevant reviews have been included in the reference list.[14,45,46,76,120,123,149,165,193,198,251]

Nowadays, structural analysis of isolated bacterial polysaccharides comprises a number of steps. Monosaccharide analysis is generally carried out using GLC and GLC-EIMS after solvolysis of the polysaccharide. Frequently used derivatives are alditol acetates and trimethylsilylated methyl glycosides.[149] Also absolute configurations are determined by GLC, mainly using trimethylsilylated (+)- or (−)-2-butyl glycosides.[149] For

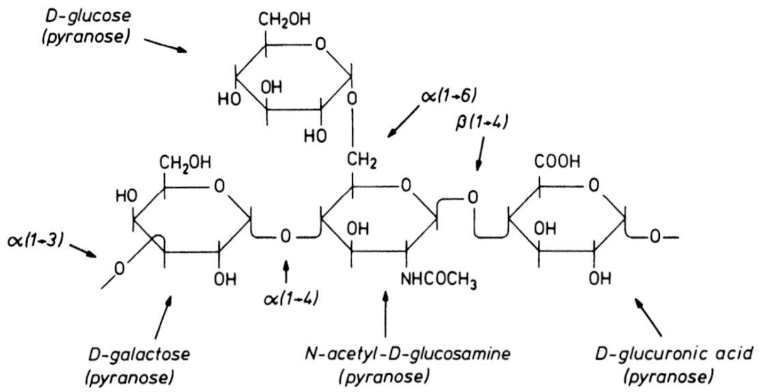

FIG. 1. Schematic presentation of the parameters, which define the primary structure of a carbohydrate chain.

the determination of substitution patterns methylation analysis is applied using different protocols, whereby GLC-EIMS plays a major role.[45,123,149,198] Frequently used derivatives are the partially methylated alditol acetates. To generate (overlapping) fragments, specific degradation techniques such as partial solvolysis, acetolysis, periodate oxidation, uronic acid degradation, and de-N-acetylation/deamination are applied.[193] When possible, to generate fragments also endo-glycosidases are used. Fragments are analyzed by monosaccharide and methylation analysis. In case of mass spectrometry, besides electron impact ionization,[149,165,198] also other ionization techniques are applied such as chemical ionization (CI),[149] fast-atom bombardment (FAB),[76,284] electrospray ionization (ESI),[256] and matrix-assisted laser desorption ionization (MALDI).[104] Especially the soft ionization techniques are of great importance in analyzing oligosaccharide fragments. Mass analyzers relevant for MS of carbohydrates are sector instruments (magnetic and electrostatic deflection), quadrupole (Q) mass filters, time-of-flight (TOF) analyzers, and Fourier transform ion cyclotron resonance mass spectrometers (FT-ICR). In this context also techniques such as mass-analyzed ion kinetic energy spectrometry (MIKES), collision induced dissociation (CID) and single/multiple-stage tandem mass spectrometry (MS-MS; MS^n)[318] have to be mentioned. Quite often ^{1}H, ^{13}C, and ^{31}P NMR spectroscopy play a major role, and 2D techniques such as correlated spectroscopy (COSY), total correlation spectroscopy (TOCSY), heteronuclear multiple quantum coherence spectroscopy (HMQC), heteronuclear multiple bond correlation spectroscopy (HMBC), nuclear Overhauser enhancement spectroscopy (NOESY), and rotating frame nuclear Overhauser enhancement spectroscopy (ROESY) are of utmost importance.

PRIMARY STRUCTURES OF PNEUMOCOCCAL CAPSULAR POLYSACCHARIDES

For the pneumococcal polysaccharides, it may be clear that the first analyses were carried out following more traditional protocols than applying MS and NMR spectroscopy, and a first comprehensive survey of structures has been published in 1964,[121] followed by a reexamination in 1976.[177] In this context, it is worthwhile to mention that the first CPS analyzed, that of serotype 3 (1941), has stood the test of time. In several

reviews[132–135,156,316] that have appeared after 1976, updated surveys of primary structures have been included, thereby not only paying attention to data of polysaccharide structures not reviewed before, but also to revisions of earlier published structures. Of course, reinvestigations were always carried out using techniques more advanced than those available to earlier investigators. In Table 2, a more updated and revised survey (1998) of primary structures of CPSs of *S. pneumoniae* is presented. It should be noted that the way of presentation of repeating units in Table 2 has not in mind to reflect their way of biosynthesis (chemical versus biological repeating units). For those who are interested in structural studies, besides the reference describing the final structure, also references have been included giving insight into the history of the structural analysis of a specific CPS, including deviating elder proposals.

As mentioned already, at the moment 90 different types of *S. pneumoniae* are known,[111] each elaborating its own, type-specific capsular polysaccharide, deposited on the outer surface of the cell wall of the specific strain. They are divided into 46 types/groups numbered 1–48 (numbers 26 and 30 are not in use; see Table 1).

Although not always, the purification of CPSs may be difficult. Especially the contamination with small amounts of C-polysaccharide can be confusing in the interpretation of initial analytical results. The CPSs are built up from repeating oligosaccharide units and are of high molecular mass. For a series of CPSs (serotypes 4, 6B, 9V, 14, 18C, 19F, 23F) molar mass and molar mass distribution measurements have been reported.[34] The most frequently detected monosaccharides, occurring in different combinations in the CPSs (Table 2), comprise α/β-D-glucose, α/β-D-galactose, α/β-L-rhamnose, N-acetyl-α/β-D-glucosamine, N-acetyl-α/β-D-galactosamine, N-acetyl-β-D-mannosamine, N-acetyl-α-L-fucosamine, and α/β-D-glucuronic acid. In addition to these monosaccharides also α-L-fucose (serotype 19A), β-D-ribose (serotype 7B, 19B, 19C), α-D-galacturonic acid (serotype 1), N-acetyl-β-D-mannosaminuronic acid (serotype 12F, 12A), N-acetyl-α-L-pneumosamine (serotype 5), 2-acetamido-4-amino-2,4,6-trideoxy-α-D-galactose (serotype 1) and 2-acetamido-2,6-dideoxy-D-xylo-hexos-4-ulose (serotype 5) can be present. In all cases, except D-galactose and D-ribose, only pyranose rings occur; D-galactose occurs in both pyranose and furanose ring forms, and D-ribose in the furanose form only.

TABLE 2. UPDATED AND REVISED SURVEY OF PRIMARY STRUCTURES OF CAPSULAR POLYSACCHARIDES OF *Streptococcus pneumoniae*

Serotype[a]		Primary structure[b]	References	Year/reference (final structure)
Danish	American			
1	1	→3)-AAT-α-D-Galp-(1→4)-α-D-GalpA-(1→3)-α-D-GalpA-(1→ +0.3 OAc	103 195	1980[195]
2	2	→4)-β-D-Glcp-(1→3)-α-L-Rhap-(1→3)-α-L-Rhap-(1→3)-β-L-Rhap-(1→ 2 ↑ 1 α-D-GlcpA-(1→6)-α-D-Glcp	28,30 130,158 178,179	1988[130]
3	3	→3)-β-D-GlcpA-(1→4)-β-D-Glcp-(1→	119,255	1941[255]
4	4	→3)-β-D-ManpNAc-(1→3)-α-L-FucpNAc-(1→3)-α-D-GalpNAc-(1→4)-α-D-Galp2,3(S)Pyr-(1→	109 113,114 124,140 143,191	1990[140]
5	5	→4)-β-D-Glcp-(1→4)-α-L-FucpNAc-(1→3)-β-D-Sugp-(1→ 3 ↑ 1 α-L-PnepNAc-(1→2)-β-D-GlcpA	26,27 29,50 126	1985[126]
6A	6	→2)-α-D-Galp-(1→3)-α-D-Glcp-(1→3)-α-L-Rhap-(1→3)-D-Rib-ol-(5→P→	26,177 253,254	1976[177]
6B	26	→2)-α-D-Galp-(1→3)-α-D-Glcp-(1→3)-α-L-Rhap-(1→4)-D-Rib-ol-(5→P→	159	1979[159]
7F	51	→6)-α-D-Galp-(1→3)-β-L-Rhap2Ac-(1→4)-β-D-Glcp-(1→3)-β-D-GalpNAc-(1→ 4 ↑ 1 2 α-D-GlcpNAc-(1→2)-α-L-Rhap ↑ 1 β-D-Galp	60 213,314	1988[213]
7A	7	→6)-α-D-Galp-(1→3)-β-L-Rhap2Ac-(1→4)-β-D-Glcp-(1→3)-β-D-GalpNAc-(1→ 4 ↑ 1 α-D-GlcpNAc-(1→2)-α-L-Rhap	24	1990[24]

(cont.)

TABLE 2. (continued)

Serotype[a]		Primary structure[b]	References	Year/reference (final structure)
Danish	American			
7B	48	→6)-α-D-GlcpNAc-(1→2)-α-L-Rhap-(1→2)-β-L-Rhap-(1→4)-β-D-Glcp-(1→4)-α-D-Glcp-(1→P→ 　　　　　　　　　　　　3 　　　　　　　　　　　　↑ 　　　　　　　　　　　　1 　　　　　　β-D-Ribf-(1→4)-α-L-Rhap	131	1991[131]
7C	50	No information		
8	8	→4)-β-D-GlcpA-(1→4)-β-D-Glcp-(1→4)-α-D-Glcp-(1→4)-α-D-Galp-(1→	146	1957[146]
9A	33	→4)-α-D-GlcpA-(1→3)-α-D-Galp-(1→3)-β-D-ManpNAc-(1→4)-β-D-Glcp-(1→4)-α-D-Glcp-(1→	38 258,275	1988[258]
9L	49	→4)-α-D-GlcpA-(1→3)-α-D-Galp-(1→3)-β-D-ManpNAc-(1→4)-β-D-Glcp-(1→4)-α-D-GlcpNAc-(1→	261	1984[261]
9N	9	→4)-α-D-GlcpA-(1→3)-α-D-Glcp-(1→3)-β-D-ManpNAc-(1→4)-β-D-Glcp-(1→4)-α-D-GlcpNAc-(1→	44,73 116,144 225,270 305	1985[144]
9V	68	→4)-α-D-GlcpA-(1→3)-α-D-Galp-(1→3)-β-D-ManpNAc-(1→4)-β-D-Glcp-(1→ 　　　　　　　　　　　　　　　　　　　　　　　　2Ac (3%) 　　　　　　　　　　　　　　　　　　　　　　　　3Ac (4%) 　　　2Ac (17%)　　　4Ac (6%) 　　　3Ac (25%)　　　6Ac (55%)	237,275	1991[275]
10F	10	→6)-β-D-Galf-(1→3)-α-D-Galp-(1→4)-β-D-GalpNAc-(1→3)-α-D-Galp-(1→2)-D-Rib-ol-(5→P→ 　　　　　　　　　　　　　　　　　　　6 　　　　　　　　　　　　　　　　　　　↑ 　　　　　　　　　　　　　　　　　　　1 　　　　　　　　　　　　　　　　β-D-Galf β-D-Galp 1 ↓ 6	316	1990[316]
10A	34	→5)-β-D-Galf-(1→3)-β-D-Galp-(1→4)-β-D-GalpNAc-(1→3)-α-D-Galp-(1→2)-D-Rib-ol-(5→P→ 　　　　　　　　　　　　　　　　　3 　　　　　　　　　　　　　　　　　↑ 　　　　　　　　　　　　　　　　　1 　　　　　　　　　　　　　　β-D-Galf	141 248,249	1995[141]

10B	No information		
10C	No information		
11F	→6)-α-D-Glc$p$NAc3Ac$_{0.5}$-(1→4)-α-D-Gal$p$2Ac-(1→3)-β-D-Gal$p$-(1→4)-β-D-Glc$p$-(1→ $\quad\quad$ 4 $\quad\quad$ ↑ $\quad$ Rib-ol-(1→P $\quad\quad\quad$ +0.5 OAc	262,263	1985[262]
11A	→6)-α-D-Glc$p$2/3Ac-(1→4)-α-D-Gal$p$-(1→3)-β-D-Gal$p$-(1→4)-β-D-Glc$p$-(1→ $\quad\quad$ 4 $\quad\quad$ ↑ $\quad$ Gro-(1→P $\quad\quad\quad$ +OAc	160,263	1988[263]
11B	→6)-α-D-Glc$p$NAc3Ac$_{0.9}$-(1→4)-α-D-Gal$p$-(1→3)-β-D-Gal$p$-(1→4)-β-D-Glc$p$-(1→ $\quad\quad$ 4 $\quad\quad$ ↑ $\quad$ Rib-ol-(1→P $\quad\quad\quad$ +0.5 OAc	262,263	1985[262]
11C	→6)-α-D-Glc$p$NAc3Ac-(1→4)-α-D-Gal$p$-(1→3)-β-D-Gal$p$-(1→4)-β-D-Glc$p$-(1→ $\quad\quad$ 4 $\quad\quad$ ↑ $\quad$ Gro-(1→P	262,263	1985[262]
11D	No information		
12F	→4)-α-L-Fuc$p$NAc-(1→3)-β-D-Gal$p$NAc-(1→4)-β-D-Man$p$NAcA-(1→ $\quad\quad$ 3 $\quad\quad$ ↑ $\quad\quad$ 1 $\quad$ α-D-Gal$p$ $\quad\quad\quad$ α-D-Glc$p$-(1→2)-α-D-Glc$p$	67,83 100,189	1981[189]
12A	→4)-α-L-Fuc$p$NAc-(1→3)-β-D-Glc$p$NAc-(1→4)-β-D-Man$p$NAcA-(1→ $\quad\quad$ 3 $\quad\quad$ ↑ $\quad\quad$ 1 $\quad$ α-D-Gal$p$NAc $\quad\quad\quad$ α-D-Glc$p$-(1→2)-α-D-Glc$p$	190	1983[190]
12B	No information		
13	→4)-β-D-Gal$p$-(1→4)-β-D-Glc$p$2/3Ac-(1→3)-β-D-Gal$f$-(1→4)-β-D-Glc$p$NAc-(1→4)-D-Rib-ol-(5→P→	285,329	1972[329]

(cont.)

TABLE 2. (continued)

Serotype[a]		Primary structure[b]	References	Year/reference (final structure)
Danish	American			
14	14	→6)-β-D-GlcpNAc-(1→3)-β-D-Galp-(1→4)-β-D-Glcp-(1→ 　　　4 　　　↑ 　　　1 　β-D-Galp	26,194	1977[194]
15F	15	→3)-α-D-Galp-(1→2)-β-D-Galp-(1→4)-β-D-GlcpNAc-(1→3)-β-D-Galp-(1→4)-β-D-Glcp-(1→ 　　　　　　　　　　3　　　　　　　+2 OAc 　　　　　　　　　　↑ 　　　　　　　Cho$_{0.2}$→P	238	1982[238]
15A	30	→3)-α-D-Galp-(1→2)-β-D-Galp-(1→4)-β-D-GlcpNAc-(1→3)-β-D-Galp-(1→4)-β-D-Glcp-(1→ 　　　　　　　　　　3 　　　　　　　　　　↑ 　　　　　　　Gro$_{0.7}$-(2→P	57	1984[57]
15B	54	→6)-β-D-GlcpNAc-(1→3)-β-D-Galp-(1→4)-β-D-Glcp-(1→ 　　　4　　　　　　+0.7 OAc 　　　↑ 　　　1 α-D-Galp-(1→2)-β-D-Galp 　　　　　　　　　　3 　　　　　　　　　　↑ 　　　　　　　Cho$_{0.2}$→P	127	1987[127]
15C	77	→6)-β-D-GlcpNAc-(1→3)-β-D-Galp-(1→4)-β-D-Glcp-(1→ 　　　4 　　　↑ 　　　1 α-D-Galp-(1→2)-β-D-Galp 　　　　　　　　　　3 　　　　　　　　　　↑ 　　　　　　　Cho$_{0.2}$→P	127	1987[127]
16F	16	Constituents: Glc, Gal, Rha, GlcN, GalN, and Gro-P	285	
16A	85	No information		

17F 17 →3)-β-L-Rha$p$-(1→4)-β-D-Glc$p$-(1→3)-α-D-Gal$p$-(1→3)-β-L-Rha$p$2Ac-(1→4)-α-L-Rha$p$-(1→2)-D-Ara-ol-(1→P→ 1996[134] 125
   4   134
   ↑
   1
α-D-Gal$p$

17A 78 →3)-β-D-Glc$p$-(1→3)-α-D-Gal$p$-(1→3)-β-L-Rha$p$2Ac-(1→4)-α-L-Rha$p$-(1→4)-β-D-Glc$p$A-(1→3)-β-D-Gal$f$-(1→ 1983[125] 125
   4   2
   ↑   ↑
   1   1
β-D-Gal$p$ α-D-Glc$p$

18F 18 →4)-β-D-Glc$p$-(1→4)-α-D-Glc$p$-(1→3)-β-L-Rha$p$2Ac-(1→ 1988[128] 85,128
Gro-(1→P
   ↓
   3
   2
   ↑
   1
α-D-Glc$p$6Ac

18A 44 →4)-β-D-Glc$p$-(1→4)-α-D-Glc$p$NAc-(1→3)-β-L-Rha$p$-(1→ 1988[129,274] 108
D-Gro-(1→P 129,274
   ↓
   3
   2
   ↑
   1
α-D-Glc$p$

18B 55 →4)-β-D-Glc$p$-(1→4)-α-D-Glc$p$-(1→3)-β-L-Rha$p$-(1→ 1997[150] 150
D-Gro-(1→P
   ↓
   3
   2
   ↑
   1
α-D-Glc$p$

18C 56 →4)-β-D-Glc$p$-(1→4)-α-D-Glc$p$-(1→3)-β-L-Rha$p$-(1→ 1990[196] 196
Gro-(1→P 199,239
   ↓
   3
   2
   ↑
   1
α-D-Glc$p$6Ac$_{0.3}$

(cont.)

TABLE 2. *(continued)*

Serotype Danish	Serotype American	Primary structure[b]	References	Year/reference (final structure)
19F	19	→4)-β-D-Man*p*NAc-(1→4)-α-D-Glc*p*-(1→2)-α-L-Rha*p*-(1→P→	137 181,210 224,336	1980[137,224]
19A	57	→4)-β-D-Man*p*NAc-(1→4)-α-D-Glc*p*-(1→3)-α-L-Rha*p*-(1→P→ α-L-Fuc*p*-(1→P at 3	152,181	1983[152]
		→4)-β-D-Man*p*NAc-(1→4)-α-D-Glc*p*-(1→2)-α-L-Rha*p*-(1→P→ β-D-Glc*p*NAc-(1→3)-β-D-Gal*p*-(1→P at 2	181,183	1980[181]
19B	58	→4)-β-D-Man*p*NAc-(1→4)-β-D-Glc*p*-(1→4)-β-D-Man*p*NAc-(1→4)-α-L-Rha*p*-(1→P→ β-D-Rib*f*-(1→4)-α-L-Rha*p* (3←1) β-D-Glc*p*	41	1992[41]
19C	59	→4)-β-D-Man*p*NAc-(1→4)-β-D-Glc*p*-(1→4)-β-D-Man*p*NAc-(1→4)-α-L-Rha*p*-(1→P→ β-D-Glc*p* (1→6) β-D-Rib*f*-(1→4)-α-L-Rha*p* (3←1)	41	1992[41]
20	20	→6)-α-D-Glc*p*-(1→6)-β-D-Glc*p*-(1→3)-β-D-Glc*p*-(1→3)-β-D-Gal*f*5,6Ac₂-(1→3)-β-D-Glc*p*-(1→3)-α-D-Glc*p*NAc-(1→P→ β-D-Gal*f* (4←1)	43,259	1997[43]
21	21	Constituents: Glc, Gal, and GlcN	285	
22F	22	→4)-β-D-Glc*p*A-(1→4)-β-L-Rha*p*2Ac₀.₈-(1→4)-α-D-Glc*p*-(1→3)-α-D-Gal*f*-(1→2)-α-L-Rha*p*-(1→ α-D-Glc*p* (3←1)	58,59 264	1989[264]

22A	63	No information		
23F	23	Gro-(2→P) ↓ 3 →4)-β-D-Glcp-(1→4)-β-D-Galp-(1→4)-β-L-Rhap-(1→ 2 ↑ 1 α-L-Rhap	139 257,271	1988[257]
23A	46	No information		
23B	64	No information		
24F	24	Constituents: Glc, Rha, GlcN, Rib, and Rib-ol-P	285	
24A	65	Constituents: Cho-P	296	
24B	60	No information		
25F	25	Constituents: Gal, GalA, GlcN, and GalN	74	
25A	27	No information		
27	27	→3)-β-D-GlcpNAc4,6(S)Pyr-(1→3)-α-D-Galp-(1→4)-β-L-Rhap-(1→4)-β-D-Glcp-(1→ 2 ↑ Cho→P	36,37 109	1977[36,37]
28F	28	Constituents: Glc, Rha, Gro, and Cho-P	285,296	
28A	79	Constituents: Cho-P	296	
29	29	→4)-β-D-GalpNAc-(1→6)-β-D-Galf-(1→3)-β-D-Galp-(1→6)-β-D-Galf-(1→1)-D-Rib-ol-(5→P→	157 249,250	1988[157]
31	31	→2)-β-L-Rhap-(1→3)-β-D-Galf-(1→3)-β-L-Rhap-(1→4)-β-D-GlcpA-(1→3)-β-D-Galf-(1→	32 272,313	1983[32]
32F	32	→4)-β-D-Glcp-(1→3)-α-D-Glcp-(1→4)-β-L-Rhap2Ac-(1→ 2 3 ↑ ↑ α-L-Rhap-(1→P) Cho→P	151 234,296	1998[151]

(cont.)

TABLE 2. (continued)

Serotype[a]		Primary structure[b]	References	Year/reference (final structure)
Danish	American			
32A	67	→4)-β-D-Glcp-(1→3)-α-D-Glcp4Ac-(1→4)-β-L-Rhap2Ac-(1→ $\underset{\uparrow}{3}$ Cho→P α-L-Rhap-(1→P $\underset{\uparrow}{2}$	151,296	1998[151]
33F	70	→3)-β-D-Galp-(1→3)-α-D-Galp-(1→3)-β-D-Galf2Ac$_{0.4}$-(1→3)-β-D-Glcp-(1→5)-β-D-Galf-(1→ $\underset{\overset{\uparrow}{1}}{2}$ α-D-Galp	260	1984[260]
33A	40	No information		
33B	42	→6)-β-D-Glcp-(1→5)-β-D-Galf-(1→3)-β-D-GalpNAc-(1→4)-α-D-Galp-(1→2)-D-Rib-ol-(5→P→ $\underset{\overset{\uparrow}{1}}{2}$ α-D-Galp +OAc	327	1974[327]
33C 33D	39	No information No information		
34	41	→3)-β-D-Galf-(1→3)-α-D-Glcp-(1→2)-β-D-Galf6Ac$_{0.5}$-(1→3)-α-D-Galp-(1→2)-D-Rib-ol-(5→P→	64,80 81,273	1968[64]
35F	35	No information		
35A	47/62	→3)-β-D-Galp-(1→3)-β-D-Galf5,6Ac$_2$-(1→3)-β-D-Glcp-(1→6)-β-D-Galf2Ac-(1→1)-Man-ol-(6→P→	43	1997[43]
35B	66	→4)-β-D-GalpNAc-(1→6)-β-D-Galf-(1→3)-β-D-Glcp-(1→6)-β-D-Galf2Ac$_{0.7}$-(1→1)-Rib-ol-(5→P→	42	1995[42]
35C 36	61 36	No information No information		

		Structure	Ref.	Year
37	37	→3)-β-D-Glcp-(1→ 2 ↑ 1 β-D-Glcp	1,164	1988[1]
38	71	No information		
39	69	No information		
40	45	No information		
41F	38	No information		
41A	74	No information		
42	80	No information		
43	75	No information		
44	81	No information		
45	72	Gro-(1→P→6)-β-D-GlcpNAc 1 ↓ 4 →3)-α-D-Galp-(1→3)-α-L-FucpNAc-(1→3)-β-D-GalpNAc-(1→2)-α-L-Rhap-(1→ 6 ↑ 1 α-D-Galp	72,212	1988[212]
46	73	Constituents: D-Gal, D-GalNAc, D-GlcNAc, and L-FucNAc	39	
47F	52	No information		
47A	84	No information		
48	82	No information		

[a]Taken from Kauffmann et al.[153]

[b]AATGal, 2-acetamido-4-amino-2,4,6-trideoxygalactose; Ara-ol, arabinitol; Fuc, fucose; FucNAc, N-acetylfucosamine; Gal, galactose; GalA, galacturonic acid; GalN, galactosamine; GalNAc, N-acetylgalactosamine; Glc, glucose; GlcA, glucuronic acid; GlcN, glucosamine; GlcNAc, N-acetylglucosamine; Gro, glycerol; ManNAc, N-acetylmannosamine; ManNAcA, N-acetylmannosaminuronic acid; Man-ol, mannitol; PneNAc, N-acetylpneumosamine, 2-acetamido-2,6-dideoxytalose; Rha, rhamnose; Rib, ribose; Rib-ol, ribitol; Sug, 2-acetamido-2,6-dideoxy-xylo-hexos-4-ulose; Ac, acetate; Cho, choline; P, phosphate; Pyr, pyruvate; p, pyranose; f, furanose. For earlier reviews that include lists of polysaccharide structures, see refs.[121,132-135,156,177,316]

Phosphate groups can occur as a phosphodiester bridge between the oligosaccharide repeats, thereby connecting two monosaccharide residues (serotypes 7B, 19F, 19A, 19B, 19C, 20) or a monosaccharide and an alditol (ribitol, arabinitol, mannitol) (teichoic acid type; serotypes 6A, 6B, 10F, 10A, 13, 17F, 29, 33B, 34, 35A, 35B). However, phosphate groups can also occur as a backbone substituent (free phosphate, glycerol-1-phosphate, glycerol-2-phosphate, ribitol phosphate, phosphorylcholine, rhamnosyl phosphate, fucosyl phosphate, galactosyl phosphate). In the structural analysis of the teichoic acid type CPSs, alkaline treatment followed by alkaline phosphatase digestion has been frequently used to generate oligosaccharide repeating units, e.g., in serotypes 6A,[254] 10A,[248] 13,[329] 29,[250] and 33B.[327]

All polysaccharides of which the structure has been elucidated, except those from serotype 7F, 7A, 14, 33F, and 37, are anionic biopolymers due to the presence of uronic acid, phosphate, and/or pyruvate. The CPS of serotype 37 is the only homoglycan found so far.[1]

O-Acetyl functions have been detected in several serotypes. Quite often it has been found that the *O*-acetyl groups are immunologically important, e.g., in serotype 1,[103] serotype 11A,[160] serotype 15F,[238] and serotype 34.[64] For serotype 20, it has been reported that the *O*-acetyl groups can be removed without significant loss of activity towards type 20 pneumococcal antisera.[259]

Pyruvate substituents have only been found in the CPSs of the serotypes 4 and 27. Both the 2,3-pyruvate (serotype 4)[140] and the 4,6-pyruvate (serotype 27)[37] have the *S*-stereoconfiguration. The pyruvate group is an immunological determinant of the CPS of serotype 4. Its removal gives rise to marked changes in immunological specificity. Here, the depyruvated CPS resembles the C-polysaccharide closely immunologically; apparently, the removal of pyruvic acid from adjacent sugars unmasks GalNAc residues which must be linked and spaced much as are those in C-polysaccharide.[115] Also the pyruvate group in the CPS of serotype 27 is an immunological determinant.[36]

In the CPS of serotype 5, 2-acetamido-2,6-dideoxy-D-*xylo*-hexos-4-ulose (D-Sug) accounts for the lability of the CPS towards alkali, a chemical phenomenon without knowing the structure already detected in 1939.[27,121] Because of the problems with D-Sug on storage of the polysaccharide, it has been suggested to reduce the CPS if it should be used as a vaccine.[126]

Comparison of the CPSs of the serotypes 6A and 6B shows that the only difference is the presence of 3-substituted D-ribitol in 6A and 4-substituted D-ribitol in 6B. As ribitol phosphate is most probably transferred to the repeating unit from CDP-ribitol, in which phosphate is linked to O-5 of D-ribitol,[25] it was assumed[177] that it is linked to the same position in 6A (and 6B).

Considering the similarity in the antigenic formula of the serotypes 7F and 7A (Table 1), it was expected that the CPSs of these serotypes should have similar structures. Structural analysis (Table 2) demonstrated that the only difference between 7F and 7A forms is the presence or absence of a terminal side-chain β-D-galactose residue. The CPS of serotype 7B has only one antigenic component in common with serotypes 7F and 7A. It is suggested that the structural basis for the common antigenic formula (7a) in the group 7

serotypes is the disaccharide element α-D-Glc*p*NAc-(1 → 2)-α-L-Rha*p*, occurring in the backbone or in the side chain (Table 2). Estimation of the minimum energy conformations of the repeating units of the CPSs of 7F, 7A and 7B using the GESA program,[131] indicated that the disaccharide element which is well exposed in 7F and 7A is also exposed to a considerable extent in 7B. Another disaccharide element, β-L-Rha*p*-(1 → 4)-β-D-Glc*p*, is also present in each of these CPSs but only as an internal fragment, and is thus less likely to be the common factor. Note that the CPS of serotype 7B does not contain *O*-acetyl groups.

Comparison of the CPS structures of the serotypes 9L and 9N shows only one difference on the monosaccharide level: the α-D-galactose residue in 9L is an α-D-glucose residue in 9N. Comparison of the CPS structures of the serotypes 9L and 9A makes clear that only one difference exists on the monosaccharide level: the *N*-acetyl-α-D-glucosamine residue in 9L is an α-D-glucose residue in 9A. The de-*O*-acetylated CPS of serotype 9V is identical to that of 9A. In the CPS of serotype 9V, there is no evidence that any residue is di-*O*-acetylated. A study discussing the complex *O*-acetylation pattern of the CPS of serotype 9V in relation to immunogenicity has appeared,[206] and it was found that *O*-acetyl groups are not absolutely required.

For the CPS of serotype 10F, a complete structure has been included in a review,[316] based on the data from an abstract without experimental details.

When neglecting the *O*-acetylation patterns, the CPSs of serotypes 11F, 11B, and 11C have identical repeating tetrasaccharide backbones.[262] However, the ribitol phosphate substituent at *N*-acetyl-α-D-glucosamine in 11F and 11B has been replaced by a glycerol phosphate substituent in 11C. The structural difference between 11F and 11B can be the 2-*O*-acetylation of the α-D-galactose unit, but confusion exists.[262,263] In the CPS of serotype 11A α-D-glucose is present instead of *N*-acetyl-α-D-glucosamine; the glucose residue bears a glycerol phosphate substituent.[263]

Comparing the CPS structures of serotypes 12F and 12A, two monosaccharide mutations are observed. In 12F the side chain at *N*-acetyl-α-L-fucosamine is α-D-galactose, and in 12A *N*-acetyl-α-D-galactosamine. The *N*-acetyl-β-D-galactosamine unit in the backbone of 12F has been interchanged by *N*-acetyl-β-D-glucosamine in 12A.

Interestingly, although the pentasaccharide repeating units of the CPSs of serotypes 15F/15A and 15B/15C contain the same monosaccharide sequence, their arrangements are different. For the serotypes 15F and 15A a linear arrangement has been reported,[57,238] and for the serotypes 15B and 15C a branched arrangement.[127] It has been suggested that probably two different routes exist for the polymerization of the pentasaccharide. Comparing the CPSs of serotypes 15F and 15A shows that the phosphate group of β-D-galactose-3-phosphate is partially substituted by choline in 15F and by glycerol in 15A. Another difference forms the *O*-acetylation, being present in the CPS of serotype 15F, but absent in that of serotype 15A. Comparison of the CPS structures of the serotypes 15B and 15C indicates that the CPS of serotype 15B is an *O*-acetylated variant of that of serotype 15C.

Remarkably, the difference between the CPSs of the serotypes 17F and 17A is far more profound than usual between serotypes, the former being of the teichoic acid type and the latter being a polysaccharide proper.[125,134] However, it should be noted that some confusion exists with respect to the structure of the CPS of serotype 17F,[125,134] as a detailed study is not available in the literature.

The non-acetylated CPS structures of the serotypes 18F, 18B and 18C are identical.[128,150,196] They vary only in their *O*-acetylation patterns: the CPS of serotype 18B is not *O*-acetylated, that of 18C partly 6-*O*-acetylated at the α-D-glucose side chain, and that of 18F completely 6-*O*-acetylated at the α-D-glucose side chain. The location of the *O*-acetyl group at C-6 of the glucose residue is tentative only. Furthermore, 18F has a 2-*O*-acetylated β-L-rhamnose residue. The CPS of serotype 18A differs from those of the other serotypes in mutating the backbone α-D-glucose residue (18F/18B/18C) to an *N*-acetyl-α-D-glucosamine residue (18A); *O*-acetylation has not been found. In the case of 18A the absolute configuration of glycerol has been established to be D (D-glycerol-1-phosphate, (2R)-glycerol-1-phosphate or *sn*-glycerol-3-phosphate).[274]

The trisaccharide repeating units of the reported CPS structures of the serotypes 19F and 19A differ only in the substitution pattern of the rhamnose residue: 2-substituted (19F) versus 3-substituted (19A).[152,224] In the case of 19A a second structure has been included in Table 2, because it has been shown that the monosaccharide composition of 19A seemed to vary according to the type of culture medium used to grow the serotype 19A organisms.[183] Such an observation is interesting as the CPS of 19A is a component of the regular polysaccharide vaccine (Table 1). When compared with those of 19F/19A, the structures of the CPSs of serotypes 19B/19C are quite different;[41] the difference between 19B and 19C is the extra branching (extra β-D-glucose unit) of the *N*-acetyl-β-D-mannosamine residue in 19C. The only common structural feature shared by all the four serotypes is the region about the phosphate diester bridge: α-L-Rha*p*-(1 → P → 4)-β-D-Man*p*NAc-(1 → 4)-D-Glc*p*.

Inspection of the structures of the CPSs of the serotypes 20 and 35A shows that an identical disaccharide element occurs,[43] namely, → 3)-β-D-Gal*f*5,6Ac₂-(1 → 3)-β-D-Glc*p*-(1 → . It has been suggested that this structure probably explains the serological cross-reactivity (antigenic determinant 20b).

Comparison of the CPS structures of serotypes 29 and 35B shows a single monosaccharide replacement: a β-D-galactose residue in serotype 29[157] for a β-D-glucose residue in serotype 35B.[42] Furthermore, the CPS of serotype 29 is not *O*-acetylated.

The structures of the CPSs of serotypes 32F and 32A only differ in the *O*-acetylation pattern.[151] The branched α-D-glucose residue in 32A is *O*-acetylated at C-4.

Finally, a reference to a statement[255] made in 1941, incorporated in a study on the structure determination of the CPS of serotype 3, is of interest: "It is hoped that further work in this field will eventually give us more thorough understanding of the chemical basis underlying the specificity of the many types of pneumococci." However, it should be said that, although many primary structures are known nowadays, multidisciplinary programs, including instrumental approaches such as NMR spectroscopy and x-ray diffraction, theoretical calculations and synthetic efforts, focused on the unraveling of the relation between cross-serological properties and molecular features (structural biology) have not got much attention.

MOLECULAR BIOLOGY AND BIOSYNTHESIS OF CAPSULAR POLYSACCHARIDES

Until very recently, the organization and function of the genes required for the biosynthesis of the capsular polysaccharides in *S. pneumoniae* remained completely unexplored. Unraveling the biosynthetic pathways could lead to the design of inhibitors capable of blocking the expression of the CPSs. So far, reports are available about the molecular organization of the capsular loci of the serotypes 1,[218] 3,[13,78,79,94] 14,[169–171] 19F,[102,215] 19B,[214] and 23F[247] and about the biosynthetic pathways of the CPSs of the serotypes 3,[79] 14,[171] and 19F.[215] Recently, a short review on the molecular biology of the capsular genes of *S. pneumoniae* has appeared.[93] Of interest are also recent studies exploring the genetic diversity of *cps* loci in various pneumococcal serotypes. To this end individual *cps*14 genes were used for cross-hybridization with chromosomal DNA from 26 different pneumococcal serotypes.[172] In this way interesting information has been generated among others with respect to potential monosaccharides linked to lipid carriers, being starters for CPS biosynthesis, for several serotypes. Similar approaches were followed for individual *cps19f* genes and chromosomal DNA from 19 different pneumococcal serotypes,[215] and for individual *cps23f* genes and chromosomal DNA from 21 different pneumococcal serotypes.[247] In this context, see another source.[69] These studies show that knowledge of the genetic determinants of different CPSs can assist in primary structure determinations, and be helpful in elucidating structure-chemical controversies.

In Fig. 2 the biosynthetic pathway of the CPS of serotype 3 (Table 2) is presented.[79] The biosynthesis seems to proceed by successive monomer addition making use of UDP-Glc and UDP-GlcA (monomeric mechanism).

In the case of the biosynthesis of the CPS of serotype 14 (Table 2), as depicted in Fig. 3,[171] use is made of the polymerization of lipid-linked intermediates (block mechanism). The proposed biological repeating unit is Gal-GlcNAc-Gal-Glc. A similar proposal is shown in Fig. 4 for the biosynthesis of the CPS of serotype 19F (Table 2).[215] Here, the biological repeating unit is Rha-P-ManNAc-Glc.

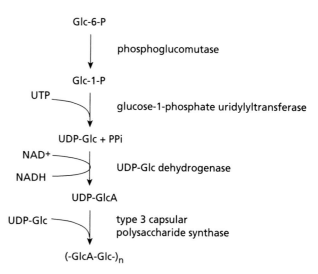

FIG. 2. Proposed biosynthetic pathway for type 3 CPS.[79]

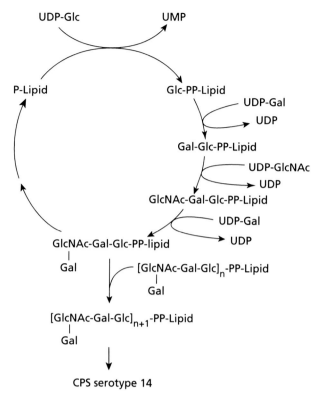

FIG. 3. Proposed biosynthetic pathway for type 14 CPS.[171]

PREPARATION OF CAPSULAR POLYSACCHARIDE FRAGMENTS

Nowadays it is possible, using multistep organic synthesis in combination with glycosyltransferases, to prepare fragments of pneumococcal polysaccharides. It will be even possible in several cases to synthesize fragments several repeating units in length. Depending on the primary structure of the polysaccharides, also degradation studies can generate specific fragments. Although the structures obtained via synthesis from monosaccharides or via degradation from polysaccharides are of lower mass than the natural polysaccharides, there are indications that they are often long enough to function very well as immunogenic components of conjugate vaccines.

A survey of synthetic fragments of CPSs of *S. pneumoniae* (Table 2) prepared so far is presented in Table 3: serotype 1, 2, 3, 4, 6A, 6B, 7F, 8, 9A, 9V, 14, 17F, 18C, 19F, 19A, 22F, 23F, 27, and 29. Free, methyl glycosidated as well as spacered oligosaccharides have been synthesized. In the case of serotype 3, the copolymerization of allyl glycosides with acrylamide is of interest.[62,63] In the case of serotype 14, a polysaccharide with a degree of polymerization of about 10 has been synthesized in a stereo- and regiospecific polycondensation reaction of a suitably protected tetrasaccharide repeating unit.[166] Note that in a few cases oligosaccharides have been synthesized taking into account a structure which has been revised in the meantime (these structures have been marked in Table 3).

In several studies reporting the primary structure of the serotype-specific polysaccharides partial acid hydrolysis played an important role. In a number of cases such an approach turned

out to be valuable to prepare higher amounts of oligosaccharides, to be used in immunological research programs. One of the classical examples is the partial acid hydrolysis of the CPS of serotype 3 (Table 2), making use of the greater stability of the glucuronosyl → glucose linkage, when compared with the glucosyl → glucuronic acid linkage, leading to a series of cellobiuronic acid oligomers, H [→ 3)-β-D-GlcpA-(1 → 4)-β-D-Glcp-(1 →]$_n$OH.[56,203,292] When the CPS of serotype 8 (Table 2) is subjected to partial acid hydrolysis, a tetrasaccharide, β-D-GlcpA-(1 → 4)-β-D-Glcp-(1 → 4)-α-D-Glcp-(1 → 4)-D-Galp, can be isolated.[146]

Partial acid hydrolysis was also used to create pools of "oligosaccharides" with definite dimensions. To give an impression of such an approach, for the CPS of serotype 3 three pools were generated with an average number of repeating units of 8, 16, and 27 (native, 37); for the CPS of 6A three pools (11, 18, 27; native, 140); for the CPS of 18C three pools (6, 11, 16); for the CPS of 19F four pools (13, 17, 26, 40; native, 160); and for the CPS of 23F three pools (10, 14, 21).[175]

Alkaline treatment (NaOH) of the CPS of serotype 6B (Table 2) yields α-D-Galp2P-(1 → 3)-α-D-Glcp-(1 → 3)-α-L-Rhap-(1 → 4)-D-Rib-ol5P. Acidic treatment (HF) affords α-D-Galp-(1 → 3)-α-D-Glcp-(1 → 3)-α-L-Rhap-(1 → 4)-D-Rib-ol and α-D-Galp-(1 → 3)-α-D-Glcp-(1 → 3)-α-L-Rhap-(1 → 4)-D-Rib-ol-(5 → P → 2)-α-D-Galp-(1 → 3)-α-D-Glcp-(1 → 3)-α-L-Rhap-(1 → 4)-D-Rib-ol.[315] Detailed NMR studies of these three oligosaccharides have been reported.[315]

De-*N*-acetylation followed by nitrous acid deamination of the *N*-acetylglucosamine residue in the CPS of serotype 14 (Table 2) gives rise to a cleavage in the CPS backbone at the anomeric center of this residue, thereby converting *N*-acetylglucosamine via glucosamine into 2,5-anhydromannose.[194] In this way a chemical repeating unit of the CPS of serotype 14 is formed with a transformed *N*-acetylglucosamine (2,5-anhydromannose) residue at the "reducing end." This principle has also been used for the generation of longer oligosaccharide fragments (up to 6 repeating units), replacing the complete alkaline de-*N*-acetylation by a partial alkaline de-*N*-acetylation.[176] The free aldehyde group of the 2,5-anhydromannose can be used directly for further conjugation of the oligosaccharides to a carrier protein by reductive amination.

Specific cleavage of the β-(1 → 4) linkage between glucuronic acid and glucose in the CPS of serotype 3 (Table 2) by enzymatic depolymerization with a *Bacillus palustris* derived endo-β-glucuronidase leads to oligosaccharides of the type H [→ 4)-β-D-Glcp-(1 → 3)-β-D-GlcpA-(1→)$_n$OH.[56,203]

Incubation of the CPS of serotype 8 (Table 2) with a *Bacillus palustris* derived depolymerase yields β-Hex-4-enepA-(1 → 4)-β-D-Glcp-(1 → 4)-α-D-Glcp-(1 → 4)-D-Galp, thereby demonstrating that the depolymerase is in fact a lyase. The enzyme transforms during cleavage of the backbone the β-D-glucuronosyl unit into its 4,5-unsaturated analogue.[33,56]

An endo-β-galactosidase from *Cytophaga keratolytica* (formerly called *Flavobacterium keratolyticus*), which catalyzes the hydrolysis of the β-(1 → 4) linkage between galactose and glucose in lactose, has been applied to the CPS of serotype 14 (Table 2) for the generation of oligosaccharides consisting of one or more repeating units depending on the conditions (e.g. β-D-Glcp-(1 → 6)-[β-D-Galp-(1 → 4)]-β-D-GlcpNAc-(1 → 3)-D-Galp and β-D-Glcp-(1 → 6)-[β-D-Galp-(1 → 4)]-β-

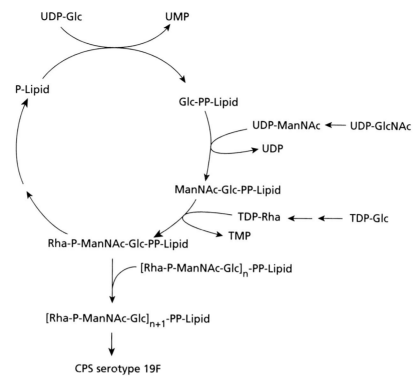

FIG. 4. Proposed biosynthetic pathway for type 19F CPS.[215]

D-GlcpNAc-(1 → 3)-β-D-Galp-(1 → 4)-β-D-Glcp-(1 → 6)-[β-D-Galp-(1 → 4)]-β-D-GlcpNAc-(1 → 3)-D-Galp).[330,331] In this context, the possible suitability of endo-β-galactosidase from *Citrobacter freundii* is mentioned.[228]

For the modification of polysaccharides containing galactose residues, such as the CPS of serotype 14 (Table 2), the use of D-galactose oxidase has been evaluated.[86]

Finally, most of the synthesized polysaccharide fragments so far have been used in inhibition studies, but the number of studies, whereby free or spacered oligosaccharides are converted into oligosaccharide-protein conjugates is growing.

CONFORMATIONAL ANALYSIS OF CAPSULAR (POLY)SACCHARIDES

For a number of capsular polysaccharides and fragments thereof, conformational studies based on NMR or x-ray analyses and theoretical calculations have been published.

A synthetic disaccharide fragment of serotype 1 (Table 2), α-D-GalpA-(1 → 3)-AAT-α-D-Galp-(1 → OCH₃ (Table 3), was studied by NMR spectroscopy and hard-sphere exoanomeric effect (HSEA) calculations.[47] For the synthetic trisaccharide fragments β-D-ManpNAc-(1 → 4)-α-D-Glcp-(1 → 2)-α-L-Rhap-(1 → OCH₃ and β-D-ManpNAc-(1 → 4)-α-D-Glcp-(1 → 3)-α-L-Rhap-(1 → OCH₃ (Table 3), representing the repeating units of the CPSs of the serotypes 19F and 19A (Table 2), respectively, NMR studies combined with HSEA and MM2 calculations have been reported.[68]

With respect to serotype 4, detailed NMR and energy calculation (MM2CARB) studies have been carried out on the in-

tact CPS (Table 2), its depyruvated form, and a tetrasaccharide derived by Smith degradation of the depyruvated CPS, β-D-ManpNAc-(1 → 3)-α-L-FucpNAc-(1 → 3)-α-D-GalpNAc-(1 → 2)-Threitol.[145] The dynamics of the polysaccharide systems and the influence of the pyruvate group were investigated using ¹³C-NMR relaxation measurements. From the constructed models it was concluded that the presence of the pyruvate group has only minor effects on the local and overall conformation of the chain in solution; only the GalNAc hydroxymethyl group is sterically hindered in the intact polymer.

An NMR study has also been carried out on the CPS of serotype 9N (Table 2),[276] and nuclear Overhauser enhancement (NOE) data were combined with energy minimizations and molecular dynamics calculations to determine the most favored conformation in solution. The optimum model is a flexible extended ribbon conformation. In a subsequent study the aqueous solution conformations of the cross-reacting polysaccharides of three serogroup 9 strains (9N, 9L, and 9A) (Table 2) were compared,[277] and turned out to be very similar. It is suggested that the antigenic specificity for group 9 polysaccharides is determined by local structural variation rather than by conformational differences.

X-ray diffraction studies on oriented fibers have been carried out for CPS serotype 3 (Table 2).[205] It turned out that the chain consists of a three-fold helix, with a repeat of 0.923 nm; conformational analyses are in favor of a left-handed helix, but a choice between two possible models could not be made. Introductory x-ray diffraction studies on oriented fibers and conformational modelling have also been described for the CPSs of the serotypes 3 and 8 (Table 2)[333] and the serotypes 1, 5, and 18 (Table 2).[334] The crystalline neutral tetrasaccharide α-

TABLE 3. SYNTHESIZED NONSPACERED AND SPACERED FRAGMENTS OF CAPSULAR POLYSACCHARIDES OF *Streptococcus pneumoniae*[a]

Serotype	Product	References
1	α-D-Gal*p*A-(1→3)-AAT-α-D-Gal*p*-(1→OCH₃	197
2	β-L-Rha*p*-(1→4)-β-D-Glc*p*-(1→3)-α-L-Rha*p*-(1→OCH₂)₃NH₂	323
3[b]	β-D-Glc*p*A-(1→4)-β-D-Glc*p*-(1→OCH₂CH=CH₂	62
	β-D-Glc*p*-(1→3)-β-D-Glc*p*A-(1→OCH₂CH=CH₂	62
	β-D-Glc*p*A-(1→4)-β-D-Glc*p*-(1→3)-β-D-Glc*p*A-(1→OCH₂CH=CH₂	63
	β-D-Glc*p*-(1→3)-β-D-Glc*p*A-(1→4)-β-D-Glc*p*-(1→OCH₂CH=CH₂	63
	β-D-Glc*p*A-(1→4)-β-D-Glc*p*-(1→3)-β-D-Glc*p*A-(1→4)-β-D-Glc*p*-(1→OCH₂CH=CH₂	63
4	β-D-Man*p*NAc-(1→3)-α-L-Fuc*p*NAc-(1→3)-D-Gal*p*NAc	117
6A	α-D-Gal*p*-(1→3)-α-D-Glc*p*-(1→3)-α-L-Rha*p*-(1→3)-D-Rib-ol	289
	α-D-Gal*p*-(1→3)-α-D-Glc*p*-(1→3)-α-L-Rha*p*-(1→3)-D-Rib-ol-(5→P→2)-α-D-Gal*p*-(1→3)-α-D-Glc*p*-(1→3)-L-Rha*p*	290
6B	α-D-Glc*p*-(1→3)-L-Rha*p*	289
	α-D-Gal*p*-(1→3)-α-D-Glc*p*-(1→3)-L-Rha*p*	289
	α-D-Gal*p*-(1→3)-α-D-Glc*p*-(1→3)-α-L-Rha*p*-(1→4)-D-Rib-ol	289
	α-D-Gal*p*-(1→3)-α-D-Glc*p*-(1→3)-α-L-Rha*p*-(1→4)-D-Rib-ol-(5→P→2)-α-D-Gal*p*-(1→3)-α-D-Glc*p*-(1→3)-L-Rha*p*	290
	α-L-Rha*p*-(1→4)-D-Rib-ol-(5→P→(CH₂)₃NH₂	307
	D-Rib-ol-(5→P→2)-α-D-Gal*p*-(1→O(CH₂)₃NH₂	307
	α-L-Rha*p*-(1→4)-D-Rib-ol-(5→P→2)-α-D-Gal*p*-(1→O(CH₂)₃NH₂	307
	D-Rib-ol-(5→P→2)-α-D-Gal*p*-(1→3)-α-D-Glc*p*-(1→O(CH₂)₃NH₂	307
	D-Rib-ol-(5→P→2)-α-D-Gal*p*-(1→3)-α-D-Glc*p*-(1→3)-α-L-Rha*p*-(1→O(CH₂)₃NH₂	308
	α-L-Rha*p*-(1→4)-D-Rib-ol-(5→P→2)-α-D-Glc*p*-(1→O(CH₂)₃NH₂	308
	α-D-Glc*p*-(1→3)-α-L-Rha*p*-(1→4)-D-Rib-ol-(5→P→2)-α-D-Gal*p*-(1→O(CH₂)₃NH₂	308
	α-D-Gal*p*-(1→3)-α-D-Glc*p*-(1→3)-α-L-Rha*p*-(1→4)-D-Rib-ol-(5→P→(CH₂)₃NH₂	306,308
7F	β-L-Rha*p*-(1→4)-β-D-Glc*p*-(1→3)-β-D-Gal*p*NAc-(1→O(CH₂)₃NH₂	323
8[c]	β-D-Glc*p*A-(1→4)-β-D-Glc*p*-(1→4)-D-Glc*p*	167
	β-D-Glc*p*-(1→4)-α-D-Glc*p*-(1→4)-D-Gal*p*	167
	α-D-Gal*p*-(1→4)-β-D-Glc*p*A-(1→O(CH₂)₂CH₃	167
9A	β-D-Man*p*NAc-(1→4)-α-D-Glc*p*-(1→4)-D-Glc*p*[d]	233
9V	β-D-Man*p*NAc-(1→4)-β-D-Glc*p*-(1→4)-D-Glc*p*	233
	α-D-Gal*p*-(1→3)-β-D-Man*p*NAc-(1→4)-β-D-Glc*p*-(1→4)-α-D-Glc*p*-(1→O(CH₂)₈CO₂CH₃	232

Serotype	Structure	Reference
14	β-D-Gal$p$-(1→4)-β-D-Glc$p$NAc-(1→3)-D-Gal$p$	188
	β-D-Gal$p$-(1→4)-β-D-Glc$p$-(1→6)-[β-D-Gal$p$-(1→4)]-D-Glc$p$NAc	337
	β-D-Gal$p$-(1→4)-β-D-Glc$p$-(1→6)-[β-D-Glc$p$NAc-(1→3)-β-D-Gal$p$-(1→4)]-D-Glc$p$	168
	β-D-Glc$p$NAc-(1→3)-β-D-Gal$p$-(1→4)-β-D-Glc$p$NAc-(1→OCH$_3$	71
	β-D-Glc$p$NAc-(1→3)-β-D-Gal$p$-(1→OCH$_3$	71
	β-D-Gal$p$-(1→4)-β-D-Glc$p$NAc-(1→3)-β-D-Gal$p$-(1→OCH$_3$	71
	β-D-Gal$p$-(1→4)-β-D-Glc$p$NAc-(1→3)-β-D-Gal$p$-(1→4)-β-D-Glc$p$-(1→OCH$_3$	71
	β-D-Gal$p$-(1→4)-β-D-Glc$p$NAc-(1→6)-[β-D-Gal$p$-(1→4)]-β-D-Glc$p$NAc-(1→OCH$_3$	166,168
	β-D-Gal$p$-(1→4)-β-D-Glc$p$NAc-(1→6)-[β-D-Glc$p$NAc-(1→3)-β-D-Gal$p$-(1→4)]-β-D-Glc$p$-(1→OCH$_3$	168
	β-D-Gal$p$-(1→4)-β-D-Glc$p$NAc-(1→O(CH$_2$)$_2$CH$_3$	244
	β-D-Glc$p$-(1→6)-[β-D-Gal$p$-(1→4)]-β-D-Glc$p$NAc-(1→O(CH$_2$)$_2$CH$_3$	244
	β-D-Gal$p$-(1→6)-[β-D-Gal$p$-(1→4)]-β-D-Glc$p$NAc-(1→O(CH$_2$)$_2$CH$_3$	244
	β-D-Gal$p$-(1→4)-β-D-Glc$p$NAc-(1→3)-β-D-Gal$p$-(1→O(CH$_2$)$_8$CO$_2$CH$_3$	188
	β-D-Gal$p$-(1→6)-β-D-Glc$p$NAc-(1→OCH$_2$CH=CH$_2$	221
	β-D-Gal$p$-(1→4)-β-D-Glc$p$-(1→4)-β-D-Glc$p$-(1→OCH$_2$C$_6$H$_5$	240
	β-D-Gal$p$-(1→4)-β-D-Glc$p$-(1→6)-[β-D-Gal$p$-(1→4)]-β-D-Glc$p$NAc-(1→OMD^e	7
	β-D-Gal$p$-(1→4)-β-D-Glc$p$-(1→6)-[β-D-Gal$p$-(1→4)]-β-D-Glc$p$NAc-(1→OAD^e	7
	β-D-Gal$p$-(1→4)-β-D-Glc$p$-(1→6)-[β-D-Gal$p$-(1→4)]-β-D-Glc$p$NAc-(1→O(CH$_2$)$_3$S(CH$_2$)$_2$NH$_2$	221
	β-D-Gal$p$-(1→4)-β-D-Glc$p$-(1→6)-[β-D-Gal$p$-(1→4)]-β-D-Glc$p$NAc-(1→O(CH$_2$)$_3$O→4)-β-D-Glc$p$-(1→O(CH$_2$)$_3$S(CH$_2$)$_2$NH$_2^f$	222
	β-D-Gal$p$-(1→4)-β-D-Glc$p$NAc-(1→O(CH$_2$)$_3$O→4)-β-D-Gal$p$-(1→6)-[β-D-Gal$p$-(1→4)]-β-D-Glc$p$NAc-(1→O(CH$_2$)$_3$O→4)-β-D-Glc$p$-(1→O(CH$_2$)$_3$S(CH$_2$)$_2$NH$_2^f$	222
17F	α-L-Rha$p$-(1→2)-D-Ara-ol-(1→P→(CH$_2$)$_3$NH$_2$	324
	α-L-Rha$p$-(1→2)-D-Ara-ol-(1→P→4)-α-L-Rha$p$-(1→O(CH$_2$)$_3$NH$_2^d$	324
	α-L-Rha$p$-(1→2)-D-Ara-ol-(1→P→4)-α-L-Rha$p$-(1→4)-β-D-Glc$p$-(1→O(CH$_2$)$_3$NH$_2^d$	324
18C	β-D-Gal$p$-(1→4)-α-D-Glc$p$-(1→3)-α-L-Rha$p$-(1→OCH$_3^d$	321
	sn-Gro-(3→P→3)-β-D-Gal$p$-(1→4)-α-D-Glc$p$-(1→3)-α-L-Rha$p$-(1→OCH$_3^d$	321
	α-D-Glc$p$-(1→2)-[β-D-Glc$p$-(1→4)]-β-D-Gal$p$-(1→OCH$_3$	321
	α-D-Glc$p$-(1→2)-[sn-Gro-(3→P→3)][β-D-Glc$p$-(1→4)]-β-D-Gal$p$-(1→OCH$_3$	321
	α-D-Glc$p$-(1→2)-[β-D-Glc$p$-(1→4)]-β-D-Gal$p$-(1→4)-α-D-Glc$p$-(1→3)-L-Rha$p$	322
19F	β-D-Man$p$NAc-(1→4)-D-Glc$p$	233
	β-D-Man$p$NAc-(1→4)-α-D-Glc$p$-(1→2)-L-Rha$p$	48,147,148,226,233,304
	β-D-Man$p$NAc-(1→4)-α-D-Glc$p$-(1→OCH$_3$	207
	β-D-Man$p$NAc-(1→4)-α-D-Glc$p$-(1→2)-α-L-Rha$p$-(1→OCH$_3$	68
	β-D-Man$p$NAc-(1→4)-α-D-Glc$p$-(1→2)-α-L-Rha$p$-(1→P→4)-β-D-Man$p$NAc-(1→4)-α-D-Glc$p$-(1→2)-α-L-Rha$p$-(1→P→4)- -β-D-Man$p$NAc-(1→4)-α-D-Glc$p$-(1→2)-α-L-Rha$p$-(1→P→(CH$_2$)$_2$NH$_2$	223
19A	β-D-Man$p$NAc-(1→4)-α-D-Glc$p$-(1→3)-L-Rha$p$	227,233
	β-D-Man$p$NAc-(1→4)-α-D-Glc$p$-(1→3)-α-L-Rha$p$-(1→OCH$_3$	68

(cont.)

TABLE 3. (*continued*)

Serotype	Product	References
22F	β-L-Rhap-(1→4)-α-D-Glcp-(1→3)-α-D-Galf-(1→O(CH₂)₃NH₂	323
23F	α-L-Rhap-(1→2)-β-D-Galp-(1→OCH₃	252
	β-D-Glcp3P-(1→4)-[α-L-Rhap-(1→2)]-β-D-Galp-(1→OCH₃[d]	319
	α-L-Rhap-(1→2)-β-D-Galp-(1→4)-β-L-Rhap-(1→OCH₃	319
	β-D-Glcp-(1→4)-[α-L-Rhap-(1→2)]-β-D-Galp-(1→OCH₃	252
	β-D-Glcp3P-(1→4)-[α-L-Rhap-(1→2)]-β-D-Galp-(1→4)-β-L-Rhap-(1→OCH₃[d]	319
	β-L-Rhap-(1→4)-β-D-Glcp-(1→4)-β-D-Galp-(1→O(CH₂)₃NH₂	323
	β-D-Glcp-(1→4)-[α-L-Rhap-(1→2)][Gro-(2→P→3)]-β-D-Galp-(1→4)-β-L-Rhap-(1→O(CH₂)₃NH₂	320
27	β-D-Glcp-(1→3)-β-D-GlcpNAc4,6(S)Pyr-(1→3)-α-D-Galp-(1→4)-β-L-Rhap-(1→O(CH₂)₅NH₂	282
29	β-D-Galf-(1→3)-β-D-Galp-(1→6)-β-D-Galf-(1→OCH₃	65

[a]For abbreviations of monosaccharides, see Table 2.
[b]For a protected disaccharide fragment of the CPS of serotype 3, see Garegg et al.[95]
[c]For two protected fragments of the CPS of serotype 8, see Chernyak and Antonov.[61]
[d]The structures of these synthesized oligosaccharides are based on polysaccharide structures, revised in the meantime (Table 2).
[e]MD, 7-methoxycarbonyl-3,6-dioxaheptyl; AD, 8-azido-3,6-dioxaoctyl.
[f]Mimics of fragments of the CPS of serotype 14.

D-Gal*p*-(1 → 3)-α-D-Glc*p*-(1 → 3)-α-L-Rha*p*-(1 → 4)-D-Rib-ol derived from the CPS of serotype 6B has been studied by x-ray, and a linear planar chain is suggested.[254]

PRIMARY STRUCTURE OF C-POLYSACCHARIDE AND F-ANTIGEN

The pneumococcal common antigens teichoic acid (C-polysaccharide) and lipoteichoic acid (F-antigen) have identical primary polysaccharide structures (Table 4),[35,91,162,173,245] which is a unique situation because in other Gram-positive bacteria these compounds are structurally unrelated. With respect to the two phosphocholine substituents in the F-antigen, it has to be mentioned that a minor fraction of apparently short chain length seems to be composed of phosphocholine-free repeating units.[35] For the moment it is unclear whether chains with both substituted and unsubstituted repeating units are also present. An earlier reported primary structure of the C-polysaccharide, wherein the ribitol-bound 6-O-substituted (phosphocholine) *N*-acetyl-β-D-galactosamine was found to be a β-D-galactosamine residue, and the *N*-acetyl-α-D-galactosamine residue not substituted at O-6,[136,156,316] has been revised.[173] For reports with earlier structural data of C-polysaccharide, see refs.[52,121,177,243,328]

Efforts focused on the organic synthesis of fragments of the C-polysaccharide have also been reported. The oligosaccharide fragments comprise β-D-Gal*p*NAc-(1 → 1)-D-Rib-ol-(5 → P → 6)-β-D-Glc*p*-(1 → O(CH₂)₃NH₂[112] and D-Rib-ol-(5 → P → 6)-β-D-Glc*p*-(1 → 3)-AAT-α-D-Gal*p*-(1 → 4)-α-D-Gal*p*NAc-(1 → OCH₃.[291]

CONJUGATES

Focusing on the preparation of covalently-linked pneumococcal polysaccharide-protein and oligosaccharide-protein conjugates, important factors in relation to vaccine development are (i) the knowledge of the primary structures of pneumococcal polysaccharides; (ii) the purity of capsular polysaccharides, of generated or synthesized oligosaccharides (polysaccharide fragments), and of carrier proteins; (iii) the choice of the carrier protein; (iv) the chemistry employed for the (poly)saccharide and/or protein random/single point activation; (v) the selection of a suitable spacer (if aimed) between the (poly)saccharide and the carrier protein; (vi) the coupling procedure; (vii) the ratio of (poly)saccharide to protein in the conjugate; (viii) the optimal chain length of saccharide fragments; (ix) the possible disturbance of the (poly)saccharide conformation; (x) the reproducibility in preparing separate batches. General reviews, discussing the preparation of conjugates can be found in refs.[11,161,185,186,211,303]

One of the severe problems in the native capsular polysaccharide production for conjugates is the contamination with C-polysaccharide. Most, if not all, isolated capsular polysaccharides contain a certain percentage of C-polysaccharide. Nowadays, the purity of capsular polysaccharide batches is controlled by NMR spectroscopic methods. With respect to synthetic oligosaccharides, the usual quality control protocols for application in humans have to be followed.

For the evaluation of their immunological properties in various animal models and humans, capsular polysaccharides and fragments thereof have been conjugated to various carrier proteins. Typical examples are tetanus toxoid,[40,66,77,175,176,208,235,236,269,279,292] diphtheria toxoid,[9,40,87,88] pertussis toxoid,[281] pneumolysin toxoid (pneumolysoid),[174,184,208,231] meningococcal outer membrane protein complex from *Neisseria meningitidis* serotype B,[8,96,97,204,325] CRM₁₉₇ (a nontoxic variant of diphtheria toxin; CRM = cross reacting material),[2,75,241,242,288,301] *Salmonella* protein,[317] small peptides selected on the basis of T-cell stimulating properties, and the laboratory models bovine[40,192,292,317,326] and human[175] serum albumin and keyhole limpet hemocyanin.[3–5,292]

With respect to polysaccharide-protein conjugates it may be clear that in a random activation protocol several complexities can arise when a polyfunctional polysaccharide of polydisperse molecular mass is conjugated to a polyfunctional carrier protein. Different conjugate forms including complex networks (cross-linking) can be the result. Typical functional groups for random activation of polysaccharides are hydroxyl groups, (generated) amino groups, carboxyl groups, and generated carbonyl (aldehyde) groups. On the protein, typical functional groups for random activation are amino groups, carboxyl groups, and thiol groups. It means that, sometimes depending on the specific polysaccharide structure, in theory a panel of chemical reactions (coupling technologies) can be applied, whereby one should keep in mind not to degrade the repetitive immunogenic epitope completely. For single point activation of polysaccharides, a reducing end must be present or generated via solvolysis (neoglycoconjugates). Spacers, usually containing terminal amino functions, carboxyl groups and/or thiol functions, can be used to overcome steric hindrance problems in reaction protocols, but also to obtain better presentations of epitopes.

Activation of hydroxyl functions can be carried out using cyanogen bromide (vicinal hydroxyl groups) or carbonyldiimidazole. Carboxyl functions are activated with carbodiimides. In the case of the presence of vicinal hydroxyl functions, periodate oxidation creates aldehyde functions that can be used in coupling protocols based on reductive amination. Amino groups can be attacked via activated carboxyl-group-containing agents. For reactions with thiol functions, frequently haloacetyl-containing agents are used. In all these approaches a careful control of the chemistry, including the neutralization of non-reacted activated groups, is necessary.

Many protocols follow the random activation of polysaccharides with cyanogen bromide and the subsequent introduction of bifunctional spacer molecules such as adipic acid dihydrazide,[4,5,66,279,281,317,326] 6-aminohexanoic acid,[184,231,236] cystamine,[77,269] or *N,N'*-bis(glycyl)cystamine.[77] The adipic acid hydrazide derivative can be coupled with side-chain carboxyl functions of glutamic acid or aspartic acid residues of the protein backbone in a carbodiimide-mediated reaction (Fig. 5a). It has been found that addition of *N*-hydroxysulfosuccinimide enhances the yield of carbodiimide-mediated coupling reactions.[4,5,299,326] The sequence of the coupling reactions can also be started with the carbodiimide activation of the protein.[204] The 6-aminohexanoic acid derivative can be coupled in a carbodiimide-mediated reaction to side-chain amino groups of lysine residues of the protein backbone (Fig. 5a). The cystamine (or *N,N'*-bis(glycyl)cystamine) derivatives are reduced and the

TABLE 4. PRIMARY STRUCTURES[a] OF THE C-POLYSACCHARIDE AND F-ANTIGEN OF *Streptococcus pneumoniae*

Primary structure

C

$$Cho \rightarrow P \qquad Cho \rightarrow P$$
$$\downarrow \qquad\qquad \downarrow$$
$$6 \qquad\qquad 6$$

H[→6)-β-D-Glc*p*-(1→3)-AAT-α-D-Gal*p*-(1→4)-α-D-Gal*p*NAc-(1→3)-β-D-Gal*p*NAc-(1→1)-D-Rib-ol-(5→P→]$_n$........peptidoglycan

F[b]

$$Cho \rightarrow P \qquad Cho \rightarrow P$$
$$\downarrow \qquad\qquad \downarrow$$
$$6 \qquad\qquad 6$$

H[→6)-β-D-Glc*p*-(1→3)-AAT-α-D-Gal*p*-(1→4)-α-D-Gal*p*NAc-(1→3)-β-D-Gal*p*NAc-(1→1)-D-Rib-ol-(5→P→]$_{2-8}$→6)-β-D-Glc*p*-(1→3)-β-D-Glc*p*-(1→3)-
-AAT-β-D-Gal*p*-(1→3)-α-D-Glc*p*-(1→3)-acyl$_2$Gro

[a]For abbreviations of monosaccharides, see Table 2.
[b]Identified fatty acids in the diacylglycerol moiety are 12:0, 14:0, 16:0, 18:0, Δ7-16:1, Δ9-16:1, Δ9-18:1, Δ11-18:1.[35]

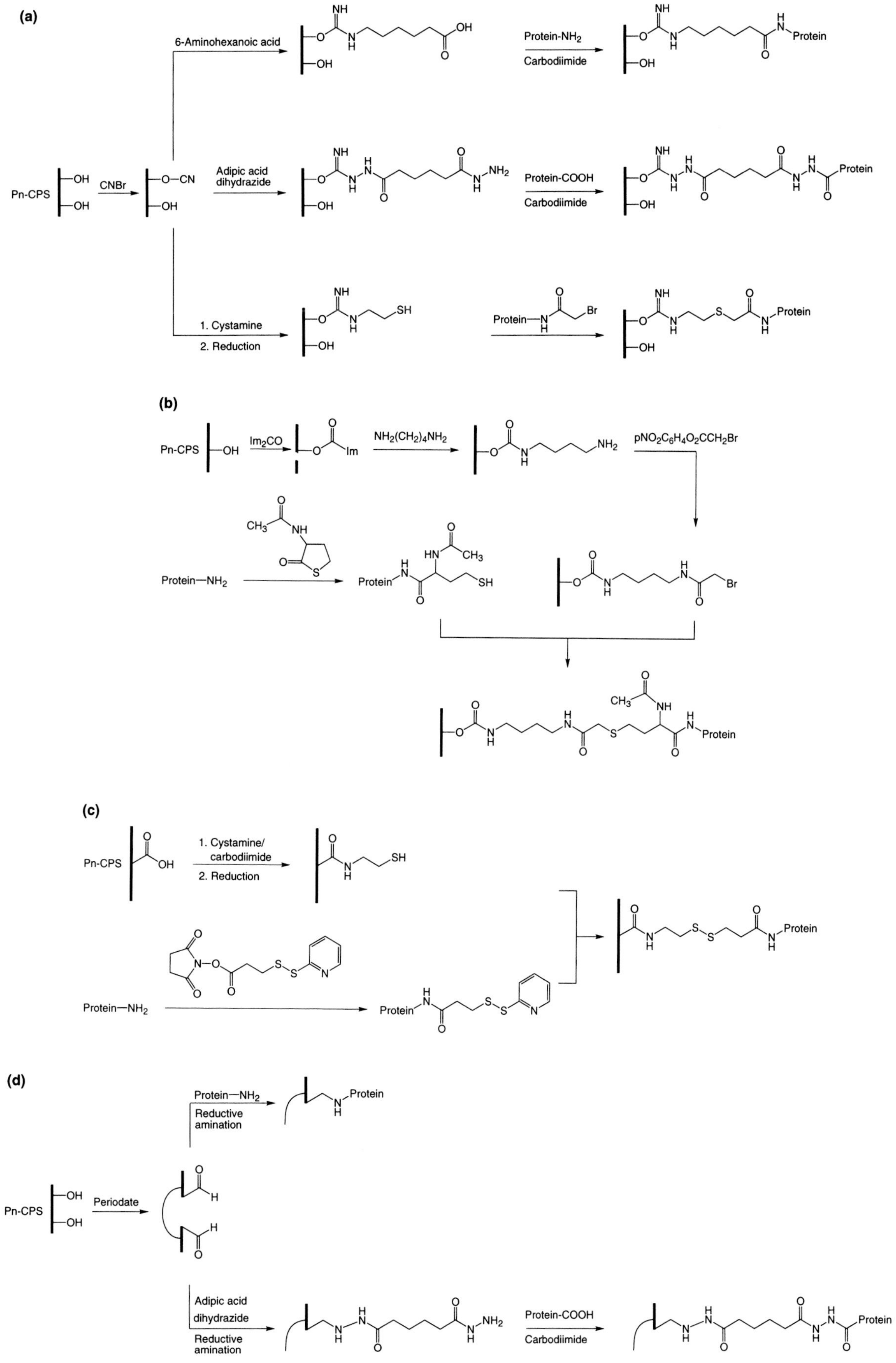

FIG. 5. Chemistry of some conjugation protocols (I).

cysteamine products are coupled with bromoacetylated (using *N*-succinimidyl bromoacetate) carrier protein to give the thioether-linked conjugates (Fig. 5a).

Another possibility is to functionalize each reaction partner separately with a bifunctional spacer molecule (Fig. 5b).[204] To this end the polysaccharide is derivatized with carbonyldiimidazole followed by a reaction with the spacer molecule 1,4-diaminobutane. Before coupling with the protein partner, the free amino function of the polysaccharide derivative is bromoacetylated with 4-nitrophenyl bromoacetate. The carrier protein (lysine) is derivatized with *N*-acetylhomocysteine using *N*-acetylhomocysteine thiolactone to attach pendant thiol groups. Coupling of both polymeric reactants yields a thioether linkage, whereby the polysaccharide-protein conjugate can be evaluated by amino acid analysis (e.g. determination of *S*-(carboxymethyl)homocysteine).[96,97,325]

In the case of uronic-acid-containing polysaccharides, sulfhydryl groups can be introduced at carboxyl functions using cystamine in a carbodiimide-mediated reaction followed by reduction (Fig. 5c). Then, the cysteamine derivative can be linked to the carrier protein using the heterobifunctional cross-linking reagent *N*-succinimidyl-3-(2-pyridyldithio)propionate.[87,88] Also a more direct approach has been reported, whereby carbodiimide-activated uronic acid-containing polysaccharide was directly coupled to carrier protein (lysine).[40]

Additionally, polysaccharides (sometimes partially depolymerized[174]) have been subjected to limited periodate oxidation to create free aldehyde functions for conjugation to carrier protein lysine residues using sodium cyanoborohydride in a reductive amination step (Fig. 5d).[75,174,175,283] A similar approach was followed in combination with adipic acid dihydrazide as a spacer, whereby conjugation to carrier protein glutamic acid or aspartic acid residues was aimed.[174]

The quality control of polysaccharide-protein conjugates is not always an easy task. Possibilities may include liquid chromatography techniques for sizing, purity and integrity, NMR characterization of polysaccharides and conjugates, amino acid analysis to determine linkages, peptide mapping for glycosylation sites, and circular dichroism for denaturing and/or unfolding of proteins and conjugates.

In the case of free oligosaccharides several protocols have been reported,[2–5,9,10,75,175,176,208,235,236,241,242,288,292] mainly based on reductive amination (single point activation), and in the following some insight is presented.

"Oligosaccharide" mixtures of definite but relatively large dimensions (small polysaccharides), obtained via partial acid hydrolysis of polysaccharides, have been conjugated directly to carrier protein lysine residues by reductive amination in the presence of sodium cyanoborohydride (Fig. 6a).[10,242,288] Such mixtures have also been treated with ammonium chloride and sodium

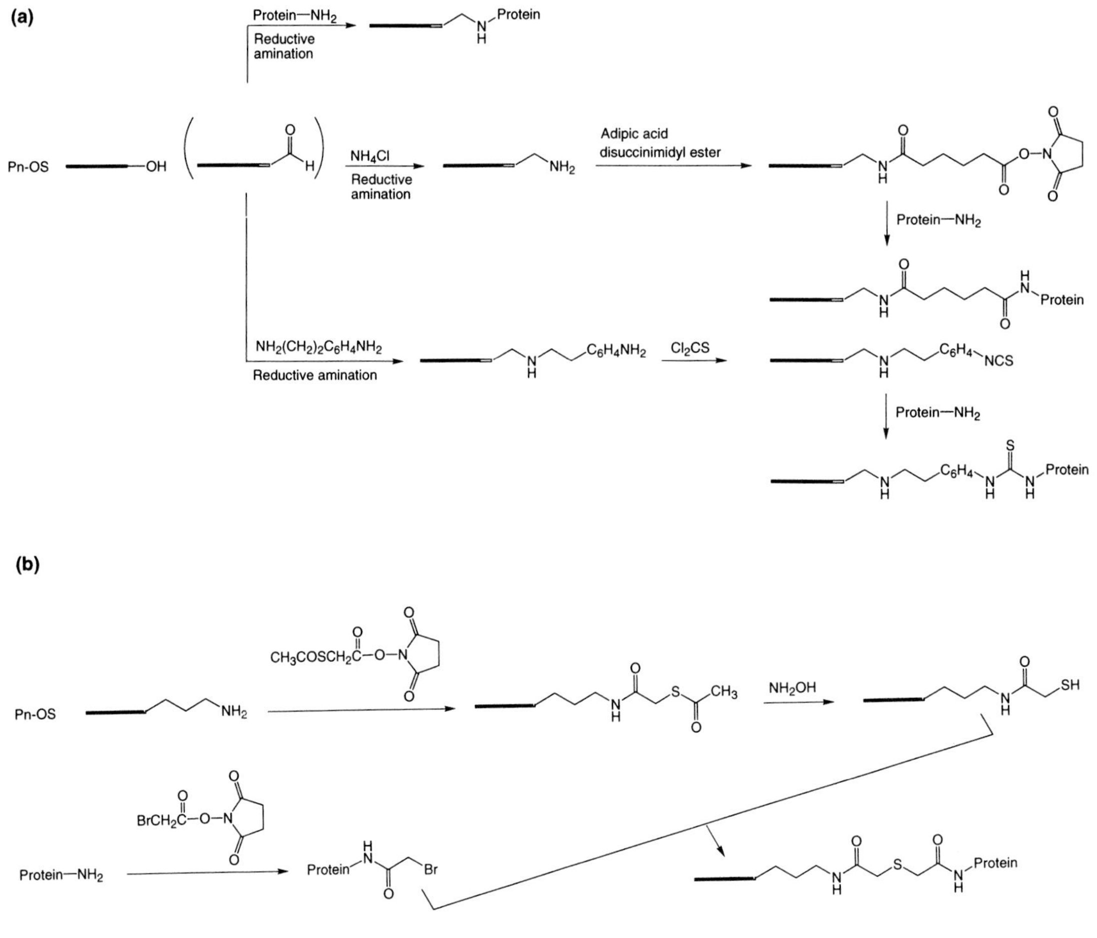

FIG. 6. Chemistry of some conjugation protocols (II).

cyanoborohydride (Fig. 6a). Here, the introduced amino groups at the "reducing end" were converted into the corresponding active esters via reaction with the disuccinimidyl ester of adipic acid, followed by coupling with the carrier protein lysine residues.[241] In another protocol "oligosaccharide" mixtures have been subjected to a limited periodate oxidation to introduce randomly aldehyde functional groups (Fig. 5d). Coupling of the generated derivatives with the carrier protein (lysine) was carried out by reductive amination using sodium cyanoborohydride.[75,208] Depolymerized polysaccharides have also been reduced with sodium borohydride before mild periodate oxidation.[175]

"Oligosaccharide" mixtures of definite dimensions, prepared via limited periodate oxidation of polysaccharides, have been activated with cyanogen bromide (Fig. 5a) and coupled to the spacer molecule 6-aminohexanoic acid, and the formed derivatives were condensed with the carrier protein (lysine) in a carbodiimide-mediated reaction.[235,236]

Coupling of the reducing end of a free oligosaccharide with 2-(4-aminophenyl)-ethylamine in the presence of sodium cyanoborohydride (reductive amination) yields an arylamine, which can be converted with thiophosgene into the corresponding phenylisothiocyanate (Fig. 6a). The latter derivative can be linked to the carrier protein via lysine residues.[292]

Oligosaccharides with a terminal 2,5-anhydrohexose residue having a free aldehyde function, derived from N-acetylhexosamine-containing polysaccharides via partial de-N-acetylation/nitrous acid deamination, have been coupled directly to the carrier protein via lysine residues using a reductive amination protocol with sodium cyanoborohydride.[176]

Synthetically prepared oligosaccharides (small polysaccharide fragments) having a spacer at the anomeric center of the "reducing end" monosaccharide have also been conjugated with carrier proteins. Anomeric 3-aminopropyl groups[306–308, 320,323,324] have been S-acetylated with N-succinimidyl S-acetylthioacetate (Fig. 6b). In this protocol the carrier protein (lysine) is bromoacetylated with N-succinimidyl bromoacetate. After removal of the acetyl group from the oligosaccharide using hydroxylamine, the free SH-containing oligosaccharides are coupled to the bromoacetylated carrier protein.[3–5] Anomeric allyl groups can be easily converted into 3-(2-aminoethylthio)propyl functions,[221,222] to be used in similar type of coupling procedures as mentioned for the 3-aminopropyl derivatives.

The coupling of pure oligosaccharides via their free anomeric centers or via the anomerically introduced spacers to carrier proteins may be better controlled and be more specific. Loading of carrier proteins can be followed using modern analytical approaches such as mass spectrometry. The degree of conjugation of smaller carbohydrate chains with carrier proteins is influenced by many factors. It means that the percentage of loading has to be optimized for each conjugate, not only in terms of applied chemistry but also in terms of immunological results.

REFERENCES

1. **Adeyeye, A., P.-E. Jansson, B. Lindberg, and J. Henrichsen.** 1988. Structural studies of the capsular polysaccharide from *Streptococcus pneumoniae* type 37. Carbohydr. Res. **180**:295–299.

2. **Åhman, H., H. Käyhty, P. Tamminen, A. Vuorela, F. Malinoski, and J. Eskola.** 1996. Pentavalent pneumococcal oligosaccharide conjugate vaccine PncCRM is well-tolerated and able to induce an antibody response in infants. Pediatr. Infect. Dis. J. **15**:134–139.

3. **Alonso de Velasco, E., A.F.M. Verheul, G.H. Veeneman, L.J.F. Gomes, J.H. van Boom, J. Verhoef, and H. Snippe.** 1993. Protein-conjugated synthetic di- and trisaccharides of pneumococcal type 17F exhibit a different immunogenicity and antigenicity than tetrasaccharide. Vaccine **11**:1429–1436.

4. **Alonso de Velasco, E., A.F.M. Verheul, A.M.P. van Steijn, H.A.T. Dekker, R.G. Feldman, I.M. Fernández, J.P. Kamerling, J.F.G. Vliegenthart, J. Verhoef, and H. Snippe.** 1994. Epitope specificity of rabbit immunoglobulin G (IgG) elicited by pneumococcal type 23F synthetic oligosaccharide- and native polysaccharide-protein conjugate vaccines: comparison with human anti-polysaccharide 23F IgG. Infect. Immun. **62**:799–808.

5. **Alonso de Velasco, E., H.A.T. Dekker, A.F.M. Verheul, R.G. Feldman, J. Verhoef, and H. Snippe.** 1995. Anti-polysaccharide immunoglobulin isotope levels and opsonic activity of antisera: relationships with protection against *Streptococcus pneumoniae* infection in mice. J. Infect. Dis. **172**:562–565.

6. **Alonso de Velasco, E., A.F.M. Verheul, J. Verhoef, and H. Snippe.** 1995. *Streptococcus pneumoniae*: virulence factors, pathogenesis, and vaccines. Microbiol. Rev. **59**, 591–603.

7. **Amvam-Zollo, P.-H., and P. Sinaÿ.** 1986. *Streptococcus pneumoniae* type XIV polysaccharide. Synthesis of a repeating branched tetrasaccharide with dioxa-type spacer-arms. Carbohydr. Res. **150**:199–212.

8. **Anderson, E.L., D.J. Kennedy, K.M. Geldmacher, J. Donnelly, and P.M. Mendelman.** 1996. Immunogenicity of heptavalent pneumococcal conjugate vaccine in infants. J. Pediatr. **128**: 649–653.

9. **Anderson, P., and R. Betts.** 1989. Human adult immunogenicity of protein-coupled pneumococcal capsular antigens of serotypes prevalent in otitis media. Pediatr. Infect. Dis. J. **8**:S50–S53.

10. **Anderson, P., M. Pichichero, and R.A. Insel.** 1985. Immunogens consisting of oligosaccharides from the capsule of *Haemophilus influenzae* type b coupled to diphtheria toxoid or the toxin protein CRM₁₉₇. J. Clin. Invest. **76**:52–59.

11. **Aplin, J.D., and J.C. Wriston.** 1981. Preparation, properties and applications of carbohydrate conjugates of proteins and lipids. Crit. Rev. Biochem. **5**:259–307.

12. **Appelbaum, P.C.** 1992. Antimicrobial resistance in *Streptococcus pneumoniae*: an overview. Clin. Infect. Dis. **15**:77–83.

13. **Arrecubieta, C., R. López, and E. García.** 1996. Type 3-specific synthase of *Streptococcus pneumoniae* (Cap3B) directs type 3 polysaccharide biosynthesis in *Escherichia coli* and in pneumococcal strains of different serotypes. J. Exp. Med. **184**: 449–455.

14. **Aspinall, G.O.** 1982. Chemical characterization and structure determination of polysaccharides. *In* G.O. Aspinall (ed.), The polysaccharides, vol. 1. Academic Press, New York, pp. 35–131.

15. **Austrian, R.** 1952. Observations on the transformation of pneumococcus in vivo. Bull. Johns Hopkins Hosp. **91**:189–195.

16. **Austrian, R.** 1981. Pneumococcus: the first one hundred years. Rev. Infect. Dis. **3**:183–189.

17. **Austrian, R.** 1981. Some observations on the pneumococcus and on the current status of pneumococcal disease and its prevention. Rev. Infect. Dis. **3(Suppl)**:S1–S17.

18. **Austrian, R.** 1989. Pneumococcal polysaccharide vaccines. Rev. Infect. Dis. **11(Suppl 3)**:S598–602.

19. **Austrian, R.** 1996. Bacterial polysaccharide vaccines. *In* S. Plotkin and B. Fantini (eds.), Vaccinia, vaccination and vaccinology: Jenner, Pasteur and their successors. Elsevier, Paris, pp. 127–133.

20. **Avery, O.T., and M. Heidelberger.** 1925. Immunological relationships of cell constituents of pneumococcus. Second paper. J. Exp. Med. **42**:367–376.

21. **Avery, O.T., and W.F. Goebel.** 1929. Chemo-immunological studies on conjugated carbohydrate-proteins. II. Immunological specificity of synthetic sugar-protein antigens. J. Exp. Med. **50**:533–550.

22. **Avery, O.T., and W.F. Goebel.** 1931. Chemo-immunological studies on conjugated carbohydrate-proteins. V. The immunological specificity of an antigen prepared by combining the capsular polysaccharide of type III pneumococcus with foreign protein. J. Exp. Med. **54**:437–447.

23. **Avery, O.T., C.M. MacLeod, and M. McCarty.** 1944. Studies on the chemical nature of the substance inducing transformation of pneumococcal types. J. Exp. Med. **79**:137–157.

24. **Backman-Marklund, I., P.-E. Jansson, B. Lindberg, and J. Henrichsen.** 1990. Structural studies of the capsular polysaccharide from *Streptococcus pneumoniae* type 7A. Carbohydr. Res. **198**:67–77.

25. **Baddiley, J., J.G. Buchanan, and B. Carss.** 1957. The configuration of the ribitol phosphate residue in cytidine diphosphate ribitol. J. Chem. Soc. 1869–1876.

26. **Barker, S.A., and P.J. Somers.** 1970. Bacterial and fungal polysaccharides. *In* W. Pigman and D. Horton (eds.), The carbohydrates, vol. IIb. Academic Press, New York, pp. 581–583.

27. **Barker, S.A., M. Stacey, and J.M. Williams.** 1960. New data about the structure of antigenic polysaccharides of *Pneumococcus*. Bull. Soc. Chim. Biol. **42**:1611–1618.

28. **Barker, S.A., P.J. Somers, M. Stacey, and J.W. Hopton.** 1965. Arrangement of the L-rhamnose units in *Diplococcus pneumoniae* type II polysaccharide. Carbohydr. Res. **1**:106–115.

29. **Barker, S.A., S.M. Bick, J.S. Brimacombe, M.J. How, and M. Stacey.** 1966. Structural studies on the capsular polysaccharide of *Pneumococcus* type V. Carbohydr. Res. **2**:224–233.

30. **Barker, S.A., P.J. Somers, and M. Stacey.** 1967. Sequence studies on *Diplococcus pneumoniae* type II polysaccharide. Carbohydr. Res. **3**:261–270.

31. **Barnes, D.M., S. Whittier, P.H. Gilligan, S. Soares, A. Tomasz, and F.W. Henderson.** 1995. Transmission of multidrug-resistant serotype 23F *Streptococcus pneumoniae* in group day care: evidence suggesting capsular transformation of the resistant strain in vivo. J. Infect. Dis. **171**:890–896.

32. **Batavyal, L., and N. Roy.** 1983. Structure of the capsular polysaccharide of *Diplococcus pneumoniae* type 31. Carbohydr. Res. **119**:300–302.

33. **Becker, G.E., and A.M. Pappenheimer, Jr.** 1966. Lyase activity of inducible S8-depolymerases from *Bacillus palustris*. Biochim. Biophys. Acta **121**:343–348.

34. **Bednar, B., and J.P. Hennessey, Jr.** 1993. Molecular size analysis of capsular polysaccharide preparations from *Streptococcus pneumoniae*. Carbohydr. Res. **243**:115–130.

35. **Behr, T., W. Fischer, J. Peter-Katalinic, and H. Egge.** 1992. The structure of pneumococcal lipoteichoic acid; improved preparation, chemical and mass spectrometric studies. Eur. J. Biochem. **207**:1063–1075.

36. **Bennett, L.G., and C.T. Bishop.** 1977. Structure of the type XXVII *Streptococcus pneumoniae* (pneumococcal) capsular polysaccharide. Can. J. Chem. **55**:8–16.

37. **Bennett, L.G., and C.T. Bishop.** 1977. The pyruvate ketal as a stereospecific immunodeterminant in the type XXVII *Streptococcus pneumoniae* (pneumococcal) capsular polysaccharide. Immunochemistry **14**:693–696.

38. **Bennett, L.G., and C.T. Bishop.** 1980. Structure of the type XXXIII *Streptococcus pneumoniae* (pneumococcal) capsular polysaccharide. Can. J. Chem. **58**:2724–2727.

39. **Benzing, L., D.J. Carlo, and M.B. Perry.** 1981. Specific capsular polysaccharide of type 46 *Streptococcus pneumoniae* (American type 73). Infect. Immun. **32**:1024–1027.

40. **Beuvery, E.C., F. van Rossum, and J. Nagel.** 1982. Comparison of the induction of immunoglobulin M and G antibodies in mice with purified pneumococcal type 3 and meningococcal group C polysaccharides and their protein conjugates. Infect. Immun. **37**:15–22.

41. **Beynon, L.M., J.C. Richards, M.B. Perry, and P.J. Kniskern.** 1992. Antigenic and structural relationships within group 19 *Streptotcoccus pneumoniae*: chemical characterization of the specific capsular polysaccharides of types 19B and 19C. Can. J. Chem. **70**:218–232.

42. **Beynon, L.M., J.C. Richards, M.B. Perry, and P.J. Kniskern.** 1995. Characterization of the capsular antigen of *Streptococcus pneumoniae* serotype 35B. Can. J. Chem. **73**:41–48.

43. **Beynon, L.M., J.C. Richards, and M.B. Perry.** 1997. Identification of the common antigenic determinant shared by *Streptococcus pneumoniae* serotypes 35A and 20 capsular polysaccharides. Structural analysis of the *Streptococcus pneumoniae* serotype 35A capsular polysaccharide. Eur. J. Biochem. **250**:163–167.

44. **Bhattacharya, S.B., and C.V.N. Rao.** 1981. A reinvestigation on the structure of the capsular polysaccharide from *Pneumococcus* type IX. J. Chem. Soc., Perkin Trans. 1:278–283.

45. **Björndal, H., C.G. Hellerqvist, B. Lindberg, and S. Svensson.** 1970. Gas-Flüssigkeits-Chromatographie und Massenspektrometrie bei der Methylierungsanalyse von Polysacchariden. Angew. Chem. **82**:643–652.

46. **Bock, K., C. Pedersen, and H. Pedersen.** 1984. Carbon-13 nuclear magnetic resonance data for oligosaccharides. Adv. Carbohydr. Chem. Biochem. **42**:193–225.

47. **Bock, K., H. Lönn, and T. Peters.** 1990. Conformational analysis of a disaccharide fragment of the polysaccharide antigen of *Streptococcus pneumoniae* type 1 using n.m.r. spectroscopy and HSEA calculations. Carbohydr. Res. **198**:375–380.

48. **Bousquet, E., M. Khitri, L. Lay, F. Nicotra, L. Panza, and G. Russo.** 1998. Capsular polysaccharide of *Streptococcus pneumoniae* type 19F: synthesis of the repeating unit. Carbohydr. Res. **311**:171–181.

49. **Breiman, R.F., J.C. Butler, F.C. Tenover, J.A. Elliott, and R.R. Facklam.** 1994. Emergence of drug-resistant pneumococcal infections in the United States. JAMA **271**:1831–1835.

50. **Brimacombe, J.S., and M.J. How.** 1962. *Pneumococcus* type V capsular polysaccharide: characterisation of pneumosamine as 2-amino-2,6-dideoxy-L-talopyranose. J. Chem. Soc. 5037–5040.

51. **Broome, C.V.** 1982. Efficacy of pneumococcal polysaccharide vaccines. Rev. Infect. Dis. **3**:582–596.

52. **Brundish, D.E., and J. Baddiley.** 1968. Pneumococcal C-substance, a ribitol teichoic acid containing choline phosphate. Biochem. J. **110**:573–582.

53. **Bruyn, G.A.W., and R. van Furth.** 1991. Pneumococcal polysaccharide vaccines: indications, efficacy and recommendations. Eur. J. Clin. Microbiol. Infect. Dis. **10**:897–910.

54. **Bruyn, G.A.W., B.J.M. Zegers, and R. van Furth.** 1992. Mechanisms of host defence against infection with *Streptococcus pneumoniae*. Clin. Infect. Dis. **14**:251–262.

55. **Butler, J.C., R.F. Breiman, H.B. Lipman, J. Hofmann, and R.R. Facklam.** 1995. Serotype distribution of *Streptococcus pneumoniae* infections among preschool children in the United States, 1978–1994: implications for development of a conjugate vaccine. J. Infect. Dis. **171**:885–889.

56. **Campbell, J.H., and A.M. Pappenheimer, Jr.** 1966. Quantitative studies of the specificity of anti-pneumococcal polysaccharide antibodies, types III and VIII. I. Isolation of oligosaccharides from acid and from enzymatic hydrolysates of S3 and S8. Immunochemistry **3**:195–212.

57. **Caroff, M., and M.B. Perry.** 1984. The specific capsular polysaccharide of *Streptococcus pneumoniae* type 15A (American type 30). Can. J. Biochem. Cell Biol. **62**:151–161.

58. **Chatterjee, B.P., and C.V.N. Rao.** 1975. Some structural features of Pneumococcus type XXII capsular polysaccharide. J. Chem. Soc., Perkin Trans. 1:985–988.

59. **Chatterjee, B.P., S. Purkayastha, and C.V.N. Rao.** 1976. Structure of *Pneumococcus* type XXII capsular polysaccharide. Indian J. Chem. **14B:**914–918.

60. **Chaudhari, A.S., C.T. Bishop, and R.J. Fielder.** 1972. Structural studies on the specific type VII pneumococcal polysaccharide. Carbohydr. Res. **25:**161–172.

61. **Chernyak, A.Ya., and K.V. Antonov.** 1992. Synthesis of protected fragments of the capsular polysaccharide from *Streptococcus pneumoniae* type 8. Bioorg. Khim. **18:**716–725.

62. **Chernyak, A.Ya., K.V. Antonov, N.K. Kochetkov, L.N. Padyukov, and N.V. Tsvetkova.** 1985. Two synthetic antigens related to *Streptococcus pneumoniae* type 3 capsular polysaccharide. Carbohydr. Res. **141:**199–212.

63. **Chernyak, A.Ya., K.V. Antonov, and N.K. Kochetkov.** 1987. Synthesis of oligosaccharide fragments of the capsular polysaccharide of *Streptococcus pneumoniae*, type 3. Bioorg. Khim. **13:**958–966.

64. **Chittenden, G.J.F., W.K. Roberts, J.G. Buchanan, and J. Baddiley.** 1968. The specific substance from *Pneumococcus* type 34 (41). Biochem. J. **109:**597–602.

65. **Choudhury, A.K., I. Mukherjee, and N. Roy.** 1998. Synthesis of a trisaccharide related to the K-antigen from *Streptococcus pneumoniae* type 29. Synth. Commun. **28:**3115–3120.

66. **Chu, C.-Y., R. Schneerson, J.B. Robbins, and S.C. Rastogi.** 1983. Further studies on the immunogenicity of *Haemophilus influenzae* type b and pneumococcal type 6A polysaccharide-protein conjugates. Infect. Immun. **40:**245–256.

67. **Cifonelli, J.A., P. Rebers, M.B. Perry, and J.K.N. Jones.** 1966. The capsular polysaccharide of pneumococcus type XII, SXII. Biochemistry **5:**3066–3072.

68. **Ciuffreda, P., D. Colombo, F. Ronchetti, and L. Toma.** 1992. Conformational analysis of the trisaccharide components of the repeating units of the capsular polysaccharides of *Streptococcus pneumoniae* types 19F and 19A. Carbohydr. Res. **232:**327–339.

69. **Coffey, T.J., M.C. Enright, M. Daniels, J.K. Morona, R. Morona, W. Hryniewicz, J.C. Paton, and B.G. Spratt.** 1998. Recombinatorial exchanges at the capsular polysaccharide biosynthetic locus lead to frequent serotype changes among natural isolates of *Streptococcus pneumoniae*. Mol. Microbiol. **27:**73–83.

70. **Cross, A.S.** 1990. The biologic significance of bacterial encapsulation. Curr. Topics Microbiol. Immun. **150:**87–95.

71. **Dahmén, J., G. Gnosspelius, A.-C. Larsson, T. Lave, G. Noori, K. Pålsson, T. Frejd, and G. Magnusson.** 1985. Synthesis of di-, tri-, and tetra-saccharides corresponding to receptor structures recognised by *Streptococcus pneumoniae*. Carbohydr. Res. **138:**17–28.

72. **Daoust, V., D.J. Carlo, J.Y. Zeltner, and M.B. Perry.** 1981. Specific capsular polysaccharide of type 45 *Streptococcus pneumoniae* (American type 72). Infect. Immun. **32:**1028–1033.

73. **Das, A., J.D. Higginbotham, and M. Heidelberger.** 1972. Oxidation of the capsular polysaccharide of pneumococcal type IX by periodate. Biochem. J. **126:**233–236.

74. **Das, A., M. Heidelberger, and R. Brown.** 1976. Identification of D-galacturonic acid in the specific capsular polysaccharide of pneumococcal type XXV. Carbohydr. Res. **48:**304–305.

75. **Daum, R.S., D. Hogerman, M.B. Rennels, K. Bewley, F. Malinoski, E. Rothstein, K. Reisinger, S. Block, H. Keyserling, and M. Steinhoff.** 1997. Infant immunization with pneumococcal CRM$_{197}$ vaccines: effect of saccharide size on immunogenicity and interactions with simultaneously administered vaccines. J. Infect. Dis. **176:**445–455.

76. **Dell, A.** 1987. FAB-mass spectrometry of carbohydrates. Adv. Carbohydr. Chem. Biochem. **45:**19–72.

77. **De Weers, O., M. Beurret, L. van Buren, L.A. Oomen, J.T. Poolman, and P. Hoogerhout.** 1998. Application of cystamine and N,N'-bis(glycyl)cystamine as linkers in polysaccharide-protein conjugation. Bioconjugate Chem. **9:**309–315.

78. **Dillard, J.P., and J. Yother.** 1994. Genetic and molecular characterization of capsular polysaccharide biosynthesis in *Streptococcus pneumoniae* type 3. Mol. Microbiol. **12:**959–972.

79. **Dillard, J.P., M.W. Vandersea, and J. Yother.** 1995. Characterization of the cassette containing genes for type 3 capsular polysaccharide biosynthesis in *Streptococcus pneumoniae*. J. Exp. Med. **181:**973–983.

80. **Dixon, J.R., J.G. Buchanan, and J. Baddiley.** 1966. The specific substance from *Pneumococcus* type 34. The configuration of the glycosidic linkages. Biochem. J. **100:**507–511.

81. **Dixon, J.R., W.K. Roberts, G.T. Mills, J.G. Buchanan, and J. Baddiley.** 1968. The O-acetyl groups of the specific substance from *Pneumococcus* type 34 (U.S. type 41). Carbohydr. Res. **8:**262–265.

82. **Dochez, A.R., and O.T. Avery.** 1917. The elaboration of specific soluble substance by pneumococcus during growth. J. Exp. Med. **26:**477–493.

83. **Duke, J.L., I.J. Goldstein, and J.A. Cifonelli.** 1974. Structural studies of capsular polysaccharide of type XII *Diplococcus pneumoniae*. Carbohydr. Res. **37:**81–88.

84. **Eby, R., M. Koster, D. Hogerman, and F. Malinoski.** 1994. Pneumococcal conjugates. *In* E. Norrby, F. Brown, R.M. Chanock, and H.S. Ginsberg (eds.), Vaccines 94: modern approaches to new vaccines including prevention of AIDS. Cold Spring Harbor Laboratory Press, Cold Spring Harbor, pp. 119–124.

85. **Estrada-Parra, S., and M. Heidelberger.** 1963. The specific polysaccharide of type XVIII pneumococcus. III. Biochemistry **2:**1288–1294.

86. **Estrada-Parra, S., and I. Gómez.** 1972. Immunochemistry of type XIV pneumococcus capsular polysaccharide oxidized by D-galactose oxidase. Immunochemistry **9:**1095–1101.

87. **Fattom, A., W.F. Vann, S.C. Szu, A. Sutton, X. Li, D. Bryla, G. Schiffman, J.B. Robbins, and R. Schneerson.** 1988. Synthesis and physicochemical and immunological characterization of pneumococcus type 12F polysaccharide-diphtheria toxoid conjugates. Infect. Immun. **56:**2292–2298.

88. **Fattom, A., C. Lue, S.C. Szu, J. Mestecky, G. Schiffman, D. Bryla, W.F. Vann, D. Watson, L.M. Kimzey, J.B. Robbins, and R. Schneerson.** 1990. Serum antibody response in adult volunteers elicited by injection of *Streptococcus pneumoniae* type 12F polysaccharide alone or conjugated to diphtheria toxoid. Infect. Immun. **58:**2309–2312.

89. **Fedson, D.S.** 1998. Pneumococcal vaccination in the United States and 20 other developed countries, 1981–1996. Clin. Infect. Dis. **26:**1117–1123.

90. **Feldman, C., and K. Klugman.** 1997. Pneumococcal infections. Curr. Opin. Infect. Dis. **10:**109–115.

91. **Fischer, W., T. Behr, R. Hartmann, J. Peter-Katalinic, and H. Egge.** 1993. Teichoic acid and lipoteichoic acid of *Streptococcus pneumoniae* possess identical chain structures—a reinvestigation of teichoic acid (C-polysaccharide). Eur. J. Biochem. **215:**851–857.

92. **Friedländer, C.** 1883. Die Mikrokokken der Pneumoniae. Fortschr. Medicin **1:**715–733.

93. **García, E., and R. López.** 1997. Molecular biology of the capsular genes of *Streptococcus pneumoniae*. FEMS Microbiol. Lett. **149:**1–10.

94. **García, E., P. García, and R. López.** 1993. Cloning and sequencing of a gene involved in the synthesis of the capsular polysaccharide of *Streptococcus pneumoniae* type 3. Mol. Gen. Genet. **239:**188–195.

95. **Garegg, P.J., S. Oscarson, and U. Tedebark.** 1998. Synthesis of the repeating unit of the capsular polysaccharide of *Streptococcus pneumoniae* type 3 as a building block suitable for formation of oligomers. J. Carbohydr. Chem. **17:**587–594.

96. **Giebink, G.S., M. Koskela, P.P. Vella, M. Harris, and C.T. Le.** 1993. Pneumococcal capsular polysaccharide-meningococcal outer membrane protein complex conjugate vaccines: immunogenicity and efficacy in experimental pneumococcal otitis media. J. Infect. Dis. **167:**347–355.

97. **Giebink, G.S., J.D. Meier, M.K. Quartey, C.L. Liebeler, and C.T. Le.** 1996. Immunogenicity and efficacy of *Streptococcus pneumoniae* polysaccharide-protein conjugate vaccines against homologues and heterologues serotypes in the chinchilla otitis media model. J. Infect. Dis. **173:**119–127.

98. **Gillespie, S.H.** 1994. The diagnosis of *Streptococcus pneumoniae* infections. Rev. Med. Microbiol. **5:**224–232.

99. **Goebel, W.F., T. Shedlovski, G.I. Lavin, and M.H. Adams.** 1943. The heterophile antigen of pneumococcus. J. Biol. Chem. **148:**1–15.

100. **Goldstein, I.J., J.A. Cifonelli, and J. Duke.** 1974. Interaction of concanavalin A with the capsular polysaccharide of pneumococcus type XII and isolation of kojibiose from the polysaccharide. Biochemistry **13:**867–870.

101. **Griffith, F.** 1928. The significance of pneumococcal types. J. Hyg. **27:**113–159.

102. **Guidolin, A., J.K. Morona, R. Morona, D. Hansman, and J.C. Paton.** 1994. Nucleotide sequence analysis of genes essential for capsular polysaccharide biosynthesis in *Streptococcus pneumoniae* type 19F. Infect. Immun. **62:**5384–5396.

103. **Guy, R.C.E., M.J. How, M. Stacey, and M. Heidelberger.** 1967. The capsular polysaccharide of type I Pneumococcus. I. Purification and chemical modification. J. Biol. Chem. **242:**5106–5111.

104. **Harvey, D.J., B. Kuster, and T.J.P. Naven.** 1998. Perspectives in glycosciences—matrix-assisted laser desorption/ionization (MALDI) mass spectrometry of carbohydrates. Glycoconjugate J. **15:**333–338.

105. **Heffron, R.** 1939. Pneumonia with special reference to pneumococcus lobar pneumonia. Harvard University Press, Cambridge.

106. **Heidelberger, M.** 1983. Precipitating cross-reactions among pneumococcal types. Infect. Immun. **41:**1234–1244.

107. **Heidelberger, M., and O.T. Avery.** 1923. The soluble specific substance of pneumococcus. J. Exp. Med. **38:**73–79.

108. **Heidelberger, M., S. Estrada-Parra, and R. Brown.** 1964. The specific polysaccharide of type XVIIIA pneumococcus. Biochemistry **3:**1548–1550.

109. **Heidelberger, M., W.F. Dudman, and W. Nimmich.** 1970. Immunochemical relationships of certain capsular polysaccharides of Klebsiella, pneumococci and Rhizobia. J. Immun. **104:**1321–1328.

110. **Henrichsen, J.** 1979. The pneumococcal typing system and pneumococcal surveillance. J. Infect. **1(suppl 2):**31–37.

111. **Henrichsen, J.** 1995. Six newly recognized types of *Streptococcus pneumoniae*. J. Clin. Microbiol. **33:**2759–2762.

112. **Hermans, J.P.G., C.E. Dreef, P. Hoogerhout, G.A. van der Marel, and J.H. van Boom.** 1988. Synthesis of two analogues of a fragment of the complex polysaccharide C substance from *Streptococcus pneumoniae* type 1. Recl. Trav. Chim. Pays-Bas **107:**600–606.

113. **Higginbotham, J.D., and M. Heidelberger.** 1972. The specific capsular polysaccharide of *Pneumococcus* type IV. Carbohydr. Res. **23:**165–173.

114. **Higginbotham, J.D., and M. Heidelberger.** 1973. Oxidation of the capsular polysaccharide of pneumococcal type IV by periodate. Carbohydr. Res. **27:**297–302.

115. **Higginbotham, J.D., M. Heidelberger, and E.C. Gotschlich.** 1970. Degradation of a pneumococcal type-specific polysaccharide with exposure of group-specificity. Proc. Natl. Acad. Sci. U.S.A. **67:**138–142.

116. **Higginbotham, J.D., A. Das, and M. Heidelberger.** 1972. Immunochemical studies on the capsular polysaccharide of pneumococcal type IX. Biochem. J. **126:**225–231.

117. **Horito, S., J.P. Lorentzen, and H. Paulsen.** 1986. Bausteine von Oligosacchariden. LXXVII. Synthese einer Trisaccharideinheit des Kapselpolysaccharides von *Streptococcus pneumoniae* Typ 4. Liebigs. Ann. 1880–1890.

118. **Horne, D., and A. Tomasz.** 1985. Pneumococcal Forssman antigen: enrichment in mesosomal membranes and specific binding to the autolytic enzyme of *Streptococcus pneumoniae*. J. Bacteriol. **161:**18–24.

119. **Hotchkiss, R.D., and W.F. Goebel.** 1937. Chemo-immunological studies on the soluble specific substance of pneumococcus. III. The structure of the aldobionic acid from the type III polysaccharide. J. Biol. Chem. **121:**195–203.

120. **Hounsell, E.F. (ed.).** 1998. Glycoscience protocols. Methods in molecular biology series. Humana Press, New York.

121. **How, M.J., J.S. Brimacombe, and M. Stacey.** 1964. The pneumococcal polysaccharides. Adv. Carbohydr. Chem. **19:**303–358.

122. **Jacobs, M.R.** 1992. Treatment and diagnosis of infections caused by drug-resistant *Streptococcus pneumoniae*. Clin. Infect. Dis. **15:**119–127.

123. **Jansson, P.-E., L. Kenne, H. Liedgren, B. Lindberg, and J. Lönngren.** 1976. A practical guide to the methylation analysis of carbohydrates. Chem. Commun. Univ. Stockholm **8:**1–75.

124. **Jansson, P.-E., B. Lindberg, and U. Lindquist.** 1981. Structural studies of the capsular polysaccharide from *Streptococcus pneumoniae* type 4. Carbohydr. Res. **95:**73–80.

125. **Jansson, P.-E., B. Lindberg, U. Lindquist, and D.J. Carlo.** 1983. Structural studies of the capsular polysaccharide from *Streptococcus pneumoniae* type 17A. Carbohydr. Res. **118:**157–171.

126. **Jansson, P.-E., B. Lindberg, and U. Lindquist.** 1985. Structural studies of the capsular polysaccharide from *Streptococcus pneumoniae* type 5. Carbohydr. Res. **140:**101–110.

127. **Jansson, P.-E., B. Lindberg, U. Lindquist, and J. Ljungberg.** 1987. Structural studies of the capsular polysaccharide from *Streptococcus pneumoniae* types 15B and 15C. Carbohydr. Res. **162:**111–116.

128. **Jansson, P.-E., B. Lindberg, J. Lindberg, and J. Henrichsen.** 1988. Structural studies of the capsular polysaccharide from *Streptococcus pneumoniae* type 18F. Carbohydr. Res. **173:**217–225.

129. **Jansson, P.-E., N.S. Kumar, B. Lindberg, G. Widmalm, and J. Henrichsen.** 1988. Structural studies of the capsular polysaccharide from *Streptococcus pneumoniae* type 18A. Carbohydr. Res. **173:**227–233.

130. **Jansson, P.-E., B. Lindberg, M. Andersson, U. Lindquist, and J. Henrichsen.** 1988. Structural studies of the capsular polysaccharide from *Streptococcus pneumoniae* type 2, a reinvestigation. Carbohydr. Res. **182:**111–117.

131. **Jansson, P.-E., J. Lindberg, K.M. Swarna Wimalasiri, and J. Henrichsen.** 1991. The structure of the capsular polysaccharide from *Streptococcus pneumoniae* type 7B. Carbohydr. Res. **217:**117–180.

132. **Jennings, H.J.** 1983. Capsular polysaccharides as human vaccines. Adv. Carbohydr. Chem. Biochem. **41:**155–208.

133. **Jennings, H.J.** 1990. Capsular polysaccharides as vaccine candidates. Curr. Topics Microbiol. Immun. **150:**97–127.

134. **Jennings, H.J., and R.A. Pon.** 1996. Polysaccharides and glycoconjugates as human vaccines. *In* S. Dumitriu (ed.), Polysaccharides in medicinal applications. Marcel Dekker, New York, pp. 443–479.

135. **Jennings, H.J., and R.K. Sood.** 1994. Synthetic glycoconjugates as human vaccines. *In* Y.C. Lee and R. Lee (eds.), Neoglycoconjugates: preparation and applications. Academic Press, New York, pp. 325–371.

136. **Jennings, H.J., C. Lugowski, and N.M. Young.** 1980. Structure of the complex polysaccharide C-substance from *Streptococcus pneumoniae* type 1. Biochemistry **19:**4712–4719.

137. **Jennings, H.J., K.-G. Rosell, and D.J. Carlo.** 1980. Structural determination of the capsular polysaccharide of *Streptococcus pneumoniae* type-19 (19F). Can. J. Chem. **58:**1069–1074.

138. **Johnston, R.B., Jr.** 1991. Pathogenesis of pneumococcal pneumoniae. Rev. Infect. Dis. **13(Suppl 6):**S509–S517.

139. **Jones, C.** 1985. Identification of the tetrasaccharide repeating-unit of the *Streptococcus pneumoniae* type 23 polysaccharide by high-field proton n.m.r. spectroscopy. Carbohydr. Res. **139:**75–83.

140. **Jones, C.** 1990. A novel method for the determination of the stereochemistry of pyruvate acetal substituents applied to the capsular polysaccharide from *Streptococcus pneumoniae* type 4. Carbohydr. Res. **198:**353–357.

141. **Jones, C.** 1995. Full assignment of the NMR spectrum of the capsular polysaccharide from *Streptococcus pneumoniae* serotype 10A. Carbohydr. Res. **269:**175–181.

142. **Jones, C.** 1998. Capsular polysaccharides from *Neisseria meningitidis* and *Streptococcus pneumoniae*. Carbohydr. Eur. **21:**10–16.

143. **Jones, C., and F. Currie.** 1988. The pneumococcal polysaccharide S4: a structural reassessment. Carbohydr. Res. **184:**279–284.

144. **Jones, C., B. Mulloy, A. Wilson, A. Dell, and J.E. Oates.** 1985. Structure of the capsular polysaccharide from *Streptococcus pneumoniae* type 9. J. Chem. Soc., Perkin Trans. 1:1665–1673.

145. **Jones, C., F. Currie, and M.J. Forster.** 1991. N.m.r. and conformational analysis of the capsular polysaccharide from *Streptococcus pneumoniae* type 4. Carbohydr. Res. **221:**95–121.

146. **Jones, J.K.N., and M.B. Perry.** 1957. The structure of the type VIII pneumococcus specific polysaccharide. J. Am. Chem. Soc. **79:**2787–2793.

147. **Kaji, E., F.W. Lichtenthaler, Y. Osa, K. Takahashi, E. Matsui, and S. Zen.** 1992. A practical, highly stereoselective synthesis of the trisaccharide repeating unit of a *Streptococcus pneumoniae* polysaccharide. Chem. Lett. 707–710.

148. **Kaji, E., F.W. Lichtenthaler, Y. Osa, K. Takahashi, and S. Zen.** 1995. A practical synthesis of mannosaminyl-β(1 → 4)-glucosyl-α(1 → 2)-rhamnose, the trisaccharide repeating unit of a *Streptococcus pneumoniae* capsular polysaccharide. Bull. Chem. Soc. Jpn. **68:**2401–2408.

149. **Kamerling, J.P., and J.F.G. Vliegenthart.** 1989. Carbohydrates. *In* A.M. Lawson (ed.), Mass spectrometry/clinical biochemistry—principles, methods, applications. Walter de Gruyter, Berlin, pp. 175–263.

150. **Karlsson, C., P.-E. Jansson, G. Widmalm, and U.B.S. Sørensen.** 1997. Structural elucidation of the capsular polysaccharide from *Streptococcus pneumoniae* type 18B. Carbohydr. Res. **304:**165–172.

151. **Karlsson, C., P.-E. Jansson, and U.B. Sørensen.** 1998. The chemical structures of the capsular polysaccharides from *Streptococcus pneumoniae* types 32F and 32A. Eur. J. Biochem. **255:**296–302.

152. **Katzenellenbogen, E., and H.J. Jennings.** 1983. Structural determination of the capsular polysaccharide of *Streptococcus pneumoniae* type 19A (57). Carbohydr. Res. **124:**235–245.

153. **Kauffmann, F., E. Lund, and B.E. Eddy.** 1960. Proposal for a change in the nomenclature of *Diplococcus pneumoniae* and a comparison of the Danish and American type designations. Int. Bull. Bacteriol. Nomencl. Taxonom. **10:**31–40.

154. **Käyhty, H., and J. Eskola.** 1996. New vaccines for the prevention of pneumococcal infections. Emerg. Infect. Dis. **2:**289–298.

155. **Kelly, T., J.P. Dillard, and J. Yother.** 1994. Effect of genetic switching of capsular type on virulence of *Streptococcus pneumoniae*. Infect. Immun. **62:**1813–1819.

156. **Kenne, L., and B. Lindberg.** 1983. Bacterial polysaccharides. *In* G.O. Aspinall (ed.), The polysaccharides, vol. 2. Academic Press, New York, pp. 287–363.

157. **Kenne, L., and B. Lindberg.** 1988. The structure of *Streptococcus pneumoniae* type 29 polysaccharide: a re-examination. Carbohydr. Res. **184:**288–291.

158. **Kenne, L., B. Lindberg, and S. Svensson.** 1975. The structure of capsular polysaccharide of the pneumococcus type II. Carbohydr. Res. **40:**69–75.

159. **Kenne, L., B. Lindberg, and J.K. Madden.** 1979. Structural studies of the capsular antigen from *Streptococcus pneumoniae* type 26. Carbohydr. Res. **73:**175–182.

160. **Kennedy, D.A., J.G. Buchanan, and J. Baddiley.** 1969. The type-specific substance from *Pneumococcus* type 11A (43). Biochem. J. **115:**37–45.

161. **Klein, D.L., and R.W. Ellis.** 1997. Conjugate vaccines against *Streptococcus pneumoniae*. *In* M.M. Levine, G.C. Woodrow, J.B. Kaper, and G.S. Cobon (eds.), New generation vaccines. Marcel Dekker, New York, pp. 503–525.

162. **Klein, R.A., R. Hartmann, H. Egge, T. Behr, and W. Fischer.** 1994. The aqueous solution structure of the tetrasaccharide-ribitol repeat-unit from the lipoteichoic acid of *Streptococcus pneumoniae* strain R6 determined using a combination of NMR spectroscopy and computer calculations. Carbohydr. Res. **256:**189–222.

163. **Klugman, P.** 1990. Pneumococcal resistance to antibiotics. Clin. Microbiol. Rev. **3:**171–196.

164. **Knecht, J.C., G. Schiffman, and R. Austrian.** 1970. Some biological properties of pneumococcus type 37 and the chemistry of its capsular polysaccharide. J. Exp. Med. **132:**475–487.

165. **Kochetkov, N.K., and O.S. Chizhov.** 1966. Mass spectrometry of carbohydrate derivatives. Adv. Carbohydr. Chem. **21:**39–94.

166. **Kochetkov, N.K., N.E. Nifant'ev, and L.V. Backinowsky.** 1987. Synthesis of the capsular polysaccharide of *Streptococcus pneumoniae* type 14. Tetrahedron **43:**3109–3121.

167. **Koeman, F.A.W., J.P. Kamerling, and J.F.G. Vliegenthart.** 1993. Synthesis of structural elements of the capsular polysaccharide of *Streptococcus pneumoniae* type 8. Tetrahedron **49:**5291–5304.

168. **Koeman, F.A.W., J.W.G. Meissner, H.R.P. van Ritter, J.P. Kamerling, and J.F.G. Vliegenthart.** 1994. Synthesis of structural elements of the capsular polysaccharide of *Streptococcus pneumoniae* type 14. J. Carbohydr. Chem. **13:**1–25.

169. **Kolkman, M.A.B., D.A. Morrison, B.A.M. van der Zeijst, and P.J.M. Nuijten.** 1996. The capsule polysaccharide synthesis locus of *Streptococcus pneumoniae* serotype 14: identification of the glycosyltransferase gene cps14E. J. Bacteriol. **178:**3736–3741.

170. **Kolkman, M.A.B., B.A.M. van der Zeijst, and P.J.M. Nuijten.** 1997. Functional analysis of glycosyltransferases encoded by the capsular polysaccharide biosynthesis locus of *Streptococcus pneumoniae* serotype 14. J. Biol. Chem. **272:**19502–19508.

171. **Kolkman, M.A.B., W. Wakarchuk, P.J.M. Nuijten, and B.A.M. van der Zeijst.** 1997. Capsular polysaccharide synthesis in *Streptococcus pneumoniae* serotype 14: molecular analysis of the complete cps locus and identification of genes encoding glycosyltransferases required for the biosynthesis of the tetrasaccharide subunit. Mol. Microbiol. **26:**197–208.

172. **Kolkman, M.A.B., B.A.M. van der Zeijst, and P.J.M. Nuijten.** 1998. Diversity of capsular polysaccharide synthesis gene clusters in *Streptococcus pneumoniae*. J. Biochem. **123:**937–945.

173. **Kulakowska, M., J.-R. Brisson, D.W. Griffith, N.M. Young, and H.J. Jennings.** 1993. High-resolution NMR spectroscopic analysis of the C-polysaccharide of *Streptococcus pneumoniae*. Can. J. Chem. **71:**644–648.

174. **Kuo, J., M. Douglas, H.K. Ree, and A.A. Lindberg.** 1995. Characterization of a recombinant pneumolysin and its use as a protein carrier for pneumococcal type 18C conjugate vaccines. Infect. Immun. **63:**2706–2713.

175. **Laferrière, C.A., R.K. Sood, J.-M. de Muys, F. Michon, and H.J. Jennings.** 1997. The synthesis of *Streptococcus pneumoniae* polysaccharide-tetanus toxoid conjugates and the effect of chain length on immunogenicity. Vaccine **15:**179–186.

176. **Laferrière, C.A., R.K. Sood, J.-M. De Muys, F. Michon, and H.J. Jennings.** 1998. *Streptococcus pneumoniae* type 14 polysaccharide-conjugate vaccines: length stabilization of opsonophagocytic conformational polysaccharide epitopes. Infect. Immun. **66:**2441–2446.

177. **Larm, O., and B. Lindberg.** 1976. The pneumococcal polysaccharides: a reexamination. Adv. Carbohydr. Chem. Biochem. **33:**295–322.

178. **Larm, O., B. Lindberg, S. Svensson, and E.A. Kabat.** 1972. Structural studies on Pneumococcus type II capsular polysaccharide. Carbohydr. Res. **22:**391–397.

179. **Larm, O., B. Lindberg, and S. Svensson.** 1973. Further studies of the capsular polysaccharide of Pneumococcus type II. Carbohydr. Res. **31:**120–126.

180. **Lee, C.-J.** 1996. Bacterial capsular polysaccharides: immunogenicity and vaccines. In S. Dumitriu (ed.), Polysaccharides in medicinal applications. Marcel Dekker, New York, pp. 411–442.

181. **Lee, C.-J., and B.A. Fraser.** 1980. The structures of the cross-reactive types 19 (19F) and 57 (19A) pneumococcal capsular polysaccharides. J. Biol. Chem. **255:**6847–6853.

182. **Lee, C.-J., and T.R. Wang.** 1994. Pneumococcal infection and immunization in children. Crit. Rev. Microbiol. **20:**1–12.

183. **Lee, C.-J., B.A. Fraser, R.A. Boykins, and J.P. Li.** 1987. Effect of culture conditions on the structure of Streptococcus pneumoniae type 19A (57) capsular polysaccharide. Infect. Immun. **55:**1819–1823.

184. **Lee, C.-J., R.A. Lock, P.W. Andrew, T.J. Mitchell, D. Hansman, and J.C. Paton.** 1994. Protection of infant mice from challenge with Streptococcus pneumoniae type 19F by immunization with a type 19F polysaccharide-pneumolysoid conjugate. Vaccine **12:**875–878.

185. **Lee, Y.C., and R.T. Lee (eds.).** 1994. Neoglycoconjugates. Part A. Synthesis. Methods in enzymology, vol. 242, Academic Press, San Diego.

186. **Lee, Y.C., and R.T. Lee (eds.).** 1994. Neoglycoconjugates. Part B. Biomedical applications. Methods in enzymology, vol. 247, Academic Press, San Diego.

187. **Leggiadro, R.J., F.F. Barrett, P.J. Chesney, Y. Davis, and F.C. Tenover.** 1994. Invasive pneumococci with high level penicillin and cephalosporin resistance at a mid-South children's hospital. Pediatr. Infect. Dis. J. **13:**320–322.

188. **Lemieux, R.U., S.Z. Abbas, and B.Y. Chung.** 1982. Syntheses of core chain trisaccharides related to human blood group antigenic determinants. Can. J. Chem. **60:**68–75.

189. **Leontein, K., B. Lindberg, and J. Lönngren.** 1981. Structural studies of the capsular polysaccharide from Streptococcus pneumoniae type 12F. Can. J. Chem. **59:**2081–2085.

190. **Leontein, K., B. Lindberg, J. Lönngren, and D.J. Carlo.** 1983. Structural studies of the capsular polysaccharide from Streptococcus pneumoniae type 12A. Carbohydr. Res. **114:**257–266.

191. **Lew, J.Y., and M. Heidelberg.** 1976. Linkage of pyruvyl groups in the specific capsular polysaccharide of Pneumococcus type IV. Carbohydr. Res. **52:**255–258.

192. **Lin, K.T., and C.-J. Lee.** 1982. Immune response of neonates to pneumococcal polysaccharide-protein conjugate. Immunology **46:**333–342.

193. **Lindberg, B., J. Lönngren, and S. Svensson.** 1975. Specific degradation of polysaccharides. Adv. Carbohydr. Chem. Biochem. **31:**185–240.

194. **Lindberg, B., J. Lönngren, and D.A. Powell.** 1977. Structural studies on the specific type-14 pneumococcal polysaccharide. Carbohydr. Res. **58:**177–186.

195. **Lindberg, B., B. Lindqvist, J. Lönngren, and D.A. Powell.** 1980. Structural studies of the capsular polysaccharide from Streptococcus pneumoniae type 1. Carbohydr. Res. **78:**111–117.

196. **Lindberg, J.** 1990. Structural studies of bacterial polysaccharides using NMR spectroscopy and mass spectrometry. Thesis Stockholm University, Sweden.

197. **Lönn, H., and J. Lönngren.** 1984. Synthesis of a disaccharide component of the capsular polysaccharide antigen of Streptococcus pneumoniae type 1. Carbohydr. Res. **132:**39–44.

198. **Lönngren, J., and S. Svensson.** 1974. Mass spectrometry in structural analysis of natural carbohydrates. Adv. Carbohydr. Chem. Biochem. **29:**41–106.

199. **Lugowski, C., and H.J. Jennings.** 1984. Structural determination of the capsular polysaccharide of Streptococcus pneumoniae type 18C (56). Carbohydr. Res. **131:**119–129.

200. **Lund, E.** 1970. On the nomenclature of the pneumococcal types. Int. J. Syst. Bacteriol. **20:**321–323.

201. **Lund, E., and J. Henrichsen.** 1978. Laboratory diagnosis, serology and epidemiology of Streptococcus pneumoniae. Methods Microbiol. **12:**241–262.

202. **MacLeod, C.M., R.G. Hodges, M. Heidelberger, and W.G. Bernhard.** 1945. Prevention of pneumococcal pneumonia by immunization with specific capsular polysaccharides. J. Exp. Med. **82:**445–465.

203. **Mage, R.G., and E.A. Kabat.** 1963. The combining regions of the type III pneumococcus polysaccharide and homologous antibody. Biochemistry **2:**1278–1287.

204. **Marburg, S., D. Jorn, R.L. Tolman, B. Arison, J. McCauley, P.J. Kniskern, A. Hagopian, and P.P. Vella.** 1986. Biomolecular chemistry of macromolecules: synthesis of bacterial polysaccharide conjugates with Neisseria meningitidis membrane protein. J. Am. Chem. Soc. **108:**5282–5287.

205. **Marchessault, R.H., K. Imada, T.L. Bluhm, and P.R. Sundararajan.** 1980. Conformation of crystalline type III pneumococcal polysaccharide. Carbohydr. Res. **83:**287–302.

206. **McNeely, T.B., J.M. Staub, C.M. Rusk, M.J. Blum, and J.J. Donnelly.** 1998. Antibody responses to capsular polysaccharide backbone and O-acetate side groups of Streptococcus pneumoniae type 9V in humans and rhesus macaques. Infect. Immun. **66:**3705–3710.

207. **Micheli, E., F. Nicotra, L. Panza, F. Ronchetti, and L. Toma.** 1985. A new approach to the synthesis of β-glycosidically linked oligosaccharides containing 2-acetamido-2-deoxy-D-mannose residues. Carbohydr. Res. **139:**C1–C3.

208. **Michon, F., P.C. Fusco, C.A.S.A. Minetti, M. Laude-Sharp, C. Uitz, C.-H. Huang, A.J. D'Ambra, S. Moore, D.P. Remeta, I. Heron, and M.S. Blake.** 1998. Multivalent pneumococcal capsular polysaccharide conjugate vaccines employing genetically detoxified pneumolysin as a carrier protein. Vaccine **16:**1732–1741.

209. **Mitchell, T.J., and P.W. Andrew.** 1995. Vaccines against Streptococcus pneumoniae. In D.A.A. Ala'Aldeen and C.E. Hormaeche (eds.), Molecular and clinical aspects of bacterial vaccine development. Wiley, Chichester, pp. 93–117.

210. **Miyazaki, T., and T. Yadomae.** 1971. Polysaccharides of type XIX Pneumococcus. Part II. The type specific polysaccharide and its chemical behaviour. Carbohydr. Res. **16:**153–159.

211. **Moreau, M.** 1996. Conjugation technologies. In S. Plotkin and B. Fantini (eds.), Vaccinia, vaccination and vaccinology: Jenner, Pasteur and their successors. Elsevier, Paris, pp. 145–149.

212. **Moreau, M., J.C. Richards, M.B. Perry, and P.J. Kniskern.** 1988. Structural analysis of the specific capsular polysaccharide of Streptococcus pneumoniae type 45 (American type 72). Biochemistry **27:**6820–6829.

213. **Moreau, M., J.C. Richards, M.B. Perry, and P.J. Kniskern.** 1988. Application of high-resolution n.m.r. spectroscopy to the elucidation of the structure of the specific capsular polysaccharide of Streptococcus pneumoniae type 7F. Carbohydr. Res. **182:**79–99.

214. **Morona, J.K., R. Morona, and J.C. Paton.** 1997. Molecular and genetic characterization of the capsule biosynthesis locus of Streptococcus pneumoniae type 19B. J. Bacteriol. **179:**4953–4958.

215. **Morona, J.K., R. Morona, and J.C. Paton.** 1997. Characterization of the locus encoding the Streptococcus pneumoniae type 19F capsular polysaccharide biosynthetic pathway. Mol. Microbiol. **23:**751–763.

216. Moxon, E.R., and J.S. Kroll. 1990. The role of bacterial poly-saccharide capsules as virulence factors. Curr. Topics Microbiol. Immun. **150:**65–86.

217. Munoz, R., J.M. Musser, M. Crain, D.E. Briles, A. Marton, A.J. Parkinson, U. Sorensen, and A. Tomasz. 1992. Geographic distribution of penicillin-resistant clones of *Streptococcus pneumoniae*: characterization by penicillin-binding protein profile, surface protein A typing, and multilocus enzyme analysis. Clin. Infect. Dis. **15:**112–118.

218. Munoz, R., M. Mollerach, R. López, and E. García. 1997. Molecular organization of the genes required for the synthesis of type 1 capsular polysaccharide of *Streptococcus pneumoniae*: formation of binary encapsulated pneumococci and identification of cryptic dTDP-rhamnose biosynthesis genes. Mol. Microbiol. **25:**79–92.

219. Musher, D.M. 1992. Infections caused by *Streptococcus pneumoniae*: clinical spectrum, pathogenesis, immunity, and treatment. Clin. Infect. Dis. **14:**801–807.

220. Nesin, M., M. Ramirez, and A. Tomasz. 1998. Capsular transformation of a multidrug-resistant *Streptococcus pneumoniae* in vivo. J. Infect. Dis. **177:**707–713.

221. Niggemann, J., J.P. Kamerling, and J.F.G. Vliegenthart. 1998. β-1,4-Galactosyltransferase-catalyzed synthesis of the branched tetrasaccharide repeating unit of *Streptococcus pneumoniae* type 14. Bioorg. Med. Chem. **6:**1605–1612.

222. Niggemann, J., J.P. Kamerling, and J.F.G. Vliegenthart. 1998. Application of β-1,4-galactosyltransferase in the synthesis of complex branched-chain oligosaccharide mimics of fragments of the capsular polysaccharide of *Streptococcus pneumoniae* type 14. J. Chem. Soc., Perkin Trans. 1:3011–3020.

223. Nilsson, M., and T. Norberg. 1998. Synthesis of a spacer-containing nonsaccharide fragment of *Streptococcus pneumoniae* 19F capsular polysaccharide. J. Chem. Soc., Perkin Trans. 1:1699–1704.

224. Ohno, N., T. Yadomae, and T. Miyazaki. 1980. The structure of the type-specific polysaccharide of *Pneumococcus* type XIX. Carbohydr. Res. **80:**297–304.

225. Pal, J., S.B. Bhattacharya, and C.V.N. Rao. 1981. Graded hydrolysis studies on *Pneumococcus* type IX capsular polysaccharide. J. Chem. Soc., Perkin Trans. 1:1393–1396.

226. Panza, L., F. Ronchetti, G. Russo, and L. Toma. 1987. Synthesis of the trisaccharide component of the repeating unit of the capsular polysaccharide of *Streptococcus pneumoniae* type 19F. J. Chem. Soc., Perkin Trans. 1:2745–2747.

227. Panza, L., F. Ronchetti, and L. Toma. 1988. *Streptococcus pneumoniae* type 19A polysaccharide. Synthesis of the trisaccharide component of the repeating unit. Carbohydr. Res. **180:**242–245.

228. Paoletti, L.C., D.L. Kasper, F. Michon, J. Di Fabio, K. Holme, H.J. Jennings, and M.R. Wessels. 1990. An oligosaccharide-tetanus toxoid conjugate vaccine against type III Group B *Streptococcus*. J. Biol. Chem. **265:**18278–18283.

229. Pasteur, L. 1881. Note sur la maladie nouvelle provoquée par la salive d'un enfant mort de la rage. Bull. Acad. Méd. (Paris) **10:**94–103.

230. Paton, J.C. 1993. Molecular analysis of the pathogenicity of *Streptococcus pneumoniae*: the role of pneumococcal proteins. Annu. Rev. Microbiol. **47:**89–115.

231. Paton, J.C., R.A. Lock, C.-J. Lee, J.P. Li, A.M. Berry, T.J. Mitchell, P.W. Andrew, D. Hansmann, and G.J. Boulnois. 1991. Purification and immunogenicity of genetically obtained pneumolysin toxoids and their conjugation to *Streptococcus pneumoniae* type 19F polysaccharide. Infect. Immun. **59:**2297–2304.

232. Paulsen, H., and B. Helpap. 1989. Synthese einer Tetrasaccharideinheit des Kapselpolysaccharides von *Streptococcus pneumoniae* Type 9V. Carbohydr. Res. **186:**189–205.

233. Paulsen, H., B. Helpap, and J.P. Lorentzen. 1988. Synthese von Trisaccharid-Einheiten der Kapselpolysaccharide von *Streptococcus pneumoniae*. Carbohydr. Res. **179:**173–197.

234. Pazur, J.H., M.S. Erikson, M.E. Tay, and P.Z. Allen. 1983. Isomeric, anti-rhamnose antibodies having specificity for rhamnose-containing, streptococcal heteroglycans. Carbohydr. Res. **124:**253–263.

235. Peeters, C.C.A.M., A.-M. Tenbergen-Meekes, D.E. Evenberg, J.T. Poolman, B.J.M. Zegers, and G.T. Rijkers. 1991. A comparative study of the immunogenicity of pneumococcal type 4 polysaccharide and oligosaccharide tetanus toxoid conjugates in adult mice. J. Immun. **146:**4308–4314.

236. Peeters, C., A.-M. Tenbergen-Meekes, J. Poolman, B. Zegers, and G. Rijkers. 1992. Induction of anti-pneumococcal cell wall polysaccharide antibodies by type 4 pneumococcal polysaccharide-protein conjugates. Med. Microbiol. Immun. **181:**35–42.

237. Perry, M.B., V. Daoust, and D.J. Carlo. 1981. The specific capsular polysaccharide of *Streptococcus pneumoniae* type 9V. Can. J. Biochem. **59:**524–533.

238. Perry, M.B., D.R. Bundle, V. Daoust, and D.J. Carlo. 1982. The specific capsular polysaccharide of *Streptococcus pneumoniae* type 15F. Mol. Immun. **19:**235–246.

239. Phillips, L.R., O. Nishimura, and B.A. Fraser. 1983. The structure of the repeating oligosaccharide unit of the pneumococcal capsular polysaccharide type 18C. Carbohydr. Res. **121:**243–255.

240. Ponpipom, M.M., R.L. Bugianesi, and T.Y. Shen. 1978. Synthesis of paragloboside analogs. Tetrahedron Lett. 1717–1720.

241. Porro, M., P. Costantino, S. Viti, F. Vannozzi, A. Naggi, and G. Torri. 1985. Specific antibodies to diphtheria toxin and type 6A pneumococcal capsular polysaccharide induced by a model of semi-synthetic glycoconjugate antigen. Mol. Immun. **22:**907–919.

242. Powers, D.C., E.L. Anderson, K. Lottenbach, and C.A.M. Mink. 1996. Reactogenicity and immunogenicity of a protein-conjugated pneumococcal oligosaccharide vaccine in older adults. J. Infect. Dis. **173:**1014–1018.

243. Poxton, I.R., E. Tarelli, and J. Baddiley. 1978. The structure of C-polysaccharide from the walls of *Streptococcus pneumoniae*. Biochem. J. **175:**1033–1042.

244. Pozsgay, V., J.-R. Brisson, and H.J. Jennings. 1990. Synthesis of a tri- and a tetra-saccharide fragment of the capsular polysaccharide of type III group B *Streptococcus*. Carbohydr. Res. **205:**133–146.

245. Qin, H., and T.B. Grindley. 1998. Determination of the configuration of ribitol in the C-polysaccharide of *Streptococcus pneumoniae*. *In* Abstracts of the XIX International Carbohydrate Symposium. San Diego, p. BP065.

246. Rahav, G., Y. Toledano, D. Engelhard, A. Simhon, A.E. Moses, T. Sacks, and M. Shapiro. 1997. Invasive pneumococcal infections: a comparison between adults and children. Medicine **76:**295–303.

247. Ramirez, M., and A. Tomasz. 1998. Molecular characterization of the complete 23F capsular polysaccharide locus of *Streptococcus pneumoniae*. J. Bacteriol. **180:**5273–5278.

248. Rao, E.V., J.G. Buchanan, and J. Baddiley. 1966. The type-specific substance from *Pneumococcus* type 10A (34); structure of the dephosphorylated repeating unit. Biochem. J. **100:**801–810.

249. Rao, E.V., J.G. Buchanan, and J. Baddiley. 1966. The type-specific substance from *Pneumococcus* type 10A (34); the phosphodiester linkages. Biochem. J. **100:**811–814.

250. Rao, E.V., M.J. Watson, J.G. Buchanan, and J. Baddiley. 1969. The type-specific substance from *Pneumococcus* type 29. Biochem. J. **111:**547–556.

251. Rauvala, H., J. Finne, T. Krusius, J. Kärkkäinen, and J. Järnefelt. 1981. Methylation techniques in the structural analysis of glycoproteins and glycolipids. Adv. Carbohydr. Chem. Biochem. **38:**389–416.

252. **Ray, A.K., U.B. Maddali, A. Roy, and N. Roy.** 1990. Synthesis of di- and trisaccharides related to the polysaccharide from *Streptococcus pneumoniae* type 23 and a study of their inhibition in the precipitin reaction. Carbohydr. Res. **197**:93–100.

253. **Rebers, P.A., and M. Heidelberger.** 1959. The specific polysaccharide of type VI pneumococcus. I. Preparation, properties and reactions. J. Am. Chem. Soc. **81**:2415–2419.

254. **Rebers, P.A., and M. Heidelberger.** 1961. The specific polysaccharide of type VI pneumococcus. II. The repeating unit. J. Am. Chem. Soc. **83**:3056–3059.

255. **Reeves, R.E., and W.F. Goebel.** 1941. Chemoimmunological studies on the soluble specific substance of pneumococcus. V. The structure of the type III polysaccharide. J. Biol. Chem. **139**:511–519.

256. **Reinhold, V.N., B.B. Reinhold, and S. Chan.** 1996. Carbohydrate sequence analysis by electrospray ionization mass spectrometry. High Resolut. Sep. Anal. Biol. Macromol. A **270**:377–402.

257. **Richards, J.C., and M.B. Perry.** 1988. Structure of the specific capsular polysaccharide of *Streptococcus pneumoniae* 23F (American type 23). Biochem. Cell Biol. **66**:758–771.

258. **Richards, J.C., and M.B. Perry.** 1988. Structural comparisons of *Streptococcus pneumoniae* specific polysaccharides of group 9 (9N, 9V, 9L, 9A) related to the choice of vaccine components. *In* A.M. Wu (ed.), The molecular immunology of complex carbohydrates. Plenum, New York, pp. 593–594.

259. **Richards, J.C., M.B. Perry, and D.J. Carlo.** 1983. The specific capsular polysaccharide of *Streptococcus pneumoniae* type 20. Can. J. Biochem. Cell Biol. **61**:178–190.

260. **Richards, J.C., M.B. Perry, and P.J. Kniskern.** 1984. The specific capsular polysaccharide of *Streptococcus pneumoniae* type 33F. Can. J. Biochem. Cell Biol. **62**:666–677.

261. **Richards, J.C., M.B. Perry, and P.J. Kniskern.** 1984. Structural analysis of the specific polysaccharide of *Streptococcus pneumoniae* type 9L (American type 49). Can. J. Biochem. Cell Biol. **62**:1309–1320.

262. **Richards, J.C., M.B. Perry, and P.J. Kniskern.** 1985. The structure of the specific capsular polysaccharide of *Streptococcus pneumoniae* type 11F (American type 11). Can. J. Biochem. Cell Biol. **63**:953–968.

263. **Richards, J.C., M.B. Perry, and M. Moreau.** 1988. Elucidation and comparison of the chemical structures of the specific capsular polysaccharides of *Streptococcus pneumoniae* groups 11 (11F, 11B, 11C, and 11A). *In* A.M. Wu (ed.), The molecular immunology of complex carbohydrates. Plenum, New York, pp. 595–596.

264. **Richards, J.C., M.B. Perry, and P.J. Kniskern.** 1989. Structural analysis of the specific capsular polysaccharide of *Streptococcus pneumoniae* type 22F. Can. J. Chem. **67**:1038–1050.

265. **Rijkers, G.T., E.A.M. Sanders, M.A. Breukels, and B.J.M. Zegers.** 1996. Responsiveness of infants to capsular polysaccharides: implications for vaccine development. Rev. Med. Microbiol. **7**:3–12.

266. **Robbins, J.B., and R. Schneerson.** 1990. Polysaccharide-protein conjugates: a new generation of vaccines. J. Infect. Dis. **161**:821–832.

267. **Robbins, J.B., R. Austrian, C.-J. Lee, S.C. Rastogi, G. Schiffman, J. Henrichsen, P.H. Mäkelä, C.V. Broome, R.R. Facklam, R.H. Tiesjema, and J.C. Parke, Jr.** 1983. Considerations for formulating the second-generation pneumococcal polysaccharide vaccine with emphasis on the cross-reactive types within groups. J. Infect. Dis. **148**:1136–1159.

268. **Robbins, J.B., R. Schneerson, S.S. Szu, and V. Pozsgay.** 1996. Polysaccharide-protein conjugate vaccines. *In* S. Plotkin and B. Fantini (eds.), Vaccinia, vaccination and vaccinology: Jenner, Pasteur and their successors. Elsevier, Paris, pp. 135–143.

269. **Rodriguez, M.E., G.P.J.M. van den Dobbelsteen, L.A. Oomen, O. de Weers, L. van Buren, M. Beurret, J.T. Poolman, and P. Hoogerhout.** 1998. Immunogenicity of *Streptococcus pneumoniae* type 6B and 14 polysaccharide-tetanus toxoid conjugates and the effect of uncoupled polysaccharide on the antigen-specific immune response. Vaccine **16**:1941–1949.

270. **Rosell, K.-G., and H.J. Jennings.** 1983. Structural elucidation of the capsular polysaccharide of *Streptococcus pneumoniae* type 9N. Can. J. Biochem. Cell Biol. **61**:1102–1107.

271. **Roy, A., and N. Roy.** 1984. Structure of the capsular polysaccharide from *Streptococcus pneumoniae* type 23. Carbohydr. Res. **126**:271–277.

272. **Roy, N.** 1978. Structural studies of the capsular polysaccharide of *Diplococcus pneumoniae* type 31. Carbohydr. Res. **63**:333–336.

273. **Roy, N., and C.P.J. Glaudemans.** 1968. The specific substance from *Diplococcus pneumoniae* type 34 (U.S. type 41): the location of the *O*-acetyl groups. Carbohydr. Res. **8**:214–218.

274. **Rundlöf, T., and G. Widmalm.** 1996. A method for determination of the absolute configuration of chiral glycerol residues in natural products using TEMPO oxidation and characterization of the glyceric acids formed. Anal. Biochem. **243**:228–233.

275. **Rutherford, T.J., C. Jones, D.B. Davies, and A.C. Elliott.** 1991. Location and quantitation of the sites of *O*-acetylation on the capsular polysaccharide from *Streptococcus pneumoniae* type 9V by ¹H-n.m.r. spectroscopy: comparison with type 9A. Carbohydr. Res. **218**:175–184.

276. **Rutherford, T.J., C. Jones, D.B. Davies, and A.C. Elliott.** 1994. NMR assignment and conformational analysis of the antigenic capsular polysaccharide from *Streptococcus pneumoniae* type 9N in aqueous solution. Carbohydr. Res. **265**:79–96.

277. **Rutherford, T.J., C. Jones, D.B. Davies, and A.C. Elliott.** 1994. Molecular recognition of antigenic polysaccharides: a conformational comparison of capsules from *Streptococcus pneumoniae* serogroup 9. Carbohydr. Res. **265**:97–111.

278. **Schiffman, G.** 1981. Chemistry and immunochemistry of the pneumococcal polysaccharide vaccine with special reference to cross-reactions and immunologic factors. Rev. Infect. Dis. **3(Suppl)**:S18–S26.

279. **Schneerson, R., J.B. Robbins, J.C. Parke, Jr., C. Bell, J.J. Schlesselman, A. Sutton, Z. Wang, G. Schiffman, A. Karpas, and J. Shiloach.** 1986. Quantitative and qualitative analyses of serum antibodies elicited in adults by *Haemophilus influenzae* type b and pneumococcus type 6A capsular polysaccharide-tetanus toxoid conjugates. Infect. Immun. **52**:519–528.

280. **Schneerson, R., J.B. Robbins, S.Z. Szu, and Y. Yang.** 1987. Vaccines composed of polysaccharide-protein conjugates: current status, unanswered questions, and prospects for the future. *In* R. Bell and G. Torrigiani (eds.), Towards better carbohydrate vaccines. Wiley, Chichester, pp. 307–327.

281. **Schneerson, R., L. Levi, J.B. Robbins, D.M. Bryla, G. Schiffman, and T. Lagergard.** 1992. Synthesis of a conjugate vaccine composed of pneumococcus type 14 capsular polysaccharide bound to pertussis toxin. Infect. Immun. **60**:3528–3532.

282. **Schüle, G., and T. Ziegler.** 1996. Efficient convergent block synthesis of a pyruvated tetrasaccharide 5-aminopentyl glycoside related to *Streptococcus pneumoniae* type 27. Tetrahedron **52**:2925–2936.

283. **Seid, Jr., R.C., R.A. Boykins, D.-F. Liu, K.W. Kimbrough, C.-L. Hsieh, and R. Eby.** 1989. Chemical evidence for covalent linkages of a semi-synthetic glycoconjugate vaccine for *Haemophilus influenzae* type B disease. Glycoconjugate J. **6**:489–498.

284. **Seifert, W.E., and R.M. Caprioli.** 1996. Fast atom bombardment mass spectrometry. High Resolut. Sep. Anal. Biol. Macromol. A **270**:453–486.

285. **Shabarova, Z.A., J.G. Buchanan, and J. Baddiley.** 1962. The composition of pneumococcus type-specific substances containing phosphorus. Biochim. Biophys. Acta **57:**146–148.

286. **Shapiro, E.D.** 1991. Pneumococcal vaccine. *In* S.J. Cryz, Jr. (ed.), Vaccines and immunotherapy. Pergamon Press, New York, pp. 127–139.

287. **Shapiro, E.D., A.T. Berg, R. Austrian, D. Schroeder, V. Parcells, A. Margolis, R.K. Adair, and J.D. Clemens.** 1991. The protective efficacy of polyvalent pneumococcal polysaccharide vaccine. N. Engl. J. Med. **325:**1453–1460.

288. **Shelly, M.A., H. Jacoby, G.J. Riley, B.T. Graves, M. Pichichero, and J.J. Treanor.** 1997. Comparison of pneumococcal polysaccharide and CRM$_{197}$-conjugated pneumococcal oligosaccharide vaccines in young and elderly adults. Infect. Immun. **65:**242–247.

289. **Slaghek, T.M., A.H. van Oijen, A.A.M. Maas, J.P. Kamerling, and J.F.G. Vliegenthart.** 1990. Synthesis of structural elements of the capsular polysaccharides of *Streptococcus pneumoniae* types 6A and 6B. Carbohydr. Res. **207:**237–248.

290. **Slaghek, T.M., A.A.M. Maas, J.P. Kamerling, and J.F.G. Vliegenthart.** 1991. Synthesis of two phosphate-containing "heptasaccharide" fragments of the capsular polysaccharides of *Streptococcus pneumoniae* types 6A and 6B. Carbohydr. Res. **211:**25–39.

291. **Smid, P., M. de Zwart, W.P.A. Jörning, G.A. van der Marel, and J.H. van Boom.** 1993. Stereoselective synthesis of a tetrameric fragment of *Streptococcus pneumoniae* type 1 containing an α-linked 2-acetamido-4-amino-2,4,6-trideoxy-D-galactopyranose (Sug*p*) unit. J. Carbohydr. Chem. **12:**1073–1090.

292. **Snippe, H., A.-J. van Houte, J.E.G. van Dam, M.J. de Reuver, M. Jansze, and J.M.N. Willers.** 1983. Immunogenic properties in mice of hexasaccharide from the capsular polysaccharide of *Streptococcus pneumoniae* type 3. Infect. Immun. **40:**856–861.

293. **Sørensen, U.B.S.** 1995. Pneumococcal polysaccharide antigens: capsules and C-polysaccharide, an immunochemical study. Dan. Med. Bull. **42:**47–53.

294. **Sørensen, U.B.S., and J. Henrichsen.** 1987. Cross-reactions between pneumococci and other streptococci due to C polysaccharide and F antigen. J. Clin. Microbiol. **25:**1854–1859.

295. **Sørensen, U.B.S., and J. Blom.** 1992. Capsular polysaccharide is linked to the outer surface of type 6A pneumococcal cell walls. APMIS **100:**891–893.

296. **Sørensen, U.B.S., R. Agger, J. Bennedsen, and J. Henrichsen.** 1984. Phosphorylcholine determinants in six pneumococcal capsular polysaccharides detected by monoclonal antibody. Infect. Immun. **43:**876–878.

297. **Sørensen, U.B.S., J. Blom, A. Birch-Andersen, and J. Henrichsen.** 1988. Ultrastructural localization of capsules, cell wall polysaccharide, cell wall proteins, and F antigen in pneumococci. Infect. Immun. **56:**1890–1896.

298. **Sørensen, U.B.S., J. Henrichsen, H.-C. Chen, and S.C. Szu.** 1990. Covalent linkage between the capsular polysaccharide and the cell wall peptidoglycan of *Streptococcus pneumoniae* revealed by immunochemical methods. Microbial Pathogenesis **8:**325–334.

299. **Staros, J.V., R.W. Wright, and D.M. Swingle.** 1986. Enhancement by *N*-hydroxysulfosuccinimide of water-soluble carbodiimide-mediated coupling reactions. Anal. Biochem. **156:**220–222.

300. **Stein, K.E.** 1994. Glycoconjugate vaccines. What next? Int. J. Technol. Assess. Health Care **10:**167–176.

301. **Steinhoff, M.C., K. Edwards, H. Keyserling, M.L. Thoms, C. Johnson, D. Madore, and D. Hogerman.** 1994. A randomized comparison of three bivalent *Streptococcus pneumoniae* glycoprotein conjugate vaccines in young children: effect of polysaccharide size and linkage characteristics. Pediatr. Infect. Dis. J. **13:**368–372.

302. **Sternberg, G.M.** 1881. A fatal form of septicaemia in the rabbit, produced by subcutaneous injection of human saliva. An experimental research. Nat. Board Health Bull. **2:**781–783.

303. **Stowell, C.P., and Y.-C. Lee.** 1980. Neoglycoproteins. The preparation and application of synthetic glycoproteins. Adv. Carbohydr. Chem. Biochem. **37:**225–281.

304. **Sugawara, T., and K. Igarashi.** 1988. Synthesis of a trisaccharide component of the capsular polysaccharide of *Streptococcus pneumoniae* type 19F. Carbohydr. Res. **172:**195–207.

305. **Szu, S., C.-J. Lee, D. Carlo, and J. Henrichsen.** 1981. Immunochemical characterization of cross-reactivity of pneumococcal group 9 capsular polysaccharide types 9N, 9A, 9L, and 9V. Infect. Immun. **31:**371–379.

306. **Thijssen, M.-J.L., K.M. Halkes, J.P. Kamerling, and J.F.G. Vliegenthart.** 1994. Synthesis of a spacer-containing tetrasaccharide representing a repeating unit of the capsular polysaccharide of *Streptococcus pneumoniae* type 6B. Bioorg. Med. Chem. **2:**1309–1317.

307. **Thijssen, M.-J.L., M.N. van Rijswijk, J.P. Kamerling, and J.F.G. Vliegenthart.** 1998. Synthesis of spacer-containing di- and tri-saccharides that represent parts of the capsular polysaccharide of *Streptococcus pneumoniae* type 6B. Carbohydr. Res. **306:**93–109.

308. **Thijssen, M.-J.L., M.H.G. Bijkerk, J.P. Kamerling, and J.F.G. Vliegenthart.** 1998. Synthesis of four spacer-containing "tetrasaccharides" that represent four possible repeating units of the capsular polysaccharide of *Streptococcus pneumoniae* type 6B. Carbohydr. Res. **306:**111–125.

309. **Tillett, W.S., and T. Francis, Jr.** 1930. Serological reactions in pneumoniae with a nonprotein somatic fraction of pneumococcus, J. Exp. Med. **52:**561–571.

310. **Tomasz, A.** 1981. Surface components of *Streptococcus pneumoniae*. Rev. Infect. Dis. **3:**190–211.

311. **Tomasz, A., A. Corso, E.P. Severina, G. Echániz-Aviles, M.C. de Cunto Brandileone, T. Camou, E. Castaneda, O. Figueroa, A. Rossi, and J.L. Di Fabio.** 1998. Molecular epidemiologic characterization of penicillin-resistant *Streptococcus pneumoniae* invasive pediatric isolates recovered in six Latin-American countries: an overview. Microbial. Drug Resist. **4:**195–207.

312. **Tuomanen, E.I.** 1997. The biology of pneumococcal infection. Pediatr. Res. **42:**253–258.

313. **Tyler, J.M.** 1982. Type-specific pneumococcal polysaccharides: concerning the anomeric configuration of the $(1 \rightarrow 3)$-D-galactofuranosyl residues in S-31. Carbohydr. Res. **99:**75–77.

314. **Tyler, J.M., and M. Heidelberger.** 1968. The specific capsular polysaccharide of type VII *Pneumococcus*. Biochemistry **7:**1384–1392.

315. **Van Dam, J.E.G., J. Breg, R. Komen, J.P. Kamerling, and J.F.G. Vliegenthart.** 1989. Isolation and structural studies of phosphate-containing oligosaccharides from alkaline and acid hydrolysates of *Streptococcus pneumoniae* type 6^B capsular polysaccharide. Carbohydr. Res. **187:**267–286.

316. **Van Dam, J.E.G., A. Fleer, and H. Snippe.** 1990. Immunogenicity and immunochemistry of *Streptococcus pneumoniae* capsular polysaccharides. Antonie van Leeuwenhoek **58:**1–47.

317. **Van de Wijgert, J.H.H.M., A.F.M. Verheul, H. Snippe, I.J. Check, and R.L. Hunter.** 1991. Immunogenicity of *Streptococcus pneumoniae* type 14 capsular polysaccharide: influence of carriers and adjuvants on isotype distribution. Infect. Immun. **59:**2750–2757.

318. **Van Setten, D.C., G.J. ten Hove, E.J.H.J. Wiertz, J.P. Kamerling, and G. van de Werken.** 1998. Multiple-stage tandem mass spectrometry for structural characterization of saponins. Anal. Chem. **70:**4401–4409.

319. **Van Steijn, A.M.P., M. Jetten, J.P. Kamerling, and J.F.G. Vliegenthart.** 1989. Syntheses of tri- and tetrasaccharide fragments of the capsular polysaccharide of *Streptococcus pneumoniae* type 23F. Recl. Trav. Chim. Pays-Bas **108:**374–383.

320. **Van Steijn, A.M.P., J.P. Kamerling, and J.F.G. Vliegenthart.** 1991. Synthesis of a spacer-containing repeating unit of the capsular polysaccharide of *Streptococcus pneumoniae* type 23F. Carbohydr. Res. **211:**261–277.

321. **Van Steijn, A.M.P., J.P. Kamerling, and J.F.G. Vliegenthart.** 1992. Synthesis of trisaccharide methyl glycosides related to fragments of the capsular polysaccharide of *Streptococcus pneumoniae* type 18C. Carbohydr. Res. **225:**229–245.

322. **Van Steijn, A.M.P., J.G.M. van der Ven, P. van Seeventer, J.P. Kamerling, and J.F.G. Vliegenthart.** 1992. Synthesis of a repeating pentasaccharide fragment of the capsular polysaccharide of *Streptococcus pneumoniae* type 18C. Carbohydr. Res. **229:**155–160.

323. **Van Steijn, A.M.P., J.P. Kamerling, and J.F.G. Vliegenthart.** 1992. Synthesis of four spacer-containing trisaccharides with the 4-*O*-(β-L-rhamnopyranosyl)-D-glucopyranose unit in common, representing fragments of capsular polysaccharides from *Streptococcus pneumoniae* types 2, 7F, 22F, and 23F. J. Carbohydr. Chem. **11:**665–689.

324. **Veeneman, G.H., L.J.F. Gomes, and J.H. van Boom.** 1989. Synthesis of fragments of a *Streptococcus pneumoniae* type-specific capsular polysaccharide. Tetrahedron **45:**7433–7448.

325. **Vella, P.P., S. Marburg, J.M. Staub, P.J. Kniskern, W. Miller, A. Hagopian, C. Ip, R.L. Tolman, C.M. Rusk, L.S. Chupak, and R.W. Ellis.** 1992. Immunogenicity of conjugate vaccines consisting of pneumococcal capsular polysaccharide types 6B, 14, 19F, and 23F and a meningococcal outer membrane protein complex. Infect. Immun. **60:**4977–4983.

326. **Verheul, A.F.M., A.A. Versteeg, M.J. de Reuver, M. Jansze, and H. Snippe.** 1989. Modulation of the immune response to pneumococcal type 14 capsular polysaccharide-protein conjugates by the adjuvant Quil A depends on the properties of the conjugates. Infect. Immun. **57:**1078–1083.

327. **Watson, M.J.** 1974. The type-specific substance from *Pneumococcus* type 33B. Biochem. J. **137:**603–606.

328. **Watson, M.J., and J. Baddiley.** 1974. The action of nitrous acid on C-teichoic acid (C-substance) from the walls of *Diplococcus pneumoniae.* Biochem. J. **137:**399–404.

329. **Watson, M.J., J.M. Tyler, J.G. Buchanan, and J. Baddiley.** 1972. The type-specific substance from *Pneumococcus* type 13. Biochem. J. **130:**45–54.

330. **Wessels, M.R., and D.L. Kasper.** 1989. Antibody recognition of the type 14 pneumococcal capsule. Evidence for a conformational epitope in a neutral polysaccharide. J. Exp. Med. **169:**2121–2131.

331. **Wessels, M.R., V. Pozsgay, D.L. Kasper, and H.J. Jennings.** 1987. Structure and immunochemistry of an oligosaccharide repeating unit of the capsular polysaccharide of type III group B *Streptococcus.* A revised structure for the type III group B streptococcal polysaccharide antigen. J. Biol. Chem. **262:**8262–8267.

332. **White, B.** 1938. The biology of pneumococcus. Harvard University Press, Cambridge.

333. **Winter, W.T., and I. Adelsky.** 1981. Pneumococcal polysaccharide conformations. Biopolymers **20:**2691–2694.

334. **Winter, W.T., M. Kaneko, and K. Borzilleri.** 1998. Conformational features of *Streptococcus pneumoniae* serotypes 5, 1 and 18 capsular antigens. *In* Abstracts of the XIX International Carbohydrate Symposium, San Diego, p. AP046.

335. **Wright, A.E., W. Morgan, L. Colbrook, and R.W. Dodgson.** 1914. Observations on prophylactic inoculations against pneumococcus infection, and on the results which have been achieved by it. Lancet **1:**1–10, 87–95.

336. **Yadomae, T., N. Ohno, and T. Miyazaki.** 1979. On the phosphate linkages and the structure of a disaccharide unit of the type-specific polysaccharide of Pneumococcus type XIX. Carbohydr. Res. **75:**191–198.

337. **Zurabyan, S.E., V.A. Nesmeyanov, and A.Ya. Khorlin.** 1976. Synthesis of a branched tetrasaccharide. 2-Acetamido-4-*O*-β-D-galactopyranosyl-6-*O*-[*O*-β-D-galactopyranosyl-(1 → 4)-β-D-glucopyranosyl]-2-deoxy-D-glucose. Izv. Akad. Nauk SSSR Ser. Khim. **6:**1421–1423.

Address reprint requests to:
Johannis P. Kamerling
Bijvoet Center
Department of Bio-Organic Chemistry
Utrecht University
P.O. Box 80.075
3508 TB Utrecht
The Netherlands

Capsule Genetics in *Streptococcus pneumoniae* and a Possible Role for Transposition in the Generation of the Type 3 Locus

MELISSA J. CAIMANO,[1,2] GAIL G. HARDY,[1] and JANET YOTHER[1]

ABSTRACT

The capsule genes of *Streptococcus pneumoniae* have a cassette-like organization in which the type-specific biosynthetic genes are flanked by genes shared among the different capsular serotypes. This general organization has been identified in the capsule loci of all serotypes analyzed to date, but significant differences that may help explain novel capsule type formation are beginning to emerge. In particular, analysis of the type 3 locus has revealed its most striking feature to be a preponderance of partial genes that have homology to sequences involved in polysaccharide biosynthesis and transposition. The predicted proteins of *cps3M*, the most downstream type 3-specific gene, and *tnpA* and *plpA*, the non-type-specific flanking sequences downstream of *cps3M*, have homologies with phosphomutases, transposases, and peptide permeases, respectively. All three of these sequences are truncated when compared to their respective homologs. Mutation and transcription analyses of these partial sequences showed that none of these sequences is essential for type 3 polysaccharide synthesis but that all are transcribed. Partial sequences were also identified in the region upstream of the type 3-specific genes. The type 3 locus structure is conserved among independent type 3 isolates but similar deletions are not apparent in the common, non-type-specific flanking sequences in other capsular types. A role for transposition-mediated events in the generation of the type 3 locus, and possibly other pneumococcal capsule loci, is suggested by these findings.

INTRODUCTION

THE POLYSACCHARIDE CAPSULE of *Streptococcus pneumoniae* is significant for both its role in pathogenesis and its role in the development of molecular genetics. In the laboratory, the inter-strain transformation of pneumococcal capsular polysaccharide biosynthetic genes was a central step in demonstrating that the "transforming principle," and hence the genetic material, is DNA.[12] In nature, the genetic exchange of DNA among *S. pneumoniae* strains is likely to have played a major role in the generation of new strains and in the evolution of capsular serotypes, of which 90 have now been described.[33,59] The significance of the capsule in virulence, antiphagocytosis, and protective immunity has long been recognized.[11,31,40,43,45,55,61,62] However, the molecular mechanisms underlying capsule expression, the generation of serotype diversity, and the apparent differences in virulence associated with capsular serotype[18,34,37,60] are only now being addressed.

Early genetic and biochemical studies of pneumococcal capsules provide the foundation on which much of the current research concerning this complex system is built. Among the significant observations arising from those studies [8,9,21,26,31,42,44,49] are: a) the type-specific genes, i.e., those involved in the biosynthesis of a specific polysaccharide, are linked on the chromosome; b) the type-specific genes for different capsular types may occupy identical sites in the chromosome; c) the type-specific genes are transferred as a unit during genetic transformation and are integrated into a recipient chromosome by recombination between homologous sequences flanking the type-specific regions in a mechanism since referred to as a cassette[41]; d) there is little homology between type-specific genes from different capsular types; e) unlinked genes are probably involved in the regulation of capsule expression; and f) only one set of type-specific genes is present in a given strain. An exception to the latter observation occurs with binary encapsulated strains, which occur only rarely and apparently only between specific combinations of donors and recipients. Binary encapsulated strains occur when

[1]Department of Microbiology, University of Alabama at Birmingham, Birmingham, AL 35294.
[2]Present address: Department of Internal Medicine, University of Texas—Southwestern Medical Center, Dallas, TX 75235-9113.
Reprinted from *Microbial Drug Resistance*, Vol. 4, No. 1, 1998.

the transfer of type-specific capsule gene cassettes results in the maintenance and expression of both the donor and recipient type-specific genes, rather than in the replacement of the recipient's type-specific genes with those of the donor.[8,14,15]

Recent studies using molecular genetics techniques have confirmed and have begun to extend the earlier observations. Sequence, hybridization, and linkage analyses have demonstrated the expected organization of the capsule loci in which type-specific genes are flanked by sequences common to strains of, apparently, all capsular types (Fig. 1). These types of analyses have also shown that the type-specific biosynthetic genes for a given polysaccharide occur only in strains expressing that polysaccharide.[25,28,32] In addition, direct evidence for a cassette-like transfer of capsule loci between strains of different capsular types has been obtained.[23,25]

Despite the high degree of overall similarity between loci of different capsular types, important differences have begun to be recognized. In particular, analysis of the type 3 locus has yielded some unexpected findings that may help explain the emergence of new capsular types and the apparent correlation between serotype and virulence. The type 3 locus contains the type-specific biosynthetic genes *cps3D* and *cps3S* that are required for type 3 capsule production.[24,25] *cps3D* encodes a UDP-glucose (UDP-Glc) dehydrogenase that converts UDP-Glc to UDP-glucuronic acid (UDP-GlcUA). *cps3S* encodes the type 3 synthase that catalyzes formation of the linkages required to form the $(GlcUA-Glc)_n$ type 3 polysaccharide. The functions encoded by these genes were originally demonstrated in mutant and functional analyses[6,24,25] and have been confirmed by expression of the cloned genes in *E. coli* (*cap3A* and *cap3B*[4,7]). Two additional type 3-specific genes, *cps3U* and, as further described here, *cps3M*, are present and are predicted to encode proteins with homology to UDP-Glc-1-P uridylyltransferases (Glc-1-P → UDP-Glc) and phosphomutases (Glc-6-P → Glc-1-P), respectively.[24] The UDP-Glc-1-P uridylyltransferase function has been demonstrated through complementation of an *E. coli galU* mutant (*cap3C*[5]) but expression of the gene is not required for type 3 capsule production in *S. pneumoniae*.[24]

The type 3 locus differs from the other capsule loci thus far described in that the biosynthetic type-specific genes are separated from the common upstream flanking sequences by an additional 1 kb region of DNA that is not found in other capsular types (this study and [24]). Unlike the situation in type 19F, where both the common and the type-specific capsule genes appear to be contained in a single operon,[32] the type 3-specific genes can be transcribed independently of the upstream common region.[24] *cps3D* and *cps3S* were shown in genetic analyses to be transcribed as part of the same operon[24] which, as demonstrated in Northern analyses, also includes at least *cps3U* (*cap3C*[5]). In addition, the upstream common sequences of type 3 that are homologous to the type 19F genes *cps19fA* and *cps19fB* contain deletions and the common sequences do not appear to be transcribed in type 3.[5] Further characterization of the type 3 locus, described herein, shows additional deviations from what appears to be the norm for *S. pneumoniae* capsule loci. Some of the unique features of this locus appear to lend support to the hypothesis that a transposition-like event might explain the occurrence of binary encapsulated strains and might provide a possible mechanism for novel capsule type formation.[24]

MATERIALS AND METHODS

Bacterial strains and plasmids

The strains and plasmids are described in Table 1. *S. pneumoniae* strains were grown in Todd-Hewitt broth (Difco, Detroit, MI) supplemented with 0.5% yeast extract (THY), or on Blood Agar Base #2 (Difco) supplemented with 3% sheep red blood cells. *E. coli* derivatives were grown in L-broth or on L-agar. Antibiotic concentrations (μg/ml) for *S. pneumoniae/E. coli* were: erythromycin, 0.3/250; kanamycin, 10/50; and ampicillin, −/100.

Isolation and cloning of the type 3 locus DNA from S. pneumoniae WU2

Cloning of the 3.1 kb *Hin*dIII fragment containing the downstream type 3-specific genes has been described.[24] The 3′ end of the type 3 *plpA* was obtained as a PCR product using primers P5 and P6 (see Table 2). The region upstream of *cps3D* was obtained from JD1008 by cloning the 2.2 kb *Hin*dIII fragment flanking the pJD396 insertion (see Table 1).

DNA techniques and sequence analysis

Plasmid DNA, isolated by the alkaline lysis method[17] was purified by CsCl centrifugation[48] when necessary. Chromosomal DNA from *S. pneumoniae* was prepared essentially as described by Hotchkiss.[35] *S. pneumoniae* was transformed as pre-

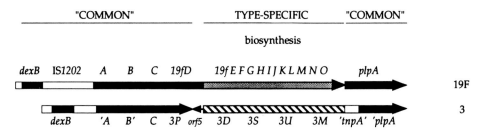

FIG. 1. Conserved structure of the capsule loci. The maps are derived from sequence data of the type 19F[32] and type 3 loci.[5,24,25] A similar organization is apparent in type 14, where the upstream common sequences and the type-specific genes have been identified.[38] The common downstream sequence containing *plpA* has also been identified adjacent to the type 2, 5, 6B, and 14 loci.[24,25,37] ■, homologous sequences; ◫ ▦, type-specific sequences; □, non-homologous sequences; ′, deleted sequence.

TABLE 1. BACTERIAL STRAINS AND PLASMIDS

Strain/plasmid	Derivation and properties	Reference
Strain		
S. pneumoniae		
WU2	Type 3 encapsulated; parent strain for sequencing and mutation analyses	19
JD770	Type 3 encapsulated derivative of WU2 containing insertion-duplication of '*cps3DSU*', identical to WU2 in capsule production and virulence, Em^R	25, 37
L82006	Type 1 encapsulated	46
D39	Type 2 encapsulated	12
A66	Type 3 encapsulated	18
ATCC6303	Type 3 encapsulated	18
EF3113	Type 3 encapsulated	18
L8 1995	Type 3 encapsulated	18
DBL5	Type 5 encapsulated	65
DBL1	Type 6B encapsulated	18
L82231	Type 14 encapsulated	18
JD867	pJD355 × WU2, insertion-duplication of '*cps3DSU*', type 3 encapsulated, Em^R	24
JD899	pJD361 × WU2, Cps3U$^-$, type 3 encapsulated, Em^R	24
JD908	pJD369 × WU2, Cps3S$^-$, non-encapsulated, Em^R	25
JD981	pJD392 × WU2, upstream insertion duplication, type 3 encapsulated, Em^R	24
JD982	pJD390 × WU2, Cps3DS$^-$, non-encapsulated, Em^R	24
JD1008	pJD396 × WU2, ORF5$^-$, type 3 encapsulated, Km^R	24
JY1200	pJY5006 × WU2, Cps3C$^-$, type 3 encapsulated, Em^R	This work
MC1032	pMC107 × WU2, PlpA$^-$, type 3 encapsulated, Em^R	This work
MC1077	pMC159 × WU2, insertion-duplication of '*cps3DS*' terminating in *S-U* intergenic region, type 3 encapsulated, Em^R	This work
MC1092	pMC123 × WU2, Cps3M$^-$, type 3 encapsulated, Em^R	This work
MC1098	pMC186 × WU2, Cps3C$^-$, type 3 encapsulated, Em^R	This work
MC1114	pMC205 × WU2, Cps3M$^-$, type 3 encapsulated, Em^R	This work
MC1119	pMC180 × WU2, insertion-duplication of '*tnpA-plpA*', type 3 encapsulated, Em^R	This work
E. coli		
DH5α	*endA1 hsdR17* (r$_k$$^-m_k$$^+$) *supE44 thi-1 recA1 gyrA relA1* Δ(*lacZYA-argF*)$_{U169}$ (φ80Δ*lacZX*Δ*M15*)	10
LE392	*hsdR514* (r$_k$$^-m_k$$^+$) *supE44 supF58* Δ(*lacIZY*)6 *galK2 galT22 metB1 trpR55* λ$^-$	58
Plasmids*		
pJY4163 and pJY4164	Lack of origin of replication for *S. pneumoniae*; promoterless *cat* gene downstream of multiple cloning site (opposite orientations in pJY4163 and pJY4164), Em^R	66
pSF151	Lacks origin of replication for *S. pneumoniae*; Km^R	56
pJD355	pJY4164::2.0 kb *Sau*3A1-*Pst*I ('*cps3D-cps3S-cps3U*')	24
pJD361	pJY4164::0.47 kb *Xba* I-*Pst*I ('*cps3S-cps3U*')	25
pJD369	pJY4164::0.58 kb *Pvu*II-*Rsa* I ('*cps3D-cps3S*')	25
pJD364	pJY4164::3.2 kb *Hin*dII ('*cps3UM-tnpA-plpA*', bp 3905-7220, Fig. 2B)	25
pJD374	pJY4163::1.4 kb *Sau*3A1 ('*cps3M-tnpA*', bp 4734-6108, Fig. 2B)	25
pJD377	pJY4164::1.2 kb *Sac*I-*Hin*dIII ('*tnpA-plpA*', bp 6121-7220, Fig. 2B)	25
pJD390	pJY4164::0.35 kb *Hin*dIII-*Mun*I ('*cps3D*')	24
pJD392	pJY4164::0.6 kb *Ecl*136II-*Hin*dIII (between *orf5* and *cps3D*)	24
pJD396	pSF151::0.26 kb *Ecl*136II-*Msc*I ('*orf5*', bp 709-965, Fig. 5)	24
pJY5006	pJY4163::0.8 kb *Sac*I-*Pst*I ('*cps3C*', upstream *Sac*I to bp 120, Fig. 5)	This work
pMC107	pJY4163::0.27 kb *Ssp*I-*Pst*I ('*plpA*', bp 6941-7211, Fig. 2B)	This work
pMC123	pJY4164::0.36 kb *Pvu*II ('*cps3M*', bp 4822-5190, Fig. 2B)	This work
pMC135	pJY4163::0.36 kb *Pvu*II ('*cps3M*', bp 4822-5190, Fig. 2B)	This work
pMC159	pJY4164::1.9 kb PCR product ('*cps3D-cps3S*; terminates in *cps3S-cps3U* intergenic region, Fig. 9)	This work
pMC180	pJY4164::0.3 *Sac*I-*Rsa*I ('*tnpA-plpA*', bp 6121-6419, Fig. 2B)	This work
pMC186	pJY4164::0.8 kb *Sac*I-*Pst*I ('*cps3C*', upstream *Sac*I to bp 120, Fig. 5)	This work
pMC205	pJY4164::0.48 kb *Eco*RI-*Xmn*I ('*cps3M*', bp 4983-5458, Fig. 2B)	This work

*Most of the restriction sites are shown in Figs. 2, 3, and 9. The gene(s), or part(s) thereof, contained in the clone and the location of the fragment (for sequence presented here) are given in parentheses.

TABLE 2. PRIMER SEQUENCES

	Sequence	Source[a]	Position[b]	Reference
IS2	5'-GCCTCAGTTAACAAGTCAAA-3'	WU2	6035–6054	Fig. 2B
M1	5'-GTGGACACCTATGAATTGTATAG-3'	WU2	4682–4704	Fig. 2B
M3	5'-GTCACCAAAATTGCGGAAAG-3'	WU2	5775–5794	Fig. 2B
M5	5'-GGCAGATTCAAAAGCGAA-3'	WU2	5003–4986	Fig. 2B
Orf1	5'-ATCAAAAGGGCGTTAGGGTA-3'	WU2	834–854	Fig. 3
Orf2	5'-AATAATTGATTAGCGCCATT-3'	WU2	1107–1088	Fig. 3
P1	5'-GCCGTAGATGATGACAACCA-3'	WU2	6326–6307	Fig. 2B
P3	5'-TTGCTGTCTGGTCAACTGGC-3'	WU2	6833–6814	Fig. 2B
P4	5'-GCATGCTCTGGATCAGGTTC-3'	R6x	13–32	47
P5	5'-CAAGAGAAATACTAAATC-3'	R6x	1971–1953	47
P6	5'-GTTGCTAAACGATATGAT-3'	WU2	7181–7198	Fig. 2B
P8	5'-TGCATTTGGATTTGACCG-3'	WU2	6523–6540	Fig. 2B

[a]Denotes strain from which primer sequence was taken.

[b]Positions of primers are numbered according to nucleotide sequence published here for WU2 in Figure 2 or 3 as indicated, and previously for R6x.[47]

viously described.[67] *E. coli*, washed in water and resuspended in 10% glycerol, was electroporated using a BTX Electro Cell Manipulator 600 (Biotechnologies and Experimental Research, Inc., San Diego, CA). *Taq* polymerase (Fisher Scientific, Pittsburgh, PA) was used for PCR amplifications. The Genius System (Boehringer Mannheim, Indianapolis, IN) was used for DIG-dUTP labeling of probes and chemiluminescent detection in blotting experiments.

Sanger dideoxy sequencing of plasmid DNA was performed using the Sequenase 2.0 kit (US Biochemicals, Cleveland, OH). Sequencing of PCR products was performed using the Sequenase PCR Product Sequencing kit (US Biochemicals). Greater than 98% of the sequence was obtained for each strand of the *cps3U-cps3M-tnpA-plpA* and the *orf5* regions. The sequence from the *cps3CPE* region (80% single-stranded) was compared to the published sequence for type 19F.[32] Differences between the two were verified in the type 3 sequence. Sequence analyses and data base searches were performed using the programs of The University of Wisconsin Genetics Computer Group (GCG)[29] and the NCBI BLAST server.[2] The sequences presented here have been assigned GenBank accession numbers U66845 (see Fig. 2) and U66846 (see Fig. 3).

Transcription analyses

Gene fusions with the *cat* reporter gene were constructed using the insertion-duplication vectors pJY4163 and pJY4164 (see

Table 1) to target insertions into the *S. pneumoniae* chromosome. Sites of the insertions were confirmed in Southern blot analyses. Due to low levels of chloramphenicol acetyltransferase activity in the standard enzyme assay,[53] levels of resistance to chloramphenicol (μg/ml) were used to assess *cat* expression. Levels of resistance were determined by growth on blood agar medium containing erythromycin (0.3 μg/ml) and chloramphenicol (1 to 8 μg/ml, in 1 μg/ml increments). The level of resistance was defined as the highest concentration permitting the formation of single colonies.

For Northern analyses, *S. pneumoniae* cultures (500 ml) were grown in THY to an $OD_{620} = 0.05$, iced, and the cells pelleted by centrifugation at 4000 $\times$ g for 15 min at 4°C. RNA was prepared according to the procedure of Pearce et al.[47] Residual chromosomal DNA was removed by RQ1 DNase digestion (Promega Corporation, Madison, WI) followed by extraction twice with phenol/chloroform/isoamyl alcohol (25:24:1), once with chloroform/isoamyl alcohol (24:1), and then precipitation overnight in ethanol. The pellet was resuspended in 50 μl DEPC-treated water containing 10 mM Ribonucleoside-Vanadyl Complex (New England Biolabs, Beverly, MA) and stored at −20°C. Yield and purity were determined by spectrophotometry and agarose gel electrophoresis. For blotting experiments, RNA was denatured at 65°C for 10 min and electrophoresed on a 1.0% agarose/2.2 M formaldehyde gel with DIG-labeled and unlabeled RNA markers (Boehringer-Mannheim or Gibco-BRL, Gaithersburg, MD). The Genius Sys-

FIG. 2. (A) Map of type 3 capsule locus. Restriction sites: Bg, *Bgl*II; Ev, *Eco*RV; H, *Hind*III; P, *Pst*I; Pv, *Pvu*II; S, *Sac*I; Sp, *Sph*I; St, *Stu*I; X, *Xba*I. Triangles, with strain names denoted in Fig. 2B, indicate the points of insertion mutations: △, insertions that do not affect capsule production; ▲, insertions that result in a capsule-negative phenotype. Descriptions of bacterial strains and plasmids are in Table 1. The insertions in *cps3DSU* have been described.[24] Mutated homologs of *cps19fA* and *cps19fB* (*cps3A* and *cps3B*, respectively) are located upstream of *cps3C* ([5] and unpublished data). Arrowheads indicate the directions of open reading frames. (B) DNA sequence of the region containing the 3' end of *cps3U*, *cps3M*, *tnpA*, and *plpA* from strain WU2. Numbering of nucleotide sequence is based on the previously reported *cps3DSU* sequence.[24] The putative *cps3M* −35 and −10 sequences and the putative Cps3M ribosome binding site (RBS) are indicated. Lower case letters are used to denote amino acid sequence that is not expected to be expressed due to lack of translational signals and/or a frameshift mutation. Underlined amino acids in PlpA indicate differences from the type 2 PlpA sequence.[47] Overlined amino acids indicate sequences conserved in phosphomutases. Symbols: ●, 1 bp deletion in *plpA* sequence; <,>, direction of translation.

A

common   type 3-specific   common

St Sp   H S   PPv S HEv   H Bg Pv   X PHHEvPvPv   S   EvPH Bg   Sp

cps3C P orf5 cps3D cps3S cps3U cps3M 'tnpA''plpA   1 kb

B

```
     Cps3U>
      I L E T Q K P G A G N E I Q L T D A I D T L N K T Q S V F A R E F V G K R Y D V
4430 CTATATTAGAAACCCAAAAGCCAGGAGCAGGTAATGAAATTCAATTGACAGATGCTATTGATACATTGAATAAGACACAGAGTGTTTTTGCGCGTGAATTTGTGGGCAAACGTTACGATG
                                                    -35            -10
      G D K F N F M K T S I D Y A L Q H P Q I K E S L K N Y V I A L G K Q L E K L D D
4550 TTGGTGATAAGTTTAATTTTATGAAAACATCAATTGATTATGCTCTTCAACATCCTCAGATTAAAGAGAGTTTAAAAAATTACGTTATTGCACTTGGTAAGCAATTGGAGAAGCTAGATG

      C S S S G H L *                Cps3M>  M N C I E S Y Q K W L N V P D L P A Y L K D E L L S M D D K T K E
4670 ACTGTTCGTCAAGTGGACACCTATGAATTGTATAGAAAGTTATCAAAAATGGCTAAATGTCCTGATCTTCCAGCTTATTTAAAAGATGAATTGCTCAGCATGGATGACAAACAAAAGA
             RBS                                                Sau3AI
      D A F Y T N L E F G T A G M R G Y I C A G T N R I N I Y V V R Q A H R S L A K L
4790 AGACGCCTTTTACACAAACCTTGAATTCGGAACAGCTGGTATGCGTGGTTATATTGGTACGGGACAAACCGTATTAATATCTATGTGGTGCGTCAAGCACACAGAAGCCTTGCCAAATT
                  PvuII

      V E S K G E T A K K A G V A I A Y D S R H F S P E F A F E S A Q V L A A H G I K
4910 AGTTGAATCAAAAGGCGAAACGGCCAAAAAGCTGGGGTTGCTATTGCCTATGACTCGCGACATTTTCACCAGAATTGCTTTTGAATCTGCCCAAGTATTAGCGGGCCCATGGCATTAA
                                                                GAATTC
                                                                EcoRI
      S Y V F E S L R P T P E L S F A V R H L G A F A G I M V T A S H T P A P F N G Y
5030 ATCTTATGTTTTTGAAAGCCTACGCCCTACTCCTGAGCTGTCTTTTGCTGTTCGTCATCTCGGAGCATTTGCTGGTATTATGGTAACCGCCAGTCATACCCCTGCTCCTTTTAATGGTTA

      K V Y G S D G G Q M L P A D A D A L T D Y I R A I D N P F A V V L A D L E E A K
5150 TAAAGTTTACGGTTCTGATGGTGGGCAAATGCTTCAGCTGATGCTGATGCTTTAACTGACTATATTCGTGCGATTGATAACCCATTTGCTGTAGTCCTTGCTGACTTAGAAGAAGCTAA
                                            CAGCTG
                                            PvuII △ MC1056/MC1092
      S T G L I E V I G E T L D A A Y L E E V K S V N I N Q D L I D Q Y G R D M Q I V
5270 ATCAACTGGTCTTATTGAAGTAATTGGTGAAACTCTCGATGCTGCCTACCTTGAAGAGGTTAAAAGCGTTAATATCAATCAAGATTTGATTGACCAATACGGTCGCGATATGCAAATTGT

      Y T P L H G T G E M L A R R A L A Q A G F E S V Q V V E A Q A K P D P D F S T V
5390 CTACACACCTCTTCATGGTACTGGAGAAATGCTAGCACGTCGAGCTTTAGCACAAGCTGGTTTCGAATCTGTTCAAGTTGTCGAAGCTCAAGCAAACCAGACCCAGACTTCTCAACAGT
                                                     GAATCTGTT
                                                     XmnI △ MC1114
      A S P N P E S Q A A F A L A E E L G R Q V D A D V L V A T D P D A D R L G V E I
5510 TGCATCACCAAACCCTGAAAGTCAAGCCGCCTTTGCCTTAGCTGAAGAACTAGGGCGTCAAGTCGATGCTGATGTATTAGTGGCGACTGACCCTGATGCTGACCGTCTCGGTGTTGAAAT

      R Q A D G S Y W N L S G N Q I G A L I A K Y I L E A H K Q A G T L P K N A A L A
5630 TCGTCAAGCTGATGGCAGTTATTGGAACCTTTCTGGTAACCAAATCGGTGCTCTTATCGCCAAATACATTTTAGAAGCTCACAAACAAGCTGGGACACTCCCAAAGAATGCTGCATTGGC

      K S I V S T E L V T K I A E S Y G A T M F N V L T G F K F I A E K I Q E F E E K
5750 AAAATCAATAGTATCAACTGAATTAGTCACCAAAATTGCGGAAAGCTATGGTGCAACCATGTTTAACGTGTTAACAGGTTTCAAATTCATCGCTGAGAAAATTCAAGAATTTGAAGAAAA
                                                                   ('TnpA')* r q s f e l i q l f
      H N H T Y M F G F E E S *
5870 ACATAACCATACCTACATGTTTGGGTTTGAAGAAAGCTGATGAGTTTATTGATTGCCTCCAGCTTGGAGTTAGAATAGGGCATCTGGATGGCATTTGTCACGTATTTTCTGTAGCGCACC
                                                                v y g y r c t q t q l f s i l k n i a e l k s n s y p m q i a n t v y k r y r v
                                                                                                    JD879 ▽ Sau3A
5990 AGCGTGCTAAGACAGTTCTAAAGGCTTGATTGAGTTGGGGAAAGCCTCAGTTAACAAGTCAAAGAAATGGTCGGCATTCTTTTCTTGCAGGTGGAAAAGCAAGGCTGGTAAAGATCG
      l t s l a t r f a q n l q p f a e t l l d f f h d a n k e q l h f l l l q y l d
          . SacI
6110 TCATAATAGTGGAGCTCATCTGAGAAAGCTAAGGTTTTATTGACGATTTCTCGAGGTGTCAGTGTCTGTCTAAAAGTTCTTGAGTAGAAGGCCTTATCAGACAGTTTTCGGCTATCCTTT
      d y y h l e d s f a l t k n v i e r p t l t q r f t r s y f a k d s l k r s i k

6230 TGGAAAATTCGCCAGTGATTTTTCATGGCCGCGATAGGAAAGTGATTGCTTGTCAAAATTCTTCATGATGACAATTCTGGTTGTCATCATCTCACGGCTTAGGTGCTGGATGATATGAAT
      q f i r w h n k m a r y s l s q k d f n k m i v i r t t m m e r s l h q i i h f

                     ('PlpA>)  q d s i t y l v g t n i d r q s y k y t s k t s g e .
6350 CTATCAAGGACGATTTGTGCATTTGGAAATAGGCATTTAATCACAAGACTCTATTACGTATCTAGTTGGTACAAATATTGACCGTCAGTCCTATAAATATACATCTAAGCACAGTGAAGA
      r d l v i q a n p f l c k i (<'TnpA')
                       frameshift PlpA
      q k t s t k k a l l n k d f r q ⇓ i a f g f d r t a y a s q l n g q t g a s k i
6470 ACAAAAACATCTACGAAAAGGCTCTCTTAAACAAGGATTTCCGTCAGCTATTGCATTTGGATTTGACCGTACAGCCTATGCCTCTCAGTTGAATGGACAAACTGGAGCAAGCAAAATC

      l r n l f v p p t f v q a d g k n f g d m v k e k l v t y g d e w k d v n l a d
6590 TTACGTAATCTCTTTGTTCCACCAACATTTGTTCAAGCAGATGGTAAAAACTTTGGCGATATGGTCAAAGAGAAATTGGTCACTTATGGGGATGAATGGAAGGATGTTAATCTTGCAGAT

      s q d g l y n p e k a t a e f a k a k l a l q a e g v g f p i h l d m p v d q t
6710 TCTCAGGATGGTCTTTACAATCCAGAAAAAGCCACGGCTGAATTTGCTAAAGCTAAATTAGCCTTACAAGCAGAAGGAGTCCAATTCCCAATTCATTTAGATATGCCAGTTGACCAGACA

      a t t k v q r v q s m k q s l e v t l g a d n v i i d i q q l q k d e v n n i t
6830 GCAACTACAAAAGTTCAGCGCGTCCAATCTATGAAACAATCCTTGGAAGTAACTTTAGGAGCTGATAATGTCATTATTGATATCCAACAACTACAAAAAGACGAAGTAAACAATATTACA
                                                                              SspI
      y f a e n a a g e d w d l s d n v g w g p d f a d p s t y l d i i k p s v g e s
6950 TATTTTGCTGAAAATGCTGCTGGCGAAGACTGGGATTTATCAGATAATGTCGGTTGGGGTCCAGACTTTGCCGATCCATCAACCTACCTTGATATCATCAAACCATCTGTAGGAGAAAGT
                                                                       EcoRV
      t k t y l g f d s g e d n v a a k k v g l y d y e k l v t e a g d e a t d v a k
7070 ACTAAACATATATTTAGGGTTTGACTCAGGGGAAGATAATGTAGCTGCTAAAAAAGTAGGTCTATATGACTACGAAAAATTGGTTACTGAGGCTGGTGATGAGGCTACAGATGTTGCTAAA

      r y d k y a a a q a w l t d s a l i i p t t s r t g r p i l s k m v p f t i p f
7190 CGCTATGATAAATACGCTGCAGCCCAAGCTTGGTTGACAGATAGTGCTTTGATTATTCCAACTACATCTCGTACAGGGCGTCCAATCTTGTCTAAGATGGTACCATTTACAATACCATTT
                   MC1032 PstI △ HindIII                                       KpnI
      a l s g n k g t s e p i l y k y l e l q d k a v t v d e y q k a q e k w m k e k
7310 GCATTGTCAGGAAATAAAGGTACAAGTGAACCAATCTTATATAAATACTTGGAACTTCAAGACAAGGCAGTCACTGTAGATGAATACCAAAAAGCTCAGGAAAAATGGATGAAAGAAAAA

      e e s n k k a q e d l a k h v k *
7430 GAAGAGTCTAATAAAAAGGCTCAAGAAGATCTCGCAAAACATGTGAAATAACTGTTGCAAAATATAAG  7497
                          BglII
```

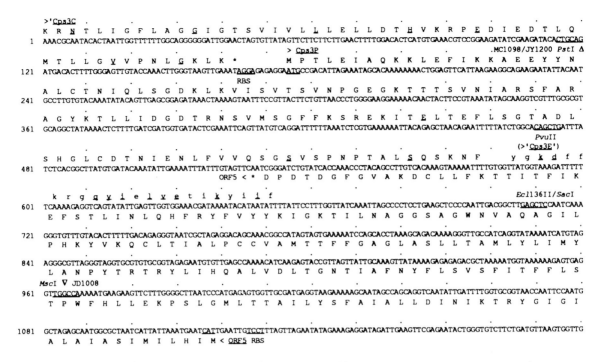

FIG. 3. Sequence of the flanking region upstream of the type 3-specific genes. The sequence begins in the 3' end of *cps3C*. Sequences homologous to *cps19fA, B,* and *C* are present upstream of this sequence (not shown and [5], GenBank accession number Z47210). The promoter for *cps3D*, the first type 3-specific gene, begins 442 bp downstream of the last nucleotide shown here. Underlined amino acids in the Cps3C, Cps3P, and Cps3E sequences indicate differences from the homologous type 19F sequences.[32] The *cps3C, cps3P,* and *cps3E* sequences shown are 95%, 99%, and 65% identical to their type 19F homologs over the regions present in both sequences. The Cps3P ORF extends an additional 19 aa but this region is not homologous to Cps19fD. The Cps3E amino acids in lower case are not expected to be translated. Symbols are as in Fig. 2. The sequence contains an additional "A" at bp 972 that was not noted in the previously reported sequence.[24]

tem (Boehringer-Mannheim) was used for labeling of probes and for chemiluminescent detection. Probes were derived by PCR amplification of: a) the cloned inserts from pJD390 (*cps3D*), pJD362 (*cps3S*), and pJD357 (*cps3U*); b) an internal fragment from pJD364 (*cps3M*) using the M-specific primers M1 and M5 (see Table 2); and c) internal fragments from pJD377 using the IS2/P1 (*tnpA*) and P8/P3 (*plpA*) primers.

Capsule determinations

Capsular serotypes were confirmed by slide agglutination using type-specific antisera (Statens Seruminstitut, Copenhagen, Denmark). For use in ELISA determinations, cultures of *S. pneumoniae* were grown to mid-exponential phase ($OD_{600} = 0.5$) in THY and were then heat killed (65°C, 20 min). Supernatant fluids from centrifuged (12,000 × g, 10 min) cultures were filtered and the cell pellets were washed and resuspended in the original culture volume with PBS (50 mM sodium phosphate pH 7.4, 100 mM NaCl). Type 3 capsule was quantitated in competitive-inhibition ELISA assays[10] using microtiter plates coated with purified type 3 polysaccharide (0.25 µg/ml PBS; ATCC, Rockville, MD) coupled to poly-L-lysine.[30] Ascites fluid containing the type 3-specific monoclonal antibody 16.3[19] was used to detect polysaccharide. Purified type 3 polysaccharide was used as the standard. Samples were diluted either 125-fold (whole cells and sonicates) or 625-fold (supernatant fluids). For each strain, the percent inhibition was

determined as the mean from at least two independent cultures, with at least four replicates performed for each culture. Statistical significance was determined using Student's t-test.

RESULTS

The loci of different capsular serotypes are designated by the locus name followed by the number of the serotype, e.g., type 3 is indicated as *cps3*.[24,32] For type 3, the type-specific genes and the genes downstream are named based on expected function.[25] Common sequences that are located upstream of the type 3-specific genes have been given the designation of their type 19F homolog when the two are identical, e.g., *cps3C* is equivalent to *cps19fC*. The type 3 locus is shown in Fig. 2A.

Truncated sequences associated with the type 3 locus

Cps3M. The putative translational start codon of Cps3M, the most downstream of the type 3-specific open reading frames, overlaps the putative stop codon of Cps3U (see Fig. 2B). Cps3M has homology to phosphoglucomutases (PGM) and phosphomannomutases (PMM) from both gram-positive and gram-negative bacteria, as well as phosphomutases from rabbit and yeast. Several regions conserved among PGMs and PMMs, and expected to be important in their function, are present within Cps3M (see Fig. 4). However, a stop codon located immedi-

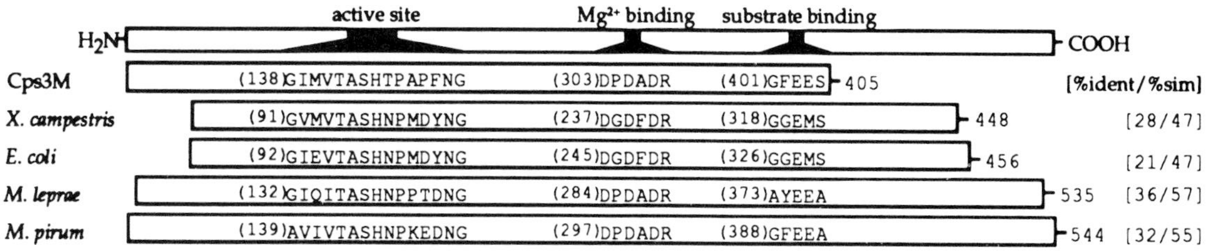

	active site	Mg²⁺ binding	substrate binding		[%ident/%sim]
Cps3M	(138)GIMVTASHTPAPFNG	(303)DPDADR	(401)GFEES	405	
X. campestris	(91)GVMVTASHNPMDYNG	(237)DGDFDR	(318)GGEMS	448	[28/47]
E. coli	(92)GIEVTASHNPMDYNG	(245)DGDFDR	(326)GGEMS	456	[21/47]
M. leprae	(132)GIQITASHNPPTDNG	(284)DPDADR	(373)AYEEA	535	[36/57]
M. pirum	(139)AVIVTASHNPKEDNG	(297)DPDADR	(388)GFEEA	544	[32/55]

FIG. 4. Comparison of Cps3M with phosphomutases. Amino acid positions are given in parentheses with the total number of amino acids given at the end. The proteins shown are *Xanthomonas campestris* XanA (PGM/PMM),[39] *E. coli* CpsG (PMM),[3] *Mycobacterium leprae* cosmid clone L308 ORF (GenBank accession # U00022), and *Mycoplasma pirum* ORF5.[57] The putative active site regions contain a serine which is thought to be phosphorylated to form the active enzyme.[51] The reported Mg²⁺ binding site sequence in yeast and rabbit muscle PGMs is DGDGDR.[20] The putative substrate binding site is homologous to that reported for PGMs and PMMs.[20]

ately after the last amino acid in the putative substrate binding site of Cps3M results in a truncated molecule that has lost over 100 amino acids when compared to the other proteins (see Fig. 2B and Fig. 4). The alteration is apparently due to a deletion rather than to a frameshift mutation as sequences homologous to phosphomutases were not detected downstream of the Cps3M stop codon. Four domains (I–IV), which together form the floor and sides of the enzymatic active site crevice, were identified in the rabbit muscle PGM crystal structure.[20] The sequence of Cps3M indicates that this protein lacks sequences which would be involved in the formation of structural domain IV.

'TnpA'. Overlapping the C-terminus of Cps3M, but of opposite orientation, is 'TnpA' (see Fig. 2B). Although *'tnpA'* extends for 555 bp and has the potential to encode a polypeptide of 22,169 Da, it lacks any apparent transcriptional or translational signals, including a methionine start codon. 'TnpA' has homology with putative transposases of insertion sequences (IS) from several gram-positive bacteria, including IS*1167* of *S. pneumoniae*, and one gram-negative bacterium. Compared to the other transposases, however, 'TnpA' represents only an internal portion of a larger ORF (see Fig. 5). No inverted or direct nucleotide repeat sequences were identified within the *'tnpA'* region. A 23 amino acid region of 'TnpA' that overlaps Cps3M is most probably coincidental, as it includes the potential sugar substrate binding site of the latter molecule (see Fig. 2B) and has no homology to other transposases.

'PlpA'. The region adjacent to *'tnpA'* contains sequence that is essentially identical to that of *plpA* from derivatives of the *S. pneumoniae* serotype 2 strain D39 (*plpA*, permease-like protein A,[47] also named *aliA*[1]).[24] PlpA has homology with several bacterial permeases involved in the transport of oligopeptides, including AmiA, the substrate binding protein member of the Ami ABC transporter in *S. pneumoniae*.[1,47] In both gram-positive and gram-negative organisms, proteins belonging to the ABC transporter family of ATP-dependent membrane transport proteins have been found to be involved in the transport of exopolysaccharides.[27] Completion of the type 3 *plpA* sequence has revealed 98% DNA identity with bp 843 to 1949 of the type 2 *plpA*. However, two striking differences between the *plpAs* are apparent. First, the type 3 *plpA* has undergone a deletion at the 5' terminus that resulted in loss of the first 281 amino acids present in the type 2 sequence. The site of the deletion is immediately adjacent to the beginning of *'tnpA'*. Second, a one bp deletion in the type 3 *plpA* (see Fig. 2B, position 6519) results in a frameshift mutation at amino acid position 43 of the type 3 PlpA. Correcting for the frameshift, the predicted amino acid sequence of the type 3 PlpA differs from that found in this region of the type 2 PlpA by only 8 amino acids (see Fig. 2B). Sequencing of PCR products was used to confirm the one bp deletion in the type 3 chromosome.

Upstream common sequences. Upstream of the type 3-specific locus are sequences that are also present upstream of the type-specific genes in a type 19F isolate,[32] a type 14 isolate,[38] and another type 3 isolate.[5] The predicted protein sequences of these genes have homology to proteins involved in polysaccharide export.[13,32] As with the downstream region, however, partial genes are apparent in the type 3 sequences. The type 3 *cps19fD* homolog, *cps3P*, lacks 279 bp found at the 3' end of

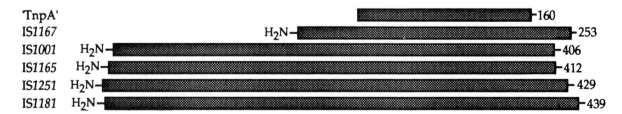

FIG. 5. Comparison of 'TnpA' with transposases. Sizes of the transposases are indicated in amino acids at the C-terminal ends. The sequences shown and their homologies (% identity/% similarity) with 'TnpA' (over the region present in each sequence) are: IS*1167*, *S. pneumoniae* (48/71, [69]); IS*1001*, *Bordetella parapertussis* (19/41, [68]); IS*1165*, *Leuconostoc mesenteroides* (31/56, [36]); IS*1251*, *Enterococcus faecium* (34/61, GenBank accession # L34675); IS*1181*, *Staphylococcus aureus* (29/53, [22]).

the type 19F gene. The Cps3P ORF is 154 amino acids long but the last 19 amino acids are not homologous to Cps19fD, whereas the first 135 amino acids are 98% identical (see Fig. 3). A shift in reading frame 5 bp past the end of the homology identifies a 23 amino acid peptide ('Cps3E'; see Fig. 3) that has 57% identity with a peptide encoded by the 5' end of cps19fE, the next downstream type 19F capsule gene. The region deleted in the type 3 strain extends 453 bp from the point of truncation in cps19fD to the start of the 23 amino acid peptide encoded by cps19fE. The remaining 1,119 bp of cps19fE have not been identified in the type 3 sequence. The complete Cps19fE homolog is present in the type 14 strain, where glycosyltransferase activity has been demonstrated.[38] Comparison of the sequences from the two characterized type 3 strains, WU2 (our data) and 406 (Arrecubieta, et al.[5] GenBank accession #Z47210) revealed only two nucleotide differences and a single amino acid difference in a 639 bp region containing the cps19fD homolog and the 3' end of the cps19fC homolog. Thus, both strains contain the partial sequence structures identified in WU2.

ORF5

Sequencing of the region between cps3D and the common upstream region, along with a correction in the previously reported partial nucleotide sequence, identified an open reading frame (ORF5) of 197 amino acids that reads in the direction opposite to Cps3DSUM (see Fig. 3). No extensive homologies with known protein sequences are apparent in this ORF. The protein predicted from the orf5 sequence is highly hydrophobic, with at least 3 potential membrane spanning regions present (data not shown). Southern blot analyses using a probe specific for orf5 detected only a single copy of this sequence in strains of capsule types 2 and 6B, but two copies were present in the type 3 strain (see Fig. 6). Based on restriction fragment sizes, the unique copy of orf5 in type 3 is the one upstream of cps3DSUM. From our previous linkage analyses[24] and the present data, it can be concluded that the type 2 and type 6B copies of this gene are not linked to their respective capsule loci. It also is not present in the capsule loci of type 19F[32] or type 14[38] (GenBank accession # X85787).

Confirmation of plpA deletion in the type 3 WU2 chromosome and identification of full length plpA in other capsular serotypes

In contrast to the type 3 plpA, the plpA identified in derivatives of the serotype 2 D39 strain is a complete gene.[1,47] To confirm the 5' deletion of plpA in the type 3 WU2 chromosome, and to determine whether this gene is intact in strains of other capsular types, PCR analyses using primers expected to permit amplification of the 5' end, the 3' end, and the full length plpA were performed (see Fig. 7A). A 997 bp PCR product corresponding to the 3' end of plpA was obtained from strains of capsular types 1, 2, 3, 5, 6B, and 14. A 1,272 bp product corresponding to the 5' end and a 1,959 bp product corresponding to the full length plpA were obtained from strains of types 1, 2, 5, 6B and 14. However, neither the 1,272 bp or 1,959 bp products was obtained from the type 3 strain. Using the 5' end plpA PCR product from the type 6B strain as a probe in Southern blot analyses, we did not detect the 5' end of plpA in type

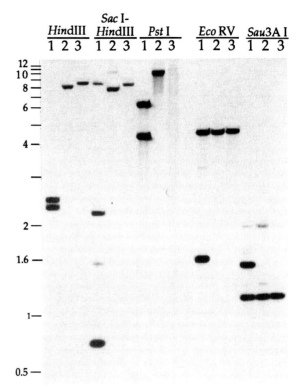

FIG. 6.   orf5 Southern analyses. Hybridization with orf5-specific probe generated using primers Orf1 and Orf2. Lanes 1, WU2 (type 3); 2, D39 (type 2); 3, DBL1 (type 6B).

3 WU2 (see Fig. 7B). Thus, the 5' end of plpA has been lost from the type 3 chromosome and the deletion may be unique to type 3 strains.

Conservation of the type 3 locus structure among different type 3 strains and in Rx1

To determine whether the deletions observed in strain WU2 are conserved among type 3 strains, we examined the capsule loci of four additional independent clinical isolates by RFLP and PCR analyses. The type 3 strains used—WU2, A66, L8 1995, ATCC 6303, and EF3113—differ with respect to PspA serotypes, virulence properties, and sites of isolation.[18] In Southern blot analyses using 14 restriction enzymes, the fragment sizes obtained with 12 enzymes were identical for all strains (see Fig. 8A). A PvuII polymorphism was noted for one strain and two strains exhibited the same StuI polymorphism (data not shown). The area examined extends >14 kb from the StuI site upstream of cps3C to the SphI site downstream of plpA (see Fig. 2A). To more precisely determine whether the cps3M-tnpA-plpA deletions are characteristic of all type 3 chromosomes, PCR analysis was performed using primers located within cps3M and plpA. The amplified products were identical for all five type 3 strains (see Fig. 8B). No amplification product was detected using a type 6B strain as a negative control.

The common laboratory strain Rx1 was derived as a nonencapsulated mutant of the type 2 strain D39, was then transformed to type 3 encapsulation, again selected for nonencapsulation, and finally selected as a highly transformable mutant.[50,54] This strain retains the type 3 capsule locus and makes a small amount of type 3 polysaccharide. It can be restored to normal type 3 encapsulation by the repair of a point mutation in *cps3D*.[24] PCR analyses confirmed that the *cps3M-tnpA-plpA* region of Rx1 contains the same deletions observed in type 3 strains (data not shown).

tnpA *is present in single copy and is linked to* plpA *in other capsule types*

IS1167, with which *tnpA* has homology (see Fig. 5), is present in multiple copies in the pneumococcal chromosome.[69]

However, only a single copy of *tnpA* was detected in strains of types 2, 3, and 6B (see Fig. 7C). The sequences detected using *tnpA* as a probe are not likely to be copies of IS*1167*, as the two sequences are only 53% homologous and hybridizations were done at >95% stringency. Thus, these two transposases represent distinct members of a family of transposases.

Probes specific for *plpA* also revealed only a single copy of this gene (see Fig. 7B). Restriction mapping with either *tnpA*- or *plpA*-specific probes yielded maps identical to those determined using a single probe containing both sequences ([24], Fig. 7B, Fig. 7C, and data not shown). Thus, *tnpA* is present in strains of other capsule types and both it and *plpA* are located on the same restriction fragments.

Transcription of the type 3 locus

Insertion-duplication mutations using vectors that yield transcriptional *cat* fusions (pJY4163 and pJY4164, see Table 1) were constructed in the genes of the type 3 locus. As shown in Fig. 9, *cps3D* and *cps3S* are transcribed at approximately equivalent levels. *cps3U* is transcribed at approximately one-half the level of *cps3DS*, whereas transcription through *cps3M* and *plpA* is about one-sixth of the *cps3DS* level. A low but detectable level of transcription was apparent through the regions flanking the type 3-specific genes (see Fig. 9).

Northern blot analyses using probes for the type 3-specific genes showed that *cps3D, S, U,* and *M* are present on the same transcripts (see Fig. 10A). Although multiple transcripts are apparent, all four probes detected an approximate 6,700 nt transcript. The remaining transcripts may result from transcription initiations at additional promoters or they may be the result of processing of the larger transcript. Utilization of the promoter identified upstream of *cps3D*[4,24] and of a potential transcription termination sequence identified downstream of *plpA*[47] would result in an approximate 6,500 nt transcript that would contain *cps3DSUM-tnpA-plpA*. Hybridization with *tnpA*- and *plpA*-specific probes showed that these sequences are contained on the same transcripts as *cps3DSUM* (see Fig. 10A). These results confirm the previous genetic observations showing that *cps3D* and *cps3S* are transcribed as part of the same operon[24] and extend the observations of Arrecubieta et al.,[4] showing that a single transcript contains at least *cps3D, cps3S,* and *cps3U* (*cap3A, cap3B, cap3C*).

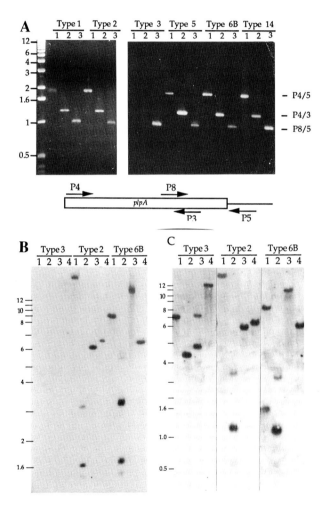

Effect of mutations on type 3 capsule production

Strains containing mutations in either *cps3D* or *cps3S* do not make detectable type 3 polysaccharide.[24,25] With these exceptions, there are no apparent requirements for expression of the genes in the type 3 locus for capsule production under standard laboratory growth conditions. The strains examined contained insertion-duplication mutations in *cps3C* (JY1200), *orf5* (JD1008), *cps3U* (JD900), *cps3M* (MC1092), and *plpA*, (MC1032). Capsule production was assessed by inspection of colony morphology for cells grown on blood agar medium and in competitive-inhibition ELISA assays using whole cells, culture supernatants, and cell sonicates of THY-grown cultures (data not shown).

FIG. 7. *plpA* and *tnpA* in strains of different capsular types. (A) PCR analysis of *plpA*. Chromosomal DNA was amplified using primers at the 5' (P4) and 3' (P5) extremes and internal (P3, P8) to *plpA*. Lanes: 1, P4/P5; 2, P4/P3; 3, P8/P5. (B) Hybridization with *plpA*. Southern blots were hybridized with the 5' end of *plpA* obtained from DBL1 (type 6B) by PCR amplification using primer combination P4/P3 and followed by digestion of the product with *Bam*HI. Lanes: 1, *Bgl*II; 2, *Hind*III; 3, *Sac*I; 4, *Sph*I. Strains: WU2 (type 3), D39 (type 2), DBL1 (type 6B). (C) Hybridization with *tnpA*. The 1.6 kb band which appears in lane 1 of type 6B is the result of contamination from an adjacent lane containing the molecular size standards. Lanes and strains are as in (B).

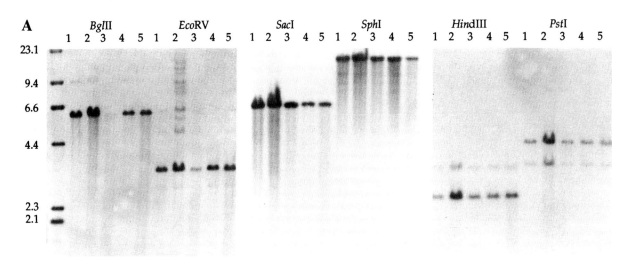

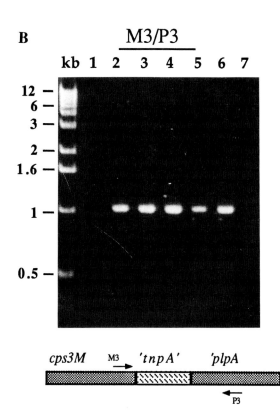

FIG. 8. Conservation of type 3 locus structure among independent type 3 isolates. (A) RFLP analysis. Restriction digests were probed with pJD351[25] which contains a 2.4 kb Sau3AI fragment extending from the 3' end of cps3D through the middle of cps3U. Results from six of the fourteen tested enzymes are shown. Not shown are the results with BstXI, ClaI, HhaI, PvuII, ScaI, StuI, StyI, and XcmI. Lanes: 1, WU2; 2, A66; 3, EF 3113; 4, L8 1995; 5, ATCC 6303. (B) PCR analysis. Chromosomal DNA was amplified using primers within the 3' end of cps3M (M3) and internal to plpA (P3). Lanes: 1, No DNA; 2, WU2; 3, A66; 4, ATCC 6303; 5, L8 1995; 6, EF3113; 7, DBL1 (type 6B).

DISCUSSION

The structure of the type 3 locus is distinct from that of other pneumococcal capsule types thus far described. The deletions identified throughout the locus, together with the presence of a partial transposase sequence, suggest that this locus is the result of an aberrant transposition event. We previously proposed a transposition-like event to explain the occurrence of binary encapsulated strains and as a possible mechanism involved in novel capsule type formation.[24] Possibly, the deletions in this locus occurred during insertion of the type 3-specific genes into the chromosome. Alternatively, the type 3 locus may have resulted from transposition-induced deletions of a locus encoding a more complex capsular structure. An examination of known pneumococcal polysaccharide structures[59] for sugar compositions and linkages does not immediately identify a likely progenitor. However, not all of the structures of the 90 known serotypes have been described, and further rearrangements may have occurred after an initial transposition-induced deletion. In addition, if the progenitor were relatively avirulent, it probably would have been selected against and either lost or only rarely isolated from the human host. Although at present there is no genetic evidence that TnpA has played a role in the evolution of pneumococcal capsular types, examples of insertion-mediated types of evolution have been described in other systems, e.g., the rfb O-antigen gene clusters in *Salmonella enterica* group D2[63] and *Vibrio cholerae* O139[16] are apparently the result of transposition and recombination events.

Whatever the origins of the type 3 locus, its structure is highly conserved among independent type 3 isolates and has thus either evolved only recently or holds importance for functions presumably associated with the type 3 capsule genes. Intact versions of several of the deleted genes (cps3P, cps3E, and plpA) are expected to encode proteins potentially involved in polysaccharide synthesis. While these common functions may be necessary for synthesis of more complex structures, the simplicity of the type 3 polysaccharide argues for an equally simple mechanism of synthesis that may not, for example, involve lipid intermediates or require additional

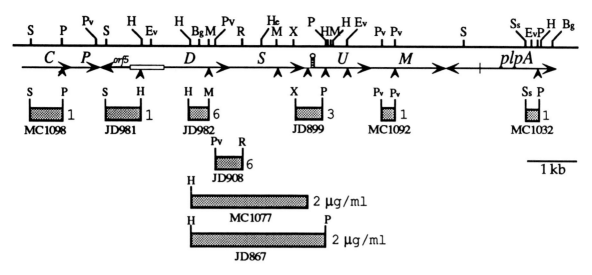

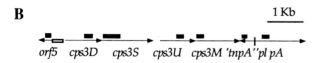

FIG. 9. Transcriptional analysis of the type 3 locus using *cat* fusions. Positions of fragments used to construct gene fusions are indicated. Levels of resistance to chloramphenicol (μg/ml) are given to the right of each fragment to indicate the direction of transcription. Insertion of *cat* fusions in the orientation opposite to that indicated for transcription results in resistance to 0.5 μg/ml. Symbols: ▲, points of *cat* fusions; ⌿, potential stem-loop structure (bp 3732 to 3771 in [24]). Restriction sites (in addition to those indicated in Fig. 2): M, *Mun*I; He, *Hae*III; R, *Rsa*I; Ss, *Ssp*I.

transport proteins. Type 3 synthesis would, however, be expected to require the functions of a phosphoglucomutase and a UDP-Glc-1-P uridylyltransferase for conversion of Glc-6-P to Glc-1-P, and Glc-1-P to UDP-Glc, respectively. Clearly,

A Probe *D   S   U   M   tnpA   plpA   pspA*

7.40 -
5.30 -

2.90 -

1.90 -
1.50 -
1.00 -
0.60 -

B   1 Kb

orf5   cps3D   cps3S   cps3U   cps3M 'tnpA''pl pA

FIG. 10. Northern analysis of the type 3 locus. Each lane contains 20 μg denatured RNA isolated from strain WU2. The probe used is indicated above each lane. (A) Hybridization with probes from the type 3 locus and an unlinked gene. The *pspA* probe recognizes the transcript for pneumococcal surface protein A (major transcript expected to be ~2 kb,[64] and unpublished data) and was used to confirm the integrity of the RNA preparation. (B) Map of the type 3 capsule locus indicating the locations of the probes.

the type 3-specific genes expected to encode these functions are not required under laboratory culture conditions and these roles must be fulfilled by essential cellular proteins such as those involved in cell wall and teichoic acid synthesis. Furthermore, it is not clear that Cps3M actually functions as a phosphomutase, as it lacks a domain expected to be important for this activity[20,52] and we have not been able to demonstrate such a function (unpublished data). Nonetheless, both *cps3U* and *cps3M* are maintained as open reading frames and are transcribed. Likewise, *tnpA* and *plpA*, which are not expected to encode proteins, are transcribed and are contained on the same transcript with *cps3DSUM*. No transcription termination sequences are apparent in either the type 3-specific genes or at the junction with downstream flanking sequences. Possibly, such sequences were deleted as a result of rearrangements in the type 3 locus and the co-transcribed flanking sequences may be required to stabilize the transcript that does not end until a termination sequence is encountered following *plpA*.

An alternative explanation for the retention of the apparently non-functional flanking sequences lies in the evolutionary advantage of being able to transfer the capsule genes during genetic transformation. The immediate flanking sequences may be essential for the exchange of capsule cassettes either because of limited DNA homology in more distant regions or because sequences located between the type-specific genes and the outlying genes are essential in certain genetic backgrounds. The variations observed in the flanking sequences are also likely to be significant in regard to the apparent correlations between virulence and the type of capsule expressed,[18,37] as these closely linked genes are expected to be transferred with the type-specific genes during DNA exchanges. The genetic analysis of the capsule loci is thus an important step toward understanding the origins of *S. pneumoniae* capsular serotypes, their role in virulence, and the complex biochemistry of their synthesis.

ACKNOWLEDGMENTS

This work was supported by Public Health Service grants AI28457, T32 AI07041, and T32 HL07553 from the National Institutes of Health. Access to the Genetics Computer Group sequence analysis programs was made available through the University of Alabama at Birmingham Center for Aids Research (P30 AI27767).

We thank Tracy Hampton and Shannon Acton for their help in cloning the upstream region and in RFLP analyses, David Briles for providing *S. pneumoniae* strains, and Joseph Dillard, William Benjamin, Alexis Brooks-Walter, and Sanford Lacks for their assistance and helpful discussions concerning these studies.

REFERENCES

1. **Alloing, G., P. dePhilip, and J.-P. Claverys.** 1994. Three highly homologous membrane-bound lipoproteins participate in oligopeptide transport by the *ami* system of the gram-positive *Streptococcus pneumoniae*. J. Mol. Biol. **241:**44–58.

2. **Altschul, S.F., W. Gish, W. Miller, E.W. Myers, and D.J. Lipman.** 1990. Basic local alignment search tool. J. Mol. Biol. **215:**403–410.

3. **Aoyama, K., A.M. Haase, and P.R. Reeves.** 1994. Evidence for effect of random genetic drift on G+C content after lateral transfer of fucose pathway genes to *Escherichia coli* K-12. Mol. Biol. Evol. **11:**829–838.

4. **Arrecubieta, C., E. Garcia, and R. Lopez.** 1996. Demonstration of UDP-Glucose dehydrogenase activity in cell extracts of *Escherichia coli* expressing the pneumococcal *cap3A* gene required for the synthesis of type 3 capsular polysaccharide. J. Bacteriol. **178:**2971–2974.

5. **Arrecubieta, C., E. Garcia, and R. Lopez.** 1995. Sequence and transcriptional analysis of a DNA region involved in the production of capsular polysaccharide in *Streptococcus pneumoniae* type 3. Gene. **167:**1–7.

6. **Arrecubieta, C., R. Lopez, and E. Garcia.** 1994. Molecular characterization of *cap3A*, a gene from the operon required for the synthesis of the capsule of *Streptococcus pneumoniae* type 3: Sequencing of mutations responsible for the unencapsulated phenotype and localization of the capsular cluster on the pneumococcal chromosome. J. Bacteriol. **176:**6375–6383.

7. **Arrecubieta, C., R. Lopez, and E. Garcia.** 1996. Type 3-specific synthase of *Streptococcus pneumoniae* (Cap3B) directs type 3 polysaccharide biosynthesis in *Escherichia coli* and in pneumococcal strains of different serotypes. J. Exp. Med. **184:**449–455.

8. **Austrian, R., H.P. Bernheimer, E.E.B. Smith, and G.T. Mills.** 1959. Simultaneous production of two capsular polysaccharides by pneumococcus. II. The genetic and biochemical bases of binary capsulation. J. Exp. Med. **110:**585–602.

9. **Austrian, R.A.** 1952. Observations on the transformation of pneumococcus in vivo. Bull. Johns Hopkins Hosp. **91:**189–196.

10. **Ausubel, F.M., R. Brent, R.E. Kingston, D.D. Moore, J.G. Seidman, J.A. Smith, and K. Struhl.** 1987. Current Protocols in Molecular Biology. John Wiley & Son, New York.

11. **Avery, O.T., and R. Dubos.** 1931. The protective action of a specific enzyme against type III pneumococcus infection in mice. J. Exp. Med. **54:**73–89.

12. **Avery, O.T., C.M. MacLeod, and M. McCarty.** 1944. Studies on the chemical nature of the substance inducing transformation of pneumococcal types. Induction of transformation by a desoxyribonucleic acid fraction isolated from pneumococcus type III. J. Exp. Med. **79:**137–158.

13. **Becker, A., K. Niehaus, and A. Puhler.** 1995. Low-molecular weight succinoglycan is predominantly produced by *Rhizobium meliloti* strains carrying a mutated ExoP protein characterized by a periplasmic N-terminal domain and a missing C-terminal domain. Mol. Microbiol. **16:**191–203.

14. **Bernheimer, H., I.E. Wermundsen, and R. Austrian.** 1967. Qualitative differences in the behavior of pneumococcal deoxyribonucleic acids transforming to the same capsular type. J. Bacteriol. **93:**320–333.

15. **Bernheimer, H.P., and I.P. Wermundsen.** 1969. Unstable binary capsulated transformants in pneumococcus. J. Bacteriol. **98:**1073–1079.

16. **Bik, E.M., A.E. Bunschoten, R.D. Gouw, and F.R. Mooi.** 1995. Genesis of the novel epidemic *Vibrio cholerae* O139 strain: Evidence for horizontal transfer of genes involved in polysaccharide synthesis. EMBO J. **14:**209–216.

17. **Birnboim, H.C., and J. Doly.** 1979. A rapid alkaline extraction procedure for screening recombinant plasmid DNA. Nucl. Acids Res. **7:**1513–1523.

18. **Briles, D.E., M. Crain, B.M. Gray, C. Forman, and J. Yother.** 1992. Strong association between capsule type and virulence for mice among human isolates of *Streptococcus pneumoniae*. Infect. Immun. **60:**111–116.

19. **Briles, D.E., M. Nahm, K. Schoroer, J. Davie, P. Baker, J. Kearney, and R. Barletta.** 1981. Antiphosphocholine antibodies found in normal mouse serum are protective against intravenous infection with type 3 *Streptococcus pneumoniae*. J. Exp. Med. **153:**694–705.

20. **Dai, J.-B., Y. Liu, W.J. Ray, Jr., and M. Konno.** 1992. The crystal structure of muscle phosphoglucomutase refined at 2.7-angstrom resolution. J. Biol. Chem. **267:**6322–6337.

21. **Dawson, M.H., and R.H.P. Sia.** 1931. In vitro transformation of pneumococcal types. I. A technique for inducing transformation of pneumococcal types in vitro. J. Exp. Med. **54:**681–699.

22. **Derbise, A., K.G.H. Dyke, and N.E. Solh.** 1994. Isolation and characterization of IS*1181*, an insertion sequence from *Staphylococcus aureus*. Plasmid. **31:**251–263.

23. **Dillard, J.D., M. Caimano, T. Kelly, and J. Yother.** 1995. Capsules and cassettes: Genetic organization of the capsule locus of *Streptococcus pneumoniae*. Dev. Biol. Stand. **85:**261–265.

24. **Dillard, J.P., M.W. Vandersea, and J. Yother.** 1995. Characterization of the cassette containing genes for type 3 capsular polysaccharide biosynthesis in *Streptococcus pneumoniae*. J. Exp. Med. **181:**973–983.

25. **Dillard, J.P., and J. Yother.** 1994. Genetic and molecular characterization of capsular polysaccharide biosynthesis in *Streptococcus pneumoniae* type 3. Mol. Microbiol. **12:**959–972.

26. **Ephrussi-Taylor, H.** 1951. Genetic aspects of transformations of pneumococci. Cold Spr. Harb. Symp. Quant. Biol. **16:**445–456.

27. **Fath, M.J., and R. Kolter.** 1993. ABC transporters: Bacterial exporters. Microbiol. Rev. **57:**995–1017.

28. **Garcia, E., P. Garcia, and R. Lopez.** 1993. Cloning and sequencing of a gene involved in the synthesis of the capsular polysaccharide of *Streptococcus pneumoniae* type 3. Mol. Gen. Genet. **239:**188–195.

29. **Genetics Computer Group.** 1991. Program Manual for the GCG Package, Version 8 ed. Genetics Computer Group, Madison.

30. **Gray, B.M.** 1979. ELISA methodology for polysaccharide antigens: Protein coupling of polysaccharides for adsorption to plastic tubes. J. Immunol. Methods. **28:**187–192.

31. **Griffith, F.** 1928. The significance of pneumococcal types. J. Hygiene. **27:**113–159.

32. **Guidolin, A., J.K. Morona, R. Morona, D. Hansman, and J.C. Paton.** 1994. Nucleotide sequence analysis of genes essential for capsular polysaccharide biosynthesis in *Streptococcus pneumoniae* type 19F. Infect. Immun. **62:**5384–5396.

33. **Henrichsen, J.** 1995. Six newly recognized types of *Streptococcus pneumoniae*. J. Clin. Microbiol. **33**:2759–2762.

34. **Hostetter, M.K.** 1986. Serotypic variation among virulent pneumococci in deposition and degradation of covalently bound C3b: Implications for phagocytosis and antibody production. J. Infect. Dis. **153**:682–693.

35. **Hotchkiss, R.D.** 1957. Isolation of sodium deoxyribonucleate in biologically active form from bacteria. Methods Enzymol. **3**:692–696.

36. **Johansen, E., and A. Kibenich.** 1992. Isolation and characterization of *IS1165*, an insertion sequence of *Leuconostoc mesenteroides* subsp. *cremoris* and other lactic acid bacteria. Plasmid. **27**:200–206.

37. **Kelly, T., J.P. Dillard, and J. Yother.** 1994. Effect of genetic switching of capsular type on virulence of *Streptococcus pneumoniae*. Infect. Immun. **62**:1813–1819.

38. **Kolkman, M.A.B., D.A. Morrison, B.A.M. van der Zeijst, and P.J.M. Nuijten.** 1996. The capsule polysaccharide synthesis locus of *Streptococcus pneumoniae* serotype 14: Identification of the glycosyl transferase gene *cps14E*. J. Bacteriol. **178**:3736–3741.

39. **Koplin, R., W. Arnold, B. Hotte, R. Simon, G. Wang, and A. Puhler.** 1992. Genetics of xanthan production in *Xanthomonas campestris*: the *xanA* and *xanB* genes are involved in UDP-glucose and GDP-mannose biosynthesis. J. Bacteriol. **174**:191–199.

40. **Kruse, W., and S. Pansini.** 1891. Untersuchungen uber den *Diplococcus pneumoniae* und verwandte Streptokokken. Ztschr. f. Hyg. u. Infektionskr. **11**:279–280.

41. **Lacks, S., B. Mannarelli, S. Springhorn, and B. Greenberg.** 1986. Genetic basis of the complementary *Dpn*I and *Dpn*II restriction systems of *S. pneumoniae*: An intracellular cassette mechanism. Cell. **46**:993–1000.

42. **Langvad-Nielson, A.** 1944. Change of capsule in the pneumococcus. Acta. Path. et Microbiol. Scand. **21**:362–369.

43. **MacLeod, C.M., R.G. Hodges, M. Heildeberger, and W.G. Bernhard.** 1945. Prevention of pneumococcal pneumonia by immunization with specific capsular polysaccharides. J. Exp. Med. **82**:445–465.

44. **MacLeod, C.M., and M.R. Krauss.** 1956. Control by factors distinct from the S transforming principle of the amount of capsular polysaccharide produced by type III pneumococci. J. Exp. Med. **97**:767–771.

45. **MacLeod, C.M., and M.R. Krauss.** 1950. Relation of virulence of pneumococcal strains for mice to the quantity of capsular polysaccharide formed in vitro. J. Exp. Med. **92**:1–9.

46. **McDaniel, L.S., J.S. Sheffield, E. Swaitlo, J. Yother, M.J. Crain, and D.E. Briles.** 1992. Molecular localization of variable and conserved regions of *pspA* and identification of additional *pspA* homologous sequences in *Streptococcus pneumoniae*. Microb. Pathog. **13**:261–269.

47. **Pearce, B.J., A.M. Naughton, and H.R. Masure.** 1994. Peptide permeases modulate transformation in *Streptococcus pneumoniae*. Mol. Microbiol. **12**:881–892.

48. **Radloff, R., W. Bauer, and J. Vinograd.** 1967. A dye-buoyant-density method for the detection and isolation of closed circular duplex DNA: The closed circular DNA in HeLa cells. Proc. Natl. Acad. Sci. USA. **57**:1514–1521.

49. **Ravin, A.W.** 1960. Linked mutations borne by deoxyribonucleic acid controlling the synthesis of capsular polysaccharide in pneumococcus. Genetics. **45**:1387–1403.

50. **Ravin, A.W.** 1959. Reciprocal capsular transformations of pneumococci. J. Bacteriol. **77**:296–309.

51. **Ray, W.J., Jr., M.A. Hermodson, J.M. Puvathingal, and W.C. Mahoney.** 1983. The complete amino acid sequence of rabbit muscle phosphoglucomutase. J. Biol. Chem. **258**:9166–9174.

52. **Sandlin, R.C., and D.C. Stein.** 1994. Role of phosphoglucomutase in lipooligosaccharide biosynthesis in *Neisseria gonorrhoeae*. J. Bacteriol. **176**:2930–2937.

53. **Shaw, W.V.** 1975. Chloramphenicol acetyltransferase from chloramphenicol-resistant bacteria. Meth. Enzymol. **43**:737–755.

54. **Shoemaker, N.B., and W.R. Guild.** 1974. Destruction of low efficiency markers is a slow process occurring at a heteroduplex stage of transformation. Mol. Gen. Genet. **128**:283–290.

55. **Stryker, L.M.** 1916. Variations in the pneumococcus induced by growth in immune serum. J. Exp. Med. **24**:49–68.

56. **Tao, L., D.J. LeBlanc, and J.J. Ferretti.** 1992. Novel streptococcal-integration shuttle vectors for gene cloning and inactivation. Gene. **120**:105–110.

57. **Tham, T.N., S. Ferris, R. Kovacic, L. Montagnier, and A. Blanchard.** 1993. Identification of *Mycoplasma pirum* genes involved in the salvage pathways for nucleosides. J. Bacteriol. **175**:5281–5285.

58. **Tilghman, S.M., D.C. Tiemeier, P. Polisky, M.H. Edgell, J.G. Seidman, A. Leder, L.W. Endquist, B. Norman, and P. Leder.** 1977. Cloning specific segments of the mammalian genome: bacteriophage lambda containing mouse globin and surrounding gene sequences. Proc. Natl. Acad. Sci. USA. **74**:4406–4410.

59. **van Dam, J.E.G., A. Fleer, and H. Snippe.** 1990. Immunogenicity and immunochemistry of *Streptococcus pneumoniae* polysaccharides. Antonie van Leeuwenhoek. **58**:1–47.

60. **Walter, A.W., V.H. Guerin, M.W. Beattie, H.Y. Cotler, and H.B. Bucca.** 1941. Extension of the separation of types among pneumococci: description of 17 types in addition to types 1 to 32 (Cooper). J. Immunol. **41**:279.

61. **White, B.** 1938. The biology of pneumococcus. The Commonwealth Fund, New York.

62. **Wood, W.B., Jr., and M.R. Smith.** 1949. The inhibition of surface phagocytosis by the capsular "slime layer" of pneumococcus type III. J. Exp. Med. **90**:85–96.

63. **Xiang, S.-H., M. Hobbs, and P.R. Reeves.** 1994. Molecular analysis of the *rfb* gene cluster of a group D2 *Salmonella enterica* strain: Evidence for its origin from an insertion sequence-mediated recombination event between group E and D1 strains. J. Bacteriol. **176**:4357–4365.

64. **Yother, J., and D.E. Briles.** 1992. Structural properties and evolutionary relationships of PspA, a surface protein of *Streptococcus pneumoniae*, as revealed by sequence analysis. J. Bacteriol. **174**:601–609.

65. **Yother, J., C. Forman, B.M. Gray, and D.E. Briles.** 1982. Protection of mice from infection with *Streptococcus pneumoniae* by anti-phosphocholine antibody. Infect. Immun. **36**:184–188.

66. **Yother, J., G.L. Handsome, and D.E. Briles.** 1992. Truncated forms of PspA that are secreted from *Streptococcus pneumoniae* and their use in functional studies and cloning of the *pspA* gene. J. Bacteriol. **174**:610–618.

67. **Yother, J., L.S. McDaniel, and D.E. Briles.** 1986. Transformation of encapsulated *Streptococcus pneumoniae*. J. Bacteriol. **168**:1463–1465.

68. **Zee, A.V.D., C. Agterberg, M.V. Agterveld, M. Peeters, and F.R. Mooi.** 1993. Characterization of *IS1001*, an insertion sequence element of *Bordetella parapertussis*. J. Bacteriol. **175**:141–147.

69. **Zhou, L., F.M. Hui, and D.A. Morrison.** 1995. Characterization of *IS1167*, a new insertion sequence in *Streptococcus pneumoniae*. Plasmid. **33**:127–138.

Address reprint requests to:
Dr. Janet Yother
Department of Microbiology
BBRB 661/12
University of Alabama at Birmingham
Birmingham, AL 35294-2170

Characterization of the Capsular Polysaccharide Biosynthesis Locus of *Streptococcus pneumoniae* Type 19F

JAMES C. PATON,[1] JUDY K. MORONA,[1] and RENATO MORONA[2]

ABSTRACT

We have used a combination of plasmid insertion/rescue and inverse polymerase chain reaction (PCR) to clone the region of the *Streptococcus pneumoniae* type 19F chromosome encoding biosynthesis of type 19F capsular polysaccharide (*cps19f*), which was then subjected to sequence analysis. The *cps19f* locus is located in the *S. pneumoniae* chromosome between *dexB* and *aliA*, and consists of 15 open reading frames (ORFs), designated *cps19fA* to *cps19fO*, that appear to be arranged as a single transcriptional unit. Insertion-duplication mutants in 13 of the 15 ORFs have been constructed in a smooth type 19F strain, all of which resulted in a rough (unencapsulated) phenotype, confirming that the operon is essential for capsule production. Comparison with sequence databases has allowed us to propose functions for 12 of the *cps19f* gene products, and a biosynthetic pathway for type 19F capsular polysaccharide. Southern hybidization analysis indicated that *cps19fA* and *cps19fB* were the only *cps* genes found in all 17 *S. pneumoniae* serotypes/groups tested. The region from *cps19fG* to *cps19fK* was found only in members of serogroup 19 and, within this *cps19fI*, was unique to type 19F.

INTRODUCTION

KNOWLEDGE OF THE FACTORS mediating capsule biosynthesis and expression is likely to provide new insights into the mechanism of pathogenesis of pneumococcal disease, and more importantly, may provide alternative targets for antimicrobial therapy. There are 90 recognized serotypes of *S. pneumoniae*, each of which produces a structurally distinct CPS. Capsule production requires a complex pathway including transport into the cell and/or synthesis of the component monosaccharides, activation of each to a nucleotide precursor, coordinated transfer of each sugar, in sequence, to the repeating oligosaccharide and subsequent polymerization, export and attachment to the cell surface. Thus, the loci encoding capsule production would be expected to consist of a large number of genes. Classical genetic studies carried out by Austrian *et al.*[3] demonstrated that the *S. pneumoniae* genes required for biosynthesis and expression of CPS are closely linked on the pneumococcal chromosome. This fact has simplified recent attempts to isolate and characterize *cps* loci of *S. pneumoniae* serotypes most commonly associated with human disease. To date, our studies have concentrated on *S. pneumoniae* type 19F, because it is one of the commonest causes of invasive disease in children. Moreover, type 19F CPS, a linear polysaccharide with a chemical repeat unit consisting of $\rightarrow$ 4)-β-D-Man$p$NAc-(1 $\rightarrow$ 4)-α-D-Glc$p$-(1 $\rightarrow$ 2)-α-L-Rha$p$-(1-PO$_4^-$ $\rightarrow$,[20] is one of the poorest immunogens in this group.[9] We have previously reported the nucleotide sequence of the first six genes of the type 19F capsule operon (designated *cps19f*)[11] and recently we have reported the isolation and characterization of the remainder of this gene cluster.[31] We have been able to assign probable functions to all but three of the ORFs and we have proposed a biosynthetic pathway for type 19F CPS.

ISOLATION AND SEQUENCE ANALYSIS OF THE COMPLETE TYPE 19F *CPS* LOCUS

We have previously isolated and sequenced a novel pneumococcal insertion element (designated IS*1202*; Genbank accession number U04047), which was shown by transformation studies to be closely linked to the *S. pneumoniae* type 19F CPS locus.[30] Attempts to isolate cosmid clones containing sequences flanking IS*1202* were unsuccessful due to the instability of large pneumococcal DNA fragments in *E. coli*, even when a low copy number cosmid was employed. We therefore used chromoso-

---

[1]Molecular Microbiology Unit, Women's and Children's Hospital, North Adelaide, S.A., Australia.
[2]Department of Microbiology and Immunology, University of Adelaide, Adelaide, S.A., Australia.

mal walking techniques (inverse PCR and plasmid insertion/rescue) to isolate smaller (2–4 kb) overlapping DNA fragments both upstream and downstream of IS*1202*. These DNA fragments were cloned into *E. coli* DH5α using either pBluescript SK or pGEM-7Zf(+) as vectors, generating a series of clones, as shown in Fig. 1. Both strands of the pneumococcal DNA inserts of each of the above plasmids (or nested deletion derivatives thereof) were then subjected to sequence analysis. Analysis of the compiled sequence showed that the putative pneumococcal *dexB* gene was located upstream of IS*1202*. The 16-kb downstream region contained a series of 15 potential open reading frames (ORFs), which we have designated *cps19fA* to *cps19fO*, as shown in Fig. 1 (the complete nucleotide sequence has been deposited with Genbank; accession number U09239). An almost perfect consensus promoter sequence (TAGACA–17bp–TATAAT) is situated 30 bp upstream of *cps19fA*. Each ORF is preceded by a ribosome binding site and the majority are very closely linked. The only potentially significant intergenic gaps occur between *cps19fJ* and *cps19fK* (63 nucleotides) and between *cps19fN* and *cps19fO* (65 nucleotides). However, potential stemmed-loop structures were not found immediately downstream of *cps19fJ* or *cps19fN* and no obvious promoter sequences were seen immediately upstream of *cps19fK* or *cps19fO*. Thus, translational coupling of

the entire locus remains a distinct possibility. A large region (1458 nucleotides) downstream of *cps19fO* did not appear to contain any significant ORFs on either DNA strand, but the region from nucleotides 15390-15630 contained numerous stemmed-loop structures reminiscent of transcription terminators. There was, however, an additional ORF commencing at nucleotide 16446, which was preceded by a ribosome binding site and by −10 and −35 promoter sequences. Comparison of our sequence data for this gene with those deposited on GenBank indicated 97.3% DNA homology with that reported for the pneumococcal *aliA* gene, which encodes an oligopeptide binding protein,[1] and so is unrelated to CPS biosynthesis. Thus, we conclude that, in *S. pneumoniae* type 19F, the *cps* locus is located between *dexB* and *aliA* in the chromosome, as shown in Fig. 1.

INSERTION-DUPLICATION MUTAGENESIS OF *CPS19F* GENES

In order to confirm the involvement of the 15 ORFs designated *cps19fA* to *cps19fO* in type 19F capsule production, we attempted to individually disrupt the chromosomal copies of the respective genes in the encapsulated strain Rx1-19F. To achieve

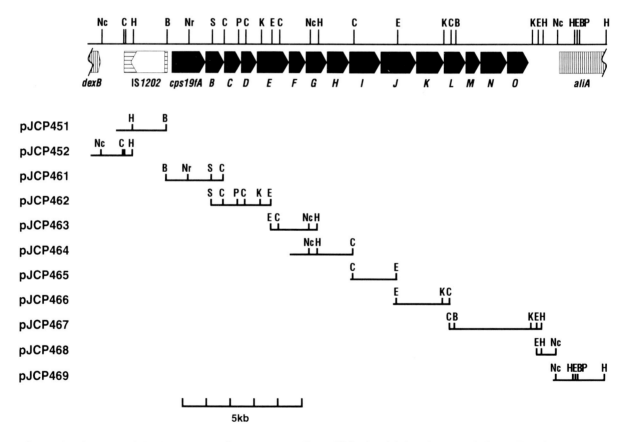

FIG. 1. Physical map of the chromosome of *S. pneumoniae* Rx1-19F in the vicinity of the *cps19f* locus. Boxed arrows represent potential ORFs and the closed box represents the insertion element IS*1202*. Gene designations are indicated below the map; *cps19fB-O* are abbreviated to *B-O*, respectively. Restriction sites are as follows: B, *Bam*HI; C, *Cla*I; E, *Eco*RI; H, *Hind*III; K, *Kpn*I; Nc, *Nco*I; Nr, *Nru*I; P, *Pst*I; S, *Sph*I. The regions of DNA subcloned into various recombinant plasmids are shown below the map.

this a small internal segment of each ORF (nucleotides 895–1221 for *cps19fA*, 1944–2258 for *cps19fB*, 2380–2998 for *cps19fC*, 3126–3519 for *cps19fD*, 3941–4544 for *cps19fE*, 5225–5725 for *cps19fF*, 6317–6603 for *cps19fG*, 7054–7247 for *cps19fH*, 8179–8440 for *cps19fI*, 9651–10165 for *cps19fJ*, 10708–11177 for *cps19fK*, 11600–11958 for *cps19fL*, 12549–12893 for *cps19fM*, 13148–13961 for *cps19fN*, and 14270–14679 for *cps19fO*) was cloned into the plasmid pVA891.[27] Recombinant plasmids were then transformed into Rx1-19F and the cells were plated onto blood agar containing erythromycin. As the pVA891 replicon cannot function in pneumococci, erythromycin-resistant transformants are the result of a homologous recombination event directed by the cloned fragment of pneumococcal DNA that leads to the integration of the pVA891 plasmid into the host chromosome, and consequent disruption of the gene of interest. Furthermore, the cloned segment of pneumococcal DNA is duplicated and flanks the integrated copy of pVA891.

Erythromycin-resistant *S. pneumoniae* Rx1-19F transformants were obtained for all except the *cps19fM*- and *cps19fO*-containing pVA891 derivatives. Correct disruption of the respective chromosomal ORF was confirmed by Southern hybridization analysis of each insertion-duplication mutant generated (data not shown). All the mutants exhibited a rough phenotype and did not produce a type 19F capsule, as judged by quellung reaction, confirming that all are part of the *cps19f* locus. On the other hand, insertion of pVA891 into IS*1202* or into the apparent non-coding region downstream of *cps19fO* (nucleotides 15149–15444 were used as the target) did not prevent type 19F capsule expression in *S. pneumoniae* Rx1-19F.

CHARACTERIZATION OF *CPS19FA-O*

The locations and several properties of each of the ORFs designated *cps19fA-O* are summarized in Table 1. Significant similarities with other known proteins, revealed by comparison with sequence databases, are described below.

The *cps19fA* gene encodes a putative 53.6-kDa protein. A central region of 177 aa exhibits significant homology (30% identity, 54% similarity) to part of the *Bacillus subtilis lytR* gene product, a membrane-bound protein which acts as a transcriptional regulator of the *lytABC* (autolysin) operon.[19] Cps19fA has a positively charged N-terminus, followed by two large hydrophobic regions, features strongly suggestive of transmembrane domains. Therefore, like LytR, Cps19fA may be a membrane-bound regulatory protein.

The *cps19fB* gene encodes a putative 28.4-kDa protein, which has a high degree of homology (63% identity, 81% similarity) to the *S. agalactiae cpsA* gene product, but the function of this is not known.[34]

The *cps19fC* gene encodes a putative 25.5-kDa protein, which exhibits significant homology (47% identity, 73% similarity) to the *S. agalactiae cpsB* gene product (the function of this protein is also not known). Cps19fC also exhibits lesser but significant homology (23% identity) with the N-terminal portion of the *Rhizobium meliloti exoP* gene product, a protein thought to be involved in the export of succinyl glycan.[10] It also exhibits homology to CLD proteins of Gram-negative bacteria, which are O-antigen chain length determinants.[4] Thus, Cps19fC could be involved in regulation of CPS chain length and/or export of CPS.

The *cps19fD* gene encodes a putative 24.9-kDa protein, which has strong homology (58% identity, 72% similarity) to the *S. agalactiae cpsC* gene product. It also exhibits 30% identity to the C-terminal portion of the *R. meliloti exoP* gene product, and so also may be involved in export of CPS.

The *cps19fE* encodes a putative 52.6-kDa protein with significant homology (45.6% identity) to the *S. agalactiae cpsD* gene product, which is a galactosyl transferase.[34] Cps19fE also has strong homology (60% identity, 70% similarity in a 111 aa region towards the C-terminus; 31% overall identity) to the *Sal-*

TABLE 1. SUMMARY OF ORFs *cps19fA-O*

ORF	Location in sequence	Predicted MW	Number of amino acids	Hydrophobicity index[a]	Predicted pI	Percentage G + C content[b]
cps19fA	169-1615	53,527	481	0.04	8.86	38.1
cps19fB	1616-2347	28,352	243	−0.46	7.58	38
cps19fC	2356-3048	25,497	230	0.11	9.34	38.2
cps19fD	3058-3741	24,947	227	−0.13	8.69	34.5
cps19fE	3751-5124	52,595	455	0.14	9.51	33.2
cps19fF	5128-5871	28,155	247	−0.19	8.93	33.6
cps19fG	5883-6693	31,647	269	−0.39	8.43	36.3
cps19fH	6694-7572	34,474	292	−0.54	7.80	30.3
cps19fI	7573-8910	51,734	445	0.68	9.59	29.7
cps19fJ	8933-10354	55,055	473	0.81	9.83	29.7
cps19fK	10418-11506	40,950	362	−0.30	5.48	35.2
cps19fL	11545-12414	32,215	289	−0.21	4.69	42.3
cps19fM	12415-13011	22,379	198	−0.40	5.05	41.5
cps19fN	13021-14070	39,053	349	−0.45	5.16	42.1
cps19fO	14136-14986	32,330	283	−0.50	4.71	41.5

[a]According to Kyte and Doolittle,[18] as implemented in PROSIS.
[b]Percent guanine plus cytosine (G + C) of coding region.
MW, molecular weight; pI, isoelectric point.

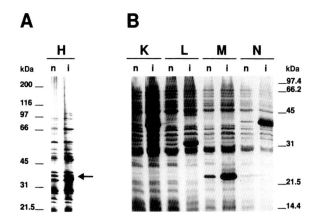

FIG. 2. T7-expression of *cps19f* genes in *E. coli*. *E. coli* DH5(pGP1-2) was transformed with various pGEM-7Zf(+) derivatives containing individual *cps19fH* (H), *cps19fK* (K), *cps19fL* (L), *csp19fM* (M), or *cps19fN* (N) ORFs. Lysates of cultures incubated at 42°C for 2 h to induce expression of T7 RNA polymerase (i) and noninduced cultures (n) were separated by SDS-PAGE and stained with Coomassie Brilliant Blue. The mobilities of molecular size markers are shown separately for **A** and **B**. (Reproduced with permission from *Molecular Microbiology*.[31])

monella *rfbP* gene product. Moreover, the hydrophobicity plots for the two proteins are very similar indeed.[11] RfbP is a undecaprenyl-phosphate galactose-phosphotransferase, catalyzing the initial step in O-antigen biosynthesis. The type 19F CPS lacks galactose and mutagenesis of *cps19fE* blocks incorporation of ^{14}C-UDP-glucose into glycolipid by isolated membranes. Thus, we believe Cps19fE catalyzes the first step in capsule biosynthesis, namely transfer of glucose-1-phosphate to a lipid carrier (presumably undecaprenyl phosphate).

The *cps19fF* gene encodes a putative 28.2-kDa protein. It has homology (33% identity, 50% similarity over 191 aa) with the *E. coli rffM* gene product, which is a putative *N*-acetyl-D-mannosaminuronic acid transferase, involved in the synthesis of enterobacterial common antigen.[7] It also has a similar degree of homology to the TagA protein of *Bacillus subtilis*, which is a putative *N*-acetyl-D-mannosamine transferase involved in cell wall teichoic acid biosynthesis.[28] Since type 19F CPS contains *N*-acetyl-D-mannosamine, we propose that Cps19fF is the transferase which catalyzes the addition of this sugar to the Glc-PP-lipid.

The *cps19fG* gene encodes a putative 31.6-kDa protein which exhibits 25.9% identity with the LicD protein of *Haemophilus influenzae*, which is encoded by the *licD* gene of its lipopolysac-

charide locus.[39] However, the precise function of LicD is unknown.

The *cps19fH* gene encodes a putative 34.5-kDa protein, assuming that translation is initiated at a TTG codon, located one nucleotide downstream from the termination codon of the preceding ORF. The nearest in-frame ATG codon is a further 90 codons downstream (the expected translation product would be approximately 20 kDa) and unlike the TTG codon, is not preceded by a ribosome binding site. To examine the expression of *cps19fH* in *E. coli*, one of the nested deletion derivatives of pJCP464, containing nucleotides 6578-7846 downstream from the vector T7 promoter, was transformed into *E. coli* DH5(pGP1-2) in which the T7 RNA polymerase gene is under the control of lambda P_L/cI_{857}.[38] Induction of cultures at 42°C for 2 h resulted in the expression of how levels of a 34–35-kDa protein in cells containing the pJCP464 derivative, which was not seen in uninduced cultures (see arrow, Fig. 2A). Both the size of the translation product and the low level of expression of *cps19fH* is consistent with initiation at the TTG codon. Cps19fH has a limited degree of homology with rhamnosyl transferases from *Yersinia enterocolitica* and *Shigella flexneri*, the alignment of which is shown in Fig. 3. Interestingly, the most conserved regions correspond to a motif previously identified in a number of rhamnosyl and other 6-deoxyhexosyl transferases.[33] This suggests that Cps19fH is likely to be the rhamnosyl transferase involved in incorporation of rhamnose into the type 19F CPS repeat unit.

The *cps19fI* gene encodes a putative 51.7-kDa protein, which has homology with Rfc proteins (O-antigen polymerases) from a variety of Gram-negative bacteria, as shown in Table 2. Although the overall homology between Cps19fI and the various Rfc proteins is low (14.0–20.1% identity) it is as strong as the degree of identity within the Gram-negative species (15.5–19.8%). The relationship between Cps19fI and Rfc proteins is even more apparent when similar as well as identical amino acids are considered, and the hydropathy plots for the various proteins are also very similar, each having at least 12 hydrophobic, potentially membrane-spanning domains.[31] It therefore seems probable that Cps19fI is the polysaccharide polymerase.

The *cps19fJ* gene encodes a putative 55.1-kDa protein with homology to RfbX proteins of *E. coli*, *Shigella* sp., and *Yersinia* sp., as well as to the CapF protein of *Staphylococcus aureus*, as shown in Table 3. The RfbX proteins are known to be involved in export of O-antigen.[24,26] Again, the overall homology between Cps19fJ and the various Gram-negative proteins is low (15.7–19.4% identity), but the degree of identity within the Gram-negative species is similar (16.1–31.4%). Moreover, the hydropathy plots for the Cps19fJ and the various RfbX-re-

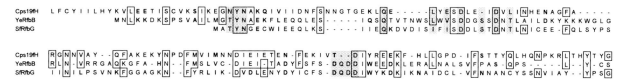

FIG. 3. Alignment of Cps19fH, from amino acid position 1 to 143, with *Yersinia enterocolitica* RfbB (YeRfbB)[40] and *Shigella flexneri* RfbG (SfRfbG)[33] using the default settings of the program CLUSTAL[12] and enhanced by manual adjustment. Identical residues are boxed; similar residues are shown in boldface; –, absence of a residue. The shaded regions correspond to those found to be most conserved amongst a variety of Gram-negative rhamnosyl and 6-deoxy-hexosyl transferases.[33] (Reproduced with permission from *Molecular Microbiology*.[31])

TABLE 2. SIMILARITY OF *cps19fl* TO OTHER PROTEINS

	Percentage identity[a]						
	Cps19fl[b]	K12Rfc[c]	SdRfc[d]	StRfc[e]	SfRfc[f]	M67Rfc[g]	M40Rfc[h]
Cps19fl	100	16.5 [394]	19.6 [382]	15.6 [417]	14 [350]	18.3 [394]	20.1 [318]
K12Rfc		100	17.5 [382]	19.1 [397]	19.4 [309]	16.5 [358]	17 [335]
SdRfc			100	15.5 [381]	16.5 [315]	18.5 [211]	16.5 [363]
StRfc				100	18.8 [308]	19.7 [269]	17.5 [341]
SfRfc					100	17.5 [331]	19.8 [349]
M67Rfc						100	17.5 [360]
M40Rfc							100

[a]Percentage of identical amino acids determined with FASTA as implemented in PROSIS. Numbers in parentheses indicate the number of amino acids over which the percentage identity occurs.
[b]*S. pneumoniae* Cps19fl.
[c]*E. coli* K12 Rfc.[37]
[d]*Shigella dysenteriae* type 1 Rfc.[16]
[e]*Salmonella typhimurium* Rfc.[6]
[f]*Shigella flexneri* Rfc.[32]
[g]*Salmonella enterica* serovar *muenchen* strain M67 Rfc.[5]
[h]*Salmonella enterica* serovar *montevideo* strain M40 Rfc.[22]

lated proteins are very similar.[31] Thus, Cps19fJ is probably the polysaccharide trisaccharide repeat unit transporter.

The *cps19fK* gene encodes a putative 40.9-kDa protein. To determine whether *cps19fK* is expressed in *E. coli*, a deletion derivative of pJCP466 (designated pJCP470), which placed nucleotides 10304–11720 downstream from the vector T7 pro-

moter, was transformed into *E. coli* DH5(pGP1-2). Induction of genes under T7 control resulted in the expression of a polypeptide or approximately 41 kDa, as predicted from the DNA sequence (Fig. 2B). Cps19fK has a high degree of homology (49% to 63% identity) with a family of proteins including the *E. coli rffE* gene product.[31] RffE is a UDP-*N*-acetyl-

TABLE 3. SIMILARITY OF *cps19fJ* TO OTHER PROTEINS

	Percentage identity[a]						
	Cps19fJ[b]	SfRfbX[c]	K12RfbX[d]	SdRfbX[e]	YeTrsA[f]	YpRfbX[g]	SaCapF[h]
Cps19fJ	100	19.2 [421]	18.1 [414]	19.4 [402]	19.2 [416]	15.7 [396]	16.4 [397]
SfRfbX		100	19.7 [396]	22.5 [409]	19.8 [424]	19.9 [403]	19 [410]
K12RfbX			100	31.4 [401]	28.3 [406]	17.4 [373]	21.5 [395]
SdRfbX				100	28.4 [401]	18.6 [269]	21.1 [393]
YeTrsA					100	20.8 [394]	20.4 [401]
YpRfbX						100	16.1 [367]
SaCapF							100

[a]Percentage of identical amino acids determined with FASTA as implemented in PROSIS. Numbers in parentheses indicate the number of amino acids over which the percentage identity occurs.
[b]*S. pneumoniae* Cps19fJ.
[c]*Shigella flexneri* RfbX.[26]
[d]*E. coli* K12 RfbX.[37]
[e]*Shigella dysenteriae* RfbX.[16]
[f]*Yersinia enterocolitica* TrsA.[36]
[g]*Yersinia pseudotuberculosis* RfbX.[14]
[h]*Staphylococcus aureus* CapF.[23]

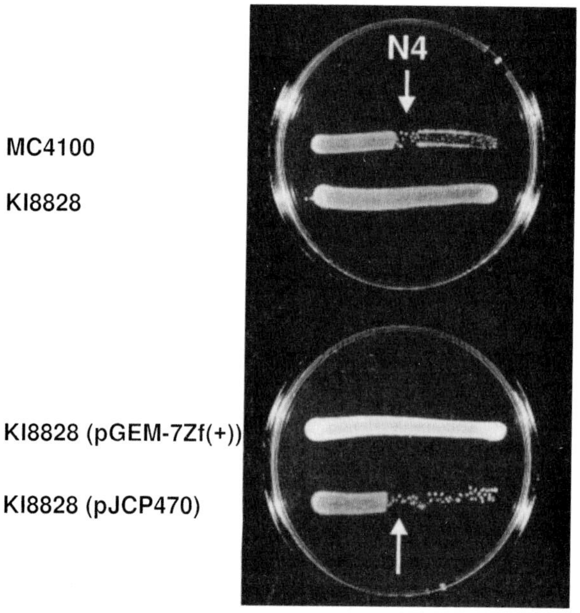

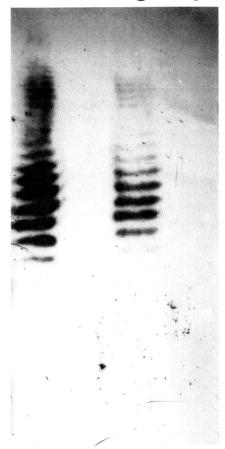

FIG. 4. N4 bacteriophage susceptibility. A suspension of bacteriophage N4 (10^9 pfu/ml) was streaked vertically on both plates as indicated by the arrows. The indicated *E. coli* strain was then streaked from left to right across the phage streak and incubated for 18 h at 37°C. (Reproduced with permission from *Molecular Microbiology*.[31])

glucosamine-2-epimerase, and functions in the synthesis of UDP-*N*-acetylmannosamine, a component of the enterobacterial common antigen.[29] Whilst the precise mechanism is not understood, *E. coli rffE* (*nfrC*) mutants are known to be resistant to infection with bacteriophage N4.[15] To examine whether *cps19fK* is capable of complementing *rffE* mutations, we transformed the *rffE* mutant K18828[15] with pJCP470 (which contains only the complete *cps19fK* ORF), or with pGEM-7Zf(+). The various strains, including the *rffE* wild-type parent *E. coli* MC4100,[35] were then examined for susceptibility to infection with N4 phage (Fig. 4). Transformation with pJCP470, but not pGEM-7Zf(+), clearly conferred susceptibility to N4 on *E. coli* KI8828. Thus, we conclude that Cps19fK is a functional RffE homologue and is therefore likely to be a UDP-N-acetylglucosamine-2-epimerase.

The *cps19fL*, *cps19fM*, *cps19fN*, and *cps19fO* genes encode proteins of 32.2, 22.4, 39.1, and 32.3 kDa, respectively. This was confirmed by T7 expression studies in *E. coli* for *cps19fL*, *cps19fM*, and *cps19fN*, as shown in Fig. 2B. These four genes have extensive homology with a portion of the *Shigella flexneri rfb* gene cluster (*rfbBDAC*), which encodes enzymes involved with rhamnose biosynthesis (dTDP-glucose-4,6-dehydratase, dTDP-L-rhamnose synthase, glucose-1-phosphate thymidylyl transferase, and dTDP-4-keto-6-deoxyglucose-3,5-epimerase, respectively).[31] The homology is strongest for *cps19fL* which exhibits 67% and 69.8% identity to *Shigella flexneri rfbA* at the DNA and deduced amino acid sequence level, respectively. Overall amino acid identities between Cps19fM, N and O and the nearest Gram-negative homologue were 34.6%, 46.3%, and 35%, respectively. Interestingly, the G+C content of this portion of the *cps19F* locus (approximately 42%) is higher than

the remainder of the locus, and this suggests that *S. pneumoniae* may have acquired these genes from a different bacterial source. To examine whether *cps19fLMNO* can substitute for *rfbBDAC*, we used PCR to amplify this portion of the *S. pneumoniae* Rx1-19F chromosome (equivalent to nucleotides 11351–15449) and cloned it into pK194. The recombinant plasmid (designated pJCP471), or pK194, was then transformed into *E. coli* Sϕ874 containing pPM2716. The latter plasmid is a derivative of pPM2213 (which contains the complete *Shigella flexneri* 4 *rfb* region and directs the expression of *Shigella flexneri* 4 O-antigen in *E. coli*) from which *rfbBDAC* has been deleted.[25] Lysates of *E. coli* Sϕ874 containing pPM2213, pPM2716, pPM2716 + pJCP471, or pPM2716 + pK194 were then subjected to Western blot analysis using a rabbit antiserum raised against *S. flexneri* 4 O-antigen (Fig. 5). Immunoreactive O-antigen can be seen in both the pPM2213 and the

FIG. 5. Complementation of *Shigella flexneri rfbBDAC* by *cps19fLMNO*. *E. coli* lysates were separated by SDS-PAGE, electroblotted onto nitrocellulose, probed with anti–*Shigella flexneri* 4 O-antigen and developed as described in the experimental procedures. Lanes: 1, *E. coli* Sϕ874 containing pPM2213; 2, *E. coli* Sϕ874 containing pPM2716; 3, *E. coli* Sϕ874 containing pPM2716 + pJCP471; 4, *E. coli* Sϕ874 containing pPM2716 + pK194.

pPM2716 + pJCP471 tracks, indicating that *cps19fLMNO* can complement the *S. flexneri* 4 *rfbBDAC* deletion in *E. coli*. Thus, we conclude that Cps19fL is a glucose-1-phosphate thymidylyl transferase, Cps19fM is a dTDP-4-keto-6-deoxyglucose-3,5-epimerase, Cps19fN is a dTDP-glucose-4,6-dehydratase, and Cps19fO is a dTDP-L-rhamnose synthase.

The above information enables us to propose that the trisaccharide biological repeat unit of type 19F CPS is → 2)-α-L-Rhap-(1-PO$_4^-$ → 4)-β-D-ManpNAc-(1 → 4)-α-D-Glcp-(1 → , i.e., the first sugar in the repeat unit is Glc, not Rha. We have also proposed a biosynthetic pathway for type 19F CPS, as shown in Fig. 6. However, definitive assignment of functions to some of the *cps19f* genes must await further phenotypic characterization of defined mutants.

CONSERVATION OF PNEUMOCOCCAL *CPS* LOCI

To examine the relationship between *cps19f* and encapsulation loci of other *S. pneumoniae* serotypes, individual *cps19f* genes were labelled with digoxigenin and used to probe (at high stringency) Southern blots of restricted chromosomal DNA from representative pneumococci belonging to 17 other serotypes, as well as other members of serogroup 19 (Table 4). Large variations in the hybridization patterns were obtained with the different gene-specific probes. Probes specific for se-

quences flanking *cps19f* (*dexB*, the 5' intergenic region, the 3' intergenic region, and *aliA*) hybridized with all serotypes tested. However, within the *cps* loci, only *cps19fA* and *cps19fB* were common to all serotypes. To date, Cps19fA and Cps19fB homologues have only been found in ORFs from genes cloned from Gram-positive bacteria.

Within serogroup 19, types 19B and 19C hybridized with all the *cps19f* probes except *cps19fI* and *cps19fJ*. Also, hybridization to *cps19fH* and *cps19fK* was weak, suggesting a lesser degree of homology. However, type 19A does not appear to have sequences closely related to *cps19fC*, *cps19fD*, *cps19fE*, *cps19fF*, *cps19fI*, *cps19fK*, and *cps19fL*, and has only limited homology to *cps19fG*, *cps19fH*, and *cps19fJ*. The apparent dissimilarity of the type 19A and type 19F *cps* loci is intriguing given the immunological relationship between the two polysaccharides. Analysis of purified type 19A CPS has yielded two distinct putative structures. One is the same as type 19F except for a 1 → 3 linkage (rather than 1 → 2) between Glc and Rha.[13] This difference would necessitate an alteration in the specificity of the polysaccharide polymerase (Cps19fI). The alternative structure involves the same trisaccharide backbone as type 19F, but with additional β-D-GlcpNAc-(1 → 3)-β-D-Galp-(1-PO$_4^-$ and α-L-Fucp-(1-PO$_4^-$ side chains attached to the Glc and Rha, respectively.[20] This would necessitate a number of additional enzyme activities not found in type 19F strains. Interestingly, individual type 19A strains were subsequently shown to be capable of producing either structural type, depending on the

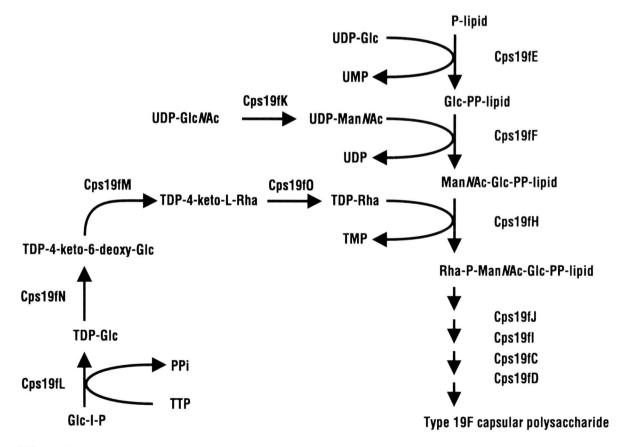

FIG. 6. Putative biosynthetic pathway for *S. pneumoniae* type 19F CPS. (Reproduced with permission from *Molecular Microbiology*.[31])

growth conditions.[21] Sequence analysis of the type 19A *cps* locus may provide a molecular explanation for this phenomenon.

Outside of serogroup 19, types 7F, 16, 18C, and 24 were the most similar to type 19F, hybridizing to 9 of the 15 *cps19f* gene probes. The least similar was type 12, which hybridized only with *cps19fA* and *cps19fB*. Sequences closely related to *cps19fL*, *cps19fM*, *cps19fN* and *cps19fO* were found in all serotypes tested whose CPS contains L-rhamnose, except for type 19A, which only hybridized to the *cps19fL* probe at low stringency, and type 2, which hybridized weakly to the same probe at high stringency. This suggests that there may be an alternative gene (or one with a diverged sequence) encoding glucose-1-phosphate thymidylyl transferase in these *S. pneumoniae* serotypes.

Four of the CPS serotypes outside of group 19 that we tested contain ManNAc (types 4, 9N, 9V, and 12). However, only types 9N and 9V contain a gene hybridizing to *cps19fF*, which encodes the putative UDP-*N*-acetyl-D-mannosamine transferase. This is consistent with the fact that only types 9N and 9V have the same β-D-Man$p$NAc-$(1 \rightarrow 4)$-α-D-Glc$p$ linkage seen in group 19. It was surprising, however, that none of these four serotypes contained genes homologous to *cps19fK*, which encodes a UDP-*N*-acetylglucosamine-2-epimerase. This enzyme activity is likely to be essential for synthesis of UDP-

ManNAc, and is probably encoded by an unrelated gene(s) in types 4, 9N, 9V, and 12. Of the various CPS serotypes tested, all but type 4 contain Glc. However, types 2, 3, 6A, 6B, 8, 12, 17, 19A, 22, and 23F also lack sequences which hybridize to *cps19fE*, which encodes the type 19F glucosyl transferase. It is possible that Glc may not be the start of the biological repeat unit in some or all of these serotypes. Whereas, Cps19fE homologues add Glc to the lipid carrier, unrelated transferases are presumably responsible for adding this sugar at subsequent positions within the repeat units.

CONCLUSION

We have used sequential rounds of inverse PCR and plasmid insertion-rescue to isolate the region of the *S. pneumoniae* type 19F chromosome responsible for CPS biosynthesis. The data presented here, combined with that which we have described previously,[11,30,31] indicates that the *cps19f* locus consists of 15 genes, which are tightly clustered on the chromosome. We have also demonstrated that *cps19f* is flanked by *dexB* and IS*1202* at the 5' end and by *aliA* at the 3' end.

TABLE 4.   HYBRIDIZATION OF TYPE 19F *cps* GENES AND NEIGHBORING SEQUENCES
WITH CHROMOSOMAL DNA FROM OTHER PNEUMOCOCCAL SEROTYPES

| | | | DIG-labeled DNA probes[a] | | | | | | | | | | | | | | | | | | Presence of sugar in capsule[b] | | |
| | | | cps19fA-O | | | | | | | | | | | | | | | | | | | | |
Type/group	dexB	IG 5'	A	B	C	D	E	F	G	H	I	J	K	L	M	N	O	IG 3'	aliA	Glc	ManNAc	Rha
19F	+	+	+	+	+	+	+	+	+	+	+	+	+	+	+	+	+	+	+	*	*	*
19A	+	+	+	+	−	−	−	−	±	±	−	±	−	−	+	+	+	+	+	*	*	*
19B	+	+	+	+	+	+	+	+	±	−	−	−	±	+	+	+	+	+	+	*	*	*
19C	+	+	+	+	+	+	+	+	±	−	−	−	±	+	+	+	+	+	+	*	*	*
2	+	+	+	+	−	−	−	−	−	−	−	−	±	+	+	+	+	+	+	*		*
3	+	+	+	+	+	+	−	−	−	−	−	−	−	−	−	−	−	±	+	*		
4	+	+	+	+	+	+	−	−	−	−	−	−	−	−	−	−	−	+	+		*	
6A	+	+	+	+	−	−	−	−	−	−	−	−	−	+	+	+	+	+	+	*		*
6B	+	+	+	+	−	−	−	−	−	−	−	−	−	+	+	+	+	+	+	*		*
7F	+	+	+	+	+	+	+	−	−	−	−	−	−	+	+	+	+	+	+	*		*
8	+	+	+	+	−	−	−	−	−	−	−	−	−	−	−	−	−	+	+	*		
9N	+	+	+	+	+	+	+	+	−	−	−	−	−	−	−	−	−	+	+	*	*	
9V	+	+	+	+	−	−	−	+	−	−	−	−	−	−	−	−	−	+	+	*	*	
12	+	+	+	+	−	−	−	−	−	−	−	−	−	−	−	−	−	+	+	*	*	
14	+	+	+	+	+	+	+	+	−	−	−	−	−	−	−	−	−	+	+	*		
16	+	+	+	+	+	+	+	−	−	−	−	−	−	+	+	+	+	+	+	*		*
17	+	+	+	+	−	−	−	−	−	−	−	−	−	+	+	+	+	+	+	*		*
18C	+	+	+	+	+	+	+	−	−	−	−	−	−	+	+	+	+	+	+	*		*
22	+	+	+	+	−	−	−	−	−	−	−	−	−	+	+	+	+	+	+	*		*
23F	+	+	+	+	−	−	−	−	−	−	−	−	−	+	+	+	+	+	+	*		*
24	+	+	+	+	+	+	+	−	−	−	−	−	−	+	+	+	+	+	+	*		*

[a]The following DNA fragments were labeled with digoxigenin and used as probes at high stringency: 0.5-kb *Nco*-I-*Eco* RI and 0.9-kb *Cla*I-*N* restriction fragments from previously published sequence[30] for *dexB* and the 5' intergenic region (IG 5'), respective;y. nucleotides 336–1468, 1571–2380, 2380–2998, 3126–3739, 3682–4979, 5225–5725, 6015–6630, 6674–7731, 7789–8965, 9013–10278, 10530–11539, 11539–12493, 12456–13139, 13139–14134, and 14134–14955 for *cpsA-O* genes, respectively, nucleotides 14955–15449 for the 3' intergenic region (IG 3') and 1.2-kb *Hin* dIII restriction fragment for *aliA*. Strong, weak and no hybridization are indicated by +, ± and −, respectively.

[b]The presence of the sugars glucose (Glc), *N*-acetyl mannosamine (Man*N*Ac), and rhamnose (Rha) in the capsule of each pneumococcal type is indicated by an asterisk.

Dillard et al.[8] also described the sequence of a 4.7-kb region of the cps3 locus, which was shown to contain three genes (cps3D, cps3S, and cps3U), which encode a UDP-glucose dehydrogenase, a polysaccharide synthase, and a glucose-1-phosphate uridyltransferase, respectively. An additional gene located downstream from cps3U (cps3M) encoded a phospho-glucomutase, although the sequence was not presented. As might be predicted from the type 3 polysaccharide structure, there is no obvious homology between these genes and any component of the cps19f locus. Arrecubieta et al.[2] have also reported the sequence of cps3D, cps3S, and cps3U homologues from another type 3 strain (which they designated cap3A, cap3B, and cap3C, respectively) and found a high degree of homology (97.6–99.7%) with that reported by Dillard et al.[8] The sequence of the region upstream of cap3A (the cps3D homologue) was also determined and shown to have extensive homology to our previously reported sequence for the 5′ portion of cps19f.[11] This portion of the cps3 locus includes two ORFs corresponding to cps19fC and cps19fD, which in type 19F probably encode proteins involved in chain length regulation and export of polysaccharide.[11] Interestingly, cps3 contains sequences with a high degree of DNA homology to cps19fA and cps19fB, but there were no type 3 ORFs corresponding to these two genes. This was due to two separate frame-shifts (with respect to csp19f) resulting in premature termination, and a deletion of 280 nucleotides at the 5′ end of the cps19fA-related region. Arrecubieta et al.[2] also reported that insertion-duplication mutagenesis of this region did not affect encapsulation of type 3 pneumococci. In contrast, mutagenesis of either cps19fA or cps19fB conferred a nonencapsulated phenotype on S. pneumoniae type 19F.[11] The only other published data for capsule loci for other pneumococcal serotypes is that of Kolkman et al.[17] for type 14. They demonstrated that cps14E, which is 98% homologous to cps19fE, encoded by glycosyl transferase. The next downstream gene (cps14F) had no significant homologies to any known genes. They also referred to unpublished sequence data for several ORFs upstream of cps14E which were almost identical to cps19f genes, but it is not known whether cps19fA or cps19fB homologues are essential for type 14 CPS biosynthesis.

From the studies of Dillard et al.[8] and Arrecubieta et al.,[2] it appears that the cps3 locus consists of 6 ORFs, four of which are serotype-specific. The cps19f locus is considerably more complex, consisting of 15 genes. The additional complexity is presumably a consequence of the more complex CPS structure and the need to coordinate sequential assembly of repeat units, immobilized on a lipid carrier. A further distinction between cps3 and cps19f relates to transcriptional organization. The four type-specific cps3 genes are transcribed as a single operon from a promoter immediately upstream of cps3D (cap3A). However, Arrecubieta et al.[2] found that there is a 1.1-kb upstream noncoding region (between cap3A and the ORFs with homology to cps19fC and cps19fD), which includes a transcription termination sequence. In contrast, no such noncoding region is found anywhere within the cps19f locus (the intergenic distances range from 1 to 65 nucleotides). The only concensus promoter sequence is immediately upstream of cps19fA.[11] Moreover, the only stemmed-loop structures likely to function as transcription terminators are found downstream of cps19fO.

Clues as to the likely function of the cps19f gene products have been provided by comparisons with known proteins whose sequences have been deposited with databases (as described above). Moreover, for cps19fK, cps19fL, cps19fM, cps19fN, and cps19fO, the function of gene products has been confirmed by complementation of mutations in E. coli. This information has been used to propose a biosynthetic pathway for type 19F CPS. However, experimental confirmation of the function of the remaining proteins encoded by cps19f will require characterization of the phenotypic impact of mutagenesis of the respective ORFs. Interpretation of phenotypic data obtained with the insertion-duplication mutants generated in our studies[11,31] is complicated by the possibility of polar effects. To date we have studied the effects of insertion-duplication mutagenesis of the first 5 cps19f ORFs on the expression of cps19fE, the product of which can be assayed by following incorporation of [14C]-UDP-glucose into glycolipid in membrane extracts of the various mutant pneumococci. Interestingly, mutagenesis of cps19fD has no effect on expression of cps19fE (these two genes are separated by only 15 nucleotides). This demonstrates that insertion of the pVA891 sequences into one ORF does not necessarily prevent transcription of downstream genes (presumably a consequence of promoter activity within the vector sequences). On the other hand, Cps19fE activity was significantly reduced by insertion-duplication mutagenesis of cps19fA, cps19fB or cps19fC (unpublished observations). Barring the possibility of polar effects, this implies that the products of these genes are required either for optimal expression of cps19fE or optimal functioning of Cps19fE. Generation of in-frame deletion mutations in each of the cps19f ORFs would simplify interpretation of these studies.

REFERENCES

1. **Alloing, G., P. de Philip, and J.-P. Claverys.** 1994. Three highly homologous membrane-bound lipoproteins participate in oligopeptide transport by the Ami system of the Gram-positive. *Streptococcus pneumoniae.* J. Mol. Biol. **241:**44–58.

2. **Arrecubieta, C., E. García, and R. López.** 1995. Sequence and transcriptional analysis of a DNA region involved in the production of capsular polysaccharide in *Streptococcus pneumoniae* type 3. Gene **167:**1–7.

3. **Austrian, R., H.P. Bernheimer, E.E.B. Smith, and G.T. Mills.** 1959. Simultaneous production of two capsular polysaccharides by pneumococcus. II. The genetic and biochemical bases of binary capsulation. J. Exp. Med. **110:**585–602.

4. **Bastin, D.A., G. Stevenson, P.K. Brown, A. Haase, and P.R. Reeves.** 1993. Repeat unit polysaccharides of bacteria: a model for polymerization resembling that of ribosomes and fatty acid synthetase, with a novel mechanism for determining chain length. Mol. Microbiol. **7:**725–734.

5. **Brown, P.K., L.K. Romana, and P.R. Reeves.** 1992. Molecular analysis of the *rfb* cluster of *Salmonella* serovar meunchen (strain M67): the genetic basis of the polymorphism between groups C2 and B. Mol. Microbiol. **6:**1385–1394.

6. **Collins, L.V., and J. Hackett.** 1991. Molecular cloning, characterization, and nucleotide sequence of the *rfc* gene, which encodes an O-antigen polymerase of *Salmonella typhimurium.* J. Bacteriol. **173:**2521–2529.

7. **Daniels, D.L., G.D. Plunkett, III, V. Burland, and F.R. Blattner.** 1992. Analysis of the *Escherichia coli* genome: DNA sequence of the region from 84.5 to 86.5 minutes. Science **257:**771–778.

8. **Dillard, J.P., M.W. Vandersea, and J. Yother.** 1995. Characterization of the cassette containing genes for type 3 capsular polysaccharide biosynthesis in *Streptococcus pneumoniae*. J. Exp. Med. **181:**973–983.

9. **Douglas, R.M., J.C. Paton, S.J. Duncan, and D. Hansman.** 1983. Antibody response to pneumococcal vaccination in children younger than five years of age. J. Infect. Dis. **148:**131–137.

10. **Glucksmann, M.A., T.L. Reuber, and G.C. Walker.** 1993. Genes needed for the modification, polymerization, export and processing of succinoglycan by *Rhizobium meliloti*: a model for succinoglycan biosynthesis. J. Bacteriol. **175:**7045–7055.

11. **Guidolin, A., J.K. Morona, R. Morona, D. Hansman, and J.C. Paton.** 1994. Nucleotide sequence of an operon essential for capsular polysaccharide biosynthesis in *Streptococcus pneumoniae* type 19F. Infect. Immunol. **62:**5384–5396.

12. **Higgins, D.G., and P.M. Sharp.** 1988. CLUSTAL: a package for performing multiple sequence alignments on a microcomputer. Gene **73:**237–244.

13. **Katzenellenbogen, E., and H.R. Jennings.** 1983. Structural determination of the capsular polysaccharide of *Streptococcus pneumoniae* type 19A (57). Carbohydr. Res. **124:**235–245.

14. **Kessler, A.C., A. Haase, and P.R. Reeves.** 1993. Molecular analysis of the 3,6-dideoxyhexose pathway genes of *Yersinia pseudotuberculosis* serogroup IIA. J. Bacteriol. **175:**1412–1422.

15. **Kiino, D.R., R. Licudine, K. Wilt, D.H.C. Yang, and L.B. Rothman-Denes.** 1993. A cytoplasmic protein, NfrC, is required for bacteriophage N4 adsorption. J. Bacteriol. **175:**7074–7080.

16. **Klena, J.D., and C.A. Schnaitman.** 1993. Function of the *rfb* gene cluster and the *rfe* gene in the synthesis of O-antigen by *Shigella dysenteriae* 1. Mol. Microbiol. **9:**393–402.

17. **Kolkman, M.A.B., D.A. Morrison, B.A.M. van der Zeijst, and P.J.M. Nuitjen.** 1996. The capsule polysaccharide synthesis locus of *Streptococcus pneumoniae* serotype 14: identification of the glycosyl transferase gene *cps14E*. J. Bacteriol. **178:**3736–3741.

18. **Kyte, J., and R.F. Doolittle.** 1982. A simple method for displaying the hydrophobic character of a protein. J. Mol. Biol. **157:**105–132.

19. **Lazarevic, V., P. Margot, B. Soldo, and D. Karamata.** 1992. Sequencing and analysis of the *Bacillus subtilis lytRABC* divergon: a regulatory unit encompassing the structural genes of the *N*-acetylmuramoyl-L-alanine amidase and its modifier. J. Gen. Microbiol. **138:**1949–1961.

20. **Lee, C.-J., and B.A. Fraser.** 1980. Structure of the cross-reactive type 19 (19F) and 57 (19A) pneumococcal capsular polysaccharides. J. Biol. Chem. **255:**6847–6853.

21. **Lee, C.-J., B.A. Fraser, R.A. Boykins, and J.P. Li.** 1987. Effect of culture conditions on the structure of *Streptococcus pneumoniae* type 19A (57) capsular polysaccharide. Infect. Immunol. **55:**1819–1823.

22. **Lee, S.J., L.K. Romana, and P.R. Reeves.** 1992. Sequence and structural analysis of the *rfb* (O antigen) gene cluster from a group C1 *Salmonella enterica* strain. J. Gen. Microbiol. **138:**1843–1855.

23. **Lin, W.S., T. Cunneen, and C.Y. Lee.** 1994. Sequence analysis and molecular characterization of genes required for the biosynthesis of type 1 capsular polysaccharide in *Staphylococcus aureus*. J. Bacteriol. **176:**7005–7016.

24. **Liu, D., R.A. Cole, and P.R. Reeves.** 1996. An O-antigen processing function for Wzx (RfbX): a promising candidate for O-unit flippase. J. Bacteriol. **178:**2102–2107.

25. **Macpherson, D.F., P.A. Manning, and R. Morona.** 1994. Characterization of the dTDP-rhamnose biosynthetic genes encoded in the *rfb* locus of *Shigella flexneri*. Mol. Microbiol. **11:**281–292.

26. **Macpherson, D.F., P.A. Manning, and R. Morona.** 1995. Genetic analysis of the *rfbX* gene of *Shigella flexneri*. Gene **155:**9–17.

27. **Macrina, F.L., R.P. Evans, J.A. Tobian, D.L., Hartley, D.B. Clewell, and K.R. Jones.** 1983. Novel shuttle plasmid vehicles for *Escherichia-Streptococcus* transgeneric cloning. Gene **25:**145–150.

28. **Mauel, C., M. Young, and D. Karamata.** 1991. Genes concerned with synthesis of poly(glycerol phosphate), the essential teichoic acid in *Bacillus subtilis* strain 168, are organized in two divergent transcriptional units. J. Gen. Microbiol. **137:**929–941.

29. **Meier-Dieter, U., R. Starman, K. Barr, H. Mayer, and P.D. Rick.** 1990. Biosynthesis of enterobacterial common antigen in *Escherichia coli*. Biochemical characterisation of Tn*10* insertion mutants defective in enterobacterial common antigen synthesis. J. Biol. Chem. **265:**13490–13497.

30. **Morona, J.K., A. Guidolin, R. Morona, D. Hansman, and J.C. Paton.** 1994. Isolation, characterization and nucleotide sequence of IS*1202*, an insertion sequence of *Streptococcus pneumoniae*. J. Bacteriol. **176:**4437–4443.

31. **Morona, J.K., R. Morona, and J.C. Paton.** 1997. Characterization of the locus encoding the *Streptococcus pneumoniae* type 19F capsular polysaccharide biosynthetic pathway. Mol. Microbiol. **23:**751–763.

32. **Morona, R., M. Mavris, A. Fallarino, and P.A. Manning.** 1994. Characterization of the *rfc* region of *Shigella flexneri*. J. Bacteriol. **176:**733–747.

33. **Morona, R., D.F. Macpherson, L. Van den Bosch, N.I.A. Carlin, and P.A. Manning.** 1995. Lipopolysaccharide with an altered O-antigen produced in *Escherichia coli* K-12 harbouring mutated, cloned *Shigella flexneri rfb* genes. Mol. Microbiol. **18:**209–223.

34. **Rubens, C.E., L.M. Heggen, R.F. Haft, and M.R. Wessels.** 1993. Identification of *cpsD*, a gene essential for type III capsule expression in group B streptococci. Mol. Microbiol. **8:**843–855.

35. **Silhavy, T.J., M.L. Berman, and L.W. Enquist.** 1984. Experiments with gene fusions. Cold Spring Harbor Laboratory, Cold Spring Harbor.

36. **Skurnik, M., R. Venho, P. Toivanen, and A. Al-Hendy.** 1995. A novel locus of *Yersinia enterocolitica* serotype O:3 involved in lipopolysaccharide outer core biosynthesis. Mol. Microbiol. **17:**575–594.

37. **Stevenson, G., B. Neal, D. Liu, M. Hobbs, N.H. Packer, M. Batley, J.W. Redmond, L. Lindquist, and P. Reeves.** 1994. Structure of the O antigen of *Escherichia coli* and the sequence of its *rfb* gene cluster. J. Bacteriol. **176:**4144–4156.

38. **Tabor, S., and C.C. Richardson.** 1985. A bacteriophage T7 RNA polymerase/promoter system for controlled exclusive expression of specific genes. Proc. Natl. Acad. Sci. U.S.A. **82:**1074–1078.

39. **Weiser, J.N., J.M. Love, and E.R. Moxon.** 1989. The molecular mechanism of phase variation of *H. influenzae* lipopolysaccharide. Cell **59:**657–665.

40. **Zhang, L., A. Al-Hendy, P. Toivanen, and M. Skurnik.** 1993. Genetic organization and sequence of the *rfb* gene cluster of *Yersinia enterocolitica* serotype O:3:similarities to the dTDP-rhamnose biosynthetic pathway of *Salmonella* and to the bacterial polysaccharide transport system. Mol. Microbiol. **9:**309–321.

Address reprint requests to:
James C. Paton
Molecular Microbiology Unit
Women's and Children's Hospital
North Adelaide, S.A., 5006
Australia

A Functional Analysis of the *Streptococcus pneumoniae* Genes Involved in the Synthesis of Type 1 and Type 3 Capsular Polysaccharides

ERNESTO GARCÍA,[1] CARLOS ARRECUBIETA,[1] ROSARIO MUÑOZ,[1] MARTA MOLLERACH,[2] and RUBENS LÓPEZ[1]

ABSTRACT

Type 3 pneumococci produce a capsule composed of cellobiuronic acid units connected in a $\beta(1 \rightarrow 3)$ linkage. Cellobiuronic acid is a disaccharide consisting of D-glucuronic acid (GlcA) $\beta(1 \rightarrow 4)$ linked to D-glucose (Glc). The genes implicated in the biosynthesis of the type 3 capsule have been cloned, expressed, and biochemically characterized. The three type 3-specific genes—designated as *cap3ABC*—are transcribed together. However, the two complete open reading frames located upstream of *cap3A* are not transcribed and, consequently, are not required for capsule formation. The promoter of the *cap3* operon was localized by primer extension analysis. The products of *cap3A*, *cap3B*, and *cap3C* were biochemically characterized as a UDP-Glc dehydrogenase, the type 3 polysaccharide synthase, and a Glc-1-P uridyltransferase, respectively. The Cap3B synthase was expressed in *Escherichia coli,* and pneumococcal type 3 polysaccharide was synthesized in this heterologous system. When a recombinant plasmid (pLSE3B) containing *cap3B* was introduced by transformation into encapsulated pneumococci of types 1, 2, 5, or 8, the lincomycin-resistant transformants displayed a binary type of capsule, this is, they showed a type 3 capsule in addition to that of the recipient type. Unencapsulated (S2) laboratory strains of *S. pneumoniae* also synthesized a type 3 capsule when transformed with pLSE3B. On the other hand, we have cloned and sequenced seven type 1-specific genes (designated as *cap1A–G*), and their functions have been preliminarily assigned based on sequence similarities.

INTRODUCTION

BACTERIAL SURFACE POLYSACCHARIDES play an important role in determining the virulence of a number of bacterial species including Gram-positive and Gram-negative microorganisms. Much of the interest in the genetics and control of synthesis of these polysaccharides stem from this fact. Proposed functions of capsular polysaccharides include adhesion to mucosal surfaces[66] or protection against bacteriophage[19,109] although the main function of the capsule is to prevent or reduce the ability of polymorphonuclear leukocytes from engulfing and digesting bacteria (for reviews, see reference 26 and 84). In spite of the fact that *Streptococcus pneumoniae* produces many virulence factors,[2,78,103] as early as in 1928, Griffith reported that unencapsulated pneumococcal variants were avirulent.[47] Loss of the capsule is accompanied by a 100,000-fold reduc-

tion of the virulence of *S. pneumoniae*[13] and it was found that nonencapsulated pneumococci are readily phagocytized when added to a suspension of leukocytes in normal serum, whereas mucoid, capsulated organisms are resistant to phagocytosis and multiply rapidly.[34,110] Furthermore, addition of an antiserum prepared against the type-specific polysaccharide causes both loss of virulence and increased sensitivity to phagocytosis,[14] and if animals are infected with type 3 pneumococci together with an enzyme specifically hydrolyzing its type-specific polysaccharide, no infection develops.[13] More recently, a reduction of virulence was achieved by transposon mutagenesis of one gene apparently essential for pneumococcal type 3 capsular biosynthesis.[107] A quantitative relationship between the amount of type-specific polysaccharide and virulence has been reported,[63,64] although the chemical composition of the capsule appears to play an important role. In fact, type 37 pneumococci

[1]Centro de Investigaciones Biológicas (CSIC), Madrid (Spain).
[2]Facultad de Farmacia y Bioquímica, Universidad de Buenos Aires, Buenos Aires (Argentina).
Reprinted from *Microbial Drug Resistance*, Vol. 3, No. 1, 1997.

produce large capsules (like those of type 3 strains) but are only slightly virulent.[57] Although most of the 90 known pneumococcal capsular polysaccharides[53] lack toxic properties, intraabdominal abscesses have been reported when tested some charged polysaccharides of *S. pneumoniae*.[104]

Transformation of the pneumococcal types was first described by F. Griffith in 1928[52] who inoculated mice subcutaneously with a mixture of live unencapsulated pneumococci and a vaccine of heat-killed encapsulated pneumococci. The mice developed an infection due to encapsulated pneumococci of the same type as the strain from which the vaccine had been prepared.[47] Later, it was shown that type transformation could occur in vitro[28] and could be induced by a cell-free extract of the donor organisms.[1] However, it was not until 1944 when Avery and co-workers reported that DNA was responsible for inducing genetic transformations.[15] Most of the results on pneumococcal transformation reported before 1960 can be found in several comprehensive, classic reviews.[8,35,37,68,69,82] More recently, in vivo transformation events involving capsular genes have been observed.[76,77] In addition, clinical isolates of *S. pneumoniae* that differ only in the capsular polysaccharide have been recovered in different countries and serotype transformation has been suggested as the most likely explanation for this finding.[17,25,55,89]

Genetic evidence indicated that the genes responsible for capsular polysaccharide biosynthesis were closely linked in the pneumococcal chromosome and could be transferred as a unit during transformation.[12,81,102] Since transformation of pneumococci to heterologous type (inter-type transformation) implies the substitution of the capsular polysaccharide of the recipient cell by that of the donor type (see reference 65, for a review), this kind of transformation event should involve the exchange of large pieces of DNA containing the genes responsible for the synthesis of the sugar components of the corresponding capsular polysaccharide as well as the transferase(s) implicated in the polymerization step.[21] A significant variation of this general rule has been reported. When unencapsulated type 3 mutants (S3⁻) deficient in UDP-glucose dehydrogenase (UDP-GlcDH) activity were transformed with DNA prepared from a capsulated type 1 strain (S1⁺), a minority of the transformants were of binary type, this is, they reacted with both anti-S3 and anti-S1 sera and produce both kinds of capsule.[9-11] Subsequent studies indicated that binary transformants retain the recipient type 3 capsular genes and, in addition, possess the capsular gene cluster of the donor DNA which includes a gene encoding the UDP-GlcDH. In addition, transformation experiments using DNA prepared from binary cells showed that the supernumerary capsular genome was inserted in the chromosome of the recipient strain in a region different from the usual capsular-polysaccharide-determining one.[12] Bernheimer and Wermundsen[20] also characterized some unusual binary transformants showing linkage between the donor and the recipient capsular genes. Binary transformants were isolated not only from S3 × S1 crosses but also in transformation experiments implicating DNAs prepared from pneumococci of other serotypes that also contain uronic acids[12,23] and, in some cases, even when unencapsulated mutants of the groups 6 or 7 (that do not contain uronic acids in their capsules) were used as recipient cells.[22]

Most of our current knowledge on the organization of genes responsible for the synthesis of capsular polysaccharide comes from studies carried out in Gram-negative bacteria (for a recent review, see reference 108). In *Escherichia coli* there is a gene cluster containing three distinct regions implicated in the expression of type II capsular polysaccharide. Region 1 is needed for the transport of mature, lipid-linked polysaccharide across the outer membrane and its assembly into a capsule. Region 2 is serotype-specific, encodes the enzymes responsible for the synthesis and polymerization of the polysaccharide, and its length is directly proportional to the chemical complexity of the capsule. Region 3 contains 2 genes (*kpsM* and *kpsT*) that are involved in the translocation of the polysaccharide through the inner membrane. Serotype-specific genes are flanked by genes common to all serotypes which appear to be involved in common functions. A similar organization had been suggested for the capsular genes of *S. pneumoniae* on the basis of transformation experiments[12,21,36] although a direct evidence for a role of the common genes on polysaccharide transport is missing. On the other hand, it has been reported that the capsules of serotypes 2, 4, 6A, 6B, 7F, 8, 14, 19F, and 23F are covalently linked to the cell wall peptidoglycan whereas those of type 3 are not.[98,99] Nothing is known about the cellular functions implicated in capsule transport and assembly in Gram-positive bacteria.

ISOLATION OF ISOGENIC, TRANSFORMABLE UNENCAPSULATED SEROTYPE 3⁻ MUTANTS OF *S. PNEUMONIAE*

We decided to investigate serotype 3 (S3) since it has a relatively simple chemical structure. It is composed of cellobiuronic acid units connected in a $\beta(1 \rightarrow 3)$ linkage.[83] Cellobiuronic acid is a disaccharide consisting of D-glucuronic acid (GlcA) $\beta(1 \rightarrow 4)$ linked to D-glucose (Glc). Furthermore, type 3 pneumococci are the most frequently isolated from clinical samples both in Spain[40] and throughout the world[75] and a great number of genetic and biochemical studies were carried out with *S. pneumoniae* strains belonging to this serotype until the early seventies (for reviews, see references 70–72 and 93).

Since many of the natural, encapsulated pneumococcal isolates are poorly transformable apparently due to a defect involving the synthesis and/or export of the activator protein (competence factor)[51,111] we decided to construct an isogenic, highly transformable S3⁻ strain that could be used as recipient in transformation experiments.[43] It should be kept in mind that when strains of different serotypes were transformed to the type 3 capsule, the corresponding transformants behaved identically with respect to capsule expression in subsequent rounds of transformation indicating that the chromosomal background of the recipient is not relevant.[21] To construct the S3⁻ strain, we first introduced by transformation the $\Delta lytA32$ mutation[62] into an R6 derivative (S2⁻) laboratory strain. The presence of this mutation should allow long periods of incubation at 37°C with no risk of autolysis and facilitates the screening of transformed clones for capsules. Afterwards, this LytA⁻ strain was transformed with DNA obtained from a clinical type 3 isolate of *S. pneumoniae* (strain 406). The capsular phenotype of all the strains reported in this paper was first determined visually on the plates and subsequently confirmed by the Quellung test. A capsulated S3$^+$ transformant (strain M23) was incubated in semisynthetic medium for 24–36 hours, and periodically tested on blood agar plates for the appearance of spontaneous unencapsulated mutants. A rough (S3$^-$) mutant (strain M24) was isolated after several culture cycles. When competent M24 cells were transformed with chromosomal DNA from strain 406, 1% to 3% of the cells showed an S3$^+$ phenotype. Although isolation of unencapsulated mutants by growing capsulated pneumococci in the presence of type-specific antiserum had been already employed by Griffith,[47] the procedure described here allowed us to easily isolate many different rough mutants (see page 76).

CLONING AND SEQUENCING OF A DNA FRAGMENT CONTAINING PART OF A TYPE 3 CAPSULAR GENE

A *Sca*I library of DNA fragments prepared from *S. pneumoniae* 406 was prepared in pUC18 and screened by transformation using competent cells of M24 as the recipient. From about 300 recombinant clones, one transformant was isolated, which contained a plasmid (hereafter pLGL1) harboring a pneumococcal DNA insert of 4.5 kb.[44] Transformation experiments using the M24 strain as recipient and different restriction fragments of that insert as donor DNAs localized the mutation responsible of the rough phenotype to a 0.24-kb *Dra*I-*Bst*YI fragment. Sequencing of a 781-bp *Eco*RV fragment of 406 DNA revealed the presence of two putative open reading frames (ORF), oppositely orientated. The one containing the *Dra*I-*Bst*YI fragment mentioned above was preceded by consensus −10 (TATAAT) and −35 (TTGACA) promoter boxes located 64 nucleotides upstream of the ATG initiation codon.[44] This ORF was preliminarily named *cap3-1* following a minor modification of the nomenclature firstly employed by Bernheimer and Wermundsen (*capIII*) to designate the capsular genes of *S. pneumoniae* type 3.[21] This gene was subsequently renamed *cap3A* (see page 76). Sequence comparison of the deduced amino acid sequence of *cap3-1* suggested that the gene product might be a dehydrogenase as it was very similar to the amino-terminus of the GDP-mannose dehydrogenase of *Pseudomonas aeruginosa* (AlgD)[30] and contains a consensus NAD$^+$ binding site characteristic of many dehydrogenases. Classical studies[70,94] revealed that at least one NAD-requiring dehydrogenase, namely UDP-GlcDH, is directly involved in the metabolic pathway of type 3 capsule polysaccharide biosynthesis, being the key enzyme for converting UDP-Glc to UDP-GlcA. In addition, 20 out of 21 unencapsulated mutants of type 3 were deficient in UDP-GlcDH activity whereas the remaining strain was a deletion mutant affecting both the gene encoding UDP-GlcDH and that concerned with polysaccharide polymerization.[23] All these data led us to infer that *cap3-1* might be the gene coding for UDP-GlcDH.[44]

Dot blot hybridization analysis showed that *cap3-1* only hybridized with DNA prepared from type 3 strains, which is in agreement with previous genetic studies which had indicated that the gene encoding the type 3 UDP-GlcDH is not homologous to the corresponding gene of other serotypes that also contain uronic acids in their capsular polysaccharide.[20] On the contrary, sequences located upstream of *cap3-1* hybridized with all

of the DNAs purified from pneumococci belonging to the most frequent serogroups (or serotypes), namely, 1, 2, 4–9, 14, 19, 23, and 33.

LOCALIZATION OF THE CAPSULAR GENES IN THE PNEUMOCOCCAL GENOME

Southern blot hybridizations and additional sequence analysis indicated that the insert of pLGL1 was in fact the consequence of a cloning artifact, this is, it resulted from the abnormal ligation of two nonadjacent *Sca*I fragments of type 3. The smaller *Sca*I fragment (2.3 kb) turned out to be unrelated with capsule formation but codes for a protein highly similar to the human glutamate decarboxylase[45] and, consequently, has a potential pathogenic interest.

Preliminary studies using Southern blot and transformation experiments had indicated that the insert of plasmid pLGL1 mentioned above was part of a 10-kb *Eco*RI fragment of DNA from strain 406. To reach a broader view on the genetic organization of type 3 capsular genes, we tried to clone this fragment in *E. coli* using pBR325 as the vector plasmid. To do that, recombinant plasmids from an *Eco*RI library of strain 406 DNA were used to transform M24 and 12 additional S3$^-$ pneumococcal mutants to the S3$^+$ phenotype.[6] This experimental design allowed us to isolate a recombinant plasmid (pKER1) (Fig. 1) able to transform 7 rough mutants to the smooth phenotype. Restriction enzyme analysis showed that pKER1 has suffered a deletion of about 2.3 kb at the right end of the 2.5-kb *Sca*I fragment previously cloned.[44] The plasmid pKER2 that contain the DNA region deleted in pKER1 was constructed by cloning the 2.3-kb *Sca*I-*Eco*RI fragment in pUC18. Those S3$^-$ mutants that were not transformed with pKER1 produced S3$^+$ colonies when transformed with pKER2. Several rough mutants (NR3-7, NR3-8, NR3-9, NR3-13, NR3-14, and NR3-16) could be transformed to S3$^+$ either with pKER1 or pKER2 indicating that the corresponding mutations were located in the 272 nucleotide-long fragment where the inserts of both plasmids overlap. Determination of the nucleotide sequence showed that the overlapping region corresponds to *cap3-1* and allowed the determination of the complete sequence of this gene (renamed as *cap3A*, hereafter).[6] On the other hand, since *cap3C* is a type 3-specific gene (see below) it seemed convenient to clone DNA fragments located downstream of this gene. This objective was accomplished by transforming the M23 strain (S3$^+$) with pUCEK2, a pUCE191 derivative containing an internal fragment of *cap3C*.[4] DNA prepared from a lincomycin-resistant transformant was digested with *Bcl*I, ligated and used to transform competent cells of *E. coli* TG1. The recombinant plasmid pUCEK21 contains, in addition to part of the *cap3C* gene, a 4.5-kb fragment of additional DNA (Fig. 1).

Dot blot analysis of DNA prepared from strains of *S. pneumoniae* expressing different capsular antigens provided information on those regions that may contain genes common to different pneumococcal serogroups and those that were type 3-specific. Figure 2 shows that genes located in pKER2 only hybridized with type 3 pneumococci whereas all the *S. pneumoniae* DNAs tested gave a hybridization signal with pKER7. On the contrary, pLGL9, that contains part of *orf1* (see page 77),

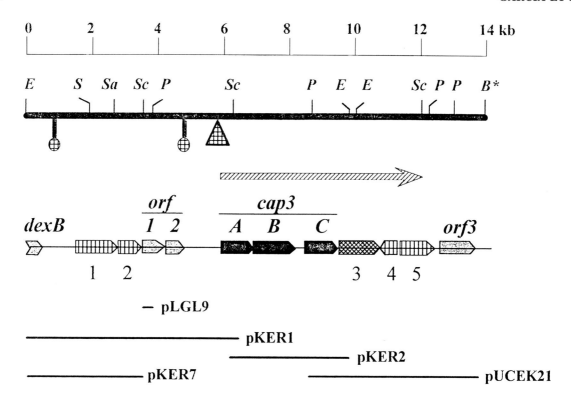

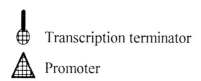

FIG. 1. Genetic organization of the 14,056-bp DNA region of the *S. pneumoniae* strain 406 containing the type 3 *cap* genes. The orientation and localization of the ORFs are indicated by arrowed boxes. 1 to 5 indicate interrupted, putative reading frames. Location of the promoter of the *cap3* operon is indicated by an upward triangle. Putative transcription terminators are also shown. The dashed arrows shows the direction and length of the mRNA transcript corresponding to the *cap3* operon. Relevant plasmids are indicated, as are pertinent restriction sites (*B, BclI; E, EcoRI; P, PstI; S, SalI; Sa, SacII; Sc, ScaI*). The asterisk indicates that only one of the *BclI* sites present in this fragment is represented.

hybridized only with DNAs prepared from serogroups 1, 3, 5, 6, 7, 14, and 19 but not with groups 2, 8, 9, 23, or 33. It should be pointed out that *S. oralis* DNA, which has 56% overall homology with *S. pneumoniae* DNA, did not hybridize with any of the probes used. Additional experiments using different subclones of pUCEK21[3] showed that DNA sequences located downstream of *cap3C* (namely those marked as 5 in Fig. 1) are common to all the pneumococci tested, in agreement with previous results.[32]

The recent development of the physical map of *S. pneumoniae* R6[46] provides a useful framework for gene localization. Pulsed-field gel electrophoresis (PFGE) and Southern blot experiments (Fig. 3) using the restriction endonucleases *SmaI* showed that type 3-specific capsular genes are located in fragment 3 (290 kb) of the physical map of strain R6.[6] It was also determined that those genes reside in the *SacII* fragment 12 (60 kb) and in the *ApaI* fragment 13 (59 kb). We observed that the

DNA sequences located immediately upstream of *cap3A* are present in all the serogroups tested and cross-hybridized with the 52-kb *SmaI* fragment 12, where the *recP* gene is located. Confirmation of this finding has been obtained independently in a similar study.[31] On the other hand, other genes (or part of them) located far upstream of the type 3-specific genes are also present in a 25-kb *SmaI* fragment of R6 DNA (Fig. 3) although a more precise mapping of this fragment has not been possible so far.

SEQUENCE ANALYSIS OF THE DNA REGIONS COMMON TO PNEUMOCOCCAL ISOLATES OF SEVERAL SEROTYPES

Sequence analysis of a 14,056 bp DNA fragment from strain 406[3] revealed the presence of six complete ORFs (Fig. 1). An incomplete ORF corresponds to a gene designated as *dex*B since

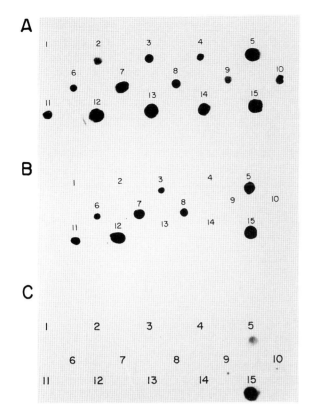

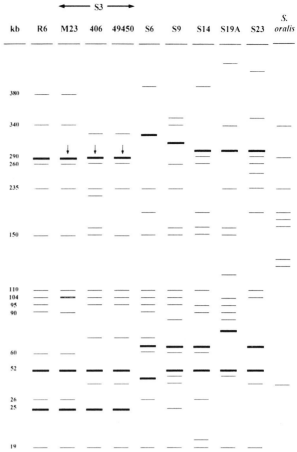

FIG. 2. Dot blot analysis obtained from various strains of *S. pneumoniae* expressing different capsular antigens. The filters were incubated with pKER7 (A), pLGL9 (B) or pKER2 (C). DNA samples from: 1, *S. oralis*; 2, *S. pneumoniae* R6; 3-14, clinical pneumococcal isolates belonging to serotypes or serogroups 1, 2, 3, 5, 6, 7, 8, 9, 14, 19, 23, and 33, respectively. 15, plasmid used as a probe in each case.

FIG. 3. Schematic representation of a hybridization experiment using *Sma*I digests of DNAs, separated by PFGE, prepared from pneumococcal isolates belonging to different serogroups. Thin lines correspond to fragments that did not hybridize with any of the probes tested (pKER1, pKER2, and pKER7) (see Fig. 1); thick lines indicate the fragments that hybridize with pKER1 and pKER7. pKER2 hybridized only with those thick bands indicated by arrows. (Reprinted with permission from Arrecubieta et al.[6])

the deduced amino acid sequence of this gene shows 65% identity with a glucan 1,6-α-glucosidase of *S. mutans* and *S. equisimilis*.[4] Inactivation of *dexB* by insertion-duplication mutagenesis indicated that this gene is involved in capsule formation neither in type 19F[48] nor in type 3. The predicted gene products of *orf1* and *orf2* were virtually identical (more than 93% identity) to those coded by *cps19fC* and *cps19fD* of *S. pneumoniae* type 19F, respectively[48] and, possibly, to those of serotype 14.[58] This result is in agreement with those obtained using DNA/DNA hybridization (see above). Guidolin and coworkers[48] also reported that two additional, complete ORFs are located between *dexB* and *cps19fC* in type 19F DNA. A global analysis of this region of type 3 DNA did not reveal the presence of any ORF although comparison between the nucleotide sequence of this region and the corresponding of type 19F showed that they were more than 95% identical.[4] However, several important differences were identified: (*i*) no insertion sequence was found downstream of *dexB* although a putative recognition sequence for the IS*1202* element[73] could be identified; (*ii*) an approximately 280-bp region corresponding to the 5′ end of the gene *cps19fA* of type 19F DNA has been deleted in type 3 DNA; (*iii*) several additional, minor deletions have been also observed. Agarose gel electrophoresis of the polymerase chain reaction (PCR) products showed that the re-

gion located between *dexB* and that corresponding to the 5′ end of *cps19fA* gene is highly variable in size among *S. pneumoniae* isolates.[4] Similar observations have been recently reported by Hall *et al.*[50] On the other hand, insertion-duplication mutagenesis of a region equivalent to *cps19fB* did not eliminate type 3 capsule formation.[4]

The analysis of the deduced amino acid sequence (373 residues) of the product of *orf3* (Fig. 1) showed that, at the amino-terminal end of the protein, there is a 38-residue sequence with the characteristics of a signal peptide suggesting that this protein is exported across the pneumococcal membrane. The putative signal peptidase cleavage site, VLA ↓, is located at positions 36 to 38. Search for similarities showed that the first 200 amino acid residues are 24% and 22% identical to those of the NanA neuraminidase of *S. pneumoniae*,[24] and the IgA-binding β antigen (Bag) of group B streptococci.[54] No other obvious similarities were found and the possible function of this protein remains unknown.

The 3-kb DNA region located between *cap3C* and *orf3* contains several incomplete reading frames. Dillard *et al.*[31] reported the existence of a fourth type 3-specific gene that was named as *cps3M* and suggested that it was homologous to phosphoglucomutases (PGM) from several bacterial species. This assumption is not completely supported by the analysis of the sequence located immediately downstream of *cap3C* (identified as 3 in Fig. 1). In fact, the predicted amino acid sequence of the reading frame from the type 3 strain 406 was similar (from 30 to 35% identity over 350–400 amino acid overlap) to several hypothetical ORFs from *Haemophilus influenzae* (Accession number U32758), *Mycoplasma pirum* (L13289), *Mycobacterium leprae* (U00022), and *Saccharomyces cerevisiae* (Z49704). When analyzed with the MOTIFS program (Wisconsin Genetics Computer Group, Madison, Wis.) using the PROSITE database[16] all these proteins showed to possess a PGM and phosphomannomutase (PMM) phosphoserine signature [(GA)-(LIVM)-X-(LIVM)-(ST)-(PGA)-<u>S</u>-H-X-P-X(4)-(GNHE) where <u>S</u> is the phosphoserine residue]. The catalytic mechanism of both PGM and PMM involves the formation of a phosphoserine intermediate. Hybridization experiments (not shown) confirmed that this reading frame is type 3-specific although dispensable for capsule biosynthesis, as previously reported for *cps3M*.[31] This is in agreement with our finding that the corresponding reading frame in strain 406 is interrupted by an incomplete reading frame that turned out to be a 622-bp fragment of an insertion sequence related to IS*1167*[112] (55% identical nucleotides) (marked as 4 in Fig. 1). The deduced amino acid sequence of this fragment showed a significant similarity with the C-moiety of the transposase encoded by IS*1167* (Fig. 4). The IS fragment should be transcribed in the opposite direction with respect to all other genes shown in Figure 1. Finally, the 1.1-kb DNA fragment located between the IS fragment and *orf3* (marked as 5 in Fig. 1) is 98% identical to the *plpA* gene of *S. pneumoniae*[79] although the reading frame of this gene in the strain 406 is truncated at its 5' end and two additional frameshift mutations were found.[3] The existence of a deleted form of the *plpA* gene in this region of type 3 strains had been reported previously.[31]

SEQUENCE ANALYSIS OF THE TYPE 3-SPECIFIC CAPSULAR GENES

It has been reported that the DNA regions located downstream of *cps19fD* contains the group 19-specific genes.[48] A noticeable difference between serotypes 3 and 19F DNAs is the existence in the former of an intergenic space of about 1100 bp between *orf2* and *cap3A* (Fig. 1) that contains sequences common to other pneumococcal serotypes (see page 76). Sequences characteristic of a consensus promoter had been located upstream of *cap3A*.[44]

As discussed above, several spontaneous, S3⁻ isolates of *S. pneumoniae* were characterized as *cap3A* mutants and three different mutations have been sequenced.[6] More recently, point as well as insertion mutations affecting *cpsD* (*cap3A*) have been reported by Dillard *et al.*[31] and all of them also conferred an unencapsulated phenotype. The 45-kDa Cap3A protein was suggested to correspond to the type 3-specific UDP-GlcDH of *S. pneumoniae* since it is homologous (57% identity and 74% similarity) to the UDP-GlcDH (HasB) of *S. pyogens*.[33] The *cap3A*⁺ allele restored the capsular synthesis in mutants previ-

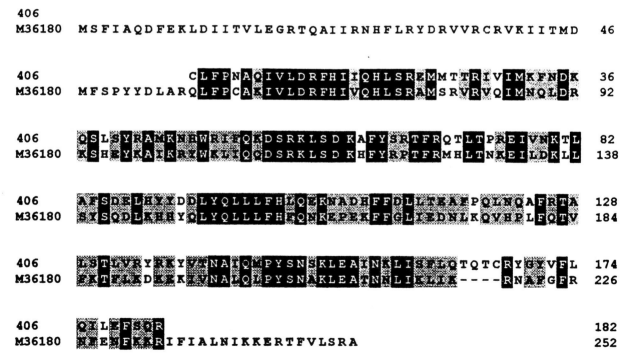

FIG. 4. Alignment of the deduced amino acid sequences of the interrupted reading frame 4 (Fig. 1) with part of the putative transposase coded by the IS*1167* element (M36180). Identical amino acid and conserved substitutions are shown in black and shaded boxes, respectively.

ously characterized as deficient in UDP-GlcDH[12] which supports the conclusion that cap3A codes for UDP-GlcDH.[6,32]

The cap3B and cap3C genes encoded proteins of approximately 49 and 34 kDa, respectively.[4] These genes are practically identical to those previously designed as cps3S and cps3U, respectively[31,32] employing the pneumococcal strain WU2 which is unrelated to the 406 strain used in our lab. Sequence comparison showed that Cap3B is similar to several polysaccharide synthases previously characterized, and in vitro capsule synthesis assays suggested that Cps3S (Cap3B) was the type 3 capsule polysaccharide synthase.[31]

Computer searches revealed that Cap3C (Cps3U) is most probably a UDP-Glc pyrophosphorylase, the enzyme responsible for the synthesis of UDP-Glc from Glc-1-P and UTP.[4,31] The cap3C gene was capable of reverting the galU defect when expressed in an E. coli mutant, i.e., the transformants were capable of fermenting galactose and manifested as red colonies on MacConkey-galactose plates, and grew in a minimal medium of elevated osmotic strength. This confirmed that Cap3C is a UDP-Glc uridylyltransferase.[4]

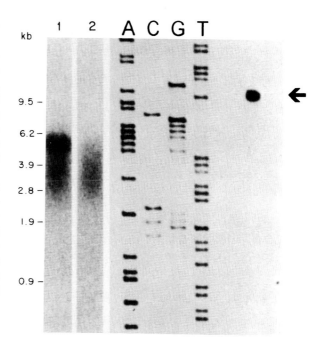

FIG. 5. Northern blot (left) and primer extension (right) analysis of total RNA of *S. pneumoniae* strain 406. The RNA was hybridized with a probe containing part of *cap3A* and *cap3B* (lane 1). Lane 2 corresponds to the same RNA preparation hybridized with a probe containing *orf1* and *orf2*. The arrow at the right indicates the extended product in the primer extension experiment. (Reprinted with permission from Arrecubieta et al.[4])

FUNCTIONAL ORGANIZATION OF CAPSULAR GENES

Based on sequence data, Guidolin et al.[48] suggested that capsular genes in type 19F pneumococci are arranged as an operon (cps19fABCDEFG) and reported that insertion-duplication mutagenesis of any of the six potential ORFs produced transformants that exhibited a rough phenotype. However, a definite conclusion on the functional organization of the type 19F capsular cluster still awaited the characterization of in-frame deletions rather than insertion mutations that most probably exhibit polar effects.

Direct molecular evidence on the involvement of certain genes in capsule formation of type 3 pneumococci has been recently achieved by the use of point mutations, and we have determined the sequence defect of three different cap3A mutants[6] that confirmed previous results obtained by biochemical and genetic means (see reference 65, for a review). In addition, a transcriptional analysis has been helpful to outline the functional organization of the type 3 capsular genes.[4] Northern blot and primer extension analyses (Fig. 5) showed an mRNA band of about 5.8 kb that includes at least cap3A, B, and C and demonstrated that transcription of type 3-specific genes starts 59 nucleotides upstream of the ATG initiation codon of the cap3A gene.[4] The length of the capsular transcript is sufficient to include the truncated ORF located downstream of cap3C (Fig. 1) and that should have represented the fourth gene of the cap3 operon. In addition, our results indicated that the genes located between dexB and cap3A are not apparently transcribed. On the other hand, insertion-duplication experiments showed that cps3U (cap3C) is not required for type 3 capsular biosynthesis[4,31] suggesting that the function of Cap3C is compensated for by another enzyme.

Recently, Watson et al.[106] reported that a region of the pneumococcal chromosome located downstream of the lytA gene encoding the major autolysin (an N-acetylmuramoyl-L-alanine amidase) was essential for encapsulation. This conclusion was reached by sequencing a region of DNA surrounding the insertion of transposon Tn916 that resulted in a lack of type 3 capsule expression.[107] An unidentified ORF (ORF1) and two copies of the putative regulator BOX element[67] were found in this region (Fig. 6A). Since the Tn916 insertion site in the mutant strain was located far away from the type 3-specific genes[6,46] it was suggested that this region might be involved in some kind of regulation of capsule biosynthesis. Taking into account that the chromosomal region claimed to be essential for capsule formation is deleted in the M31 strain (an S2⁻ strain) isolated some years ago in our laboratory,[87] we transformed this strain to the S3⁺ phenotype, and the combined use of PFGE and Southern blot hybridizations (Fig. 6B) revealed that the encapsulated transformant of M31 still harbored a deletion identical to that of the parental strain demonstrating that the region that lies just 3' of the lytA gene is not essential for the synthesis of type 3 capsule.[42]

BIOCHEMICAL CHARACTERIZATION OF Cap3A AND Cap3B

As reported above, several lines of evidence had been achieved suggesting that cap3A coded for a UDP-GlcDH. Nevertheless, only very recently, direct biochemical evidence has been provided. Repeated attempts to clone the entire cap3A gene in E. coli together with its own promoter were unsuccessful and only deleted recombinant plasmids were obtained. A similar situation was experienced during the cloning of hasB

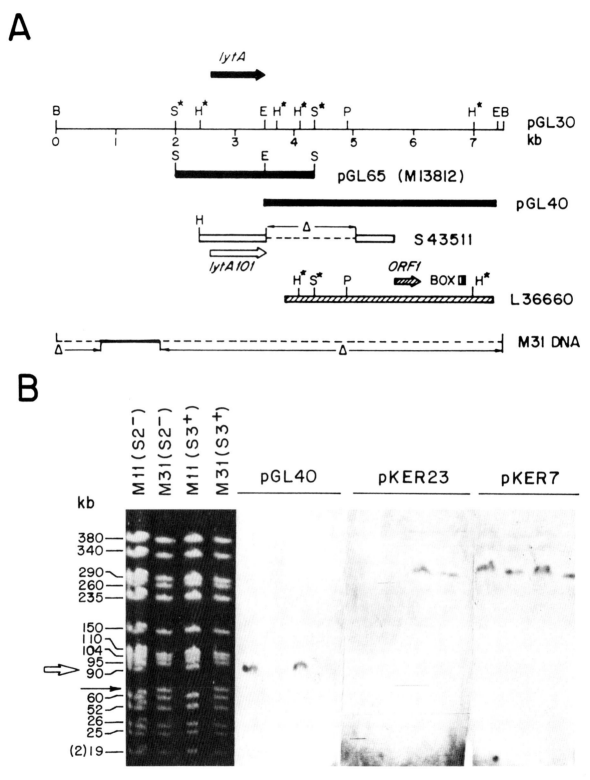

FIG. 6. Physical map of the 7.5-kb *Bcl*I DNA fragment containing the *lytA* gene and PFGE of the DNA prepared from S3[+] transformants of the Δ*lytA* strain M31. (**A**) The region shown corresponds to the *S. pneumoniae* DNA insert of the recombinant plasmid pGL30.[87] M13812, S43511, and L36660 correspond to the accession numbers reporting the sequences of the indicated regions. The *lytA* and the *lytA101* genes are indicated by black and white arrows, respectively. The location of ORF1 and the BOX element are also shown. Δ corresponds to deleted regions. Symbols: B, *Bcl*I; E, *Eco*RI; H, *Hind*III; P, *Pvu*II; S, *Sau*3AI. An asterisk indicates that only some of the restriction sites present are represented. Reprinted with permission from.[42] (**B**) PFGE of the DNAs obtained from the indicated strains digested with *Sma*I and blotted and hybridized with the indicated probes. pKER23, that contains part of *cap3A* and *cap3B*, has been described elsewhere.[4]

encoding the UDP-GlcDH from *S. pyogenes*[33] suggesting that overproduction of this enzyme might be toxic for the host cells. In order to clone *cap3A* in the absence of its own promoter, this gene was first PCR amplified and then cloned under the control of a T7 RNA polymerase-inducible promoter. Upon addition of isopropyl-β-D-thiogalactopyranoside (IPTG) the *cap3A* gene was overexpressed in *E. coli* as a 46-kDa protein[5] which is in agreement with the M_r (44,646) deduced from the nucleotide sequence of *cap3A*.[6,31] The identity of this protein with Cap3A was ascertained by the determination of the N-terminal amino acid sequence. Spectrophotometric determinations and high-performance liquid chromatography analysis of the reaction products demonstrated that *E. coli* extracts containing Cap3A exhibit UDP-GlcDH activity. In contrast with previous results,[70] Mg^{2+} was apparently not required for full pneumococcal UDP-GlcDH activity, since the addition of 10 mM EDTA did not inhibit the reaction. The optimal pH for activity appeared to be about 9.0 and iodoacetic acid inhibited the enzyme activity, indicating that a cysteine residue is involved in the catalytic activity of the pneumococcal UDP-GlcDH, as previously suggested.[6,70]

Classical genetic studies of pneumococcal capsular type 3 strains suggested that all but one of the spontaneous mutations that alter the formation of type 3 polysaccharide were located in *cap3A* and only a deletion affecting simultaneously *cap3A* and *cap3B*[23] or insertion mutations[31] affecting *cap3B* have been reported so far. Since polar effects are likely to occur as a consequence of plasmid or transposon insertion, we attempted to obtain a definite conclusion on the role of Cap3B on capsular biosynthesis by analyzing a *cap3B* point mutant (NR3-10) that produced, approximately, 10% of the capsular polysaccharide found in the wild-type parental strain.[7] Sequence analysis revealed that the leaky phenotype of the NR3-10 strain was the consequence of a frameshift mutation in the *cap3B* gene that might be partially overwhelmed during translation of the mRNA of the mutant.

The Cap3B protein was expressed in *E. coli* following a strategy consisting of amplifying the *cap3B* gene by PCR and cloning the product under the control of the φ10 promoter (a T7 RNA polymerase-inducible promoter). The presence of the plasmid pLys[100] in the recipient *E. coli* strain appears to be essential for the successful cloning of *cap3B*. This requirement is possibly due to the fact that pLysS encodes the lytic enzyme of the T7 bacteriophage which is known to inhibit the viral RNA polymerase thus reducing further the expression of the inducible φ10 promoter. The Cap3B protein was expressed in *E. coli* harboring pTBP3 as a 49-kDa protein upon the addition of IPTG.[7] More importantly, sonicated extracts prepared from induced cultures of *E. coli* (pTBP3) contained highly polymerized, type 3 polysaccharide. Uninduced cultures also synthesized pneumococcal polysaccharide although at a lower rate (10–25% of that found in induced cultures). These results demonstrated that Cap3B is the type 3-specific synthase of *S. pneumoniae* and that it has both UDP-Glc and UDP-GlcA glycosyltransferase activities and possibly synthesizes the type 3 polysaccharide in a processive manner by monomer addition as is the case of the hyaluronan synthase (HasA) of group A streptococci.[29] On the other hand, subcellular fractionation studies revealed that as much as 40% of the type 3 pneumococcal polysaccharide synthesized was located in the periplasmic space of *E. coli*. At least

two genes responsible for the translocation of the polysaccharide across the cytoplasmic membrane, namely, *kpsM* and *kpsT* have been characterized in *E. coli* and other capsulated Gram-negative species. The KpsMT proteins belong to the family of the ABC transporters.[38] It is still uncertain whether the mechanism for the transport of pneumococcal polysaccharide is the same as that used for the transport of the homologous polysaccharide. In Gram-positive bacteria, the mechanism of polysaccharide transport has not been characterized so far although in type III capsule of group B streptococci[86] and type 19F pneumococci[48] has been suggested that some of the genes located upstream of the specific capsular cluster might be responsible for the transport of the intracellularly synthesized capsular polysaccharide. Nevertheless, the DNA region corresponding to the reading frames suggested to participate in the transport of the polysaccharide of group B streptococci and 19F pneumococci are not functional in type 3 pneumococci as reported elsewhere,[4] strongly suggesting that another still unknown mechanism may be responsible for the export of the capsular polysaccharide through the cytoplasmic membrane.

The *cap3B* gene was also cloned into a shuttle plasmid capable of replicating both in *E. coli* and *S. pneumoniae*, and the recombinant plasmid (pLS3B) was introduced by transformation into pneumococcal strains of capsular types 1, 2, 5, and 8, all of them containing hexuronic acids.[105] Quellung reaction and immunodiffusion analysis (Fig. 7) demonstrated that the corresponding transformants were of the binary type and expressed a type 3 capsule together with that of the recipient cell, and strongly suggested that the mechanism of polysaccharide transport of the recipient cells is used for the formation of a type 3 capsule in binary transformants. Furthermore, when two S2− laboratory derivatives of the rough strain R36A were transformed with pLS3B, the transformants expressed a type 3 capsule (but not type 2). In every case, the type 3 polysaccharide produced was of high M_r.[7] In conclusion, provided that the corresponding sugar nucleotide precursors (UDP-Glc and UDP-GlcA) are present, *cap3B* appears to be the only gene required to direct type 3 polysaccharide biosynthesis in pneumococcal strains or in *E. coli*.

PHYSICAL MAP AND SEQUENCE ANALYSIS OF THE TYPE 1 CAPSULAR GENOME OF *S. PNEUMONIAE*

Type 1 polysaccharide is composed of trisaccharide repeating-units having the structure: → 3)-α-Sug*p*-(1 → 4)-α-D-Gal*p*A-(1 → 3)-α-D-Gal*p*A-(1 →, in which GalA is galacturonic acid and Sug denotes 2-acetamido-4-amino-2,4,6-trideoxy-D-galactose.[61] The latter compound is also a structural component of the teichoic[41] and lipoteichoic acids[18] of *S. pneumoniae* and has also been identified in the side chains of the *Shigella sonnei* phase I lipopolysaccharide.[56] On the other hand, it has been found that type 1 pneumococcal polysaccharide contains a nonstoichiometric amount of *O*-acetyl groups per repeating unit that are immunologically important.[39,49] It has been demonstrated that UDP-GalA is synthesized from UDP-GlcA through the action of a specific epimerase rather than through oxidation of UDP-Gal[95,97] and unencapsulated type 1 mutants deficient in either the epimerase or in the UDP-GlcDH have been described.[70–72,94]

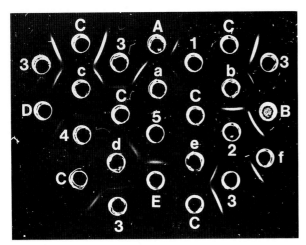

FIG. 7. Double immunodiffusion in agarose of capsulated pneumococci. 1 to 5 indicate antisera against pneumococcal polysaccharides of types 1, 2, 3, 5, and 8, respectively. A to E designate capsular polysaccharides purified from the *S. pneumoniae* strains of serotypes 1, 2, 3, 5, and 8, respectively. a to d correspond to binary transformants of the following serotypes: 1/3, 2/3, 5/3, and 8/3, respectively. e and f contain polysaccharide prepared from S3[+] transformants of M11 and M31, respectively. (Reprinted with permission from Arrecubieta et al.[7])

On the other hand, type 1 polysaccharide has been synthesized in vitro from crude pneumococcal extracts and identified immunologically.[91,92]

Cloning of the DNA region containing the genes responsible for the synthesis of type 1 polysaccharide was carried out by probing a library of pneumococcal type 1 DNA with the genes *orf1* and *orf2* from type 3 pneumococcus which are conserved in type 1 DNA (Fig. 2) and subsequent chromosome walking. An schematic representation of the organization of type 1 genes is shown in Fig. 8. The general arrangement of type 1 genes appears to be more similar to that of type 19F than that of type 3: (*i*) common and specific genes seem to be or-

ganized as an operon with no or only small intergenic spaces; (*ii*) a close relative of the IS*1167* insertion element (112) is located downstream of *dex*B. Nevertheless, as in type 3, another copy of the same IS element is also located downstream of *cap1G*. (*iii*) Four complete ORFs (*orf1* to *orf4*) are located immediately upstream of the *cap1* genes (as in type 19F DNA) and, apparently, form an operon with the specific genes. Sequence comparison between the preliminary sequences determined for the *cap1* genes and those compiled in the databanks strongly suggested that *cap1A* and *cap1B* correspond to genes encoding a glycosyl transferase and an *O*-acetylase, respectively, whereas no convincing evidence exists so far on the function of *cap1C* to *cap1F*.

Several data support the assumption that *cap1G* gene encodes the type 1 UDP-GlcDH: (*i*) sequence comparison revealed that Cap3A and Cap1G are 61% identical (77% similar) although Cap3A is smaller (394 amino acids) than Cap1G (410 amino acids); (*ii*) when *cap1G* was cloned into pLSE1[85] and used to transform a *cap3A* mutant, the lincomycin-resistant transformants produced a type 3 capsule; (*iii*) UDP-GlcDH activity could be demonstrated in crude sonicated extracts prepared from the *E. coli* C600 strain transformed with the same recombinant plasmid (not shown). Most of our current knowledge on the genetics of type 1 capsular polysaccharide biosynthesis came from studies on binary transformants produced by crosses implicating strains of different serotypes that synthesize hexuronic acids (see page 74). One of the main conclusions reached in those studies was that the genes coding for the UDP-GlcDH of types 1 and 3 were not homologous since recombination among them was never found.[20] This statement was fully confirmed by sequence determination, this is, *cap1G* and *cap3A* only are 65% identical. Phylogenetic analysis indicated that Cap1G is equally distant from Cap3A than, for instance, from *S. pyogenes* HasB, *E. coli* KfiD, or *S. flexneri* Udg (not shown).

When we performed searches for Cap1G homologues in the databanks, we found a remarkably high similarity between Cap1G and several proteins from Gram-negative organisms (Fig. 9). It was somehow unexpected that *kfiD*, a gene en-

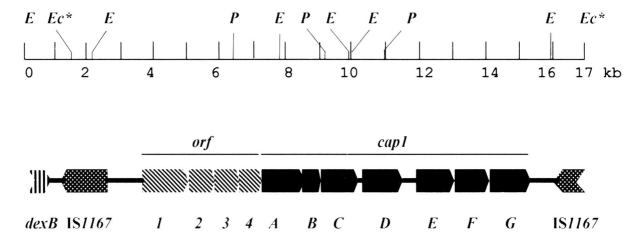

FIG. 8. Genetic organization of the 17-kb DNA region of the *S. pneumoniae* strain 13868 containing the type 1 *cap* genes. The orientation and localization of the ORFs are indicated by arrowed boxes. Some restriction sites are indicated (E, *Eco*RI; Ec, *Eco*47III; P, *Pst*I). The asterisks indicate that only some of the *Eco*47III sites present in this fragment are represented.

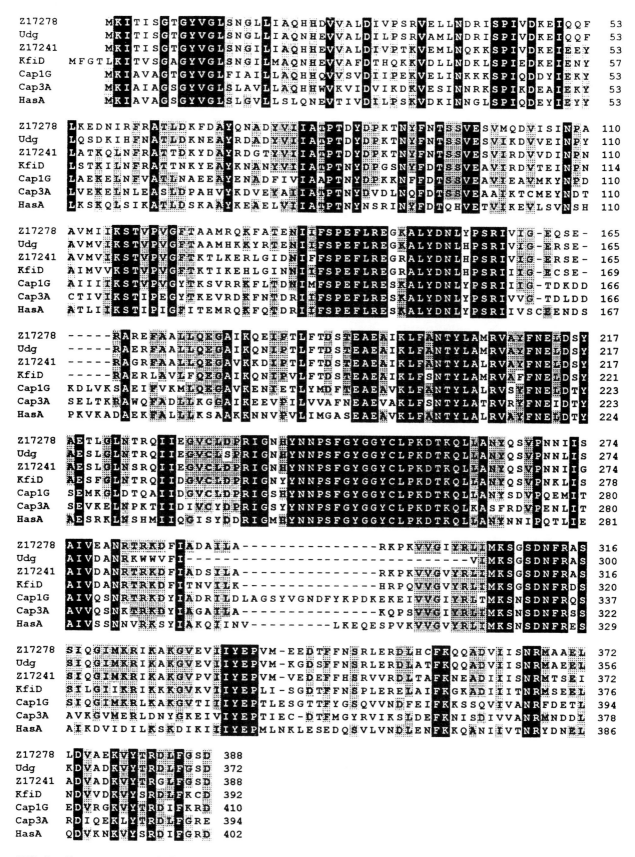

FIG. 9. Computer-generated alignment (PILEUP) of Cap1G with the UDP-GlcDH of *S. pneumoniae* type 3 (Cap3A), *S. pyogenes* (HasA), *E. coli* K5 (KfiD), *Salmonella enterica* LT2 (Z17278), *S. flexneri* (Udg), and *E. coli* O111 (Z17241). Residues on black or shaded boxes indicate amino acids identical in all or in at least five of the seven proteins shown, respectively.

Table 1. G + C Content of Several Gram-positive and Gram-negative Genes Encoding UDP-GlcDH

Species	Total mol % G + C	Gene (accession no.)	mol % G + C
S. pneumoniae type 1	38.5–39	*cap1G* (—)	32.5
S. pneumoniae type 3	38.5–39	*cap3A* (Z47210)	33.9
S. pyogenes WF50	34.5–38.5	*hasB* (L08444)	31.1
E. coli K5	49.9	*kfiD* (X77617)	35.6
E. coli O111 M92	49.9	— (Z17241)	46.0
S. enterica LT2	51.6	*orf1* (Z17278)	44.1
S. flexneri 2a	49–53	*udg* (X71970)	43.9

coding the UDP-GlcDH implicated in the synthesis of the K5 capsular polysaccharide of *E. coli*,[80,90] had a low G + C content (35.6%) closer to that found in *S. pneumoniae* (38.5%) than that reported for *E. coli* (49.9%) (Table 1). Other genes from Gram-negative species were also similar to *cap1G* although their G + C content was similar to that of their respective hosts. Furthermore, the codon usage of the *kfiD* gene (Table 2) resembled more that of pneumococci than that of *E. coli*.[74] All these results taken together support the hypothesis suggesting that *E. coli* may have acquired some genes through horizontal transformation events from Gram-positive species.[101]

Table 2. Codon Usage for Pneumococcal and *E. coli* UDP-GlcDH

Aa	Codon	Cap1G	Cap3A	KfiD	S. pneumoniae[a]	E. coli[b]
Gly	GGG	1	2	3	505	20398
	GGA	7	9	5	1230	15593
	GGU	11	5	12	1392	48818
	GGC	1	1	3	532	5546
Thr	ACG	0	0	5	364	25605
	ACA	11	10	8	1181	14546
	ACU	10	11	7	1114	18356
	ACC	2	0	2	764	43917
Asn	AAU	19	17	22	2038	34184
	AAC	2	4	8	832	42066
Ser	AGU	8	6	4	887	16409
	AGC	0	2	1	482	29318
	UCG	0	1	0	2391	16005
	UCA	4	2	9	873	14566
	UCU	10	12	12	1065	18534
	UCC	2	2	0	400	17432
Leu	UUG	5	7	10	1564	23991
	UUA	10	11	8	887	24608
	CUG	1	3	2	483	98957
	CUA	2	5	3	574	7454
	CUU	9	3	7	891	21023
	CUC	2	1	2	494	19793
Pro	CCG	3	2	3	203	43573
	CCA	4	4	8	880	15926
	CCU	7	7	3	706	13359
	CCC	0	1	1	184	9610
Gln	CAG	1	3	3	805	55658
	CAA	11	4	5	1435	26856
Val	GUG	3	5	6	650	48359
	GUA	11	10	3	823	21645
	GUU	16	17	15	1405	36901
	GUC	2	1	4	820	27784
Ala	GCG	5	3	4	454	61590
	GCA	13	8	8	995	38809
	GCU	9	13	7	1598	31580
	GCC	2	2	4	905	47668

[a]Data compiled from 141 complete genes (74).
[b]Data compiled from 6068 complete genes (74).

CONCLUSION

Classic studies using genetic transformation allowed the coining of the term capsular genome meaning the closely linked genes controlling the production of capsular polysaccharide.[22] Inter-type transformation takes place when the donor DNA displaces the resident capsular genome and it was assumed that this interchange was mediated by homologous sequences flanking the type-specific gene cluster. Our current knowledge on the organization of capsular genes at the molecular level, although limited, fully confirms those early interpretations. In types 19F, 3, and 1 (and possibly also in type 14) the genes responsible for the synthesis of the corresponding activated sugars and the specific glycosyl transferases (synthases) are clustered together in the *S. pneumoniae* chromosome not far from genes encoding the penicillin-binding proteins PBP1a and PBP2x. The putative functions attributed to different gene products have been deduced mostly by sequence comparison except for genes *cap3ABC*, *cps14E*, and *cap1G* where direct experimental evidence of their role in capsule biosynthesis has been recently obtained. It is of particular interest that expression of only one gene (*cap3B*) was required for the synthesis of high molecular size, type 3 polysaccharide in *E. coli* and *S. pneumoniae* strains that produce UDP-GlcA. It is noteworthy that approximately 50% of the pneumococcal type 3 polysaccharide synthesized in *E. coli* appears in the periplasmic space, although the mechanism for this transport remains to be elucidated. A type 3 capsule was assembled both in capsulated and in unencapsulated pneumococcal strains when transformed with a plasmid expressing the Cap3B synthase. It can be postulated that the mechanism of polysaccharide transport of the recipient cell is used for the formation of a type 3 capsule.

Sequence comparison suggested that some of the genes located upstream of the type-specific ones might be implicated in polysaccharide transport and/or assembly, as has been shown to occur in Gram-negative microorganisms. In types 1 and 19F DNAs, the capsule-specific genes are apparently organized forming an operon that also includes four genes located upstream. However, this is not the case in the DNA of type 3 pneumococcal strain where has been possible to demonstrate that the promoter of the capsule-specific genes is located immediately before *cap3A*. In addition, sequence determination and Northern blot analysis strongly suggested that the DNA sequences located upstream of the type 3-specific genes represent pseudogenes that are not transcribed. It is yet to be determined whether the common genes are actually required for capsule formation or the transport of polysaccharide and its assembly into a capsule is driven by other still-unknown genes. Alternatively, we can not rule out the possibility that diverse functional organizations of the capsular genes may exist in different pneumococcal serotypes.

There is increasing evidence suggesting that capsular biosynthetic genes can be transferred among different clinical isolates of *S. pneumoniae*. It is tempting to speculate that the IS-like elements located at one (type 3 and 19F) or both sides (type 1) of the capsular genes might have been involved in horizontal transfer of the pneumococcal capsular genome. Interestingly, it has been recently reported that the type 1 capsule-encoding genes (*cap1*) of *Staphylococcus aureus* are located in a discrete genetic element of about 34 kb terminated, at one end, by an IS-like element,[60] and it is also well established that the type b capsule genes of *Haemophilus influenzae* are located in a 17-kb compound transposon.[59]

ACKNOWLEDGMENTS

We thank P. García and J. L. García for helpful comments and for the critical reading of the manuscript, and M. Sheehan for correcting the English version. The technical assistance of E. Cano and M. Carrasco, and the skillful work by A. Hurtado and V. Muñoz is greatly acknowledged. This work was supported by grant PB-93-0115-C02-01 from the Programa Sectorial de Promoción General del Conocimiento. C. A. is a beneficiary of a predoctoral fellowship from Eusko Jaurlaritza.

REFERENCES

1. **Alloway, J.L.** 1933. Further observations on the use of pneumococcus extracts in effecting transformation of type *in vitro*. J. Exp. Med. **57**:265–278.

2. **Alonso De Velasco, E., A.F. Verheul, J. Verhoef, and H. Snippe.** 1995. *Streptococcus pneumoniae*: Virulence factors, pathogenesis, and vaccines. Microbiol. Rev. **59**:591–603.

3. **Arrecubieta, C.** 1996. Ph.D. thesis. Universidad Complutense, Madrid.

4. **Arrecubieta, C., E. García, and R. López.** 1995. Sequence and transcriptional analysis of a DNA region involved in the production of capsular polysaccharide in *Streptococcus pneumoniae* type 3. Gene **167**:1–7.

5. **Arrecubieta, C., E. García, and R. López.** 1996. Demonstration of UDP-glucose dehydrogenase activity in cell extracts of *Escherichia coli* expressing the pneumococcal *cap3A* gene required for the synthesis of type 3 capsular polysaccharide. J. Bacteriol. **178**:2971–2974.

6. **Arrecubieta, C., R. López, and E. García.** 1994. Molecular characterization of *cap3A*, a gene from the operon required for the synthesis of the capsule of *Streptococcus pneumoniae* type 3: Sequencing of mutations responsible for the unencapsulated phenotype and localization of the capsular cluster on the pneumococcal chromosome. J. Bacteriol. **176**:6375–6383.

7. **Arrecubieta, C., R. López, and E. García.** 1996. Type 3-specific synthase of *Streptococcus pneumoniae* (Cap3B) directs type 3 polysaccharide biosynthesis in *Escherichia coli* and in pneumococcal strains of different serotypes. J. Exp. Med. **184**:449–455.

8. **Austrian, R.** 1952. Bacterial transformation reactions. Bacteriol. Rev. **16**:31–50.

9. **Austrian, R., and H.P. Bernheimer.** 1955. Some biological properties of doubly encapsulated pneumococci. J. Clin. Invest. **34**:920–921.

10. **Austrian, R., and H.P. Bernheimer.** 1959. Simultaneous production of two capsular polysaccharides by pneumococcus. I. Properties of a pneumococcus manifesting binary capsulation. J. Exp. Med. **110**:571–584.

11. **Austrian, R., H.P. Bernheimer, E.E.B. Smith, and G.T. Mills.** 1958. Acquisition of new capsular type by pneumococcus, a multifactor transformation. Cold Spring Harbor Symp. Quant. Biol. **23**:99–100.

12. **Austrian, R., H.P. Bernheimer, E.E.B. Smith, and G.T. Mills.** 1959. Simultaneous production of two capsular polysaccharides by pneumococcus. II. The genetic and biochemical bases of binary capsulation. J. Exp. Med. **110**:585–602.

13. **Avery, O.T. and R. Dubos.** 1931. The protective action of a specific enzyme against type III pneumococcus infection in mice. J. Exp. Med. **54:**73–89.

14. **Avery, O.T., and W.F. Goebel.** 1931. Chemo-immunological studies on conjugated carbohydrate-proteins. V. The immunological specificity of an antigen prepared by combining the capsular polysaccharide of type III pneumococcus with foreign protein. J. Exp. Med. **54:**437–447.

15. **Avery, O.T., C.M. MacLeod, and M. McCarty.** 1944. Studies on the chemical nature of the substance inducing transformation of pneumococcal types. Induction of transformation by a deoxyribonucleic acid fraction isolated from pneumococcus type III. J. Exp. Med. **79:**137–158.

16. **Bairoch, A., P. Bucher, and K. Homann.** 1996. The PROSITE database, its status in 1995. Nucleic Acids Res. **24:**189–196.

17. **Barnes, D.M., S. Whittier, P.H. Gilligan, S. Soares, A. Tomasz, and F.W. Henderson.** 1995. Transmission of multidrug-resistant serotype 23F *Streptococcus pneumoniae* in group day care: Evidence suggesting capsular transformation of the resistant strain in vivo. J. Infect. Dis. **171:**890–896.

18. **Behr, T., W. Fischer, J. Peter-Katalinic, and H. Egge.** 1992. The structure of pneumococal lipoteichoic acid. Improved preparation, chemical and mass spectrometric studies. Eur. J. Biochem. **207:**1063–1075.

19. **Bernheimer, H.P., and J.-G. Tiraby.** 1976. Inhibition of phage infection by pneumococcus capsule. Virology **73:**308–309.

20. **Bernheimer, H.P., and I.E. Wermundsen.** 1969. Unstable binary capsulated transformants in pneumococcus. J. Bacteriol. **98:**1073–1079.

21. **Bernheimer, H.P., and I.E. Wermundsen.** 1972. Homology in capsular transformation reactions in *Pneumococcus*. Mol. Gen. Genet. **116:**68–73.

22. **Bernheimer, H.P., I.E. Wermundsen, and R. Austrian.** 1967. Qualitative differences in the behavior of pneumococcal deoxyribonucleic acids transforming to the same capsular type. J. Bacteriol. **93:**320–333.

23. **Bernheimer, H.P., I.E. Wermundsen, and R. Austrian.** 1968. Mutation in pneumococcus type III affecting multiple cistrons concerned with the synthesis of capsular polysaccharide. J. Bacteriol. **96:**1099–1102.

24. **Cámara, M., G.J. Boulnois, P.W. Andrew, and T.J. Mitchell.** 1994. A neuraminidase from *Streptococcus pneumoniae* has the features of a surface protein. Infect. Immun. **62:**3688–3695.

25. **Coffey, T.J., C.G. Dowson, M. Daniels, J. Zhou, C. Martin, B.G. Spratt, and J.M. Musser.** 1991. Horizontal transfer of multiple penicillin-binding protein genes, and capsular biosynthetic genes, in natural populations of *Streptococcus pneumoniae*. Mol. Microbiol. **5:**2255–2260.

26. **Cross, A.S.** 1990. The biological significance of bacterial encapsulation. Curr. Topics Microbiol. Immunol. **150:**87–95.

27. **Dai J.B., Y. Liu, W.J. Ray Jr., and M. Konno.** 1992. The crystal structure of muscle phosphoglucomutase refined at 2.7-angstrom resolution. J. Biol. Chem. **267:**6322–6337.

28. **Dawson, M.H., and R.H.P. Sia.** 1931. A technique for inducing transformation of pneumococcal types *in vitro*. J. Exp. Med. **54:**681–699.

29. **DeAngelis, P.L., and P.H. Weigel.** 1994. Immunochemical confirmation of the primary structure of streptococcal hyaluronan synthase and synthesis of high molecular weight product by the recombinant enzyme. Biochemistry **33:**9033–9039.

30. **Deretic, V., J.F. Gill, and A.M. Chakrabarty.** 1987. *Pseudomonas aeruginosa* infection in cystic fibrosis: Nucleotide sequence and transcription regulation of the *algD* gene. Nucleic Acids Res. **15:**4567–4581.

31. **Dillard, J., M.W. Vandersea, and J. Yother.** 1995. Characterization of the cassette containing genes for the type 3 capsular polysaccharide biosynthesis in *Streptococcus pneumoniae*. J. Exp. Med. **181:**973–983.

32. **Dillard, J.P., and J. Yother.** 1994. Genetic and molecular characterization of capsular polysaccharide biosynthesis in *Streptococcus pneumoniae* type 3. Mol. Microbiol. **12:**959–972.

33. **Dougherty, B., and I. van de Rijn.** 1993. Molecular characterization of *hasB* from an operon required for hyaluronic acid synthesis in group A streptococci. Demonstration of UDP-glucose dehydrogenase activity. J. Biol. Chem. **268:**7118–7124.

34. **Enders, J.F., M.F. Shaffer, and C.-J. Wu.** 1936. Correlation of the behavior *in vivo* of pneumococci type III varying in their virulence for rabbits with certain differences observed *in vitro*. J. Exp. Med. **64:**307–331.

35. **Ephrussi-Taylor, H.** 1951. Genetic aspects of transformations of pneumococci. Cold Spring Harbor Symp. Quant. Biol. **16:**445–456.

36. **Ephrussi-Taylor, H.** 1951. Transformations allogènes du pneumocoque. Exp. Cell Res. **2:**589–607.

37. **Ephrussi-Taylor, H.** 1955. Current status of bacterial transformation. Adv. Virus Res. **3:**275–307.

38. **Fath, M.J., and R. Kolter.** 1993. ABC transporters: bacterial exporters. Microbiol. Rev. **57:**995–1017.

39. **Felton, L., and B. Prescott.** 1939. Studies on immunizing substances in pneumococci. X. The relationship between the acetyl group on type I pneumococcus polysaccharide and antigenicity. J. Bacteriol. **38:**579–593.

40. **Fenoll, A., C. Martín-Bourgon, R. Muñoz, D. Vicioso, and J. Casal.** 1991. Serotype distribution and antimicrobial resistance of *Streptococcus pneumoniae* isolates causing systemic infections in Spain, 1979-1989. Rev. Infect. Dis. **13:**56–60.

41. **Fischer, W., T. Behr, R. Hartmann, J. Peter-Katalinic, and H. Egge.** 1993. Teichoic acid and lipoteichoic acid of *Streptococcus pneumoniae* possess identical chain structures. A reinvestigation of teichoic acid (C polysaccharide). Eur. J. Biochem. **215:**851–857.

42. **García, E., C. Arrecubieta, and R. López.** 1996. The *lytA* gene and the DNA region located downstream of this gene are not involved in the formation of the type 3 capsular polysaccharide of *Streptococcus pneumoniae*. Curr. Microbiol. **33:**133–135.

43. **García, E., P. García, and R. López.** 1992. Clonación de genes capsulares de *Streptococcus pneumoniae*. Rev. Esp. Quimioter. **5 (Suppl. 1):**38–43.

44. **García, E., P. García, and R. López.** 1993. Cloning and sequencing of a gene involved in the synthesis of the capsular polysaccharide of *Streptococcus pneumoniae* type 3. Mol. Gen. Genet. **239:**188–195.

45. **García, E., and R. López.** 1995. *Streptococcus pneumoniae* type 3 encodes a protein highly similar to the human glutamate decarboxylase (GAD$_{65}$). FEMS Microbiol. Lett. **133:**113–118.

46. **Gasc, A.-M., L. Kauc, P. Barraillé, M. Sicard, and S. Goodgal.** 1991. Gene localization, size, and physical map of the chromosome of *Streptococcus pneumoniae*. J. Bacteriol. **173:**7361–7367.

47. **Griffith, F.** 1928. The significance of pneumococcal types. J. Hyg. **27:**113–159.

48. **Guidolin, A., J.K. Morona, R. Morona, D. Hansman, and J.C. Paton.** 1994. Nucleotide sequence analysis of genes essential for capsular polysaccharide biosynthesis in *Streptococcus pneumoniae* type 19F. Infect. Immun. **62:**5384–5396.

49. **Guy, R.C.E., M.J. How, M. Stacey, and M. Heidelberger.** 1967. The capsular polysaccharide of type I pneumococcus. I. Purification and chemical modification. J. Biol. Chem. **242:**5106–5111.

50. **Hall, L.M.C., R.A. Whiley, B. Duke, A. Efstratiou, J.P. Maskell, and C.A. Arias.** 1995. Genetic relationships among UK invasive pneumococci of common serotypes, with preliminary data on dihydropteroate synthase and capsule synthesis genes, p. 9. *In* Abstracts of the Third European Meeting on the Molecular

Biology of the Pneumococcus. September 16–18, 1995. University of Leicester.

51. **Håvarstein, L.S., G. Coomaraswamy, and D.A. Morrison.** 1995. An unmodified heptadecapeptide pheromone induces competence for genetic transformation in *Streptococcus pneumoniae.* Proc. Natl. Acad. Sci. USA **92:**11140–11144.

52. **Hayes, W.** 1966. Genetic transformation: a retrospective appreciation. J. Gen. Microbiol. **45:**385–397.

53. **Henrichsen, J.** 1995. Six newly recognized types of *Streptococcus pneumoniae.* J. Clin. Microbiol. **33:**2759–2762.

54. **Jerlström, P.G., G.S. Chatwal, and K.N. Timmis.** 1991. The IgA-binding β antigen of the c protein complex of group B streptococci: Sequence determination of its gene and detection of two binding regions. Mol. Microbiol. **5:**843–849.

55. **Kell, C.M., J.Z. Jordens, M. Daniels, T.J. Coffey, J. Bates, J. Paul, C. Gilks, and B.G. Spratt.** 1993. Molecular epidemiology of penicillin-resistant pneumococci isolated in Nairobi, Kenya. Infect. Immun. **61:**4382–4391.

56. **Kenne, L., B. Lindberg, K. Petersson, E. Katzenellenbogen, and E. Romanowska.** 1990. Structural studies of the O-specific side-chains of the *Shigella sonnei* phase I lipopolysaccharide. Carbohydr. Res. **78:**119–126.

57. **Knecht, J.C., G. Schiffman, and R. Austrian.** 1970. Some biological properties of pneumococcus type 37 and the chemistry of its capsular polysaccharide. J. Exp. Med. **132:**475–487.

58. **Kolkman, M.A.B., D.A. Morrison, B.A.M. van der Zeijst, and P.J.M. Nuijten.** 1996. The capsule polysaccharide synthesis locus of *Streptococcus pneumoniae* serotype 14: Identification of the glycosyl transferase gene *cps14E.* J. Bacteriol. **178:**3736–3741.

59. **Kroll, J.S., B.M. Loynds, and E.R. Moxon.** 1991. The *Haemophilus influenzae* capsulation gene cluster: a compound transposon. Mol. Microbiol. **5:**1549–1560.

60. **Lee, C.Y.** 1995. Association of staphylococcal type-1 capsule-encoding genes with a discrete genetic element. Gene **167:**115–119.

61. **Lindberg, B., B. Lindqvist, J. Lönngren, and D.A. Powell.** 1980. Structural studies of the capsular polysaccharide from *Streptococcus pneumoniae* type 1. Carbohydr. Res. **78:**111–117.

62. **López, R., J.M. Sánchez-Puelles, E. García, J.L. García, C. Ronda, and P. García.** 1986. Isolation, characterization and physiological properties of an autolytic defective mutant of *Streptococcus pneumoniae.* Mol. Gen. Genet. **204:**237–242.

63. **MacLeod, C.M., and M.R. Krauss.** 1950. Relation of virulence of pneumococcal strains for mice to the quantity of capsular polysaccharide formed *in vitro.* J. Exp. Med. **92:**1–9.

64. **MacLeod, C.M., and M.R. Krauss.** 1953. Control by factors distinct from the S transforming principle of the amount of capsular polysaccharide produced by type III pneumococci. J. Exp. Med. **97:**767–771.

65. **Mäkelä, P.H., and B.A.D. Stocker.** 1969. Genetics of polysaccharide biosynthesis. Annu. Rev. Genet. **3:**291–322.

66. **Mandrell, R.E., M.A. Apicella, R. Lindstedt, and H. Leffler.** 1994. Possible interaction between animal lectins and bacterial carbohydrates. Methods Enzymol. **236:**231–254.

67. **Martin, B., O. Humbert, M. Cámara, E. Guenzi, J. Walker, T. Mitchell, P. Andrew, M. Prudhomme, G. Alloing, R. Hakenbeck, D.A. Morrison, G.J. Boulnois, and J.P. Claverys.** 1992. A highly conserved repeated DNA element located in the chromosome of *Streptococcus pneumoniae.* Nucleic Acids Res. **20:**3479–3483.

68. **McCarty, M.** 1946. Chemical nature and biological specificity of the substance inducing transformation of pneumococcal types. Bacteriol. Rev. **10:**63–71.

69. **McCarty, M., H.E. Taylor, and O.T. Avery.** 1946. Biochemical studies of environmental factors essential in transformation of pneumococcal types. Cold Spring Harbor Symp. Quant. Biol. **11:**177–182.

70. **Mills, G.T.** 1960. Genetic and biochemical lesions of polysaccharide synthesis in the pneumococcus. Fed. Proc. **19:**991–995.

71. **Mills, G.T., and E.E.B. Smith.** 1962. Biosynthetic aspects of capsule formation in the pneumococcus. Brit. Med. Bull. **18:**27–30.

72. **Mills, G.T., and E.E.B. Smith.** 1965. Biosynthesis of capsular polysaccharides in the pneumococcus. Bull. Soc. Chim. Biol. **47:**1751–1765.

73. **Morona, J.K., A. Guidolin, R. Morona, D. Hansman, and J.C. Paton.** 1994. Isolation, characterization, and nucleotide sequence of IS*1202,* an insertion sequence of *Streptococcus pneumoniae.* J. Bacteriol. **176:**4437–4443.

74. **Nakamura, Y., K. Wada, Y. Wada, H. Doi, S. Kanaya, T. Gojobori, and T. Ikemura.** 1996. Codon usage tabulated from the international DNA sequence databases. Nucleic Acids Res. **24:**214–215.

75. **Nielsen, S.V., and J. Henrichsen.** 1992. Capsular type of *Streptococcus pneumoniae* isolated from blood and CSF during 1982–1987. Clin. Infect. Dis. **15:**794–798.

76. **Ottolenghi-Nightingale, E.** 1969. Spontaneously occurring bacterial transformation in mice. J. Bacteriol. **100:**445–452.

77. **Ottolenghi-Nightingale, E.** 1972. Competence of pneumococcal isolates and bacterial transformation in man. Infect. Immun. **6:**785–792.

78. **Paton, J.C., P.W. Andrew, G.J. Boulnois, and T.J. Mitchell.** 1993. Molecular analysis of the pathogenicity of *Streptococcus pneumoniae*: The role of pneumococcal proteins. Annu. Rev. Microbiol. **47:**89–115.

79. **Pearce, B.J., A.M. Naughton, and H.R. Masure.** 1994. Peptide permeases modulate transformation in *Streptococcus pneumoniae.* Mol. Microbiol. **12:**881–892.

80. **Petit, C., G.P. Rigg, C. Pazzani, A. Smith, V. Sieberth, M. Stevens, G. Boulnois, K. Jann, and I.S. Roberts.** 1995. Region 2 of the *Escherichia coli* K5 capsule gene cluster encoding proteins for the biosynthesis of the K5 polysaccharide. Mol. Microbiol. **17:**611–620.

81. **Ravin, A.W.** 1960. Linked mutations borne by deoxyribonucleic acid controlling the synthesis of capsular polysaccharide in pneumococcus. Genetics **45:**1387–1403.

82. **Ravin, A.W.** 1961. The genetics of transformation. Adv. Genet. **10:**61–163.

83. **Reeves, R.E., and W.F. Goebel.** 1941. Chemoimmunological studies on the soluble specific substance of pneumococcus. V. The structure of the type III polysaccharide. J. Biol. Chem. **139:**511–519.

84. **Roberts, I.S., F.K. Saunders, and G.J. Boulnois.** 1989. Bacterial capsules and interactions with complement and phagocytes. Biochem. Soc. Trans. **17:**462–464.

85. **Ronda, C., J.L. García, and R. López.** 1988. Characterization of genetic transformation in *Streptococcus oralis* NCTC 11427. Expression of pneumococcal amidase in *S. oralis* using a new shuttle vector. Mol. Gen. Genet. **215:**53–57.

86. **Rubens, C.E., L.M. Heggen, R.F. Haft, and M.R. Wessels.** 1993. Identification of *cpsD,* a gene essential for type III capsule expression in group B streptococci. Mol. Microbiol. **8:**843–855.

87. **Sánchez-Puelles, J.M., C. Ronda, J.L. García, P. García, R. López, and E. García.** 1986. Searching for autolysin functions. Characterization of a pneumococcal mutant deleted in the *lytA* gene. Eur. J. Biochem. **158:**289–293.

88. **Shibaev, V.N.** 1986. Biosynthesis of bacterial polysaccharide chains composed of repeating units. Adv. Carbohydr. Chem. Biochem. **44:**277–339.

89. **Sibold, C., J. Wang, J. Henrichsen, and R. Hakenbeck.** 1992. Genetic relationship of penicillin-susceptible and -resistant *Streptococcus pneumoniae* strains isolated on different continents. Infect. Immun. **60:**4119–4126.

90. **Sieberth, V., G.P. Rigg, I.S. Roberts, and K. Jann.** 1995. Expression and characterization of UDPGlc dehdyrogenase (KfiD) which is encoded in the type-specific region 2 of the *Escherichia coli* K5 capsule genes. J. Bacteriol. **177:**4562–4565.

91. **Smith, E.E.B., B. Galloway, and G.T. Mills.** 1961. The enzymic synthesis by a pneumococcal extract of a serologically reactive polymer from uridine diphosphate galacturonic acid. Biochem. Biophys. Res. Commun. **4:**420–424.

92. **Smith, E.E.B., and G.T. Mills.** 1962. Experiments on the biosynthesis of type I pneumococcal capsular polysaccharide. Biochem. J. **82:**42P.

93. **Smith, E.E.B., and G.T. Mills.** 1966. Formation of type 3 pneumococcal capsular polysaccharide. Methods Enzymol. **8:**446–450.

94. **Smith, E.E.B., G.T. Mills, R. Austrian, and H.P. Bernheimer.** 1960. Uridine pyrophosphoglucose dehydrogenase in capsulated and non-capsulated strains of pneumococcus type I. J. Gen. Microbiol. **22:**265–271.

95. **Smith, E.E.B., G.T. Mills, H.P. Bernheimer, and R. Austrian.** 1958. The presence of an uronic acid epimerase in a strain of pneumococcus type I. Biochim. Biophys. Acta **29:**640–641.

96. **Smith, E.E.B., G.T. Mills, H.P. Bernheimer, and R. Austrian.** 1960. The synthesis of type III pneumococcal capsular polysaccharide from uridine nucleotides by a cell-free extract of *Diplococcus pneumoniae* type III. J. Biol. Chem. **235:**1876–1880.

97. **Smith, E.E.B., G.T. Mills, and E.M. Harper.** 1957. The isolation of uridine pyrophosphogalacturonic acid from a type I pneumococcus. Biochim. Biophys. Acta **23:**662–663.

98. **Sørensen, U.B.S. and J. Blom.** 1992. Capsular polysaccharide is linked to the outer surface of type 6A pneumococcal cell walls. APMIS **100:**891–893.

99. **Sørensen, U.B.S., J. Henrichsen, H.-C. Chen, and S.C. Szu.** 1990. Covalent linkage between the capsular polysaccharide and the cell wall peptidoglycan of *Streptococcus pneumoniae* revealed by immunochemical methods. Microb. Pathog. **8:**325–334.

100. **Studier, F.W.** 1991. Use of bacteriophage T7 lysozyme to improve an inducible T7 expression system. J. Mol. Biol. **219:**37–44.

101. **Syavanen, M.** 1994. Horizontal gene transfer: evidence and possible consequences. Annu. Rev. Genet. **28:**237–261.

102. **Taylor, H.E.** 1949. Additive effects of certain transforming agents from some variants of pneumococcus. J. Exp. Med. **89:**399–424.

103. **Tuomanen, E.I., R. Austrian, and H.R. Masure.** 1995. Pathogenesis of pneumococcal infection. N. Engl. J. Med. **332:**1280–1284.

104. **Tzianabos, A.O., A.B. Onderdonk, B. Bosner, R.L. Cisneros, and D.L. Kasper.** 1993. Structural features of polysaccharides that induce intra-abdominal abscesses. Science **262:**416–419.

105. **van Dam, J.E.G., A. Fleer, and H. Snippe.** 1990. Immunogenicity and immunochemistry of *Streptococcus pneumoniae* capsular polysaccharides. A. van Leeuwenhoek **58:**1–47.

106. **Watson, D.A., V. Kapur, D.M. Musher, J.W. Jacobson, and J.M. Musser.** 1995. Identification, cloning, and sequencing of DNA essential for encapsulation of *Streptococcus pneumoniae*. Curr. Microbiol. **31:**251–259.

107. **Watson, D.A., and D.M. Musher.** 1990. Interruption of capsule production in *Streptococcus pneumoniae* serotype 3 by insertion of transposon Tn*916*. Infect. Immun. **58:**3135–3138.

108. **Whitfield, C., and M.A. Valvano.** 1993. Biosynthesis and expression of cell-surface polysaccharides in Gram-negative bacteria. Adv. Microb. Physiol. **35:**135–246.

109. **Wilkinson, J.F.** 1958. The extracellular polysaccharides of bacteria. Bacteriol. Rev. **22:**46–73.

110. **Wood, W.B. Jr., and M.R. Smith.** 1949. The inhibition of surface phagocytosis by the capsular "slime layer" of pneumococcus type III. J. Exp. Med. **90:**85–96.

111. **Yother, J., L.S. McDaniel, and D.E. Briles.** 1986. Transformation of encapsulated *Streptococcus pneumoniae*. J. Bacteriol. **168:**1463–1465.

112. **Zhou, L., F.M. Hui, and D.A. Morrison.** 1995. Characterization of IS*1167*, a new insertion sequence in *Streptococcus pneumoniae*. Plasmid **33:**127–138.

Address reprint requests to:
Ernesto García
Departamento de Microbiología Molecular
Centro de Investigaciones Biológicas
Consejo Superior de Investigaciones Científicas
Velázquez 144, 28006 Madrid, Spain

Pneumococcal Lipoteichoic and Teichoic Acid

WERNER FISCHER

INTRODUCTION

Lipoteichoic acids (LTAs) and teichoic acids (TAs) are widespread polymers of the cell wall membrane complex in a large number of gram-positive bacteria. LTAs possess a glycolipid anchor and are hydrophobically anchored in the outer layer of the cytoplasmic membrane. TAs are covalently attached, usually through a linkage unit, by a phosphodiester bond to part of the *N*-acetylmuramyl residues of peptidoglycan (Fig. 1).[18,37,79] Pneumococci are so far unique because their teichoic acid (TA) and lipoteichoic acid (LTA) possess identical repeat and chain structures, whereas, in other gram-positive bacteria, TAs and LTAs are structurally and biosynthetically distinct entities.

In 1930, long before LTAs and TAs had been discovered and defined, pneumococcal TA was described as pneumococcal C-polysaccharide by Tillet *et al.*[75] Thirteen years later, pneumococcal LTA was isolated by Goebel *et al.*[33] and named lipocarbohydrate or pneumococcal F-antigen owing to its fatty acid content and immunological properties. In these early studies, a structural relationship between C-polysaccharide and lipocarbohydrate was suggested and in contrast to the various strain-specific capsular polysaccharides, lipocarbohydrate and C-polysaccharide were considered pneumococcal common antigens.[32,33] This was recently confirmed by serological methods which showed that all 83 known capsular types of *Streptococcus pneumoniae* possess C-polysaccharide and F-antigen.[72] The two polymers differ immunologically, as Forssman antigenicity is associated with the LTA.[4,6,32,33] Immunoelectron microscopy showed that C-polysaccharide is uniformly distributed on both the inside and outside of the cell walls, and LTA on the surface of the cytoplasma membrane[73] (Fig. 2).

Landmarks of structural studies were the discovery of *N*-acetylgalactosamine phosphate as a component of C-polysaccharide,[27,44] followed by the detection of choline as another component.[76] Choline had long been known as an essential growth factor of pneumococci.[3]

Further progress in structural analysis was achieved by Brundish and Baddiley[9,10] who released the C-polysaccharide from the cell wall with 10% TCA and, after several steps, including anion exchange chromatography, obtained a pure compound which was composed of phosphate, *N*-acetylgalactosamine, glucose, *N*-acetyldiaminotrideoxyhexose, and choline. Choline phosphate and ribitol phosphate were identified as units in the polymer and the presence of ribitol phosphate and sugar residues led to a change in name from C-polysaccharide to teichoic acid. Subsequent structural studies by Watson and Baddiley[80] led to a partial structure of teichoic acid in which a trisaccharide-ribitol phosphate repeat was proposed with D-glucose as a major component. In later work, the structure was modified essentially to a disaccharide which did not include D-glucose as a major constituent, despite the fact that the presence of four anomeric resonances in the ^{13}C NMR spectrum of the teichoic acid strongly suggested additional hexosyl residues.[62] In 1980, Jennings *et al.*[43] published a complete structure of the teichoic acid, which will be discussed next.

Until 1992, there were no structural studies of LTA. Fatty acids[10,33] galactosamine, glucose, ribitol, and phosphorus[24] were reported as components of LTA, but quantitative data and linkage analyses were missing. The presence of 2-acetamido-4-amino-2,4,6-trideoxygalactose (AATGal) was not demonstrated, the nature of the lipid anchor remained obscure, and in all experiments Forssman antigenicity was used as a measure of LTA concentrations.

The structure of LTA was clarified in 1992 after a novel more effective isolation procedure had been developed.[4] In 1993, the identity of the chain structures of LTA and TA was demonstrated.[21] In view of this identity, basic studies into structure and conformation were performed with LTA because intact TA is more difficult to prepare.

LIPOTEICHOIC ACID

Figure 3 shows the classical LTA structure, in which a 1,3-linked poly(glycerophosphate) chain is attached by a phosphodiester bond to a glycolipid which also occurs in the free state as a membrane component. This classical LTA type is most wide spread and occurs in bacilli, enterococci, lactobacilli, lactococci, listeria, staphylococci and some streptococci.[16,18]

The structure of pneumococcal LTA is quite different[4]: Glycerophosphate is replaced by ribitol phosphate and between the ribitol phosphate residues, a tetrasaccharide is intercalated. The tetrasaccharide contains D-glucose, the positively charged 2-acetamido-4-amino-2,4,6-trideoxy-D-galactose (AATGal), and two *N*-acetyl-D-galactosaminyl residues which, in the ex-

Institute of Biochemistry, Faculty of Medicine, University Erlangen-Nürnberg, Erlangen, Germany.

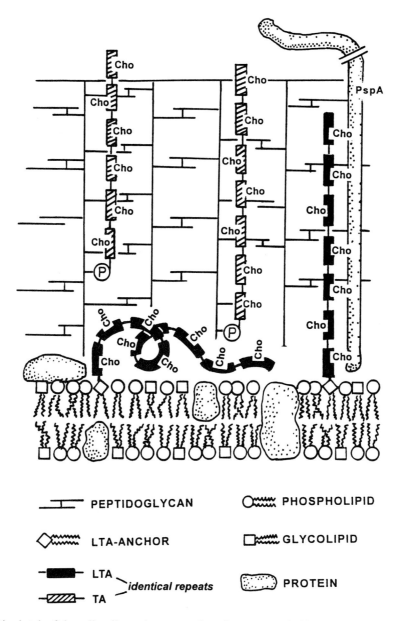

PEPTIDOGLYCAN   PHOSPHOLIPID

LTA-ANCHOR   GLYCOLIPID

LTA   PROTEIN
              identical repeats
TA

FIG. 1. Diagrammatic sketch of the cell wall membrane complex of pneumococci. Cho, phosphocholine; ℗, phosphodiester; Pneumococcal surface protein (PspA) is shown as an example of a choline-binding protein that is noncovalently attached to phosphocholine residues of LTA.[85]

ample shown, carry at O6 each a zwitterionic phosphocholine residue. All sugars belong to the D-series and are in the pyranose form. The repeats are connected to each other by phosphodiester bonds between O5 of the ribitol and O6 of the D-glucopyranosyl residue of adjacent repeats. The chain is attached by a phosphodiester bond to O6 of the terminal glucosyl residue of D-Glc$p$(β1-4)-D-AATGal$p$(β1-3)-D-Glc$p$(α1-3)acyl$_2$Gro, a so far unique glycolipid that contains the positively charged AATGal residue intercalated between two D-glucopyranosyl residues. In contrast to other LTAs, the glycolipid anchor of pneumococcal LTA cannot be detected in the free form among membrane lipids which contain as major glycolipid D-Gal$p$(α1-2)-D-Glc$p$(α1-3)acyl$_2$Gro (Fig. 4).

Classification of pneumococcal lipoteichoic acid and related amphiphiles

The classification as LTA was based on the definition that LTAs are lipid macroamphiphiles that contain aditolphosphates as integral part of the hydrophilic chain.[18] If the definition is based on the mode of biosynthesis, LTAs are classified as being synthesized from lipid precursors, whereas TAs are synthesized from nucleotide-activated precursors (Table 1).[19] As ribitol phosphate is activated as CDP-ribitol, pneumococcal LTA may be classified as glycolipid-linked TA. Moreover, this classification would also take into account the hypothesis of common steps in the biosynthesis of the identical chain structures of pneumococcal LTA and TA.

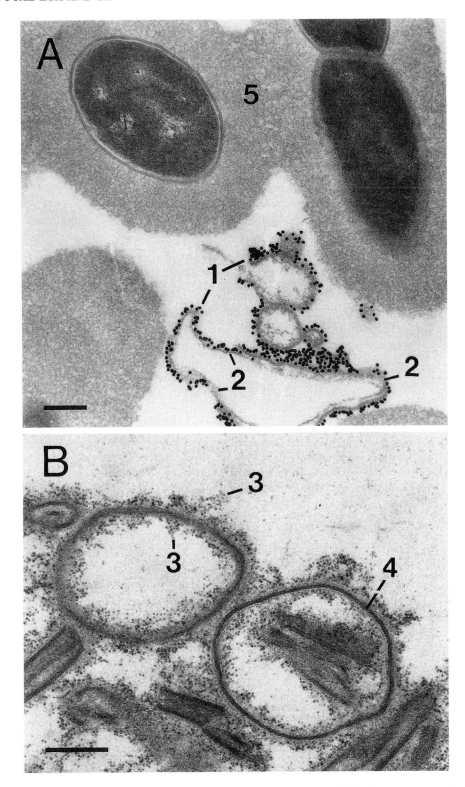

FIG. 2. Visualization of LTA (**A**) and TA (**B**) by immunoelectron microscopy. 1, LTA (Forssman antigen); 2, plasma membrane; 3, TA (C-polysaccharide); 4, peptidoglycan; 5, capsular layer. In A, antibodies were marked with gold particles; in B, ferritin-labeled antibodies were used. Bar = 0.2 μm (for details, see Sørensen et al.[73]). By courtesy of Dr. U.B.S. Sørensen.

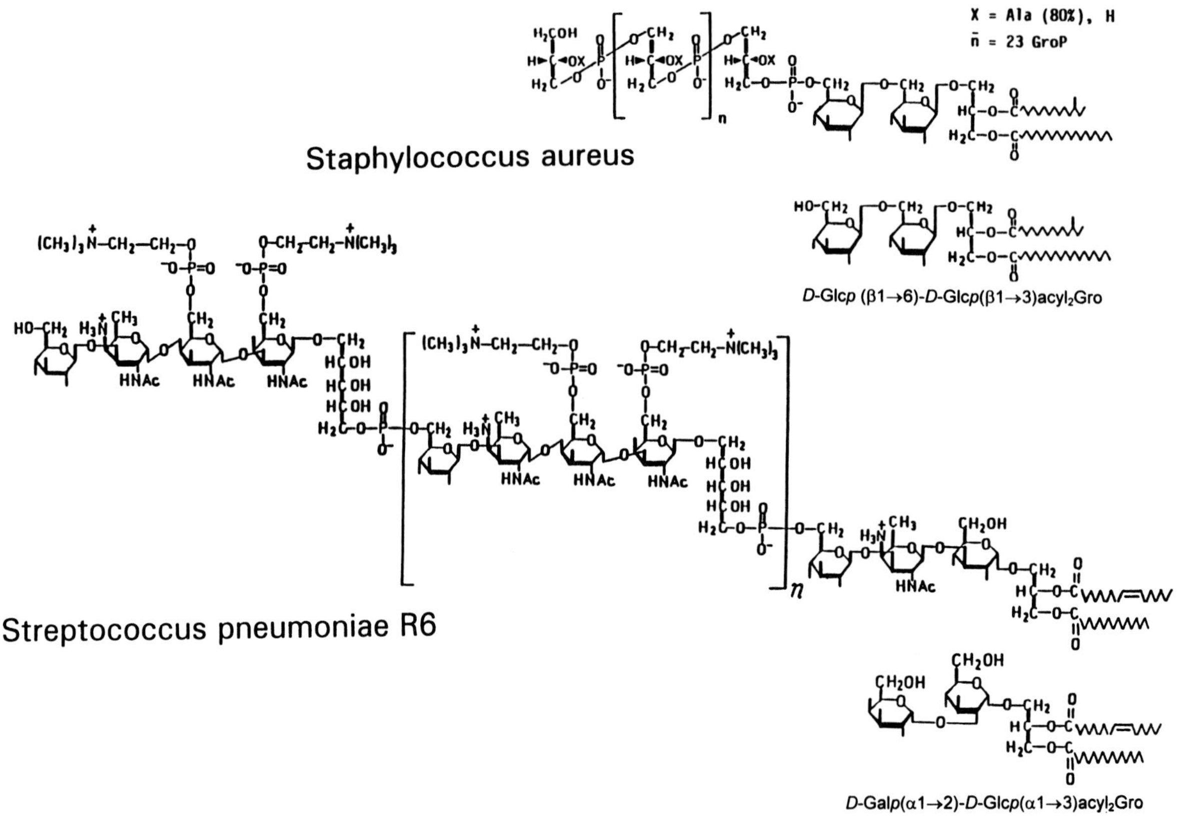

FIG. 3. Structure of pneumococcal LTA[4] in comparison with a classical phosphodiester-linked poly(glycerophosphate) LTA. The major membrane glycolipids of the two bacteria are depicted below the respective lipid anchors.

LTA containing ribitol phosphate and phosphocholine has been suggested to occur in *Streptococcus oralis*,[41] which is genetically closely related to *S. pneumoniae*.[44] A similar LTA may be expected to occur in the *S. oralis* group comprising the formerly named *Streptococcus sanguis* II, *Streptococcus viridans* I, II, IV, and *Streptococcus "mitior,"* which all possess ribitol phosphate and phosphocholine in their TAs.[44] From the TA of *S. oralis*, HF released an oligomer of equimolar amounts of ribitol, galactose and galactosamine.[44] Lipid macroamphiphiles, consisting of oligosaccharide-substituted poly(ribitol phosphate), were reported for *Streptococcus defectivus* and *Streptococcus adjacens*.[31,70,71]

Extraction and purification of lipoteichoic acid

For extraction of pneumococcal LTA from mechanically disintegrated cells, the classical hot phenol/water procedure, used for the preparation of other LTAs, proved inappropriate because pneumococcal LTA partitions into the phenol layer along with the membrane lipids.[4] Instead a Bligh-Dyer procedure has been found appropriate: LTA and lipids are first extracted into a monophasic system (CHCl₃/MeOH/H₂O; 1:2:1, by volume), the cell walls are removed by centrifugation, and to the supernatant water and CHCl₃ are added to achieve phase separation (CHCl₃/MeOH/H₂O; 1:1:0.9, by volume). LTA is recovered from the aqueous layer and without any enzymatic treatment effectively purified by hydrophobic interaction chro-

matography (HIC). This one-step procedure is also the method of choice for the purification of LTAs and lipoglycans from other gram-positive bacteria, which are extracted by the hot phenol/water procedure.[17,20] Crude preparations are dissolved in 0.05 M sodium acetate, pH 4.7, containing 10–15% n-propanol and applied to octyl Sepharose columns, preequilibrated, and first eluted with this solvent. Nucleic acids, polysaccharides and proteins, being not hydrophobic, are eluted by this step. Lipid macroamphiphiles require to be eluted a propanol gradient, which continuously weakens the hydrophobic interaction between the hydrocarbon chains of the amphiphile and the octyl groups of the matrix. As a consequence of this separation principle, LTAs and lipoglycans elute in the order of increasing hydrophobicity, i.e. in the order of decreasing size of the headgroup[50] and, if present, increasing number of fatty acids.[20,51] The elution profile of pneumococcal LTA is shown later (see Fig. 16).

Structural analysis of lipoteichoic acid

The structure of lipoteichoic acid was accomplished by chemical analysis and fast atom bombardment mass spectrometry (FAB-MS). Independently, the whole structure was established by ^{1}H, ^{13}C, and ^{31}P NMR spectroscopy.[4]

These procedures made it possible to derive the structure from the analysis of the chain and three key products. Two of these key products, the acylated glycolipid and the dephos-

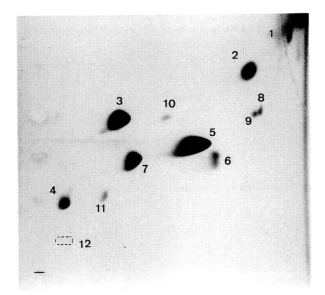

FIG. 4. TLC of crude membrane lipids of *Streptococcus pneumoniae* Rx1, grown on choline-containing medium (W. Fischer, unpublished data). Identification: 1, nonpolar lipids; 2, D-Glcp(α1 → 3)acyl$_2$Gro; 3, D-Galp(α1 → 2)-D-Glcp(α1 → 3)acyl$_2$Gro; 4, phosphoglucolipid; 5, bis(phosphatidyl)glycerol; 6, polyprenolphosphate; 7, phosphatidyl glycerol; 8–11, not identified; 12, location of the lipid anchor (when added to the lipid extract). Silica gel (Merck 60); first development (upward): CHCl$_3$/MeOH/H$_2$O (65:25:4, by vol.); second development: CHCl$_3$/AcOH/MeOH/H$_2$O (80:14:10:3, by vol.). Visualization: phosphomolybdic acid and charring.

phorylated repeat, were released by hydrolysis with 48% HF (2–4°C, 36 h). Under these conditions HF cleaves phosphodiester and phosphomonoester bonds releasing choline and the total phosphorus as inorganic phosphate. The β-glycosidic linkage between D-GalNAcp and ribitol is unexpectedly susceptible to acid hydrolysis, so that, dependent on the duration of treatment with HF, increasing amounts of this cleavage product are formed. The water-soluble chain fragments and the glycolipid anchor are separated by phase partitioning.

Structure of the lipid anchor and the dephosphorylated repeat. Figure 5 shows the positive ion FAB-MS of the peracetylated derivatives of the lipid anchor (Fig. 5A) and the dephosphorylated tetrasaccharide-ribitol (Fig. 5B). The components were N-acetylated, using (C^{2}H$_3$CO)$_2$O, and then peracetylated with (CH$_3$CO)$_2$. Primary fragmentation occurs at the glycosidic bonds, so that in Fig. 5A,B the resulting primary ions (marked by asterisks) reveal the sugar sequence from the nonreducing terminus: at m/z = 331, glucosyl; at m/z = 562 the disaccharide containing the AATGal residue; at m/z = 850 and 849, the trisaccharide containing an additional glucosyl in the glycolipid and an additional N-acetylgalactosaminyl residue in the repeat. In the spectrum of the repeat, the ions at m/z = 303, 608 and 1123 show the sugar sequence from the reducing terminus of the molecule (marked by a solid square). The molecular ion [M+H$^+$] at m/z = 1456 (1453) confirms the overall structure. The spectrum of the repeat also illustrates how the number of non–N-acetylated aminogroups in the native compound can be determined. When before peracetylation, the free

aminogroups are N-acetylated, using a mixture of acetic anhydride and its deuterated analogue, pairs of fragments are observed, whereby each free aminogroup contributes an increase by three mass units. The difference by three mass units between the ion pairs in the repeat of LTA therefore indicates one free amino group in the native compound, and the ion pairs at m/z 1453/1456, 846/849, and 559/562 along with the single ion at m/z 331 locate it on the AATGal residue.

In the glycolipid moiety, the major fatty acid combinations are 18:1/16:0 and 16:1/16:0 differing by 28 mass units. They are recognized in the molecular ions [M + H$^+$] at m/z = 1416/1444, the ions at m/z = 1086/1114 (from which the terminal glucose was lost), and in the diacylglycerol ions themselves at m/z = 549/577 (Fig. 5).

Structure of the bis(phosphocholine)-containing repeat. The third key product, used for analysis, is the repeat which retained the bis(phosphocholine) substituents and lost the intrachain phosphodiester (Fig. 6). It was obtained by alkaline hydrolysis, which selectively breaks the intrachain phosphodiester bonds via a cyclic intermediate, leaving isomeric phosphomonoester at O4 and O5 of the ribitol moiety,[2] which are readily removed with phosphomonoesterase. Negative ion FAB-MS of the N-acetylated derivative revealed a molecular ion [M + Cl$^-$] at m/z = 1313, which indicates the presence of two phosphocholine residues, consistent with chemical measurements. The fragments at m/z = 1263 (M − 15), 1245 (M' − 15), and m/z = 1192 (M − 87 + 1), 1174 (M' − 87 + 1) are characteristic for choline residues, reflecting the loss of CH$_3$ and (CH$_2$)$_2$N$^+$(CH$_3$)$_3$, respectively. The fragments at m/z = 923 (887 + 36) and m/z = 873 (923 − 50) may be ascribed to the bis(phosphocholine) di(N-acetylgalactosaminyl) ribitol moiety. The fragments at m/z 1295 (1313 − 18) and 1245 (1263 − 18) indicate repeats terminating in 2,5-anhydroribitol which is formed on alkali hydrolysis by a side reaction.[2] The fragmentation pattern did not allow to decide whether the phosphocholine residues are attached to separate N-acetylgalactosaminyl residues or to the same. The location at O6 of the two N-acetylgalactosaminyl residues was achieved by methylation analysis[4] and ^{31}P-^{1}H correlation spectroscopy[46]: the ^{31}P-resonances at 1.45 and 1.85 ppm could be assigned to O6 of ring C and D, respectively (for designations, see Fig. 8).

Connection between the repeats. The connection between the repeats was established by periodate oxidation.[4] Per repeat it re-

TABLE 1. BIOSYNTHETIC PRECURSORS OF LTA[16,19] AND THE TA-LINKAGE UNIT-COMPLEX[1,37,61a,79]

Precursor	LTA	TA
Lipid anchor	Glycolipid	None
Polyol-*P*-donor	Phosphatidyl glycerol	CDP-glycerol
		CDP-ribitol
Glycosyl donor	Prenol-*P*-Gal	UDP-Gal
	Prenol-*P*-Glc	UDP-Glc
		UDP-GlcNAc
		UDP-ManNAc

For biosynthetic schemes of LTA[19] and the TA-linkage unit-complex,[19,61a] see the references given. In the synthesis of the TA-linkage unit-complex, C$_{55}$-P serves as an intermediate lipid carrier. Prenol, undecaprenol (C$_{55}$-OH).

48% HF-DEGRADATION OF LTA

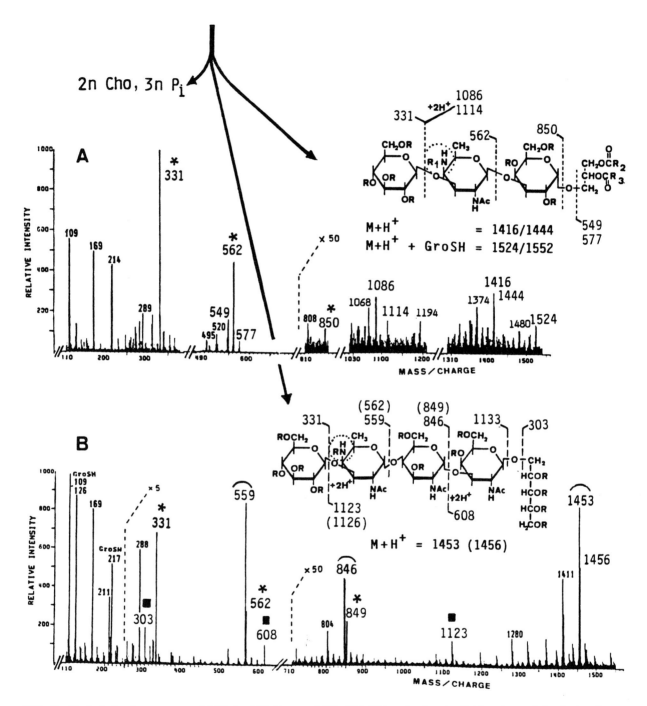

FIG. 5. Hydrolysis of pneumococcal LTA by 48% (by mass) HF, 4°C, 36 h, releasing the lipid anchor and the dephosphorylated repeats whereby choline is liberated and total phosphorus released as inorganic phosphate. Positive-ion FAB mass spectrum of the N-deuteroacetylated and peracetylated lipid anchor (R = CH$_3$CO; R$_1$ = C^{2}H$_3$CO; R$_2$, R$_3$, hydrocarbon chains of fatty acids) **(A)** and the dephosphorylated repeats that were before peracetylation N-acetylated using a mixture of (CH$_3$CO)$_2$O and (C^{2}H$_3$CO)$_2$O **(B)**. For fragmentation, see text. (Modified from data in Behr et al.[4])

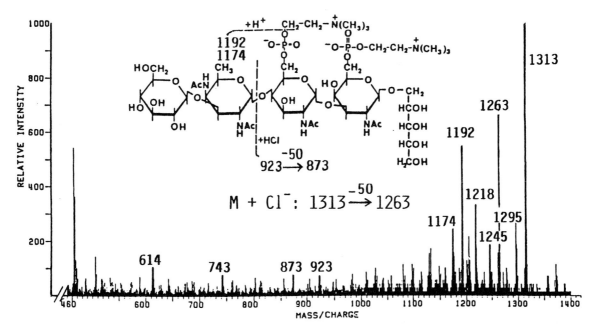

FIG. 6. Negative-ion FAB-mass spectrum of the *N*-acetylated bis(phosphocholine)-containing repeat-unit and its fragmentation scheme.

sulted in the reduction of 4-mol equivalent periodate and concomitant formation of 2-mol equivalents formate, one derived from C3 of the ribitol and one from C3 of the D-glucopyranosyl moiety. The carbonyl groups formed were reduced with NaBH₄ and finally the acetal bonds were split by mild acid hydrolysis (0.1 M HCl, 37°C, 24 h). This procedure led to ethyleneglycolphosphoryl glycerol, which contains C4 and C5 of the ribitol and C4 to C6 of the adjacent D-glucopyranosyl moiety, indicating, consistent with the data of periodate oxidation, that the phosphodiester links ribitol 5-phosphate to O6 of the adjacent glucosyl moiety. The same was shown to be true for the attachment of the chains to the terminal glucose of the glycolipid moiety.

Controlled periodate oxidation of LTA cleft the ribitol residues but left the glucopyranosyl rings intact. The carbonyl groups were reduced with NaBH₄ and the derivative, purified by column chromatography on Sephadex G25, was peracetylated. Analysis by (+) FAB-MS yielded only the molecular ion [M + H⁺] at mz 1607. Therefore, on the molecular ion a high energy collision-induced dissociation experiment (MS/MS) was performed. Assignments of the fragment ions, depicted in Fig. 7, confirm the proposed linkage between the repeats and made it possible to locate the two phosphocholine residues at O6 of the galactosaminyl moieties.

Molecular weight. A sample of lipoteichoic acid was de–*O*-acylated, *N*-acetylated, and analyzed by positive-ion ultraviolet laser-induced desorption/ionization MS.[4] The molecular ion area [M + Na⁺]⁺ revealed three peaks at m/z = 7027.2, 8337.2 (major) and 9623.5 corresponding to species carrying on the deacylated glycolipid chains of five, six, and seven repeats (calculated nominal values 7056, 8334, and 9612, respectively).

Nuclear magnetic resonance spectroscopy

Confirmation of structure. Independent proof of the proposed structure and information concerning the conformation was ob-

tained by NMR spectroscopy.[46] Using 500-MHz ¹H¹H-COSY and ¹H-detected C,H-COSY (HMQC), it was possible to assign unequivocally all proton resonances for the four hexopyranosyl residues of the bis(phosphocholine)-containing tetrasaccharide-ribitol repeat. Figure 9 compares the 2D-NOESY spectra of (a) the isolated N-acetylated (Cho*P*)₂-substituted repeat and (b) the per–*N*-acetylated oligomeric chain of five to seven (Cho*P*)₂-substituted repeats, attached to the de-acylated glycolipid anchor (for structures and alphabetical sugar ring labeling, see Fig. 8). The signals for α-anomeric protons at 4.99 ppm (³J_{H,H} 4.0 Hz) and 5.21 ppm (³J_{H,H} 3.9 Hz) are assigned to ring B and C, the β-anomeric protons at 4.61 ppm (³J_{H,H} 7.8) and 4.67 ppm (³J_{H,H} 8.6 Hz) to ring A and D, respectively (Fig. 9). The 6-methyl group resonance at 1.07 ppm, belonging to ring B with its anomeric proton at 4.99 ppm, served to differentiate between the two α-D-galactopyranosyl spin systems. The β-sugars were distinguishable based upon the absence of the glycosylation shift for the glucopyranosyl ring in the isolated repeat. For the oligomeric chain, the anomeric resonances of both β-glucosyl residues, one being part of the repeat (A), and the other of the deacylated lipid anchor (F), coincide. An additional anomeric resonance (A′) of low intensity is ascribed to the non-phosphorylated β-D-glucopyranosyl residue at the end of the chain. The anomeric resonances of the two other sugars of the deacylated lipid anchor, the β-2,4-diacetamido-2,4,6-trideoxygalactose (G) and the α-glucose (H), are of the expected low intensity.

In the 2D-NOESY spectra of Fig. 9, five interresidue cross peaks are observed. Cross-peaks 1, 3 and 4 represent the connectivities between the protons at both sites of the glycosidic bond, A1 → B3, B1 → C4, C1 → D3. Cross-peaks 2 and 5 also are interproton through space connectivities, connecting A1 → B4 and C1 → D4, i.e., proton 1 of the glycon and the equatorial proton 4 on the Gal ring of the aglycon, which provide ad-

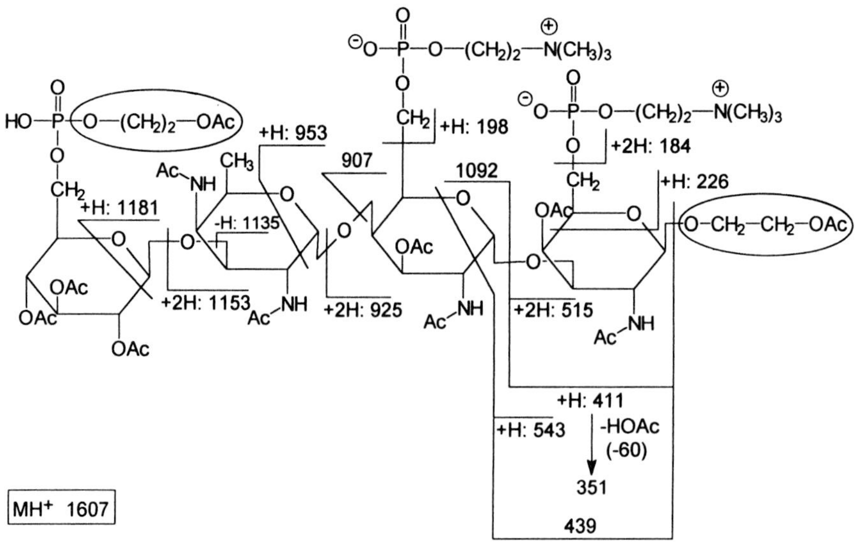

FIG. 7. Assignment of daughter ions obtained by MS/MS of the peracetylated (ChoP)$_2$ repeat containing the NaBH$_4$-reduced fragments of the periodate-oxidized ribitol phosphate moieties. The two ethyleneglycol residues derived from ribitol phosphates are highlighted by ellipses. The starting material in this experiment was the LTA of *S. pneumoniae* R6 (Fischer, W. and G. Pohlentz, unpublished data).

ditional conformational information for these glycosidic linkages. Accordingly, the sugar sequence and the attachment sites of the glycosidic bonds at the aglycon follow directly from the assignment of the cross peaks (Table 2).

Conformation of N-acetylated lipoteichoic acid. Comparing the spectra of the isolated tetrasaccharide ribitol-unit and the oligomeric chain in Fig. 9, it is quite clear that they are very similar and that the chemical shifts of the conformational important cross peaks are practically identical. This observation means that in aqueous solution the conformation of the bis(phosphocholine)-containing tetrasaccharide ribitol is the

same, whether it is present as isolated repeat or incorporated by phosphodiester bonds into a chain of five to seven repeats.

Figure 10 shows a three-dimensional model of the bis(phosphocholine)-containing tetrasaccharide-ribitol which is based on the NOE-derived distance constraints. Computer calculations by CHARMm, molecular mechanic dynamic methods, and Monte Carlo simulation were used to take account of charge, hydrogen bonding and solvent effects. The glycosidic linkages between the sugar residues appear to be relatively stiff, probably due to substituent steric effects. The linkage between the β-GalNAc (D) and the ribitol residue (E) is rather mobile but

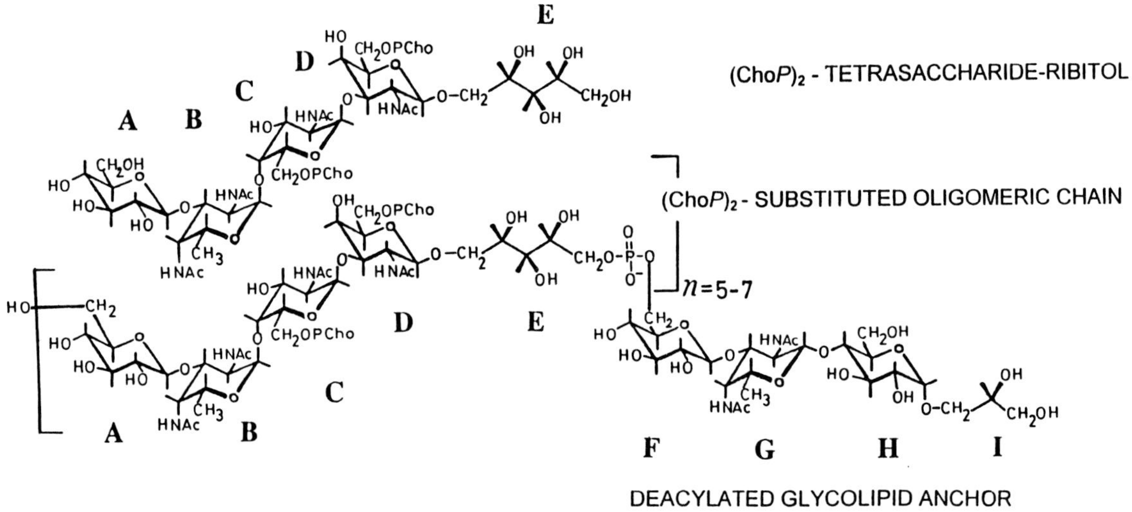

FIG. 8. Pneumococcal LTA (per-*N*-acetylated): Isolated (ChoP)$_2$-tetrasaccharide-ribitol repeat and (ChoP)$_2$-substituted oligomeric chain (5-7 phosphodiester-linked repeats), attached to the deacylated glycolipid anchor. **A–I:** Sugar-unit labeling of components. Alphabetical labeling indicates the following components: β-D-Glucopyranosyl (A); 2-acetamido-4-amino-2,4,6-trideoxy-α-D-galactopyranosyl (B); 2-*N*-acetyl-α-D-galactopyranosyl-6-phosphocholine (C); 2-*N*-acetyl-β-D-galactopyranosyl-6-phosphocholine (D); ribitol (E); β-D-glucopyranosyl (F); 2-acetamido-4-amino-2,4,6-trideoxy-β-D-galactopyranosyl (G); α-D-glucopyranosyl (H); glycerol (I).

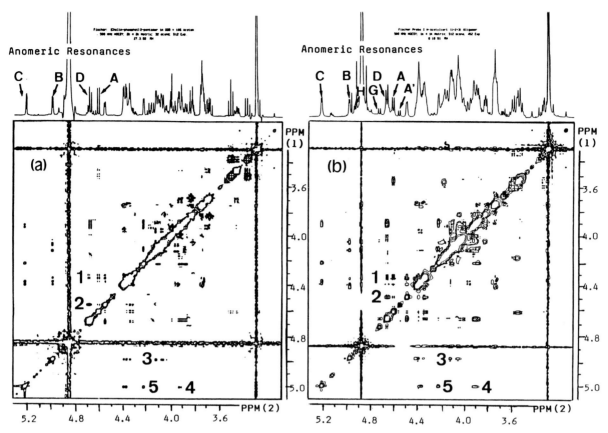

FIG. 9. 2D-NOESY spectra for the *N*-acetylated (Cho*P*)₂-substituted tetrasaccharide-ribitol repeat (**a**) and the oligomeric per-*N*-acetylated (Cho*P*)₂-substituted chain, attached to the deacylated glycolipid anchor (**b**). The anomeric protons A–D, A′, G, and H are indicated using the same alphabetical sugar-unit labeling as in Fig. 8. 1–5, NOESY cross-peaks, that are the conformationally important ones; for the definition of their numbering, see Table 2. The spectra were recorded at 500 MHz in aqueous solution at 300 K. (Reprinted with permission from *Carbohydrate Research.*[46])

the ribitol itself is unexpectedly immobile. Figure 11 shows the three-dimensional structure of a bis(phosphocholine)-containing chain in which the stretched ribitol moieties are readily recognized. Molecular dynamic simulations show that on heating and cooling two adjacent chains, lying next to one another, may interact to form condensed helical-like complexes. Such complexes may occur in LTA micelles (see Fig. 18) rather than on the surface of the cytoplasma membrane.

Conformational mobility induced by the positively charged AATGal residue. A conformational role of the AATGal residue

(Fig. 8, ring B) became apparent on ³¹P-NMR spectroscopy (Fig. 12).[47] When the AATGal residue of the isolated bis(phosphocholine)-containing tetrasaccharide ribitol-repeat is *N*-acetylated, two sharp resonances are seen at 1.45 and 1.85 ppm, one for each phosphocholine residue (Fig. 12a). These two resonances are also seen with the *N*-acetylated oligomer, where at lower field at 3.60 ppm another sharp resonance comes from the phosphodiester-group, interlinking the repeats (Fig. 12b). When, however, the AATGal residue is in its native positively charged form, all resonances are broadened, in particular that

TABLE 2.   NOE Cross-Peaks Observed in the 500 MHz 2D-NOESY Spectrum of Bis(phosphocholine)-Containing Tetrasaccharide-Ribitol, Measured in D₂O at 303K

NOE cross-peaks	PPM(1)	PPM(2)	Distance Å	Assigned H(1)→H(x)
1	4.625	4.363	2.48	A-1→B-3
2	4.625	4.507	2.72	A-1→B-4
3	5.012	4.142	2.26	B-1→C-4
4	5.222	3.922	2.33	C-1→D-3
5	5.222	4.230	2.35	C-1→D-4

H–H distances were calculated using the H-1–H-3–H-5 distances in Gal*N*Ac and the H-1–H-5 distance in sugar residue B (AATGal). For designation of sugar residues (A–C), see Fig. 8.
From Klein et al.[47]

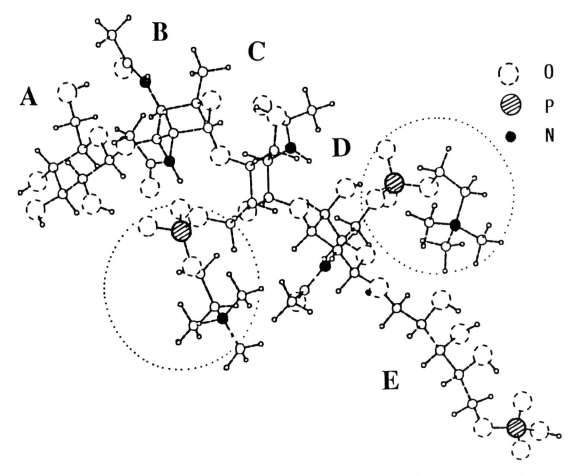

FIG. 10. The three-dimensional structure of the *N*-acetylated bis(phosphocholine)-containing tetrasaccharide-ribitol repeat-unit with NOE-derived distance constraints applied during minimization. The NOE effects were measured in the *N*-acetylated repeat-unit and in the intact per-*N*-acetylated oligomeric chain consisting of five to seven repeat units (mole weights: 7056, 8334, and 9612). The phosphocholine residues are encircled. For A–E, see Fig. 8. O, P, and N represent atoms. (Reprinted with permission from *Carbohydrate Research.*[46])

of the intrachain phosphate group (Fig. 12c,d). These findings suggest that the positively charged aminogroup of AATGal interacts electrostatically or by hydrogen bonding with the negative charge of the phosphate group on the adjacent glucosyl residue.

In Fig. 13, 2D-NOESY spectra are compared for the bis(phosphocholine)-substituted oligomer with *N*-acetylated AATGal residues and its bis(phosphocholine)-containing native analog, in which the AATGal residues are positively charged. The dotted lines, which are in right angles to the diagonal, connect cross peaks of the two spectra whose chemical shifts are not affected by acetylation of the amino group. The heavy lines, which are not in right angles to the diagonal, connect those cross-peaks that exhibit substantial substitution shifts. They generally involve the protons of ring B, the AAT-Gal residue. Moreover, the cross peak volumes for these H-H interactions also show marked differences—highlighted by the rectangles. These volume differences indicate changes of the inter-proton distances and, as shown in Table 3, the largest effect is seen for the relative distance between proton 3 and 5.

These changes of interproton distances can only be explained by considering different ring conformations of the AATGal residue.

Apart from the most stable $^4C_1$ chair conformation, other conformations, such as boat, skew, or even inverted $_4C^1$ chair, are possible for hexopyranoses. If we express the various ring conformations in terms of ring torsion tor2 (C-1–C-2–C-3–C-4) and plot them against the distance between proton 3 and 5 (Fig. 14), then we find these distances an appropriate measure for differentiating between the various conformers.

Molecular dynamic simulations using model compounds reveal pure chair conformation, if the AATGal residue is *N*-acetylated. But, if it is in the positively charged native form, equal populations in the ($^4C_1$)-chair and the energetically less favored ($^5S_1$) skew conformation are observed (Fig. 15). The change in conformation is induced by the strong interaction between the positively charged 4-aminogroup of the AATGal residue and the phosphate group on the adjacent glucosyl moiety, which compels the aminogroup from the axial into the equatorial position (Fig. 15). Accordingly, pure chair conformation is

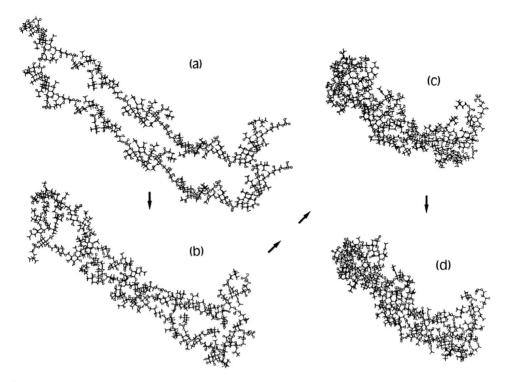

FIG. 11. The copolymerized complex of two adjacent per-*N*-acetylated oligomeric chains is shown after different stages in molecular dynamic simulation: starting conformation (**a**); after 10-ps simulation at 600 K (**b**); after a further 50-ps simulation (**c**); and after cooling (simulated annealing) from 600 K to absolute zero (**d**). The final copolymer is stabilized by hydrogen bonds, 157 in total, mainly between saccharide ring hydroxyl groups. (Reprinted with permission from *Carbohydrate Research*.[46])

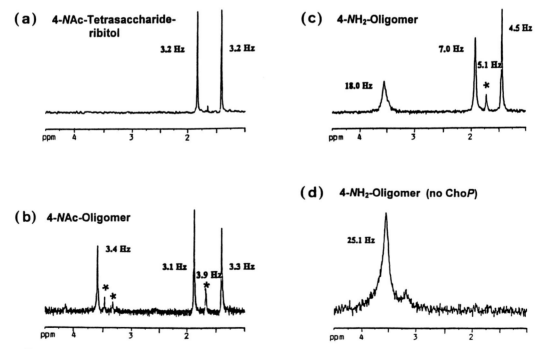

FIG. 12. ^{31}P spectra at 202.45 MHz for (Cho$P$)$_2$-tetrasaccharide ribitol repeat with a 4-*N*-acetylated AATGal-residue (**a**); per-*N*-acetylated (Cho$P$)$_2$-oligomeric chain (**b**); native (Cho$P$)$_2$-oligomeric chain, with positively charged 4-NH_2-groups on the AAT-Gal-residues (**c**); and Cho$P$-free oligomeric chain with positively charged 4-NH_2 groups on the AATGal-residues (**d**). The small peaks marked with an asterisk are those originating from terminal repeat units. All chemical shifts are referred to Na$_3$PO$_4$ as an internal standard at 6.0 ppm. (Reprinted with permission from *Carbohydrate Research*.[47])

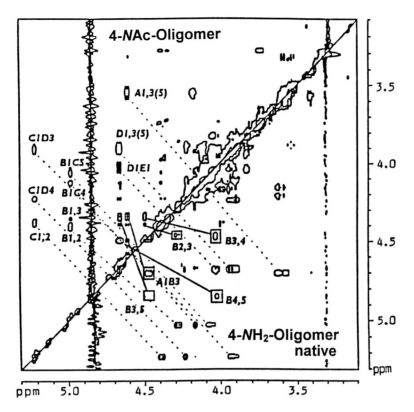

FIG. 13. Comparison of the 2D-NOESY spectra for deacylated LTA in the 4-*N*-acetylated form (upper left) and in the native form containing the positively charged 4-*N*H₂ groups (lower right). Both interresidue (e.g., A1B3) and intraresidue [e.g., A1,3(5)] cross-peaks are shown, with dotted lines indicating equivalent peaks in the two spectra. Cross-peaks that are shifted by *N*-acetylation are connected by solid lines. They are generally associated with the B residues and highlighted by rectangles for the native 4-*N*H₂ oligomeric chain. (Reprinted with permission from *Carbohydrate Research.*[47])

reestablished when the phosphate group is removed, in spite of the positively charged AATGal residue.

Due to the presence of AATGal in each repeat, the conformation of the whole chain will be affected which possibly may explain the unusual behavior on phenol/water extraction.[4] Of particular future interest is the interaction of the native zwitterionic teichoic acids and their artificial negatively charged *N*-acetylated derivatives with the various proteins that are able to recognize and interact with pneumococcal teichoic acids.

Forssman antigenicity

Among the properties of crude LTA preparations is Forssman antigenicity.[32] Forssman antigens, defined by the ability to induce rabbits to form hemolytic antibodies to sheep

red blood cells, have been reported for a wide variety of animal organs and bacteria (for references, see Fraser and Mallette[19]). The Forssman hapten sphingolipids from horse spleen and kidney,[69] canine intestine and kidney,[74] sheep erythrocytes,[23] as well as Forssman reactive streptococcal group C polysaccharide[11] have in common the nonreducing terminus D-Gal*N*Ac(α1-3)-D-Gal*N*Ac(β1 → .., which has been established to be the immunodeterminant of Forssman reactivity.

When crude LTA preparations are subjected to hydrophobic interaction chromatography, the elution profiles of LTA phosphorus and Forssman antigenicity do not coincide (Fig. 14). Forssman antigenicity is highest at the lower descending part of the phosphate elution profile, where shorter-chain LTA species with decreasing phosphocholine content elute.

TABLE 3.   RELATIVE INTER-PROTON DISTANCES WITHIN THE HEXAPYRANOSE RING B USING THE H-3–H-4 DISTANCE AS THE REFERENCE (=1.00), DETERMINED FROM THE INTEGRATED CROSS-PEAK VOLUMES IN THE 2D-NOESY SPECTRA

Cross-peaks (NOE)	2-NAc-4-NH₂ oligomer	2,4-di-NAc oligomer	2,4-di-NAc tetrasaccharide ribitol
B1,2	0.92	0.95	0.96
B3,4	1.00	1.00	1.00
B4,5	1.04	0.92	0.94
B3,5	1.25	1.05	1.06

From *Carbohydrate Research.*[47]

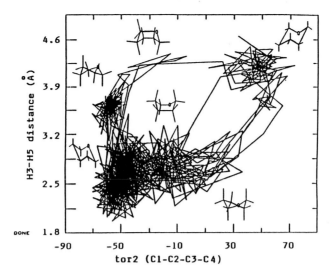

FIG. 14. A plot of tor2 (C-1–C-2–C-3–C-4) against the interproton distance H-3–H-5 for the 2-acetamido-4-amino-2,4,6-trideoxygalactopyranose ring illustrating its use for determining the ring conformation. (Reprinted with permission from *Carbohydrate Research.*[47])

Although the repeat

$$\begin{array}{cc} \text{Cho}P & \text{Cho}P \\ | & | \end{array}$$

—[6-D-Glc(β1-3)-D-α-AATGal(α1-4)-D-GalNAc(α1-3)-

D-GalNAc(β1-1)-ribitol-5-*P*-]—

contains D-GalNAc(α1-3)-D-GalNAc(β1 → , but not terminal and substituted with phosphocholine residues, it is unlikely to possess Forssman antigenicity. We rather expect Forssman antigenicity to be associated with incomplete biosynthetic inter-

mediates or decomposed species, possessing phosphocholine-free disaccharide as nonreducing terminus. These suggestions are supported by the observation that 152 out of 164 pneumococcal isolates cross-reacted with antiserum against streptococcal group C polysaccharide,[72] which contains as immunodeterminant D-GalNAc(α1-3)-D-Gal(β1 → as side branches.[11]

Other properties of Forssman antigen, such as the effect on the activity[39,40] or cellular distribution[5] of pneumococcal autolytic enzyme, and the activation of the mammalian complement cascade[42,82] require the presence of phosphocholine

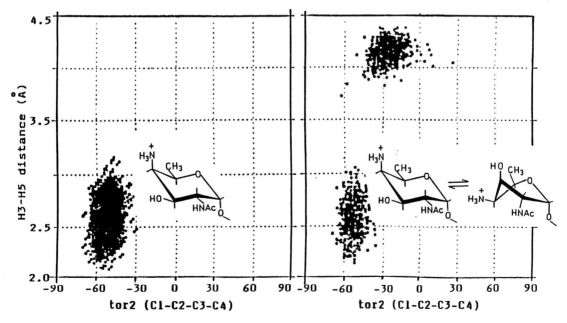

FIG. 15. The ring torsion tor2 (C-1–C-2–C-3–C-4) plotted against the H-3–H-5 distance for the negatively charged partial trisaccharide Me-β-D-glucose-6-phosphate-(1 → 3)-2,4-diacetamido-2,4,6-trideoxy-α-D-galactose-[6-Cho*P*]-(1 → 4) *N*-acetyl-α-D-galactosamine (left) and analog plot for the zwitterionic 2-acetamido-4-amino-2,4,6-trideoxy-α-D-galactose analog (right). (Redrawn with permission from *Carbohydrate Research.*[47])

residues and may, in contrast to Forssman antigenicity, represent biological activities of the LTA itself.

Microheterogeneity

From octyl Sepharose macroamphiphiles elute in the order of increasing hydrophobicity, i.e., decreasing length of the hydrophilic chain. As can be seen from Fig. 16, the chain length of this LTA preparation varied between five and two repeats. Mass spectrometry of another sample showed mostly chains with six repeats, accompanied by smaller amounts of species with five and seven.[4] Microheterogeneity is also seen on SDS PAGE where LTAs yield a ladder-like pattern of up to six or seven bands, each differing from the next by one repeat. Species with one phosphocholine per repeat are distinguished from species with two by higher mobility of the individual bands.[88]

Supramolecular structure of lipoteichoic acid

The unusually complex zwitterionic chain structure and the positively charged lipid anchor of pneumococcal LTA initiated a study by x-ray small angle scattering of its supramolecular organization in aqueous dispersion. We found earlier that variously substituted poly(glycerophosphate) LTAs as well as a lipoglycan formed very similar globular micelles over a wide range of temperature at various salt concentrations.[49]

Figure 17 shows the x-ray scattering equivalent electron density profile of pneumococcal LTA[22] in comparison with that obtained earlier with staphylococcal LTA.[49] Keeping in mind that the profile obtained is just a scattering equivalent to the real structure and that there may exist other scattering equivalents, an interpretation of the fine-structure of the profile, especially of the modulations in its outer part, can only be speculative. Nevertheless, the model profiles seem to demonstrate

the lipid core of the micelles: in the center of the micelle, electron densities lower than the water level (0.0) with a rapid increase of density towards the hydrophilic head of the lipid anchor. Starting 3 and 4 nm from the center of the micelle a strong decline in electron density is observed followed by a subsequent gradual and modulated decrease until the density reaches water level at about 11–12 nm from the center. The density modulations are more exaggerated with staphylococcal LTA, and the differences may be due to differences in the hydrophilic chain structures. Theoretical calculations and NMR measurements suggested a certain stiffness of the pneumococcal chain[46] which may leave less space for coiling and result in a more continous decrease of electron density. As depicted in Fig. 18, the dimensions of the two micelles are similar: The lipid core has a diameter of 5 nm and a surface area of 78.5 nm[2], providing space for 160 LTA molecules (surface area of diacylglycerol molecule 0.5 nm[2]). In the hydrophilic shell of a thickness of 8.5 nm, the hydrophilic chains of *Staphylococcus aureus* LTA, measuring in stretched conformation 18.8 nm (25 glycerophosphate residues) are more tightly packed than the chains of pneumococcal LTA, measuring in stretched conformation 17.3 nm (7.2 repeats).[22]

From these and previous observations we may conclude that, independent of the greatly varying hydrophilic chain structures, the critical structural element that is responsible for the micellar organization is the diacylglycerol moiety of lipoteichoic acids and lipoglycans. It renders the ratios of the cross sectional areas of the hydrophilic to the hydrophobic moiety larger than one, resulting in a conical molecular shape. This behavior discriminates LTAs from most membrane lipids and from LPS of gram-negatigve bacteria which, due to their cylindrical shape, preferentially adopt lamellar structures.[48,59,60] Accordingly, pneumococcal lipoteichoic acid is expected to share with other

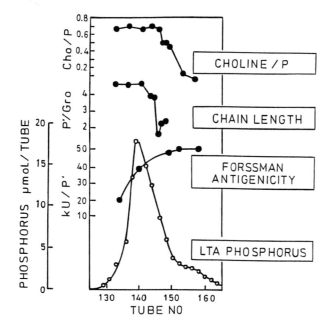

FIG. 16. Elution profile of LTA phosphorus from a column of octyl-Sepharose plotted against the molar ratio of choline/phosphorus, the chain length (molar ratio of intrachain-phosphorus/glycerol), and Forssman antigenicity (kU/μmol intrachain-phosphorus). P, total phosphorus; P′, intrachain phosphorus (total phosphorus − phosphocholine-phosphorus). (Modified from data in Behr et al.[4])

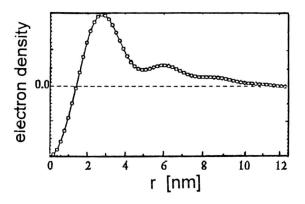 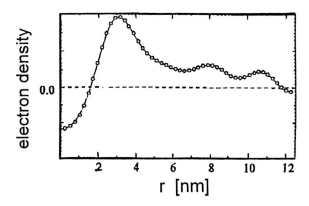

FIG. 17. X-ray scattering analysis of the supramolecular structure in aqueous dispersion. Depicted is the scattering equivalent electron density profile of a micelle of pneumococcal lipoteichoic acid (left) in comparison with a micelle of *S. aureus* lipoteichoic acid (right). The profiles were obtained by a least-square fit of the corresponding distance-distribution function with respect to the experimental distribution function. The graph shows the electron-density profiles (arbitrary units) along a line from the center of the micelle ($r = 0$ nm) to its outside boundary ($r \approx 11.5$ nm).[22] Electron density of water set zero. Values for *S. aureus* LTA were taken from Labischinski *et al.*[49]

lipoteichoic acids the inability to form stable monolayers and to require *in vivo* membranes of lamellar phase lipids to be inserted.[19,36]

The different arrangement of LTA in aqueous dispersion and in association with the cytoplasmic membrane should be considered when the results of experiments on biological activities are interpreted. Pneumococcal TA, which forms monomolecular solutions, has the capacity to activate the alternative complement pathway,[82] but LTA, present as micelles, acquires this capacity not before binding to the surface of erythrocytes.[42] This binding occurs through insertion of the acyl chains into the lipid bilayer and predictably results in an oriented presentation of single chains.

LTA in aqueous dispersion possesses the capacity to block the activity of pneumococcal autolysin in a dose-dependent and specific manner: pneumococcal TA and ethanol-amine-containing LTA were not inhibitory.[5,39] The inhibitory capacity is apparently dependent on the micellar organization because it was lost through binding of LTA to Sepharose, deacylation, or embedding it into detergent micelles.[5,39] On the surface of the micelle, the accumulation of phosphocholine residues apparently effects a particularly firm binding of autolysin and thus prevents its access to the cell wall substrate.[5] As in pneumococcal cells LTAs are present in the cytoplasmic membrane presumably as monomeric chains, the proposed regulation of the autolytic activity by LTA is unlikely.

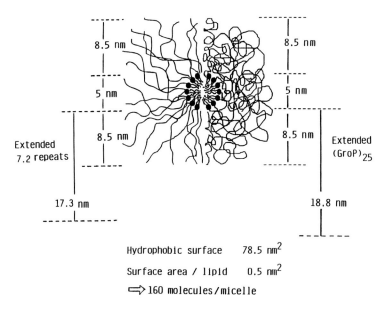

FIG. 18. Schematic view of a cross-section through a tentative micelle of pneumococcal LTA (left) and staphylococcal LTA (right). (Redrawn from Fischer et al.[22])

TEICHOIC ACIDS

Preparation of cell walls and teichoic acid

Purified cell walls are prepared by standard procedures.[38] Immediately after harvesting, the cells are heated in 2–4% boiling sodium dodecyl sulfate (SDS) to inactivate degradative enzymes, and after cooling, SDS is removed by several washings with water. The inactivated cells are mechanically disintegrated. Nucleic acids and proteins are removed by successive treatment with nucleases and trypsin. After a second extraction with SDS, follows successive centrifugation with water, 5.8 M LiCl, and 10 mM EDTA.

The release of TA chains from cell walls by repeated treatment with 10% TCA at 4°C is rather ineffective, but so far the only procedure available.[10,21,43] TAs of other gram-positive bacteria which are attached to peptidoglycan by a linkage unit can be released by mild acid and mild alkaline treatment.[1,37] These classical procedures proved inappropriate with pneumococcal TA because mild acid hydrolysis led to a cleavage of the glycosidic bond between GalNAc and ribitol, and the anchoring of TA to the cell wall resisted mild alkaline treatment (W. Fischer, unpublished data). Nevertheless, the formation of MurNAc-6-P on acid hydrolysis[34,53] indicates the existence of a linkage unit, because the direct attachment of TA via its terminal ribitol phosphate to muramic acid would leave the phosphomonoester on the ribitol residue instead on MurNAc. ManNAc and glycerophosphate, typical components of the linkage units in other gram-positive bacteria,[1,37] could not be detected which may explain the observed resistance to mild alkaline treatment.

Identical chain structures of lipoteichoic acid and teichoic acid

The LTA chain structure, depicted in Fig. 3,[4] was similar to, but not identical with the TA structure proposed by Jennings et al.,[43] which contained only a single phosphocholine residue attached to the ribitol-linked galactosamine, and this galactosamine, being not N-acetylated, was positively charged. This difference prompted us to isolate the teichoic acid from Streptococcus pneumoniae R6,[21] from which we had previously isolated the LTA. The chromatogram in Fig. 19 shows that the phosphorylated repeats of TA are in number, chromatographic mobility, and intensity identical with those of LTA. The pattern of TA suggests major repeats with two phosphocholine residues and precludes a positively charged galactosaminyl residue. Chemical and NMR analyses confirmed these conclusions.[21]

The identical chain structures have two important consequences: (i) The conformational considerations, discussed for LTA, are also relevant for TA, and (ii) LTA and TA may share at least certain initial steps in biosynthesis. All so far known about biosynthesis is that the phosphocholine residues of LTA or the completed phosphocholine-containing LTA are not precursors of TA.[7]

In favor of common biosynthetic steps is also the similar chain length of LTA and TA and, for a given strain, the identical number of phosphocholine residues per repeat. From the data in Table 4, it can be calculated that in LTA and TA of S. pneumoniae R6 on the average 78% of the repeats are substi-

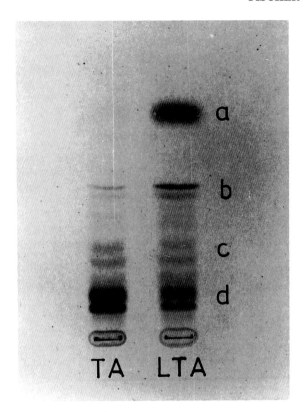

FIG. 19. TLC analysis of the alkaline hydrolysis products of teichoic acid and lipoteichoic acid, both isolated from S. pneumoniae R6.[21] Alkaline hydrolysis cleaves selectively the intrachain phosphate groups, leaving the phosphocholine residues intact. Via a cyclic phosphate intermediate at the ribitol moiety. O4 and O5-phosphomonoesters arise, leading to the double bands in the chromatogram. Before TLC, the samples were desalted and re-N-acetylated. Identification: repeat, containing two phosphocholine residues (**d**); one phosphocholine residue (**c**); no phosphocholine residue (**b**); lipid anchor (**a**). TLC, silica gel (Merck 60); solvent, propanol/25% (by mass) ammonia/H₂O (6:3:1, by vol.). Visualization: 1-naphthol/H₂SO₄.

tuted with two phosphocholine residues, 22% with one. In strain Rx1 the reverse is true: on the average 85% of the repeats carry one phosphocholine residue per repeat, 15% two. If the repeat is substituted with a single phosphocholine, this is attached to O6 of the non–ribitolphosphate-linked GalNAc residue (ring C in Fig. 8).

Cell wall composition and distribution of teichoic acids in the peptidoglycan network

The cell wall components of pneumococcus Rx1 and JY2190, a choline-independent derivative of it (see below) are shown in Table 5. The ratio of muramic acid-6-phosphate to total muramic acid indicates that in the peptidoglycan on average 19% of the muramic acid residues are substituted with TA. Similar values can be calculated from previous data[52,58] but in some preparations values up to 30% were observed (W. Fischer, K. Leopold, and C. Emilius, unpublished data). There is obviously a variation of the teichoic acid content associated

TABLE 4.   LTA AND TA OF *S. pneumoniae*
R6 AND *S. pneumoniae* Rx1

Strain	Component	Chain length (repeats/chain)	Cho/P	Cho/Repeat
R6	LTA	7.1 ± 0.7	0.63	1.70
	TA	n.d.	0.65	1.86
Rx1	LTA	6.7 ± 0.4	0.53	1.13
	TA	7.1 ± 1.5	0.54	1.17

Chain length of LTA, molar ratio of intrachain phosphorus to the lipid anchor glycerol; chain length of TA, molar ratio of intrachain phosphorus to *N*-acetylmuramyl-6-*P*; Cho/*P*, molar ratio of choline to total phosphorus; Cho/repeat, molar ratio of choline to intrachain phosphorus.

Rx1: for all structural studies, the nonlytic derivative Rx1/AL[-4a] was used.

with the reversible spontaneous phase variation between transparent and opaque phenotypes.[81] Compared with opaque variants, the transparent incorporate 1.5- to 4-fold more choline into their cell walls and, as measured by an ELISA, contain 2- to 3.8-fold higher amounts of cellular TA, whereas in the opaque phenotype the cellular content of capsular polysaccharide is higher. By testing the phase variants in animal models, it could be shown that pneumococcus varies between an avirulent transparent form, adapted for carriage, and a virulent opaque form, deficient in the ability to colonize the nasopharynx.[45] On the other hand it was shown that only transparent pneumococci possess the ability to transcytose through brain microvascular endothelial cells.[64a]

Insight into the distribution of TA within the peptidoglycan network has been obtained by cleavage of pneumococ-

cal cell walls with muramidases, followed by separation of TA-substituted and nonsubstituted muropeptides on molecular sieve columns[25,27] or by anion exchange chromatography (Fig. 20). As judged from the distribution of muropeptide markers (muramic acid, glutamic acid, radiolabeled lysine), 30–40% of the muropeptides are present in the TA-containing fraction.

Cleavage with muramidases of distinct substrate specificity led to the characterization of the TA-substituted muropeptides, depicted in Fig. 21. Noteworthy are muropeptides III and IV; they were released by a muramidase that does not cleave the glycosidic bond of TA-substituted muraminyl residues. The fact that by this enzyme mostly the depicted short-chain muropeptides were formed, precludes clustering of TA in the peptidoglycan network. On the other hand, muropeptides II and IV suggest a more or less regular distribution in so far as crosslinks seem to connect preferentially TA-substituted with nonsubstituted muropeptides.

Phosphocholine residues are also exposed on the surface of pneumococci. Live cells of various serotypes had similar amounts of surface phosphocholine accessible to antiphosphocholine antibody, and antiphosphocholine antibody protected mice against fatal pneumococcal infection.[86] Another example is the binding of wild-type pneumococci to CRP (C-polysaccharide reactive protein, an acute phase reactant) which can be completely inhibited by phosphocholine.[57] In addition, surface-exposed phosphocholine plays a role as an adhesive ligand for pneumocytes and peripheral endothelial cells,[30] and phosphocholine-specific binding was demonstrated to involve also the platelet-activating-factor receptor which enhances pneumococcal adherence and penetration of host cells.[12,64a]

TABLE 5.   COMPONENTS OF PURIFIED CELL WALLS
FROM STRAIN Rx1 AND THE MUTANT JY2190

Component	Concentration (μmol/mg[dry wt])	
	Rx1	JY2190
Teichoic acid		
Phosphate	1.11	0.58
Intrachain phosphate	0.56	0.58
Galactosamine	1.06	1.04
Glucose	0.63	0.63
Ribitol + 2,5-anhydroribitol	0.64	0.61
Choline	0.55	0
Peptidoglycan		
Muramic acid	0.34	0.38
Muramic acid–6–phosphate	0.07	0.09
Glucosamine	0.30	0.32
Glutamic acid	0.52	0.54
Serine	0.07	0.02
Alanine	0.85	0.83
Lysine	0.51	0.55

Rx1: see Table 4.
Intrachain-phosphate = total phosphate − choline phosphate.
Adapted from Yother et al.[87]

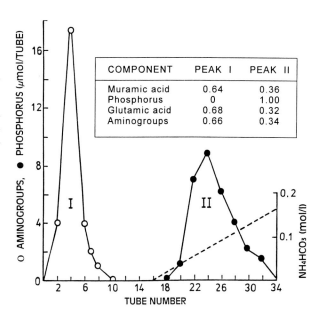

COMPONENT	PEAK I	PEAK II
Muramic acid	0.64	0.36
Phosphorus	0	1.00
Glutamic acid	0.68	0.32
Aminogroups	0.66	0.34

FIG. 20.   Separation of nonsubstituted muropeptides (I) and TA-containing muropeptides (II) on DEAE-Sephadex. **Inset:** Distribution of individual components between peak I and II. Muropeptides were released from cell walls of pneumococcus Rx1 with CPL (muramidase of pneumococcal bacteriophage Cp-1).[27,87]

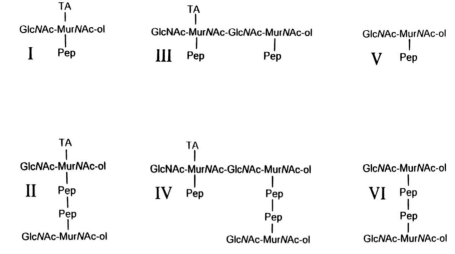

FIG. 21. Teichoic acid–containing muropeptides. Muropeptides I and II were released by a muramidase that cleaves the glycosidic bonds of TA-substituted and nonsubstituted MurNAc-residues; III and IV, were released by a muramidase that selectively cleaves the glycosidic bonds of nonsubstituted MurNAc-residues. The TA-free muropeptides V and VI were released by both enzymes. After enzymatic hydrolysis, cleavage points were marked by reduction with borohydride. Pep, stem peptides.

ROLE OF CHOLINE IN PNEUMOCOCCAL PHYSIOLOGY

Pneumococci are not able to synthesize the choline required for the synthesis of LTA and TA. Moreover, choline is an essential growth factor[3,63] but can be substituted in this function by nutritional ethanolamine.[77] Although ethanolaminephosphate is incorporated into LTA and TA at the same positions as phospocholine (W. Fischer, Hartmann R., and G. Pohlentz, unpublished data), it is not able to replace phosphocholine functionally. Ethanolamine-grown cells lack transformability,[77] and there is an increasing number of pneumococcal proteins that specifically recognize and bind to phosphocholine residues. The N-terminal domains of these proteins are distinct and responsible for the respective biological activity, whereas the C-terminal domains are highly homologous and contain 6 to 10 choline-recognizing repeats of 20 amino acids each. The question whether there are differences in the choline-binding domains in strains that contain two, respectively one phosphocholine per repeat has not yet been addressed.

Recently a genetic *lic* locus was identified that is required for phosphocholine metabolism in *S. pneumoniae*.[88] It contains eight genes, five of which are proposed to encode a choline permease and the enzymes that catalyze the activation of choline and the incorporation of phosphocholine into TA and LTA.

Cell wall lytic enzymes

N-Acetylmuramyl-L-alanine-amidase, the major autolytic enzyme (LytA) of pneumococci was the first reported protein to contain a C-terminal choline-binding domain of six choline-recognizing repeats.[28,54,67] LytA might be required for separation of daughter cells during cell division and is responsible for stationary phase, penicillin- and deoxycholate-induced cell lysis.[54,65,77] Binding of the amidase to the phosphocholine residues of TA[68] is prerequisite for peptidoglycan hydrolysis.[35,40] Phosphocholine on TA or LTA is also required for the conversion of the inactive E-form, in which LytA is synthe-

sized, into the active C-form.[5,78] Pneumococci possess an additional minor autolysin, characterized as endo-β-1,4-*N*-acetyl-glucosaminidase, which also requires phosphocholine-TA on its cell wall substrate.[29,54]

Since in ethanolamine-grown cells both autolysins are inactive, these cells form long chains, and are resistant to all kinds of autolysis. However, the requirement of LytA for built-in phosphocholine residues is no longer seen when cell walls are degraded to muropeptides[25] or when TA is removed from peptidoglycan.[68] Accordingly, also the TA-free cell walls of *Escherichia coli*, transfected with *lytA* are hydrolyzed *in vivo*.[14] These observations suggest that TA prevents the access of autolysin to its substrate and that this effect may be overcome by binding of the enzyme to the phosphocholine residues. The activity of LytA must be strictly regulated in growing cells. At the present time, however, the cellular location of LytA, the mechanism that keeps the enzyme inactive, and the mode of triggering its activity are still a matter of debate.[5,13,14,85]

Phosphocholine-recognizing C-terminal domains, similar to that of the host's autolysin, are found in amidases and muramidases of pneumococcal-specific bacteriophages.[27,26,54] These lytic enzymes are also dependent on cell wall–linked phosphocholine-substituted TA.

Pneumococcal surface protein A

Another well characterized protein that contains a C-terminal domain of 10 choline-recognizing repeats is pneumococcal surface protein A (PspA).[84] In contrast to surface proteins of other gram-positive bacteria, PspA is anchored to the outer layer of the plasma membrane with choline-mediated interaction between membrane-associated LTA and its C-terminal repeat region (Fig. 1).[85] Accordingly, in ethanolamine-grown cells or in mutants that lack phosphocholine on LTA (see later), PspA is no longer retained and is lost into the surrounding medium.[85,87] The function of PspA is unknown. Yet it is important in pneumococcal virulence; it is the immunodeterminant protein antigen on *S. pneumoniae* cells and capable of eliciting protective

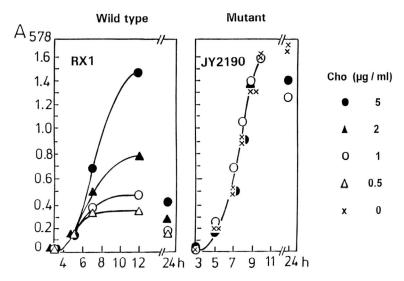

FIG. 22. Effect of choline on growth of the parent strain Rx1 and the mutant JY 2190 of *S. pneumoniae*. The strains were grown in chemically defined medium, containing no or the indicated choline (Cho) additions. (Reprinted with permission from Yother et al.[87])

immunity in animal models of pneumococcal infection.[8,55,56] Interestingly, intranasal immunization of mice with PspA did not only prevent colonization of the nasopharynx but also subsequent invasive disease,[83] and mice could be also protected from fatal infections by oral immunization with an avirulent live recombinant *Salmonella* strain, producing PspA.[61] PspC is another surface protein of unknown function whose choline-binding domain is 90% homologous to that of PspA.[8]

Other choline-binding proteins

Recently, in pneumococcal lysates at least eight novel choline-binding proteins (CBP) were identified by use of a choline affinity matrix.[66] Four of these proteins could be located at the bacterial surface, and five reacted with human reconvalescent sera. Antisera to these proteins passively protected mice, challenged with a lethal dose of pneumococci in the peritoneum. CbpA, the predominant component of this mixture, was characterized as an adhesin and a determinant of virulence. The deduced amino acid sequence from the corresponding gene showed a particular N-terminal region and a conserved C-terminal domain consisting of 10 repeated choline-binding domains, nearly identical to PspA. CbpA is involved in adherence of pneumococci to cytokine-activated human cells, plays an important role in nasopharyngeal colonization,[66] and is involved in pneumococcal transvesiculation through brain microvascular endothelial cells.[64a]

PNEUMOCOCCAL STRAINS THAT DO NOT REQUIRE CHOLINE OR ANALOGS FOR GROWTH

None of the functions of phosphocholine in pneumococcal cells, discussed above, is of vital necessity, and all functions together can not explain the strict nutritional requirement of choline. Of great interest are therefore two recently described

strains that acquired the capacity to grow in the absence of choline and analogs.

One strain, the mutant JY 2190, was isolated by serial passage of strain Rx1 in chemically defined medium (CDM)[64] containing decreasing concentrations of ethanolamine with each passage.[87] The ability to grow in the absence of choline is illustrated in Fig. 22. Whereas the parent strain stopped growing when the limited amount of choline was consumed, the growth rate of the mutant was unaffected whether choline was absent or present at various concentrations. The decrease of optical density after 24 h indicates that stationary phase lysis had occurred in the parent strain whereas the mutant strain showed no or little lysis. Grown in the absence of choline or analogs, the mutant formed long chains of >100 cells. The same picture was obtained with the mutant grown on ethanolamine. Under both growth conditions, cells were resistant to all kinds of autolysis and lost PspA into the surrounding medium. However, when the mutant was grown at low concentrations of choline, cell

TABLE 6. COMPOSITIONAL ANALYSIS OF TA FROM *S. pneumoniae* R6, *S. pneumoniae* Rx1, AND THE MUTANT STRAIN *S. pneumoniae* JY 2190

Component	R6	Rx1	JY2190
Phosphorus	1.00	1.00	1.00
Choline	0.65	0.54	0
Intrachain phosphate	0.35	0.48	1.00
Glucose	0.31	0.55	1.05
GalNAc	0.70	0.98	1.90
Ribitol + 2,5-anhydroribitol	0.35	0.48	1.10
Quinovosamine	+	+	+

Rx1: see Table 4.

Values are molar ratios to phosphorus. Quinovosamine is indicative for AATGal.[4]

Adapted from Yother et al.[87]

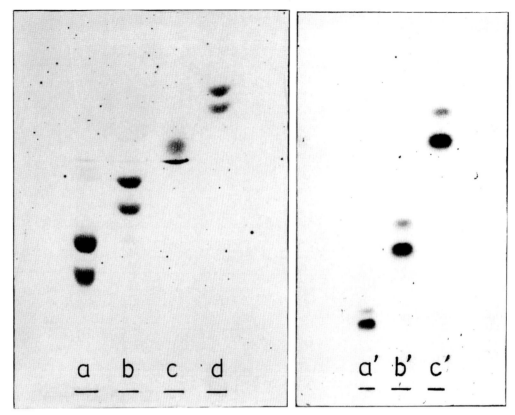

FIG. 23. Variously substituted LTAs/TAs, visualized by TLC of the alkali hydrolysis products (for mode of cleavage, desalting and N-acetylation, see Fig. 19). **a–d:** Repeats with phosphomonoesters at O4 and O5 of the ribitol residue. **a′–c′:** Repeats after phosphomonoester cleavage. Substitution: two phosphocholine residues (a,a′); one phosphocholine residue (b,b′); no substituent (c,c′); two N-acetylated phosphoethanolamine residues (d). The minor components in front of a′–c′ are the respective tetrasaccharide 2,5-anhydroribitol derivatives in which O2 of the ribitol moiety eliminated the phosphate group from O5; for mechanism, see Archibald and Baddiley[2]. Provenance: prepared from LTA of *S. pneumoniae* R6 (a), from TA of *S. pneumoniae* Rx1 (AL⁻) (b), from a mixture of LTA and TA of the mutant strain *S. pneumoniae* JY2190 grown in CDM (c), from TA of *S. pneumoniae* R6 grown in CDM containing 400 μg/ml ethanolamine (d). TLC: Silica gel (Merck 60); solvent, propanol/25% (by mass) ammonia/H$_2$O (60:40:15, by vol.). Visualization: 1-naphthol/H$_2$SO$_4$.

separation was normalized, PspA remained cell associated and cells were again susceptible to penicillin- and deoxycholate-induced lysis. Under these conditions choline phosphate was detected on LTA and TA.

Two alternatives were considered to explain these observations: Either the mutant had acquired the ability to decarboxylate serine, thus producing ethanolamine itself, or growth did actually occur in spite of unsubstituted LTA and TA. Search for ethanolamine failed and compositional analysis revealed only one phosphate equivalent per repeat, proving LTA and TA to be indeed unsubstituted (Table 6). The lack of any substituent became also evident on TLC of the alkaline hydrolysis products (Fig. 23). In spite of the absence of phosphocholine, LTA and TA were structurally unaltered and there was also no change in cell wall composition, except that the phosphate content was half that of the parent strain (Table 5). In contrast to ethanolamine-grown cells,[60] the choline-free mutant cells retained the capability to undergo genetic transformation, but, compared to Rx1, with lower frequency and at an earlier stage of growth. The properties of the mutant could be transferred to the parent strain by DNA of the mutant.

Another choline-independent *S. pneumoniae* strain, R6Cho⁻,

was recovered from a heterologous cross with DNA of *Streptococcus oralis*.[68] *S. oralis*, genetically closely related to *S. pneumoniae*,[44] also incorporates phosphocholine into TA and possibly LTA, but, in contrast to pneumococci, *S. oralis* does not have an absolute requirement for choline or analogs.[41] Grown in the absence of choline, R6Cho⁻ formed long chains, did not lyse in the stationary phase, and was resistant against penicillin- and deoxycholate-induced lysis. Cell walls, isolated from these cells, did not contain choline, had a reduced phosphate content but the stem peptide profile was quite similar to that of the parent strain R6. Growth in the presence of choline normalized cell separation and restored all kinds of LytA-catalyzed cell lysis.

The gene, affected by the mutation in strain JY2190 has not yet been identified. The evidence of *in vitro* experiments that peptidoglycan synthesis, the basis of cell growth, was inhibited by choline deprivation, suggested interdependence of TA and peptidoglycan metabolism.[15] If one assumes that pneumococcal TA, like TA of other gram-positive bacteria,[37] is synthesized in linkage to polyprenol phosphate and that only completed phosphocholine- or phosphoethanolamine-substituted TA is transferred to peptidoglycan, polyprenol-linked TA lacking these substituents would not be transferred, but would trap polyprenolphosphate rendering it unavailable for peptidoglycan synthesis. In this hypothesis, the nutritional requirement for choline resides in a recognition site of the TA-transferase for phosphoaminoalcohols on TA. Accordingly, the mutation in JY2190 may have rendered the activity of the TA-transferase independent of this regulation. Strain R6Cho⁻ may have acquired by the heterologous cross the TA-transferase from *Streptococcus oralis*, which, due to the choline-independent growth of *S. oralis*, is apparently not under this kind of control.

ACKNOWLEDGMENTS

I gratefully acknowledge the contribution of my coworkers and the invaluable help by all colleages who are named as coauthors in the reference list. Part of the work in my laboratory was financially supported by Deutsche Forschungsgemeinschaft (DFG grants Fi-218/4-7,8) and Bundesministerium für Bildung und Forschung (BMBF grant 01K1940/1-3).

REFERENCES

1. **Araki, Y., and E. Ito.** 1989. Linkage units in cell walls of gram-positive bacteria. Crit. Rev. Microbiol. **17:**121–135.
2. **Archibald, A.R., and J. Baddiley.** 1966. The teichoic acids. *In* M.L. Wolfrom and R.S. Tipson (eds.), Advances in carbohydrate chemistry, vol. 21. Academic Press, New York, pp. 323–375.
3. **Badger, E.** 1944. The structural specificity of choline for the growth of type III pneumococcus. J. Biol. Chem. **153:**183–191.
4. **Behr, T., W. Fischer, J. Peter Katalinic, and H. Egge.** 1992. The structure of pneumococcal lipoteichoic acid. Improved preparation, chemical and mass spectrometric studies. Eur. J. Biochem. **207:**1063–1075.
4a. **Berry, A.M., R.A. Lock, D. Hansman, and J.C. Paton.** 1989. Contribution of autolysin to virulence of *Streptococcus pneumoniae.* Infect. Immun. **57:**2324–2330.
5. **Briese, T., and R. Hakenbeck.** 1985. Interaction of the pneumococcal amidase with lipoteichoic acid and choline. Eur. J. Biochem. **146:**417–427.
6. **Briles, E.B., and A. Tomasz.** 1973. Pneumococcal Forssman antigen. A choline-containing LTA. J. Biol. Chem. **248:**6394–6397.
7. **Briles, E.B., and A. Tomasz.** 1975. Membrane lipoteichoic acid is not a precursor to wall teichoic acid in pneumococci. J. Bacteriol. **122:**335–337.
8. **Briles, D.E., S.K. Hollingshead, E. Swiatlo, A. Brooks-Walter, A. Szalai, A. Virolainen, L.S. McDaniel, K.A. Benton, P. White, K. Prellner, A. Hermansson, P.C. Aerts, H. van Dijk, and M.J. Crain.** 1997. PspA and PspC: their potential for use as pneumococcal vaccines. Med. Drug Resist. **3:**401–408.
9. **Brundish, D.E., and J. Baddiley.** 1967. The characterization of pneumococcal C–polysaccharide as a ribitol teichoic acid. Biochem. J. **105:**30c–31c.
10. **Brundish, D.E., and J. Baddiley.** 1968. Pneumococcal C–substance, a ribitol teichoic acid containing choline phosphate. Biochem. J. **110:**573–582.
11. **Coligan, J.E., B.A. Fraser, and T.J. Kindt.** 1977. A disaccharide hapten from streptococcal group C carbohydrate that cross-reacts with the Forssman glycolipid. J. Immunol. **118:**6–11.
12. **Cundell, D.R., N.P. Gerard, C. Gerard, I. Idanpaan-Helkklia, and E.I. Tuomanen.** 1995. *Streptococcus pneumoniae* anchor to activated human cells by the receptor for platelet-activating factor. Nature **377:**435–438.
13. **Diaz, E., E. Garcia, C. Ascaso, E. Méndez, R. López, and J.L. Garcia.** 1989. Subcellular localization of the major pneumococcal autolysis: a peculiar mechanism of secretion in *Escherichia coli.* J. Biol. Chem. **264:**1238–1244.
14. **Díaz, E., M. Munthali, H. Lünsdorf, J.-V. Höltje, and K.N. Timmis.** 1996. The two-step lysis system of pneumococcal bacteriophage EJ-1 is functional in Gram-negative bacteria: triggering of the major pneumococcal autolysin in *Escherichia coli.* Mol. Microbiol. **19:**667–681.
15. **Fischer, H., and A. Tomasz.** 1984. Production and release of peptidoglycan and wall teichoic acid polymers in pneumococci treated with beta-lactam antibiotics. J. Bacteriol. **157:**507–513.
16. **Fischer, W.** 1990. Bacterial phosphoglycolipids and lipoteichoic acids. *In* M. Kates (ed.), Glycolipids, phosphoglycolipids and sulfoglycolipids. Handbook of lipid research, vol. 6. Plenum Press, New York, pp. 123–234.
17. **Fischer, W.** 1991. One-step purification of bacterial lipid macroamphiphiles by hydrophobic interaction chromatography. Anal. Biochem. **194:**353–358.
18. **Fischer, W.** 1994. Lipoteichoic acids and lipoglycans. *In* J.-M. Ghuysen and R. Hakenbeck (eds.), Bacterial cell wall. New comprehensive biochemistry, vol. 27. Elsevier Science, Amsterdam, pp. 199–215.
19. **Fischer, W.** 1994. Lipoteichoic acid and lipids in the membrane of *Staphylococcus aureus.* Med. Microbiol. Immunol. **183:**61–76.
20. **Fischer, W.** 1996. Molecular analysis of lipid macroamphiphiles by hydrophobic interaction chromatography. J. Microbiol. Methods **25:**129–144.
21. **Fischer, W., T. Behr, R. Hartmann, J. Peter Katalinic, and H. Egge.** 1993. Teichoic acid and lipoteichoic acid of *Streptococcus pneumoniae* possess identical chain structures. A reinvestigation of teichoic acid (C polysaccharide). Eur. J. Biochem. **215:**851–857.
22. **Fischer, W., S. Markwitz, and H. Labischinski.** 1997. Small-angle x-ray scattering analysis of pneumococcal lipoteichoic acid phase structure. Eur. J. Biochem. **244:**913–917.
23. **Fraser, B.A., and M.F. Mallette.** 1974. Structure of Forssman hapten glycosphingolipid from sheep erythrocytes. Immunochemistry **11:**581–593.
24. **Fujiwara, M.** 1967. The Forssman antigen of *Pneumococcus.* Jpn. J. Exp. Med. **37:**581–592.
25. **Garcia-Bustos, J.F., and A. Tomasz.** 1987. Teichoic acid-containing muropeptides from *Streptococcus pneumoniae* as substrates for the pneumococcal autolysin. J. Bacteriol. **169:**447–453.
26. **García, E., J.L. García, P. García, A. Arrarás, J.M. Sanchez-Puelles, and R. López.** 1988. Molecular evolution of lytic enzymes of *Streptococcus pneumoniae* and its bacteriophages. Proc. Natl. Acad. Sci. U.S.A. **85:**914–918.
27. **Garcia, J.L., E. Garcia, A. Arras, P. Garcia, C. Ronda, and R. López.** 1987. Cloning, purification, and biochemical characterization of the pneumococcal bacteriophage Cp-1 lysin. J. Virol. **61:**2573–2580.
28. **Garcia, P., J.L. Garcia, E. Garcia, and R. López.** 1986. Nucleotide sequence and expression of pneumococcal autolysin from its own promotor in *Escherichia coli.* Gene **43:**265–272.
29. **García, P., J.L. García, E. García, and R. López.** 1989. Purification and characterization of the autolytic glucosaminidase of *Streptococcus pneumoniae.* Biochem. Biophys. Res. Commun. **158:**251–256.
30. **Geelen, S., C. Battacharyya, and E. Tuomanen.** 1993. Cell wall mediates pneumococcal attachment and cytopathology to human endothelial cells. Infect. Immun. **61:**1538–1543.
31. **George, M., and I. van de Rijn.** 1988. Nutritionally variant streptococcal serotype I antigen. Characterization as a lipid-substituted poly(ribitol phosphate). J. Immun. **140:**2008–2015.
32. **Goebel, W.F., and M.H. Adams.** 1943. The immunological properties of the heterophile antigen and somatic polysaccharide of *Pneumococcus.* J. Exp. Med. **77:**435–448.
33. **Goebel, W.F., T. Shedlovsky, G.I. Lavin, and M.H. Adams.**

1943. The heterophil antigen of *Pneumococcus*. J. Biol. Chem. **148**:1–15.

34. **Gotschlich, E.C., and T.-Y. Liu.** 1967. Structural and immunological studies on the pneumococcal C polysaccharide. J. Biol. Chem. **242**:463–470.

35. **Guidicelli, S., and A. Tomasz.** 1984. Attachment of pneumococcal autolysin to wall teichoic acids, an essential step in enzymatic degradation. J. Bacteriol. **158**:1188–1190.

36. **Gutberlet, T., S. Markwitz, H. Labischinski, and H. Bradaczek.** 1991. Monolayer investigations on the bacterial amphiphile lipoteichoic acid and on lipoteichoic acid/dipalmitoyl glycerol mixtures. Macromol. Chem. Macromol. Symp. **46**:283–287.

37. **Hancock, I.C., and J. Baddiley.** 1985. Biosynthesis of the bacterial envelope polymers teichoic acid and teichuronic acid. *In* A.N. Martonosi (ed.), The enzymes of biological membranes. Biosynthesis and metabolism, vol. 2. Plenum Press, New York, pp. 279–307.

38. **Heumann, D., C. Barras, A. Severin, M.P. Glauser, and A. Tomasz.** 1994. Gram-positive cell walls stimulate synthesis of tumor necrosis factor alpha and interleukin-6 by human monocytes. Infect. Immun. **62**:2715–2721.

39. **Höltje, J.-V., and A. Tomasz.** 1975. Lipoteichoic acid: a specific inhibitor of autolysin activity in *pneumococcus*. Proc. Natl. Acad. Sci. U.S.A. **72**:1690–1694.

40. **Höltje, J.-V., and A. Tomasz.** 1975. Specific recognition of choline residues in the cell wall of teichoic acid by the *N*-acetylmuramyl-L-alanine amidase of pneumococci. J. Biol. Chem. **250**:6072–6076.

41. **Horne, D.S., and A. Tomasz.** 1993. Possible role of a choline-containing teichoic acid in the maintenance of normal cell shape and physiology in *Streptococcus oralis*. J. Bacteriol. **175**:1717–1722.

42. **Hummel, D.S., A.J. Swift, A. Tomasz, and J.A. Winkelstein.** 1985. Activation of alternative complement pathway by pneumococcal lipoteichoic acid. Infect. Immun. **47**:384–387.

43. **Jennings, H.J., C. Lugowski, and N.M. Young.** 1980. Structure of the complex polysaccharide C-substance from *Streptococcus pneumoniae* type I. Biochemistry **19**:4712–4719.

44. **Kilpper-Bälz, R., P. Wenzig, and K.H. Schleifer.** 1985. Molecular relationships and classification of some viridans streptococci as *Streptococcus oralis* and emended description of *Streptococcus oralis* (Bridge and Sneath, 1982). Int. J. System. Bacteriol. **35**:482–488.

45. **Kim, J.O., and J.N. Weiser.** 1998. Association of intrastrain phase variation in quantity of capsular polysaccharide and teichoic acid with the virulence of *Streptococcus pneumoniae*. J. Infect. Dis. **177**:368–377.

46. **Klein, R.A., R. Hartmann, H. Egge, T. Behr, and W. Fischer.** 1994. The aqueous solution structure of the tetrasaccharide-ribitol repeat unit from the lipoteichoic acid of *Streptococcus pneumoniae* strain R6 determined using a combination of NMR spectroscopy and computer calculations. Carbohydr. Res. **256**:189–222.

47. **Klein, R.A., R. Hartmann, H. Egge, T. Behr, and W. Fischer.** 1996. The aqueous solution structure of a lipoteichoic acid from *Streptococcus pneumoniae* strain R6 containing 2,4-diamino-2,4,6-trideoxy-galactose: evidence for conformational mobility of the galactopyranose ring. Carbohydr. Res. **281**:79–98.

48. **Labischinski, H., G. Barnickel, H. Bradaczek, D. Naumann, E.T. Rietschel, and P. Giesbrecht.** 1985. High state of order of isolated bacterial lipopolysaccharide and its possible contribution to the permeation barrier property of the outer membrane. J. Bacteriol. **162**:9–20.

49. **Labischinski, H., D. Naumann, and W. Fischer.** 1991. Small and medium angle x-ray analysis of bacterial lipoteichoic acid phase structure. Eur. J. Biochem. **202**:1269–127.

50. **Leopold, K., and W. Fischer.** 1992. Hydrophobic interaction chromatography fractionates lipoteichoic acid according to the size of the hydrophilic chain: a comparative study with anion-exchange and affinity chromatography for suitability in species analysis. Anal. Biochem. **201**:350–355.

51. **Leopold, K., and W. Fischer.** 1993. Molecular analysis of the lipoglycans of *Mycobacterium tuberculosis*. Anal. Biochem. **208**:57–64.

52. **Liu, T.-Y., and E.C. Gotschlich.** 1963. The chemical composition of pneumococcal C-polysaccharide. J. Biol. Chem. **238**:1928–1934.

53. **Liu, T.-Y., and E.C. Gotschlich.** 1967. Muramic acid phosphate as a component of the muropeptide of Gram-positive bacteria. J. Biol. Chem. **242**:471–476.

54. **Lopez, R., E. García, P. García, and J.L. García.** 1997. The pneumococcal cell wall degrading enzymes: a modular design to create new lysins? Microbial Drug Res. **3**:199–211.

55. **McDaniel, L.S., G. Scott, K. Widenhofer, J. Carroll, and D.E. Briles.** 1986. Analysis of a surface protein of *Streptococcus pneumoniae* recognized by protective monoclonal antibodies. Microbial Pathog. **1**:519–531.

56. **McDaniel, L.S., J.S. Sheffield, P. Delucchi, and D.E. Briles.** 1991. PspA, a surface protein of *Streptococcus pneumoniae*, is capable of eliciting protection against pneumococci of more than one capsular type. Infect. Immun. **59**:222–228.

57. **Mold, C., C.P. Rodgers, R.L. Kaplan, and H. Gewurz.** 1982. Binding of human C-reactive protein to bacteria. Infect. Immun. **38**:392–395.

58. **Mosser, J.L., and A. Tomasz.** 1970. Choline-containing teichoic acid as a structural component of pneumococcal cell wall and its role in sensitivity to lysis by an autolytic enzyme. J. Biol. Chem. **245**:287–298.

59. **Naumann, D., C. Schultz, J. Born, H. Labischinski, K. Brandenburg, G. von Busse, H. Brade, and U. Seydel.** 1987. Investigations into the polymorphism of lipid A from lipopolysaccharides of *Escherichia coli* and *Salmonella minnesota* by Fourier-transform infrared spectroscopy. Eur. J. Biochem. **164**:159–169.

60. **Naumann, D., C. Schultz, A. Sabisch, M. Kastowsky, and H. Labischinski.** 1989. New insights into the phase behavior of a complex anionic amphiphile: architecture and dynamics of bacterial deep rough lipopolysaccharide membranes as seen by FTIR, x-ray, and molecular modeling techniques. J. Mol. Struct. **214**:213–246.

61. **Nayak, A.R., S.A. Tinge, R.C. Tart, L.S. McDaniel, D.E. Briles, and R. Curtiss III.** 1998. A live recombinant avirulent oral *Salmonella* vaccine expressing pneumococcal surface protein A induces protective responses against *Streptococcus pneumoniae*. Infect. Immun. **66**:3744–3751.

61a. **Pooley, H.M., and D. Karamata.** 1994. Teichoic acid synthesis in *Bacillus subtilis*: genetic organization and biological roles. *In* J.-M. Ghuysen and R. Hakenbeck (eds.), Bacterial cell wall. New comprehensive biochemistry, vol. 27. Elsevier Science, Amsterdam, pp. 187–198.

62. **Poxton, I.R., E. Tarelli, and J. Baddiley.** 1978. The structure of C-polysaccharide from the walls of *Streptococcus pneumoniae*. Biochem. J. **175**:1033–1042.

63. **Rane, L., and Y. Subbarow.** 1940. Nutritional requirements of the pneumococcus. 1. Growth factors for types I, II, V, VII, VIII. J. Bacteriol. **40**:695–704.

64. **Rijn, van de, I., and R.E. Kessler.** 1980. Growth characteristics of group A streptococci in a new chemically defined medium. Infect. Immun. **27**:444–448.

64a. **Ring, A-,J.N. Weiser, and E.I. Tuomanen.** 1998. Pneumococcal trafficking across the blood-brain barrier. Molecular analysis of a novel bidirectional pathway. J. Clin. Invest. **102**:347–360.

65. **Ronda, C., J.L. García, E. García, J.M. Sánchez-Puelles, and R. López.** 1987. Biological role of the pneumococcal amidases.

Cloning of the *lytA* gene in *Streptococcus pneumoniae*. Eur. J. Biochem. **164**:621–624.

66. **Rosenow, C., P. Ryan, J.N. Weiser, S. Johnson, P. Fontan, A. Ortqvist, and H.R. Masure.** 1997. Contribution of novel choline-binding proteins to adherence, colonization and immunogenicity of *Streptococcus pneumoniae*. Mol. Microbiol. **25**:819–829.

67. **Sanchez-Puelles, J.M., J.M. Sanz, J.L. García, and E. García.** 1990. Cloning and expression of gene fragments encoding the choline-binding domain of pneumococcal murein hydrolases. Gene **89**:69–75.

68. **Severin, A., Horne, D. and Tomasz, A.** 1997. Autolysis and cell wall degradation in a choline-independent strain of *Streptococcus pneumoniae*. Microbial Drug Resist. **3**:391–400.

69. **Siddiqui, B., and S.I. Hakomori.** 1971. A revised structure for the Forssman hapten glycolipid hapten. J. Biol. Chem. **246**:5766–5769.

70. **Sieling, P.A., and I. van de Rijn.** 1991. Purification and characterization of *Streptococcus adjacens* (nutritionally variant streptococcus serotype II) group antigen. Infect. Immun. **59**:592–599.

71. **Sieling, P.A., M.J. Thomas, and I. van de Rijn.** 1992. Characterization of the *Streptococcus adjacens* group antigen structure. J. Bacteriol. **174**:349–354.

72. **Sørensen, U.B.S., and J. Henrichsen.** 1987. Cross reaction between pneumococci and other streptococci due to C polysaccharide and F antigen. J. Clin. Microbiol. **25**:1854–1859.

73. **Sørensen, U.B.S., J. Blom, A. Birch-Andersen, and J. Henrichsen.** 1988. Ultrastructural localization of capsules, cell wall polysaccharide, cell wall proteins, and F antigen in pneumococci. Infect. Immun. **56**:1890–1896.

74. **Sung, S.J., W.J. Esselman, and C.C. Sweeley.** 1973. Structure of a pentahexosyl ceramide (Forssman hapten) from canine intestine and kidney. J. Biol. Chem. **248**:6528–6533.

75. **Tillet, W.S., W.F. Goebel, and O.T. Avery.** 1930. Chemical and immunological properties of a species-specific carbohydrate of pneumococci. J. Exp. Med. **52**:895–900.

76. **Tomasz, A.** 1967. Choline in the cell wall of a bacterium novel type of polymer-linked choline in *pneumococcus*. Science **157**:694–697.

77. **Tomasz, A.** 1968. Biological consequences of the replacement of choline by ethanolamine in the cell wall of pneumococcus: chain formation, loss of transformability, and loss of autolysin. Proc. Natl. Acad. Sci. U.S.A. **59**:86–93.

78. **Tomasz, A., and M. Westphal.** 1971. Abnormal autolytic enzyme in a pneumococcus with altered teichoic acid composition. Proc. Natl. Acad. Sci. U.S.A. **68**:2627–2630.

79. **Ward, J.B.** 1981. Teichoic and teichuronic acids: biosynthesis, assembly, and location. Microbiol. Rev. **45**:211–243.

80. **Watson, M.J., and J. Baddiley.** 1974. The action of nitrous acid on C-teichoic acid (C-substance) from the walls of *Diplococcus pneumoniae*. Biochem. J. **137**:399–404.

81. **Weiser, J.N., R. Austrian, P.K. Sreenivasan, and H.R. Masure.** 1994. Phase variation in pneumococcal opacity: relationship between colonial morphology and nasopharyngeal colonization. Infect. Immun. **62**:2582–2589.

82. **Winkelstein, J.A., and Tomasz, A.** 1978. Activation of the alternative complement pathway by pneumococcal cell wall teichoic acid. J. Immunol. **120**:174–178.

83. **Wu, H.Y., M.H. Nahm, Y. Guo, M.W. Russell, and D.E. Briles.** 1997. Internasal immunization with PspA (Pneumococcal surface protein A) can prevent carriage and infection with *Streptococcus pneumoniae*. J. Infect. Dis. **175**:839–846.

84. **Yother, J., and D.E. Briles.** 1992. Structural properties and evolutionary relationships of PspA, a surface protein of *Streptococcus pneumoniae*, as revealed by sequence analysis. J. Bacteriol. **174**:601–609.

85. **Yother, J., and White, J.M.** 1994. Novel surface attachment mechanism of the *Streptococcus pneumoniae* protein PspA. J. Bacteriol. **176**:2976–2985.

86. **Yother, J., C. Forman, B.M. Gray, and D.E. Briles.** 1982. Protection of mice from infection with *Streptococcus pneumoniae* by anti-phosphocholine antibody. Infect. Immun. **36**:184–188.

87. **Yother, J., K. Leopold, J. White, and W. Fischer.** 1998. Generation and properties of a *Streptococcus pneumoniae* mutant which does not require choline or analogs for growth. J. Bacteriol. **180**:2093–2101.

88. **Zhang, J.-R., I. Idanpaan-Heikkila, W. Fischer, and E.I. Tuomanen.** 1999. Pneumococcal *lic*D2 is involved in phosphorylcholine metabolism. Molec. Microbiol. **31**:1477–1488.

Address reprint requests to:
Werner Fischer
Inst. Biochem., Med. Fak.
Fahrstrasse 17
D-91054 Erlangen
Germany

The Peptidoglycan of *Streptococcus pneumoniae*

ANATOLY SEVERIN and ALEXANDER TOMASZ

INTRODUCTION

INTEREST IN UNIQUE CHEMICAL and immunologically important components of *Streptococcus pneumoniae* antedates the recognition that these were covalently linked components of the pneumococcal cell wall. Thus, the pneumococcal C-polysaccharide or "common antigen," first described in 1930,[32] the unusual amino sugar 2,4,6-trideoxy-2,4,diamino hexose,[2] galactosamine phosphate,[21] and phosphorylcholine[33] were eventually all shown to be components of a complex teichoic acid with ribitol phosphate and glycosidic bonds representing its backbone, which was attached covalently to some of the muramic acid residues of the peptidoglycan in the pneumococcal cell wall.[7,19] The polymer containing galactosamine phosphate as well as *N*-acetyl glucosamine and *N*-acetyl muramic acid together with alanine, glutamic acid, and lysine isolated from deoxycholate extracts of pneumococci,[22] have turned out to be incomplete degradation products of the pneumococcal cell wall, solubilized by the pneumococcal autolytic enzyme first described by Dubos[5] and subsequently identified as an *N*-acetyl muramic acid L-alanine amidase (amidase).[18] The relationship of these components to one another and to the pneumococcal cell wall was clarified in 1970 when the methods used for the preparation of cell walls of other bacteria were applied to the commonly used laboratory strain R36A of pneumococci.[25] Extraction with hot sodium dodecyl sulfate (SDS) followed by mechanical breakage and treatments with proteolytic enzymes, lithium chloride, and other solvents yielded pure preparations of pneumococcal cell walls free of contamination by other cellular components. Observation of such preparations in the electron microscope showed the presence of structures with the size and pointed "football shape" typical of whole pneumococcal cells. Chemical analysis indicated that these structures were composed in roughly equal proportions of a lysine-containing peptidoglycan and a complex wall teichoic acid containing phosphorylcholine[25] (Fig. 1). The chemistry and some of the biological activities of this teichoic acid are described in Fischer (this volume). Here we shall describe properties of the pneumococcal peptidoglycan.

Structure and species-specific composition of peptidoglycan

The pneumococcal autolytic amidase was used to solubilize the pneumococcal cell wall under conditions that led to the quantitative splitting of the covalent bond between the L-alanine residue of the stem peptides and the *N*-acetyl muramic acid residue of the glycan. Fractionation on a size exclusion column allowed the separation of peptide-free glycan chains to four size classes of stem peptides: oligomeric, trimeric, and dimeric components, and monomeric stem peptides, of which the fraction containing dimeric components was by far the most abundant.[10] The relative rarity of components with a polymerization grade higher than 3 is in striking contrast to the case of the peptidoglycan of staphylococci, in which over 65% of all peptides are represented by oligomers composed of more than nine stem peptide units.[3]

The four size classes of stem peptides were next fractionated by reverse-phase high performance liquid chromatography (RP-HPLC), which resulted in the resolution of the peptidoglycan to over 19 unique stem peptide components.[11] These were identified subsequently through the determination of amino acid composition, amino termini, partial sequencing by Edman degradation, and mass spectrometry. In the structural assignments for these stem peptides it was assumed that they had an alternating sequence of L- and D-amino acids, beginning with L-alanine followed by D-isoglutamine and L-lysine. Stem peptides containing two D-alanine residues at the carboxyl terminus were rare. The two most abundant stem peptides were a monomeric tripeptide and the directly crosslinked tri-tetrapeptide, which was the most frequent dimeric component of the peptidoglycan. Another interesting feature of the peptide network was the presence of both directly and indirectly crosslinked peptide components, thus allowing the classification of pneumococcal cell wall either as an A1-α or A3-α,[26] depending on which particular dimer one considers. Indirectly crosslinked stem peptides contained alanyl-serine or alanyl-alanine interpeptide bridges.

A large number of *S. pneumoniae* isolates recovered over a time period of several decades and, expressing a large number of different capsular serotypes, all produced a unique peptidoglycan when the cell walls were prepared from bacteria grown in the common laboratory medium and harvested in the middle of exponential growth. This common stem peptide composition therefore appears to be specific for the species.[28]

When screening large numbers of pneumococcal isolates, several naturally occurring peptidoglycan variants were also identified in which the proportions of the various muropeptide components deviated from the species-specific composition.[28]

The Rockefeller University, New York, NY 10021.

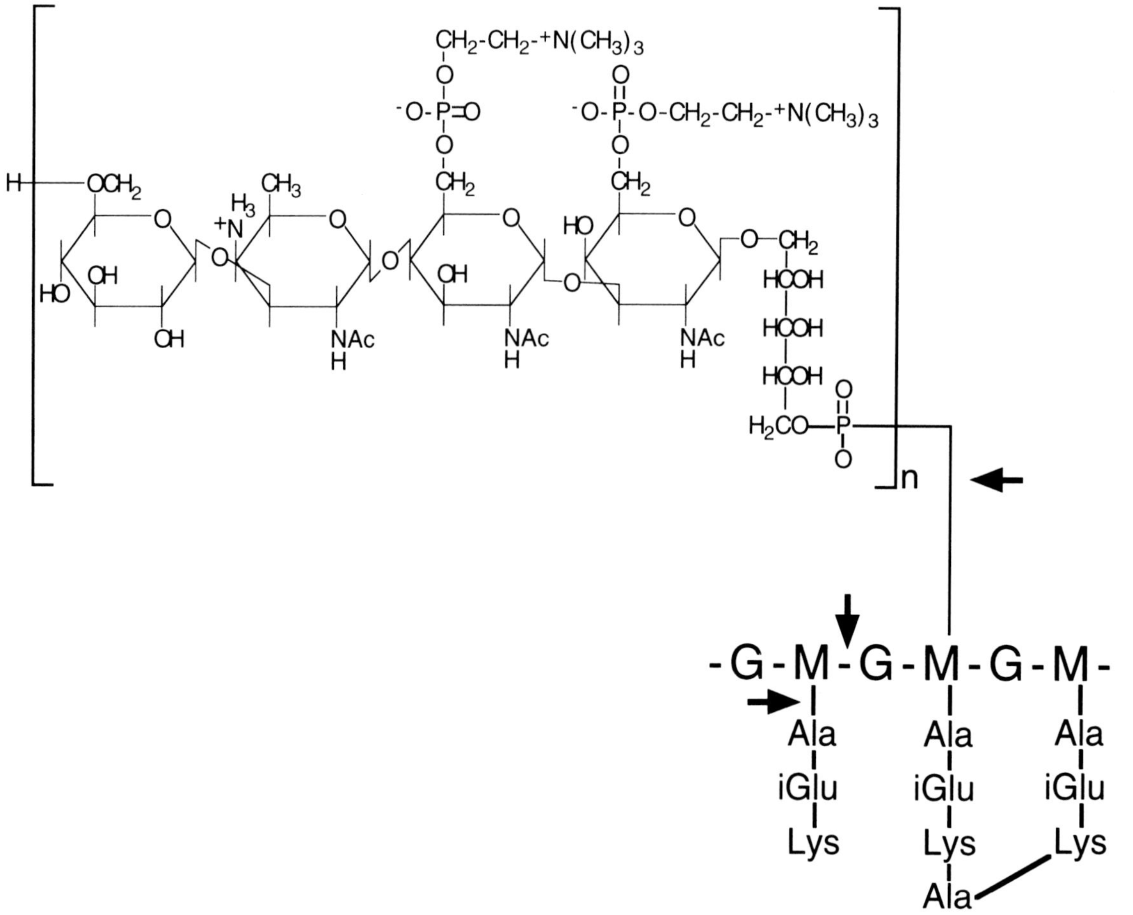

FIG. 1. Basic structure of the teichoic acid and peptidoglycan units making up the pneumococcal cell wall. Symbols: G, *N*-acetylglucosamine residues; M, *N*-acetyl muramic acid residues; -G-M-, represent the 1,4 β-glycosidic bonds that constitute the backbone of the glycan strand. The three arrows indicate the cutting sites of the pneumococcal amidase (between M and Ala), and the M1 muramidase (between M and G). The third arrow points to the HF-sensitive bond connecting some as yet unidentified residue in the wall teichoic acid and a muramic acid.

Interestingly, all such peptidoglycan variants identified so far were resistant to penicillin and the particular peptidoglycan type, recognized by the HPLC pattern, were unique to the particular pneumococcal clone.

Figure 2 shows HPLC profiles of the penicillin-susceptible laboratory strain R36A, which represents the species-specific stem peptide profile of pneumococci. Also shown is one of the naturally occurring peptidoglycan variants isolated from the penicillin-resistant clone HUN663, HUN665, and HUN963. Both the species-specific peptide pattern as well as the pattern of stem peptides characteristic of the peptidoglycan variants shown in the HUN clone were stable: They were reproduced precisely even after several thousand generations of growth in the test tube *in vitro* (see HUN663 tp) and also during passage *in vivo*, *i.e.*, after sublethal peritoneal inoculation of mice and recovery of bacteria from the spleen (HUN663 mp). Figure 2 also shows the precise reproduction of these HPLC patterns in independent isolates belonging to the same pneumococcal clone, as defined by pulsed-field gel electrophoresis (PFGE) or multilocus enzyme analysis (see HUN663, HUN665, and HUN963). The proposed chemical structures corresponding to the peaks numbered in Fig. 2 are shown in Fig. 3. A shift in

the penicillin-resistant clone toward the higher representation of indirectly crosslinked stem peptides is evident.

The degree of reproducibility of these stem peptide patterns through the analytical technique of RP-HPLC is shown for strain R36A (species-specific peptidoglycan), for five independent cell wall preparations in Table 1. Table 2 shows the means of stem peptide concentrations in several of the pneumococcal peptidoglycan variants and Table 3 shows in detail the reproducibility of the extremely abnormal stem peptide pattern identified in the penicillin-resistant clone from Hungary (HUN663). These three tables also illustrate two outstanding features of these peptidoglycans: (i) in spite of the differences in stem peptide composition, the ratio of monomeric to crosslinked (dimeric and trimeric) stem peptides was remarkably constant in all of the peptidoglycans examined; and (ii) the tables show the quantitative distortion of peptidoglycan composition from the predominance of linear peptides, which is characteristic of the species-specific peptidoglycan, toward the predominance of branched peptides, which is a feature of the peptidoglycan variants. A graphic illustration of these distortions is shown in Fig. 4 in which the percentage representation of various stem peptides is shown as barograms for strain R36A and for two peptidoglycan variants, one represented by the Hungarian penicillin-resistant clone and a second penicillin-resistant clone identified in the Czech Republic.[6]

Penicillin resistance and peptidoglycan composition

The mechanism of penicillin resistance in clinical isolates and also in laboratory mutants involves remodeling of the high-molecular-size penicillin-binding proteins in such a manner that their affinity for the drug molecule is reduced.[16] In clinical isolates, this mechanism appears to be linked to the acquisition of DNA fragments carrying sequences of penicillin-binding protein (*pbp*) genes originating from heterologous sources, the results of which are "mosaic" *pbp* genes in pneumococci, which

carry stretches of the foreign *pbp* genes that replace sequences native to the pneumococcus.[4,13] In laboratory-derived penicillin-resistant mutants, the tuning down of penicillin affinities is the result of the accumulation of point mutations.[15] The penicillin molecule is a close structural analog of the carboxy terminal D-alanyl-D-alanine residue of the muropeptide cell wall building blocks, which are substrates of the transpeptidase reactions catalyzed by the bacterial PBPs. Reduced affinity for the substrate analog, therefore, may result in a diminished catalytic efficiency of the remodeled penicillin-resistant PBPs toward their natural substrates as well. Therefore, it was conceivable that the often drastic shift in muropeptide composition seen in penicillin-resistant clinical isolates reflects an attempt by the penicillin-resistant bacteria to overcome this handicap

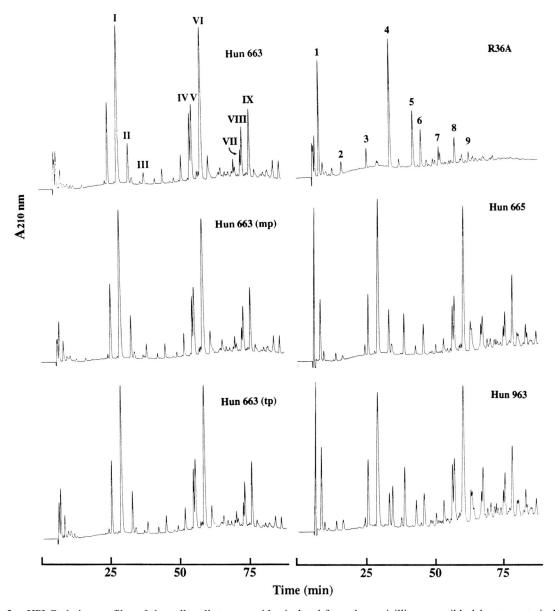

FIG. 2. HPLC elution profiles of the cell wall stem peptides isolated from the penicillin-susceptible laboratory strain R36A and several isolates belonging to the penicillin-resistant Hungarian clone. HUN663, HUN665, and HUN963 represent clinical isolates; mp, cell walls of HUN663 after mouse passage of the strain; tp, cell walls of HUN663 after over 1,000 generations of passage *in vitro* in test tube cultures. Arabic and roman numerals mark the various major stem peptide peaks. (Reproduced with permission from *Journal of Bacteriology*.[28])

Penicillin susceptible (R36A)   **Penicillin resistant (Hun 663)**

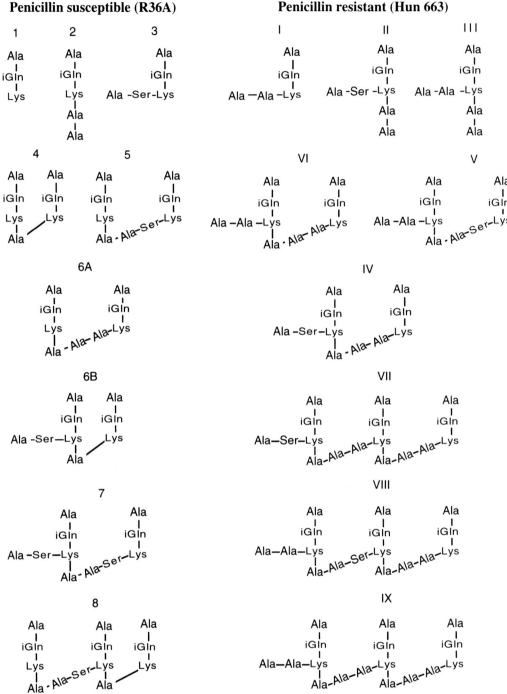

FIG. 3. Chemical structures proposed for the major cell wall stem peptides identified in penicillin-susceptible and penicillin-resistant (Hungarian clone) strains of *S. pneumoniae.* (Reproduced with permission from *Journal of Bacteriology.*[28])

by the preferential utilization of branched muropeptides, which might show a better fit with the altered catalytic site of the penicillin-resistant PBPs (Fig. 5). Thus, it was proposed that the distorted muropeptide composition identified in several clinical isolates of penicillin-resistant pneumococci may be the "biological price" of penicillin resistance.[9]

Initial experiments with genetic crosses provided support for this model. When DNA from a highly penicillin-resistant South

African pneumococcus was used to transfer penicillin resistance into the penicillin-susceptible laboratory strain, it was shown that the gradual increase in penicillin resistance level of the transformants was accompanied by a shift toward the abnormal cell wall composition approaching that of the DNA donor strain.[9] This situation is illustrated by Fig. 6, which shows, in barogram form, stem peptide patterns of the penicillin-susceptible recipient strain R6(Hex⁻), the penicillin-resistant DNA

TABLE 1. REPRODUCIBILITY OF CELL WALL STEM PEPTIDE COMPOSITION IN FIVE SEPARATE CELL WALL PREPARATIONS OF *Streptococcus pneumoniae* R36A

R36A prep#	Peptide material (%)																Recovery (%)	Monomer (%)	Dimer and trimer (%)	Total peptide (%)		
	1	2	3	I	II	4	III	5	6	7	IV	V	8	VI	9	VII VIII XI				Linear (L)	Branched (B)	B/L
1	21.1	6.5	2.6	1.7	—	31.2	2.5	13.3	6.2	5.1	0.7	0.7	6.1	—	2.1	—	68	34	66	72	28	0.4
2	20.5	5.7	2.6	1.7	—	33.7	2.1	12.3	6.2	4.5	0.5	0.5	5.1	—	2.1	—	79	32	68	72	28	0.4
3	23.6	3.6	4.5	1.3	—	30.9	2.2	15.8	5.4	4.2	0.6	0.6	5.2	—	1.7	—	72	35	65	69	31	0.45
4	24.1	3.6	4.6	1.6	—	31.0	2.2	16.1	4.6	4.4	0.7	0.7	5.4	—	1.9	—	71	36	64	69	31	0.45
5	22.4	3.3	4.2	1.3	—	29.4	2.0	14.4	6.1	4.4	1.1	1.1	6.9	—	3.1	—	61	34	66	68	32	0.5
Mean	22.3	4.5	3.7	1.5	—	31.2	2.2	14.4	5.7	4.5	0.7	0.7	5.7	—	2.2	—		34	66	70	30	0.4
Standard deviation	1.55	1.46	1.01	0.20	—	1.55	0.19	1.62	0.70	0.34	0.23	0.23	0.76	—	0.54	—		1.48	1.48	1.87	1.87	0.04

(Reproduced with permission from *Journal of Bacteriology*.[28])

TABLE 2. CELL WALL STEM PEPTIDE COMPOSITION OF *STREPTOCOCCUS PNEUMONIAE* AND TWO OF ITS NATURAL PEPTIDOGLYCAN VARIANTS

Strain (origin)	No. of isolates	Serotype	Peptide material (%)																		Monomer (%)	Dimer and trimer (%)	Total peptide (%)		
			1	2	3	I	II	4	III	5	6ᵃ	7	IV	V	8	VI	9	VII	VIII	IX			Linear (L)	Branched (B)	B/L
R36A (USA)	1	—	22.3 ᵇ	4.5	3.7	1.5	—	31.2	2.2	14.4	5.7	4.5	0.7	0.7	5.7	—	2.2	—	—	—	34	66	70	30	0.4
			1.55ᶜ	1.46	1.01	0.20	—	1.55	0.19	1.62	0.70	0.34	0.23	0.23	0.76	—	0.54	—	—	—	1.48	1.48	1.87	1.87	0.04
USA	7	6B	24.6	1.6	4.6	2.9	0.9	28.6	2.4	9.6	7.7	5.8	0.8	2.2	3.7	2.9	1.4	—	—	—	37	63	64	36	0.6
			1.33	0.63	1.02	0.61	0.48	4.31	0.79	2.26	0.95	0.61	0.37	0.89	0.56	0.52	0.44	—	—	—	1.58	1.89	4.36	4.36	0.11
Northern Europe	5	6B	28.3	2.0	5.0	3.5	0.4	28.0	0.2	12.0	10.2	1.9	0.6	0.8	3.5	2.3	1.9	—	—	—	39	61	69	31	0.5
			1.24	0.86	0.98	0.49	0.06	2.33	0.04	1.96	1.63	0.62	0.19	0.14	0.10	0.73	0.31	—	—	—	1.17	1.17	1.64	1.64	0.03
Hungary (PG variant 1)	1	19A	1.9	0.3	8.1	23.6	4.4	0.9	1.2	0.5	1.5	2.6	6.3	9.1	0.6	23.3	0.3	2.2	5.4	8.0	40	60	4	96	24.0
			0.16	0.10	0.19	0.41	0.32	0.05	0.20	0.06	0.17	0.22	0.32	0.25	0.10	0.41	0.11	0.13	0.16	0.28	0.55	0.55	0	0	0
Czech 2 (PG variant 2)	6	14	16.0	0.4	16.4	5.6	0.6	7.7	1.0	15.4	8.3	14.6	3.0	2.8	2.0	1.9	4.4	—	—	—	40	60	35	65	1.9
			2.07	0.12	1.40	0.67	0.12	0.89	0.19	0.78	1.01	1.55	0.46	0.44	0.63	0.28	0.56	—	—	—	2.23	2.23	2.90	2.90	0.24

ᵃPeptides 6A and 6B were not separated.

ᵇMean.

ᶜStandard deviation.

(Reproduced with permission from *Journal of Bacteriology*.[28])

TABLE 3.   REPRODUCIBILITY OF CELL WALL STEM PEPTIDE COMPOSITION IN FIVE SEPARATE CELL WALL PREPARATIONS OF *Streptococcus pneumoniae* HUN 663

Hun 663 prep#	Peptide material (%)																		Recovery (%)	Monomer (%)	Dimer and trimer (%)	Total peptide (%)		
	1	2	3	I	II	4	III	5	6	7	IV	V	8	VI	9	VII	VIII	XI				Linear (L)	Branched (B)	B/L
1	2.0	0.1	7.9	23.4	4.8	0.8	1.3	0.6	1.9	2.3	6.2	9.0	0.6	23.8	0.1	2.1	5.2	8.0	79	40	60	4	96	24.0
2	1.7	0.4	7.9	24.1	4.7	0.9	1.4	0.5	1.5	2.4	5.9	8.8	0.7	22.8	0.4	2.3	5.6	8.4	77	40	60	4	96	24.0
3	1.9	0.3	8.1	23.0	4.2	0.9	1.3	0.5	1.5	2.6	6.5	9.4	0.8	23.5	0.3	2.3	5.5	7.6	79	39	61	4	96	24.0
4	2.1	0.4	8.3	23.9	4.3	0.8	1.1	0.5	1.4	2.7	6.4	9.3	0.5	22.9	0.4	2.0	5.4	7.8	83	40	60	4	96	24.0
5	1.8	0.3	8.3	23.6	4.0	0.7	1.0	0.5	1.4	2.7	6.6	9.1	0.6	23.5	0.1	2.2	5.5	8.2	75	39	61	4	96	24.0
Mean	1.9	0.3	8.1	23.6	4.4	0.9	1.2	0.5	1.5	2.6	6.3	9.1	0.6	23.3	0.3	2.2	5.4	8.0		40	60	4	96	24.0
Standard deviation	0.16	0.10	0.19	0.41	0.32	0.05	0.20	0.06	0.17	0.22	0.32	0.25	0.10	0.41	0.11	0.13	0.16	0.28		0.55	0.55	0	0	0

(Reproduced with permission from *Journal of Bacteriology*.[28])

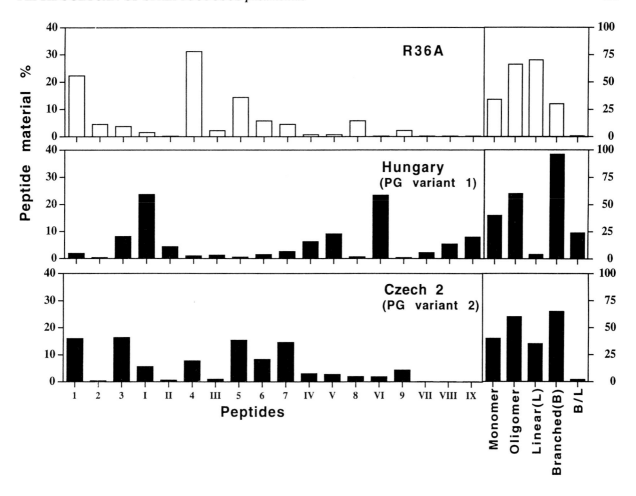

FIG. 4. Stem peptide patterns characteristic of the species-specific (R36A) and penicillin-resistant cell walls. Barograms represent the percentage molar proportion of the particular stem peptide species, the structures of which are shown in Fig. 3.

donor HUN663, and a genetic transformant, HUN663tr.1 isolated from the cross. The barogram shows that HUN663tr.1, which has reached the penicillin resistance level of the DNA donor, also appeared to have inherited a stem peptide composition similar to that of the DNA donor strain. However, when one of these transformants, HUN663tr.4, was used as DNA donor to backcross penicillin resistance into the original penicillin-susceptible strain R6(Hex⁻), the highly penicillin-resistant transformants recovered from this second genetic cross showed a peptidoglycan composition that resembled much more that of the penicillin-susceptible recipient strain than that of the first transformant, HUN663tr.1, or that of the original penicillin-resistant DNA donor (Fig. 7). Thus, this two-step genetic cross has managed to dissociate the penicillin-resistant phenotype from the peptidoglycan abnormality,[27] which was a unique and stable property firmly associated with the penicillin resistance trait of the Hungarian clone.

The results of these genetic crosses suggest that the abnormality of cell wall composition is not an obligatory consequence of penicillin resistance. Nevertheless, the reasons why in several penicillin-resistant clones the resistant phenotype is closely linked to abnormal peptidoglycan structure remains an open question. It is conceivable that genetic determinants encoding

for the synthesis of branched peptides may also be introduced into pneumococci from heterologous sources similar to the manner envisioned for the origin of mosaic *pbp* genes. Such determinants of branched muropeptide synthesis may even be genetically linked to *pbp* genes in some of the heterologous donor organisms. It should be remembered, however, that the capacity to produce both branched and directly interlinked stem peptides is already present in the penicillin-susceptible pneumococci (see Fig. 3). The quantitative shift from dominance of linear toward dominance of the branched component may be the effect of some regulatory mutation. The possibility that such branched peptides may be preferred substrates of low-affinity PBPs has reappeared in the results of experiments in which the peptidoglycan composition of penicillin-resistant laboratory mutants was examined.[31] In mutant 220m (penicillin MIC 2.0 μg/ml), which was derived from strain 220 (penicillin MIC 0.02 μg/ml) in the laboratory by serial passage on gradually increasing concentrations of penicillin, the peptidoglycan of the mutants showed massive reduction in the proportion of the directly crosslinked tritetrapeptides (stem peptide 4), and an increase in two monomeric stem peptides, one carrying an alanyl-serine site branch (stem peptide 3) and another carrying an alanyl-alanine branch (stem peptide I) on the ε-amino group of

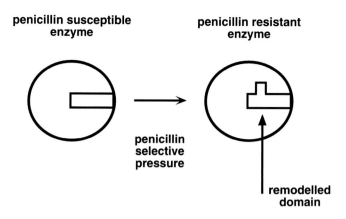

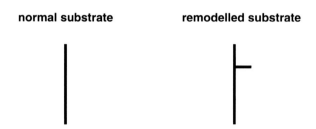

FIG. 5. Model for the relationship between penicillin-resistant PBPs and the structure of cell wall stem peptides. It is assumed that the remodeling of penicillin-binding proteins (penicillin-susceptible enzymes) in the direction of reduced affinity as seen in the penicillin-resistant isolates produces a remodeled active site domain in these enzymes, for which the remodeled (branched) muropeptide cell wall precursors are preferred substrates over that of the linear muropeptides.

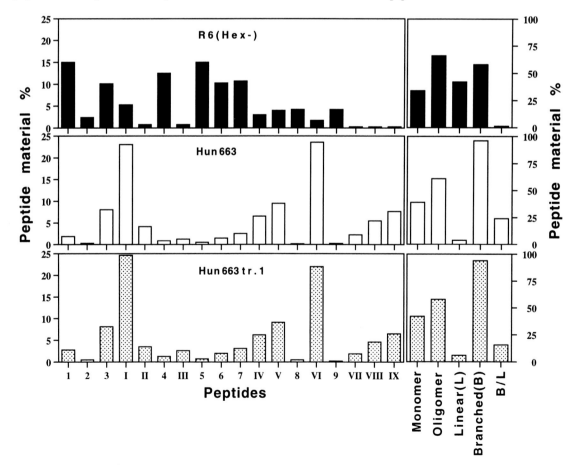

FIG. 6. Inheritance of the abnormal cell wall muropeptide pattern in the first-order genetic transformants selected for penicillin resistance. Symbols as in Fig. 4.

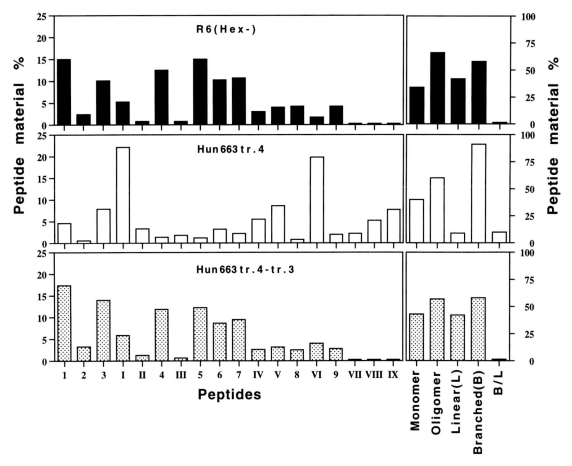

FIG. 7. Separation of abnormal cell wall muropeptide pattern from the penicillin-resistant phenotype in the second order genetic transformants. Symbols as in Fig. 4. (Reproduced with permission from *Antimicrobial Agents Chemotherapy.*[30])

the lysine residues (see Fig. 8). In this respect alone, the laboratory mutants resembled penicillin-resistant clinical isolates. On the other hand, and in sharp contrast to the penicillin-resistant clinical strains, the laboratory mutant seemed to be unable to retain the dominance of oligomeric to monomeric muropeptides. This latter fact highlights what seems to be one of the critical differences between penicillin-resistant pneumococci emerging in the clinical environment and penicillin-resistant mutants constructed in the laboratory. Whereas the basic mechanism (construction of PBPs of low drug affinity) appears to be similar, the laboratory mutants resistant to penicillin appear to contain PBPs of poor transpeptidase activity, as indicated by the inverse relationship between oligomeric and monomeric components of their peptidoglycan. Additional abnormalities in cell morphology, growth rate, and autolytic behavior are also characteristic of the laboratory-generated penicillin-resistant mutants and are all missing from penicillin-resistant strains that emerge in the clinical environment. It was suggested that this difference reflects the presence of separate "fitness" genes in the clinical isolates,[31] possibly obtained from heterologous sources by genetic recombination which compensate, in some manner, the "handicap" inherent in the performance of PBPs with altered active sites (Table 4).

Role of PBP3 in peptidoglycan composition

The dominance of monomeric tripeptides in the peptidoglycan of *S. pneumoniae* suggests the presence of powerful L,D- and D,D-carboxypeptidase activities in this bacterium. PBP3 of pneumococci was shown to have strong homologies to D,D-carboxypeptidases.[14] A pneumococcal mutant in which the PBP3 gene was interrupted in such a manner that this protein was not retained in the plasma membrane was analyzed for the composition of its cell walls. Extensive alterations in the stem peptide composition were noted,[29] which were consistent with the decrease in a functional carboxypeptidase activity in the mutants. The role of PBP3 in the composition of the peptidoglycan was reexamined using selective inhibition of PBP3. Laboratory strain R36A as well as two clinical strains—Ala50 (penicillin MIC 0.2 μg/ml) and HUN665 (penicillin MIC 4.0 μg/ml)—were grown in the presence of clavulanic acid at sub-MIC concentrations sufficient to inhibit PBP3 completely and selectively without interference with bacterial growth. Peptidoglycan isolated from these bacteria grown with or without one-third of their MICs of clavulanic acid were analyzed by HPLC and the elution profiles are shown in Fig. 9. In each case, extensive and unique distortion of the peptidoglycan patterns characteristic of

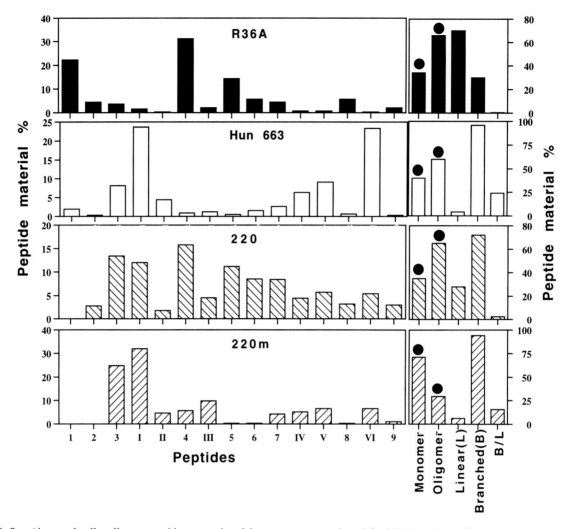

FIG. 8. Abnormal cell wall muropeptide pattern in a laboratory mutant selected for high-level penicillin resistance. Solid circles (●) point to the distorted ratio of monomeric to oligomeric stem peptides in the laboratory mutant 220m.

the particular strains when grown without the antibiotic are seen in the antibiotic-treated cultures.[30] The stem peptide components marked with arabic and roman numerals or with capital letters were eluted from the HPLC and their chemical structures determined by chemical analysis and mass spectrometry. Figure 10

shows that clavulanic acid inhibition of PBP3 resulted in the production of peptidoglycans in which all acceptor peptides carried intact D-alanyl-D-alanine carboxyl termini. A biosynthetic scheme rationalizing the reactions that must have led to this altered peptidoglycan composition is shown in Fig. 11.

TABLE 4. PENICILLIN RESISTANCE IN *STREPTOCOCCUS PNEUMONIAE:*
SAME BASIC MECHANISM WITH AND WITHOUT "FITNESS"

	Laboratory mutants	*Clinical isolates*
Original (parental) MIC (μg/ml)	0.02	0.005 to 0.001
Resistant MIC	2.0	2.0 up to 16.0
Reduced penicillin affinity in all high-molecular-weight PBPs	Yes	Yes
Polymorphism of PBPs	?	Yes
Peptidoglycan abnormal	Yes	Yes
High degree (normal) cross-linking of muropeptides in cell wall	No ($\leq$0.3)	Yes (3.0)
Morphology	Abnormal	Normal
Cell growth rate	Reduced	Normal
Autolysis in stationary phase	Premature	Normal or slow

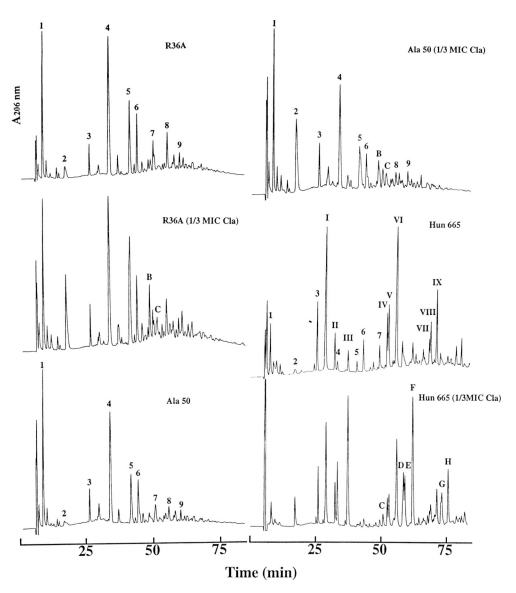

FIG. 9. HPLC elution profiles of cell wall stem peptides produced in pneumococci grown in the presence of clavulanic acid. Strains R36A (penicillin-susceptible laboratory strain) and strains Ala50 (penicillin MIC = 0.2 μg/ml) and HUN665 (penicillin MIC 4.0 μg/ml) were grown with and without one-third of the MIC of clavulanic acid in the growth medium. Cell walls were isolated and analyzed by RP-HPLC, as described. Arabic and roman numerals and capital letters refer to stem peptide species, the tentative structures of which are shown in Fig. 10. (Reproduced with permission from *Antimicrobial Agents Chemotherapy.*[30])

Maturation of peptidoglycan during biosynthesis

A simple model for some of the key reactions catalyzed by penicillin-binding proteins in the polymerization of the pneumococcal peptidoglycan is shown in Fig. 12. The unique dependence of the activity of the pneumococcal autolytic amidase on the presence of choline residues in the cell wall teichoic acids has allowed the development of an experimental system in which nascent, *i.e.*, newly incorporated material could be selectively released from the cell wall by the amidase, while the rest of the biosynthetically "old" material remained intact.[34] The experimental design involved growing pneumococci in a medium in which the normal choline component is replaced by ethanolamine. Bacteria growing under these conditions incor-porate ethanolamine into their cell wall teichoic acids in positions normally occupied by choline. It was shown earlier that the attachment of the autolytic amidase to the cell wall[12] and its hydrolytic activity[17] has an absolute requirement for the presence of choline residues in the cell wall teichoic acid. Bacteria in which choline is replaced in the teichoic acid with ethanolamine residues produce cell walls that are totally resistant to the hydrolytic action of the amidase. Introducing even minute quantities of choline into the growth medium of a culture growing in ethanolamine-containing medium results in an immediate shift to choline utilization, production of choline-containing wall teichoic acids, and their incorporation into the single growth zone of the cell wall of *S. pneumoniae*, which is located in the equatorial area of the cell surface.[1] Exposing such

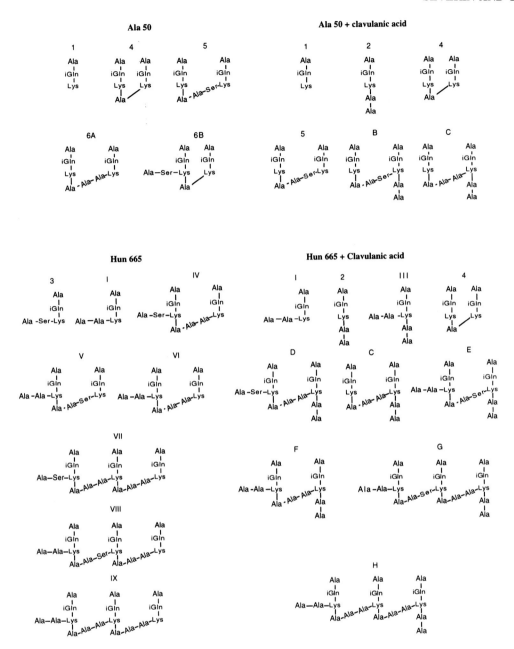

FIG. 10. Structures of the major cell wall stem peptide species produced in strains Ala50 and HUN665 grown in the presence of low concentrations of clavulanic acid. (Reproduced with permission from *Antimicrobial Agents Chemotherapy*.[30])

bacteria to exogenous autolysin results in the rapid and selective removal of the recently made choline-containing cell wall polymers, while the rest of the cell wall containing the ethanolamine residues remains insoluble (Fig. 13). Varying the time of exposure of such cultures to the "pulse" of choline and/or following the choline pulse with a shift back to ethanolamine in the growth medium in combination with using radioactive tracers such as lysine to mark the peptidoglycan produced in the choline versus ethanolamine phases of the experiment allows one to examine the composition of pneumococcal cell wall as a function of its biosynthetic age. The design of such an experimental system is reproduced in Fig. 14. This

system was applied to the examination of the composition of newly incorporated pneumococcal peptidoglycan (*i.e.*, material synthesized during a 1-min period of combined exposure to choline and radioactive lysine), which was then compared to the composition of the same material after it was allowed to "age" after the bacteria were shifted back to the ethanolamine-containing medium. In both the newly made and "aged" cell wall material, application of the pneumococcal amidase allowed the selective solubilization of stem peptides that were synthesized while the bacteria were producing choline-containing teichoic acid. The results of this experiment indicated that the nascent peptidoglycan was greatly enriched in monomeric

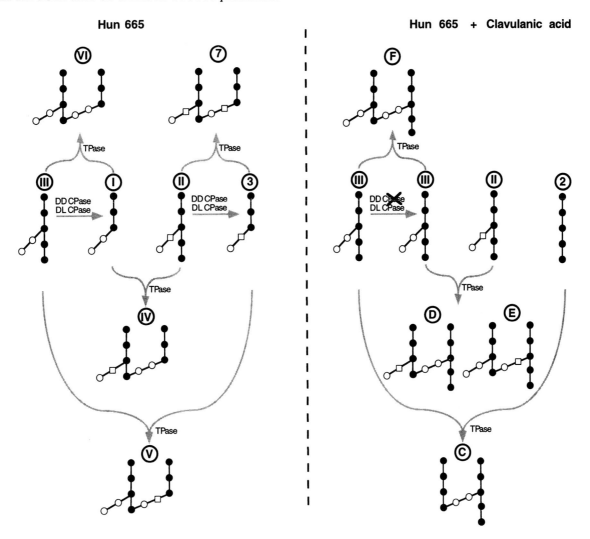

FIG. 11. Biosynthetic scheme proposed to explain the origin of prominent cell wall stem peptide species in strain HUN665 grown with or without clavulanic acid in the growth medium. Arabic and roman numerals and capital letters identify prominent stem peptide species, as described in Fig. 10. Transpeptidase (TPase), D,D- and D,L-carboxypeptidase (CPase) are assumed to catalyze the particular set of enzymatic reactions. Solid circles (●) refer to the amino acid residues in the backbone of the linear stem peptide; open circles (○) and open squares (□) identify alanine and/or serine residues in the crosslinking peptides.

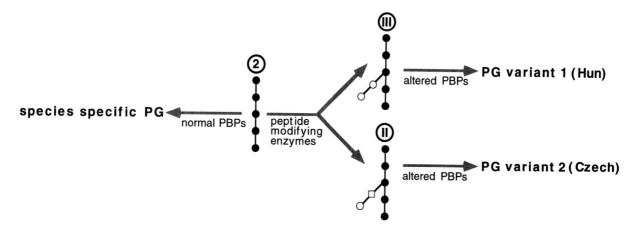

FIG. 12. The role of PBPs and peptide modifying enzymes in the generation of species-specific cell wall and its peptidoglycan variants in *S. pneumoniae*. (Reproduced with permission from *Journal of Bacteriology*.[28])

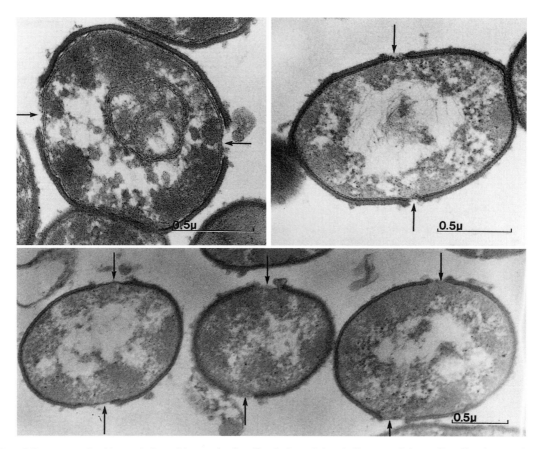

FIG. 13. "Microsurgery" with autolytic amidase: selective dissolution of the choline-containing cell wall polymers that incorporated in the equatorial zone of *S. pneumoniae* during a 1-min pulse. Arrows indicate the equatorial portion of cell wall removed during autolysin treatment. (Reproduced with permission from *Journal of Bacteriology.*[20])

tripeptide components, and during the "aging" process the proportion of monomers declined from 60–70% to 35–45% of all stem peptides, accompanied by a parallel increase in the dimeric peptides, which represented about 30–35% of stem peptides in the nascent material and increased to 45–50% during the "aging" process.[20]

The increase in the amount of the dipeptide component (tri-tetra) during the "aging" or maturation process raises the question of where the tetrapeptide component of these compounds is coming from? The decline in the proportion of monomeric tripeptides and the parallel increase in the dimeric tri-tetrapeptides during maturation suggests that the source of the tripeptide component of the dimeric peptides is most likely the tripeptide monomer. As to the source of the tetrapeptide component, we can only speculate. Clearly, the source of the tetrapeptide component must be a precursor capable of serving as a donor in a transpeptidase reaction; therefore, it must carry an intact D-alanyl-D-alanine terminus. It is possible that the direct source of the tetrapeptide is stem peptide 2, *i.e.*, the monomeric pentapeptide, which has high metabolic turnover in the cell wall. Nevertheless, the concentration of this peptide in the peptidoglycan is rather low. As an alternative hypothesis it has been proposed that the source of the tetrapeptide component may be the bactoprenol-linked disaccharide pentapeptide.[31] In this model, newly made peptidoglycan units incorporate into the pneumococcal cell wall by a transglycosylase, either as tripep-

tide monomers (converted from the pentapeptide to the tripeptide already on the precursor level) or as pentapeptides that are then rapidly converted to tripeptides by the combined action of D,D- and L,D-carboxypeptidases. Such a process would prime a newly made cell wall for equatorial growth, *i.e.*, it would enrich the newly made cell wall in peptides that can only serve as acceptors.[24] The peptide partners need for crosslinking would then arrive in a slower maturation process that may involve a heterogeneous-phase transpeptidation process between tripeptides already in the cell wall and wall precursor bactoprenol-linked pentapeptides acting as donors. Such a mechanism would fit the pattern of streptococcal cell wall enlargement that occurs primarily through equatorial growth.[1]

Degradation of the peptidoglycan in vitro and in vivo

One of the most frequently observed phenomena in pneumococcal microbiology is the rapid dissolution of cells when treated with detergents or cell wall-acting antimicrobial agents. Most strains of pneumococci also show a similar self-induced disintegration (autolysis) in the stationary phase of growth. Several experiments have shown that these autolytic phenomena are the result of the action of the pneumococcal autolytic enzyme, the product of the *lytA* gene,[23] *i.e.*, the very enzyme that has been used extensively in the elucidation of the chemical structure of pneumococcal peptidoglycan.

Purified pneumococcal cell walls exposed *in vitro* to pure autolytic enzyme rapidly solubilize such cell walls through the hydrolysis of amide bonds between the muramic acid and L-alanine residues. Under *in vitro* conditions, the activity of the amidase is not selective to a particular type of stem peptide: only during very short (less than 1 min) exposures of cell walls to the amidase could one observe a relative enrichment of the solubilized material for monomeric stem peptide components. This is understandable because liberation of monomeric components requires the hydrolysis of only a single covalent bond. *In vitro* autolytic degradation beyond these very short time periods always produced the entire family of muropeptides present in the mature pneumococcal peptidoglycan.[8]

A completely different pattern of hydrolysis was observed when the pneumococcal autolysin was triggered *in vivo* by adding bacteriolytic concentrations of penicillin to the growth medium of cells that carried radioactively labeled lysine in their cell walls. Addition of penicillin resulted in the rapid drop of optical density in such cultures, indicating dissolution of the bacterial cells. Analysis of the supernatants of such lysing cultures showed that the radiolabeled peptidoglycan released into the medium was still covalently linked to the glycan and to the choline-containing wall teichoic acids, even at times when more than half of the optical density of the culture was already lost. Passing such lysates through an antiphosphocholine affinity column capable of retaining material bound to choline-containing

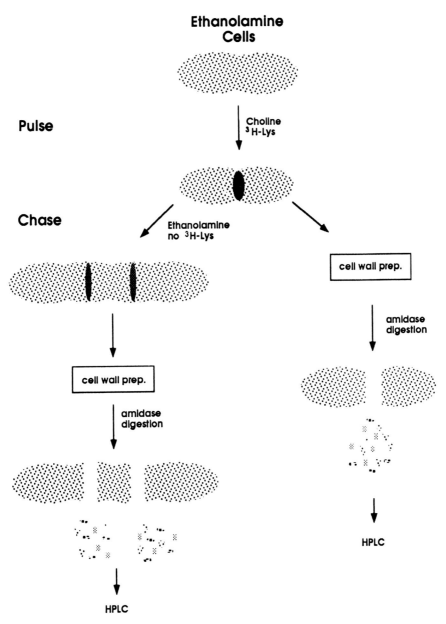

FIG. 14. Physical separation of newly made (nascent) cell wall from "old" portions of the cell wall using the "microsurgery" experiment described in Fig. 13.

teichoic acids showed that more than 90% of the solubilized peptidoglycan was still part of a covalently interlinked macromolecular structure that had the same composition as the intact cell wall except that it was in solution.[8] Appearance of free stem peptides in the medium only occurred after a prolonged time lag, indicating that under these conditions of *in vivo* autolysis the release of stem peptides from the cell wall was a secondary process. The data suggest that *in vivo* triggering of the autolytic enzyme would preferentially attack some strategically located bonds, possibly amide bonds in stem peptides that connect parallel layers of peptidoglycan in the pneumococcal cell wall.

REFERENCES

1. **Briles, E.B., and A. Tomasz.** 1970. Radioautographic evidence for equatorial wall growth in a gram positive bacterium: segregation of choline ^{3}H-labeled teichoic acid. J. Cell. Biology **47**:786–790.

2. **Brundish, D.E., and J. Baddiley.** 1967. The characterization of pneumococcal C-polysaccharide as a ribitol teichoic acid. Biochem. J. **105**:30c–31c.

3. **De Jonge, B.L.M., Y.-S. Chang, D. Gage, and A. Tomasz.** 1992. Peptidoglycan composition of a highly methicillin-resistant *Staphylococcus aureus* strain: the role of penicillin binding protein 2A. J. Biol. Chem. **267**:11248–11254.

4. **Dowson, C.G., A. Hutchison, J.A. Brannigan, R.C. George, D. Hansman, J. Liñares, A. Tomasz, J. Maynard Smith, and B.G. Spratt.** 1989. Horizontal transfer of penicillin-binding protein genes in penicillin-resistant clinical isolates of *Streptococcus pneumoniae*. Proc. Natl. Acad. Sci. USA **86**:8842–8846.

5. **Dubos, R.J.** 1937. Mechanism of the lysis of pneumococci by freezing and thawing, bile, and other agents. J. Exp. Med. **66**:101–112.

6. **Figueiredo, A.M.S., R. Austrian, P. Urbaskova, L.A. Teixeira, and A. Tomasz.** 1995. Novel penicillin-resistant clones of *Streptococcus pneumoniae* in the Czech Republic and in Slovakia. Microb. Drug Resist. **1**:71–78.

7. **Fischer, W., T. Behr, R. Hartmann, J.P. Katalinic, and H. Egge.** 1993. Teichoic acid and lipoteichoic acid of *Streptococcus pneumoniae* possess identical chain structures. A reinvestigation of teichoic acid (C polysaccharide). Eur. J. Biochem. **215**:851–857.

8. **Garcia-Bustos, J., and A. Tomasz.** 1989. Mechanism of pneumococcal cell wall degradation *in vitro* and *in vivo*. J. Bacteriol. **171**:114–119.

9. **Garcia-Bustos, J., and A. Tomasz.** 1990. A biological price of antibiotic resistance: major changes in the peptidoglycan structure of penicillin-resistant pneumococci. Proc. Natl. Acad. Sci. USA **87**:5414–5419.

10. **Garcia-Bustos, J.F., B.T. Chait, and A. Tomasz.** 1987. Structure of the peptide network of pneumococcal peptidoglycan. J. Biol. Chem. **262**:15400–15405.

11. **Garcia-Bustos, J.F., B.T. Chait, and A. Tomasz.** 1988. Altered peptidoglycan structure in a pneumococcal transformant resistant to penicillin. J. Bacteriol. **170**:2143–2147.

12. **Giudicelli, S., and A. Tomasz.** 1984. Attachment of pneumococcal autolysin to wall teichoic acids, an essential step in enzymatic wall degradation. J. Bacteriol. **158**:1188–1190.

13. **Hakenbeck, R., A. Konig, I. Kern, M. van der Linden, W. Keck, D. Billot-Klein, R. Legrand, B. Schoot, and L. Gutmann.** 1998. Acquisition of five high-M_r penicillin-binding protein variants during transfer of high-level β-lactam resistance from *Streptococcus mitis* to *Streptococcus pneumoniae*. J. Bacteriol. **180**:1831–1840.

14. **Hakenbeck, R., and M. Kohiyama.** 1982. Purification of penicillin-binding protein 3 from *Streptococcus pneumoniae*. Eur. J. Biochem. **127**:231–236.

15. **Hakenbeck, R., C. Martin, C.G. Dowson, and T. Grebe.** 1994. Penicillin-binding protein 2b of *Streptococcus pneumoniae* in piperacillin-resistant laboratory mutants. J. Bacteriol. **176**:5574–5577.

16. **Handwerger, S., and A. Tomasz.** 1986. Alterations in kinetic properties of penicillin-binding proteins of penicillin-resistant *Streptococcus pneumoniae*. Antimicrob. Agents Chemother. **30**:57–63.

17. **Holtje, J.-V., and A. Tomasz.** 1975. Specific recognition of choline residues in the cell wall teichoic acid by the N-acetylmuramyl-L-alanine amidase of pneumococcus. J. Biol. Chem. **250**:6072–6076.

18. **Holtje, J.-V., and A. Tomasz.** 1976. Purification of the pneumococcal N-acetylmuramyl-L-alanine amidase to biochemical homogeneity. J. Biol. Chem. **251**:4199–4207.

19. **Jennings, H.J., C. Lugowski, and N.M. Young.** 1980. Structure of the complex polysaccharide C-substance from *Streptococcus pneumoniae* type 1. Biochemistry **19**:4712–4719.

20. **Laitinen, H., and A. Tomasz.** 1990. Changes in composition of peptidoglycan during maturation of the cell wall in pneumococci. J. Bacteriol. **172**:5961–5967.

21. **Liu, T.-Y., and E.C. Gotschlich.** 1963. The chemical composition of pneumococcal C-polysaccharide. J. Biol. Chem. **238**:1928–1934.

22. **Liu, T.-Y., and E.C. Gotschlich.** 1967. Muramic acid phosphate as a component of the muropeptide of Gram-positive bacteria. J. Biol. Chem. **242**:471–476.

23. **Lopez, R., E. Garcia, P. Garcia, and J.L. Garcia.** 1997. The pneumococcal cell wall degrading enzymes: a modular design to create new lysins? Microb. Drug Resist. **3**:199–211.

24. **Mirelman, D.** 1981. Assembly of wall peptidiglycan polymers, pp. 67–86. *In* M. Salton and G.D. Shockman (ed.). β-Lactam Antibiotics. Academic Press, Inc., New York.

25. **Mosser, J.L., and A. Tomasz.** 1970. Choline-containing teichoic acid as a structural component of pneumococcal cell wall and its role in sensitivity to lysis by an autolytic enzyme. J. Biol. Chem. **245**:287–298.

26. **Schleifer, K.H., and O. Kandler.** 1972. Peptidoglycan types of bacterial cell walls and their taxonomic implications. Bacteriol. Rev. **36**:407–477.

27. **Severin, A., A.M.S. Figueiredo, and A. Tomasz.** 1996. Separation of abnormal cell wall composition from penicillin resistance through genetic transformation of *Streptococcus pneumoniae*. J. Bacteriol. **178**:1788–1792.

28. **Severin, A., and A. Tomasz.** 1996. Naturally occurring peptidoglycan variants of *Streptococcus pneumoniae*. J. Bacteriol. **178**:168–174.

29. **Severin, A., C. Schuster, R. Hakenbeck, and A. Tomasz.** 1992. Altered murine composition in a DD-carboxypeptidase mutant of *Streptococcus pneumoniae*. J. Bacteriol. **174**:5152–5155.

30. **Severin, A., E. Severina, and A. Tomasz.** 1997. Abnormal physiological properties and altered cell wall composition in *Streptococcus pneumoniae* grown in the presence of clavulanic acid. Antimicrob. Agents Chemother. **41**:504–510.

31. **Severin, A., M.V. Vaz Pato, A.M. Sa Figueiredo, and A. Tomasz.** 1995. Drastic changes in the peptidoglycan composition of penicillin resistant laboratory mutants of *Streptococcus pneumoniae*. FEMS Microbiol. Lett. **130**:31–35.

32. **Tillet, W.S., W.F. Goebel, and O.T. Avery.** 1930. Chemical and

immunological properties of a species-specific carbohydrate of pneumococci. J. Exp. Med. **52:**895–900.

33. **Tomasz, A.** 1967. Choline in the cell wall of a bacterium: novel type of polymer-linked choline in pneumococcus. Science **157:**694–697.

34. **Tomasz, A., E. Zanati, and R. Ziegler.** 1971. DNA uptake during genetic transformation and the growing zone of the cell envelope. Proc. Natl. Acad. Sci. USA **68:**1848–1852.

Address reprint requests to:
Dr. Alexander Tomasz
Laboratory of Microbiology
The Rockefeller University
1230 York Avenue
New York, NY 10021

The Pneumococcal Cell Wall Degrading Enzymes: A Modular Design to Create New Lysins?

RUBENS LÓPEZ, ERNESTO GARCÍA, PEDRO GARCÍA, and JOSÉ LUIS GARCÍA

ABSTRACT

Autolysins are enzymes that degrade different bonds in the peptidoglycan and, eventually, cause the lysis and death of the cell. *Streptococcus pneumoniae* contains a powerful autolytic enzyme that has been characterized as an *N*-acetylmuramoyl-L-alanine amidase. We have cloned the *lytA* gene coding for this amidase and studied in depth the genetics and expression of this gene, which represented the first molecular analysis of a bacterial autolysin. Two observations have been fundamental in revealing further knowledge on the lytic systems of pneumococcus: (a) The well-documented dependence of the pneumococcal autolysin on the presence of choline in the cell wall for activity, and (b) the early observation that most pneumococcal phages also required the presence of this amino-alcohol in the growth medium to achieve a successful liberation of the phage progeny. We concluded that choline would serve as an element of strong selective pressure to preserve certain structures of the host and phage lytic enzymes which should lead to sequence homologies. We constructed active chimeras between the lytic enzymes of *S. pneumoniae* and its bacteriophages using genes that share sequence homology as well as genes that completely lack homologous regions. In this way, we demonstrated that the pneumococcal lytic enzymes are the result of the fusion of two independent functional modules where the carboxy-terminal domain might be responsible for the specific recognition of choline-containing cell walls whereas the active center of these enzymes should be localized in the N-terminal part of the protein. The modular design postulated for the pneumococcal lysins seems to be a widespread model for many types of microbial proteins and the construction of functional chimeric proteins between the lytic enzymes of pneumococcus and those of several gram-positive microorganisms, like *Clostridium acetobutylicum* or *Lactococcus lactis*, provided interesting clues on the modular evolution of proteins. The study of several genes coding for the lytic enzymes of temperate phages of pneumococcus also highlighted on some evolutionary relationships between microorganisms. We suggest that lysogenic relationships may represent a common mechanism by which pathogenic organisms like pneumococcus should undergo a rapid adaptation to an evolving environment.

BACTERIAL AUTOLYSINS are endogenous enzymes that specifically cleave covalent bonds of the cell wall and eventually cause the lysis and the death of the cell. These enzymes show both substrate and bond specificities. The former characteristic is related to their interaction with the insoluble substrate whereas the latter determines the site of action. The bond specificity allows their classification as muramidases (lysozymes), glucosaminidases, *N*-acetylmuramoyl-L-alanine amidase (amidase, hereafter), and endopeptidases.[32]

Most organisms contain one or more lytic enzymes. The wide distribution of these enzymes has led to the generalized idea that the lysins participate in a variety of fundamental biological functions such as the synthesis of the cell wall, the separa-

tion of the daughter cells at the end of the cell division, cell motility, the development of natural genetic transformation, etc.[45] It has also been suggested that the autolytic enzymes are responsible for the irreversible effects caused by the β-lactam antibiotics (bacteriolytic and bactericidal effects) that turn out to be the most relevant from the clinical point of view.[66] Nevertheless, the elucidation of the physiological roles of these enzymes has been a matter of continuous debate due to the difficulties in obtaining deletion mutations in the genes encoding the lytic enzymes.

Streptococcus pneumoniae contains a powerful autolytic enzyme, an amidase.[30] Probably, this amidase (LytA) is the best characterized autolysin described so far.[29,68] The activity of this

Centro de Investigaciones Biológicas (CSIC), Madrid, Spain.
Reprinted from *Microbial Drug Resistance*, Vol. 3, No. 2, 1997.

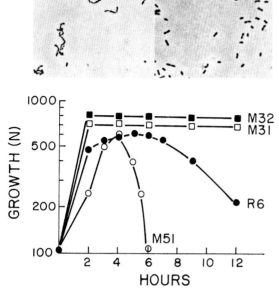

FIG. 1. Growth curves of the pneumococcal strain M51 and two *lytA* mutants. Growth was monitored by nephelometry. The photographs correspond to exponentially growing cultures of M31 (A) and of M51 (B) strains. (Reprinted with permission from Ronda et al.[49])

murein hydrolase is strongly dependent on the presence of choline residues in the cell wall teichoic acid of this bacterium. In this sense, *S. pneumoniae* is one of the rare microorganisms that contains choline in the cell envelope and replacement of the choline by its analog ethanolamine causes a series of dramatic changes in the cell physiology (e.g., growth in long chains, loss of competence for transformation, resistance to lysis, etc.). All these alterations have been attributed to the fact that ethanolamine-grown cells contain an inactive form (E-form) of the amidase (see ref. 67 for a review). This inactive form can be "converted" to the active form (C-form) by incubation at low temperature with choline-containing cell walls.[69]

As a fundamental step to isolate autolysin-defective mutants and to achieve a better knowledge of the genetics of this enzyme, we developed a new procedure to guarantee the rapid identification of the Lyt phenotype,[25] which opened up the possibility of cloning and sequencing, for the first time, a gene (*lytA*) coding for a bacterial autolysin.[24] The cloning of *lytA* also facilitated the isolation of the genes encoding the cell wall lytic enzymes from pneumococcal bacteriophages based on sequence homologies.[17,18,19,47] These initial findings have been fundamental for: (a) ascribing precise biological functions to the autolytic enzymes; (b) providing direct experimental proofs on the modular organization of these lytic enzymes; (c) gaining information on the appearance of repeating units in the primary structure of these proteins that seem to be involved in the recognition of their polymeric substrates (i.e., the cell wall); (d) to analyze the relationships and evolutionary origin of the lytic genes of phages and bacteria.

M31: A PNEUMOCOCCAL MUTANT DELETED IN THE *LYTA* GENE. BIOLOGICAL FUNCTIONS OF THE PNEUMOCOCCAL AMIDASE

The molecular characterization of the *lytA* gene made the genetics of this pneumococcal autolysin accessible for investigation. Several pneumococcal strains containing different point mutations in this gene were isolated and characterized leading to the construction of a genetic map of the *lytA* gene.[21,26,40] However, a more definitive answer to the question of the biological role(s) of the amidase was only obtained through the isolation of a mutant strain (M31) completely deleted in the *lytA* gene.[53] This mutant shows a normal growth rate, development of the competent state for genetic transformation and, apparently (Fig. 1), the most remarkable consequence of the absence of amidase are the formation of small chains (6 to 8 cells), the absence of lysis in the stationary phase of growth and its tolerant response against β-lactam antibiotics. The construction of a recombinant plasmid containing the *lytA* gene (pRG2) and the availability of competent M31 cells provided the tools to study

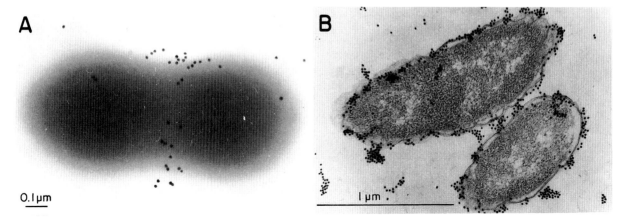

FIG. 2. Immunochemical localization of the pneumococcal amidase in intact cells of *S. pneumoniae* and in ultrathin sections of *E. coli*. *S. pneumoniae* M51 grown in medium containing choline (A) or ultrathin sections of *E. coli* (B) were labeled with anti-amidase serum. (Reprinted with permission from Diaz et al.[10])

the consequences of the reintroduction of the amidase gene in the appropriate background. The exclusive presence of this gene (as a pneumococcal DNA insert in the recombinant plasmid) in *S. pneumoniae* (strain M51) restored the synthesis of the lytic enzyme and, in turn, the capacity to form 'diplo' cells (Fig. 1), and to autolyse in the stationary growth phase or upon addition of penicillin.[49]

Although the expression of pneumococcal genes in heterologous systems has been a difficult task, the *lytA* gene was over-expressed in *Escherichia coli*[22,24] and we have demonstrated that the primary translation product of this gene is the low-activity E-form of the enzyme.[24] The abundant expression of the pneumococcal amidase in *E. coli* allowed the localization of this enzyme in the cell envelope of *E. coli* by using immuno-chemical labeling on ultrathin sections using an antiserum against the autolytic amidase. On the other hand, intact cells of strain M51 of pneumococcus showed the labeling to be localized mainly[10] in the septal region (Fig. 2), a result that confirmed the previous finding that the functional role of the amidase was the separation of the daughter cells.[49] This experimental approach also suggested that the pneumococcal autolysin should be associated initially to the inner face of the membrane probably through the interaction between the negatively charged phospholipids and some of the 42 positively charged amino acid residues present in the amidase.[10,19] Then, the protein is translocated to the outer side of the membrane

where its interaction with the lipoteichoic acid (LTA) should contribute to stabilizing its association to the membrane. The autolysin, that is synthesized without any N-terminal signal sequence was not processed during translocation.[10] Physiological events, like metabolic changes produced during formation of a nascent cross-wall, should release the amidase locally which could explain the postulated role of the pneumococcal autolysin in daughter cell separation providing a more scientific background to our previous findings.[49,67]

Another interesting biological property of the main pneumococcal autolysin has been related to alterations in its primary structure. These alterations in the LytA amidase seem to be responsible for the characteristics exhibited by some strains of *S. pneumoniae* (i.e., strain 101/87) that have been classically misclassified and should now be considered as atypical pneumococcal strains.[13] The activity of the main autolytic enzyme of strain 101/87 (LytA101 amidase) has been studied and we detected that, in remarkable contrast with the wild-type LytA amidase, LytA101 was inhibited by sodium deoxycholate, the test used to identify *S. pneumoniae* (bile solubility). Furthermore, we found some alterations in the DNA region flanking the *lytA101* gene of strain 101/87 when compared to that of the wild-type strain R6. Our findings illustrate how alterations in the activity of the main autolytic enzyme or in its regulation can give rise to dramatic changes affecting the phenotypic characteristics of a clinical isolate of pneumococcus. In turn, it might also influence the pathogenic properties of such strains, as recently emphasized,[71] autolysis plays a role *in vivo* because strains that exhibit alterations in their lytic systems appear to contribute to higher morbidity and mortality from this type of infection. To summarize, the atypical pneumococcal strains are clinically important because they are frequently associated with more invasive types of diseases such as meningitis.[51]

Finally, taking advantage of the great affinity of LytA to choline, we also observed the interaction between the pneumococcal amidase and several choline-analogs, such as diethylaminoethanol (DEAE), which suggested the possibility of using DEAE-cellulose as an affinity chromatography matrix. This observation has led to the development of a rapid and striking procedure for the purification of the pneumococcal lysin as illustrated in Fig. 3. This procedure has been later extended to the purification of several lysins of the pneumococcal phages as well the C-terminal moiety of these enzymes which has reported advantages for the use of these proteins with biotechnological properties (see following).

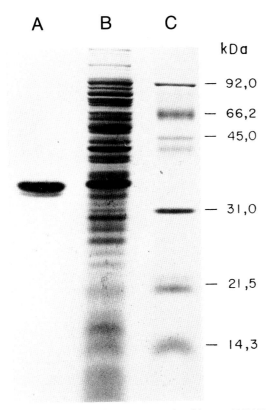

FIG. 3. Purification of pneumococcal amidase on DEAE-cellulose. (A). Purified pneumococcal amidase obtained by affinity chromatography on DEAE-cellulose. (B). Total extract obtained from *E. coli* RB791(pGL100).[22] (C). Protein standards. Molecular masses are indicated in kDa. (Reprinted with permission from Sanz et al.[61])

A SECOND PEPTIDOGLYCAN HYDROLASE IN *STREPTOCOCCUS PNEUMONIAE*

As just pointed out, strain M31 grows normally and does not lyse upon long incubation at 37°C. Nevertheless, M31 suffers a slow lysis when incubated at 30°C which suggested the presence of another lysin in pneumococcus.[54] This new lytic enzyme has been purified showing a M_r of 64000 and has been characterized as an *endo-β-1,4-N*-acetylglucosaminidase that also requires choline in the teichoic acid of the cell wall substrate for catalytic activity.[20] This hydrolase behaves as an autolysin causing the lysis of the cultures upon incubation at 30°C

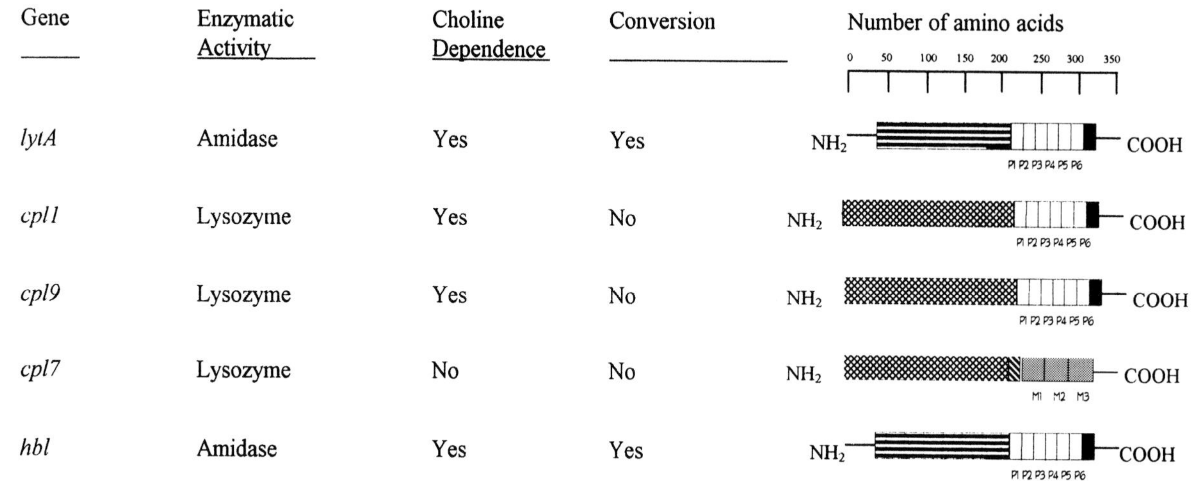

Gene	Enzymatic Activity	Choline Dependence	Conversion	Number of amino acids
				0 50 100 150 200 250 300 350
lytA	Amidase	Yes	Yes	NH₂ — [====] [||||] [■] — COOH P1 P2 P3 P4 P5 P6
cpl1	Lysozyme	Yes	No	NH₂ — [▒▒▒▒] [||||] [■] — COOH P1 P2 P3 P4 P5 P6
cpl9	Lysozyme	Yes	No	NH₂ — [▒▒▒▒] [||||] [■] — COOH P1 P2 P3 P4 P5 P6
cpl7	Lysozyme	No	No	NH₂ — [▒▒▒▒] [ ] — COOH M1 M2 M3
hbl	Amidase	Yes	Yes	NH₂ — [====] [||||] [■] — COOH P1 P2 P3 P4 P5 P6

FIG. 4. Modular organization of the lytic enzymes of *S. pneumoniae* and its bacteriophages. The most relevant properties of the lytic muramidases of phages Cp-1, Cp-7, and Cp-9, and the amidases of phage HB-3 and the host pneumococcus are compared. The amino acid sequences showing a *z* value higher than 4.7 according to Lipman and Pearson[36] are represented by identical shading. P1–P6 and M1–M3 represent the motifs found in the C-terminal domains of the pneumococcal lytic enzymes (see text).

although we can not exclude a more subtle activity of this enzyme at 37°C, the optimal growth temperature for *S. pneumoniae*. Preliminary experiments have suggested that the pneumococcal glucosaminidase may also participate in the process of daughter cell separation. In fact, this suggestion is supported by the finding that a mutant strain of pneumococcus lacking the LytA amidase grew at 37°C forming small chains and changed this morphology for the typical 'diplo' cells when incubated at 30°C, the optimal temperature for catalytic activity of the pneumococcal glucosaminidase.[39] Finally, the irreversible effects (lysis and killing) caused by β-lactam antibiotics have been postulated to be the secondary consequences of the inhibition of penicillin-sensitive enzymes (i.e., PBPs) and are provoked by the uncontrolled activity of the pneumococcal amidase.[66] With the use of the pneumococcal strain having mutations in the amidase, we found that the two autolytic enzymes are directly involved in the penicillin-induced killing of *S. pneumoniae*.[39]

MODULAR ORGANIZATION OF THE CELL WALL LYTIC ENZYMES OF PNEUMOCOCCI

The study of several families of pneumococcal phages has proven useful as an instrument for expanding our knowledge of the mechanisms of interchange in pneumococcus, as well as to gain information on the relationship between host and parasite.[37,38] The successful infection of M31, the ΔlytA strain with the pneumococcal phage Cp-1 indicated the existence of a phage-coded lytic activity (Cpl1). *In vitro* transcription–translation experiments with Cp-1 DNA as a template showed that this DNA synthesized an enzyme that specifically lysed pneumococcal cell walls containing choline in their teichoic acids. This enzyme was purified and biochemically characterized as a lysozyme.[17] The striking choline-dependence of the pneumococcal lysins suggested that the presence of this amino alcohol in the cell wall of pneumococcus might act as an element

of strong selective pressure reducing the evolutionary drifting of *cpl1* and *lytA,* the genes coding for the phage lysozyme and for the host amidase, respectively. This was demonstrated by the fact that Cp-1 DNA hybridized with *lytA* and this gene was used as a probe to map and clone the gene *cpl1* encoding the Cpl1 lysozyme.[17]

This experimental approach was also used to analyze the lytic genes of other phages of the Cp family, and the comparison of the nucleotide sequences of the host and phage lytic genes showed that the 3' regions of these genes were quite similar and the C-terminal domains of these lysins were virtually identical (Fig. 4). In contrast, the N-terminal halves of the LytA amidase and the Cpl1,7 and 9 lysozymes were completely different.[23] Interestingly, no homology was detectable in Southern blot analysis with the DNA of another phage of the same family, Cp7, that also coded for a lysozyme.[23] Biological analyses of this phage showed that it was capable of lysing pneumococcal cells containing either choline or ethanolamine (the analog of choline that is not recognized by the host amidase and the other Cp lysins). In addition, the lysin coded by Cp-7 (Cpl7) has also lost the dependence on choline for activity as revealed by biochemical assays.[23] Remarkably, the comparison of the deduced amino acid sequences of the lysozymes coded by the phages of the Cp family revealed that only 10 amino acids were different between Cpl1 and Cpl9 and 9 of these changes resided in the N-terminal moiety of the protein, whereas the comparison of Cpl1 and Cpl7 revealed that 34 out of the first 204 amino acids were different. Interestingly, two acidic amino acids (Asp and Glu) that have been proposed to be involved in the catalytic process by lysozymes[32] are conserved in the three phage lysozymes of pneumococcus.[18,19] The role of amino acids Asp-9 and Glu-36 in the activity of Cpl1 lysozyme was investigated by site-directed mutagenesis and we concluded that amino acid replacements at position 9 turned out to be more critical for activity than those at position 36.[59]

Additional comparisons of the host amidase, and the Cpl1

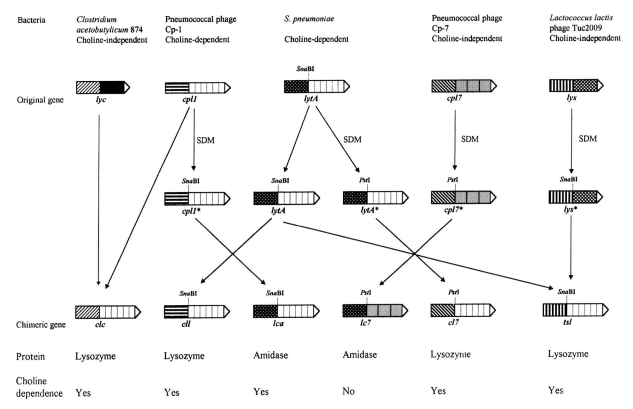

FIG. 5. Diagrammatic representation of the constructions of the plasmids coding for the chimeric pneumococcal murein-hydrolases, the pneumococcal-clostridial, or the pneumococcal-lactococcal cell wall lytic chimeras (bottom row). The headed arrows (upper and central rows) represent the lytic genes and the direction of transcription. Asterisks indicate a new restriction sequence introduced by site-directed mutagenesis (SDM). The relevant characteristics of the enzymes are also indicated.

and Cpl9 lysozymes, revealed that the C-terminal domains of these choline-dependent enzymes present a set of six modular repetitions (P1–P6), each about 20-amino acid long, as previously observed for the host amidase.[18] Notably, the C-terminal moiety of Cpl7 was completely different and the set of six modular repetitions was replaced by a 2.8 perfect tandem repeats (Fig. 4), each 48-amino acid long (M1–M3). This characteristic, apparently, parallels with the aforementioned observation that the Cpl7 lysozyme has lost its dependence on the presence of choline for activity.

Further experimental data on the organization of the lysins of the pneumococcal systems was achieved through the analysis of the primary sequence of the amidases coded by two temperate phages of *S. pneumoniae* (HB–3 and EJ–1), two enzymes that also require choline for activity.[14,46,47] It was found that 287 out of the 318 amino acid residues of host and the HB–3 amidases were identical (90.2%) and 31 of the nonidentical amino acids were conservative substitutions. The C-terminal half of the phage amidases also contains the set of six repeated sequences (P1 to P6), each about 20-amino acid residues long (Fig. 4).

A global analysis of the sequence comparison led us to propose that pneumococcal cell wall lytic enzymes could be the result of the fusion of two independent functional domains, one containing the active center (N-terminal domain) and the other responsible for the recognition of the choline present in the teichoic acids of the cell wall (C-terminal domain).[18,23,47] This

hypothesis was based on the observation that the host LytA and phage Hbl amidases and the phage Cpl1 and Cpl9 lysozymes which depend on the presence of choline in the teichoic acids for activity, have homologous C-terminal domains. However, the phage Cpl7 lysozyme that has lost this dependence contains a completely different C-terminal domain.[23] On the other hand, the N-terminal domains of the Cpl1, Cpl9, and Cpl7 lysozymes are homologous but different to the N-terminal domains of the LytA and Hbl amidases. These observations prompted us to test whether the fusion of these domains might create active chimeric enzymes with novel properties. This experimental approach should allow us to confirm our theory about the modular organization of the pneumococcal cell wall lytic enzymes, opening up new insights in the evolutionary design of these proteins.

INTERCHANGE OF FUNCTIONAL DOMAINS OF THE LYTIC ENZYMES OF *S. PNEUMONIAE* AND ITS BACTERIOPHAGES SWITCHES ENZYME SPECIFICITY

Based on the knowledge of the known DNA sequences of the *lytA* and *cpl1* genes,[18,19] we constructed chimeric proteins between host and phage lytic enzymes that share sequence similarity. The alignment of these sequences enzymes allowed us to identify possible equivalent points on the two genes. Consequently, the new proteins were generated through *in vitro* recombination at these points, at sites approximating the junction zone of the N- and C-terminal domains of the enzymes.[11] We created by site-directed mutagenesis a single *Sna*BI site in the *cpl1* gene to facilitate the construction (Fig. 5). We found that the introduction of this new site was neutral with respect to the reading frame of the gene and to the enzymatic activity, a fundamental requirement for the successful construction of the novel chimeric enzymes. The new recombinant plasmids generated, pCL and pLC, contain the gene coding for a pair of chimeric proteins between the phage lysozyme and the pneumococcal amidase. The biochemical characterization of the extracts prepared from *E. coli* HB101 transformed with pCL or pLC, demonstrated the presence of active lytic enzymes, named as Cll and Lca, respectively, that degraded only choline-containing pneumococcal cell walls. These chimeric enzymes présent novel properties that were, as expected, a combination of those showed by the parental enzymes.

Nevertheless, a general acceptance of our proposal on the modular organization of the pneumococcal lytic enzymes required the construction of active chimeric enzymes by *in vitro* recombination between nonhomologous genes. To do that, we performed the fusion of *lytA* and *cpl7* gene. In this case, we created by site-directed mutagenesis the appropriate restriction site in both genes (Fig. 5). We generated a *Pst*I site within the sequence that had been postulated to be the junction region of the N- and C-terminal modules.[12] Again, the introduction of this site was neutral with respect to the reading frames and to their catalytic activities. Using this strategy, we created two recombinant plasmids, pCL7 and pLC7, containing two new chimeric genes named *lc7* and *cl7,* respectively. As expected, extracts prepared from *E. coli* HB101 (pCL7) showed a lytic activity that hydrolyzed pneumococcal cell walls containing either choline or ethanolamine in the teichoic acid and was biochemically characterized as an amidase.[12] In contrast, the extract obtained from *E. coli* HB101 (pLC7) corresponded to a lysozyme that was only capable of degrading choline-containing pneumococcal cell walls.

A critical review of the current literature reveals that only a limited number of active multienzyme systems has been obtained by gene fusion.[3,35,70] To collect further information on the catalytic modules of the pneumococcal systems, we have described the construction of a trifunctional pneumococcal murein hydrolase (Chl) that contains a choline binding domain (ChbD) and two catalytic domains (lysozyme and amidase). The chimeric enzyme behaves as a choline-dependent enzyme and its activity is comparable to that of the parent enzymes.[60] Combined genetic and biochemical analyses of Chl suggested that the lysozyme catalytic module confers 88% of the total activity whereas 12% of the activity can be ascribed to the amidase module. Recently, Oshida et al.[42] reported the existence of an open reading frame in the chromosome of *Staphylococcus aureus* coding for a hybrid protein with an amidase domain and an endo-β-*N*-acetylglucosaminidase domain that is processed after synthesis, leading to the separation of the two activities, although no information is shown on the possible bifunctionality of the nonprocessed polypeptide. The preference of an organism to possess different activities in different polypeptide chains or to include them in the same protein like Chl, depends on the advantage that any of the systems might provide to the host. Our results reinforce the theory that many proteins may have evolved

by the fusion of DNA fragments encoding functional polypeptides (domains) which can fold independently[27] and the extension of these observations to other bacterial systems should provide further experimental support as discussed next.

CLONING AND EXPRESSION OF GENE FRAGMENTS ENCODING THE N-TERMINAL AND THE C-TERMINAL DOMAINS OF THE PNEUMOCOCCAL MUREIN HYDROLASES: STRUCTURAL ORGANIZATION OF THE LytA AMIDASE

We have also cloned in *E. coli* the 3′ moieties of the *lytA* and *cpl1* genes and expressed the C-terminal domains of the pneumococcal amidase and of the Cpl1 lysozyme without their N-terminal domains.[55] Biochemical and circular dichroism analyses indicated that these are the domains responsible for the specific recognition of the choline-containing pneumococcal cell walls by the lytic enzymes and suggested that these ChbDs can function independently of their catalytic domains.[58] Taking advantage of the strong affinity of these polypeptides to choline or some choline analogs such as DEAE (see earlier), we developed a new single-step system to immobilize and/or purify fusion proteins containing the ChbD of the pneumococcal murein hydrolases.[56] The viability of this approach has been illustrated by fusing our binding domain to proteins of interest, like the acid fibroblast growth factor, with a peptide containing the cleaving sequence recognized by blood coagulation factor Xa. Then, the binding moiety can be removed to yield proteins in a totally unmodified form suitable for clinical and functional studies.[41] More recently, a similar approach has been used to engineer a fusion protein ActA (a protein coded by *Listeria monocytogenes* that induces the assembly of host actin) with the C-terminal domain of the LytA.[63] The fusion protein has been used to coat uniformly *S. pneumoniae* cells and this experimental design has been useful to demonstrate that ActA is sufficient to direct mobility in the absence of other *L. monocytogenes* gene products, a characteristic that enhances the virulence of this bacteria. The use of the C-terminal ChbD of the pneumococcal murein hydrolases as a tag polypeptide also presents another advantage of technological interest because it al-

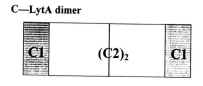

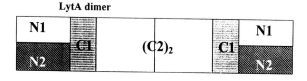

FIG. 6. Schematic drawing of the C-LytA and LytA structural organization in cooperative domains. (Reprinted with permission from Usobiaga et al.[72])

lows the purification of small peptides or proteins which may otherwise be degraded by cell proteases.

The development of these experimental tools permitted the realization of studies on the structural organization of the LytA amidase and its isolated C-LytA domain as well as the variations induced by choline binding by using differential scanning calorimetry and analytical ultracentrifugation.[72] Calorimetric analyses revealed a folding of the polypeptide chain in several independent or quasi-independent cooperative subdomains and that the N-terminal region of the protein is important for attaining the native tertiary fold of the C-terminus. Analytical ultracentrifugation studies have shown that the LytA exhibits a monomer ↔ dimer association equilibrium, through the C-terminal part of the molecule (Fig. 6). Dimerization is regulated by choline interaction and involves the preferential binding of two molecules of choline per dimer. The LytA amidase appears to be an elongated molecule consisting of at least four subdomains per subunit (two per module) designed as N1, N2, C1, and C2. Thermodinamic analysis have also revealed that the suppression of the N-terminal region results in a loosening of the structure of the isolated C-terminal module. In addition, cooperativity between monomers through the C2 domain is always observed in LytA, whereas the C-LytA saturation of the lower affinity binding sites is required. In spite of the homology between sequences of the C-terminal modules of the LytA amidase and the Cpl1 lysozyme,[18] there are great differences between their structural organization in cooperative subdomains.[58] Although both choline-binding modules are designed to improve the attachment of the enzyme to the cell wall, it is obvious that the host-encoded lytic enzyme should exhibit a more efficient regulatory mechanism. LytA is involved in cell division, as already discussed, and its activity should be under time and space regulation, whereas the regulation of Cpl1 lysozyme, a phage-encoded protein, is restricted to the phage cycle.

On the other hand, we have also constructed recombinant plasmids that express in E. coli the DNA regions encoding the N-terminal domains of the choline-dependent LytA amidase and Cpl1 lysozyme and of the choline-independent Cpl7 lysozyme, respectively, showing that these domains also adopt an active conformation even in the absence of their C-terminal domains.[57] Nevertheless, the lower activity shown by the catalytic domains when compared with that of the complete enzymes suggests that the acquisition of a substrate-binding domain represents a noticeable evolutionary advantage for enzymes that interact with polymeric substrates, allowing them to achieve a higher catalytic efficiency. Again, this finding strongly supports the hypothesis that the pneumococcal murein hydrolases have evolved by the fusion of different modules,[23] opening up the possibility of new examples of cell wall hydrolytic domains in nature, derived from the ancestral precursor of the pneumococcal enzymes.

ACTIVITY OF THE CHIMERIC ENZYME LC7 ON PNEUMOCOCCAL CELLS: SOME HINTS ON REGULATORY MECHANISMS

The information collected from the results discussed show that the C-terminal domain of LytA, composed of six repeat units and a short tail, acts as a binding arm attaching the enzyme to the choline residues of pneumococcal cell walls.[55] We have demonstrated that the amino acids located at the C terminus are involved in the choline activation process (conversion) from the E-form to the C-form[52] whereas the functional changes produced in the LytA amidase, analyzed by serial deletions of its C-terminal repeats, have revealed that the enzyme must contain at least four units to efficiently recognize the choline residues of pneumococcal cell walls. The loss of an additional unit dramatically reduced its hydrolytic activity as well as the binding affinity, suggesting that the catalytic efficiency of this enzyme can be considerably improved by keeping the protein attached to the cell wall substrate, as already suggested.[16] This behavior strongly supports the model proposed by Knowles' group[65] to explain the role of cellulase-binding domains postulating that the catalytic efficiency of these enzymes can be considerably improved by keeping the protein attached to the substrate, because in this way, the local concentration of the putative cleavage sites is increased. This model, that can be extended to enzymes acting on other polymeric substrates as the LytA amidase, implies that the existence of several binding sites could allow the protein to "walk" along the surface of the substrate. Remarkably, proteins lacking one or two repeat units were more sensitive to the inhibition by free choline than the wild type enzyme, whereas the N-terminal catalytic domain was insensitive to this inhibition.[16]

Interestingly, the truncated proteins were inhibited by deoxycholate (DOC), and the expression of the LytA amidase lacking the last 11 amino acids in strain M31 conferred to the cell an atypical phenotype (Lyt+ DOC−) (i.e., the cells autolyzed at the end of the stationary phase but were not sensitive to DOC-induced lysis, as just discussed for some clinical isolates of pneumococci).

The purified Lc7 amidase, the chimeric enzyme that has lost the dependence of choline for activity (Fig. 5), was also used to determine whether this enzyme was active when tested in vivo. To carry out this experiment, we grew the pneumococcal strain M31 in the presence of Lc7 amidase. As noted, S. pneumoniae M31 has a complete deletion of the lytA gene and it did not autolyze at the end of the stationary phase of growth but it has been well established that this strain can be "cured" by the addition of LytA amidase to the culture medium.[53] When the lc7 gene was transferred to a shuttle plasmid capable of replication in S. pneumoniae, a derivative of the pLSE1,[53] and the resulting recombinant plasmid (pNLC7) was used to transform M31, we found that the newly created chimeric enzyme Lc7 was active in the homologous system and capable of restoring in M31 all of the biological properties that the pneumococcal host amidase possesses (e.g., lysis of the culture at the end of the exponential phase of growth, formation of "diplo" cells, etc.). Most important, experiments carried out in synthetic medium containing ethanolamine that leads to the formation of ethanolamine-containing pneumococcal cells, demonstrated that the wild type strain did not lyse in this medium due to the absence of an autolysin capable of hydrolyzing ethanolamine-containing cell walls whereas the cells expressing the lc7 gene did autolyse in this medium.[12]

These findings suggested that Lc7 amidase, an enzyme that has not yet been found in nature, behaves in vivo as an autolysin, and most important, the enzyme was placed under the regulatory system of the cell during the exponential phase of growth. Because the LC7 amidase is not inhibited by choline, the choline-mediated regulation of the LytA amidase by the LTA (i.e., the previously postulated specific inhibition by the choline residues of the LTA anchored in the cell membrane,[2,29] cannot be considered as the unique mechanism of control for the host autolysin. Thus, it can be concluded that an alternative regulatory mechanism must exist to prevent the autolysis of pneumococcus during cell growth. As we have reported, the LytA amidase was anchored to the inner membrane of *E. coli*, a microorganism that does not contain choline in its cellular envelope. This interaction seems to represent an intrinsic property of the amidase and it is reasonable to assume a similar regulatory mechanism for the LytA amidase in *S. pneumoniae*.

CONSTRUCTION OF CHIMERIC LYTIC ENZYMES BETWEEN DIFFERENT GRAM-POSITIVE BACTERIA AND THEIR BACTERIOPHAGES

The nucleotide sequence of the *lyc* gene coding for the autolytic enzyme (Lyc) of *Clostridium acetobutylicum* ATCC824, a gram-positive anaerobic sporeformer widely used for the industrial-scale production of acetone and butanol has recently been determined.[7] This autolytic enzyme, previously characterized as a muramidase,[6] seems to have a modular organization.[7]

As pointed out for the pneumococcal system, comparative analysis of the clostridial Lyc muramidase with other muramidases suggested the existence of a junction region located around amino acid 200 between the apparent N- and C-terminal regions of this enzyme.[7] A fusion protein was engineered using plasmids pCM18, containing a *Hind*III-*Kpn*I fragment coding for the C-terminal domain of the Cpl1 muramidase and pAC281 containing a *Kpn*I-*Eco*RI fragment coding for the N-terminal domain of the Lyc muramidase.

Taking advantage of the restriction sites, Sau3AI (*lyc*)[7] and SspI (*cpl1*),[17] located at equivalent points of both genes (codons for Asp-192 and Ile-184, respectively) as just defined, the chimeric *clc* gene was generated through *in vitro* recombination following the strategy shown in Fig. 5. Furthermore, the

construction of a recombinant plasmid, pCLC100, containing the *clc* gene placed under the control of a strong promoter of *E. coli* should facilitate the overproduction of the protein coded by this gene. Competent cells of *E. coli* DH1 were transformed with the recombinant plasmid pCLC100. The presence of a protein containing the ChbD of the Cpl1 muramidase, in the extracts prepared from this transformant was determined by affinity chromatography.[61] When crude extracts obtained by sonication of *E. coli* DH1 (pCLC100) were applied to these columns, a prominent band with an apparent M_r of 40,000, as would be expected from the deduced amino acid sequence of the chimeric gene, was found. The Clc enzyme was unable to degrade the cell walls of *C. acetobutylicum* ATCC824 but hydrolyzed pneumococcal cell walls. This chimeric enzyme, like the Cpl1 muramidase, shows an absolute requirement for the presence of choline in the pneumococcal cell wall substrate for activity. Replacement of choline by ethanolamine in the teichoic acids completely abolished the activity of the chimeric protein. Furthermore, choline, a noncompetitive inhibitor of the lytic enzymes of pneumococcus and its bacteriophages,[28] inhibited the activity of the Clc enzyme. Because the parental Lyc muramidase was choline-independent and unable to degrade pneumococcal cell walls, the formation of this active chimeric enzyme by exchanging protein domains between two enzymes that specifically hydrolyze cell walls of bacteria belonging to different genera, shows that a switch on substrate specificity has been achieved. The chimeric Clc muramidase behaved as an autolytic enzyme when it was adsorbed onto a live autolysin-defective mutant of *S. pneumoniae*.[8]

Given that the fusion of the N-terminal domain of the clostridial lysozyme and the C-terminal domain of the Cpl1 lysozyme from the Cp-1 phage demonstrated that the N-terminal domain of the Lyc lysozyme contains the catalytic domain, we carried out a new construction to determine whether the C-terminal domain of the clostridial lysozyme, a choline-independent enzyme, was also involved in cell wall recognition, as demonstrated for the lytic enzymes of the pneumococcal system. A chimeric enzyme, assembled by the fusion of the N-terminal domain of the LytA amidase and the C-terminal domain of the Lyc lysozyme (not documented), exhibited an amidase activity capable of hydrolyzing choline-containing clostridial

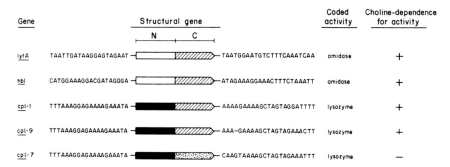

FIG. 7. Schematic representation of the lytic enzyme genes of *S. pneumoniae* and its bacteriophages and of their flanking regions. The structural genes are represented by boxes, and the direction of transcription is indicated by arrows. N and C correspond to the sequences coding for the N- and C-terminal domains, respectively, of the translated proteins, and equal shadowing represents sequence similarity. The nucleotides correspond to the flanking regions upstream of the ATG initiation codons and downstream of the TAA termination codons. (Reprinted with permission from Romero et al.[47])

cell walls with an efficiency 250-times higher than when tested on pneumococcal walls.[9] This experimental approach demonstrated the basic role of the C-terminal domain of a clostridial lytic enzyme in substrate recognition as already proven in the pneumococcal lysins.

Most recently, we have succeeded in the preparation of an active chimeric cell wall lytic enzyme by fusing the region coding for the N-terminal half of the lactococcal phage Tuc2009 lysin and that encoding the C-terminal domain of the pneumococcal host amidase.[62] On the basis of sequence comparisons, the existence of an open reading frame in the phage Tuc2009, that infects *Lactococcus lactis ssp. cremoris*[1] and exhibited a modular organization similar to that described for the lytic enzymes of pneumococcus and its bacteriophages had been proposed. On the basis of these observations and following an experimental protocol similar to those just described (Fig. 5), we constructed a new lytic gene coding for a protein showing a lytic activity on choline-containing pneumococcal cell wall that was identified as a glycosidase.[62] This finding illustrates how the construction of chimeric enzymes also provides biochemical information on enzymes that, due to technical limitations, appear rather difficult to decipher in the parental system.

The construction of these active chimeric enzymes between different bacterial systems and its bacteriophages provides further experimental support for the theory of modular evolution which assumes that novel proteins have evolved by the assembly of pre-existing polypeptide units.

REMODELLING DOMAINS IN NATURE

An interesting question posed by these observations comes from the availability of new modules that should allow the introduction of variability in the enzymes that exhibit a modular organization to report evolutionary advantages to the host and the phage. The study of several genes coding for lytic enzymes of temperate phages of pneumococcus has also highlighted some evolutionary relationships between microorganisms. We have sequenced a DNA fragment containing the *hbl* gene of the pneumococcal bacteriophage HB-3, which codes for the phage

lytic amidase and found a remarkable similarity (about 87%) between the *lytA* and *hbl* genes.[46,47] This similarity completely disappeared outside the ORF coding for both amidases (Fig. 7). The *hbl* gene transformed amidase-deficient strains of *S. pneumoniae* to the wild type phenotype and Southern blotting experiments provided evidence for the recombination between donor and recipient genes.[47] HB-3 is a temperate phage and we recently have found that another temperate pneumococcal phage, EJ-1, showing a completely different morphology, also possesses a gene (*ejl*) similar to the *lytA* gene.[14]

A global analysis of the genes coding for amidases of pneumococcus and its bacteriophages that have been sequenced so far revealed that they share two characteristics with other cell wall lytic enzymes: (a) the remarkable similarity between the structural genes was lost in their flanking regions (Fig. 7) and (b) the *hbl* and *ejl* genes seem to form part of an operon as already observed in the cases of the lytic genes of the pneumococcal phages Cp-1, Cp-7, Cp-9 that code for lysozymes.[18,47] The fact that the similarity between bacterial and phage genes encoding cell wall lytic enzymes is limited to their structural regions, reinforces the suggestion that, in this case, the coding regions define the evolutionary concept of interchangeable functional modules, whereas the flanking noncoding regions that should be involved in regulatory functions, would not be interchanged, because they are specific for bacterial and phage systems.[47] The recombination between the phage and host genes noted earlier, together with the construction of bacterial-phage chimeric genes with biological activity, strongly indicates that recombinational mechanisms should play a relevant role in the evolution of the genes coding for cell wall lytic enzymes of phages and bacteria. The lysogenic relationship of a phage, containing a cell wall lytic gene, with a host cell may provide the ideal background to establish interchanges without affecting the viability of the system, until the appearance of a viable variant of the lytic enzyme that, eventually, should report evolutionary advantages to both phage and host cell.[44]

Another interesting observation carried out in our group provided new clues on this proposal. The presence of a phage remnant (*hblR* gene), homologous to the lytic gene *hbl7* HB-3 phage, in the genome of a DpnII *S. pneumoniae* strain (8R1)

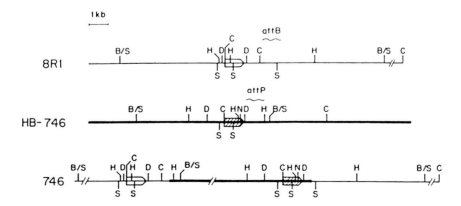

FIG. 8. Location of the *att* regions and detection of phage remnants. Partial restriction maps of the 8R1, HB-746, and 746 DNA fragments that contain the *attB* and *attP* regions are shown. Symbols: —, chromosomal DNA, —, phage DNA; ▷, the *hblR* gene (remnant); ▨, the *hbl7* gene. Abbreviations: B, *Bgl*II; C, *Cla*I; D, *Dra*I; H, *Hae*III; N, *Nco*I; S, *Sau*3AI. (Reprinted with permission from Romero et al.[48])

may be reminiscent of an ancestral interaction between phage and bacterial genomes,[48] an assumption favored by the fact that the phage HB-746 attachment site is shown to map close to gene coding for the lytic amidase of this phage that lysogenize the pneumococcal 8R1 strain (Fig. 8). This observation provides, in the pneumococcal system, an additional clue to support the view on the chimeric origin of phages, where it has been proposed that lytic genes arose from host genes whose products direct the turnover of cell envelope components.[4] It has been suggested that genes, like modules for DNA replication or lytic functions, might exist as linked gene blocks in the pool of interbreeding bacteria in nature[43] and a viable phage might enter into a lysogenic relationship with a cell that contains a repertory of "spare parts" of phages allowing occasional new phage properties to appear. Comparison of the sequences of PBP2x genes revealed an overall divergence of 0.4% in penicillin-susceptible isolates.[15] Also, the amylomaltase genes (*malP*) of several pneumococcal strains were almost identical.[15] However, the sequences of *pbp2b* and *pbp2x* genes from penicillin-resistant pneumococci differed by 7% to 18%. It has been suggested that this divergence has been introduced in these strains apparently through horizontal transfer giving rise to these type of mosaic structures.[15,33] The variability in nucleotide composition found in the cell wall lytic genes of *S. pneumoniae* and its bacteriophages (12%–19%)[14,23,47] suggests that recombination between phage and bacterial genes may be the instrument to introduce variability in the genes coding for lytic enzymes in this system. Furthermore, the presence of genetic remnants, apparently limited to the lytic genes, as revealed when the genome of strain 8R1 was hybridized with the phage genome, indicates that these "promiscuous" genes may remain in the host as a result of abnormal excisions in the course of eventual initiations of lytic cycles which might account for the presence of such remnants in locations close to the attachment sites, as illustrated by some of the pneumococcal phages.[48] In turn, the presence in the genome of most DpnII strains tested with two highly similar cell wall lytic genes, one of them corresponding to a type of "molecular fossil", should provide the ideal background to carry out such exchange between phages and the bacterial genome without altering an essential function, because otherwise most of these recombinations would result in nonviable or abortive phages[44] and should affect an essential host gene like those involved in lytic functions.

CONCLUSION

The noticeable capacity of screening of the Lyt phenotype provided by a filter technique,[25] a procedure that allowed detection of as much as a single Lyt+ colony among several thousands of Lyt−, or vice versa, was a fundamental achievement to facilitate the study of autolytic enzymes at the molecular level. The cloning of *lytA* gene coding for the major pneumococcal autolysin was the first example of cloning of bacterial autolysin gene, and its expression in *E. coli* represents a novel procedure for obtaining high amounts of the autolytic enzyme.[22,24] This approach has also provided experimental evidence demonstrating that the enzymatic activity E-form, represented the primary product of the *lytA* gene, whereas the active

C-form resulted from an activation of the E-form at a later state, as previously postulated.[69]

The isolation and characterization of a pneumococcal mutant with a complete deletion in the *lytA* gene combined with experiments of reintroduction of the *lytA* gene into a recombinant plasmid,[49,53] facilitated the direct demonstration of the role played by the pneumococcal amidase in the separation of the daughter cells. Studies on the subcellular localization of the amidase in the homologous and, in a heterologous system, confirmed the peripheral localization and the functional role of the pneumococcal autolysin.[10] Furthermore, the availability of the strain M31 allowed the identification of a new murein hydrolase,[54] later characterized as a glucosaminidase[21] that also depends on the presence of choline for activity and behaves as an autolysin when incubated at 30°C. The precise assignment of the biological role of this autolytic enzyme must wait until mutants (deleted or otherwise) in the gene coding for the pneumococcal glucosaminidase can be obtained.

The results reviewed here reveal that the specificity for binding to the cell wall substrate resides in the C-terminal domain of the pneumococcal lytic enzymes which have several repeated motifs. An overall analysis of a series of proteins from different microorganisms suggests the existence of a family of carbohydrate-binding proteins with conserved C-terminal repeats that also appear to be of modular design.[73] The N-terminal part should provide enzymatic functions. The recent finding that the N-terminal domains of the pneumococcal murein hydrolases were active and degraded choline- or ethanolamine-containing pneumococcal cell walls with similar efficiency, a result which should be expected of murein hydrolases that do not contain the ChbD, provides an experimental argument in favor of the hypothesis that the N-terminal domains of these enzymes might have constituted independent proteins during the evolution of the murein hydrolases. The lower activity shown by the catalytic domains when compared with that of the complete enzymes suggested that the acquisition of a substrate-binding domain should represent a remarkable advantage for enzymes that interact with polymeric substrates, allowing the improvement of their catalytic efficiency.[55]

We have recently shown that the existence of regions of high nucleotide similarity between phage and bacterial DNAs promotes site-specific recombination which should allow restructuring and evolution of the bacterial and phage genomes[46] as has been already suggested in other systems.[64] In addition, it has been pointed out that phage genomes probably came from the host gene pool and known mechanisms of gene rearrangement are adequate to ensure that phage genomes can acquire new genes from that pool as occasion demands.[4] Illegitimate recombination should be the dominant force that converts the phage genomes in a mosaic of genes from nonphage sources.[31] In this sense, the preparation of chimeric enzymes from the genes coding for the lytic enzymes of *S. pneumoniae* and its bacteriophages as well as the construction of chimeric genes between the cell wall lytic genes of *C. acetobutylicum* and pneumococcus and between *L. lactis* and *S. pneumoniae*[8,9,62] has provided excellent experimental support to the theory of modular evolution of proteins. Some of these chimeric constructions have been the result of fusing two genes that lack sequence similarity and belong to different bacterial genera, a result that strengthens the generally accepted view that one of the forces that drives the evolution of microorganisms is the potential of recombinant mechanisms for creating DNA fusions which allow them to adapt rapidly to new environments.

This model of organization appears to be important for the function of enzymes degrading polymeric insoluble substrates.[73] Furthermore, this modular design seems to be a widespread model for many types of microorganisms, as recently documented in the cases of *Staphylococcus aureus*,[42] *Enterococus hirae*,[5] *C. acetobutylicum*,[73] *L. lactis*[1] and of the gene encoding PspA, the pneumococcal surface protein A, that also shows the presence, in the C-terminal domain, of repeating motifs and it has been shown to bind to choline residues on the cell wall.

A two domain structural organization similar to that of the lytic enzymes of pneumococcus and its bacteriophages has been proposed for the clostridial muramidase[7,9] and for the lysin of the phage Tuc2009 of *L. lactis*.[1] Furthermore, the comparative analysis between the deduced amino acid sequences of the clostridial muramidase and muramidases of the pneumococcal phages of the Cp family revealed a significant similarity in the N-terminal portion of these enzymes. These observations, in view of the juxtaposition of *Clostridium* and *Streptococcus* genera allow questions relating to the evolutionary interrelationships between different bacterial genera and their bacteriophages to be posed. The creation of new chimeric enzymes provides a potential model to test and extend, by direct analysis, the modular theories of evolution of the peptidoglycan hydrolases.

The presence of segments with homologous sequences in the polypeptide chains and the similarity in gene organization of many proteins appear to support the view that the evolution of large proteins is favored by the interchange of pre-existing structural blocks possessing an established folding design, because this mechanism should facilitate the formation of cooperative structures.[43] The presence in the chimeric Clc muramidase of the domain that specifies the protein interaction with the pneumococcal cell wall substrate allows the catalytic domain of the clostridial muramidase to hydrolyze this substrate. This demonstrates the importance of the cooperation between the two domains to produce a functional enzyme. This type of cooperativity might be due not only to an increase in the substrate concentration with respect to the enzyme by anchoring the enzyme onto the solid substrate, but also to a role of this binding domain in the solubilization of the cell wall as has been suggested in the case of the cellobiohydrolases of the filamentous fungus *Trichoderma reesei*, that also possess two functional domains.[65] It is worthwhile to note that the specific hydrolytic activity of the chimeric Clc muramidase, estimated to be about 1% that of Cpl1 muramidase, appears to be noticeably high for a newly constructed enzyme and provides sufficient activity for further improvement by natural selection.

In summary, from the data discussed here, we suggest that the phage and bacterial lytic genes of the pneumococcal system provide examples on how both short nucleotide sequence and large DNA regions, encompassing entire domains, can be shuffled, through recombinatory events, during the evolutionary process to generate new genes coding for active but impaired proteins whose catalytic efficiencies would be improved by selective pressures in the course of evolution. This, in turn, might be a variation of the so-called short-sighted evolution that should improve the mechanisms of virulence of pathogenic microorganisms[34] such as *S. pneumoniae*.

ACKNOWLEDGMENTS

We are grateful for the scientific contribution of C. Ronda, C. Croux, J. M. Sánchez-Puelles, E. Díaz, A. Romero J. Sanz, and M. Sheehan former colaborators of our laboratory, to some part of this work. We thank M. Carrasco and E. Cano for technical assistance and A. Hurtado and V. Muñoz for the art work. This work was supported by a grant from Dirección General de Investigación Científica y Técnica (PB93–0115–C02–01).

REFERENCES

1. **Arendt, E.K., C. Daly, G.F. Fitzgerald, and M. van de Guchte.** 1994. Molecular characterization of lactococcal bacteriophage Tuc2009 and identification and analysis of genes encoding lysin, a putative holin, and two structural proteins. Appl. Environ. Microbiol. **60:**1875–1883.

2. **Briese, T., and R. Hakenbeck.** 1985. Interaction of the pneumococcal amidase with lipoteichoic acid and choline. Eur. J. Biochem. **146:**417–427.

3. **Büllow, L., and K. Mosbach.** 1991. Multienzyme systems obtained by gene fusion. Trends Biotechnol. **9:**226–231.

4. **Campbell, A.** 1988. Phage evolution and speciation. *In* R. Calendar (ed.), The bacteriophages. Plenum Publishing, New York, pp. 1–14.

5. **Chu, C.P., R. Kariyama, L. Daneo-Moore, and G. Shockman.** 1992. Cloning and sequence analysis of the muramidase-2 gene from *Enterococcus hirae*. J. Bacteriol. **174:**1619–1625.

6. **Croux, C.,B. Canard, G. Goma, and P. Soucaille.** 1992. Purification and characterization of the extracellular lytic enzyme of *Clostridium acetobutylicum* ATCC824: A novel muramidase acting on non-*N*-acetyl peptidoglycan. Appl. Environ. Microbiol. **58:**1075–1081.

7. **Croux, C., and J.L. García.** 1991. Sequence of the *lyc* gene encoding the autolytic lysozyme of *Clostridium acetobutylicum* ATTC824: Comparison with other lytic enzymes. Gene **104:**25–31.

8. **Croux, C., C. Ronda, R. López, and J.L. García.** 1993. Interchange of functional domains switches enzyme specificity: Construction of a chimeric pneumococcal–clostridial cell wall lytic enzyme. Mol. Microbiol. **9:**1019–1025.

9. **Croux, C., C. Ronda, R. López, and J.L. García.** 1993. Role of the C-terminal domain of the lysozyme of *Clostridium acetobutylicum* ATCC824 in a chimeric pneumococcal-clostridial cell wall lytic enzyme. FEBS Lett. **336:**111–114.

10. **Díaz, E., E. García, C. Ascaso, E. Méndez, R. López, and J.L. García.** 1989. Subcellular localization of the major pneumococcal autolysin: A peculiar mechanism of secretion in *Escherichia coli*. J. Biol. Chem. **264:**1238–1244.

11. **Díaz, E., R. López, and J.L. García.** 1990. Chimeric phage–bacterial enzymes, a clue in the molecular evolution of genes. Proc. Natl. Acad. Sci. USA **87:**8125–8129.

12. **Díaz, E., R. López, and J.L. García.** 1991. Chimeric pneumococcal cell wall lytic enzymes reveal important physiologycal and evolutionary traits. J. Biol. Chem. **266:**5464–5471.

13. **Díaz, E., R. López, and J.L. García.** 1992. Role of the major pneumococcal autolysin in the atypical response of a clinical isolate of *Streptococcus pneumoniae*. J. Bacteriol. **174:**5508–5515.

14. **Díaz, E., R. López, and J.L. García.** 1992. EJ-1, a temperate

phage of *Streptococcus pneumoniae* with a *Myoviridiae* morphotype. J. Bacteriol. **174**:5516–5525.

15. **Dowson, C.G., A. Hutchinson, J.A. Branningan, R.C. George, D. Hansman, J. Liñares, A. Tomasz, J. Maynard-Smith, and B.G. Spratt.** 1989. Horizontal transfer of penicillin-binding protein genes in penicillin-resistant clinical isolates of *Streptococcus pneumoniae*. Proc. Natl. Acad. Sci. USA **86**:8842–8846.

16. **García, J.L., E. Díaz, A. Romero, and P. García.** 1994. Carboxy-terminal deletion analysis of the major pneumococcal autolysin. J. Bacteriol. **176**:4066–4072.

17. **García, J.L., E. García, A. Arrarás, P. García, C. Ronda, and R. López.** 1987. Cloning, purification and biochemical characterization of the pneumococcal bacteriophage Cp-1 lysin. J. Virol. **61**:2573–2580.

18. **García, E., J.L. García, P. García, A. Arrarás, J.M. Sánchez-Puelles, and R. López.** 1988. Molecular evolution of lytic enzymes of *Streptococcus pneumoniae* and its bacteriophages. Proc. Natl. Acad. Sci. USA **85**:914–918.

19. **García, P., J.L. García, E. García, and R. López.** 1986. Nucleotide sequence and expression of the pneumococcal autolysin gene from its own promoter in *Escherichia coli*. Gene **43**:265–272.

20. **García, P., J.L. García, E. García, and R. López.** 1989. Purification and characterization of the autolytic glycosidase of *Streptococcus pneumoniae*. Biochem. Biophys. Res. Commun. **158**:251–256.

21. **García, E., J.L. García, P. García, C. Ronda, J.M. Sánchez-Puelles, and R. López.** 1987. Molecular genetics of the pneumococcal amidase: Characterization of the *lytA* mutants. *In* J.J. Ferretti and R. Curtis III (eds.), Streptococcal genetics. ASM, Washington, DC, pp. 189–192.

22. **García, J.L., E. García, and R. López.** 1987. Overproduction and rapid purification of the amidase of *Streptococcus pneumoniae*. Arch. Microbiol. **149**:52–56.

23. **García, P., J.L. García, E. García, J.M. Sánchez-Puelles, and R. López.** 1990. Modular organization of the lytic enzymes of *Streptococcus pneumoniae* and its bacteriophages. Gene **86**:81–88.

24. **García, E., J.L. García, C. Ronda, P. García, and R. López.** 1985. Cloning and expression of the pneumococcal autolysin gene in *Escherichia coli*. Mol. Gen. Genet. **201**:225–230.

25. **García, E., C. Ronda, J.L. García, and R. López.** 1985. A rapid procedure to detect the autolysin phenotype in *Streptococcus pneumoniae*. FEMS Microbiol. Lett. **29**:77–81.

26. **García, J.L., J.M. Sánchez-Puelles, P. García, R. López, C. Ronda, and E. García.** 1986. Molecular characterization of an autolysin-defective mutant of *Streptococcus pneumoniae*. Biochem. Biophys. Res. Commun. **137**:614–619.

27. **Gilbert W.** 1978. Why genes in pieces? Nature **271**:501.

28. **Giudicelli, S., and A. Tomasz.** 1984. Attachment of pneumococcal autolysin to wall teichoic acids, an essential step in enzymatic wall degradation. J. Bacteriol. **158**:1188–1190.

29. **Höltje, J.-V., and A. Tomasz.** 1976. Purification of the pneumococcal *N*-acetylmuramyl-L-alanine amidase to biochemical homogeneity. J. Biol. Chem. **251**:4199–4207.

30. **Howard, L.V., and H. Gooder.** 1974. Specificity of the autolysin of *Streptococcus (Diplococcus) pneumoniae*. J. Bacteriol. **117**:796–804.

31. **Hunkapiller, T.H., H. Huang, L. Hoong, and J.H. Campbell.** 1982. The impact of modern genetics on evolutionary theory. *In* R. Millman (ed.), Perspectives on evolution. Sinauer, Sunderland, MA, pp. 164–189.

32. **Jollès, P., and J. Jollès.** 1984. What's new in lysozyme research? Mol. Cell. Biochem. **63**:165–189.

33. **Laible, G., B.G. Spratt, and R. Hakenbeck.** 1991. Interspecies recombinal events during the evolution of altered PBP2x genes in penicillin-resistant isolates of *Streptococcus pneumoniae*. Mol. Microbiol. **5**:1993–2002.

34. **Levin, B.R., and J.J. Bull.** 1994. Short-sighted evolution and the

virulence of pathogenic microorganisms. Trends Microbiol. **2**:76–81.

35. **Lindbladh, C., M. Persson, L. Bülow, and K. Mosbach.** 1992. Characterization of a recombinant bifunctional enzyme, galactose dehydrogenase/bacterial luciferase, displaying an improved bioluminiscence in a three-enzyme system. Eur. J. Biochem. **204**:241–247.

36. **Lipman, D.J., and W.R. Pearson.** 1985. Rapid and sensitive protein similarities searches. Science **227**:1435–1441.

37. **López, R., J.L. García, E. García, C. Ronda, and P. García.** 1992. Structural analysis and biological significance of the cell wall lytic enzymes of *Streptococcus pneumoniae* and its bacteriophage. FEMS Microbiol. Lett. **100**:439–448.

38. **López, R., E. García, and C. Ronda.** 1981. Bacteriophages of *Streptococcus pneumoniae*. Rev. Infect. Dis. **3**:212–223.

39. **López, R., C. Ronda, and E. García.** 1990. Autolysins are direct involved in the bactericidal effect caused by penicillin in wild type and in tolerant pneumococci. FEMS Microbiol. Lett. **66**:317–322.

40. **López, R., J.M. Sánchez-Puelles, E. García, J.L. García, C. Ronda, and P. García.** 1986. Isolation, characterization and physiological properties of an autolytic defective mutant of *Streptococcus pneumoniae*. Mol. Gen. Genet. **204**:237–242.

41. **Ortega, S., J.L. García, M. Zazo, J. Varela, I. Muñoz-Willery, P. Cuevas, and G. Giménez-Gallego.** 1992. Single-step purification on DEAE-Sephacel of recombinant polypeptides produced in *Escherichia coli*. Biotechnology **10**:795–798.

42. **Oshida, T., M. Sugai, H. Komatsuzawa, Y.-M.H. Suginaka, and A. Tomasz.** 1995. A *Staphylococcus aureus* autolysin that has an N-acetylmuramoyl-L-alanine amidase domain and an endo-β-N-acetylglucosaminidase domain: Cloning, sequence analysis, and characterization. Proc. Natl. Acad. Sci. USA **92**:285–289.

43. **Privalov, P.L.** 1989. Thermodynamic problems of protein structure. Annu. Rev. Biophys. Biophys. Chem. **18**:47–69.

44. **Reanney, D.C., and H.W. Ackermann.** 1982. Comparative biology and evolution of bacteriophages. Adv. Virus Res. **27**:205–280.

45. **Rogers, H.J., H.R. Perkins, and J.B. Ward.** 1980. Microbial cell walls and membranes. Chapman and Hall, London.

46. **Romero, A., R. López, and P. García.** 1990. Characterization of the pneumococcal bacteriophage HB-3 amidase: Cloning and expression in *Escherichia coli*. J. Virol. **64**:137–142.

47. **Romero, A., R. López, and P. García.** 1990. Sequence of the *Streptococcus pneumoniae* bacteriophage HB-3 amidase reveals high homology with the major host autolysin. J. Bacteriol. **172**:5064–5070.

48. **Romero, A., R. López, and P. García.** 1992. The insertion site of the temperate phage HB-746 is located near the phage remnant in the pneumococcal host chromosome. J. Virol. **66**:2860–2864.

49. **Ronda, C., J.L. García, E. García, J.M. Sánchez-Puelles, and R. López.** 1987. Biological role of the pneumococcal amidase: Cloning of the *lytA* gene in *Streptococcus pneumoniae*. Eur. J. Biochem. **164**:621–624.

50. **Ronda, C., J.L. García, and R. López.** 1989. Characterization of genetic transformation in *Streptococcus pneumoniae* NCTC 11427: Expression of the pneumococcal amidase in *S. oralis* using a new shuttle vector. Mol. Gen. Genet. **215**:53–57.

51. **Salyers, A.S., and D.D. Whitt.** 1994. Bacterial pathogenesis: A molecular approach. ASM Press, Washington, DC.

52. **Sánchez-Puelles, J.M., J.L. García, R. López, and E. García.** 1987. 3'-end modifications of the *Streptococcus pneumoniae lytA* gene: Role of the carboxy terminus of the pneumococcal autolysin in the process of enzymatic activation (conversion). Gene **61**:13–19.

53. **Sánchez-Puelles, J.M., C. Ronda, J.L. García, P. García, R. López, and E. García.** 1986. Searching for autolysin functions. Characterization of a pneumococcal mutant deleted in the *lytA* gene. Eur. J. Biochem. **158**:289–293.

54. **Sánchez-Puelles, J.M., C. Ronda, E. García, E. Méndez,**

J.L. García, and R. López. 1986. A new peptidoglycan hydrolase in *Streptococcus pneumoniae*. FEMS Microbiol. Lett. **35**:163–166.

55. Sánchez-Puelles, J.M., J.M. Sanz, J.L. García, and E. García. 1990. Cloning and expression of gene fragments encoding the choline-binding domain of pneumococcal murein hydrolases. Gene **89**:69–75.

56. Sánchez-Puelles, J.M., J.M. Sanz, J.L. García, and E. García. 1992. Immobilization and single-step purification of fusion proteins using DEAE-cellulose. Eur. J. Biochem. **203**:153–159.

57. Sanz, J.M., E. Díaz, and J.L. García. 1992. Studies on the structure and function of the N-terminal domain of the pneumococcal murein hydrolases. Mol. Microbiol. **6**:921–931.

58. Sanz, J.M., and J.L. García. 1990. Structural studies of the lysozyme coded by the pneumococcal phage Cp-1: Conformational changes induced by choline. Eur. J. Biochem. **187**:409–416.

59. Sanz, J.M., P. García, and J.L. García. 1992. Role of Asp-9 and Glu-36 in the active site of the pneumococcal CPL1 lysozyme: An evolutionary perspective of lysozyme mechanism. Biochemistry **31**:8485–8499.

60. Sanz, J.M., P. García, and J.L. García. 1996. Construction of a multifunctional pneumococcal murein hydrolase by module assembly. Eur. J. Biochem. **235**:601–605.

61. Sanz, J.M., R. López, and J.L. García. 1988. Structural requirements of choline derivatives for "conversion" of pneumococcal amidase: A new single-step procedure for purification of this autolysin. FEBS Lett. **232**:308–312.

62. Sheehan, M.M., J.L. García, R. López, and P. García. 1996. Analysis of the catalytic domain of the lysin of the lactococcal bacteriophage Tuc2009 by chimeric gene assembling. FEMS Microbiol. Lett. **140**:23–28.

63. Smith, G., D.A. Portnoy, and J.A. Theriot. 1995. Asymmetric distribution of the *Listeria monocytogenes* ActA protein is required and sufficient to direct actin-based motility. Mol. Microbiol. **17**:945–951.

64. Stroynowsky, I.T. 1981. Distribution of bacteriophage φ3T homologous deoxyribonucleic acid sequences in *Bacillus subtilis* 168, related bacteriophages and other *Bacillus* species. J. Bacteriol. **148**:91–100.

65. Teeri, T.T., T. Reikainen, L. Ruhonen, T.A. Jones, and K.C. Knowles. 1992. Domain function in *Trichoderma reesei* cellobiohydrolases. J. Biotechnol. **24**:169–176.

66. Tomasz, A. 1979. The mechanism of the irreversible antimicrobial effects of penicillins: How the beta-lactam antibiotics kill and lyse bacteria. Annu. Rev. Microbiol. **33**:113–137.

67. Tomasz, A. 1981. Surface components of *Streptococcus pneumoniae*. Rev. Infect. Dis. **3**:190–211.

68. Tomasz, A. 1984. Building and breaking of bonds in the cell wall of bacteria- the role of autolysins. *In* C. Nombela (ed.), Microbial cell wall synthesis and autolysis. Elsevier, Amsterdam, pp. 3–12.

69. Tomasz, A., and M. Westphal. 1971. Abnormal autolytic enzyme in a pneumococcus with altered teichoic acid composition. Proc. Natl. Acad. Sci. USA **68**:2627–2630.

70. Tomme, P., N.R. Gilkes, R.C. Miller Jr., A.J. Warren, and D. G. Kilburn. 1994. An internal cellulose-binding domain mediates adsorption of an engineered bifunctional xylanase/cellulase. Protein Eng. **7**:117–123.

71. Tuomanen, E., H. Pollack, A. Parkinson, M. Davidson, R. Fackland, R. Rich, and O. Zak. 1988. Microbiological and clinical significance of a new property of defective lysis in clinical strains of pneumococci. J. Infect. Dis. **158**:36–43.

72. Usobiaga, P., F.J. Medrano, M. Gasset, J.L. García, J.L. Saíz, G. Rivas, J. Laynez, and M. Menéndez. 1996. Structural organization of the major autolysin from *Streptococcus pneumoniae*. J. Biol. Chem. **271**:6832–6838.

73. Wren, B.W. 1991. A family of clostridial and streptococcal ligand-binding proteins with conserved C-terminal repeat sequences. Mol. Microbiol. **5**:797–803.

Address reprint requests to:
Rubens López
Departamento de Microbiología Molecular
Centro de Investigaciones Biológicas
Consejo Superior de Investigaciones Científicas
Velázquez 144, 28006 Madrid
Spain

Bacteriophages of *Streptococcus pneumoniae:* A Molecular Approach

PEDRO GARCÍA, ANA C. MARTÍN, and RUBENS LÓPEZ

ABSTRACT

We have characterized four families of pneumococcal phages with remarkable morphological and physiological differences. Dp-1 and Cp-1 are lytic phages, whereas HB-3 and EJ-1 are temperate phages. Interestingly, Cp-1 and HB-3 have a terminal protein covalently linked to the 5' ends of their lineal DNAs. In the case of Dp-1, we have found that the choline residues of the teichoic acid were essential components of the phage receptors. We have also developed a transfection system using mature DNAs from Dp-4 and Cp-1. In the latter case, the transfecting activity of the DNA was destroyed by treatment with proteolytic enzymes, a feature also shared by the genomes of several small *Bacillus* phages. DNA replication was investigated in the case of Dp-4 and Cp-1 phages. The terminal protein linked to Cp-1 DNA plays a key role in the peculiar mechanism of DNA replication that has been coined as *protein-priming*. Recently, the linear 19,345-bp double-stranded DNA of Cp-1 has been completely sequenced, several of its gene products have been analyzed, and a complete transcriptional map has been ellaborated. Most of the pneumococcal lysins exhibit an absolute dependence of the presence of choline in the cell wall substrate for activity, and phage lysis requires, as reported for other systems, the action of a second phage-encoded protein, the holin, which presumably forms some kind of lesion in the membrane. The two lytic gene cassettes, from EJ-1 and Cp-1 phages, have been cloned and expressed in heterologous and homologous systems. The finding that some lysogenic strains of *Streptococcus pneumoniae* harbor phage remnants has provided important clues on the interchanges between phage and bacteria and supports the view of the chimeric origin of phages.

G enetic transformation between different pneumococcal capsular types, as performed by Avery and coworkers,[2] can be considered the starting point of Molecular Biology. Nevertheless, the subsequent development of this discipline in this human pathogen has been hampered by several technical problems like the requirement of complex media to grow pneumococci. This fact could largely explain the difficulties isolating and characterizing mutants in this system, which would facilitate genetic studies, as well as the lack of experimental conditions to detect phage plaques. *Streptococcus pneumoniae* phages were first isolated in 1975 from throat swabs of healthy children, by two independent groups.[41,66] These phages have represented a useful tool for expanding the knowledge of the genetic interchange mechanisms in pneumococcus as well as to gain information on the relationship between host and parasite. In recent years, several pneumococcal bacteriophages from different origins have been isolated and characterized. These have provided the much-needed approaches in collecting new detailed information that has facilitated our current studies on the molecular biology of the pneumococcal system.[14,35,53]

GENERAL CHARACTERISTICS OF PNEUMOCOCCAL PHAGES

Pneumococcal phages belong to four families and they present a great variety in morphology, including lytic and temperate phages,[32] as illustrated in Fig. 1. Dp-1 and Cp-1 are lytic phages whereas HB-3 and EJ-1 are temperate ones. It is worth noting that EJ-1 is purified from mitomycin-induced cultures of the pneumococcal strain 101/87, but repeated attempts to infect several pneumococcal strains or species taxonomically related to pneumococci (i.e., *S. oralis*) with either purified EJ-1 phage particles or crude lysates from mitomycin-treated cells

Centro de Investigaciones Biológicas, Madrid Spain.
Reprinted from *Microbial Drug Resistance*, Vol. 3, No. 2, 1997.

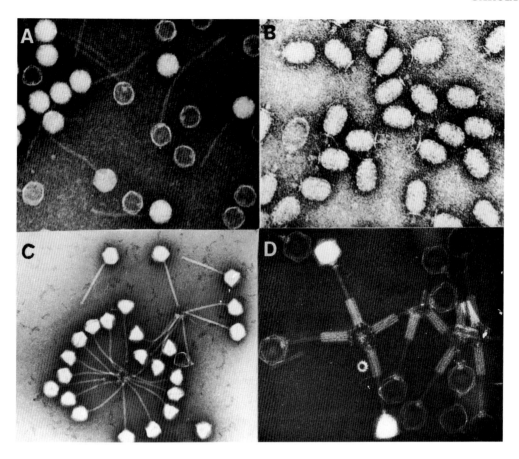

FIG. 1. Electron micrographs of negatively stained preparations of purified bacteriophages. A, Dp-1; B, Cp-1; C, HB-3; D. EJ-1 (magnifications: A, 125,000; B, 175,000; C, 83,000; D, 170,000).

TABLE 1.   SOME CHARACTERISTICS OF PNEUMOCOCCAL BACTERIOPHAGES

| Characteristics | Bacteriophage | | | |
| | Lytic | | Temperate | |
	Dp-1	*Cp-1*	*HB-3*	*EJ-1*
Family	*Siphoviridae*	*Podoviridae*	*Siphoviridae*	*Myoviridae*
Other members	Dp-4, ω-1, ω-2	Cp-5, Cp-7, Cp-9	HB-746; HB-623	
Morphology				
Head diameter (nm)	67	60 × 45	65	57
Tail length (nm)	155	20	156	130
Presence of appendages and fibers	No	Yes	No	Yes
Presence of lipid envelope	Yes	No	No	No
Main structural proteins (kDa)	38	39	34	48
	25	29.5	22	36
Phage genome				
DNA type	DS	DS	DS	DS
Melting temperature (°C)	83.5	87	ND	ND
DNA size (kb)	57	19	40	42
Transfection	Yes	Yes	No	No
Terminal protein linked to DNA (kDa)	No	Yes (26.8)	Yes (23)	No
Lysin gene (nt)	*pal* (899)	*cp11* (1,017)	*hbl3* (954)	*ejl* (948)
Lytic enzyme (kDa)	Amidase (35)	Lysozyme (39)	Amidase (36)	Amidase (36)
Presence of holin (kDa)	Yes (8)	Yes (15.4)	Yes (12.9)	Yes (10.9)

DS, Linear double stranded DNA; ND, Not determined.

GENERATION
NUMBER

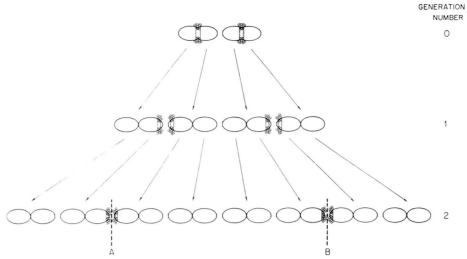

FIG. 2. Schematic representation of the localization and segregation of the choline-containing phage adsorption sites during growth of pneumococci. Immediately after the administration of a pulse of choline to the ethanolamine-grown bacteria, the phage-coated areas (indicative of the choline-containing surface areas) appear to be localized to the equatorial zone of the bacteria. After continued incubation of the bacteria (after the pulse of choline) in ethanolamine-containing medium for one or two generation times, the movement of phage receptors along the bacterial chains seemed to follow a conservative mode of segregation. The localization of phage receptors at the chain termini may have arisen by mechanical chain breakage, as shown here at points A and B. (Reprinted with permission from Lopez et al.[33])

were unsuccessful.[14] The host range of Cp-1 phage is not restricted to *S. pneumoniae,* because it can infect and replicate in *S. oralis,* which shares a common habitat with pneumococcus in humans.[54] Bernheimer[6] first reported the isolation of temperate phages from encapsulated *S. pneumoniae* and suggested that lysogeny was associated with strains of capsular types most frequently causing pediatric infections.[7]

The most relevant physicochemical characteristics of the DNAs from pneumococcal phages and some of the derived proteins are summarized in Table 1. Dp-1 contains a lipid envelope[37] and codes for a lytic enzyme (PAL) involved in the liberation of the phage progeny.[56] Dp-1, ω, and HB-3 phages belong to the family *Siphoviridae* and have long noncontractile tails, whereas EJ-1 is classified as *Myoviridae* with a long contractile tail. In contrast, Cp phages have a short tail and belong to *Podoviridae.* Another remarkable characteristic is the presence of a protein covalently linked to the 5'-ends of their DNAs in the Cp-1 and HB-3 phages. This property is, in the case of the temperate HB-3, a unique peculiarity because the protein must be lost prior to integration in the host chromosome.[51]

PHAGE RECEPTORS IN S. PNEUMONIAE

An important feature of *S. pneumoniae,* shared only by few other species, is the presence of the aminoalcohol choline as a normal constituent of the teichoic acids of the cell wall.[67] A detailed study of the pneumococcal phage receptors has been carried out with Dp-1[33] concluding that choline residues of the teichoic acid are absolutely required for the adsorption of Dp-1. Replacement of choline by structural analogs, like ethanolamine, in the culture medium provokes important morphological and biochemical changes in pneumococci and also blocks phage adsorption. The strong affinity of Dp-1 for the

choline residues has been used to demonstrate by electron microscopy the incorporation and distribution of newly synthesized molecules of the teichoic acid–peptidoglycan complex into the cell wall (Fig. 2). Another conclusion was that these choline residues are essential components of the primary Dp-1 receptors in *S. pneumoniae.*

On the other hand, Dp-1 was not capable of developing an infective cycle in *S. oralis,* probably due to the extremely rapid but reversible adsorption of Dp-1 to these cells.[54] Nevertheless, the demonstrated capacity of the Dp-1 DNA to transfect competent cells of *S. oralis* may provide an alternative procedure for the preservation of these phages when multiplying in a natural habitat.

GENETIC TRANSFECTION

Competence for genetic transformation in pneumococcus is a specialized temporary state characterized by the binding and nicking of double-stranded DNA at the cell surface, the uptake of a single-stranded fragment of DNA accompanied by the simultaneous degradation of the complementary strand, and finally, integration of that DNA at homologous regions of the chromosome.[29] This state can be reached under natural and relatively simple conditions requiring neither stationary-phase cells (as for *Haemophilus*) nor late-logarithmic-phase cells (as for *Bacillus*) but simply exponentially growing cells at a critical but rather low cell density.[68] On the other hand, transfection is the infection process of a host cell by a virus DNA to reconstitute the entire genome inside the bacteria. The first transfecting DNA used in our laboratory was that of Dp-4 and represented the necessary step to characterize the mechanism of transport and fate of this DNA. Selection of appropriate receptor cells has been a key factor in optimizing the transfection process, because the use of a nuclease-deficient mutant increased 100-fold the number of transfectants with respect to the score achieved when competent cells of the wild type strain R6 were used as receptor. Calcium ions but not magnesium ions stimulated both binding and uptake up to 45 min of incubation at 30°C and the saturation level was reached at a DNA concentration of about 10 μg/ml.[63] Our results have shown that the incorporation of 2–3 molecules of phage DNA per receptor cell are required to produce an infective phage plaque.[57] In remarkable contrast, Porter and Guild[46] using phage ω-2 DNA as donor have found that the saturation levels were reached at about 200 μg/ml when the DNA was extracted from mature phages, whereas the efficiency increased when replicative form of the DNA, this is, the DNA extracted from phage-infected cells, was employed as the donor. These authors also reported a phage-associated gene transfer system that had many of the properties of generalized transduction. They claimed that the cell DNA to be transferred is packaged in phage structures and is adsorbed by recipient cells in this form but did not enter them by the phage DNA entry process. Instead, it remained attached to the cells in a DNAse sensitive transformation pathway leading to intracellular single strands that recombine by formation of heteroduplexes that are subject to action of Hex-dependent mismatch correction system. For these unusual features, they coined this gene transfer as pseudotransduction.[45]

Another transfection system has been developed using Cp-1 DNA. In this case, the transfecting activity was destroyed by treatment of the purified DNA with proteolytic enzymes, in contrast with the situation found with Dp-4 DNA. These results strongly suggested the presence of a protein covalently linked to the DNA that should play an essential role in the intracellular development of Cp-1 (i.e., in the replication of DNA or protecting it from being degraded by the host nucleolytic enzymes).[55] Subsequent *in vitro* and *in vivo* experiments demonstrated the presence of the terminal protein involved in DNA replication as demonstrated in other linear genomes that initiate DNA replication through a protein-primed mechanism (see following).[23] It must be emphasized that the maximum yield of Cp-1 DNA transfection was achieved with monomeric forms of the DNA-protein complex. The kinetics of transfection showed a linear dose-response, suggesting the entry of an entire single DNA strand that escaped nicking or degradation by surface-bound or excreted nucleases,[55] in contrast with the situation found in *Bacillus subtilis.*[11]

DNA REPLICATION OF PNEUMOCOCCAL PHAGES

Studies of the intracellular fate of viral DNA during either infection or transfection of pneumococcal cells has allowed two mechanisms of phage replication to be considered, depending on the presence or absence of a terminal protein linked to the DNA.

Replication of Dp-4

We studied the intracellular events following Dp-4 infection of pneumococcal cells until the formation of mature virions and subsequent lysis. To perform such analyses, we selectively inhibited host DNA replication by using 6-(p-hydroxyphenylazo)-

uracil (HPUra), a specific inhibitor of the DNA polymerase III of *Escherichia coli*, without affecting Dp-4 DNA replication.[34] Radioactive assays using ^{3}H-labeled Dp-4 DNA demonstrated that phage DNA synthesis started 15 min after infection and proceeds during 45 min until 15 min before lysis. In the early period of infection, a rapidly sedimenting complex was found in detergent lysates of Dp-4-infected cells analyzed by centrifugation in neutral sucrose gradients. This complex contained labeled parental viral DNA and newly synthesized DNA.[20] In addition, treatment with alkali, pronase, or SDS released the radioactivity from the complex into a form which sediments with mature Dp-4 DNA. Moreover, results obtained from alkaline sucrose gradient analysis suggested that this DNA consists of strands of the same length as those found of mature phage DNA, and probably attached to the bacterial membrane, as it was observed in the case of the phage ϕ29 from *B. subtilis*. Both parental and newly synthesized Dp-4 DNA appeared in the rapid sedimenting complex whereas only the latter was chased into mature phage DNA, suggesting that the parental DNA that had been attached to the membrane did not participate in the progeny of phage Dp-4.[20]

Replication of Cp-1

The ability of all known nucleic acid DNA or RNA polymerases to proceed only in the 5′–3′ direction posed a problem for synthesizing DNA at the end of a linear replicon. A general mechanism to initiate replication is the formation of an RNA primer synthesized by specific enzymes, the primases; a primer can be used in the case of circular DNA molecules or linear DNAs that are converted either to circular or concatemeric molecules. An alternative mechanism for the initiation of replication is the specific nicking of one of the strands of a circular double-stranded DNA, producing a free 3′-OH group that is used for elongation. In the case of linear DNAs that remain as such for replication, RNA priming cannot be used for the initiation of replication because after removal of the RNA, it is not possible to fill the gap that would result at the 5′-ends of the newly synthesized DNA chain. Some linear DNA molecules contain a palindromic nucleotide sequence at the 3′-end which allows the formation of a hairpin structure that provides the 3′-OH group for elongation. The finding of specific proteins covalently linked to the 5′-ends of viral linear double-stranded DNAs, the so-called terminal proteins, led to the discovery of a new mechanism for the initiation of replication in which the primer, instead of being the 3′-OH group of a nucleotide provided by RNA or DNA molecules, is the -OH group of a serine, threonine, or tyrosine residue of the terminal protein. This replication system has been extensively studied in the case of adenovirus and bacteriophage ϕ29 DNAs.[59,60,65]

In the pneumococcal system, the transfection experiments just described demonstrated the key role of a terminal protein linked to the DNA of phage Cp-1 for its biological activity, as it had been documented in the case of ϕ29.[27] Later, we showed that incubation of extracts of Cp-1-infected *S. pneumoniae* with [α-^{32}P]dATP produced a labeled protein with an electrophoretic mobility corresponding to that of the Cp-1 terminal protein. The reaction product was resistant to treatment with micrococcal nuclease and sensitive to treatment with proteinase K. Incubation of the ^{32}P-labeled protein with 5 M piperidine for 4 h at 50°C released 5'-dAMP, indicating that a covalent complex between the terminal protein and 5'-dAMP was formed *in vitro*. When the four deoxynucleoside triphosphates were included in the reaction mixture, electrophoresis on SDS-polyacrylamide gels showed that a labeled complex of slower mobility than the terminal protein-dAMP complex could be elongated, indicating that it was an initiation complex.[23] Other members of the Cp phages also had terminal proteins linked to their DNAs, although these proteins had several peculiarities, in particular, that of Cp-7 phage.[36] The linkage between the terminal protein of Cp-1 and its DNA was shown to be a phosphodiester bond between the -OH group of a threonine residue of the protein and the 5'-dAMP, the terminal nucleotide at both DNA ends.[23] In contrast, these linkages have been identified as serine for $\phi29$[24] and adenovirus[13] and tyrosine for PRD1 phage.[4]

Cp-1 DNA replicates at an optimal rate when *S. pneumoniae*-infected cells were incubated at 30°C. The *in vitro* formation of the initiation complex between the terminal protein and 5'-dAMP was only partially inhibited at 37°C, whereas an almost complete inhibition of the DNA replication was found at this temperature *in vivo*.[18]

All of the genomes having a covalently linked terminal protein whose end-terminal sequences have been determined, showed an inverted terminal repeat of variable length. Cp-1 has a 236-nucleotide long inverted terminal repeat and, in addition, the 116 nucleotides following the repeat showed a 93% iden-

tity.[17] Similarly, in the case of phages Cp-5 and Cp-7, these repeats are 343 and 347 nucleotides long, respectively.[16] The similarity between the inverted terminal repeats of the three DNAs was 84%–92%, which was in the range calculated for the whole genomes from restriction enzyme analysis.[36] The first 39 base pairs are the same for the three DNAs, and the differences are concentrated between nucleotides 74 and 98 and between nucleotides 229 and 253. On the other hand, Cp-5 DNA is more related to Cp-1 DNA than Cp-7 DNA in agreement with the degree of similarity of the terminal proteins. The comparison of the DNA ends of the PRD1 family with those of the $\phi29$ and Cp-1 relatives reveals that the conserved terminal sequence of the PRD1 family and the left end of the $\phi29$ family is 17–18 base pairs long. Within this sequence, there is a homologous sequence CCCCT(A)CCC which is also found in the Cp-1 DNA termini some nucleotides upstream from the DNA end. The finding that the right end of $\phi29$ DNA does not have this sequence and that its left end is first packaged in the phage heads suggests that this sequence might be required for DNA packaging.[59]

Following a more detailed set of experiments, we studied both the initiation and the first elongation steps of Cp-1 DNA replication allowing us to conclude that: (a) formation of terminal protein-dAMP is template-instructed; (b) single-stranded DNA molecules can support protein-primed replication; (c) a specific DNA sequence at the origin is required for efficient

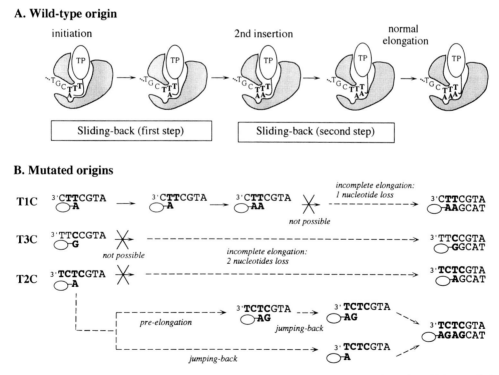

FIG. 3. (A) Stepwise sliding back model for transition from initiation to elongation. The integrity of DNA ends is maintained by two successive steps of sliding back. The third nucleotide of the 3' DNA end is used as template during the entire process. Shaded areas correspond to the polymerization domain of Cp-1 DNA polymerase, defining a cleft proposed to be used as both DNA and terminal protein (TP) binding sites. (B) Effect of mutations in the terminal reiteration. Different possibilities to explain the partial elongation products obtained with mutated oligonucleotides are depicted. Straight arrows indicate those reactions occurring as indicated in the scheme proposed in A. Broken arrows indicate alternative routes for replicating mutated oligonucleotides. (Reprinted with permission from Martin et al.[38])

template recognition; (d) terminal protein-dAMP formation is directed by the third nucleotide from the 3'-end of the template molecule, although the two terminal nucleotides are recovered during the first steps of elongation; (e) a stepwise sliding-back mechanism accounts for the maintenance of Cp-1 DNA ends (Fig. 3). These results reinforce the hypothesis that sliding-back must be a common feature in all genomes that use protein-priming to initiate replication.[38]

To summarize, the mechanism of DNA replication of linear genomes that make use of an -OH group from terminal proteins has been extensively studied only in adenovirus,[28] PRD1,[9] and φ29.[42] Nevertheless, a large variety of linear genomes containing terminal protein, including bacteriophages, eukaryotic viruses, RNA viruses, mitochondrial DNAs from male-sterile maize, plasmids from different origins, transposable elements, etc., has been found.[60] More recently, it has been reported that several bacterial chromosomes (e.g., those of *Borrelia burgdorferi* or *Streptomyces coelicolor*) are also linear and contain a terminal protein covalently linked to their ends.[26] These characteristics together with the presence of inverted-terminal repeats in the DNA ends have led to their assignment as a coherent group of genetic elements called invertrons, and to the suggestion that this replication mechanism can be more common in nature than previously thought.[58]

TEMPERATE BACTERIOPHAGES

The identification of pneumococcal temperate phages was first reported by H. Bernheimer in the mid-1970s[6] when she described the morphological and serological properties of several phages isolated from capsulated pneumococci recovered from pediatric patients. It had been suggested that lysogenized pneumococci lost their capacity to undergo genetic transformation and transformability was restored after cells were spontaneously cured of their prophage.[43] Nevertheless, several lysogenic strains are capable of transforming, although with lower efficiencies.[39] Classical restriction-modification phenomena were demonstrated *in vivo* with some of these temperate phages, and a correlation of restriction with the presence of one or the other of the two known pneumococcal restriction endonucleases was suggested.[7,44] More recently, we have also studied the physiological and molecular characteristics of the HB phages. Analysis of the polypeptide composition of the virions and the restriction endonuclease patterns of their DNAs revealed differences among three of these phages, HB-3, HB-623, and HB-746. Interestingly, the genomes of these phages, about 40 kb long, have been isolated as DNA-protein covalent complexes where the molecular weight of these proteins was about 23,000. Comparative pulsed-field gel electrophoresis and Southern hybridization of the *Sma*I restriction fragments of DNAs from one lysogenic bacteria and its parental strain revealed that the prophage genome was integrated in the host chromosome.[51] In contrast, the 42-kb genome of the temperate phage EJ-1 does not appear to contain any terminal protein.[14]

It has been speculated that the function of the terminal proteins of HB phages might be to protect the DNA molecules during their transport from the membrane to the insertion region of the host bacteria or to serve a function during integration.[51] In

this sense, note that the free linear double-stranded T-DNA molecules from *Agrobacterium tumefaciens* becomes covalently linked through the 5'-ends to the VirD2 protein before these T-DNA molecules are transferred to the genome of the host plant.[15,25] The determination of the precise role(s) of the terminal protein of the HB phages should require a detailed dissection of the mechanism of integration of phage DNA into the host DNA, most probably through the loss of the protein, as well as the precise step when the protein becomes bound to the phage DNA after induction of the prophage to initiate a lytic cycle.

To further characterize the integration process of the temperate phages, we succeeded in localizing the attachment sites of HB-746 and EJ-1 phages, *attP*, through which they integrate into the bacterial chromosome. A common interesting feature is that both *attP* sites lie downstream of the corresponding lytic genes of these phages.[14,50] Even more, in the surrounding regions of both *attP*, there are nucleotide stretches that share noticeable primary and secondary structure similarity with the sequence GGGGCA which is repeated four times along these regions. It has been suggested that this sequence participates in the binding of integrases.[31] In the particular case of the HB-746 phage, we have also mapped the bacterial attachment site *attB* in the host parental genome. This *attB* site was also located downstream of the *hblR* gene that coded for another lytic enzyme and it is almost identical to the phage lytic gene.[50] This phage remnant, present in several *S. pneumoniae* strains, might be reminiscent of an ancestral interaction between phage and bacterial genomes. Interestingly, several genes involved in the virulence of bacterial pathogens may have been derived from a bacteriophage or from an integrative plasmid which carried a bacteriophage integrase and attachment site. In several cases, the use of tRNA genes as integration sites for many bacteriophages and plasmids may favor intergeneric transmission, as tRNA genes are highly conserved.[12]

PHAGE–BACTERIAL INTERRELATIONSHIP IN THE PNEUMOCOCCAL SYSTEM

Once a DNA molecule from a temperate bacteriophage enters the cell, its final fate will depend on the vital choice to follow: the lytic cycle that will lead to cell death and liberation of the phage progeny or the lysogenic cycle with the silent integration of the DNA into the host chromosome. As we have discussed, in the pneumococcal system both lytic and temperate phages are known, but the mechanisms that govern this decision are unknown. Nevertheless, a step previous to the establishment of the lytic or lysogenic state is the restriction–modification system encoded by the receptor bacteria which determines the phage host range. In this respect, the pneumococcal system is rather peculiar because *Dpn*I cleaves only methylated DNA whereas cells lacking this enzyme possess a complementary restriction system, *Dpn*II, that cleaves the same sequence (5'-GATC-3') but when it is not methylated.[30] It has been suggested that the main purpose of the *Dpn*I and *Dpn*II restriction systems would be the protection of the cell against viral infection, and could allow the survival of a remnant of a population after infection initiated in a cell of one particular restriction phenotype. This hypothesis has been experimentally tested in the case of HB-3 phage[44], but has not been proved for

Cp-1 nor Dp-1 phages. In the former case, Cp-1 lacks the target sequence for Dpn enzymes,[40] whereas Dp phage DNAs have abnormal bases[19] which would render them resistant to these enzymes as the result of an adaptation to protect the virus against such restriction systems. On the other hand, in experiments carried out with the phage HB-746, we demonstrated that the RecA protein directly or indirectly controls prophage induction which in turn suggested the existence of an SOS repair system in *S. pneumoniae*.[39]

We emphasize the relationship between the phage-coded pneumococcal lysins and that from the host bacteria, which play important functions in the growth of host cells as well as in the liberation of the phage progeny.[56] In recent years, we have cloned and sequenced the lytic genes from EJ-1, HB-3, Cp-1, Cp-7, and Cp-9 phages, and their enzymatic products have been overexpressed and purified.[32] The comparison of phage-coded enzymes with the host *N*-acetylmuramoyl-L-alanine amidase (LytA) revealed that all but one phage lytic enzymes shared interesting properties like the absolute requirement for choline in the teichoic acids to degrade the cell wall and the noncompetitive inhibition of this activity by lipoteichoic acid, a choline-containing component of pneumococcal membrane.[14,21,48] The exception was Cp17, the lysin from Cp-7 phage, which contains a carboxy terminal domain completely different from that of the rest of the enzymes and, consequently, this lysin has lost the dependence of choline to degrade the pneumococcal cell walls.[22] The biochemical and functional similarities among these enzymes allowed us to postulate a modular organization of the pneumococcal lysins where the N-terminal domain is responsible for the catalytic activity whereas the C-terminal domain recognizes the substrate.[22] The maximum value of identity between bacterial and phage genes was 87.1% when comparing host *lyt*A and *hbl*3 from HB-3 temperate phage. This nucleotide sequence similarity allows recombination between both genomes and such recombination should permit restructuring and evolutionary adaption in both organisms.[49] Due to this homology, it is probable

that the phage-encoded amidase derived directly from the corresponding *S. pneumoniae* gene, although we cannot exclude the previous suggestion that the host genes have descended from related phage genes.[10] Nevertheless, the differences in nucleotide sequences (about 9%) revealed that evolutionary divergence has occurred between the two genes, a conclusion that supports the previous suggestion[47] that the genomes of temperate phages are part of the vertically inherited "survival kit" of bacterial DNA and that they are subjected to the same selective pressures as other chromosomal genes.

FUNCTIONAL ORGANIZATION OF THE GENOME OF CP-1

Recently, we have determined the complete nucleotide sequence of the Cp-1 genome and analyzed its functional organization by determining the transcriptional map as well as some of its main gene products.[40] Putting aside the peculiarities of the DNA ends, terminal protein and DNA replication mechanism already discussed in the aforementioned sections, we will review the more relevant results dealing with some molecule characteristics of this pneumococcal phage.

Sequence analyses

The double-stranded Cp-1 DNA has 19,345 bp and contains 29 ORFs, 23 on one strand and 6 on the opposite strand. When the amino acid sequences encoded by each ORF were compared with those compiled in the GenBank EMBL database, only the products of 10 ORFs showed significant similarity (around 28% identity and 80% similarity) to proteins of bacteriophage φ29 that infects *B. subtilis*. The similar proteins correspond to those involved in DNA replication process (terminal protein and DNA polymerase), structural and morphogenetic proteins (major head, collar, connector, tail, and encapsidation proteins), and proteins involved in lysis function (holin and lysozyme).

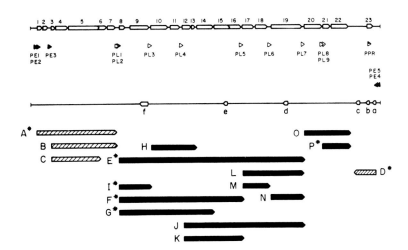

FIG. 4. Schematic transcription map of Cp-1. ORFs are represented as white arrows, indicating the direction of transcription on the two DNA strands. Early and late promoters are indicated by black and white arrowheads, respectively; the PPR promoter is indicated by a black-and-white arrowhead. Early and late transcripts are marked as stripped and black arrows, respectively, preceded by capital letters. Asterisks and double arrowheads indicate transcripts which initiate by using a tandem promoter. (Reprinted with permission from Martin et al.[40])

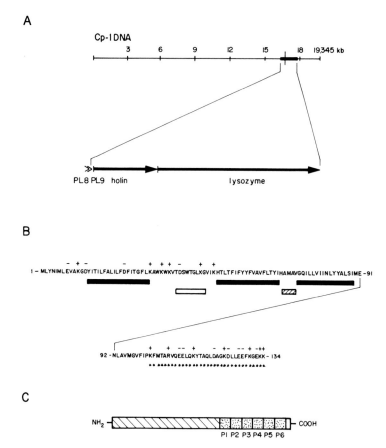

FIG. 5. Holin and lysozyme of Cp-1. (A) Localization of ORF21 and ORF22 coding for holin and lysozyme, respectively. PL8 and PL9 represented by arrowheads indicate the late tandem promoters preceding the holin gene. (B) Secondary structure prediction of the holin. Transmembrane helices are represented as black boxes and β-turns as white or stripped boxes. Positive (+) or negative (−) charges of amino acids are indicated above the sequence. Asterisks indicate the charged C-terminal domain. (C) Modular organization of lysozyme. Stripped region represents the N-terminal domain and the six dotted boxes, P1–P6, indicate choline binding domains.

Transcriptional map

On the basis of its temporal expression, transcription of the Cp-1 genome takes place in two stages: early and late. Combined Northern blot and primer extension experiments allowed us to map the 5′ initiation sites of the transcripts, and we found that only three genes were transcribed from right to left (Fig. 4). It is unlikely that the shift from early to late transcription was controlled in a unique region of DNA, in contrast with what was found in $\phi 29$.[61] Besides the translated transcripts, we have also suggested the existence of a short RNA in an early region located at the right end of the genome. Similar RNAs have been

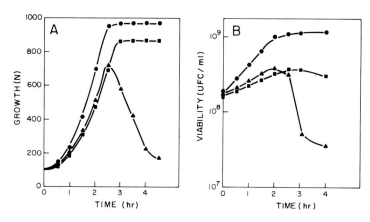

FIG. 6. Expression of *cph*1 and *cpl*1 in *S. pneumoniae.* (A) Growth curves. Cultures of M31 (pLSE1) (●), M31 (pAMR21) (■), and M31 (pAMR22) (▲), incubated at 37°C. (B) Viability of the same cultures.

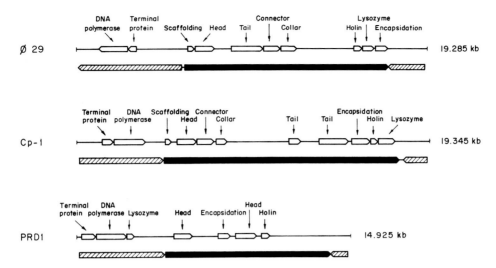

FIG. 7. Functional organization of ϕ29, Cp-1, and PRD1 genomes. White arrows indicate some of identified ORFs, stripped arrows represent early mRNAs and black arrows late mRNAs of these genomes.

found in the proheads of several phages that replicate through protein-priming mechanism, and their secondary structures are highly conserved.[3] These phage-encoded RNAs are required for DNA packaging into phage proheads in both *in vivo* and *in vitro* experiments.[1] Concerning the starting transcription signals, we have found that early promoters had a higher degree of sequence similarity between the -35 and -10 boxes and their spacing regions, whereas in the case of the late promoters, there was noticeable heterogeneity.

Proteolysis of major head protein

In the course of cloning and expression experiments of several phage genes, we observed that the major head protein suffered a posttranscriptional proteolysis of the first 49 amino acids of its corresponding primary gene product. Furthermore, this processing did not take place in *E. coli,* which suggested that the protease was specific to the pneumococcal system. By subcloning and Western experiments, we have identified this protease gene as Cp-1-encoded and showed that the corresponding gene is located in the central part of the genome corresponding to the major late transcript (unpublished results).

Lytic genes

Like most phages, Cp-1 lyses its host by the action of a cell wall-degrading enzyme (i.e., the lysozyme Cpl1). This enzyme has been purified and extensively studied under structural and functional points of view.[21,62] In the strategy of lysis, however, Cp-1 codes for a second, small membrane protein which allows the access of the lysozyme to the peptidoglycan. This protein, called holin, forms part of a group of phage-encoded proteins, characterized by sharing secondary structure traits but not similarity in their primary sequence. Common traits of the holins are: low molecular weight, several membrane-spanning helical domains linked by β-turns and a highly charged, hydrophylic carboxy-terminus (Fig. 5).[69] We have cloned both lytic genes, *cph1* and/or *cpl1,* in *E. coli* under the control of an inducible promoter. In these circumstances, the holin protein is capable of killing *E. coli* cells up to two logarithmic units after 2 h of

induction, but the culture did not lyse. Nevertheless, cells harboring a plasmid construction with holin and lysozyme genes together, did lyse after induction and the viability loss was similar to that of the culture with the holin alone. Following a similar strategy, we have cloned these lytic genes in a shuttle vector (pLSE1)[52] capable of replicating in *S. pneumoniae,* although it is worth noting that inducible promoters have not been described in pneumococci so far. Consequently, in the pneumococcal system, *cph1* and *cpl1* genes were cloned without its own promoter and downstream of the tetracycline resistance gene of pLSE1. The results, depicted in Fig. 6, showed that

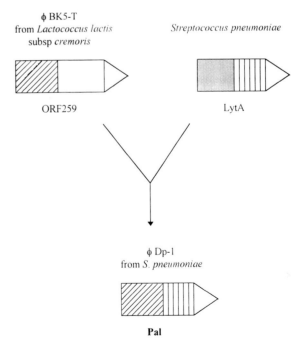

FIG. 8. Modular organization of PAL enzyme. N- and C-terminal domains of the proteins are depicted as different shadings or traits revealing the chimeric origin of the Dp-1 lytic enzyme.

both genes had the same effect as previously observed in *E. coli* cells, i.e., holin itself did not lyse the culture but the viability loss was noticeable, whereas holin and lysozyme together were capable of lysing M31, an amidase deleted mutant, with a similar loss of viability as for holin-containing cells. The regulatory controls that, presumably, are involved in the expression of the two lytic genes are unknown.

Evolutionary considerations

Cp-1 is the first pneumococcal phage whose complete sequence has been determined. As discussed, a striking morphological similarity between Cp-1 and ϕ29 is apparent and the two phages share similar protein-priming mechanisms for the initiation of replication.[60] Furthermore, the organizational similarities between Cp-1 and ϕ29 as well as the homologies between many of the proteins coded by their genes, suggest that at least part of the two genomes may have diverged from a distant common ancestor. Concerning the transcriptional organization, it is surprising that PRD1, a phage that infects several gram-negative bacteria and that also has a terminal protein, displays a genome arrangement very similar to that of Cp-1 (Fig. 7). Assuming that the genomes of Cp-1 and ϕ29 have evolved from genetic elements that have similar organizations, we can speculate that the leftmost region of one of their genomes underwent an inversion at some point during evolution. Taking into account that Cp-1 and ϕ29 are phages that infect bacterial hosts with different genetic backgrounds and that colonize quite distinct ecological niches, the comparison of the primary sequences of the two phage DNAs provides new clues to expand previous observations based on studies of 16S RNA,[64] on the phylogenetic relationships between the genera *Bacillus* and *Streptococcus*.

Finally, in the context where phages are envisaged as chimeric entities capable of recruiting their genes from different origins through evolution, we have recently cloned and sequenced the lytic gene of the pneumococcal phage Dp-1 (M. Sheehan, unpublished results), and the analyses found may strongly support this theory. This enzyme, termed PAL, constitutes a natural chimeric lytic protein, because it is clearly built up of two independent modules apparently arising from different gram-positive bacteria: the N-terminal domain has a 41.9% identity to the N-terminal part of ORF259, coding most likely for a lytic enzyme,[8] of the phage BK5-T that infects *Lactococcus lactis,* and the C-terminal part is 64.6% identical to the corresponding domain of pneumococcal amidase LytA (Fig. 8).

ACKNOWLEDGMENTS

The scientific contribution of C. Ronda, E. García, J. L. García, A. Romero, E. Díaz, and M. Sheehan to some part of this work, is greatly appreciated. We thank M. Carrasco and E. Cano for technical assistance and A. Hurtado and V. Muñoz for the art work. This work was supported by a grant from Dirección General de Investigación Científica y Técnica (PB93–0115–C02–01).

REFERENCES

1. **Anderson, D., and J.W. Bodley.** 1990. Role of RNA in bacteriophage ϕ29 DNA packaging. J. Struct. Biol. **104**:70–74.

2. **Avery, O.T., C.M. MacLeod, and M. McCarty.** 1944. Studies on the chemical nature of the substance inducing transformation of pneumococcal types: Induction of transformation by a deoxyribonucleic acid fraction isolated from pneumococcus type III. J. Exp. Med. **79**:137–157.

3. **Bailey, S., J. Wichitwechkarn, D. Johnson, B.E. Reilly, D.L. Anderson, and J.W. Bodley.** 1990. Phylogenetic analysis and secondary structure of the *Bacillus subtilis* bacteriophage RNA required for DNA packaging. J. Biol. Chem. **265**:22365–22370.

4. **Bamford, J.K.H., and L. Mindich.** 1984. Characterization of the DNA-protein complex at the termini of the bacteriophage PRD1 genome. J. Virol. **50**:309–315.

5. **Barany, F., and A. Tomasz.** 1980. Genetic transformation of *Streptococcus pneumoniae* by heterologous plasmid deoxyribonucleic acid. J. Bacteriol. **144**:698–709.

6. **Bernheimer, H.P.** 1977. Lysogeny in pneumococci freshly isolated from man. Science **195**:66–68.

7. **Bernheimer, H.P.** 1979. Lysogenic pneumococci and their bacteriophages. J. Virol. **138**:618–624.

8. **Boyce, J.D., B.E. Davidson, and A.J. Hillier.** 1995. Sequence analysis of the *Lactococcus lactis* temperate bacteriophage BK5-T and demonstration that the phage DNA has cohesive ends. Appl. Environ. Microbiol. **61**:4089–4098.

9. **Caldentey, J., L. Blanco, D.H. Bamford, and M. Salas.** 1993. *In vitro* replication of bacteriohage PRD1 DNA: Characterization of the protein-primed initiation site. Nucleic Acids Res. **21**:3725–3730.

10. **Campbell, A.** 1988. Phage evolution and speciation. *In* R. Calendar (ed.), The bacteriophages. Plenum, New York, pp. 1–14.

11. **Canosi, V., G. Morelli, and T.A. Trautner.** 1978. The relationship between molecular structure and transformation efficiency of some *S. aureus* plasmids isolated from *B. subtilis*. Mol. Gen. Genet. **166**:259–267.

12. **Cheetham, B.F., and M.E. Katz.** 1995. A role for bacteriophages in the evolution and transfer of bacterial virulence determinants. Mol. Microbiol. **18**:201–208.

13. **Desiderio, S.V., and T.J. Kelly, Jr.** 1981. Structure of the linkage between adenovirus DNA and the 55,000 molecular weight terminal protein. J. Mol. Biol. **145**:319–337.

14. **Díaz, E., R. López, and J.L. García.** 1992. EJ-1, a temperate bacteriophage of *Streptococcus pneumoniae* with a *Myoviridae* morphotype. J. Bacteriol. **174**:5516–5525.

15. **Durrenberger, F., A. Crameri, B. Hohn, and Z. Koukolikova-Nicola.** 1989. Covalently bound VirD2 protein of *Agrobacterium tumefaciens* protects the T-DNA from exonucleolytic degradation. Proc. Natl. Acad. Sci. USA **86**:9154–9158.

16. **Escarmís, C., P. García, E. Méndez, R. López, M. Salas, and E. García.** 1985. Inverted terminal repeats and terminal proteins of the genome of pneumococcal phages. Gene **36**:341–348.

17. **Escarmís, C., A. Gómez, E. García, C. Ronda, R. López, and M. Salas.** 1984. Nucleotide sequence at the termini of the DNA of *Streptococcus pneumoniae* phage Cp-1. Virology **133**:166–171.

18. **García, E., C. Ronda, P. García, and R. López.** 1986. Studies on the replication of bacteriophage Cp-1 DNA in *Streptococcus pneumoniae*. Microbiología SEM **2**:115–120.

19. **García, E., C. Ronda, and R. López.** 1979. Bacteriophages of *Streptococcus pneumoniae*: Physicochemical properties of bacteriophage Dp-4 and its transfecting DNA. Eur. J. Biochem. **101**:59–64.

20. **García, E., C. Ronda, and R. López.** 1980. Replication of bac-

teriophage Dp-4 in *Streptococcus pneumoniae*. Virology **105**:405–414.

21. **García, J.L., E. García, A. Arrarás, P. García, C. Ronda, and R. López.** 1987. Cloning, purification, and biochemical characterization of the pneumococcal bacteriophage Cp-1 lysin. J. Virol. **61**:2573–2580.

22. **García, P., J.L. García, E. García, J.M. Sánchez-Puelles, and R. López.** 1990. Modular organization of the lytic enzymes of *Streptococcus pneumoniae* and its bacteriophages. Gene **86**:81–88.

23. **García, P., J.M. Hermoso, J.A. García, E. García, R. López, and M. Salas.** 1986. Formation of a covalent complex between the terminal protein of pneumococcal bacteriophage Cp-1 and 5′-dAMP. J. Virol. **58**:31–35.

24. **Hermoso, J.M., E. Méndez, F. Soriano, and M. Salas.** 1985. Location of the serine residue involved in the linkage between the terminal protein and the DNA of phage ϕ29. Nucleic Acids Res. **13**:7715–7728.

25. **Herrera-Estrella, A., Z. Chen, M. Van Montagu, and K. Wang.** 1988. VirD proteins of *Agrobacterium tumefaciens* are required for the formation of a covalent DNA-protein complex at the 5′ terminus of T-strand molecules. EMBO J. **7**:4055–4062.

26. **Hinnebusch, J., and K. Tilly.** 1993. Linear plasmids and chromosomes in bacteria. Mol. Microbiol. **10**:917–922.

27. **Hirokawa, H.** 1972. Transfecting deoxiribonucleic acid of *Bacillus* bacteriophage ϕ29 that is protease sensitive. Proc. Natl. Acad. Sci. USA **69**:1555–1559.

28. **King, A., and P.C. Van der Vliet.** 1994. A precursor terminal protein-trinucleotide intermediate during initiation of adenovirus DNA replication: Regeneration of molecular ends *in vitro* by a jumping back mechanism. EMBO J. **13**:5786–5791.

29. **Lacks, S.A., and B. Greenberg.** 1976. Single-strand breakage on binding of DNA to cells in the genetic transformation of *Diplococcus pneumoniae*. J. Mol. Biol. **101**:255–275.

30. **Lacks, S.A., B.M. Mannarelli, S.S. Springhorn, B. Greenberg, and A.G. de la Campa.** 1987. Genetics of the complementary restriction systems *Dpn*I and *Dpn*II revealed by cloning and recombination in *Streptococcus pneumoniae*. In J.J. Ferretti, R. Curtis III (ed.) Streptococcal genetics, ASM, Washington, DC, pp. 31–41.

31. **Lee, C.Y., and S.L. Buranen.** 1989. Extent of the DNA sequence required for integration of staphylococcal bacteriophages L54a. J. Bacteriol. **171**:1652–1657.

32. **López, R., J.L. García, E. García, C. Ronda, and P. García.** 1992. Structural analysis and biological significance of the cell wall lytic enzymes of *Streptococcus pneumoniae* and its bacteriophage. FEMS Microbiol. Lett. **100**:439–448.

33. **López, R., E. García, P. García, C. Ronda, and A. Tomasz.** 1982. Choline-containing bacteriophage receptors in *Streptococcus pneumoniae*. J. Bacteriol. **151**:1581–1590.

34. **López, R., E. García, and C. Ronda.** 1980. Selective replication of diplophage Dp-4 deoxyribonucleic acid in 6-(p-hydroxyfenylazo)-uracil treated *Streptococcus pneumoniae*. FEBS Lett. **111**:66–68.

35. **López, R., E. García, and C. Ronda.** 1982. Bacteriophages of *Streptococcus pneumoniae*. Rev. Infect. Dis. **3**:212–223.

36. **López, R., C. Ronda, P. García, C. Escarmís, and E. García.** 1984. Restriction cleavage maps of the DNAs of *Streptococcus pneumoniae* bacteriophages containing protein covalently bound to their 5′ ends. Mol. Gen. Genet. **197**:67–74.

37. **López, R., C. Ronda, A. Tomasz, and A. Portolés.** 1977. Properties of "diplophage": A lipid containing bacteriophage. J. Virol. **24**:201–210.

38. **Martín, A.C., L. Blanco, P. García, M. Salas, and J. Méndez.** 1996. *In vitro* protein-primed initiation of pneumococcal phage Cp-1 DNA replication occurs at the third 3′ nucleotide of the linear

template: A stepwise sliding-back mechanism. J. Mol. Biol. **260**:369–377.

39. **Martin, B., P. García, M.-P. Castanié, and J.-P. Claverys.** 1995. The *rec*A gene of *Streptococcus pneumoniae* is part of a competence-induced operon and controls lysogenic induction. Mol. Microbiol. **15**:367–379.

40. **Martín, A.C., R. López, and P. García.** 1996. Analysis of the complete nucleotide sequence and functional organization of the genome of *Streptococcus pneumoniae* bacteriophage Cp-1. J. Virol. **70**:3678–3687.

41. **McDonnell, M., C. Ronda, and A. Tomasz.** 1975. "Diplophage": A bacteriophage of *Diplococcus pneumoniae*. Virology **63**:577–582.

42. **Méndez, J., L. Blanco, J.A. Esteban, A. Bernad, and M. Salas.** 1992. Initiation of ϕ29 DNA replication occurs at the second 3′ nucleotide of the linear template: A sliding-back mechanism for protein-primed DNA replication. Proc. Natl. Acad. Sci. USA **89**:9579–9583.

43. **Moynet, D.J., and G.J. Tiraby.** 1980. Inhibition of transformation in *Streptococcus pneumoniae* by lysogeny. J. Bacteriol. **141**:1298–1304.

44. **Muckerman, C.C., S.S. Springhorn, B. Greenberg, and S.A. Lacks.** 1982. Transformation of restriction endonuclease phenotype in *Streptococcus pneumoniae*. J. Bacteriol. **152**:183–190.

45. **Porter, R.D., N.B. Shoemaker, G. Rampe, and W.R. Guild.** 1979. Bacteriophage-associated gene transfer in pneumococcus: transduction or pseudotransduction? J. Bacteriol. **137**:556–567.

46. **Porter, R.D., and W.R. Guild.** 1978. Transfection in pneumococcus: Single-strand intermediates in the formation of infective centers. J. Virol. **25**:60–72.

47. **Reanney, D.C., and H.W. Ackermann.** 1982. Comparative biology and evolution of bacteriophages. Adv. Virus Res. **27**:205–280.

48. **Romero, A., R. López, and P. García.** 1990. Characterization of the pneumococcal bacteriophage HB-3 amidase: Cloning and expression in *Escherichia coli*. J. Virol. **64**:137–142.

49. **Romero, A., R. López, and P. García.** 1990. Sequence of the *Streptococcus pneumoniae* bacteriophage HB-3 amidase reveals high homology with the major host autolysin. J. Bacteriol. **172**:5064–5070.

50. **Romero, A., R. López, and P. García.** 1992. The insertion site of the temperate phage HB-746 is located near the phage remnant in the pneumococcal host chromosome. J. Virol. **66**:2860–2864.

51. **Romero, A., R. López, R. Lurz, and P. García.** 1990. Temperate bacteriophages of *Streptococcus pneumoniae* that contain protein covalently bound to the 5′ ends of their DNAs. J. Virol. **64**:5149–5155.

52. **Ronda, C., J.L. García, and R. López.** 1988. Characterization of genetic transformation in *Streptococcus oralis* NCTC 11427. Expression of pneumococcal amidase in *S. oralis* using a new shuttle vector. Mol. Gen. Genet. **215**:53–57.

53. **Ronda, C., R. López, and E. García.** 1981. Isolation and characterization of a new bacteriophage, Cp-1, infecting *Streptococcus pneumoniae*. J. Virol. **40**:551–559.

54. **Ronda, C., J.L. García, and R. López.** 1989. Infection of *Streptococcus oralis* NCTC 11427 by pneumococcal phages. FEMS Microbiol. Lett. **65**:187–192.

55. **Ronda, C., R. López, A. Gómez, and E. García.** 1983. Protease-sensitive transfection of *Streptococcus pneumoniae* with bacteriophage Cp-1 DNA. J. Virol. **48**:721–730.

56. **Ronda, C., R. López, A. Tapia, and A. Tomasz.** 1977. Role of the pneumococcal autolysin (murein hydrolase) in the release of the progeny bacteriophage and in the bacteriophage-induced lysis of the host cell. J. Virol. **21**:366–374.

57. **Ronda, C., R. López, A. Tomasz, and A. Portolés.** 1978. Trans-

fection of *Streptococcus pneumoniae* with bacteriophage DNA. J. Virol. **26:**221–225.

58. **Sakaguchi, K.** 1990. Invertrons, a class of structurally and functionally related genetic elements that includes linear DNA plasmids, transposable elements, and genomes of adeno-type viruses. Microbiol. Rev. **54:**66–74.

59. **Salas, M.** 1988. Phages with protein attached to the DNA ends. *In* R. Calendar (ed.), The bacteriophages. Plenum, New York, pp. 169–191.

60. **Salas, M.** 1991. Protein-priming of DNA replication. Annu. Rev. Biochem. **60:**39–71.

61. **Salas, M., and F. Rojo.** 1993. Replication and transcription of bacteriophage φ29 DNA. *In* A. Sonenshein (ed.), *Bacillus subtilis* and other gram-positive bacteria: Biochemistry, physiology, and molecular genetics. American Society for Microbiology, Washington, DC, pp. 843–857.

62. **Sanz, J.M., and J.L. García.** 1990. Structural studies of the lysozyme coded by the pneumococcal phage Cp-1. Conformational changes induced by choline. Eur. J. Biochem. **187:**409–416.

63. **Serratosa, C., R. López, E. García, and C. Ronda.** 1984. Conditions to enhance transfection in *Streptococcus pneumoniae.* Virus Res. **1:**443–453.

64. **Stackebrandt, E., W. Ludwig, M. Weizenegger, S. Dorn, T.** McGill, G.E. Fox, C.R. Woese, W. Schubert, and K.H. Schleifer. 1987. Comparative 16S rRNA oligonucleotide analyses and murein types of round-spore-forming bacilli and nonspore-forming relatives. J. Gen. Microbiol. **133:**2523–2529.

65. **Stillman, B.W.** 1983. The replication of adenovirus DNA with purified proteins. Cell **35:**7–9.

66. **Tiraby, J.G., E. Tiraby, and M. S. Fox.** 1975. Pneumococcal bacteriophages. Virology **68:**566–569.

67. **Tomasz, A.** 1967. Choline in the cell wall of a bacterium: Novel type of polymer-linked in pneumococcus. Science **157:**694–697.

68. **Tomasz, A., and R.D. Hotchkiss.** 1964. Regulation of the transformability of pneumococcal cultures by macromolecular cell products. Proc. Natl. Acad. Sci. USA **51:**480–486.

69. **Young, R.** 1992. Bacteriophage lysis: Mechanism and regulation. Microbiol. Rev. **56:**430–481.

Address reprint requests to:
Pedro Garciá
Departamento de Microbiologiá Molecular
Centro de Investigaciones Biológicas
Consejo Superior de Investigaciones Científicas
Velázquez 144
28006 Madrid Spain

Streptococcus pneumoniae
Copyright © 2000 Mary Ann Liebert, Inc., 2 Madison Avenue, Larchmont, NY 10538

Lipopolysaccharide and Peptidoglycan: CD14-Dependent Bacterial Inducers of Inflammation

ERNST TH. RIETSCHEL,[1] JENS SCHLETTER,[1] BIRGIT WEIDEMANN,[1] VOLKER EL-SAMALOUTI,[1] TAILA MATTERN,[1] ULRICH ZÄHRINGER,[1] ULRICH SEYDEL,[1] HELMUT BRADE,[1] HANS-DIETER FLAD,[1] SHOICHI KUSUMOTO,[2] DIPIKA GUPTA,[3] ROMAN DZIARSKI,[3] and ARTUR J. ULMER[1]

ABSTRACT

Surface structures of bacteria contribute to the microbial pathogenic potential and are capable of causing local and generalized inflammatory reactions. Among these factors, endotoxin and peptidoglycan are of particular medical importance. Both toxic bacterial polymers are now recognized to interact with the same cellular receptor, the CD14 molecule, which is expressed on different types of immune cells, in particular, monocytes/macrophages. The interaction between these bacterial activators and CD14 leads to the production of endogenous mediators such as tumor necrosis factor α, interleukin 1 (IL-1), and IL-6, which are ultimately responsible for phlogistic responses. The fact that CD14 recognizes not only endotoxin and peptidoglycan but also other glycosyl-based microbial polymers suggests that this cellular surface molecule represents a lectin.

LIPOPOLYSACCHARIDE

LIPOPOLYSACCHARIDES (LPS) are unique structural components of the cell envelope of gram-negative bacteria.[26,33,35,36] They exist in almost all gram-negative bacteria and constitute an indispensible component of their outer membrane. This membrane is asymmetrically constructed in that its inner leaflet contains glycerophospholipids, whereas the lipid matrix of the outer leaflet is formed primarily of the lipophilic moiety (lipid A) of the LPS molecule. The barrier provided by the LPS membrane contributes to the natural resistance of gram-negative bacteria to a number of exogenous noxes such as hydrophobic antibiotics, detergents, dyes, and bile acids.[29] Besides its functional role in the bacterial cell, a multitude of biological, often toxic effects are evoked in animal hosts by LPS when released from multiplying or desintegrating bacteria. These effects, which are collectively refered to as endotoxic activities, include fever or hypothermia, tachycardia, tachypnoe, leukopenia or leukocytosis, hypotension and disseminated intravascular coagulation, and are known as manifestations of severe gram-negative sepsis.[36] In fact, higher doses of endotoxin may result in multiorgan failure and lethal shock. There-fore, due to the clear association between LPS and sepsis, endotoxin has been implicated as a main factor involved in the pathophysiological manifestations and consequences of gram-negative bacterial sepsis.

Chemical and physical structure of lipopolysaccharide

LPS of various gram-negative bacterial families are made up according to the same architectural principle, i.e., they consist of a polysaccharide portion and a covalently bound lipid A component.[26] In the classical case of Enterobacteriaceae (e.g., *Salmonella enterica*, *Escherichia coli*), the polysaccharide portion consists of two regions, the O-specific chain and the core oligosaccharide. The O-specific chain is usually composed of a polymer of repeating oligosaccharide units. The O-specific chain is characteristic of and unique for a given LPS and its bacterial origin (serotype). In view of the existence of thousands of serotypes, comparison of different gram-negative bacteria reveals an enormous structural variability of the O-specific chain region. The core portion, consisting of the O-chain proximal outer core and the lipid A-proximal inner core, is structurally less variable.[19] In the case of *S. enterica* and *E. coli*

---

[1]Research Center Borstel, Center for Medicine and Biosciences, D-23845 Borstel, Germany.
[2]Osaka University, Faculty of Science, Department of Chemistry, Toyonaka 560, Osaka, Japan.
[3]Northwest Center for Medical Education, Indiana University, School of Medicine, Gary, IN 46408.
This review is dedicated to our esteemed colleague Prof. Dr. Hans Paulsen on the occasion of his seventy-fifth birthday (May 20, 1997).
Reprinted from *Microbial Drug Resistance*, Vol. 4, No. 1, 1998.

the outer core exhibits some variability due to different locations and linkages of its constituents. Nevertheless, common elements are recognized, such as the pyranosidic hexoses D-glucose (Glc), D-galactose (Gal), and 2-amino-2-deoxy-D-glucose (GlcN). Hexoses are also present in the outer core of *Klebsiella pneumoniae* and *Proteus mirabilis*. As a rule, the inner core of LPS contains 2-keto-3-deoxyoctonic acid (Kdo) and (in *Enterobacteriaceae* and many other families) heptose residues of the L-*glycero*-D-*manno* configuration that often are phosphorylated. Thus, the inner core region of various LPS represents a chemically similar region. The lipid A component, constituting the structurally most uniform domain, represents the covalently bound lipid component of LPS.[53] It can be separated from the polysaccharide region by treatment of LPS with mild acid, which cleaves the linkage between the lipid A-proximal Kdo residue of the inner core and lipid A preferentially. Lipid A has been identified as the endotoxic principle of LPS.[14]

With the aim of defining those structural and conformational peculiarities that endow it with endotoxic properties, lipid A has been chemically analyzed in detail. Fig. 1 shows the structure of lipid A of four different types of gram-negative bacteria that all express biologically highly active LPS (*E. coli*, *Haemophilus influenzae*, *Chromobacterium violaceum*, and *Neisseria meningitidis*). Structurally, these lipid A types share a 1,4′-bisphosphorylated β1,6-linked D-GlcN disaccharide (lipid A backbone) that is acylated by four (R)-3-hydroxy fatty acids at positions 2, 3, 2′, and 3′. Also, in all lipid A types, the hydroxy group in position 4 is free and that at position 6′ serves as the attachment site of Kdo, i.e., the polysaccharide region. In each case the acyl group at position 2′ of GlcN II carries at its 3-hydroxy group a further (fifth) fatty acid. The four structures, however, differ in the location of a sixth acyl group (R1 or R2) and the chain length of fatty acids (symbols m, n, and o). As Fig. 1 shows, lipid A of *E. coli* and *H. influenzae* carries this sixth fatty acid at GlcN II and, thus, possesses an asymmetric distribution of acyl groups over GlcN I and GlcN II (4 + 2), whereas a symmetric acyl arrangement (3 + 3) is present in lipid A of *C. violaceum* and *N. meningitidis*.[45,53] Importantly, the average length of acyl chains is smaller in the latter group (mainly 12 carbon atoms) than in the former (mainly 14 carbon atoms).

These structural examples demonstrate that lipid A of various origins exhibits a similar architecture, but that variations exist concerning the nature and location of acyl groups. More striking examples for structural variability of lipid A are found, for example, in *Rhizobium*, *Chlamydia*, and *Legionella* where very long chain (C22–C32) acyl groups, also in the form of (ω − 1)-hydroxy or oxo-derivatives, are present. In *Rhodobacter sphaeroides* and *R. capsulatus*, part of the 3-hydroxy fatty acids is replaced by 3-oxo fatty acids and, interestingly, these latter lipid A preparations are endotoxically inactive.[45] Further variations of the lipid A structure concern the substitution of phosphate groups and the nature of backbone glycosyl residues (not shown in Fig. 1). Thus, GlcN may be replaced by 2,3-diamino-2,3-dideoxy-D-glucose (GlcN3N), as is the case, for example, in *Rhodopseudomonas viridis*, *Campylobacter jejeuni*, and *L. pneumophila*.[53] Finally, phosphate groups may be absent from lipid A. This is the case, for example, in *Bacteroides fragilis* lipid A and *Rhizobium leguminosarum*, which both lack the nonglycosidic phosphate group.[32]

Based on the results of chemical analyses, *E. coli* type lipid A has been chemically synthesized.[22] The demonstration of identity of bacterial and synthetic preparations in all chemical, physicochemical, physical, and biological parameters[14] unequivocally verified the previously deduced and proposed structure of lipid A to be correct.

Lipid A and LPS represent amphiphiles and, therefore, form aggregates in aqueous medium above the critical aggregate concentration. The availability of defined and homogenous synthetic lipid A and partial structures allowed analyses as to the nature of such aggregates, i.e., their three-dimensional physical structure. These investigations showed that biologically active lipid A adopts, at physiological ambient conditions [37°C, pH 7, high (>90%) water content, presence of Mg^{2+}] exclusively nonlamellar structures.[4,5,37] These nonlamellar structures are either cubic (*S. enterica* sv. *minnesota*) or hexagonal (*R. gelatinosus*). In contrast, endotoxically nonactive lipid A (*R. capsulatus*) adopt lamellar structures.[4,5] The three-dimensional structure of lipid A multimers and the conformation of the corresponding monomers of active and nonactive lipid A is shown schematically in Fig. 2. It is likely that endotoxicity is expressed by individual LPS or lipid A molecules possessing a conformation that, at higher concentration, leads to the observed three-dimensional nonlamellar structures.[5,37] Recent studies employing disaggregated LPS[46] or LBP-mediated incorporation of LPS into membrane matrices[39,40] support the hypothesis that endotoxic activity is mediated by single molecules. It further appears that a peculiar spatial shape of lipid A is required for the expression of endotoxicity. We have termed this unique arrangement of lipid A the "endotoxic conformation".[37] The conformation of endotoxic and nontoxic lipid A is shown schematically in Fig. 2.

	Nature of		Number of Carbon Atoms		
	R^1	R^2	m	n	o
Escherichia coli	H	14:0	14	14	12
Haemophilus influenzae	H	14:0	14	14	14
Neisseria meningitidis	12:0	H	14	12	12
Chromobacterium violaceum	12:0	H	12	10	12

12:0, dodecanoic acid   14:0, tetradecanoic acid

FIG. 1. Chemical structure of the lipid A component of *Escherichia coli*, *Haemophilus influenzae*, *Chromobacterium violaceum*, and *Neisseria meningitidis*.[53]

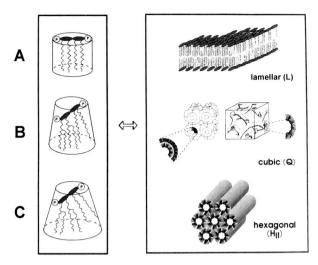

FIG. 2. Physical structure of lipid A. Shown are the schematic conformation of lipid A monomers of endotoxically active (*E. coli* and *S. enterica* sv. *minnesota*, *Rh. gelatinosa*) and nonactive LPS (*Rh.* capsulatus) and the aggregate structures that they form under physiological conditions.[4,5,37]

Biological activity of lipopolysaccharide

The initial key event in endotoxin activity can be defined as the interaction of the lipid A component of LPS with specific humoral and, notably, cellular recognition molecules.[36] It is reasonable to assume that at least two parameters determine the result of the interaction between lipid A and host cells, i.e., between individual lipid A molecules being in their endotoxic conformation and the host recognition system resulting in the activation of monocytes and the production of bioactive mediators. These parameters are the capacity of lipid A to bind specifically to the receptor and, subsequently, the ability of lipid A to activate the cell by a receptor-mediated mechanism.

Recent studies in our laboratory have shown that the hydrophilic lipid A backbone (bis-phosphorylated D-GlcN disaccharide together with two fatty acids) mediates the specific binding of lipid A or LPS to the cellular receptor.[21] On the other hand, it is the number, nature, and distribution of fatty acids, i.e., the acylation pattern that determines the activation capacity and mediator-inducing capacity of lipid A.[21] These investigations also revealed that the binding of lipid A is a necessary but not sufficient event for the activation of cells. It appears that an additional receptor-mediated triggering mechanism is required for which the acylation pattern of lipid A plays a most critical role and which provides the external signal for cellular stimulation.

The separation of the "binding" and "activation" events suggested the possibility that endotoxically inactive LPS or partial structures may bind to target cells without activating them, thus representing possible inhibitors of LPS-induced effects. Indeed, we[13,25,49] and others[27] have demonstrated that the chemically synthesized form (compound 406) of tetraacyl lipid A lacking in comparison to lipid A lauric (12:0) and myristic acid (14:0) (Fig. 1), and representing an intermediate in lipid A biosynthesis (precursor Ia), inhibits, in a dose-dependent manner, the monokine production by human monocytes induced by LPS but

not by lipoprotein, or Bacille Calmette-Guérin. As has been shown by northern blot analysis, compound 406 suppresses the LPS-induced formation of mRNA for TNFα and IL-1, indicating that monokine production is inhibited before or at the level of transcription.[13] Similar results have been reported for the isostructural natural precursor Ia (also termed lipid IVa) isolated from *S. enterica* sv. *typhimurium* and for nontoxic lipid A species of *R. sphaeroides* and *R. capsulatus*. Very recently, an LPS antagonist, the structure of which is based on that of *R. capsulatus* lipid A, was synthesized (compound E5531). This molecule protects mice from endotoxin-induced lethality and, when administered together with an antibiotic, from lethal *E. coli*-induced peritonitis.[8]

Endotoxin receptors and mediators

Intensive research on the mechanisms of endotoxin action has revealed that LPS, instead of being directly toxic to host cells or organs, exerts its biological effects indirectly through stimulation of host cells to produce endogenous mediator substances, which elicit various responses in the host.[36] Endotoxins are able to engage many different cell types, including lymphocytes, neutrophils, and endothelial cells, but the key role in endotoxin action is played by circulating and tissue macrophages. Endotoxin activity involves LPS-binding by a 60 kDa lipopolysaccharide-binding glycoprotein (LBP)[41] that circulates in the blood and by recognition of the LPS-LBP complex by a binding protein located on the surface of macrophages. This cellular binding protein is a 55 kDa leukocyte surface antigen termed CD14 and its activation by the LPS-LBP complex triggers the production of endogenous mediators.[52] This pathway is, however, only one of several plausible alternatives. Thus, it is possible that CD14 binds LPS but does not deliver the activation signal but, rather, enables LPS to activate another receptor. Moreover, high LPS doses lead to CD14-independent cell activation suggesting the existence of further receptors. In addition to CD14, other cellular receptors such as CD11c/CD18 bind endotoxin and mediate signal transduction.[20]

The mediator substances produced by endotoxin-stimulated macrophages fall into three chemically different categories, namely proteins, reduced oxygen species, and lipids.[30] The first category comprises proteins of the interleukin family (IL-1, IL-6, and IL-8), TNFα, interferon-γ, and proteases such as elastase and cathepsin G. TNFα appears to be the principal mediator of endotoxin action, as typical endotoxin effects (e.g., fever, activation of blood coagulation, lethality) can be inhibited by anti-TNFα antibodies or can be equally provoked in experimental animals by administration of TNFα. TNFα, having been recognized first as a plasma factor capable of causing hemorrhagic necrosis of tumors, is a typical example of an endotoxin-associated mediator in that it is harmful and even lethal in large concentrations, but normally functions as a part of the natural host defense against infections and as a regulator of leukocytes and endothelial cells. Receptors of TNFα are present on most cell types, and binding of TNFα results in a cascade of responses, such as apoptosis and activation including synthesis of TNFα itself. Thus, the endotoxin-induced activation process spreads and more TNFα and other cytokines, including IL-1, IL-6, and IL-8, are produced. The interleukins share many of the properties of TNFα, IL-1, for instance, representing a powerful endogenous pyrogen.

Other cellular mediator substances produced upon endotoxin stimulation include highly reactive oxygen-containing molecules such as nitric oxide (NO) and reduced oxygen radicals that have been associated with the antimicrobial action of macrophages. The lipid mediators comprise the platelet-activating factor and several products of the cyclooxygenase and lipooxygenase pathways of arachidonic acid metabolism, such as thromboxane A_2, prostaglandin E_2, and the leukotrienes. Prostaglandin E_2 appears to function as a negative feedback signal for mediator synthesis.

Thus, the array of products elaborated by macrophages and other cell types, if produced in high concentration in response to a heavy endotoxin stimulus, such as is present in septic shock, work to the host's disadvantage, leading to multiorgan failure, circulatory collapse, and death. In localized or less severe infections, the foregoing mechanisms help to eliminate the infection and serve to support recovery. In addition, it is assumed that constant low levels of the ubiquitously available endotoxin (i.e., as produced by the microbial flora of the bowel) are of importance for the maintenance of the proper functioning of the entire immune system insofar as they provide a continuous stimulus of the affected cells. Therefore, endotoxin has been visualized as a vitamine.

PEPTIDOGLYCAN

In recent years, the number of septic episodes due to gram-positive bacteria has increased.[3] Associated with their cell wall, this group of bacteria contains different classes of molecules that express biological activity and that, therefore, could play a role in the pathophysiology of gram-positive septicaemia. These structures include the M protein, lipoteichoic acids, and peptidoglycan. Peptidoglycan (PG) is especially abundant in gram-positive bacteria, where it accounts for half of the mass of the cell wall. Chemically, PG constitutes a polymer of alternating β1,4-linked D-GlcN and N-acetylmuramic acid (MurNAc) residues. These glycosyl polymers are interlinked by peptide bridges, thus forming a three-dimensional network.[38] PG, particularly if rendered water-soluble, induces a variety of biological effects that are known as manifestations of sepsis including fever, leukocytosis, and shock.[10,17,18,28,34,47] These phlogistic effects are, as in the case of LPS, mediated by monocyte/macrophage-derived soluble mediators such as TNFα, IL-1, and IL-6. It is, therefore, possible that PG fragments released from growing, multiplying, or desintegrating bacteria initiate or contribute to the pathophysiology of gram-positive septic shock.

In previous efforts to define the structural requirements for biological activity of PG, muramyl dipeptide (MDP) was identified as representing the minimal structural unit of PG expressing bioactivity.[24,44] MDP consists of muramic acid (MurNAc, the 3-O-D-lactyl ether of D-GlcN) that carries at the carboxyl group of lactate the dipeptide L-alanyl-D-isoglutamine and its structure is shown in Fig. 3. The biological analyses of fully synthetic MDP have confirmed its biological effectiveness.[1,24,44,48]

Cytokine induction by peptidoglycan

Confirming earlier findings of others, we have shown that soluble peptidoglycan (sPG), isolated from penicillin-treated *Staphylococcus aureus* induces, in human peripheral monocytes, TNFα, IL-1, and IL-6 in a dose-dependent manner.[50] As considerably higher doses (10^2 to 10^3) of sPG than of LPS are required for cytokine induction, it was speculated that sPG activity was due to contaminating endotoxin. This, however, could be ruled out by demonstrating that, in contrast to LPS, the sPG effect was independent of serum or LBP, and that it was not suppressed by polymyxin B or by bactericidal/permeability increasing protein (BPI). Unexpectedly, sPG-induced cytokine production could be inhibited by pretreatment of cells with compound 406.[50] As discussed, this compound is known to inhibit, in larger doses antagonistically, LPS-induced cytokine synthesis.[27,49] Therefore, it is possible that sPG is recognized by the same cellular surface protein as LPS, i.e., by membrane-bound CD14, indicating that CD14 also represents the receptor for sPG.

CD14 as cellular receptor for soluble peptidoglycan

In recent studies we have, in fact, demonstrated the importance of CD14 for sPG recognition by monocytes.[50,51] The anti-CD14 monoclonal antibody (mAb) MEM-18 is known to inhibit LPS reactivity toward human peripheral monocytes and this antibody is also capable of inhibiting stimulation of human peripheral mononuclear cells (MNC) by sPG. In contrast, mAb biG-4, which binds to CD14, but does not block LPS association, is also inactive against sPG, indicating that sPG may be recognized by a similar CD14 region as LPS. To further study the involvement of CD14 in binding of sPG to monocytes, sPG was labelled by FITC, and FITC-sPG conjugates were shown to exhibit an identical capacity to that of the nonlabelled preparation to induce cytokines. Using cells kept in the phagocytosis-inhibiting buffer SEPDAF, a dose- and time-dependent binding of labelled sPG was demonstrated by flow cytometry (see Fig. 4), suggesting specificity of binding.

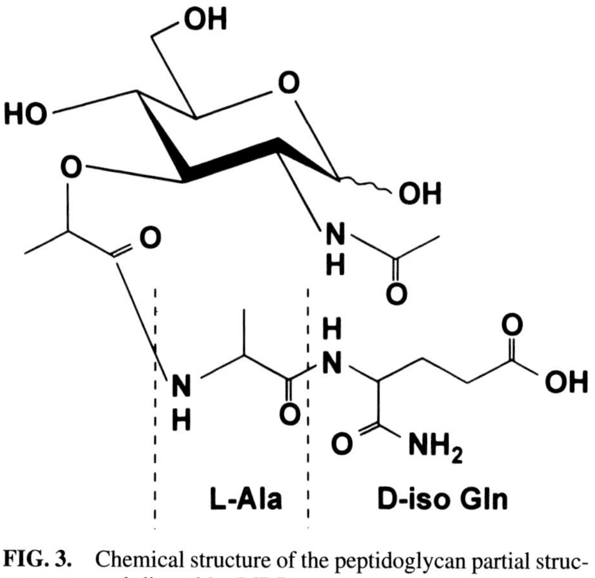

FIG. 3. Chemical structure of the peptidoglycan partial structure muramyl dipeptide (MDP).

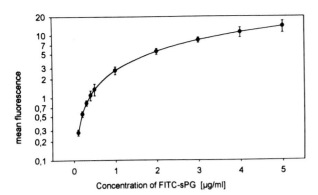

FIG. 4. Dose-dependence of binding of FITC-labelled soluble peptidoglycan to human monocytes.[51]

The specific association of sPG with monocytes was inhibited not only by nonlabeled sPG, but also by LPS and preparation 406. However, sPG association was not affected by the CD14-independent monocyte activator glycosphingolipid-4A (GSL-4A).[23] Most notably, sPG binding was also inhibited by MDP, indicating that MDP represents the minimal structure involved in sPG association with MNC (see Fig. 5). Thus, after many attempts to define a cellular binding site for MDP, CD14 has not been identified as the functional receptor.[51] It remains, however, to be shown whether MDP or other PG partial structures, such as component G(Anh)MTetra, with MurNAc in the β1.6-anhydro form, represent the in vivo-formed compound that interacts most efficiently with CD14.[9] It is of particular interest that MDP, as a partial structure of PG, may act under certain experimental conditions as an antagonist in suppressing,

for example, PG-induced acute and chronic arthritis in rats.[48] Further studies showed that binding of FITC-sPG was inhibitable by mAb MEM-18, as was FITC-sPG induced cytokine production. mAb MEM-18 also suppressed MDP-induced IL-1 formation, and, as expected, mAb biG-4 was not active in this system. Finally, the association of sPG with CD14 could be directly demonstrated. Using a gel-shift assay in native PAGE, we were able to show that sPG, like LPS, binds to sCD14 (Fig. 6).[51] Recent analyses demonstrating that sPG-induced NF-kB activation was CD14-dependent, provide additional support for the hypothesis that CD14 represents the functional receptor for sPG.[16]

The problem of the specificity of this interaction, however, needs further study. CD14, in addition to LPS and sPG, also recognizes other bacterial activators of immune cells including polymannuronic acid (mannuronan),[12] lipoarabinomannan (LAM),[2,7,16] chitosan,[31] and possibly lipoteichoic acid (LTA). These bioactive molecules differ greatly in chemical make-up, but share a glycosyl (hexosyl) region that, therefore, may be involved in the interaction of the polymers with CD14. In the case of LPS, the GlcN-containing hydrophilic backbone of lipid A mediates the binding to CD14 and cells. As *gluco-* or *manno*-configurated glycosyl residues are also constituents of sPG, LAM, LTA, and mannuronan, and as the binding of these macromolecules can be inhibited by hexose-containing partial structures, it is tempting to speculate that the D-*gluco*/D-*manno* carbohydrate region is recognized by CD14. CD14, therefore, may represent a typical lectin. The domain of CD14, through which it interacts with LPS/lipid A, is being elucidated presently. It, thus, is not yet known, whether the other bioactive structures that interact with CD14 also bind to this very epitope. Finally, it has been suggested that the PG- and mannuronan-activated cellular pathways of signal transduction in monocytes are different from those triggered by LPS.[11,15,16] It

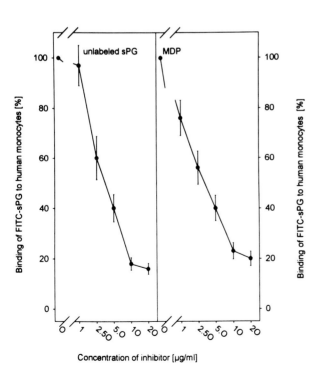

FIG. 5. Inhibition of FITC-labelled sPG binding to human monocytes by nonlabelled sPG and MDP.[51]

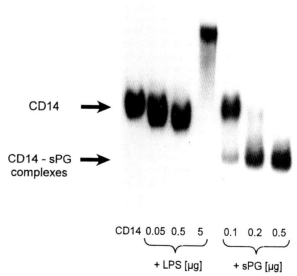

FIG. 6. Demonstration of binding of sPG to CD14 by changes in electrophoretic mobility in a native PAGE assay. Addition of LPS or sPG leads to altered mobility of CD14 as visualized by anti-CD14 antibodies.[51]

thus appears possible that CD14 recognizes a variety of bacterial immunomodulators each of which, however, initiates different extends of common or individual signal transduction pathways.

SIGNAL TRANSDUCTION PATHWAYS INDUCED BY LIPOPOLYSACCHARIDE AND PEPTIDOGLYCAN

The signal transduction events that follow interaction of LPS and PG with cells and result in activation of macrophages are beginning to be elucidated. In human monocytes, CD14 seems to associate with lyn (a tyrosine kinase that belongs to the src-family) and activation of monocytes by LPS results in an increased phosphorylation on tyrosine residues and activation of CD14-associated lyn.[42] Similar activation of lyn may also follow PG interaction with CD14, since PG induces increased tyrosine phosphorylation of lyn in mouse macrophages.[16] However, it is still not known how CD14 activates lyn and what the signal transduction events downstream from lyn are. One such possible downstream event could be activation of mitogen-activated protein (MAP) kinases and, indeed, both LPS and PG activate MAP kinases. However, the signals generated by LPS and PG are not identical, since LPS strongly activates all three families of MAP kinases (ERK, JNK, and p38), whereas PG strongly activates ERK, moderately activates JNK, and very weakly activates p38.[11] LPS also activates several transcription factors, such as NF-kB, NF-IL6, Ets, PU.1, and AP-1.[43] So far, PG has been shown only to activate NF-kB,[9,16] and this activation is mediated through CD14.[16] The NF-kB-activating function of CD14 for LPS and PG are, again, not identical, since different sequences in the N-terminal 65-amino acid region of CD14 are critical for the LPS- and PG-induced responses.[16] In summary, since different signal transduction pathways culminate in activation of various families of MAP kinases and transcription factors, LPS and PG are likely to activate multiple signal transduction pathways and the extent of activation of each pathway seems to be different for LPS and PG.

FINAL REMARKS

Lipopolysaccharide and peptidoglycan, as vital components of a functional bacterial cell wall, are both essential for microbial viability. The two bacterial polymers have also been recognized for many years as major toxins inducing inflammatory reactions in suitable host organisms. In fact, they potentiate each other in their capacity to cause local or generalized inflammation.[48] LPS has been well established as representing an important pathogenic factor in severe bacterial infections, and quantitative determinations in sera of patients suffering from meningococcal sepsis have proven a direct correlation between the levels of circulating endotoxin and the severity of the disease.[6] In recent years, PG also has emerged as a potential bacterial virulence factor. Although PG exerts potent proinflammatory activities, its significance in septic episodes remains to be established. For such studies to be successful, reliable methods for the quantitative estimation of PG in tissues or inflammatory fluids must be elaborated.

LPS and PG share initial steps of biosynthesis and they also share certain structural features. As described in this paper, both bacterial immunostimulators are recognized by the same monocyte surface antigen, the CD14 molecule. It will be of great interest to determine which pathways, similar or divergent, of signal transduction follow after this common recognition, i.e., how the host distinguishes LPS from PG. Biochemical elucidation of such intracellular events may also help to increase understanding of the molecular mechanisms involved in the synergistic toxicity of PG, MDP, and LPS and to help in the development of new intervention strategies in bacterial sepsis.

ACKNOWLEDGMENTS

The financial support of the DFG (Sonderforschungsbereich 367, projects B1, B2, B8, and C5, Sonderforschungsbereich 470, projects B4 and B5, Graduiertenkolleg GRK 288/1-96, projects A1, A2, A3, and A4), of the BMBF (grant 01KI/9471 EThR, US, UZ, and AJU), of GIF (grant I 0373-169. 13/94 UZ, EThR), and of the Fonds der Chemischen Industrie (EThR, HDF) is gratefully appreciated. We thank Mrs. F. Richter and G. Müller for typing this manuscript and for photographic work.

REFERENCES

1. Azuma, I., K. Sugimura, T. Taniyama, M. Yamawaki, Y. Yamamura, S. Kusumoto, S. Okada, and T. Shiba. 1976. Adjuvant activity of mycobacterial fractions: Immunological properties of synthetic N-acetylmuramyl dipeptide and the related compounds. Infect. Immun. 14:18.

2. Barnes, P.F., D. Chatterjee, J.S. Abrams, L. Shuzhuang, E. Wang, M. Yamamura, P.J. Brennan, and R.L. Modlin. 1992. Cytokine production induced by Mycobacterium tuberculosis lipoarabinomannan. J. Immunol. 149:541–547.

3. Bone, R.C. 1994. Gram-positive organisms and sepsis. Arch. Intern. Med. 154:26–34.

4. Brandenburg, K., H. Mayer, M.H.J. Koch, J. Weckesser, E.T. Rietschel, and U. Seydel. 1993. Influence of the supramolecular structure of free lipid A on its biological activity. Eur. J. Biochem. 218:555–563.

5. Brandenburg, K., U. Seydel, A.B. Schromm, H. Loppnow, M.H.J. Koch, and E.T. Rietschel. 1996. Conformation of lipid A, the endotoxic center of bacterial lipopolysaccharide. J. Endotoxin Res. 3:173–178.

6. Brandtzaeg, P. 1996. Significance and pathogenesis of septic shock. Curr. Top. Microbiol. Immunol. 216:15–37.

7. Chatterjee, D., A.D. Roberts, K. Lowell, P.J. Brennan, and I.M. Orme. 1992. Structural basis of capacity of lipoarabinomannan to induce secretion of tumor necrosis factor. Infect. Immun. 60:1249–1253.

8. Christ, W.J., O. Asano, A.L.C. Robidoux, M. Perez, Y. Wang, G.R. Dubuc, W.E. Gavin, L.D. Hawkins, P.D. McGuinness, M.A. Mullarkey, M.D. Lewis, Y. Kishi, T. Kawata, J.R. Bristol, J.R. Rose, D.P. Rossignol, S. Kobayashi, I. Hishnuma, A. Kimura, A. Asakawa, N. Asakawa, K. Katayama, and I. Yamatsu. 1995. E5531, a pure endotoxin antagonist of high potency. Science 268:80–83.

9. Dokter, W.H.A., A.J. Dijkstra, S.B. Koopmans, B.K. Stulp, W. Keck, M.R. Halie, and E. Vallenga. 1994. G(Anh)MTetra, a natural bacterial cell wall breakdown product, induces interleukin-1β

and interleukin-6 expression in human monocytes. J. Biol. Chem. **269:**4201–4206.

10. **Dziarski, R.** 1988. Enhancement of B-cell stimulation by muramyl dipeptide through a mechanism not involving interleukin 1 or increased Ca^{2+}. Cell. Immunol. **111:**10–27.

11. **Dziarski, R., Y.P. Jin, and D. Gupta.** 1996. Differential activation of extracellular signal-regulated kinase ERK1, ERK2, p38, and c-Jun NH_2-terminal kinase mitogen-activated protein kinases by bacterial peptidoglycan. J. Infec. Dis. **174:**778–785.

12. **Espevik, T., M. Otterlei, G. Skjak-Braek, L. Ryan, S.D. Wright, and A. Sundan.** 1993. The involvement of CD14 in stimulation of cytokine production by uronic acid polymers. Eur. J. Immunol. **23:**255–261.

13. **Feist, W., A.J. Ulmer, M.H. Wang, J. Musehold, C. Schlüter, J. Gerdes, H. Herzbeck, H. Brade, S. Kusumoto, T. Diamantstein, E.T. Rietschel, and H.-D. Flad.** 1992. Modulation of lipopolysaccharide-induced production of tumor necrosis factor, interleukin 1, and interleukin 6 by synthetic precursor Ia of lipid A. FEMS Microbiol. Immunol. **89:**73–90.

14. **Galanos, C., O. Lüderitz, E.T. Rietschel, O. Westphal, H. Brade, L. Brade, M.A. Freudenberg, F.U. Schade, M. Imoto, S. Yoshimura, S. Kusumoto, and T. Shiba.** 1985. Synthetic and natural *Escherichia coli* free lipid A express identical endotoxic activities. Eur. J. Biochem. **148:**1–5.

15. **Gupta, D., Y.-P. Jin, and R. Dziarski.** 1995. Peptidoglycan induces transcription and secretion of $TNF\alpha$ and activation of Lyn, extracellular signal-regulated kinase, and Rsk signal transduction proteins in mouse macrophages. J. Immunol. **155:**2620–2630.

16. **Gupta, D., T.N. Kirkland, S. Viriyakosol, and R. Dziarski.** 1996. CD14 is a cell-activating receptor for bacterial peptidoglycan. J. Biol. Chem. **271:**23310–23316.

17. **Heumann, D., C. Barras, A. Severin, M.P. Glauser, and A. Tomasz.** 1994. Gram-positive cell walls stimulate synthesis of tumor necrosis factor alpha and interleukin-6 by human monocytes. Infect. Immun. **62:**2715–2721.

18. **Heymer, B., and E.T. Rietschel.** 1977. Biological properties of peptidoglycans. Microbiology 1977. Am. Soc. Microbiol., Washington D.C., pp 344–349.

19. **Holst, O., and H. Brade.** 1992. Chemical structure of the core region of lipopolysaccharides. *In* D.C. Morrison and J.L. Ryan (eds.), Bacterial endotoxic lipopolysaccharides, vol. 1. Molecular biochemistry and cellular biology. CRC Press, Boca Raton, pp. 135–170.

20. **Ingalls, R.R., and D.T. Golenbock.** 1995. CD11c/CD18, a transmembrane signalling receptor for lipopolysaccharide. J. Exp. Med. **181:**1473–1479.

21. **Kirikae, T., F.U. Schade, U. Zähringer, F. Kirikae, H. Brade, T. Kusama, and E.T. Rietschel.** 1994. The significance of the hydrophilic backbone and the hydrophobic fatty acid regions of lipid A for macrophage binding and cytokine induction. FEMS Imm. Med. Microbiol. **8:**13–26.

22. **Kusumoto S.** 1992. Chemical synthesis of lipid A. *In* D.C. Morrison and J.L. Ryan (eds.), Bacterial endotoxic lipopolysaccharides, vol. 1. Molecular biochemistry and cellular biology. CRC Press, Boca Raton, pp. 81–106.

23. **Kirzwon, C., U. Zähringer, K. Kawahara, B. Weidemann, S. Kusumoto, E.T. Rietschel, H.-D. Flad, and A.J. Ulmer.** 1995. Glycosphingolipids from *Shingomonas paucimobilis* induce monokine production in human mononuclear cells. Infect. Immun. **63:**2899–2905.

24. **Lederer, E., and L. Chedid.** 1982. Immunomodulation by synthetic muramyl peptides and trehalose diesters. *In* E. Mihich (ed.), Immunological approaches to cancer therapeutics. J. Wiley & Sons, Inc., New York, pp. 107–135.

25. **Loppnow, H., H. Brade, I. Dürrbaum, C.A. Dinarello, S. Kusumoto, E.T. Rietschel, and H.-D. Flad.** 1989. Interleukin 1 induction-capacity of defined lipopolysaccharide partial structures. J. Immunol. **142:**3229–3238.

26. **Lüderitz, O., M.A. Freudenberg, C. Galanos, V. Lehmann, E.T. Rietschel, and D. Shaw.** 1982. Lipopolysaccharides of gram-negative bacteria. *In* S. Razin and S. Rottem (eds.), Current topics in membranes and transport, vol. 17. Academic Press, New York, pp. 79–151.

27. **Lynn, W.A., and D.T. Golenbock.** 1992. Lipopolysaccharide antagonists. Immunol. Today **13:**271–276.

28. **Mattsson, E., L. Verhage, J. Rollof, A. Fleer, J. Verhoef, and H. van Dijk.** 1993. Peptidoglycan and teichoic acid from *Staphylococcus epidermidis* stimulate human monocyts to release tumor necrosis factor-α, interleukin-1β and interleukin-6. FEMS Immun. Med. Microbiol. **7:**281–288.

29. **Nikaido, H., and M. Vaara.** 1987. Outer membrane. *In* C. Neidhardt, J.L. Ingraham, K. Brooks Low, B. Matgasanik, M. Schaechter, and H.E. Umbarger (eds.) *Escherichia coli* and *Salmonella typhimurium.* Cellular and molecular biology. Am. Soc. Microbiol., Washington, D.C., pp. 7–22.

30. **Nathan, C.F.** 1987. Secretory products of macrophages. J. Clin. Invest. **79:**319–323.

31. **Otterlei, M., A. Sundan, G. Skjåk-Bræk, L. Ryan, O. Smidsrød, and T. Espevik.** 1993. Similar mechanisms of action of defined polysaccharides and lipopolysaccharidese: Characterization of binding and tumor necrosis factor alpha induction. Infect. Immun. **61:**1917–1925.

32. **Price, N.P., T.M. Kelly, C.r.H. Raetz, and R.W. Carlson.** 1994. Biosynthesis of a structurally novel lipid A in *Rhizobium leguminosarum:* Identification and characterization of six metabolic steps leading from UDP-GlcNAc to 3-deoxy-D-*manno*-2-octulosonic $acid_2$-lipid IV_A. J. Bacteriol. **176:**4646–4655.

33. **Raetz, C.R.H.** 1990. Biochemistry of endotoxins. Annu. Rev. Biochem. **59:**129–170.

34. **Riesenfeld-Orn, I., S. Wolpe, J.F. Garcia-Bustos, M.K. Hoffmann, and E. Tuomanen.** 1989. Production of interleukin-1 but not tumor necrosis factor by human monocytes stimulated with pneumococcal cell surface components. Infect. Immun. **57:**1890–1893.

35. **Rietschel, E.T., T. Kirikae, F.U. Schade, U. Mamat, G. Schmidt, H. Loppnow, A.J. Ulmer, U. Zähringer, U. Seydel, F. Di Padova, M. Schreier, and H. Brade.** 1994. Bacterial endotoxin: Molecular relationships of structure to activity and function. FASEB J. **218:**217–225.

36. **Rietschel, E.T., H. Brade, O. Holst, L. Brade, S. Müller-Loennies, U. Mamat, U. Zähringer, F. Beckmann, U. Seydel, K. Brandenburg, A.J. Ulmer, T. Mattern, H. Heine, J. Schletter, H. Loppnow, U. Schönbeck, H.-D. Flad, S. Hauschildt, F.U. Schade, F. Di Padova, S. Kusumoto, and R.R. Schumann.** 1996. Bacterial endotoxin: Chemical constitution, biological recognition, host response, and immunological detoxification. Curr. Top. Microbiol. Immunol. **216:**39–81.

37. **Seydel, U., K. Brandenburg, and E.T. Rietschel.** 1994. A case for an endotoxic conformation. Progr. Clin. Biol. Res. **388:**17–30.

38. **Schleifer, K.H., and O. Kandler.** 1972. Peptidoglycan types of bacterial cell walls and their taxonomic implications. Bacteriol. Rev. **36:**407–477.

39. **Schromm, A.B., K. Brandenburg, E.T. Rietschel, and U. Seydel.** 1995. Do endotoxin aggregates intercalate into phospholipid membranes in a nonspecific, hydrophobic manner? J. Endotox. Res. **2:**313–323.

40. **Schromm, A.B., K. Brandenburg, E.T. Rietschel, H.-D. Flad, S.F. Carroll, and U. Seydel.** 1996. Lipopolysaccharide-binding protein (LBP) mediates CD14-independent intercalation of lipopolysaccharide into phospholipid membranes. FEBS Lett., **399:**267–271.

41. **Schumann, R.R., S.R. Leong, G.W. Flaggs, P.W. Gray, S.D.**

Wright, J.C. Mathison, P.S. Tobias, and R.J. Ulevitch. 1990. Structure and function of lipopolysaccharide binding protein. Science 249:1429–1431.

42. Stefanova I., M.L. Corcoran, E.M. Horak, L.M. Wahl, J.B. Bolen, and I.D. Horak. 1993. Lipopolysaccharide induces activation of CD14-associated protein tyrosine kinase p53/56[lyn]. J. Biol. Chem. 268:20725–20728.

43. Sweet, J.M., and D.A. Hume. 1996. Endotoxin signal transduction in macrophages. J. Leukoc. Biol. 60:8–26.

44. Takada, H., and S. Kotani. 1995. Muramyl dipeptide and derivatives. In D.E.S. Stewart-Tull (ed.), The theory and practical application of adjuvants. John Wiley and Sons, Chichester, pp. 171–201.

45. Takayama, K., and N. Qureshi. 1992. Chemical structure of lipid A. In D.C. Morrison and J.L. Ryan (eds.), Molecular biochemistry and cellular biology. (Bacterial endotoxin lipopolysaccharides, vol. 1). CRC Press, Boca Raton, pp. 43–60

46. Takayama, K., D.H. Mitchell, Z.Z. Din, P. Mukerjee, C. Li, and D.L. Coleman. 1994. Monomeric Re lipopolysaccharide from Escherichia coli is more active than the aggregated from in the Limulus amoebocyte lysate assay and in inducing Egr-1 mRNA in murine peritoneal macrophages. J. Biol. Chem. 269:2241–2244.

47. Timmerman, C.P., E. Mattsson, L. Martinez-Martinez, L. De Graaf, J.A.G. van Strijp, H.A. Verbrugh, J. Verhoef, and A. Fleer. 1993. Induction of release of tumor necrosis factor from human monocytes by staphylococci and staphylococcal peptidoglycans. Infect. Immun. 61:4167–4172.

48. Stimpson, S.A., J.H. Schwab, M.J. Janusz, S.K. Anderle, R.R. Brown, and W.J. Cromartie. 1986. Acute and chronic inflammation induced by peptidoglycan structures and polysaccharide complexes. In P. Seidl and K.H. Schleifer (eds.), Biological properties of peptidoglycan. W. de Gruyter (ed.), Berlin, New York, pp. 273–290.

49. Ulmer, A.J., W. Feist, H. Heine, T. Kirikae, F. Kirikae, S. Kusumoto, T. Kusama, H. Brade, F.U. Schade, E.T. Rietschel, and H.-D. Flad. 1992. Modulation of endotoxin-induced monokine release in human monocytes by lipid A partial structures inhibiting the binding of ^{125}I-LPS. Infect. Immun. 60:5145–5152.

50. Weidemann, B., H. Brade, E.T. Rietschel, R. Dziarski, V. Bažil, S. Kusumoto, H.-D. Flad, and A.J. Ulmer. 1994. Soluble peptidoglycan-induced monokine production can be blocked by anti-CD14 monoclonal antibodies and by lipid A partial structures. Infect. Immun. 62:4709–4715.

51. Weidemann, B., J. Schletter, R. Dziarski, S. Kusumoto, V. Hořejši, F. Stelter, E.T. Rietschel, H.-D. Flad, and A.J. Ulmer. 1997. Specific binding of soluble peptidoglycan and muramyl dipeptide to human monocytes is mediated by CD14. Infect. Immun. 65:858–864.

52. Wright S.D., R.A. Ramos, P.S. Tobias, R.J. Ulevitch, and J.C. Mathison. 1990. CD14, a receptor for complexes of lipopolysaccharide (LPS) and LPS binding protein. Science 249:1431–1433.

53. Zähringer, U., B. Lindner, and E.T. Rietschel. 1994. Molecular structure of lipid A, the endotoxic center of bacterial lipopolysaccharides. Adv. Carbohydr. Chem. Biochem. 50:211–276.

Address reprint requests to:
Prof. Dr. E. Th. Rietschel
Research Center Borstel
Center for Medicine and Biosciences
Parkallee 22
D-23845 Borstel
Germany

Streptococcus pneumoniae

Versatility of Choline-Binding Domain

JOSE L. GARCÍA, ANA R. SÁNCHEZ-BEATO, FRANCISCO J. MEDRANO, and RUBENS LÓPEZ

ABSTRACT

The primary reservoir of the aminoalcohol choline in nature is phosphatidylcholine, the major phospholipid in most eukaryotes, but choline is found unusually in prokaryotes. Although the presence of choline in the cell wall of bacteria was considered a peculiar characteristic of *Streptococcus pneumoniae*, this molecule has been recently found in a reduced number of bacteria. Nevertheless, the unique bacterium that has an absolute requirement of choline for growth is pneumococcus where it plays a fundamental structural role as a constituent of the lipoteichoic and teichoic acids of the cell envelope. The interaction of these compounds with different pneumococcal choline-binding proteins has been proved to have important physiological implications. The first choline-binding protein identified was the major pneumococcal autolysin, the LytA amidase. Up to now, 18 proteins of this family have been characterized in *S. pneumoniae*, *C. beijerinkii*, and several pneumococcal phages. These proteins appear to have evolved by the fusion of two independent domains, the N-terminal domain that is responsible for the specific physiological activity of the corresponding protein and the C-terminal domain that recognizes the choline residues of the cell envelope. The latter domain, known as choline-binding domain (ChBD), is built up by a variable number (4–11) of repeated motifs of about 20 amino acids. The existence of these ChBDs provides an excellent model to analyze the molecular processes involved in cassette recruitment during protein evolution, and support the concept of bacteria as adaptable chimera. We review here the state of the art of the choline-binding proteins identified so far in *S. pneumoniae* and other bacteria.

INTRODUCTION

THIS ARTICLE REVIEWS the current knowledge on the fundamental role that the aminoalcohol choline (trimethylaminoethanol) plays in the physiology of *Streptococcus pneumoniae*, one of the most important human pathogens. Our attention will be particularly focused on proteins that contain a specific domain that allows them to recognize and bind choline, and that will be referred to as the choline-binding domain (ChBD).

METABOLISM OF CHOLINE

The metabolism of choline is relatively well known for eukaryotes but very few data are available for bacteria. This section will summarize how choline is synthesized, degraded or combined with different compounds (Fig. 1).

Metabolism of choline in eukaryotes

Choline is a dietary requirement that crosses the cell membrane by way of an active transport system before being phosphorylated by choline kinase or metabolized to betaine by two mitochondrial enzymes, i.e., choline dehydrogenase and betaine aldehyde dehydrogenase.

The primary reservoir of choline is phosphatidylcholine, the major phospholipid in most eukaryotes, which is synthesized in animals, plants and fungi by one of two pathways, involving the transfer of CDP-choline to diacylglycerol or the S-adenosylmethionine-dependent methylation of phosphatidylethanolamine. This reaction is catalyzed by the phosphatidylethanolamine N-methyltransferase which generates phosphatidylcholine by successive transfers of methyl groups from S-adenosyl-L-methionine.[103] In animals, one enzyme appears to catalyze the three methylation steps, but, in yeasts, the methyltransferase reactions proceed in two steps, an enzyme controls the first methylation

Departamento de Microbiología Molecular, Centro de Investigaciones Biológicas, CSIC, Madrid, Spain.

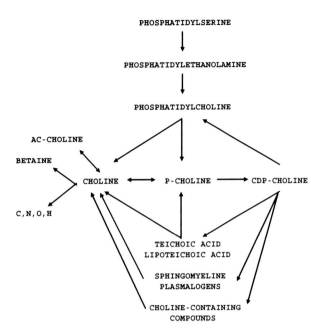

FIG. 1. Metabolism of choline. Schematic representation of the metabolism of choline in eukaryotic and prokaryotic cells.

and another the conversion of monomethylphosphatidylethanolamine into phosphatidylcholine.

The methylation of phosphatidylethanolamine represents the sole known source of choline in nature since the primary acceptor of methyl groups is phosphatidylethanolamine and not the soluble precursors of the CDP-ethanolamine pathway.[103] Since ethanolamine is produced by decarboxylation of L-serine, the backbone of choline is obtained from L-serine.

Free choline in nature is generated primarily from the catabolism of phosphatidylcholine that is carried out by phospholipases. Phospholipases A1 and A2 hydrolyze the *sn*-1 and *sn*-2 fatty acyl bonds, respectively; phospholipase C hydrolyzes the glycerophosphate ester bond, and phospholipase D the choline phosphate ester bond. Lysophosphatidylcholine is degraded by lysophospholipases, which convert it to fatty acid and glycerolphosphorylcholine. The latter can be hydrolyzed subsequently to choline and glycerolphosphate or glycerol and phosphorylcholine by a phosphodiesterase.[103]

Choline is also found in other phospholipids such as glyceryl ether phospholipids and sphingolipids. The glyceryl ether phospholipids contain an ether unit instead of an acyl unit at C1 and are synthesized starting with dihydroxyacetone phosphate. The alkyl and alkyl-1-enyl types of ether-linked phospholipids are present in mammalian cells almost exclusively as structural analogues of phosphatidylcholine and phosphatidylethanolamine. Most mammalian tissues contain at least small amounts of plasmanylcholine (alkyl type) and plasmenylcholine (alkyl-1-enyl type, plasmalogen). The alkyl type is found predominantly as choline phosphoglycerolipids, whereas the plasmalogens occur mainly as ethanolamine phosphoglycerolipids. The most significant discovery and advancement in the study of the ether-linked analogues of phosphatidylcholine was the elucidation of the chemical structure of the platelet activating factor (PAF), which was identified as 1-alkyl-2-acetyl-*sn*-glycero-3-phosphocholine. On the other hand,

the backbone of sphingolipids is sphingosine rather than glycerol. Sphingosine is transformed first into ceramide (*N*-acyl sphingosine) and then into sphingomyelin, cerebrosides or gangliosides. In sphingomyelin, the terminal hydroxyl group of ceramide is substituted by phosphorylcholine, which comes from phosphatidylcholine.

Finally, it is important to point out that an appropriate supply of choline for acetylcholine synthesis is critical for cholinergic nerve function, since the nervous system does not synthesize choline *de novo*. Acetylcholine is synthesized from choline and acetyl-CoA by a choline acyltransferase and is hydrolyzed to choline and acetate by acetylcholinesterase.

Metabolism of choline in prokaryotes

The unique bacterium that has an absolute requirement of choline (or choline analogues) for growth is *S. pneumoniae*. Although this nutritional requirement was known since 1937,[1,5,63,71] choline was not shown to be linked to a polysaccharide component of the pneumococcal cell wall until 1967.[96] Further studies showed that choline was a component of the teichoic acid[12,62] and of lipoteichoic acid.[11] The structure of these components and their metabolism as well as the recent isolation of two pneumococcal mutants that do not require choline for growth will be discussed below.

The presence of choline in the cell wall of bacteria had been considered a peculiar characteristic of pneumococcus. However, this aminoalcohol has been recently found in other bacteria (Table 1), i.e., *S. oralis*,[53] *S. mitis*,[35,36] *C. beijerinckii*,[29] and *C. saccharoperbutylacetonicum*.[66] In contrast with the case of pneumococcus *S. oralis*, *C. beijerinckii* and *C. saccharoperbutylacetonicum* do not require choline for growth, and the role of choline in *S. mitis* remains to be elucidated.

On the other hand, the diagnosis of *S. pneumoniae* infection has been attempted by methods that detect species-specific C-polysaccharide antigen which contains phosphorylcholine. Doubts about the specificity of this technique have been raised on the grounds that many other organisms share phosphorylcholine as an immunodominant epitope (Table 2). In some strains of *Haemophilus influenzae*, this antigen has been localized in the plasma membrane and near the septum, but further studies are needed to determine its nature and function.[35,36]

Choline is also found in other bacterial components. Although it has been considered, as a general rule, that bacteria do not contain phosphatidylcholine or the partially methylated intermediates, there are many exceptions to this rule. The number of bacterial strains where choline has been identified in their phospholipids is increasing along with the increasing number of analyses that are done to identify the lipid composition of

TABLE 1.   BACTERIA CONTAINING CHOLINE IN THE CELL WALL

Bacteria	References
Streptococcus pneumoniae	96
Streptococcus oralis	53,74
Streptococcus constellatus	53
Streptococcus mitis	35
Clostridium beijerinckii	29
Clostridium NI-4	29,66

TABLE 2. BACTERIA CONTAINING
PHOSPHORYLCHOLINE ANTIGENS

Bacteria	References
Streptococcus pneumoniae	22,36,38,67
Haemophilus influenzae	22
Haemophilus parainfluenzae	22
Corynebacterium jeikeium	22
Corynebacterium sp.	22
Bacillus spp.	22
Micrococcus spp.	22
Lactococcus sp.	22
Gemella haemolysans	22
Streptococcus sp. group G	22
Streptococcus oralis	35
Streptococcus mitis	35
Morganella morganii	15,56,68
Lactobacillus acidophilus	67,69
Streptococcus group O	68
Streptococcus group H	68

bacterial membranes.[3,6,39,41,50,51,95] Apparently, bacterial phosphatidylcholine is not synthesized by the CDP-choline pathway. The source of the methyl groups in bacterial phosphatidylcholine is methionine, and *S*-adenosylmethionine appears to be the direct methyl donor. A phosphatidylethanolamine *N*-methyltransferase capable of catalyzing the three methylation reactions has been characterized in *Rhodobacter sphaeroides*[2] and *Zimomonas mobilis*.[103] Some strains of *C. beijerinckii* appear to contain only *N*-methylethanolamine in their phospholipids and plasmalogens suggesting that they have a *N*-methyltransferase capable to catalyze only the first methylation reaction.[103] In addition, both types of *N*-methyltransferases have been found in *Agrobacterium tumefaciens*.[103] The fact that no choline nucleotide pathway has been identified so far for the synthesis of bacterial phosphatidylcholine would indicate that the phosphatidylethanolamine methylation is the first step to evolve in the metabolism of choline. The prevalence of monomethylated and dimethylated compounds, often in the absence of phosphatidylcholine in some bacterial strains, suggests that the choline-pathway evolved in a stepwise manner.

A novel phosphocholine-containing glycolglycerophospholipid named GGPL-1 was isolated from a *Mycoplasma fermentans*, a pathogen causing rheumatoid arthritis, and this compound appears to be a major immunological determinant.[59] Interestingly, a role in hypoosmotic adaptation has been suggested for an unusual cyclic oligosaccharide, a phosphocholine-substituted $\beta\beta$-1,3;1,6 cyclic glucan (PCCG), that has been isolated from *Bradyrhizobium japonicum*.[65] It has been proposed that phosphocholine head group of PCCG might be derived from the turnover of membrane lipids. Moreover, since phosphatidylcholine is the most abundant phospholipid in this microorganism, an important role in plant infections has been suggested for this compound.

Finally, the ability for catabolic oxidation of choline seems widespread in bacteria,[54] but some of them, like *Escherichia coli*, use choline to synthesize the osmoprotective compound glycine betaine by a choline-glycine betaine pathway that contains two enzymes.[92]

Role of choline in Streptococcus pneumoniae

Since choline is required for pneumococcal growth and this microorganism does not contain phosphatidylcholine, the aminoalcohol is exclusively incorporated into the teichoic and lipoteichoic acids of the cell envelope.[96]

The lipoteichoic acid of pneumococcus was the first lipocarbohydrate detected in Gram-positive bacteria, however, its structure has been determined very recently, showing that it contains two molecules of phosphorylcholine for each repeated unit.[8,91] The pneumococcal lipoteichoic acid is polydisperse since its chain length varies between two and eight repeated units. More recently, analyses carried out to determine the precise structure of teichoic acid have revealed that it is unusually highly related to the lipoteichoic acid since their chain structures are identical.[23]

Although the mechanism for incorporation of choline into the pneumococcal cell wall antigens is unknown, it had been suggested that it proceeds by a CDP-choline pathway.[7,70] Choline kinase and phosphate cytidyltransferase (cytidine diphosphocholine pyrophosphorylase) activities were detected in cell free extracts of pneumococcus.[7,70,105,106] Two DNA probes containing a fragment of the *cki* and *cct* genes encoding the choline kinase and the choline phosphate cytidyltransferase of *Saccharomyces cerevisiae*, respectively, hybridized with DNA of pneumococcus under low stringency conditions.[105,106] In this sense, a gene named *pck* encoding a choline kinase similar to LicA from *H. influenzae* has been recently identified in *S. pneumoniae* (GenBank accession number AF036951). A comparative analysis of this gene with the proteins of the data banks revealed that it is also highly similar to the *licA* gene from *Mycoplasma pneumoniae* (GenBank accession number AE000028) and showed a significant identity with some regions of the *cki* gene from *S. cerevisiae* in agreement with the above observation. We have located the *pck* gene within the partial pneumococcal genome sequence provided by TIGR and it appears to form together with five additional genes a single transcription unit. Two of these genes, located just downstream of *pck*, are homologous to the *licB* and *licC* genes of *H. influenzae*, two genes of the *licABCD* locus (*lic1*) that has been suggested to be involved in the incorporation of choline into lipopolysaccharide.[104] Whether the pneumococcal genes found in the *pkc* locus are responsible for the incorporation of choline into lipoteichoic or teichoic acids remains to be elucidated.

On the other hand, the *lic1* locus has been implicated in the phase variation of phosporylcholine in *H. influenzae*.[104] This phase variation was also observed in pneumococcus and has been correlated with the synthesis of teichoic acid and the incorporation of choline.[52] The pneumococcus phase varies between a virulent form with more capsular polysaccharide and less teichoic acid and an avirulent form with less capsular polysaccharide and more teichoic acid.[52] In this sense, it has been observed that lipoteichoic containing an intact phosporylcholine residue is a ligand responsible for binding of pneumococci to the receptor of asialo-GM1 of epithelial cells.[93]

Interestingly, it had been observed that ethanolamine and other aminoalcohols containing N-C-C-OH or N-C-C-C-OH linkages could satisfy the nutritional requirement of pneumococcus for choline.[5] However, the incorporation of these substances in the cell wall causes striking changes in several cell properties.[97] These experiments also showed that pneumococcus was unable to carry out the methylation of ethanolamine to choline and, in the presence of choline, the incorporation of ethanolamine is inhibited. On the other hand, phosphorylcholine is released from the pneumococcal teichoic and lipoteichoic acid by the action of a teichoic acid phosphorylcholine esterase.[44] A choline esterase able to release choline residues from the cell wall has also been detected in *S. oralis*.[74]

Most of the current knowledge about the role of choline in pneumococcus came from the study of the biological consequences of its replacement by ethanolamine.[97] The biological properties of bacteria containing ethanolamine or its mono and dimethyl derivatives in the cell walls show a trend to normality in the following order: ethanolamine < monomethylethanolamine < dimethylethanolamine. Cultures growing in the presence of ethanolamine form long chains and did not lyse at the end of the stationary phase (Fig. 2). These cells are resistant to the deoxycholate-induced lysis and are unable to undergo genetic transformation. It was also observed that a choline concentration 200 times above the average metabolic requirement caused moderate chaining of pneumococci.[97] A filamentous growth of *S. pneumoniae* in the presence of certain quaternary ammonium compounds or in the absence of divalent cations was also observed several years ago.[4,63]

Choline, as a structural component of the teichoic acid of pneumococcus, plays a key role in determining its sensitivity to the major autolytic enzyme, since walls prepared from pneumococci where choline was replaced by ethanolamine were found to be completely resistant to autolysis.[62] These cells contain an apparently abnormal form of the autolytic enzyme (low molecular weight, E-form) that can be "converted" to the normal enzyme (high molecular weight, C-form) by incubation *in vitro* with choline-containing cell walls.[100] Ethanolamine-containing cells are tolerant to extremely high doses of bacteriolytic antibiotics[98] and their cell walls cannot be solubilized by the autolytic enzyme.[40] As will be discussed below, all these properties have been correlated with the existence of a choline-dependent *N*-acetylmuramyl-L-alanine-amidase.

Although many pneumococcal cell wall subcomponents are inflammatory, teichoic acid-containing portions of the cell wall have been shown to provide the stimulus for the acute inflammatory response: they trigger the alternative complement pathway,[49,107] promotes secretion of IL-1,[72] induce leukocytosis

and increase vascular permeability.[99,101] These findings suggested that the pneumococcal teichoic and lipoteichoic acids have an unusual inflammatory potential. In this sense, it has been shown that the C-reactive protein[61] and antiphosphorylcholine antibodies of the T15 idiotype[10] are optimally protective against *S. pneumoniae* infection in mice. Moreover, when a mouse CBA/N(*xid*) was genetically modified to produce significant amounts of circulating anti-phosphorylcholine antibodies, it becomes protected against a lethal challenge with *S. pneumoniae*.[55] Immunization with different phosphocholine-containing antigens or passive transfer of antiphosphorylcholine antibodies also protected mice against *S. pneumoniae*.[22] Thus, phosphorylcholine appears to be a critical determinant of the inflammatory activity of pneumococcal teichoic and lipoteichoic acids.

Phosphorylcholine is also a basic determinant of the biological activity of PAF, a choline-containing glyceryl ether phospholipid, that is a mediator of the inflammation produced by different cells in response to injury.[14] This substance induces cellular activation after binding to a receptor that is a member of the superfamily of G proteins.[14] Although no evidence for a direct PAF-like activity of pneumococcal cell wall components was detected *in vitro*, it has been suggested that the intensity of inflammation associated with the pneumococcal infection in brain and lung is increased by the unique participation of endogenous PAF in the inflammatory response to *S. pneumoniae* cell wall components.[13] More recently, it has been shown that *S. pneumoniae* anchors to activated human cells by the PAF receptor.[17] Attachment of bacterial phosphorylcholine enhanced adherence has been coupled to invasion of endothelial and epithelial cells.[17]

Very recently, two mutants of *S. pneumoniae* that do not require choline for growth have been generated by two different methods.[88,110] Mutant JY2190 was isolated by serial passage of strain Rx1 in a medium containing decreasing concentration of ethanolamine with each passage,[110] whereas strain R6Cho⁻ was recovered from a heterologous cross with DNA from *S. oralis*.[88] Both mutants cultured in choline-free medium grew with normal generation time but formed long chains, failed to undergo stationary phase autolysis and were resistant to lysis induced by deoxycholate or penicillin. The cell wall composition was not altered except that the phosphate content was reduced due to the lack of phosphocholine. During growth in the

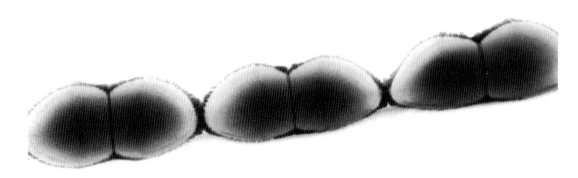

FIG. 2.   Morphology of pneumococcal cells grown in ethanolamine-containing medium.

presence of choline, the R6Cho⁻ strain reversed all the atypical properties,[88] whereas the JY2190 mutant was unable to lyse in the stationary phase and showed poor reactivity with antibody to phosphocholine.[110] Although the properties of strain JY2190 can be transferred to the parent strain by DNA of the mutant, the gene(s) involved in this process remain to be characterized.

Finally, choline-containing teichoic acids are essential for the adsorption of phage Dp-1 to pneumococci.[57]

CHOLINE-BINDING PROTEINS

As documented above, choline plays a fundamental structural role in pneumococcus as a constituent of different components of the cell envelope, but other physiological roles, through its interaction with different choline-binding proteins, have also been well characterized. This section examines the state of the art about these proteins in *S. pneumoniae* and other bacteria.

Choline-binding proteins in Streptococcus pneumoniae

Since pneumococcus only contains choline in the teichoic and lipoteichoic acids, these compounds are the ligands of the choline-binding proteins and are responsible for the role that choline and these proteins play in this microorganism. Although most of our current knowledge on choline-binding proteins in bacteria comes from the studies carried out with the major pneumococcal autolysin, the analysis of the choline-binding proteins encoded by bacteriophages has also been of great relevance to determine the molecular basis of choline recognition.

Cell wall amidase. The first protein of *S. pneumoniae* that was identified as choline-dependent was the major autolysin, since it was observed that the autolysin-catalyzed hydrolysis of the cell wall required the interaction between the enzyme and choline residues in the teichoic acid.[45] This enzyme has been purified and characterized as a *N*-acetylmuramyl-L-alanine amidase.[46,48] The lipoteichoic acid (Forssman antigen) was recognized as a powerful inhibitor of this enzyme and it was suggested that this compound may play a physiological role in the *in vivo* control of autolysin activity.[43] High choline or phosphorylcholine concentrations blocked the adsorption of pneumococcal autolytic enzyme to the cell walls and inhibit enzymatic activity in a non competitive manner.[9,37] Even *in vivo*, high choline concentrations in the culture medium led to phenotypically amidase-deficient pneumococci.[9,37] Other aminoalcohols or derivatives such as ethanolamine, monomethylethanolamine and phosphorylethanolamine have no effect on enzyme adsorption or hydrolytic activity.[37] These experiments reinforced the previous hypothesis that the enzymatic hydrolysis of cell walls requires prior adsorption of the enzyme to the insoluble substrate and that choline residues have the role of adsorption ligands in the process.[26,37] In addition, it was suggested, for the first time, that the enzyme might contain two sites, one responsible for choline recognition and the other involved in the catalytic activity.[9] It was also observed that the membrane-associated form of the amidase (C-form) could be completely released with high choline concentrations suggesting that the enzyme is bound to the membrane-attached lipoteichoic acid rather than being a membrane protein itself.[9] The interaction of the autolysin with lipoteichoic acid and choline was used to develop a rapid procedure of purification of the enzyme by affinity chromatography on lipoteichoic- or choline-Sepharose.[9]

The low molecular weight form (E-form) of the pneumococcal autolysin can be converted to the active form (C-form) not only by preincubation with choline-containing pneumococcal cell walls[100] but also with free choline. In this case, the choline-converted enzyme showed a low molecular weight, suggesting that the conversion is dependent of a specific interaction between the molecule of choline and the enzyme.[9] Further analyses demonstrated that tertiary amines appears to be the minimal structure required to convert *in vitro* the E-form to the C-form.[87] Since diethylethanolamine was one of the compounds found to activate the amidase, a new procedure was developed to purify the enzyme by affinity chromatography on DEAE-cellulose.[87]

Cell wall glucosaminidase. The isolation of the pneumococcal mutant M31 that has a complete deletion of the *lytA* gene encoding the autolytic amidase allowed the identification of a new peptidoglycan hydrolase.[81] *In vivo* experiments have demonstrated that the glucosaminidase also behaves as an autolytic enzyme.[31] The enzyme purified to electrophoretic homogeneity showed a M_r of 64,000 and has been characterized as an *endo-ββ1,4-N-acetylglucosaminidase* that requires choline in the teichoic acid of the cell wall substrate for catalytic activity.[31] In addition, the finding that the enzyme can be purified by affinity chromatography on choline-Sepharose suggested that it also contains a choline-binding site.

Phage-encoded lysins. Early experiments had indicated that the pneumococcal phase Dp-1 encoded a cell wall lytic enzyme that participates in the liberation of the phage progeny.[34] The lytic enzyme, named phage-associated lysin (PAL), was characterized as a choline-dependent amidase.[30] The *pal* gene encoding this amidase has been cloned and sequenced[90] revealing that PAL appears to be a natural chimeric enzyme of intergeneric origin, that is, the N-terminal domain was highly similar to the catalytic domain of the murein hydrolase of the lactococcus phage BK5-T, whereas the C-terminal domain was homologous to those found in the lytic enzymes of the pneumococcal system. As pointed out above, this phage should also encode a choline-receptor that is essential for its adsorption to pneumococci,[57] but the precise nature of this receptor remains to be determined.

Other lysins encoded by pneumococcal bacteriophages have been characterized,[58] e.g., the lysozymes from Cp-1, Cp-7, and Cp-9,[25,28,32] and the amidases from the temperature bacteriophages HB-3[73] and EJ-1.[20] With the sole exception of the lysozyme of Cp-7 all these enzymes are choline-dependent for activity and can be purified by affinity chromatography on choline-Sepharose or DEAE-cellulose suggesting that they contain a choline-binding site. The structural analysis of these enzymes provided the basis to establish the hypothesis on the modular evolution of the pneumococcal cell wall lytic enzymes,[32] as discussed below.

Pneumococcal surface protein A. Pneumococcal surface protein A (PspA) is the only surface protein of *S. pneumoniae* known to exhibit significant immunogenic and virulence properties.[60,109] PspA utilizes a novel mechanism for anchoring to the cell surface. In contrast to the surface proteins of other Gram-positive bacteria, its anchoring to the cell envelope requires choline-mediated interaction between the membrane-associated lipoteichoic acid and the C-terminal repeat region of PspA.[60,111] Interestingly, the protein can be released from the cell surface by a high concentration of choline. The analysis of the sequence for the gene encoding PspA revealed that it contains a ChBD similar to that found in the major autolysin.[109]

Pneumococcal surface protein SpsA. A novel pneumococcal surface protein named SpsA capable of binding specifically to human secretory immunoglobulin A has been recently described.[42] Free secretory component also binds to *S. pneumoniae*, whereas serum IgA does not, suggesting that pneumococcal binding to the secretory immunoglobulin A is mediated by the secretory component. The N-terminal domain of SpsA is responsible for the binding to the secretory component whereas the C-terminal domain was built by 9 highly conserved repeats of 20 amino acids each found in other choline-binding proteins. The protein appear to be secreted by using a typical signal sequence of 37 amino acids. It has been proposed that the interaction between *S. pneumoniae* and the secretory component via SpsA represents a novel biological interaction that might increase virulence by the impairment of bacterial clearance.[42]

Pneumococcal adhesin CbpA. The protein CbpA was characterized as the predominant component of a mixture of proteins eluted in a choline-dependent fashion from a *pspA* dependent strain of pneumococcus.[75] CbpA is a surface-exposed protein of 75 kDa that react with human convalescent antisera. The deduced sequence from the corresponding gene showed the typical chimeric architecture of choline-binding proteins. A *cbpA*-deficient mutant showed more than 50% reduction in adherence to cytokine activated human cells and failed to bind to immobilized sialic acid or lacto-*N*-neotetraose, known pneumococcal ligands on eukaryotic cells.[75] Carriage of this mutant in an animal model of nasopharyngeal colonization was reduced 100-fold. According to these observations it has been suggested that CbpA can play a relevant role as an adhesin and a determinant of virulence and could be considered as a pneumococcal vaccine candidate.[75]

PcpA protein. The PcpA protein contains 708 residues resulting in a predicted M_r of 79,000 and a calculated pI of 9.3. The deduced polypeptide showed a high content in threonine and serine (17%) almost evenly distributed within the 469 amino acids of the N-terminal region preceding a typical choline-binding domain built by 11 identical repeats.[79] Two tandem arrays of five characteristic amphipatic leucine reach repeats (LRR) of 22–26 amino acids in length that have been found in the N-terminal region fo the PcpA. These LRR showed a significant similarity to chaoptin, a surface glycoprotein found in the photoreceptor cells of the flies, and to follicle-stimulating human receptor Fshr. Since these amphipatic repeats have been proposed to be involved in protein-protein and protein-lipid interactions it has been suggested a role for PcpA in pneumococcal adhesion.[79]

Other choline-binding proteins. When crude extracts of pneumococcus were purified in choline-Sepharose columns it was observed that, apart from the amidase, at least six proteins were also specifically eluted with choline, suggesting that *S. pneumoniae* contains additional choline-binding proteins.[9] In agreement with this finding, it has been recently shown that at

least eight proteins larger than 45 kDa can be eluted with choline from a choline-containing matrix loaded with an extract prepared from a *pspA*-deficient mutant.[75] Antisera to these proteins passively protected mice challenged in the peritoneum with a lethal dose of pneumococci.[75] Some of these proteins might be the cell wall glycosidase,[31] the phosphorylcholine esterase[44] or the enzymes of the CDP-choline pathway,[105] but only the first one has been shown to be able to bind to choline-Sepharose.

Choline-binding proteins in bacteria other than Streptococcus pneumoniae

Although the enzymes that are involved in the metabolism of phosphatidylcholine might contain active sites that can bind choline, these proteins are probably not very different from those found in eukaryotes and will not be reviewed here. Most interesting is the fact that a limited number of bacteria appear to contain choline as a component of the cell wall (Table 1). Although very few data were available about the existence of choline-binding proteins in these bacteria, it was described that *C. beijerinckii* NCIB 8052 (formerly named *C. acetobutylicum*) contained several proteins that could be purified by affinity chromatography on choline-Sepharose and this microorganism grows forming long chains in the presence of 2% of choline[29] (Fig. 3). The chromatographic fraction eluted with choline from extracts prepared from *C. beijerinckii* showed a choline-dependent amidase activity capable of degrading pneumococcal walls. Although it was previously suggested that this activity

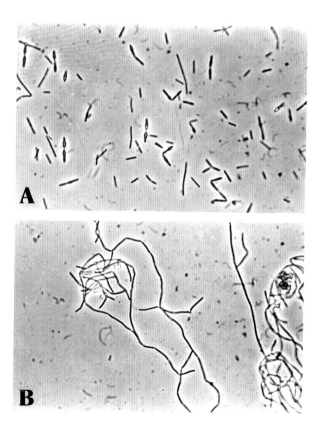

FIG. 3. Morphology of *C. beijerinckii* cells. Cells were grown in the presence (A) or absence of 2% choline (B).[29]

could be ascribed to the major protein contained in the choline fraction, further analyses have demonstrated that this major band corresponds to a secretable protein named CspA.[76,77] CspA is a member of a family of four homologous proteins of unknown function that contain a ChBD similar to that found in pneumococcal choline-binding proteins.[78]

S. oralis contains an enzyme that can remove a limited amount of choline residues when tested on purified cell walls.[74] This activity has been identified as an esterase that exhibits some biochemical properties similar to those previously found for several cell wall lytic enzymes of *S. pneumoniae*. However, there is not any evidence, at the molecular level, suggesting that this enzyme could contain a ChBD.

Genetic analyses

The *lytA* gene encoding the major pneumococcal autolysin was the first gene encoding a choline-binding protein that has been cloned.[24] Since then, several genes encoding other choline-binding proteins have been sequenced (Table 3). Nevertheless, the preliminary analysis of the LytA sequence did not provide any evidence for the assignment of a specific function to the N- or C-terminal moieties of the molecule.[33] The comparative analysis between *lytA* and the *cpl1* gene encoding the lysozyme of the Cp-1 phage reported an illuminating information on the organization of the cell wall lytic enzymes.[25] This comparison revealed that both proteins contained homologous C-terminal domains that were ascribed to the specific recognition of the choline residues of the teichoic acids. Further analyses revealed that the sequence of *cpl7*, a gene encoding a choline-independent lysozyme of the Cp-7 phage, provided a strong support to the theory of the modular evolution of the pneumococcal cell wall lytic enzymes.[32]

Southern blot analysis has shown that, under low stringency conditions, a C-terminal encoding probe of the *pspA* gene hybridized with five additional bands of a *Hin*dIII-digested DNA from the strain Rx1 of *S. pneumoniae*.[60] One of these bands corresponds to the *lytA* gene and the other bands may encode

proteins that interact with the choline residues of the cell surface. Similar experiments have shown that under low stringency conditions, the *lytA* gene hybridized with four additional bands.[105] Recent experiments carried out in our laboratory using different probes encoding ChBDs have allowed us to clone three genes that encode the proteins PcpA, PcpB and PcpC containing ChBDs[76,79] (Fig. 4). The putative role of PcpA in adherence has been discussed above whereas PcpB is homologous to different proteases.[76] All these results are in agreement with the observation that several proteins present in pneumococcal cell extracts can be eluted with choline from a choline-Sepharose column[9,75] and strongly suggest that *S. pneumoniae* possesses many other genes encoding ChBDs that may play important physiological roles. The genes *spsA*,[42] *cbpA*,[75] and *pbcA*,[47] recently isolated and sequenced clearly illustrate this hypothesis.

STRUCTURE AND EVOLUTION OF CHOLINE-BINDING DOMAIN

Although the three-dimensional structure of ChBD is not available, other experimental approaches have allowed us to obtain relevant information on the structure of this domain as well as to suggest interesting evolutionary links between proteins showing affinity by choline-containing substrates.

Structural analysis

The primary structure of ChBDs is built up by a variable number of repeated peptides containing 20–22 amino acids (Fig. 5). The first consensus sequence of this repetitive peptide was deduced from the comparison of the *lytA* and the *cpl1* genes, respectively.[25] Both proteins contain six repeated sequences in their C-termini, which might be useful for the simultaneous recognition of several molecules of choline. Although the construction of chimeric genes provided a solid support to the hypothesis that this domain would be responsible for the choline-

TABLE 3. CLONED GENES ENCODING A ChBD

Gene	Organism	Function	Activity	References
lytA	*S. pneumoniae*	Autolysin	Amidase	33
lytA101	*S. pneumoniae*	Autolysin	Amidase	21
pspA	*S. pneumoniae*	Antigen	Unknown	109
pcpA	*S. pneumoniae*	Adhesion?	Unknown	79
pcpB	*S. pneumoniae*	Unknown	Protease?	76
pcpC	*S. pneumoniae*	Unknown	Unknown	76
cbpA	*S. pneumoniae*	Adhesion	Unknown	75
spsA	*S. pneumoniae*	Binding	Unknown	42
pbcA	*S. pneumoniae*	Binding	Unknown	47
cspA	*C. beijerinckii*	Unknown	Unknown	77
cspB	*C. beijerinckii*	Unknown	Unknown	78
cspC	*C. beijerinckii*	Unknown	Unknown	78
cspD	*C. beijerinckii*	Unknown	Unknown	78
cpl1	Phage Cp-1	Lysin	Lysozyme	25
cpl9	Phage Cp-9	Lysin	Lysozyme	32
ejl	Phage EJ-1	Lysin	Amidase	20
hbl	Phage HB-3	Lysin	Amidase	73
pal	Phage Dp-1	Lysin	Amidase	90

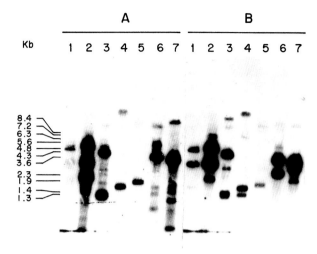

FIG. 4. Southern blot analysis of *S. pneumoniae* R6. Chromosomal DNA from *S. pneumoniae* was digested with *Eco*RV (lane 1), *Hinc*II (lane 2), *Hind*III (lane 3), *Pst*I (lane 4), *Pvu*II (lane 5), or *Ssp*I (lane 6) and hybridized under low stringent conditions with the oligonucleotides Chol1 (A) or Mod1 (B), which encode two polypeptides of seven amino acids of the consensus repeated unit of ChBD (Sánchez-Beato[76] and Fig. 5). Molecular size markers in kb are indicated at the left.

binding properties of these proteins,[18,19,58] the most relevant evidence was obtained when the region encoding this domain was independently cloned and expressed in *E. coli*.[83] The truncated polypeptides corresponding to the C-termini of the enzymes LytA and Cpl1, named C-LytA and C-Cpl1, respectively, showed a great affinity for choline, although they were devoid of cell wall-degrading activity. In contrast, when the 5′-terminal regions of these genes were expressed in *E. coli* the resulting polypeptides showed a low, but significant, cell wall hydrolytic activity.[84] The findings that the trypsin-sensitivity of the C-terminal domain diminished in the presence of choline[85] and that C-Cpl1 and C-LytA reduced the hydrolytic activity of the lytic enzymes by competing for cell wall-binding,[80] also support the hypothesis that choline interacts with the C-terminal domain of these enzymes.

Circular dichroism (CD) analysis of the CPl-1 secondary structure revealed that choline induces remarkable changes in the intensity of the bands at 210, 230, and 295 nm, with the appearance of an unusual positive band at 225 nm.[85] This band was attributed to the high content of aromatic amino acids in the Cpl1 lysozyme. Since 12 out of 15 tryptophans are located in the C-terminal region, the CD changes observed with choline were ascribed to a change in the environment of these aromatic

amino acids. The conformational change was reversible and correlated with the competitive inhibitory effect of choline on lysozyme activity, supporting, by a new experimental approach, the basic role of choline in the recognition of the cell wall substrate.

The analysis of the secondary structure prediction indicated that the ChBD has a high percentage of probable β-turn structures containing basic residues, a finding that could explain why this region is extremely sensitive to trypsin digestion. Interestingly, this analysis also shows that the six repeated sequences of this domain do not show a similar repeated secondary structure and then the overall predicted secondary structure of the ChBD would result from two sheet-bends-helix modules connected by five bend-sheet structures, probably arranged in parallel or antiparallel conformations.[85] On the other hand, the analysis of the CD data obtained in the presence of choline suggested that this molecule produces a redistribution of the ββ-sheet and ββ-turn contributions. A prediction of the secondary structure of a hypothetical ChBD formed by the fusion of four consensus repeats is shown in Fig. 6. All these data were compatible with the two-domain structure of the Cpl-1 lysozyme and reinforced the hypothesis that the C-terminal region is directly involved in the binding of the enzyme to the teichoic or lipoteichoic acids of the pneumococcal cell envelope.

The CD analyses carried out with the isolated ChBDs, i.e., C-LytA and C-Cpl1 proteins, confirmed that the changes induced by choline in the Cpl-1 lysozyme were due to the specific interaction with its C-terminal domain. Consequently, we concluded that this domain represents the major contribution to the unusual CD band observed at 225 nm that can be ascribed to the CD of the aromatic amino acids.[83]

Differential scanning calorimetry (DSC) has been used to characterize the thermal stability of the Cpl-1 lysozyme and its isolated N- and C-terminal domains.[86] The heat capacity function of Cpl-1 lysozyme shows two peaks that can be correlated with the transitions of the N- and C-terminal domains. At saturating concentration of choline the transition corresponding to the C-terminal domain is shifted to higher temperatures. Although choline does not affect the transition temperature nor the denaturation enthalpy of the isolated N-terminal domain, the analysis of the DSC curves showed that choline decreases the enthalpy corresponding to the N-terminal domain when added to the native Cpl-1 lysozyme. Under saturation concentrations of choline, Cpl-1 lysozyme unfolds as a single cooperative unit. Apparently, the linkage of both domains in Cpl-1 reduces the value for the specific enthalpy of the N-terminal transition by a factor of two without a remarkable change in transition temperature. This result suggests that the presence of the C-terminal domain enhances the microstability of the native structure of the N-terminal region. On the other hand, the independence of both domains for their folding-unfolding transitions indicates that few hydrophobic contacts are established between each domain. This conclusion is in agreement with the finding that the chimeric cell wall lytic enzymes constructed by interchange of catalytic domains are as efficient as the parental enzymes.[18,19] The Vant'Hoff plot for DSC experiments of Cpl-1 carried out in the presence of various concentrations of choline allowed us to propose the existence of five choline-binding sites per monomer.[86]

The structural organization of the LytA amidase and its iso-

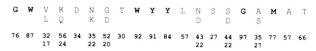

FIG. 5. Consensus sequence of the repeated unit of ChBD. Numbers indicate the probability to find the residue in the repeated units of the ChBDs sequenced so far (Table 3).

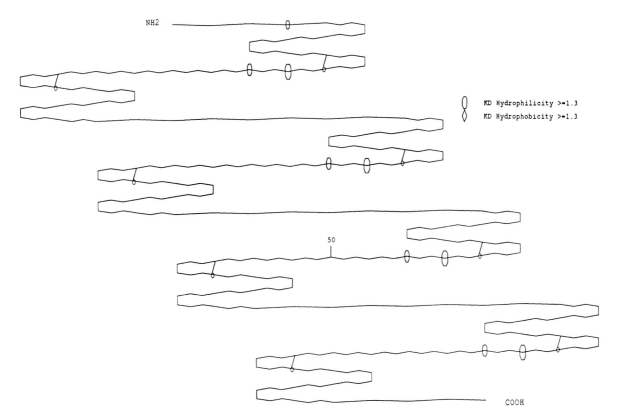

KD Hydrophilicity >=1.3
KD Hydrophobicity >=1.3

FIG. 6. Secondary structure prediction of a hypothetical ChBD containing four consensus repeated units. Prediction was carried out using the PLOTSTRUCTURE program of the University of Wisconsin Molecular Biology Package (WIMP).

lated C-LytA domain have been also examined by DSC.[102] Deconvolution of calorimetric curves has revealed a folding of the amidase in several independent or quasiindependent cooperative domains. The higher complexity found in this case suggests that the interaction between the N- and C-terminal domains of the amidase is more important than that observed in the Cpl-1 lysozyme. Analytical centrifugation studies have shown that LytA exhibits a monomer-dimer association equilibrium, through the C-terminal part of the molecule. Dimerization is regulated by choline interaction and involves the preferential binding of two molecules of choline per dimer. The LytA amidase might be described as an elongated molecule consisting of at least four subdomains, N1 and N2 contained in the N-terminal region, and C1 and C2 in the C-terminal one. The LytA dimer can be modeled as a prolate ellipsoid of about 13 × 190 Å, which can be visualized as a stalk, made of the C-terminal domains, bearing at each end a catalytic site. The dimerization is carried out through the interaction of the C2 subdomains. This shape would facilitate the diffusion of the protein through the highly cross-linked framework of the cell wall and increase the number of accessible hydrolyzable bonds per attachment site. On the other hand, the analyses of the DSC curves and sedimentation velocity of LytA and C-LytA in the presence of choline provided evidence about the existence of two types of choline-binding sites, i.e., of low and high affinity, but how these two types of sites might affect the interaction of the protein with the cell wall or whether they could be related to the

choline-activation of LytA (conversion) remain to be elucidated.

A different experimental approach to study the relationships between structure and function of the ChBDs has been carried out by generating deletions of the C-terminal domain of the LytA amidase using protein engineering techniques.[27,80] These results suggested that the 11-terminal amino acids of the amidase are important in the process of conversion from the E-form to the active C-form.[80] A serial deletion of the six repeated units of the C-terminal domain revealed that at least four units are required to efficiently recognize the choline residues of the cell walls.[27] The loss of an additional unit dramatically reduces its hydrolytic activity as well as the binding affinity to choline, suggesting that the catalytic efficiency of this enzyme is considerably improved by keeping the enzyme attached to the cell wall substrate. Interestingly, the truncated proteins were inhibited by deoxycholate (DOC), and the expression of a LytA amidase lacking the last 11 amino acids in *S. pneumoniae* M31 ($\Delta lytA$) conferred to the cells an atypical phenotype (Lyt+, DOC−) which has been previously observed in some clinical isolates of pneumococci.[21] These results are in agreement with the existence of several choline-binding sites and suggest that the stepwise acquisition of the repeat units and the tail could be considered an evolutionary advantage for the enzyme, since the presence of these motifs increases its hydrolytic activity.

The structure of the C-terminal domain of PspA resembles that of the cell wall lytic enzymes, but it contains 10 highly conserved 20 amino acid repeats.[109,112] A deletion of five out of the 10 units resulted in the release of PspA from the pneumococcal cell surface suggesting that the interaction of PspA with lipoteichoic acid is dependent of the number of repeated units.[111,112] However, the absence of the last five repeats does not mean that the protein has completely lost the choline-binding properties, since PspA molecules containing at least five repeats can be purified by affinity chromatography on DEAE-cellulose.[111] The presence of more repeated units in PspA could be justified by the fact that the function of this protein depends on its rigid attachment to the lipoteichoic acid, whereas the LytA amidase, which only contains six repeats, should be able to walk across the teichoic acids of the cell wall surface to carry out its hydrolytic function.

The number of repeats found in the ChBDs of the pneumococcal proteins appears to be rather variable. Thus, the ChBDs of the proteins SpsA, CbpA and PbcA contain nine, ten, and four motifs, respectively.[42,47,75] Up to now, the PcpA is the protein that has the largest number of repeats since its ChBD is built by 11 identical motifs of 20 amino acids and a tail of 19 amino acids that appears to be a degenerated motif.[79] The ChBD of PcpB contains acids that appears to be a degenerated motif.[79] The ChBD of PcpB contains only four repeated units although the last one was highly degenerated.[76] The complete structure of PcpC appears to be more complex since the entire protein might derive from three consensus repeats plus 12 highly degenerated repeats.

The major secreted protein of *C. beijerinckii* NCIB 8052, a choline containing strain, is a glycosylated protein named CspA that specifically recognizes the choline residues of the cell wall.[77] This protein can be purified by affinity chromatography in DEAE-cellulose since it contains 4 consensus repeat units plus one degenerated repeat in its C-terminus. Although its function is still unknown, the abundance of this protein in the culture medium suggests that it must play a relevant physiological role. Moreover, the identification in the same microorganism of three genes, namely *cspB*, *cspC*, and *cpsD* encoding homologous proteins with six, four, and four repeats, respectively, also suggests that these genes must be critical for cell subsistence.[78]

An additional observation that reinforces the assumption that the ChBD can be folded independently from the catalytic domain providing a new example of its versatility was the demonstration that it can be utilized for the construction of fusion proteins that are able to be purified in a single step by affinity chromatography in DEAE-cellulose.[64,82]

To conclude the structural analysis of the ChBD it would be interesting to establish a relationship between its high content of aromatic amino acids and its choline-binding capacity. It could be helpful to review what is already known for other choline-binding sites like that of acetylcholinesterase.[94] Since the three-dimensional structure of this protein has been established the choline-binding site is perfectly defined. This protein contains two subsites in the active site, the esteratic and the anionic sites, corresponding to the catalytic machinery and the choline-binding pocket, respectively. The anionic subsite binds the quaternary group of acethycholine, but it has been suggested that it is uncharged and lipophilic, and several studies supported the presence of aromatic residues within this site. The most remarkable feature of the enzyme structure is a deep and narrow gorge which penetrates halfway into the enzyme, named the active site gorge. Fourteen aromatic residues line a substantial portion of the surface of the gorge. These residues and their flanking regions are highly conserved in the enzymes of different species and are located primarily in the loops between $\beta\beta$-strands. At least two of these aromatic residues contribute significantly to quaternary ligand-binding. The indole ring of a tryptophan and the benzene ring of a phenylalanine make an aromatic-aromatic interaction with the ligand. It has been suggested that the interaction of acetylcholine and aromatic residues was the result of a cation-π electron interaction between the quaternary ion and the aromatic rings.

Based on these studies, it can be suggested that the three conserved aromatic residues Trp-Tyr-Tyr present in the middle of the repeat units of ChBD could be directly involved in the binding of choline.

Evolutionary considerations

Ligand-binding domains consisting of repeat units are common in proteins involved in recognition processes. The multiplicity of the repeat sequences may allow a single protein to bind several ligands.[108] These repetitive amino acid sequences have been found in a great variety of important bacterial ligand-binding proteins. Interestingly, many of them have been found to be cell wall-associated proteins.[108] A detailed analysis of the derived amino acid sequences of these proteins revealed that the choline-binding proteins of pneumococcus may be part of a great superfamily of proteins that includes several streptococcal glycosyltransferases and toxins A and B from *C. difficile*.[108] All of these proteins show repeats containing a Tyr-Phe dipeptide and a glycine 10 residues upstream of this dipeptide. Aromatic amino acids are generally conserved at certain other positions, particularly just upstream of the Tyr-Phe dipeptide. Differences in the nonconserved residues and in the arrangements of the repeats within the entire protein might be expected to account for the precise binding specificity of each individual protein.[108]

The existence of ChBDs encoded by pneumococcal phages as well as the possibility to construct highly active chimeric proteins[16,18,19,58,89] between the phage and host enzymes provides an excellent model to analyze the molecular processes involved in cassette recruitment during evolution and contributes to support the concept of bacteria as adaptable chimera. The acquisition of the C-terminal module conferring the choline specificity to the pneumococcal cell wall lytic enzymes seems to be a good example to reinforce the theory that molecular evolution may occur between genes by interchange of modules. The case of the lysin encoded by the pneumococcal phage Dp-1 represents a paradigm of a natural chimera of intergeneric origin.[90] This enzyme has resulted by a natural fusion of a typical pneumococcal ChBD with the murein hydrolase domain of the lysin encoded by the phage Bk5-T of *Lactococcus lactis*.

The high degree of similarity found between the ChBDs of several pneumococcal proteins and the ChBD of the major secretable protein of *C. beijerinckii* strongly supports the hypothesis that they have evolved from a common ancestral protein and also reinforces the postulates of the modular theory of protein evolution. How these domains have been exchanged among these bacteria, which live in different ecological habitats, is still an open question, but suggests that the trail of the ChBD can be followed in other bacteria and/or phages.

Although it appears reasonable to speculate with the possibility that the ChBDs have evolved from a common ancestral protein, there are some recent data that recommend to reconsider this hypothesis. It is obvious that the repetitive arrangement of the amino acids suggests that these domains have evolved by an intragenic duplication phenomenon. However, the high similarity of the 10 repeats of PspA and, particularly, the identity of the 11 repeats found in PcpA may indicate that they were more recently duplicated than the repeats found in other proteins. Although both proteins have been identified in the same microorganism, the repeats of PspA and PcpA are not identical, which rules out the possibility that they have evolved by the interchange of their C-terminal domains. The most plausible explanation to this finding would be that these ChBDs have evolved independently, and very recently, by several duplications of a single repeat. Hence, we are tempted to conclude that the evolutionary link between the choline-binding proteins could be the existence of an ancestral motif that has the capacity of being easily duplicated. The origin of this 'selfish' motif and the specific properties which allow it to be so easily duplicated remains to be investigated.

ACKNOWLEDGMENTS

We thank E. García and P. García for helpful comments and for the critical reading of the manuscript, and M. Sheehan for correcting the English version. The technical assistance of E. Cano, and M. Carrasco and the skillful work by A. Hurtado is greatly acknowledged. This work was supported by grant PB93-0115-C02-O1 from the Programa Sectorial de Promoción General del Conocimiento. A.R.S.-B. is a beneficiary of a predoctoral fellowship from the Comunidad Autonoma de Madrid.

REFERENCES

1. **Adams, M.H., and A.M. Roe.** 1945. A partially defined medium for cultivation of pneumococcus. J. Bacteriol. **49:**401–409.

2. **Arondel, V., C. Benning, and C.R. Somerville.** 1993. Isolation and functional expression in *Escherichia coli* of gene encoding phosphatidylethanolamine methyltransferase (EC 2.1.1.17) from *Rhodobacter sphaeroides*. J. Biol. Chem. **268:**16002–16008.

3. **Asselineau, J., and H.G. Trüper.** 1982. Lipid composition of six species of the phototrophic bacterial genus *Ectothiorhodospira*. Biochem. Biophys. Acta **712:**111–116.

4. **Austrian, R.** 1953. An analysis of the bases for morphologic variation in pneumococcus and description of hitherto undefined morphologic variants. J. Exp. Med. **98:**21–34.

5. **Badger, E.** 1944. The structural specificity of choline for the growth of type II pneumococcus. J. Biol. Chem. **153:**183–191.

6. **Barridge, J.K., and J.M. Shively.** 1968. Phospholipids of the thiobacilli. J. Bacteriol. **95:**2182–2185.

7. **Bean, B., and Tomasz, A.** 1977. Choline metabolism in pneumococci. J. Bacteriol. **130:**571–574.

8. **Behr, T., W. Fischer, W., R. Hartman, J. Peter-Katalinic, and H. Egge.** 1992. The structure of pneumococcal lipoteichoic acid. Improved preparation, chemical and mass spectrometric studies. Eur. J. Biochem. **207:**1063–1075.

9. **Briese, T., and R. Hakenbeck.** 1985. Interaction of the pneumococcal amidase with lipoteichoic acid and choline. Eur. J. Biochem. **146:**417–427.

10. **Briles, D.E., C. Forman, S. Hidak, and J.L. Chaffin.** 1982. Antiphosphorylcholine antibodies of the T15 idiotype are optimally protective against *Streptococcus pneumoniae*. J. Exp. Med. **156:**1177–1785.

11. **Briles, E.B., and A. Tomasz.** 1973. Pneumococcal Forssman antigen. A choline-containing lipoteichoic acid. J. Biol. Chem. **248:**6394–6397.

12. **Brundish, D.E., and J. Baddiley.** 1968. Pneumococcal C-substance, a ribitol teichoic acid containing choline phosphate. Biochem. J. **110:**573–582.

13. **Cabellos, C., D.E. MacIntyre, M. Forrest, M. Burroughs, S. Prasad, and E. Toumanen.** 1992. Different roles for platelet-activating factor during inflammation of the lung and subarachnoid space. The special case of *Streptococcus pneumoniae*. J. Clin. Invest. **90:**612–618.

14. **Chao, W., and M.S. Olson.** 1993. Platelet-activating factor: receptors and signal transduction. Biochem. J. **292:**617–629.

15. **Claflin, J.L., J. George, C. Dell, and J. Berry.** 1989. Patterns of mutations and selection in antibodies to the phosphocholine-specific determinant in *Proteus morganii*. J. Immunol. **143:**3054–3063.

16. **Croux, C., C. Ronda, R. López, and J.L. García.** 1993. Interchange of functional domains switches enzyme specificity: construction of a chimeric pneumococcal-clostridial cell wall lytic enzyme. Mol. Microbiol. **9:**1019–1025.

17. **Cundell, D.R., N.P. Gerard, C. Gerard, I. Idanpaan-Heikkila, and E.I. Toumanen.** 1995. *Streptococcus pneumoniae* anchors to activated human cells by the receptor for platelet-activating factor. Nature **377:**435–438.

18. **Díaz, E., R. López, and J.L. García.** 1990. Chimeric phage-bacterial enzymes: a clue to the modular evolution of genes. Proc. Natl. Acad. Sci. U.S.A. **87:**8125–8129.

19. **Díaz, E., R. López, and J.L. García.** 1991. Chimeric pneumococcal cell wall lytic enzymes reveal important physiological and evolutionary traits. J. Biol. Chem. **266:**5464–5471.

20. **Díaz, E., R. López, and J.L. García.** 1992. EJ-1, a temperate bacteriophage of *Streptococcus pneumoniae* with a *Myoviridae* morphology. J. Bacteriol. **174:**5516–5525.

21. **Díaz, E., R. López, and J.L. García.** 1992. Role of the major pneumococcal autolysin in the atypical response of a clinical isolate of *Streptococcus pneumoniae*. J. Bacteriol. **174:**5508–5515.

22. **Fischer, R.T., D.L. Longo, and J.J. Kenny.** 1995. A novel phosphocholine antigen protects both normal and X-linked immune deficient mice against *Streptococcus pneumoniae*. Comparison of the 6-*O*-phosphocholine hydroxyhexanoate-conjugate with other phosphocholine-containing vaccines. J. Immunol. **148:**3373–3382.

23. **Fischer, W., T. Behr, R. Hartman, J. Peter-Katalinic, and H. Egge.** 1993. Teichoic acid and lipoteichoic acid of *Streptococcus pneumoniae* possess identical chain structures. A reinvestigation of teichoic acid (C polysaccharide). Eur. J. Biochem. **215:**851–857.

24. **García, E., J.L. García, C. Ronda, P. García, and R. López.** 1985. Cloning and expression of the pneumococcal autolysin gene in *Escherichia coli*. Mol. Gen. Genet. **201:**225–230.

25. **García, E., J.L. García, P. García, A. Arrarás, J.M. Sánchez-Puelles, and R. López.** 1988. Molecular evolution of lytic enzymes of *Streptococcus pneumoniae* and its bacteriophages. Proc. Natl. Acad. Sci. U.S.A. **85:**914–918.

26. **García, E., J.M. Rojo, P. García, C. Ronda, R. López, and A. Tomasz.** 1982. Preparation of antiserum against pneumococcal autolysin. Inhibition of autolysin activity and some autolytic processes by the antibody. FEMS Microbiol. Lett. **14:**133–136.

27. **García, J.L., E. Díaz, A. Romero, and P. García.** 1994. Carboxy-terminal deletion analysis of the major pneumococcal autolysin. J. Bacteriol. **176:**4066–4072.

28. **García, J.L., E. García, A. Arrarás, P. García, C. Ronda, and**

R. López. 1987. Cloning, purification, and biochemical characterization of the pneumococcal bacteriophage Cp-1 lysin. J. Virol. **61**:2573–2580.

29. **García, J.L., E. García, J.M. Sánchez-Puelles, and R. López.** 1988. Identification of a lytic enzyme of *Clostridium acetobutylicum* that degrades choline-containing pneumococcal cell walls. FEMS Microbiol. Lett. **52**:133–138.

30. **García, P., E. García, C. Ronda, R. López, and A. Tomasz.** 1983. A phage-associated murein hydrolase in *Streptococcus pneumoniae* infected with bacteriophage Dp-1. J. Gen. Microbiol. **129**:489–497.

31. **García, P., J.L. García, E. García, and R. López.** 1989. Purification and characterization of the autolytic glycosidase of *Streptococcus pneumoniae*. Biochem. Biophys. Res. Commun. **158**:251–256.

32. **García, P., J.L. García, E. García, J.M. Sánchez-Puelles, and R. López.** 1990. Modular organization of the lytic enzymes of *Streptococcus pneumoniae* and its bacteriophages. Gene **86**:81–88.

33. **García, P., J.L. García, E. García, and R. López.** 1986. Nucleotide sequence and expression of the pneumococcal autolysin gene from its own promoter in *Escherichia coli*. Gene **43**:265–272.

34. **García, P., R. López, C. Ronda, E. García, and A. Tomasz.** 1983. Mechanism of phage-induced lysis in pneumococcal. J. Gen. Microbiol. **129**:479–487.

35. **Gillespie, S.H., P.H.M. McWhinney, S. Patel, J.G. Raynes, K.P.W.J. McAdam, R.A. Whiley, and J.M. Hardie.** 1993. Species of alpha-hemolytic streptococcal possessing a C-polysaccharide phosphorylcholine-containing antigen. Infect. Immun. **61**:3076–3077.

36. **Gillespie, S.H., S. Ainscough, A. Dickens, and J. Lewin.** 1996. Phosphorylcholine-containing antigens in bacteria from the mouth and respiratory tract. J. Med. Microbiol. **44**:35–40.

37. **Giudicelli, S., and A. Tomasz.** 1984. Attachment of pneumococcal autolysin to wall teichoic acids, an essential step in enzymatic wall degradation. J. Bacteriol. **158**:1188–1190.

38. **Glaudemans, C.P.J.** 1975. The interaction of homogeneous murine myeloma immunoglobulins with polysaccharide antigens. Adv. Carbohydr. Chem. Biochem. **31**:313–346.

39. **Golberg, I., and A.P. Jenssen.** 1977. Phospholipid and fatty acid composition of methanol utilizing bacteria. J. Bacteriol. **130**:535–537.

40. **Gotschlich, E.C., and T.Y. Liu.** 1967. Structural and immunological studies on the pneumococcal C polysaccharide. J. Biol. Chem. **242**:463–470.

41. **Hagen, P.O., H. Golfine, and P.J. Le B. Williams.** 1966. Phospholipids of bacteria with extensive intracytoplasmic membranes. Science **151**:1543–1544.

42. **Hammerschmidt, S., Talay, S.R., Brandtzaeg, P., and Chhatwal, G.S.** 1997. SpsA, a novel pneumococcal surface protein with specific binding to secretory immunoglobulin A and secretory component. Mol. Microbiol. **25**:1113–1124.

43. **Höltje, J.-V., and A. Tomasz.** 1975. Lipoteichoic acid: a specific inhibitor of autolysin activity in pneumococcus. Proc. Natl. Acad. Sci. U.S.A. **72**:1690–1694.

44. **Höltje, J.-V., and A. Tomasz.** 1975. Teichoic acid phosphorylcholine esterase. A novel enzyme activity in pneumococcus. J. Biol. Chem. **249**:7032–7034.

45. **Höltje, J.-V., and A. Tomasz.** 1975. Specific recognition of choline residues in the cell wall teichoic acid by the *N*-acetylmuramyl-L-alanine amidase of pneumococcus. J. Biol. Chem. **250**:6072–6075.

46. **Höltje, J.-V., and A. Tomasz.** 1976. Purification of the pneumococcal *N*-acetylmuramyl-L-alanine amidase to biochemical homogeneity. J. Biol. Chem. **251**:4199–4207.

47. **Hostetter, M.K., Cheng, Q., and Finkel, D.A.** 1998. C3-bind-

ing protein in *Streptococcus pneumoniae*. GenBank accession number AF067128 (unpublished).

48. **Howard, L.V., and H. Gooder.** 1974. Specificity of the autolysin of *Streptococcus pneumoniae*. J. Bacteriol. **117**:796–804.

49. **Hummell, D.S., A.J. Swift, A. Tomasz, and J.A. Winkelstein.** 1985. Activation of the alternative complement pathway by pneumococcal lipoteichoic acid. Infect. Immunol. **47**:384–387.

50. **Ikawa, M.** 1967. Bacterial phosphatides and natural relationships. Bacteriol. Rev. **31**:54–64.

51. **Johnston, N.C., and H. Golfine.** 1983. Lipid composition in the classification of butyric acid–producing clostridia. J. Gen. Microbiol. **129**:1075–1081.

52. **Kim, J.O., and Weiser, J.N.** 1998. Association of intrastrain phase variation in quantity of capsular polysaccharide and teichoic acid with the virulence of *Streptococcus pneumoniae*. J. Infect. Dis. **177**:386–377.

53. **Kilpper-Bälz, R., P. Wenzig, and K.H. Schleifer.** 1985. Molecular relationships and classification of some viridans streptococci as *Streptococcus oralis* and emended description of *Streptococcus oralis* (Bridge and Sneath 1982). Int. J. Syst. Microbiol. **35**:482–498.

54. **Kortstee, G.J.J.** 1970. The aerobic decomposition of choline by microorganisms. I. The ability of aerobic organisms, particularly coryneform bacteria, to utilize choline as the sole carbon and nitrogen source. Arch. Microbiol. **71**:235–244.

55. **Lim, P.L., W.F. Choy, S.T.H. Cham, D.T.M. Leung, and S.S.M. NG.** 1994. Transgene-encoded antiphosphorylcholine (T15+) antibodies protect CBA/N(*xid*) mice against infection with *Streptococcus pneumoniae* but not *Trichinella spiralis*. Infect. Immunol. **62**:1658–1661.

56. **Logan, A.C., K.-P.N. Chow, A. George, P.D. Weinstein, and J.J. Cebra.** 1991. Use of Peyer's patch and lymph node fragment cultures to compare local immune responses to *Morganella morganii*. Infect. Immunol. **59**:1024–1031.

57. **López, R., E. García, P. García, C. Ronda, and A. Tomasz.** 1982. Choline-containing bacteriophage receptors in *Streptococcus pneumoniae*. J. Bacteriol. **151**:1581–1590.

58. **López, R., J.L. García, E. García, C. Ronda, and P. García.** 1992. Structural analysis and biological significance of the cell wall lytic enzymes of *Streptococcus pneumoniae* and its bacteriophages. FEMS Microbiol. Lett. **100**:439–448.

59. **Matsuda, K., T. Kasama, I. Ishizuka, S. Handa, N. Yamamoto, and T. Taki.** 1994. Structure of a novel phosphocholine-containing glycerolipid from *Mycoplasma fermentans*. J. Biol. Chem. **269**:33123–33128.

60. **McDaniel, L.S., J.S. Sheffield, E. Swiatto, J. Yother, M.J. Crain, and D.E. Briles.** 1992. Molecular localization of variable and conserved regions of *pspA* and identification of additional *pspA* homologous sequences in *Streptococcus pneumoniae*. Microbial. Pathog. **13**:261–269.

61. **Mold, C., S. Nakayama, T.J. Holzer, H. Gewurz, and T.W. Du Clos.** 1981. C-reactive protein is protective against *Streptococcus pneumoniae* infection in mice. J. Exp. Med. **154**:1703–1708.

62. **Mosser, J.L., and A. Tomasz.** 1970. Choline-containing teichoic acid as a structural component of pneumococcal cell wall and its role in sensitivity to lysis by an autolytic enzyme. J. Biol. Chem. **245**:287–298.

63. **Okamoto, H. and T. Sharo.** 1937. Über das charakteristische Langkettenwachstum der Pneumokokken durch quaternäre Ammoniumverbindungen, insbesondere das Cholin. Zugleich über die Differenzieurung der Pneumokokken un Streptokokken durch Cholin. Jpn. J. Med. Sci. IV Pharmacol. **10**:166–167.

64. **Ortega, S., J.L. García, M. Zazo, J. Varela, I. Muñoz-Willery, P. Cuevas, and G. Giménez-Gallego.** 1992. Single-step purification on DEAE-Sephacel of recombinant polypeptides produced in *Escherichia coli*. Bio/Technology **10**:795–798.

65. **Pfeffer, P.E., G. Bécard, D.B. Rolin, J. Uknalis, P. Cooke, and**

S.-I. Tu. 1994. In vivo nuclear magnetic resonance study of the osmoregulation of phosphocholine-substituted $\beta\beta$-1,3:1,6 cyclic glucan and its associated carbon metabolism in *Bradyrhizobium japonicum* USDA 110. Appl. Env. Microbiol. **60**:2137–2146.

66. Podvin, L., G. Reysset, J. Hubert, and M. Sebald. 1988. Presence of choline in teichoic acid of *Clostridium acetobutylicum* NI-4 and choline inhibition of autolytic function. J. Gen. Microbiol. **134**:1603–1609.

67. Potter, M. 1970. Mouse IgA myeloma proteins that bind polysaccharide antigens of enterobacterial origin. Fed. Proc. **29**:85–91.

68. Potter, M. 1971. Antigen-binding myeloma proteins in mice. Ann. N.Y. Acad. Sci. **190**:306–321.

69. Potter, M., and R. Lieberman. 1970. Common individual antigen determinants in five of eight BALB/c IgA myeloma proteins that bind phosphoryl choline. J. Exp. Med. **132**:737–751.

70. Poxton, I.R., and Leak, D.J. 1977. The biosynthesis of a choline nucleotide by a cell-free extract from *Streptococcus pneumoniae*. J. Gen. Microbiol. **100**:23–29.

71. Rane, L., and Y. Subbarow. 1940. Nutritional requirements of the pneumococcus 1. Growth factors for types I, II, V, VII, VIII. J. Bacteriol. **40**:695–704.

72. Reisenfeld-Orn, I., S. Wolpe, J.F. García-Bustos, M.K. Hoffman, and E. Tuomanen. 1989. The production of interleukin-1 but not tumor necrosis factor by human monocytes stimulated with pneumococcal cell surface components. Infect. Immunol. **57**:1890–1893.

73. Romero, A., R. López, and P. García. 1990. Characterization of the pneumococcal bacteriophage HB-3 amidase: cloning and expression in *Escherichia coli*. J. Virol. **64**:137–142.

74. Ronda, C., J.L. García, and R. López. 1991. Teichoic acid choline esterase, a novel hydrolytic activity in *Streptococcus oralis*. FEMS Microbiol. Lett. **80**:289–294.

75. Rosenow, C., Ryan, P., Weiser, J.N., Johnson, S., Fontan, P., Orqvist, A. and Masure, R. 1997. Contribution of novel choline-binding protein to adherence, colonization and immunogenicity of *Streptococcus pneumoniae*. Mol. Microbiol. **25**:819–829.

76. Sánchez-Beato, A.R. 1995. Ph.D. dissertation. Universidad Complutense, Madrid.

77. Sánchez-Beato, A.R., C. Ronda, and J.L. García. 1995. Tracking the evolution of the bacterial choline-binding domain. Molecular characterization of the *Clostridium acetobutylicum* NCIB 8052 *cspA* gene. J. Bacteriol. **177**:1098–1103.

78. Sánchez-Beato, A.R., and J.L. García. 1996. Molecular characterization of a family of choline-binding proteins of *Clostridium beijerinckii* NCIB 8502. Gene **180**:13–21.

79. Sánchez-Beato, A.R., López, R., and J.L. García. 1998. Molecular characterization of PcpA: a novel choline-binding protein of *Streptococcus pneumonaie*. FEMS Microbiol. Lett. **164**:207–214.

80. Sánchez-Puelles, J.M., J.L. García, R. López, and E. García. 1987. 3′-End modification of the *Streptococcus pneumoniae lytA* gene: role of the carboxy terminus of the pneumococcal autolysin in the process of enzymatic activation (conversion). Gene **61**:13–19.

81. Sánchez-Puelles, J.M., C. Ronda, E. García, E. Méndez, J.L. García, and R. López. 1986. A new peptidoglycan hydrolase in *Streptococcus pneumoniae*. F.E.M.S. Microbiol. Lett. **35**:163–166.

82. Sánchez-Puelles, J.M., J.M. Sanz, J.L. García, and E. García. 1992. Immobilization and single-step purification of fusion proteins using DEAE-cellulose. Eur. J. Biochem. **203**:153–159.

83. Sánchez-Puelles, J.M., J.M. Sanz, J.L. García, and E. García. 1990. Cloning and expression of gene fragments encoding the choline-binding domain of pneumococcal murein hydrolases. Gene **89**:69–75.

84. Sanz, J.M., E. Díaz, and J.L. García. 1992. Studies on the structure and function of the N-terminal domain of the pneumococcal murein hydrolase. Mol. Microbiol. **6**:921–931.

85. Sanz, J.M., and J.L. García. 1990. Structural studies of the lysozyme coded by pneumococcal phage Cp-1. Conformational changes induced by choline. Eur. J. Biochem. **187**:409–416.

86. Sanz, J.M., J.L. García, J. Laynez, P. Usobiaga, and M. Menéndez. 1993. Thermal stability and cooperative domains of CPL1 lysozyme and its NH$_2$- and COOH-terminal modules. J. Biol. Chem. **268**:6125–6130.

87. Sanz, J.M., R. López, and J.L. García. 1988. Structural requirements of choline derivatives for "conversion" of pneumococcal amidase. FEBS Lett. **232**:308–312.

88. Severin, A., Horne, D., and Tomasz, A. 1997. Autolysis and cell wall degradation in choline-independent strain of *Streptococcus pneumoniae*. Microbial. Drug Res. **3**:391–400.

89. Sheehan, M.M., García, J.L., López, R., and García, P. 1996. Analysis of the catalytic domain of the lysin of the lactococcal bacteriophage Tuc2009 by chimeric gene assembling. FEMS Microbiol. Lett. **140**:23–28.

90. Sheehan, M.M., García, J.L., López, R., and García, P. 1997. The lytic enzyme of the pneumococcal phage Dp-1: a chimeric lysin of intergenic origin. Mol. Microbiol. **25**:717–725.

91. Sorensen, U.B.S., J. Blom, A. Birch-Andersen, and J. Henrichsen. 1988. Ultrastructural localization of capsules, cell wall polysaccharide, cell wall proteins, and F antigen in pneumococci. Infect. Immunol. **56**:1890–1896.

92. Styrvold, O.B., P. Falkenberg, B. Landfald, M.W. Eshoo, T. Bjornsen, and A.R. Strom. 1986. Selection, mapping, and characterization of osmoregulatory mutants of *Escherichia coli* blocked in the choline-glycine betaine pathway. J. Bacteriol. **165**:856–863.

93. Sundberg-Kovamees, M., Holme, T. and Sjogren, A. 1996. Interaction of the C-polysaccharide of *Streptococcus pneumoniae* with the receptor asialo-GM1. Microbial. Pathog. **21**:223–234.

94. Sussman, J.L., and I. Silman. 1992. Acetylcholinesterase: structure and use as a model for specific cation-protein interactions. Curr. Opin. Struct. Biol. **2**:721–729.

95. Thiele, O.W., and J. Oulevey. 1981. Occurrence of phosphatidylcholine in hydrogen-oxidizing bacteria. Eur. J. Biochem. **118**:183–186.

96. Tomasz, A. 1967. Choline in the cell wall of a bacterium: novel type of polymer-linked choline in pneumococcus. Science **157**:694–697.

97. Tomasz, A. 1968. Biological consequences of the replacement of choline by ethanolamine in the cell wall of pneumococcus: chain formation, loss of transformability, and loss of autolysis. Proc. Natl. Acad. Sci. U.S.A. **59**:86–93.

98. Tomasz, A., A. Albino, and E. Zanati. 1970. Multiple antibiotic resistance in a bacterium with suppresed autolytic system. Nature **227**:138–140.

99. Tomasz, A., and K. Saukkonen. 1989. The nature of cell wall-derived inflammatory components of pneumococci. Pediatr. Infect. Dis. J. **8**:902–903.

100. Tomasz, A. and M. Westphal. 1971. Abnormal autolytic enzyme in pneumococcus with altered teichoic acid composition. Proc. Natl. Acad. Sci. U.S.A. **68**:2627–2630.

101. Tuomanen, E., R. Rich, and O. Zak. 1987. Induction of pulmonary inflammation by components of the pneumococcal cell surface. Am. Rev. Respir. Dis. **135**:869–874.

102. Usobiaga, P., F.J. Medrano, M. Gasset, J.L. García, J.L. Sainz, G. Rivas, J. Laynez, and M. Menéndez. 1996. Structural organization of the major autolysin from *Streptococcus pneumoniae*. J. Biol. Chem. **271**:6832–6838.

103. Vance, D.E. 1989. Phosphatidylcholine metabolism. CRC Press, Boca Raton.

104. Weiser, J.N., Schepetov, and Chong, S.T.H. 1997. Decoration of lipopolysaccharide with phosphocholine: a phase-variable characteristic of *Haemophilus influenzae*. Infect. Immunol. **65**:943–950.

105. **Whiting, G.C., and S.H. Gillespie.** 1996. Incorporation of choline into *Streptococcus pneumoniae* cell wall antigen: evidence for choline kinase activity. FEMS Microbiol. Lett. **138:**141–145.

106. **Whiting, G.C., and S.H. Gillespie.** 1996. Investigation of a choline phosphate synthesis pathway in *Streptococcus pneumoniae*: evidence for choline phosphate cytdyltransferase activity. FEMS Microbiol. Lett. **143:**279–284.

107. **Winkelstein, J.A., and A. Tomasz.** 1978. Activation of the alternative complement pathway by pneumococcal cell wall teichoic acid. J. Immunol. **120:**174–178.

108. **Wren, B.W.** 1991. A family of clostridial and streptococcal ligand-binding proteins with conserved *C*-terminal repeat sequences. Mol. Microbiol. **5:**797–803.

109. **Yother, J., and D.E. Briles.** 1992. Structural properties and evolutionary relationships of PspA, a surface protein of *Streptococcus pneumoniae*, as revealed by sequence analysis. J. Bacteriol. **174:**601–609.

110. **Yother, J., Leopold, K., White, J., and Fischer, W.** 1998. Generation and properties of a *Streptococcus pneumonaie* mutant which does not require choline or analogs for growth. J. Bacteriol. **180:**2093–2101.

111. **Yother, J., and J.M. White.** 1994. Novel surface attachment mechanism of the *Streptococcus pneumoniae* protein PspA. J. Bacteriol. **176:**2976–2985.

112. **Yother, J., G.L. Handsome, and D.E. Briles.** 1992. Truncated forms of PspA that are secreted from *Streptococcus pneumoniae* and their use in functional studies and cloning of the *pspA* gene. J. Bacteriol. **174:**610–618.

Address reprint requests to:
Jose L. García
Departamento de Microbiología Molecular
Centro de Investigaciones Biológicas
CSIC
Velázquez 144
28006 Madrid
Spain

Phase Variation in Colony Opacity by
Streptococcus pneumoniae

JEFFREY N. WEISER

THIS ARTICLE DESCRIBES the current state of investigation into phenotypic variation in the Gram-positive pathogen, *Streptococcus pneumoniae*. The phenomenon to be described is complex and involves intrastrain variations affecting multiple cell-surface structures which contribute to the ability of the organism to interact with its host (summarized in Table 1).

Characteristics of phenotypic variation in the pneumococcus

Streptococcus pneumoniae, the pneumococcus, is highly proficient at colonization of its human host. Despite its narrow host range, it is capable of considerable flexibility as demonstrated by the ability of different strains to synthesize a vast repertoire unique capsular polysaccharides. The pneumococcus has, in addition, the capacity to thrive in a number of different host environments, including the bloodstream and the mucosal surface of the nasopharynx. As is the case for other respiratory tract pathogens that frequently cause invasive infection, the ability of the pneumococcus to adapt to these varied environments requires changes in the expression of specific cell-surface molecules.[8,16] The focus of this laboratory has been the identification of variably expressed cell-surface components as a means of gaining insight into the pathogenesis of pneumococcal disease at a molecular level.

Phenotypic variation in the pneumococcus can be appreciated by detailed examination of colony morphology.[17] Since a colony is an array of closely packed organisms, differences in their physical characteristics may affect the arrangement of organisms within the colony. In some cases, these differences may alter the passage of light through the colony resulting in altered colony appearance. When viewed with oblique, transmitted light and magnification on transparent medium, it is possible to observe opaque and transparent colony forms in colonies derived from an individual strain (see Fig. 1). For some strains, intermediate forms can be identified. Variation in colony morphology appears to be common to all strains, although it is more readily appreciated in isolates of certain serotypes, possibly because the capsule may act to obscure phenotypic differences. Opacity variation is not apparent on opaque medium, such as blood agar, which probably accounts for why these differences had not previously been described.

There is spontaneous, reversible variation between colony phenotypes (phase variation). It is possible to detect sectored colonies resulting from phase variation during the clonal expansion of a single organism as it forms a colony. The frequency of switching is highly variable from isolate to isolate (10^{-3} to 10^{-6}/generation) and appears to be independent of in vitro growth conditions, including pH, temperature, and osmolarity. Under standard culture conditions, pneumococcal isolates are highly heterogeneous populations. It is possible, however, to separate many strains into nearly uniform populations of opaque and transparent forms for comparison.

Correlation between opacity variation and pneumococcal infection

Animal models were used to determine whether differences in colony morphology correlated with a difference in the ability of the pneumococcus to colonize and infect a host. The relative ability of opaque and transparent variants to colonize the nasopharynx, the initial step in the pathogenesis of pneumococcal disease, was assessed in an infant rat model. This is a convenient model for obtaining washes of the nasopharynx which are plated to determine the quantity as well as the phenotype of the colonizing organisms. Following a single intranasal inoculum, the number of organisms in the nasopharynx expands rapidly and the pups remain heavily colonized for at least several weeks. Pneumococcal carriage by infant rats, furthermore, does not appear to be limited to certain serotypes. When equal inocula (10^3 CFU) of relatively uniform populations of opaque or transparent variants of the same strain were compared in this model, only the transparent organisms were able to establish dense and stable colonization of the mucosal surface of the nasopharynx. After challenge with a large inoculum (10^7 CFU) of an opaque variant, the pups gradually became colonized, but by the end of 7 days, the opaque variant had been cleared and there was heavy colonization with transparent forms. This suggested that since such a large inoculum contained a small number of transparent variants, these were selected for from among the heterogeneous inoculum.

Evidence that the transparent phenotype is selected for during nasopharyngeal colonization left in question the biologic role of the opaque phenotype. This was addressed by using intraperitoneal rather than intranasal inoculation in order to bypass the requirements of colonization. Because infant rats are

---

Departments of Pediatrics and Microbiology, Children's Hospital of Philadelphia and University of Pennsylvania School of Medicine, Philadelphia, PA 19104.
Reprinted from *Microbial Drug Resistance*, Vol. 4, No. 2, 1998.

TABLE 1. SUMMARY OF THE ASSOCIATION OF
COLONY PHENOTYPE WITH CHARACTERISTICS
AND STRUCTURES OF THE PNEUMOCOCCUS

Characteristic/structure	Phenotype	
	Opaque	Transparent
Autolysis	↓	↑
LytA	↓	↑
PspA	↑	↓
CR112 (CbpA)	↓	↑
Teichoic Acid	↓	↑
Nasopharyngeal colonization (infant rat)	↓	↑
Intraperitoneal virulence (adult mice)	↑	↓

not highly susceptible to invasive pneumococcal infection, it was necessary to perform these experiments in an adult mouse model of sepsis. This required the use of virulent serotypes for mice in which the opaque and transparent forms are easily distinguished. Equal intraperitoneal inocula of relatively uniform populations of opaque or transparent variants of the same strain (10^7 CFU) were compared in this model. All mice receiving opaque organisms died of sepsis. In contrast, of the few mice that expired following inoculation with transparent organisms, splenic cultures revealed only organisms with the opaque phenotype. This suggests that during invasive infection, there is a strong selection for organisms with the opaque morphology.

Based on the animal experiments, it appears that the pneumococcus phase varies between at least two forms—one adapted for nasopharyngeal colonization and the other for events following colonization. The animal experiments demonstrated the relevance of opacity variation to the pathogenesis of pneumococcal infection.

Genetic basis of opacity variation

Two approaches, genetic and biochemical analysis, were taken to define the bacterial characteristics that change in association with colony opacity, and may contribute to the differences observed in the animal models. The initial genetic approach relied on the ability to transform the pneumococcus at high efficiency.[11] Chromosomal DNA from an opaque isolate was used to transform a transparent recipient so as to acquire the opaque phenotype. With "opaque" DNA from some strains, the frequency of obtaining opaque colonies was far higher than in controls with "transparent" DNA in which opaque colonies were seen only as a result of background phase variation. A chromosomal library in bacteriophage lambda constructed with DNA from one such strain was then screened to identify a single clone able to transform the transparent recipient to the opaque phenotype. Analysis of this opacity locus revealed two genes, *glpD* and *glpF*, with homology to the glycerol regulon genes in other bacteria. Following these genes was a sequence with homology to repetitive pneumococcal intergenic elements, BOX A and C, upstream of an open reading frame which could encode a 126 amino acid protein. This ORF has no homology to current entries in sequence databases. Following this ORF

there is another long ORF in the opposite orientation. This ORF also lacks significant homology to current entries in sequence databases, and has a highly unusual feature located upstream, 19 tandem thymidine (T) residues. Highly repetitive features have been shown to create molecular switches associated with phase variation.[18] The number of T repeats at this site demonstrates inter- and intrastrain variation in number from 12 to 23 (unpublished data). Although the analysis of this complex region is in progress, several observations are of potential relevance. The stem-loop forming element, BOX A–C, was not present in the same locus of the recipient strain. Introduction of these elements during transformation affected colonial morphology, possibly by altering expression of the 126 amino acid ORF, a putative regulatory gene, downstream from the BOX element. Mutagenesis confirmed that this element increases the frequency of variation in opacity. Strains lacking the BOX A–C element appear to phase vary at lower rates and DNA with transforming activity contains this element. When the BOX element is incorporated into a transparent recipient, the increased frequency of variation makes it possible to detect higher numbers of opaque colonies.

A second genetic approach relied upon the construction of a chromosomal library in an *Escherichia coli*/streptococcal shuttle plasmid (pMU1328).[13] A chromosomal insert in pMU1328 able to transform *S. pneumoniae* to a more opaque phenotype was isolated. Analysis of this insert showed that it contained the 5' end of a 1964 amino acid sequence whose translation product is highly homologous to the IgA1 protease from *S. sanguis*. The deduced protein contained in LPxTGx motif which resembles the anchoring domain of Gram-positive cell-surface proteins. The LPxTGx motif, however, was located near the N-terminus rather than the typical location at the C-terminus. The

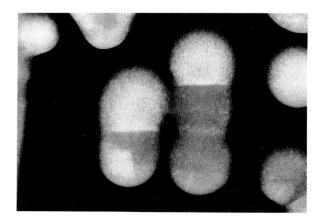

FIG. 1. Colonies of a serotype 18C clinical isolate demonstrating variation in colony opacity. Colony morphology was determined on tryptic soy plates containing 1% agar onto which 100 μL catalase (5,000 U) (Worthington Biochemical Co., Freehold, NJ) was added. Plates were grown at 37°C overnight in a candle extinction jar, which provided an atmosphere of increased CO_2 necessary for optimal growth on this medium. Following growth on transparent medium, colonies were photographed using a stereo-zoom microscope with oblique, transmitted illumination. In addition to opaque and transparent colonies, a sectored colony is shown. Magnification 60×.

contribution of this feature to the export of this protein is unknown. Interruption of the chromosomal gene resulted in loss of expression of an approximately 200 kD protein and complete elimination of detectable IgA1 protease activity. This indicated that this gene is responsible for the ability of the pneumococcus to cleave human IgA1, the principle immunoglobulin class on the mucosal surface. Mutagenesis of the chromosomal copy of the gene, however, had no discernible effect of colony morphology even though overexpression on a multicopy plasmid was associated with altered colony morphology. It was concluded, therefore, that the IgA1 protease is not the major contributing factor to opacity variation.

Variation in the expression of cell-surface proteins

The relationship of several previously identified cell-surface proteins to opacity variation has been examined. The role of cell lysis or autolysis in this phenomenon was considered because of several observations.[14] (1) Opaque colonies are dome-shaped, whereas transparent colonies are umbilicated after equivalent incubation conditions. (2) Electron micrographs of organisms grown under identical conditions suggested that there was breakdown of the cell-wall structures only in the transparent cells.[17] (3) Opaque organisms undergo spontaneous lysis more slowly and are more resistant to the detergent deoxycholate.[11] Autolysis occurs once the bacteria reaches stationary phase through the enzymatic degradation of the cell wall primarily by the major murein amidase, LytA (autolysin). It was determined whether differences in rates of autolysis were a result of differences in the peptidoglycan substrate or the amidase.[14] The hydrolysis of purified cell walls of opaque and transparent organisms as determined by HPLC analysis of stem peptides released by treatment with amidase was indistinguishable. This result made it unlikely that the peptidoglycan was responsible for the observed differences in autolysis. The expression of autolysin in opaque and transparent variants was compared using antiserum to LytA (provided by Dr. R. Lopez). Low levels of autolysis in opaque variants correlated with decreased levels of immunoreactive LytA on colony immunoblots and Western analysis. Mutants in which the *lytA* gene has been interrupted have an altered colony morphology but are still capable of displaying phenotypic variation. This indicated that LytA is only one factor contributing to opacity variation. The question of whether LytA, which is present in higher amounts on the cell surface of transparent variants, has a role in the more efficient colonization by this phenotype was examined in the infant rat model of pneumococcal carriage. LytA− mutants in encapsulated strains (provided by Dr. J. Paton) were indistinguishable when compared to LytA+ parent strains in their ability to colonize the infant rat nasopharynx.

The hypothesis that another cell-surface protein is expressed in higher amounts in transparent variants, like LytA, and contributes to colonization was examined as follows. LytA is known to anchor to the cell by binding to phosphorylcholine (ChoP) on the lipoteichoic acid. Antisera to pneumococcal proteins that adhered to a choline column (provided by Dr. R. Masure) was used to compare the differential expression of choline binding proteins. In addition to LytA, this antisera recognized at least two other proteins that could be eluted from cells by incubation in high concentrations of choline. One of these proteins was the pneumococcal surface protein, PspA, which was present in greater quantities in opaque variants. Although the function of PspA is unknown, it has been shown to contribute to the virulence of the pneumococcus in mice. Studies to determine whether the increased virulence of opaque variants in the mouse model of sepsis is caused by their increased expression of this protein are in progress. The other choline binding protein was a 112 kD protein, characterized in the Masure laboratory, which was present in higher amounts in transparent variants. Mutagenesis of the gene encoding this protein in an encapsulated strain eliminated its expression and resulted in a more than two-log decrease in the number of organisms colonizing the infant rat nasopharynx (unpublished data). The 112 kD choline binding protein, therefore, may contribute to the enhanced ability of transparent pneumococci to colonize the mucosal surface of the nasopharynx.

Relationship between opacity variation and carbohydrate containing structures

The biochemical comparison of pneumococcal variants has focused on two additional cell-surface structures, the capsular polysaccharide and the teichoic acids. The capsule is a well-recognized virulence determinant, and relatively small differences in the amount of capsular polysaccharide have been shown to have a significant effect of the ability of the pathogen to cause infection.[10] Opacity variation is present in unencapsulated mutants, which suggests that differences in the amount or composition of the capsule is not responsible for phenotypic variation.[17] It remains possible, however, that transparent and opaque variants differ with respect to capsulation and that this affects their relative virulence. Variants of the same strain are indistinguishable using type-specific antiserum by Quelling, suggesting that their capsules are antigenically related. Techniques for accurate quantification of the capsular polysaccharide of each phenotype are somewhat problematic. This was addressed using flow cytometry on bacteria fluorescently labelled with serotype specific antisera (unpublished data). This technique allows for comparison of the relative intensity of fluorescence per cell. The optical characteristics of opaque and transparent organisms were similar. Controls in which heterologous typing sera were used showed no significant fluorescence. Using antisera of the same serotype as the organisms examined, the mean intensity per detected event tended to be somewhat higher for transparent bacteria. Since this phenotype is less virulent in the animal model, it was concluded that if there is variation in amount of capsule, it is unlikely to be significant, and it does not appear to be a contributing factor in the dramatic differences noted in the animal models of infection.

Differences in the other carbohydrate structure on the cell surface, the teichoic acids, were analyzed by taking advantage of the unique structure of these molecules which contain choline in the form of covalently bound choline phosphate or phosphorylcholine. Choline, which is obtained exclusively from the nutrient medium, is essential for growth of both transparent and opaque variants. It is estimated that approximately 90% of the choline incorporated into cells is localized to the cell wall teichoic acid (C-polysaccharide) with the remainder in the lipoteichoic acid (pneumococcal Forssman antigen), which is an-

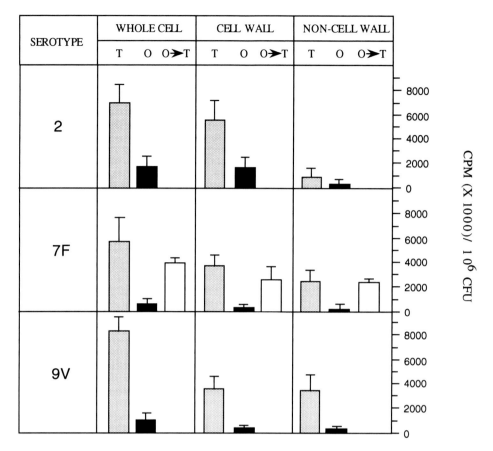

FIG. 2. Comparison of the incorporation of [³H]-choline in phenotypic variants. Teichoic acid was radiolabeled by adding [³H]-choline 0.5–1.0 μCi/mL to the growth medium. Crude cell walls were prepared by boiling for 15 min in 5% SDS as described.[7] Choline incorporation, expressed as the number of counts per minute in 10⁶ colony-forming units, was determined in whole cells, and cells fractionated into cell wall-associated (SDS-insoluble) and non-cell wall-associated (SDS-soluble) fractions. For the serotype 7F strains, a revertant of an opaque variant with a transparent phenotype was also analyzed. The values given are the mean of three separate determinations ±SD. The first row refers to opaque variant P125, and transparent variant, P126, which are unencapsulated mutants derived from the same serotype 2 isolate.

chored in the plasma membrane.[2] The pneumococcus is also atypical because the cell wall teichoic acid and the lipoteichoic acid possess identical chain structures.[6] The teichoic acids consist of polymers that contain from two to eight identical repeating units linked by ribitol phosphate. Each repeating unit includes two phosphorylcholine residues.

The quantity of teichoic acid per cell was compared in opaque and transparent variants by measuring the incorporation of [³H]-choline from the culture medium. After growth to the same density, transparent variants incorporated 3.9- to 8.7-fold more of the radiolabel per cell compared to opaque variants of the same strain (see Fig. 2). The correlation between choline incorporation and colony morphology was confirmed by showing that the level of incorporation in a spontaneous revertant of an opaque to a transparent variant was essentially equivalent to that of the transparent form of the same strain. Cells grown in the presence of [³H]-choline were fractionated to determine the cellular location of the increased choline incorporated into organisms with the transparent phenotype. The majority of the label was found in the SDS-insoluble cell fraction, which includes the crude cell wall and the cell wall-associated teichoic acid.

The amount of cell surface exposed ChoP was also compared by immunofluorescence using a MAb, TEPC-15, that reacts with phosphorylcholine and has been shown to bind to phosphorylcholine on the pneumococcus (see Fig. 3). Although both phenotypes reacted with the MAb, the greater intensity of reactivity for organisms of the transparent form suggests that there is more surface-exposed phosphorylcholine associated with this phenotype. To quantitate the difference in the level of cell-surface phosphorylcholine, opaque and transparent variants were labeled with TEPC-15 and compared using flow cytometry (see Fig. 4). There was no difference between phenotypes in optical characteristics, and both forms demonstrated increased fluorescence with TEPC-15 compared to controls. The mean intensity of fluorescence, however, was an average of 5.6-fold greater for the transparent than the opaque phenotype (mean of 1237 ± 731 *SD* vs. 218 ± 135 *SD* for 10,000 events detected).

These findings would suggest that either the structure of the teichoic acid or the amount of teichoic acid per cell is subject to variation, since the only significant reservoir of cellular choline is the teichoic acids. Differences in teichoic acid structure could account for these observations if the amount of

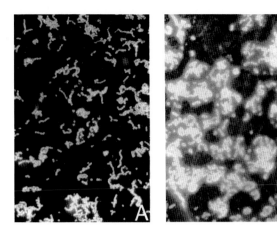

FIG. 3. Immunofluorescence of pneumococci incubated with a MAb against phosphorylcholine, TEPC-15, and labeled with fluorescein as described.[12] Magnification 3700×. (**A**) Opaque variant. (**B**) Transparent variant.

choline per teichoic acid chain varied due to either differences in the average number of repeating units per chain or the number of phosphorylcholine residues per repeating unit. Either of these differences in structure would be expected to affect the size distribution of teichoic acid chains. Western analysis us-

ing the MAb, TEPC-15, was used to visualize lipoteichoic acid (SDS-soluble fraction), and cell wall-associated teichoic acid (SDS-insoluble fraction) released by enzymatic digestion of crude cell walls with mutanolysin and proteinase K (see Fig. 5). The teichoic acids in both the SDS-soluble and crude cell wall fractions showed a ladder-like array of doublet bands, which represents chains with differing numbers of repeating units. The more slowly migrating band in each doublet appears to be lipoteichoic acid, because of its prominence in the SDS-soluble fraction and its larger molecular weight due to its terminal acyl group. The faster migrating band in each doublet appears to be the cell wall-associated teichoic acid, since it is more prominent following enzymatic digestion of the crude wall fraction. When samples from equivalent numbers of opaque and transparent organisms were compared, there was no appreciable difference in the migration of each chain or in the average chain length. The intensity of reactivity for each band, however, was greater for the transparent variant. This observation suggests that the higher amount of choline in transparent pneumococci is a result of increased numbers of teichoic acid residues per cell rather than variation in structure or average number of repeating units per chain. Since the cell wall-associated teichoic acid is covalently attached to muramic acid residues in the peptidoglycan and only a fraction of the muramic acid residues appear to be linked to a teichoic acid chain, the differences in the amount of teichoic acid observed in this

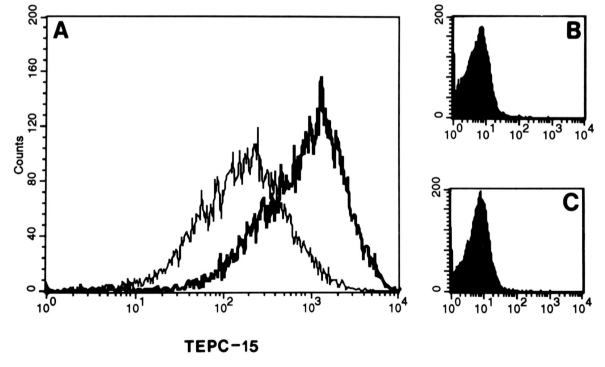

TEPC-15

FIG. 4. Histogram of flow cytometry pattern comparing the distribution of fluorescence intensity of cells labeled with TEPC-15 for an opaque variant and a transparent variant of the same strain, which is indicated in bold (**A**). Controls in which mouse ascites was substituted for TEPC-15 showed minimal flourescence (opaque variant, **B**; transparent variant, **C**). Cells were incubated in TEPC-15 (1/1000 dilution in PBS) or control mouse ascites for 1 hr at 37°C followed by R-phycoerythrin-coupled anti-mouse immunoglobulins (1/40 dilution in PBS for 1 hr at 37°C. After four washes in PBS, the cells were heated to 70°C for 10 min and fixed in 1% paraformaldehyde. Front and side-scatter characteristics were compared with fluorescence intensity on a FACScan instrument (Becton Dickinson Immunocytometry Systems, San Jose, CA). Cells were differentiated from debris by gating only on particles taking up propidium iodide.

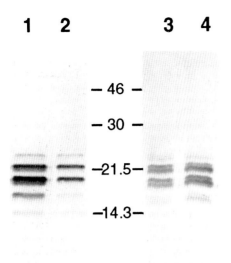

FIG. 5. Western analysis comparing the migration of teichoic acids from opaque and transparent phenotypic variants in SDS-PAGE. The SDS-soluble cell fraction of cells (lanes 1,2), or mutanolysin and proteinase K digested crude cell walls (lanes 3,4) were separated on 15% SDS-PAGE gels, transferred to membranes and immunoblotted with MAb, TEPC-15, to visualize the phosphorylcholine containing teichoic acids. Opaque phenotype (lanes 2,3); transparent phenotype (lanes 1,4). Size markers indicated in kilodaltons are protein standards.

study could be a consequence of a differing proportion of muramic acid residues having an attached teichoic acid chain.[5]

Role of phosphorylcholine in the biology of S. pneumoniae

Since teichoic acid is a major component of the cell surface, differences in amounts of ChoP that distinguish opaque and transparent phase variants might have numerous effects on the cell. The cell-surface expression of proteins binding to ChoP might be altered by variation in the quantity of this anchor. Evidence that expression of choline binding proteins varies in association with colony opacity has been presented. In addition, ChoP on the pneumococcus may interact directly with host molecules. Choline, which is generally not present in procaryotes, is a major component of eucaryotic lipids, and is found on many host structures.

Pneumococci have been shown to adhere to human buccal epithelial cells, type II pneumocytes (human lung epithelial cells in culture) and vascular endothelial cells.[4] For each of these cell types, transparent organisms bind in greater numbers compared to opaque organisms of the same strain. This result correlates with the enhanced ability of the transparent variant to colonize the nasopharynx. The adherence of transparent, but not opaque, pneumococci is augmented by stimulation of resting human cells with cytokines, interleukin-1 or tumor necrosis factor. Adherence to stimulated cells correlates with the ability of transparent variants to bind to cells transfected with the receptor for platelet activating factor (rPAF). Inflammatory cytokines activate the expression of the rPAF, which has been identified on many host tissues. It has been proposed that the

pneumococcus interacts with the rPAF by structural mimicry of PAF.[3] Since both the cell surface of the pneumococcus and PAF contain ChoP, this structure may be crucial to the binding of the bacteria to this host-cell target, an interaction that is inhibited by rPAF antagonists and high concentrations of exogenous choline. This interaction has also been shown to require the presence of choline on the organism, since pneumococci grown in the presence of ethanolamine in lieu of choline are poorly adherent. It is possible that the enhanced adherence to activated cells by transparent organisms is due to the increased expression of ChoP associated with this phenotype. This study supports this hypothesis by demonstrating that the same phenotype associated with increased adherence via the PAF receptor contains approximately fivefold more cell-surface choline.[4] Phase variation in the display of this ligand may allow the organism to switch from an adherent to nonadherent state. This may be critical to the organism's ability to exist, both in the nasopharynx where attachment to cells may be beneficial for prolonged carriage, and in the bloodstream where adherence to cells may confer a disadvantage for survival. The expression of elevated amounts of ChoP associated with the transparent phenotype may, in addition, promote clearance of the organism by the host. Human serum contains natural antibody to ChoP, and C-reactive protein appears to recognize this structure and may promote clearance of the pneumococcus.[1,9] These factors may lead to a selection of pneumococci with less cell-surface ChoP, i.e., of the opaque phenotype, once an organism has bypassed the mucosal barrier.

Phase variation in the expression of ChoP is not unique to the pneumococcus, although this structure is distinctly uncommon in prokaryotes. Recently, this laboratory has reported that another pathogen of the human respiratory tract, *Haemophilus influenzae*, a Gram-negative bacteria that has a life cycle with many similarities to that of *S. pneumoniae*, decorates its cell surface with ChoP.[15] In the case of *H. influenzae*, ChoP is found on the saccharide portion of the lipopolysaccharide (LPS). In fact, MAb TEPC-15 reacts with ChoP on the surface glycolipids of both *H. influenzae* (LPS) and *S. pneumoniae* (lipoteichoic acid) (see Fig. 6). *H. influenzae* also acquires choline from

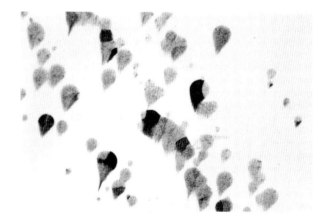

FIG. 6. Colony immunoblot showing reactivity of *H. influenzae* strain Eagan with a MAb TEPC-15, which reacts with phosphorylcholine (ChoP). There are reactive and nonreactive variants in addition to sectored colonies, which indicate phase variation in the display of this epitope. Magnification 10×.

the growth medium, although unlike the pneumococcus, it is not a nutritional requirement. The expression of ChoP on the LPS requires a previously identified chromosomal locus containing four genes, *licA–D*.[18] Phase variation is mediated a molecular switch based on multiple tandem repeats of the sequence 5'-CAAT'-3' within the open reading frame of *licA*. The gene product of *licA* has homology to eucaryotic choline kinases, suggesting that the bacterial pathway for choline incorporation has common features with that of eucaryotes. The genes involved in choline incorporation in the pneumococcus are unknown. The only other bacteria in which homology to *licA* has been described is in members of the genus Mycoplasma. Since mycoplasma, hemophilus, and streptococcus all share the ability to infect the respiratory tract, there may be a common mechanism involving ChoP in their pathogenesis.

ACKNOWLEDGMENTS

The author is indebted to Dr. R. Austrian for his expertise and advice. J.N. Weiser is a Lucille P. Markey Charitable Scholar. This work was supported by the Lucille P. Markey Charitable Trust and a grant from the Public Health Service (AI38446).

REFERENCES

1. **Briles, D.E., G. Scott, B. Gray, M.J. Crain, M. Blaese, M. Nahm, V. Scott and P. Haber.** 1987. Naturally occurring antibodies to phosphocholine as a potential index of antibody responsiveness to polysaccharides. J Infect Dis. **155:**1307–14.

2. **Briles, E.B. and A. Tomasz.** 1973. Pneumococcal Forssman antigen. A choline-containing lipoteichoic acid. J. Biol. Chem. **248:**6394–6397.

3. **Cundell, D.R., N.P. Gerard, C. Gerard, I. Idanpaan-Heikkila, and E.I. Tuomanen.** 1995. *Streptococcus pneumoniae* anchor to activated human cells by the receptor for platelet-activating factor. Nature **377:**435–438.

4. **Cundell, D.R., J.N. Weiser, J. Shen, A. Young and E.I. Tuomanen.** 1995. Relationship between colonial morphology and adherence of *Streptococcus pneumoniae*. Infect Immun. **63:**757–761.

5. **Fischer, H., and A. Tomasz.** 1985. Peptidoglycan cross-linking and teichoic acid attachment in *Streptococcus pneumoniae*. J. Bacteriol. **163:**46–54.

6. **Fischer, W., T. Behr, R. Hartmann, P. Peter-Katalinic, and H. Egge.** 1993. Teichoic acid and lipoteichoic acid of *Streptococcus pneumoniae* posses identical structures: investigation of teichoic acid (C polysaccharide). Biochem. **215:**851–857.

7. **Garcia-Bustos, J.F., B.T. Chait, and A. Tomasz.** 1987. Structure of the peptide network of pneumococcal peptidoglycan. J. Biol. Chem. **262:**15400–15405.

8. **Hammerschmidt, S., A. Muller, H. Sillmann, M. Muhlenhoff, R. Borrow, and et al.** 1996. Capsule phase variation in *Neisseria meningitidis* serogroup B by slipped-strand mispairing in the polysialyltransferase gene (siaD): Correlation with bacterial invasion and the outbreak of meningococcal disease. Mol. Microbiol. **20:**1211–1220.

9. **Horowitz, J., J.E. Volanakis, and D.E. Briles.** 1987. Blood clearance of *Streptococcus pneumoniae* by C-reactive protein. J. Immunol. **138:**2598–2603.

10. **MacLeod, C.M., and M.R. Krauss.** 1950. Relation of virulence of pneumococcal strains for mice to the quantity of capsular polysaccharide formed in vitro. J. Exp. Med. **90:**1–9.

11. **Saluja, S.K., and J.N. Weiser.** 1995. The genetic basis of colony opacity in *Streptococcus pneumoniae:* Evidence for the effect of box elements on the frequency of phenotypic variation. Mol. Microbiol. **16:**215–227.

12. **Tuomanen, E. and A. Tomasz.** 1991. Mechanism of phenotypic tolerance of nongrowing pneumococci to beta-lactam antibiotics. Scand. J. Infect. Dis. **74:**102–112.

13. **Wani, J., J. Gilbert, A. Plaut, and J. Weiser.** 1996. Identification, cloning and sequencing of the immunoglobulin A1 protease gene of *Streptococcus pneumoniae*. Infect. Immun. **64:**3967–3974.

14. **Weiser, J., Z. Markiewicz, E. Tuomanen, and J. Wani.** 1996. Relationship between phase variation in colony morphology, intrastrain variation in cell wall physiology and nasopharyngeal colonization by *Streptococcus pneumoniae*. **64:**2240–2245.

15. **Weiser, J., M. Shchepetov, and S. Chong.** 1997. Decoration of lipopolysaccharide with phosphorylcholine: A phase-variable characteristic of *Haemophilus influenzae*. Infect. Immun. **65:**943–950.

16. **Weiser, J.N.** 1993. Relationship between colony morphology and the life cycle of *Haemophilus influenzae:* The contribution of lipopolysaccharide phase variation to pathogenesis. J. Infect. Dis. **168:**672–680.

17. **Weiser, J.N., R. Austrian, P.K. Sreenivasan, and H.R. Masure.** 1994. Phase variation in pneumococcal opacity: Relationship between colonial morphology and nasopharyngeal colonization. Infect. Immun. **62:**2582–2589.

18. **Weiser, J.N., J.M. Love, and E.R. Moxon.** 1989. The molecular mechanism of phase variation of *H. influenzae* lipopolysaccharide. Cell **59:**657–665.

Address reprint requests to:
Jeffrey N. Weiser
University of Pennsylvania
301B Johnson Pavilion
Philadelphia, PA 19104-6076

Pneumococcal Proteins PspA and PspC: Their Potential for Use as Vaccines

DAVID E. BRILES,[1,2] SUSAN K. HOLLINGSHEAD,[1] EDWIN SWIATLO,[1,3] ALEXIS BROOKS-WALTER,[1] ALEX SZALAI,[2,3] ANNI VIROLAINEN,[1] LARRY S. McDANIEL,[1] KIMBERLY A. BENTON,[1] PIET C. AERTS,[4] HANS VAN DIJK,[4] and MARILYN J. CRAIN[1,2]

INTRODUCTION

ALTHOUGH CAPSULAR POLYSACCHARIDES (PS) from *Streptococcus pneumoniae* (Fig. 1) have long been considered effective immunogens against pneumococcal infection, their use has eliminated only a small fraction of the morbidity and mortality associated with this organism world-wide.[25,36] There are several reasons for this. One is that the 23-valent polysaccharide vaccine has not been used as widely as recommended. Another is that the vaccine is only about 60% effective against invasive infections caused by the 23 capsular types included in the vaccine.[48] Also, it is so poorly immunogenic in children less than 2 years of age that there are no approved indications for its use in this important at-risk group.[3,16] Moreover, recent data indicate that not all antibodies to certain PS antigens, especially capsular type 6, are always protective.[1,37,39] One way to improve the immunogenicity of capsular polysaccharides in humans is to conjugate the polysaccharides with immunogenic T cell–dependent protein carriers.[20,38,40,42] This approach has worked very well for *Haemophilus influenzae* type b polysaccharide which, when conjugated to protein carriers, becomes an effective and safe vaccine for children.[2,51]

However, the situation for pneumococcal PS-protein conjugates is different from that of the *H. influenzae* conjugate vaccine. Pneumococci have at least 90 serologically distinguishable PS types which comprise 48 cross-reactive groups.[26] The current capsular polysaccharide vaccine represents a compromise and contains a carefully chosen mixture of 23 polysaccharides from the most common capsule types. The 23 valent PS vaccine was developed for use in adults and elicits antibody against capsular types found in 85–90% of invasive infections.[43] A broadly protective PS-protein conjugate vaccine for adults would need to contain a similar number of different PS-protein conjugates. Fortunately, in children the number of predominant polysaccharide types is generally no more than 7–10.[23] Even with only seven PS-protein chemical conjugates the vaccine would be a complex synthetic formulation. Moreover, preliminary data indicate that the conjugates may not be any more immunogenic in adults than the much less expensive PS vaccine for some serotypes.[50] A major problem with use of a complex multivalent conjugate vaccine is that most pneumococcal disease occurs in children in developing countries, where it accounts for over one million deaths per year. Regardless of its efficacy, an expensive vaccine may be unlikely to be used on a large scale in the developing world.

Another consideration is that infants are frequently infected with encapsulated bacteria and would presumably benefit from protective anti-polysaccharide immune responses. Infants make strong responses to protein antigens. The fact that evolution has developed an anti-polysaccharide response in mammals with delayed maturation suggests that deleterious consequences may result from eliciting of at least certain anti-polysaccharide responses shortly after birth.[21,22,56]

In contrast to this theoretical concern, immunization of children 2 months of age and older with *H. influenzae* b polysaccharide protein conjugate vaccine has had remarkable success at eliminating *H. influenzae* b disease without causing detectable problems.[2,51] This result has provided encouragement for the continued development of other PS-protein conjugate vaccines for use in young children. However, the *H. influenzae* vaccine elicits antibody to only a single polysaccharide. In the case of a multivalent pneumococcal PS-protein conjugate vaccine, the hypothetical risk of inducing a deleterious immune outcome could be greater than for a monovalent vaccine such as *H. influenzae* type b.

These concerns are tempered, however, by the fact that millions of children's lives could be saved world wide by the development of an effective affordable pneumococcal PS-protein conjugate vaccine. Thus, our failure to understand the reasons for late development of polysaccharide responsiveness should not prevent the development of new PS-protein conjugate vaccines. To minimize the chance of a new vaccine causing possible adverse outcomes, however, it may be important to include an ongoing assessment of overall health status, including subsequent physical and mental development, in the conduct of PS-protein trials.

Departments of [1]Microbiology, [2]Pediatrics, and [3]Medicine, University of Alabama at Birmingham, Birmingham, Alabama.
[4]Department of Infectious Diseases University Children's Hospital, Utrecht, The Netherlands.

Streptococcus pneumoniae

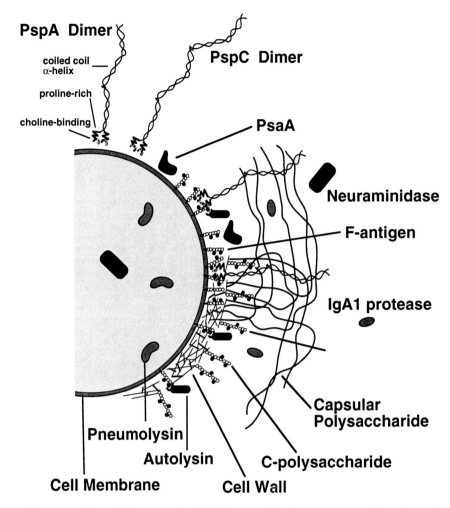

FIG. 1. Diagrammatic representation of *S. pneumoniae* depicting several surface components for which roles in virulence and/ or elicitation of protection have been established. Analysis of the structure of PspA and PspC indicate that they are coiled coil proteins. Whether they exist as linear homodimers, as depicted has not yet been determined. The figure illustrates the ahelical, proline-rich, and choline-binding domains of PspA and PspC. A fourth domain, a 17–amino acid C-terminal tail is not shown in this diagram. This diagram is based on an earlier depiction of *S. pneumoniae*.[12]

PROTEIN VACCINE CANDIDATES

The complexity of PS-protein conjugate vaccines, and the concerns regarding induction of PS responses in very young children, has led to investigations of the possibility that cross-reactive pneumococcal proteins may be able to elicit protection in young children. Such antigens might be used to broaden the protection elicited by a small number of PS-protein conjugates, or if highly successful, might be able to replace the need for a PS-protein conjugate pneumococcal vaccine. Protein antigens can be inexpensively produced by recombinant technology, and like other protein-based vaccines they would be expected to be highly immunogenic in children and in the elderly.

The capsule is the most conspicuous surface component of the pneumococcus and human antibodies to many of the capsular polysaccharides have been shown to be highly efficacious

in preventing infection.[4,25,48] Thus, for protein antigens including pneumococcal surface protein A (PspA),[12] pneumolysin[41] pneumococcal surface adhesin A (PsaA),[53] it will be necessary to rigorously establish protective efficacy in animals before they can be considered for large scale human trials.

A capsule is a highly effective adaptation to shield the pneumococcus from opsonophagocytosis. Antibodies to polysaccharide negate this effect, fix complement, and opsonize pneumococci. Although some pneumococcal proteins may have antiphagocytic effects, they may also be important for attachment, invasion, and spread of pneumococci.[55] Some proteins may have specific roles for survival of pneumococci in infection sites such as the lung, middle ear, or cerebrospinal fluid, while others may be important for survival of pneumococci in the blood. Thus, to investigate fully the roles of pneumococcal proteins it will be necessary to consider animal models in addition to a standard mouse protection test, which evaluates only bacteremia and sepsis.

Pneumolysin provides an excellent example of a pneumococcal protein that has been tested for its activities in multiple animal models including sepsis and infections gaining entry through mucosal and pulmonary surfaces.[6,45–47,52] Only through a detailed investigation of the ability of proteins to protect against natural (nasopharyngeal and pulmonary) exposure, attachment, invasion, and bacteremia will the full vaccine potential of each pneumococcal protein be determined. It will also be important to investigate the role of immunity to pneumococcal PS in these models, since studies of immunity to PS have generally been restricted to bacteremia and sepsis models.

This article focuses on studies of PspA, a surface protein found on all pneumococci. PspA is able to elicit protection against pneumococcal infection in mice. Three recent reviews describe PspA and its ability to elicit immunity to pneumococcal infections,[11–13] one of which provides a historical development of our knowledge of PspA.[12] The present article focuses on the most recent developments relating to PspA and its sister protein PspC.

PspA

PspA has been shown to be required for full virulence of pneumococci.[35,63] The protection elicited by PspA immunization is mediated by antibody; passive protection can be obtained by use of immune serum or monoclonal antibodies.[29,32,33] PspA is serologically variable.[17,35] Because of this variability a PspA-based vaccine may need to contain PspAs of more than one pneumococcus to be able to protect against all pneumococci. The fact that PspA is serologically variable supports its potential usefulness as a human vaccine. Except for rare instances,[5,19] pneumococcal infection is restricted to humans. If the variability of PspA is driven by selective pressure to escape prior immunity (as is believed to be the case for the diversity of capsular types) then immunity to PspA must be effective at eliminating colonization and/or infection in humans.[17]

PspAs contain multiple antigenic epitopes and the serological variability of PspA is a result of the different combinations of these epitopes within any one PspA.[17] Although the number of different combinations of epitopes is large, most PspAs share at least some epitopes and are cross-reactive. Indeed, using a single rabbit antiserum raised to a single PspA, it has been possible to recognize PspAs on all pneumococci examined to date.[17] An earlier review describes the serologic variability of PspA and pneumococci in detail.[12] It is important to note, however, that PspAs are sufficiently cross-reactive and that immunization with one PspA generally elicits immunity to strains of pneumococci which express different PspA serotypes.[29,33,54]

STRUCTURE OF PspA

Several different *pspA* genes have been sequenced,[27,30,61] and the exact locations of domains responsible for serological diversity have been identified.[34] From the sequence of *pspA* it is known that the mature protein product is composed of several clearly distinguishable domains.[30,61] The amino acid sequence of the N-terminal one-half of PspA predicts an α-helical coiled-coil structure. This same region of the protein is surface exposed and is recognized by virtually all MAb made against isolated or cell-associated PspA.[17,31,61] The α-helical domain is followed by a proline-rich domain where a predominant sequence pro-ala-pro-ala-pro is repeated multiple times. In other surface proteins of Gram positive bacteria, proline-rich regions are present where the protein spans the cell wall. At the C-terminal end of PspA is a 200–amino acid choline-binding domain made up of 10 repeats of 20 amino acids each. The final 17 amino acids make up a slightly hydrophilic domain whose function is, as yet, unknown.

The choline-binding region at the C-terminus of PspA has a large degree of homology to, yet is distinct from, similar choline-binding regions in the major autolysin and several phage lysins of *S. pneumoniae*[61] and to a number of other less well-characterized proteins.[8,44] It has been shown that this choline-binding region in PspA is responsible for the attachment of PspA to the pneumococcal surface.[62,64] The attachment of PspA to pneumococci is thought to be via the phosphocholine residues of the lipoteichoic acids (previously named pneumococcal F-antigen).[12,62] It is interesting that while PspA is readily able to bind choline-Sepharose columns and Sepharose columns made with other choline analogs, including phosphocholine, it can be readily eluted from these columns by choline but not by phosphocholine[10,64] (J. Russel and Dr. Briles, unpublished data).

DIVERSITY OF PspA

The entire sequence of *pspA* has been published for strains Rx1[61] and EF5668.[30] Sequences for the 5′ half of PspA, encoding the α-helical half of the protein, have been determined for 18 additional strains.[27] A comparison of these sequences shows that the proline-rich region, the choline-binding region, and the C-terminal 17 amino acids of PspA are highly conserved. Nearly all of the variation among different PspAs occurs in the α-helical domain comprising the N-terminal half of PspA. The α-helical regions of PspA/WU2 and PspA/Rx1 are 82% identical and 87% similar, but this region of PspA/EF5668 is only 61% identical and 70% similar to that of PspA/Rx1. Further sequencing has shown that the α-helical regions of PspA molecules exhibit complex mosaic patterns of conserved and variable sequences.[27]

It has been shown that the 3′-end of the variable α-helical domain is critical for eliciting cross-protective antibodies.[13,31,54] This major protection-eliciting region of PspA corresponds roughly to the region comprising amino acids 192–290 of PspA/Rx1 and is directly adjacent to the proline-rich domain. The corresponding regions of 24 different PspA molecules were sequenced to evaluate diversity. Based on sequence identities in the aligned sequences, six distinct groups called clades were observed (Fig. 2).[27,28] It was also possible to group the PspAs into clades based on the sequences of the first 100 N-terminal amino acids and the proline-rich region. What was most interesting, however, was that the relationship of the strains falling into these groups of sequence homology differed for each region of the molecule. In other words, strains that fell into a single clade based on the sequences of amino acids 192–290 were

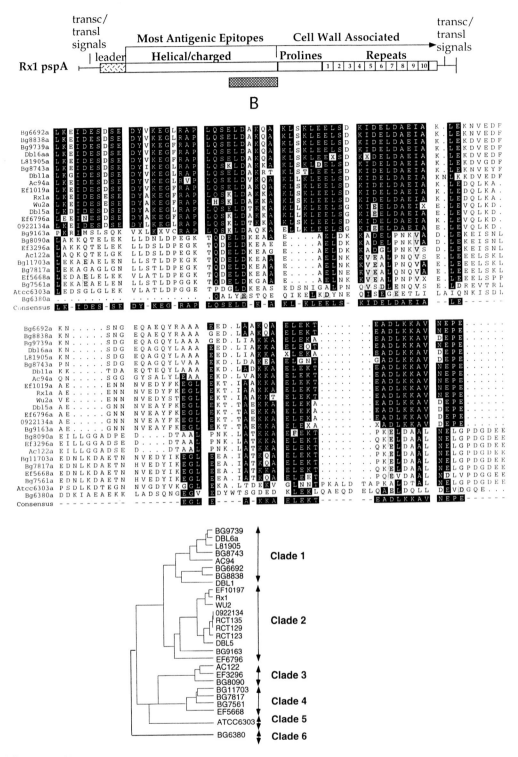

FIG. 2. Alignment of PspA sequences in the major protection-eliciting region of the molecule. The top of the figure is an outline of the pspA gene and its domain structure. The box B depicts the fragment of PspA represented in the sequence alignment in the center of the figure. Strain names from which the pspA genes were sequenced are to the left of the alignment. Sequences were aligned by Pileup with a gap penalty of 3.0 and gap-length penalty of 0.1. A dendrogram (at the bottom) represents the relationships of strains sequenced and defines groups called "clades."

often in very different clades based on the sequence of the N-terminal 100 amino acids or the proline-rich region. These results suggest that there has been significant recombination within *pspA* genes[28] and provides an explanation for how different PspAs are able to express quite different combinations of epitopes.[17]

FUNCTION of PspA

In a study using the bystander complement assay, we have observed that an encapsulated mutant strain lacking PspA expression fixed more complement than the isogenic parent strain expressing PspA (Fig. 3), even though they were found to have identical levels of capsular polysaccharide.[18] The bystander assay detects C3 activated by, but not deposited on, the pneumococcal surface. In another study, we similarly observed that infections of nonimmune mice with PspA$^-$ capsular type 3 pneumococci caused greater early activation of serum complement than did infections with a PspA$^+$ isogenic parent. The greater complement activation with the PspA$^-$ infections was evidenced by increased disappearance of antigenic C3 from the circulation. This was true, even after correcting for the difference in bacteremia following infection with the PspA$^+$ and

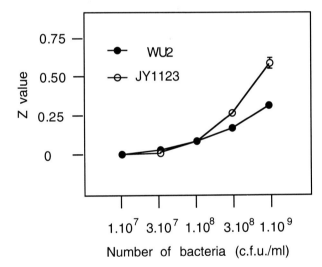

FIG. 3. Bystander complement activation by capsular type 3 strain WU2 and its PspA$^-$ mutant JY1123[62] as detected by a complement activation microassay. Chicken erythrocytes and heat-killed pneumococci in either VBS^{++} (Veronal-buffered saline with Ca^{2+} and Mg^{2+}) and normal human serum with or without trypsin. Hemoglobin release was measured by absorbance at 405 nm, and percent of lysis was determined from the formula: Y = ([I − II]/[III − IV]) × 100, where Z = number of active sites per erythrocyte Z = −ln (1 − Y/100), in which I = absorbance of the sample, II = serum control with no bacteria, and III and IV represent the absorbance values of controls for water (100% lysis) and buffer (0% lysis), respectively. Strains WU2 and JY1123 were shown to have indistinguishable amounts of type 3 capsular polysaccharide by ELISA with a specific anti–type 3 antibody. A control strain DW3.7[58] lacking capsule and PspA did not have type 3 polysaccharide by this assay. An incorrect version of this figure was published previously.[9]

PspA$^-$ pneumococci (A.-H. Tu, A. J. Szalai and D. E. Briles, unpublished data). These combined results suggest that PspA is able to reduce the consumption of complement by pneumococci, thus leading to reduced complement mediated clearance and phagocytosis of pneumococci.

The ability of antibodies to PspA to enhance blood clearance of pneumococci is not seen in mice that have been treated with cobra venom factor to deplete C3.[13] One interpretation of this finding is that anti-PspA is protective because it leads to complement dependent opsonization. It is also possible that blood clearance due to anti-PspA is the result of increased complement activation at the surface due to antibody-mediated blockage of PspA's anti-complementary function.

ADULT MOUSE CARRIAGE MODEL

An adult mouse model for carriage has been developed to study the role of PspA in carriage and the ability of a mucosal immune response to PspA to prevent infection. In this model, inbred mice are able to carry pneumococci of all seven capsular types tested.[13,62] Carriage of pneumococci in mice was independent of the capacity of the strains to cause fatal disease in mice. The strains carried in the nasopharynx included isolates of capsular types 2, 3, 4, and 6, which are rapidly lethal in mice following i.v. or i.p. infection as well as isolates of capsular types 14, 19, and 23, which are relatively avirulent in mice.

In immune-deficient CBA/N mice, which exhibit the XID phenotype, carriage could be observed with all strains except for those of capsular types 2 and 3. In XID mice, strains of capsular types 2 and 3 rapidly invade from the nasopharynx and cause fatal infections.[59,60,62] This result is consistent with observations made following i.v. infection with many of these same strains.[7] While most of our capsular types 4 and 6 strains are inevitably fatal when injected i.v. into CBA/N mice, death only occurs after at least a short period of stable bacteremia. In contrast, capsular types 2 and 3 increase in numbers in the blood of CBA/N mice in an exponential manner until death at 24–36 h after inoculation of 100 CFU.[7] Thus, the ability of the capsular type 2 and 3 strains to cause sepsis and death following intranasal inoculation may be associated with their greatly enhanced ability to cause uncontrolled bacteremia in the blood.

PROTECTION AGAINST CARRIAGE BY IMMUNIZATION WITH PspA AND PspA's ROLE IN CARRIAGE

Using the mouse carriage model it has been demonstrated that mucosal, but not systemic, immunity to PspA can prevent nasopharyngeal carriage of pneumococci in mice.[59] The ability to induce immunity to carriage is not a characteristic unique to PspA since immunity elicited by a 6B PS-protein conjugate,[59] heat killed rough pneumococci, and lysates of rough pneumococci can also protect against carriage.[9,59]

Interestingly, although antibodies to PspA can protect against carriage, mutant pneumococci lacking PspA still cause significant carriage (A. Virolainen and D.E. Briles, unpublished data). One way that antibodies to PspA could protect against carriage even though PspA is not essential for carriage, might be that the target of these antibodies is not PspA but some other cross-reacting surface protein which is essential for carriage. A candidate for such a protein is PspC.[14]

PspC

PspC, like PspA has an N-terminal α-helical domain, a central proline-rich domain, and a choline-binding domain which is 90% homologous to PspAs choline-binding domain. The proline-rich regions of PspA and PspC are also extremely similar. The major differences between the two proteins is in the α-helical domain. The α-helical domain of PspC is from 50% to 100% larger than most PspA α-helical domains and contains a large repeat of about 100 amino acids which are generally absent from PspA. In some cases, the C-terminal end of the α-helical domain is so homologous to some of the PspA clades that it could be readily assigned to one of them if it were not known to be a separate molecule. Since PspAs within the same clade cross-react immunologically, it is suspected that at least some PspA and PspC molecules may strongly cross-react.[14] Thus, it is possible that some of the protection seen after immunization with PspA may be the result of antibody binding to PspC.

The existence of a *pspC* gene (previously called the "*pspA*-like" sequence) was first established in 1992 when *pspA* was used to probe genomic digests of chromosomal DNA. The full-length *pspA* sequence identified two unlinked loci in the chromosomes of all pneumococci examined. Both genes were shown to contain elements that hybridized with both the 3' and 5' halves of *pspA*.[33,49] The PspC protein has also been named CbpA and SpsA for the ability of the protein to bind choline and secretory IgA.[24,44] An antiserum to recombinant PspC detects PspC in all pneumococci examined and weakly cross-reacts with PspA, which migrates as a smaller molecule than PspC on Western blots.[15]

ANTI-PspA IN HUMAN SERA

Based on our present information it appears that PspA is cross-reactive enough to elicit broad protection against pneumococcal infection in mice.[12,33,54] Our more recent evidence indicates that PspA can also elicit protection against carriage and subsequent invasive disease.[59] Although the ability of PspA and/or PspC to elicit similar protective immunity in man has not been determined, it is known that all adults examined to date have serum antibody to PspA in concentrations ranging from 2 to 80 μg/mL. In children, the antibody levels were one third of adult levels by two months of age and half adult levels by 3 years of age (A. Virolainen, J. Russell, and D. E. Briles, unpublished data). By examining the levels of anti-PspA in acute phase sera of children with invasive infections we obtained indirect evidence for a protective role of antibodies to PspA in man. Children with invasive pneumococcal disease had sixfold lower levels of IgG to PspA than children with invasive infections with other agents.[57] These results provide encouragement for the eventual development of pneumococcal pro-tein vaccines that can protect humans from infection and colonization with *S. pneumoniae*.

ACKNOWLEDGMENTS

These studies were supported in part by AI21548, AI27201, and AI33205 from the National Institutes of Allergy and Infectious Diseases, HL51646 from the National Heart, Lung, and Blood Institute, Respiratory Pathogens Research Unit subcontract with Baylor University, and WHO. Flora Gathof is acknowledged for assistance in preparation of the manuscript. This chapter is a revision of a review published in 1997 that summarized a presentation at the International Meeting on the Molecular Biology of *Streptococcus pneumoniae* and Its Diseases. Oeiras, Portugal, September 25–30, 1996.

REFERENCES

1. **Aaberge, I.S., B. Hvalbye, and M. Lovil.** 1996. Enhancement of *Streptococcus pneumoniae* serotype 6B infection in mice after passive immunization with human serum. Microbial Pathog. **21:**125–137.

2. **Anderson, P., M. Pichichero, R. Insel, P. Farsad, and M. Santosham.** 1985. Capsular antigens noncovalently or covalently associated with protein as vaccines to *Haemophilus influenzae* type b: comparison in two-year-old children. J. Infect. Dis. **152:**634–636.

3. **Anonymous.** 1997. Prevention of pneumococcal disease: recommendations of the advisory committee on immunization practices (ACIP). M.M.W.R. **46:**1–24.

4. **Austrian R.** 1979. Pneumococcal vaccine: development and prospects. Am. J. Med. **67:**547–549.

5. **Benson, C.E., and C.R. Sweeney.** 1984. Isolation of *Streptococcus pneumoniae* type 3 from equine species. J. Clin. Microbiol. **20:**1028–1030.

6. **Benton, K.A., M.P. Everson, and D.E. Briles.** 1995. A pneumolysin-negative mutant of *Streptococcus pneumoniae* causes chronic bacteremia rather than acute sepsis in mice. Infect. Immunol. **63:**448–455.

7. **Benton, K.A., J.C. Paton, and D.B. Briles.** 1997. Differences in virulence of mice among *Streptococcus pneumoniae* strains of capsular types 2, 3, 4, 5, and 6 are not attributable to differences in pneumolysin production. Infect. Immunol. **65:**1237–1244.

8. **Briese, T., and R. Hakenbeck.** 1985. Interaction of the pneumococcal amidase with lipoteichoic acid and choline. Eur. J. Biochem. **146:**417–427.

9. **Briles, D.E., S.K. Hollingshead, E. Swiatlo, A. Brooks-Walter, A. Szalai, A. Virolainen, L.S. McDaniel, K.A. Benton, P. White, K. Prellner, et al.** 1997. PspA and PspC: their potential for use as pneumococcal vaccines. Microbial Drug Resist. **3:**401–408.

10. **Briles, D.E., J.D. King, M.A. Gray, L.S. McDaniel, E. Swiatlo, and K.A. Benton.** 1996. PspA, a protection-eliciting pneumococcal protein: Immunogenicity of isolated native PspA in mice. Vaccine **14:**858–867.

11. **Briles, D.E., E. Swiatlo, and K. Edwards.** Vaccine strategies for *Streptococcus pneumoniae*. *In* D.L. Stevens (ed.), *Streptococci. ICAAC/IDSA*, Chicago (in press).

12. **Briles, D.E., R.C. Tart, E. Swiatlo, J.P. Dillard, P. Smith, K.A. Benton, B.A. Ralph, A. Brooks-Walter, M.J. Crain, S.K. Hollingshead, and L.S. McDaniel.** 1998. Pneumococcal diversity: considerations for new vaccine strategies with an emphasis on

pneumococcal surface protein A (PspA). Clin. Microbiol. Rev. **11**:645–657.

13. **Briles, D.E., R.C. Tart, H.-Y. Wu, B.A. Ralph, M.W. Russell, and L.S. McDaniel.** 1996. Systemic and mucosal protective immunity to pneumococcal surface protein A. N.Y. Acad Sci. **797**:118–126.

14. **Brooks-Walter, A., R.C. Tart, D.E. Briles, and S.K. Hollingshead.** 1997. The pspC gene encodes a second pneumococcal surface protein homologous to the gene encoding the protection-eliciting PspA protein of *Streptococcus pneumoniae*. ASM Annu. Mtg. **1997**:35(abst).

15. **Brooks-Walter, A., R.C. Tart, D.E. Briles, and S.K. Hollings-head.** The *pspC* gene of *Streptococcus pneumoniae* encodes a polymorphic protein PspC, which is capable of eliciting protective immunity to pneumococcal bacteremia and sepsis. Infect. Immun.(submitted).

16. **Cowan, M.J., A.J. Ammann, D.W. Wara, V.M. Howie, L. Schultz, N. Doyle, and M. Kaplan.** 1978. Pneumococcal polysaccharide immunization in infants and children. Pediatrics **62**:721–727.

17. **Crain, M.J., W.D. Waltman, II, J.S. Turner, J. Yother, D.E. Talkington, L.M. McDaniel, B.M. Gray, and D.E. Briles.** 1990. Pneumococcal surface protein A (PspA) is serologically highly variable and is expressed by all clinically important capsular serotypes of *Streptococcus pneumoniae*. Infect. Immunol. **58**: 3293–3299.

18. **deVelasco, E.A., A.F.M. Verheul, J. Verhoef, and H. Snippe.** 1995. *Streptococcus pneumoniae*: virulence factors, pathogenesis and vaccines. Microbiol. Rev. **59**:591–603.

19. **Fallon, M.T., M.K. Reinhard, B.M. Gray, T.W. Davis, and J.R. Lindsey.** 1988. Inapparent *Streptococcus pneumoniae* type 35 infections in commercial rats and mice. Lab. Anim. Sci. **38**:129–132.

20. **Fattom, A., W.F. Vann, S.C. Szu, A. Sutton, D. Bryla, G. Shiffman, J.B. Robbins, and R. Schneerson.** 1988. Synthesis and physiochemical and immunological characterization of pneumococcus type 12F polysaccharide-diphtheria toxoid conjugates. Infect. Immunol. **56**:2292–2298.

21. **Finne, J., D. Bitter-Suermann, C. Goridis, and U. Finne.** 1987. An IgG monoclonal antibody to group B meningococci cross-reacts with developmentally regulated polysialic acid units of glycoproteins in neural and extraneural tissues. J. Immunol. **138**: 4402–4407.

22. **Finne, J., M. Leinonen, and P.H. Makela.** 1983. Antigenic similarities between brain components and bacteria causing meningitis. Implications for vaccine development and pathogenesis. Lancet **2**:355–357.

23. **Gray, B.M., and H.C. Dillon.** 1986. Clinical and epidemiologic studies of pneumococcal infection in children. Pediatr. Infect. Dis. **5**:201–207.

24. **Hammerschmidt, S., S.R. Talay, P. Brandtzaeg, and G.S. Chhatwal.** 1997. SpsA, a novel pneumococcal surface protein with specific binding to secretory immunoglobulin A and secretory component. Mol. Microbiol. **25**:1113–1124.

25. **Heffron, R.** 1939. Pneumonia. Commonwealth Fund, New York.

26. **Henrichsen, J.** 1995. Six newly recognized types of *Streptococcus pneumoniae*. J. Clin. Microbiol. **33**:2759–2762.

27. **Hollingshead, S.K., R.S. Becker, and D.E. Briles.** Diversity of PspA: mosaic genes and evidence for past recombination in *Streptococcus pneumoniae* (submitted).

28. **Hollingshead, S.K., D. Bessen, and D.E. Briles.** 1998. Archeological footprints of horizontal gene transfer: mosaic cell surface proteins in *Streptococcus pyogenes* and *Streptococcus pneumoniae*. *In* M. Syvanen and C. Kado (ed.), Horizontal gene transfer: implications and consequences. Chapman and Hall, London, pp. 192–207.

29. **Langermann, S., S.R. Palaszynski, J.E. Burlein, S. Koenig, M.S.**

Hanson, D.E. Briles, and C.K. Stover. 1994. Protective humoral response against pneumococcal infection in mice elicited by recombinant Bacille Calmette-Guérin vaccines expressing PspA. J. Exp. Med. **180**:2277–2286.

30. **McDaniel, L.S., D.O. McDaniel, S.K. Hollingshead, and D.E. Briles.** 1998. Comparison of the PspA sequence from *Streptococcus pneumoniae* EF5668 to the previously identified PspA sequence from strain Rx1 and ability of PspA from EF5668 to elicit protection against pneumococci of different capsular types. Infect. Immunol. **66**:4748–4754.

31. **McDaniel, L.S., B.A. Ralph, D.O. McDaniel, and D.E. Briles.** 1994. Localization of protection-eliciting epitopes on PspA of *Streptococcus pneumoniae* between amino acid residues 192 and 260. Microbial Pathog. **17**:323–337.

32. **McDaniel, L.S., G. Scott, J.F. Kearney, and D.E. Briles.** 1984. Monoclonal antibodies against protease-sensitive pneumococcal antigens can protect mice from fatal infection with *Streptococcus pneumoniae*. J. Exp. Med. **160**:386–397.

33. **McDaniel, L.S., J.S. Sheffield, P. Delucchi, and D.E. Briles.** 1991. PspA, a surface protein of *Streptococcus pneumoniae*, is capable of eliciting protection against pneumococci of more than one capsular type. Infect. Immunol. **59**:222–228.

34. **McDaniel, L.S., J.S. Sheffield, E. Swiatlo, J. Yother, M.J. Crain, and D.E. Briles.** 1992. Molecular localization of variable and conserved regions of *pspA*, and identification of additional *pspA* homologous sequences in *Streptococcus pneumoniae*. Microbial Pathog. **13**:261–269.

35. **McDaniel, L.S., J. Yother, M. Vijayakumar, L. McGarry, W.R. Guild, and D.E. Briles.** 1987. Use of insertional inactivation to facilitate studies of biological properties of pneumococcal surface protein A (PspA). J. Exp. Med. **165**:381–394.

36. **McIntyer, P.** 1997. Epidemiology and prevention of pneumococcal disease. Commun. Dis. Intell. **21**:41–45.

37. **Nahm, M.H., J.V. Olander, and M. Magyarlaki.** 1997. Identification of cross-reactive antibodies with low opsonophagocytic activity for *S. pneumoniae*. J. Infect. Dis. **176**:698–703.

38. **O'Brien, K.L., M.C. Steinhoff, K. Edwards, H. Keyserling, M.L. Thoms, and D. Madore.** 1996. Immunologic priming of young children by pneumococcal glycoprotein conjugate, but not polysaccharide, vaccines. Pediatr. Infect. Dis. J. **15**:425–430.

39. **Park, M.K., Y. Sun, J.V. Olander, J.W. Hoffmann, and M.H. Nahm.** 1996. The repertoire of human antibodies to the carbohydrate capsule of *Streptococcus pneumoniae* 6B. J. Infect. Dis **174**:75–82.

40. **Paton, J.C., R.A. Lock, C.-J. Lee, J.P. Li, A.M. Berry, T.J. Mitchell, P.W. Andrew, D. Hansman, and G.J. Bulnois.** 1991. Purification and immunogenicity of genetically obtained pneumolysin toxoids and their conjugation to *Streptococcus pneumoniae* type 19F polysaccharide. Infect. Immunol. **59**:2297–2304.

41. **Paton, J.S.** 1996. The contribution of pneumolysin to the pathogenicity of *Streptococcus pneumoniae*. Trends Microbiol. **4**:103–106.

42. **Rennels, M.B., K.M. Edwards, H.L. Keyserling, K.S. Reisinger, D.A. Hogerman, D.V. Madore, I. Chang, P.R. Paradiso, F.J. Malinoski, and A. Kimura.** 1998. Safety and immunogenicity of heptavalent pneumococcal vaccine conjugated to CRM197 in United States infants. Pediatrics **101**:604–611.

43. **Robbins, J.B., R. Austrian, C.-J. Lee, S.C. Rastogi, G. Schiffman, J. Henrichsen, P.H. Makela, C.V. Broome, R.R. Facklam, R.H. Tiesjema, and J.C. Parke, Jr.** 1983. Considerations for formulating the second-generation pneumococcal capsular polysaccharide vaccine with emphasis on the cross-reactive types within groups. J. Infect. Dis. **148**:1136–1159.

44. **Rosenow, C., P. Ryan, J.N. Weiser, S. Johnson, P. Fontan, A. Ortqvist, and H.R. Masure.** 1997. Contribution of novel choline-

binding proteins to adherence, colonization and immunogenicity of *Streptococcus pneumoniae*. Mol. Microbiol. **25:**819–829.

45. **Rubins, J.B., D. Charboneau, C. Fashing, A.M. Berry, J.C. Paton, J.E. Alexander, P.W. Andrew, T.J. Mitchell, and E.N. Janoff.** 1996. Distinct roles for pneumolysin's cytotoxic and complement activities in pathogenesis of pneumococcal pneumonia. Am. J. Respir. Crit. Care Med. **153:**1339–1346.

46. **Rubins, J.B., P.G. Duane, D. Clawson, D. Charboneau, J. Young, and D.E. Niewoehner.** 1993. Toxicity of pneumolysin to pulmonary alveolar epithelial cells. Infect. Immunol. **61:**1352–1358.

47. **Rubins, J.B., P.G. Duane, and E.N. Janoff.** 1992. Toxicity of pneumolysin to pulmonary endothelial cells in vitro. Infect. Immunol. **60:**1740–1746.

48. **Shapiro, E.D., A.T. Berg, R. Austrian, D. Schroeder, V. Parcells, A. Margolis, R.K. Adair, and J.D. Clemmens.** 1991. Protective efficacy of polyvalent pneumococcal polysaccharide vaccine. N. Engl. J. Med. **325:**1453–1460.

49. **Sheffield, J.S., W.H. Benjamin, and L.M. McDaniel.** 1992. Detection of DNA in Southern blots by chemiluminescence is a sensitive and rapid technique. Biotechniques **12:**836–839.

50. **Shelly, M.A., H. Jacoby, G.J. Riley, B.T. Graves, M. Pichichero, and J.J. Treanor.** 1997. Comparison of pneumococcal polysaccharide and CRM$_{197}$ conjugated pneumococcal oligosaccharide vaccines in young and elderly adults. Infect. Immunol. **65:**242–247.

51. **Takala, A.K., J. Eskola, M. Leinonen, H. Kaythy, A. Nissinen, E. Pekkanen, and P.H. Makela.** 1991. Reduction of oropharyngeal carriage of *Haemophilus influenzae* type b (Hib) in children immunized with an Hb conjugate vaccine. J. Infect. Dis. **164:**982–986.

52. **Takashima, K., K. Tateda, T. Matsumoto, J. Iizawa, M. Nakao, and K. Yamaguchi.** 1997. Role of tumor necrosis factor alpha in pathogenesis of pneumococcal pneumonia in mice. Infect. Immunol. **65:**257–260.

53. **Talkington, D.F., B.G. Brown, J.A. Tharpe, A. Koening, and H. Russell.** 1996. Protection of mice against fatal pneumococcal challenge by immunization with pneumococcal surface adhesion A (Psa A). Microbial Pathog. **21:**17–22.

54. **Tart, R.C., L.S. McDaniel, B.A. Ralph, and D.E. Briles.** 1996. Truncated *Streptococcus pneumoniae* PspA molecules elicit cross-protective immunity against pneumococcal challenge in mice. J. Infect. Dis. **173:**380–386.

55. **Tuomanen, E.I., R. Austrian, and R. Masure.** 1995. Mechanisms of disease. N. Engl. J. Med. **332:**1280–1284.

56. **Vakil, M., D.E. Briles, and J.F. Kearney.** 1991. Antigen-independent selection of T15 idiotype during B-cell ontogeny in mice. Dev. Immunol. **1:**203–212.

57. **Virolainen, A., W. Russell, S. Rapola, D.E. Briles, and H. Käythy.** 1996. Human antibodies to pneumococcal surface protein A (PspA). ICAAC Abst. **36:**150.

58. **Watson, D.A., and D.M. Musher.** 1990. Interruption of capsule production in *Streptococcus pneumoniae* serotype 3 by insertion of transposon Tn*916*. Infect. Immunol. **58:**3135–3138.

59. **Wu, H.-Y., M. Nahm, Y. Guo, M. Russell, and D.E. Briles.** 1997. Intranasal immunization of mice with PspA (pneumococcal surface protein A) can prevent intranasal carriage and infection with *Streptococcus pneumoniae*. J. Infect. Dis. **175:**893–846.

60. **Wu, H.-Y., A. Virolainen, B. Mathews, J. King, M. Russell, and D.E. Briles.** 1997. Establishment of a *Streptococcus pneumoniae* nasopharyngeal model of pneumococcal carriage in adult mice. Microbial Pathog. **23:**127–137.

61. **Yother, J., and D.E. Briles.** 1992. Structural properties and evolutionary relationships of PspA, a surface protein of *Streptococcus pneumoniae,* as revealed by sequence analysis. J. Bacteriol. **174:**601–609.

62. **Yother, J., G.L. Handsome, and D.E. Briles.** 1992. Truncated forms of PspA that are secreted from *Streptococcus pneumoniae* and their use in functional studies and cloning of the *pspA* gene. J. Bacteriol. **174:**610–618.

63. **Yother, J., L.S. McDaniel, M.J. Crain, D.F. Talkington, and D.E. Briles.** 1991. Pneumococcal surface protein A: structural analysis and biological significance. *In* G.M. Dunny, P.P. Cleary, and L.L. McKay (ed.), Genetics and molecular biology of streptococci, lactococci, and enterococci. American Society for Microbiology, Washington, D.C., pp. 88–91.

64. **Yother, J., and J.M. White.** 1994. Novel surface attachment mechanism for the *Streptococcus pneumoniae* protein PspA. J. Bacteriol. **176:**2976–2985.

Address reprint requests to:
David E. Briles
University of Alabama at Birmingham
845 19th St. S., Rm. 658
Birmingham, AL 35294

Molecular Analysis of Putative Pneumococcal Virulence Proteins

JAMES C. PATON, ANNE M. BERRY, and ROBERT A. LOCK

ABSTRACT

Although the polysaccharide capsule has been recognized as a *sine qua non* of virulence, recent attention has focused on the role of pneumococcal proteins in pathogenesis, particularly in view of their potential as vaccine antigens. The contribution of pneumolysin, two distinct neuraminidases, autolysin, hyaluronidase, and the 37 kDa pneumococcal surface adhesin A has been examined by specifically mutagenizing the respective genes in the pneumococcal chromosome and examining the impact on virulence in animal models. The vaccine potential of these proteins has also been assessed by immunization of mice with purified antigens, followed by challenge with virulent pneumococci.

INTRODUCTION

In spite of the obvious importance of pneumococcal disease, until recently surprisingly little was known of the molecular mechanism whereby *Streptococcus pneumoniae* invades, damages, and in some cases, kills its host. Research in our laboratory has been aimed at understanding this process, with particular reference to the role of putative protein virulence determinants (see reference 20 for review). If such proteins were found to be essential for the invasiveness and virulence of the pneumococcus, then they might form the basis of novel vaccines. Such vaccine antigens would have two advantages; first, they may provide protection against all serotypes of *S. pneumoniae*; and second, they should be highly immunogenic in infants and young children, who generally respond well to protein antigens. The pneumococcal proteins could also be used as carriers for the less immunogenic capsular polysaccharide antigens in conjugate vaccine formulations.

The best characterized pneumococcal virulence protein is pneumolysin, a thiol-activated cytolysin, which is produced by virtually all clinical isolates of *S. pneumoniae*. The first direct evidence that pneumolysin contributes to the pathogenesis of disease was the finding that immunization of mice with purified toxin conferred a significant degree of protection against intranasal challenge with virulent *S. pneumoniae*.[21] Since then a substantial body of information on the structure and function of the toxin, its effects on human cells and tissues, and the manner in which it contributes to pathogenesis, has been assembled.[6,19] These studies, which are discussed in detail elsewhere in this volume, included examination of the effects of mutagenesis of the pneumolysin gene on virulence of *S. pneumoniae*. The fact that systemic virulence was reduced, but not abolished, indicated that although pneumolysin is an important virulence determinant, other pneumococcal products are also involved. In recent years we and others have been examining the contribution of other candidate virulence proteins by constructing strains of *S. pneumoniae* with defined mutations in the genes that encode them, and determining whether or not this has an impact on virulence in a mouse model. We have also purified some of these putative virulence proteins, from either *S. pneumoniae* or recombinant *Escherichia coli* and tested whether immunization with these antigens confers any protection against challenge with virulent pneumococci.

PNEUMOCOCCAL SURFACE PROTEIN A (PspA)

Pneumococcal surface protein A is a confirmed pneumococcal virulence protein, which has been extensively characterized at the genetic level.[29,31] Defined PspA-negative pneumococci have been shown to have significantly increased median survival time after intravenous challenge than their otherwise isogenic wild-type parents.[17] Also, immunization of mice with a purified truncated PspA confers protection against challenge with a variety of serotypes of *S. pneumoniae*.[29,30] A

Molecular Microbiology Unit, Women's and Children's Hospital, North Adelaide, S.A., 5006, Australia
Reprinted from *Microbial Drug Resistance*, Vol. 3, No. 1, 1997.

detailed examination of the genetics, structure, and function of PspA is also presented elsewhere in this volume.

AUTOLYSIN

The possible involvement of the major pneumococcal autolysin (LytA) in pathogenesis was suggested by the fact that pneumolysin is a cytoplasmic protein, that is released into the external medium when pneumococci undergo autolysis (e.g., at the end of the logarithmic phase of growth). When autolysis is blocked *in vitro* by growth of pneumococci in the presence of antibody to purified autolysin, pneumolysin activity remains cell-associated (Fig. 1). Thus, autolysin could contribute to pathogenesis by catalyzing the release of pneumolysin or other intracellular toxins in high local concentrations at the site of an infection, as well as by generating cell wall break-down products, which are highly inflammatory. To investigate this we constructed defined autolysin-negative type 2 and type 3 pneumococci and demonstrated that, like the pneumolysin-negative mutants, these strains were significantly less virulent than their otherwise isogenic parents[1,5] (Fig. 2). Also, immunization of mice with purified autolysin conferred a degree of protection against challenge with virulent pneumococci[1,14] (Fig. 3). However, immunization of mice with a combination of pneumolysin and autolysin did not increase the degree of protection from challenge with fully virulent pneumococci over that obtained by immunization with either antigen alone.[14] Also, immunization with autolysin did not provide any protection at all against challenge with high doses of pneumolysin-negative pneumococci.[14] These findings implied that the major contribution of autolysin to pneumococcal virulence in our animal model was

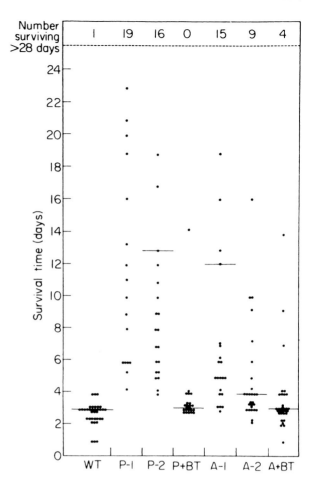

FIG. 2. Effect of mutagenesis of pneumolysin or autolysin genes on virulence of *S. pneumoniae* type 3. Groups of 36 mice were challenged intraperitoneally with 5×10^6 cfu of wild-type pneumococcus (WT), pneumolysin-negative pneumococci (P-1 and P-2), a pneumolysin-positive back-transformant of P-1 (P + BT), autolysin-negative pneumococci (A-1 and A-2), or an autolysin-positive back-transformant of A-1 (A + BT). The horizontal bar indicates median survival time for each group. (Reprinted with permission from *Microbial Pathogenesis.*[5])

to catalyze the release of pneumolysin. However, studies with the chinchilla model of otitis media, demonstrated that challenge with autolysin-negative pneumococci results in significantly lower inflammatory responses after penicillin therapy than challenge with either the wild-type or pneumolysin-negative strains.[26] Thus, it appears that the relative contribution of individual virulence factors may vary from one disease state or animal model to another.

NEURAMINIDASES

All fresh clinical isolates of *S. pneumoniae* appear to be capable of producing one or more neuraminidases. Such enzymes have the potential to cause great damage to the host by cleaving terminal sialic acid residues from a wide variety of glycolipids, glycoproteins and oligosaccharides on cell surfaces or in body fluids. Neuraminidases might also unmask potential cell

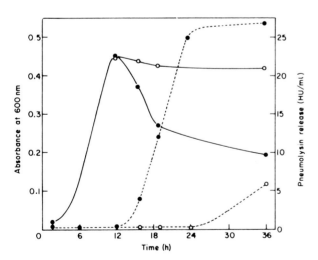

FIG. 1. Effect of anti-autolysin on cellular autolysis and release of pneumolysin. *S. pneumoniae* D39 was grown in THY medium supplemented with 0.5% control mouse serum (solid circles) or anti-autolysin serum (open circles). Growth of the culture was moniotored by Absorbance at 600 nm (unbroken line). Samples were also withdrawn at the indicated times and microfuged, prior to determination of the amount of pneumolysin in the culture supernatant by haemolysis assay (broken line). (Reprinted with permission from *Microbial Pathogenesis.*[14])

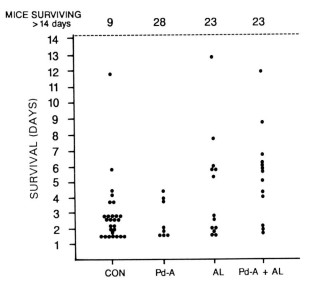

FIG. 3. Effect of immunization with autolysin (AL) and pneumolysoid (Pd-A), on survival time of mice challenged with *S. pneumoniae* D39. Mice were immunized with three doses of 20 μg of purified AL, Pd-A, or both antigens, or were sham-immunized (CON). Mice were then challenged intraperitoneally with 6.5 × 10³ cfu of D39 and their survival time was recorded. The number of mice in each group which were alive and well after 14 days is also indicated. (Reprinted with permission from *Microbial Pathogenesis*.[4])

surface receptors for putative pneumococcal adhesins.[13] A role for this enzyme in pathogenesis is also supported by an early observation that both coma and bacteremia occur significantly more often amongst patients with pneumococcal meningitis when the concentration of *N*-acetyl neuraminic acid in the cerebrospinal fluid is elevated.[18]

Direct assessment of the contribution made by neuraminidase to pneumococcal pathogenicity has been complicated by the fact that there appear to be multiple forms of the enzyme. Early studies suggested that pneumococcal neuraminidase existed as multiple isoenzymes, with sizes of approximately 70 kDa, but we have previously suggested that these are a consequence of proteolytic degradation of a parental enzyme. We purified a single 107 kDa neuraminidase species from *S. pneumoniae* lysates treated with protease inhibitors, but in the absence of these, several smaller (as low as 86 kDa) fully active forms were isolated.[15] We also demonstrated that the purified enzyme was toxic for mice when injected intraperitoneally. Interestingly, immunization with formaldehyde-treated 107 kDa neuraminidase conferred a significant degree of protection against challenge with virulent pneumococci, further suggesting a role for the enzyme in pathogenesis[16] (Fig. 4).

Camara *et al.*[7] cloned and sequenced a neuraminidase-encoding gene from *S. pneumoniae*, which they designated *nanA*. Although there is some ambiguity as to the precise translation initiation site for *nanA* (there are two in-frame ATG start codons preceded by ribosome binding sites), the most likely primary translation product would have a size of 112 kDa, including a hydrophobic signal peptide at its N-terminus. Cleavage of the signal peptide would yield a processed NanA of approximately 108 kDa, which is very close to our SDS-PAGE size estimate

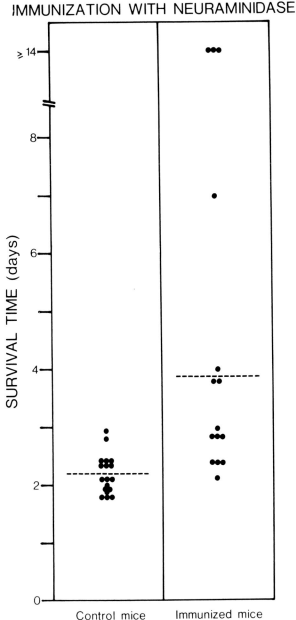

FIG. 4. Mice were immunized with three doses of 20 μg of purified 107 kDa neuraminidase (NanA), or were sham-immunized (Control). Mice were then challenged intraperitoneally with 6.5 × 10³ cfu of D39 and their survival time was recorded. The number of mice in each group which were alive and well after 14 days is also indicated. The broken line indicates median survival time for each group.

for the purified pneumococcal neuraminidase (107 kDa). Moreover, we have since subjected our purified enzyme to N-terminal amino acid sequence analysis and found the first nine residues to be QEGASEQPL, which is identical to that predicted for NanA after cleavage of the signal peptide (Lock and Paton, unpublished data). The C-terminus of NanA contains a typical Gram-positive cell surface anchorage domain (LPXTGE),[7] which is consistent with our earlier finding that the major portion of neuraminidase activity in pneumococcal cultures is cell-associated. Presumably neuraminidase could be released from the cells either by proteolytic cleavage or after cellular autolysis.

We used an internal fragment of *nanA* cloned in pVA891 to construct a derivative of *S. pneumoniae* D39 in which the *nanA* gene had been inactivated by insertion-duplication mutagenesis. In an intraperitoneal challenge model, this derivative was marginally less virulent than its D39 parent (median survival times were 1.44 days and 1.06 days, respectively; $P < 0.01$) (Fig. 5). However, although challenge of mice with a NanA-positive back-transformant of the mutant resulted in a lower median survival time (1.22 days), this difference (with respect to the NanA-negative strain) did not reach statistical significance (Fig. 5). We were also unable to detect a difference in virulence between D39 and the NanA-negative derivative in an intranasal challenge model. Interestingly, Mitchell *et al.* (unpublished studies) have also constructed a NanA-negative D39 derivative using a different mutagenesis vector, and demonstrated a significantly increased median survival time after intranasal challenge (2.7 days, compared with 2.0 days for mice challenged with D39). They also found lower numbers of pneumococci in both the blood and the lungs of mice challenged with their mutant rather than D39 (Mitchell *et al.*, unpublished studies). Differences in dose of pneumococci and susceptibility of the mouse strain may explain the apparent discrepancy.

Phenotypic characterization of our NanA-negative pneumococcus indicated that it still retained a small but significant amount of neuraminidase activity, which again raised the possibility that *S. pneumoniae* might produce more than one neuraminidase. This might also account for the rather modest impact of mutagenesis of *nanA* on virulence that we observed in our animal model. We have recently shown that there is indeed a second neuraminidase gene in *S. pneumoniae*.[2] This gene (designated *nanB*) is located on the pneumococcal chromosome approximately 4.5 kb downstream of *nanA*. *NanB* appears to be part of a large operon consisting of at least 6 open reading frames (ORFs) (Fig. 6). *NanA* is unlikely to be part of this operon, as there is a strong transcription termination sequence immediately downstream of this gene. Each of the six ORFs downstream of *nanA* have strong ribosome binding sites 6–8 bp 5′ to the initiation codon, but a consensus −10 and −35 promoter sequence was found only upstream (150–180 bp) of ORF-1. Moreover, there were no obvious transcription termination sequences downstream of any of ORFs 1–4 or *nanB*. The precise functions of ORFs 1–5 are not known, but comparison of their deduced amino acid sequences with those deposited with GenBank has provided some clues. First, ORFs 3 and 4 have a degree of homology (in both cases approximately 30% identity over 280 amino acids) with MsmF and MsmG, respectively. These are membrane proteins which form part of a

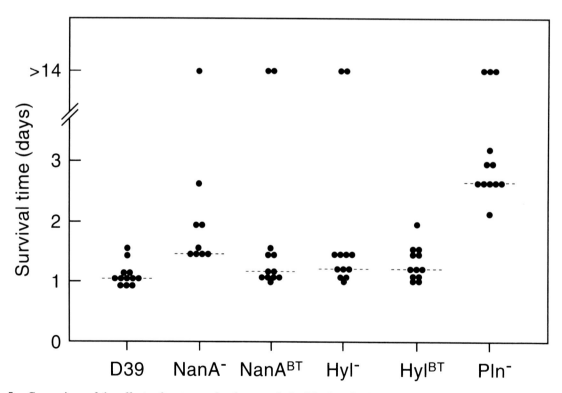

FIG. 5. Comparison of the effects of mutagenesis of pneumolysin, NanA or hyaluronidase genes on virulence of *S. pneumoniae* D39. Groups of 12-13 mice were challenged intraperitoneally with 3×10^3 cfu of wild-type D39, otherwise isogenic derivatives deficient in NanA (NanA⁻), hyaluronidase (Hyl⁻) or pneumolysin (Pln⁻), a NanA-positive back-transformant of NanA⁻ (NanA^BT), or a hyaluronidase-positive back-transformant Hyl⁻ (Hyl^BT). Survival time for each mouse, as well as the number of mice in each group which were alive and well after 14 days, was recorded. The broken line indicates median survival time for each group.

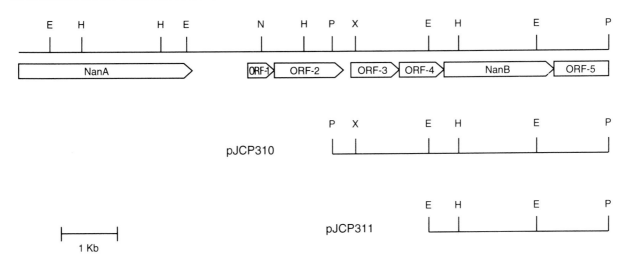

FIG. 6. Genetic map of a portion of the *S. pneumoniae* chromosome in the vicinity of *nanA* and *nanB*. The horizontal lines represent *S. pneumoniae* DNA subcloned in pBluescript (pJCP310 and pJCP311). Open reading frames (determined by sequence analysis) are indicated below the map. Restriction sites are abbreviated as follows: *E, Eco*RI; H, *Hind* III; N, *Nco*I; P, *Pst*I; X, *Xho*I. (Reprinted with permission from the *Journal of Bacteriology*.[2])

binding protein-dependent transport system in *S. mutans* responsible for multiple sugar metabolism.[24] ORF-2 contains a typical lipoprotein signal sequence and has a limited degree of homology (32% identity, 58% similarity, over 50 amino acids) with MsmE, the putative sugar-binding protein of the *msm* locus. Thus, it is possible that *nanB* is part of an operon encoding cleavage of *N*-acetyl neuraminic acid from host glycoproteins or glycolipids, as well as binding and transport of the sugar into the pneumococcus. The incomplete ORF-5 has a high degree of homology (65% identity over 347 amino acids) with a hypothetical 41.9-kDa *E. coli* protein of unknown function in the *leuX-fecE* intergenic region (GenBank accession number U14003).

NanB has a predicted size of 74.5 kDa, after cleavage of a 29 amino acid signal peptide. There is negligible amino acid homology between NanA and NanB, but NanB does exhibit limited homology (30% identity over 169 residues) with the sialidase of *Clostridium septicum*. The region of greatest homology includes an R-I-P motif that is found in the active site of other bacterial neuraminidases. NanB also contains three copies of the aspartate box consensus motif SXDXGXTW that is common to other neuraminidases.[22] NanB has been purified from recombinant *E. coli*, and found to have a pH optimum of 4.5, compared with pH 6.5 to 7.0 for NanA. SDS-PAGE analysis of purified NanB suggested that its size (approximately 65 kDa), was smaller than that predicted by the nucleotide sequence. This was not a consequence of incorrect assignment of the signal peptidase cleavage site, as this was confirmed by N-terminal amino acid sequence analysis of the purified enzyme. Neither was it an artifact of expression in *E. coli*, as Western blot analysis demonstrated that the apparent 65-kDa form was seen in both *S. pneumoniae* and recombinant *E. coli* lysates. Thus, the size discrepancy may be a consequence of anomalous behaviour on SDS-PAGE, and/or post-translational C-terminal processing. However, if C-terminal processing is taking place, cleavage must be occurring at similar sites in *S. pneumoniae* and *E. coli*. Proteolytic processing is not unprecedented for

pneumococcal neuraminidases, as we have previously reported for NanA.

At present, the benefits to the pneumococcus of production of two disctinct neuraminidases is unclear. NanA and NanB are both exported proteins with typical signal peptides, but NanB lacks the C-terminal cell surface anchorage domain found in NanA. This, combined with the widely different pH optima of the two enzymes may assist exploitation of distinct environmental niches. NanA also has a 100-fold higher specific activity than NanB when assayed using the fluorigenic substrate (2'-(4-methylumbelliferyl)-α-D-*N*-acetylneuraminic acid, but this may not hold for other potential substrates. NanA may not be more active than NanB in vivo if such differences in substrate preference exist.

In an attempt to determine whether NanB contributes to pathogenesis, we have examined whether immunization of mice with the purified enzyme confers protection against challenge with virulent pneumococci (Fig. 7). We observed a weak but significant protective effect (median survival times after intraperitoneal challenge were 2.25 days and 1.7 days for NanB-immunized and control mice, respectively, $P < 0.05$). We are currently in the process of constructing pneumococci deficient in the production of both NanA and NanB to determine the overall importance of neuraminidase in the pathogenesis of disease.

HYALURONIDASE

Virtually all strains of *S. pneumoniae* produce a hyaluronidase, which might contribute to pathogenesis by degradation of connective tissues, thereby facilitating invasion. We have characterized the hyaluronidase gene from a type 23 pneumococcus, which is sufficient to encode a 107 kDa polypeptide.[3] We also purified an active 89 kDa hyaluronidase from recombinant *E. coli* carrying this gene. N-terminal amino acid sequence analysis indicated that in *E. coli*, translation initiation was oc-

Intraperitoneal challenge: D39 (10⁵ CFU)

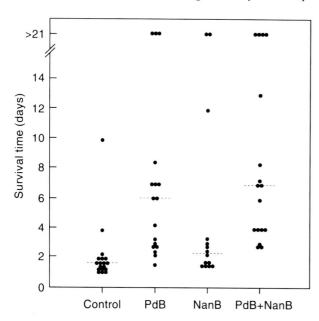

FIG. 7. Effect of immunization with NanB and pneumolysoid (PdB), on survival time of mice challenged with *S. pneumoniae* D39. Mice were immunized with three doses of 10 μg of purified NanB, PdB, or both antigens, or were sham-immunized (Control). Mice were then challenged intraperitoneally with 10^5 cfu of D39 and their survival time was recorded. The number of mice in each group which were alive and well after 21 days is also indicated. The broken line indicates median survival time for each group.

curring primarily at a TTG codon within the major ORF, thereby accounting for the smaller than expected size. Western blot analysis using antiserum raised against the purified 89 kDa hyaluronidase indicated that the *E. coli* clone also expressed the 107-kDa form of the enzyme and this antiserum labeled a 107 kDa protein in partially-purified hyaluronidase preparations from *S. pneumoniae*. The cellular location of hyaluronidase is uncertain. In fresh *S. pneumoniae* cultures, most of the enzyme activity is cell-associated, which is consistent with the presence of the Gram-positive cell surface anchorage domain (LPXTGE) near its C-terminus. However, the 107 kDa protein does not have a signal peptide at its N-terminus (assuming we have correctly assigned the translation initiation site), as would be expected for a typical exported protein. The involvement of hyaluronidase in pathogenesis also remains uncertain. To date we have not been able to demonstrate any protection in a mouse immunization/challenge model, and mutagenesis of the hyaluronidase gene in the pneumococcal chromosome does not have a detectable impact on virulence in a mouse intraperitoneal challenge model (Fig. 5). The role of hyaluronidase in a nasal colonization model is currently being assessed.

PNEUMOCOCCAL SURFACE ADHESIN A (PsaA)

The 37 kDa pneumococcal protein now referred to as PsaA (Pneumococcal surface adhesin A) was first detected by Rus-

sell *et al.*[23] using monoclonal antibodies and has attracted a lot of interest in recent years. Talkington *et al.*[28] have recently reported that immunization with purified PsaA protected mice from challenge with virulent *S. pneumoniae*. Indeed, PsaA is one of three pneumococcal proteins currently being considered as nonserotype-dependent vaccine antigens, along with pneumolysin and pneumococcal surface protein A (PspA). A clue as to the possible function of PsaA was provided by sequence analysis of the cloned *psaA* gene, which demonstrated a significant degree of homology with putative lipoprotein adhesins of *S. sanguis* and *S. parasanguis*.[25] However, the direct contribution of *psaA* to pathogenesis has not been studied previously.

In order to address this, a PCR-amplified internal region of the *psaA* gene cloned in pVA891 was used to interrupt the respective region of the chromosome of *S. pneumoniae* D39. The resultant *psaA*-negative pneumococcus (designated PsaA⁻₁) was virtually avirulent for mice in either an intraperitoneal or intranasal challenge model. The *psaA*-related genes in the oral streptococci have been shown to be part of complex operons consisting of up to 4 ORFs,[10] and Northern blot analysis has demonstrated that in *S. pneumoniae* the *psaA* transcript is at least 3 kb long.[25] Thus, although an intact *psaA* operon is clearly essential for virulence, this may be a consequence of polar effects on downstream sequences. We isolated the *S. pneumoniae* D39 *psaA*-encoding region by rescue of the pVA891 replicon, along with flanking sequences, from PsaA⁻₁. Sequence analysis of this DNA as well as additional flanking DNA isolated by inverse PCR, confirmed that there is one ORF (designated ORF3) commencing 123 nucleotides 3′ to *psaA*. There is no obvious transcription termination sequence between *psaA* and ORF3, but there is a very stable stemmed loop structure immediately downstream from ORF3. In view of this, we constructed two additional insertion-duplication mutants of *S. pneumoniae* D39, as shown in Fig. 8. The first of these (designated PsaA⁺) duplicates the 3′ end of *psaA*, thereby inserting the pVA891 sequences immediately downstream of the *psaA* termination codon, but keeping the gene itself intact. The second mutation interrupts ORF3. When the impact of these mutations on intranasal virulence was assessed, both PsaA⁺ and ORF3⁻ were as virulent as D39, in stark contrast to PsaA⁻₁ which was completely avirulent (Fig. 9). However, in the intraperitoneal challenge model, which employs much lower doses of the various *S. pneumoniae* derivatives (3×10^3 cfu [colony forming units] cf. 5×10^6 cfu for intranasal challenge), both PsaA⁺ and ORF3⁻ were less virulent than D39, as judged by survival time ($P < 0.01$ and $P < 0.001$, respectively) (Fig. 10). For ORF3⁻, the overall survival rate (6/12) was also significantly greater than that for D39 (0/12) ($P < 0.02$). Thus ORF3 appears to make a significant contribution to virulence in its own right. Nevertheless, this impact is still minor compared with PsaA⁻₁, which was significantly less virulent than D39 or the other two mutants, as judged by both survival time and overall survival rate. At higher intraperitoneal (IP) doses (10^6 cfu), PsaA⁻₁ remained avirulent, whereas ORF3⁻ was as virulent as D39 (result not presented).

The precise function of the various ORFs in the *psaA* operon are uncertain. The two ORFs upstream of *fimA*, the *psaA* homologue of *S. parasanguis*, encode an ATP-binding protein and a hydrophobic membrane protein with homology to members of a superfamily of ATP-binding membrane transport sys-

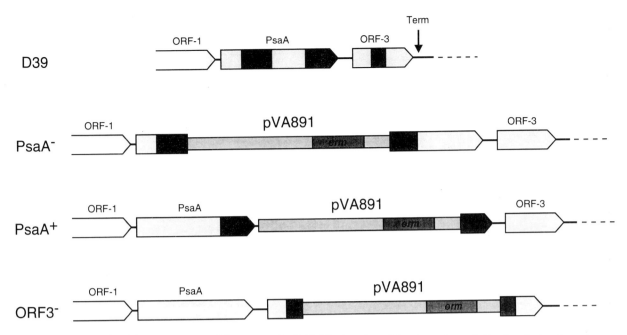

FIG. 8. Mutagenesis of the *psaA* operon of *S. pneumoniae* D39. The location of the strong transcription terminator downstream of ORF3 is shown on the map for D39, which also shows the regions subcloned into pVA891 for generation of mutants (shaded). For each of the D39 derivatives PsaA⁻, PsaA⁺ and ORF3⁻, the duplicated region of DNA is shaded. (Reprinted with permission from *Infection and Immunity.*[4])

tems.[10] However, the function of the downstream ORF3 (which shares 76% amino acid identity with *S. pneumoniae* D39 ORF3) is unknown. It is possible, however, that a functional ORF3 product is required for optimum expression of *PsaA*.

In view of the high degree of homology between PsaA and putative lipoprotein adhesins of other streptococci, we also examined the impact of mutagenesis of the psaA operon on adherence capacity of *S. pneumoniae*, using two different model systems. The first employed agglutination of neuraminidase-treated bovine erythrocytes as a model for adherence to receptors with exposed GlcNAcβ1-3Gal, the glycoconjugate implicated in attachment of pneumococci to oropharyngeal cells. No difference was observed between the degree of hemagglutination when either D39 or PsaA⁻$_1$ were tested at a concentration of 5×10^8 cfu/ml. The capacity of pneumococci to adhere directly to A549 cells (a type II pneumocyte cell line) was also examined. At a dose of 5×10^6 cfu, total adherence of *S. pneumoniae* D39 was 1090 ± 331 cfu/well, compared with 98 ± 18 cfu/well for PsaA⁻$_1$ ($P < 0.01$). Interestingly, the D39 derivative in which ORF3 had been interrupted exhibited intermediate adherence (255 ± 40 cfu/well), which was significantly different from that for both D39 ($P < 0.01$) and PsaA⁻$_1$ ($P < 0.01$). This finding is consistent with our observation that in the low dose intraperitoneal challenge model, the virulence of ORF3⁻ was intermediate between that of D39 and PsaA⁻$_1$. Interestingly, Cundell *et al.*[8] have recently reported that mutagenesis of either of two peptide permease loci (*plpA* and *ami*) significantly reduced adherence of pneumococci to both A549 cells and endothelial cells. However, these peptide permeases are unrelated to PsaA.

Sequence analysis of the *psaA* gene from the type 2 *S. pneu-* *moniae* strain D39 indicated significant deviation from that previously published for the homologue from *S. pneumoniae* R36A. The deduced amino acid sequence for the product of this gene (designated PsaA/D39) is shown in Fig. 11, aligned with

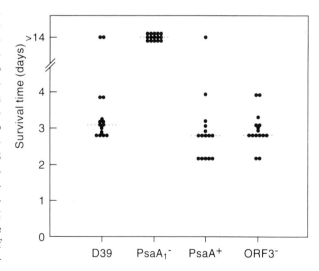

FIG. 9. Intranasal challenge. Groups of QS mice were challenged intranasally with approximately 5×10^6 cfu of the indicated strains. The survival time of each mouse is indicated. The broken lines denote the median survival time for each group. (Reprinted with permission from *Infection and Immunity.*[4])

Intraperitoneal Virulence: (3x10³ CFU)

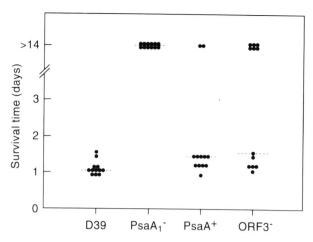

FIG. 10. Intraperitoneal challenge. Groups of QS mice were injected intraperitoneally with approximately 3×10^3 cfu of the indicated strains. The survival time of each mouse is indicated. The broken lines denote the median survival time for each group. (Reprinted with permission from *Infection and Immunity.*[4])

those published for PsaA from strain R36A (PsaA/R36A),[25] and the closely related putative fimbrial adhesins SsaB from *S. sanguis*,[11] FimA from *S. parasanguis*,[9] and ScaA from *S. gordonii*.[12] There was a similar degree of identity (77.4–79.9%) between PsaA/D39 and each of these proteins. Although substantial variation in amino acid sequence occurred in the signal peptide, the 12 residues at the N-termini of the mature polypeptides also showed minimal similarity with each other. Indeed, PsaA/D39 and PsaA/R36A have identical amino acids at only three of these 12 positions. The overall identity between mature PsaA/D39 and mature PsaA/R36A is 81%. The extent to which this may impact on the utility of PsaA as a pneumococcal vaccine antigen remains to be determined. Although immunofluorescent staining of intact pneumococci suggests that at least some epitopes are exposed on the cell surface,[23] at present there is insufficient information available to make predictions of the structure and localization of specific domains within PsaA. PsaA and the related streptococcal proteins all contain the prolipoprotein recognition sequence LXXC at the carboxyl end of their signal peptides, which might suggest that the N-terminus is closely associated with the cell membrane, anchored via an *N*-acyl glyceride cysteine. This prediction, however, is not supported by the immuno-electron micrographs of Fenno *et al.*[10] showing FimA localized at the tips of *S. parasanguis* fimbriae. Similar studies on the location of PsaA in *S. pneumoniae* are in progress.

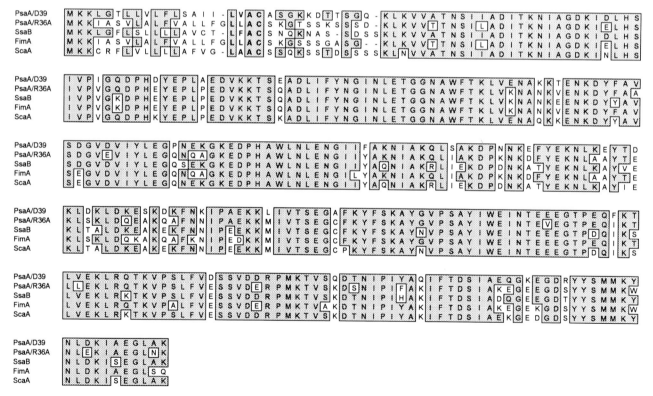

FIG. 11. Amino acid sequence alignment of PsaA/D39 and related proteins. The deduced amino acid sequence for PsaA/D39 was aligned with those published for PsaA from strain R36A (PsaA/R36A),[25] and the closely related putative fimbrial adhesins SsaB from *S. sanguis*,[11] FimA from *S. parasanguis*,[9] and ScaA from *S. gordonii*,[12] using the program CLUSTAL. Residues with identity to PsaA/D39 are boxed and shaded. The position of the consensus prolipoprotein cleavage site (LXXC) (residues 17-20 for PsaA/D39) in each of the proteins is shown in bold type. (Reprinted with permission from *Infection and Immunity.*[4])

CONCLUSIONS

Examination of the role of pneumococcal proteins in pathogenesis of disease is complicated by the fact that it is a multistep process, involving adherence to and colonization of mucosal surfaces, resistance to specific and nonspecific host defences, penetration and invasion of host tissues, and generation of tissue damage mediated either directly by toxins or indirectly via inflammatory responses. The relative contribution of specific virulence proteins may vary depending on the type of disease (e.g., pneumonia, bacteraemia, meningitis, otitis media, etc.). Interpretation may also be complicated by the degree to which a given animal model reflects the respective human condition. Notwithstanding these uncertainties, clear roles for pneumolysin, PspA, PsaA and probably NanA have been demonstrated. However, convincing evidence of a role for NanB and hyaluronidase is yet to be obtained. In addition to the above, other proteins are undoubtedly important. For example, peptide permeases encoded by *plpA* and the *ami* locus have been shown to contribute directly to adherence of pneumococci.[8] A pyruvate oxidase encoded by the *spxB* gene has also been shown to be important for adherence properties of pneumococci, and mutagenesis of *spxB* resulted in diminished virulence in animal models of colonization, pneumonia, and sepsis.[27] Analysis of the behavior of pneumococci carrying defined mutations in combinations of the above genes, in a range of animal models, is likely to provide further information on the molecular mechanism of pathogenesis of pneumococcal disease, and may well result in identification of further targets for protein-based vaccination.

REFERENCES

1. **Berry, A.M., R.A. Lock, D. Hansman, and J.C. Paton.** 1989. Contribution of autolysin to the virulence of *Streptococcus pneumoniae*. Infect. Immun. **57:**2324–2330.

2. **Berry, A.M., R.A. Lock, and J.C. Paton.** 1996. Cloning and nucleotide sequence of *nanB*, a second *Streptococcus pneumoniae* neuraminidase gene and purification of the NanB enzyme from recombinant *Escherichia coli*. J. Bacteriol. **178:**4854–4860.

3. **Berry, A.M., R.A. Lock, S.M. Thomas, D.P. Rajan, D. Hansman, and J.C. Paton.** 1994. Cloning and nucleotide sequence of the *Streptococcus pneumoniae* hyaluronidase gene and purification of the enzyme from recombinant *Escherichia coli*. Infect. Immun. **62:**1101–1108.

4. **Berry, A.M. and J.C. Paton.** 1996. Sequence heterogeneity of PsaA, a 37-kDa putative adhesin essential for virulence of *Streptococcus pneumoniae*. Infect. Immun. **64:** 5255–5262.

5. **Berry, A.M., J.C. Paton, and D. Hansman.** 1992. Effect of insertional inactivation of the genes encoding pneumolysin and autolysin on the virulence of *Streptococcus pneumoniae* type 3. Microb. Pathogen. **12:**87–93.

6. **Boulnois, G.J., J.C. Paton, T.J. Mitchell, and P.W. Andrew.** 1991. Structure and function of pneumolysin, the multifunctional, thiol-activated toxin of *Streptococcus pneumoniae*. Mol. Microbiol. **5:**2611–2616.

7. **Camara, M., G.J. Boulnois, P.W. Andrew, and T.J. Mitchell.** 1994. A neuraminidase from *Streptococcus pneumoniae* has the features of a surface protein. Infect. Immun. **62:**3688–3695.

8. **Cundell, D.R., B.J. Pearce, J. Sandros, A.M. Naughton, and H.R. Masure.** 1995. Peptide permeases from *Streptococcus pneu-

9. **Fenno, J.C., D.J. LeBlanc, and P. Fives-Taylor.** 1989. Nucleotide sequence analysis of a type 1 fimbrial gene of *Streptococcus sanguis* FW213. Infect. Immun. **57:**3527–3533.

10. **Fenno, J.C., A. Shaikh, G. Spatafora, and P. Fives-Taylor.** 1995. The *fimA* locus of *Streptococcus parasanguis* encodes an ATP-binding membrane transport system. Mol. Microbiol. **15:**849–863.

11. **Ganeshkumar, N., P.M. Hannam, P.E. Kolenbrander, and B.C. McBride.** 1991. Nucleotide sequence of a gene coding for a saliva binding protein (SsaB) from *Streptococcus sanguis* 12 and possible role of the protein in coaggregation with actinomyces. Infect. Immun. **59:**1093–1099.

12. **Kolenbrander, P.E., R.N. Andersen, and N. Ganeshkumar.** 1994. Nucleotide sequence of the *Streptococcus gordonii* PK488 coaggregation adhesin gene, *ScaA*, and ATP-binding cassette. Infect. Immun. **62:**4469–4480.

13. **Krivan, H.C., D.D. Roberts, and V. Ginsberg, V.** 1988. Many pulmonary pathogenic bacteria bind specifically to the carbohydrate sequence GalNAcβ1-4Gal found in some glycolipids. Proc. Natl. Acad. Sci. USA **85:**6157–6161.

14. **Lock, R.A., D. Hansman, and J.C. Paton.** 1992. Comparative efficacy of autolysin and pneumolysin as immunogens protecting mice against infection by *Streptotoccus pneumoniae*. Microb. Pathogen. **12:**137–143.

15. **Lock, R.A., J.C. Paton, and D. Hansman.** 1988. Purification and immunological characterization of neuraminidase produced by *Streptococcus pneumoniae*. Microb. Pathogen. **4:**33–43.

16. **Lock, R.A., J.C. Paton, and D. Hansman.** 1988. Comparative efficacy of pneumococcal neuraminidase and pneumolysin as immunogens protective against *Streptococcus pneumoniae* infection. Microb. Pathogen. **5:**461–467.

17. **McDaniel, L.S., J. Yother, M. Vijayakumur, L. McGarry, W.R. Guild, and D.E. Briles.** 1987. Use of insertional inactivation to facilitate studies of biological properties of pneumococcal surface protein A (PspA). J. Exp. Med. **165:**381–394.

18. **O'Toole, R.D., L. Goode, and C. Howe.** 1971. Neuraminidase activity in bacterial meningitis. J. Clin. Invest. **50:**979–985.

19. **Paton, J.C.** 1996. The contribution of pneumolysin to the pathogenicity of *Streptococcus pneumoniae*. Trends in Microbiology **4:**103–106.

20. **Paton, J.C., P.W. Andrew, G.J. Boulnois, and T.J. Mitchell.** 1993. Molecular analysis of the pathogenicity of *Streptococcus pneumoniae*: The role of pneumococcal proteins. Annu. Rev. Microbiol. **47:**89–115.

21. **Paton, J.C., R.A. Lock, and D. Hansman.** 1983. Effect of immunization with pneumolysin on survival time of mice challenged with *Streptococcus pneumoniae*. Infect. Immun. **40:**548–552.

22. **Roggentin, P., B. Rothe, J.B. Kaper, J. Galen, L. Lawrisuk, E.R. Vimr, and R. Schauer.** 1989. Conserved sequences in bacterial and viral sialidases. Glycoconjugate J. **6:**349–353.

23. **Russell, H., J.A. Tharpe, D.E. Wells, E.H. White, and J.E. Johnson.** 1990. Monoclonal antibody recognizing a specific protein from *Streptococcus pneumoniae*. J. Clin. Microbiol. **28:**2191–2195.

24. **Russell, R.R.B., J. Aduse-Opoku, I.C. Sutcliffe, L. Tao, and J.J. Ferretti.** 1992. A binding protein-dependent transport system in *Streptococcus mutans* responsible for multiple sugar metabolism. J. Biol. Chem. **267:**4631–4637.

25. **Sampson, J.S., S.P. O'Connor, A.R. Stinson, J.A. Tharpe, and H. Russell.** 1994. Cloning and nucleotide sequence analysis of psaA, the *Streptococcus pneumoniae* gene encoding a 37-kilodalton protein homologous to previously reported *Streptococcus* sp. adhesins. Infect. Immun. **62:**319–324.

26. **Sato, K., M.K. Quartey, C.L. Liebeler, C.T. Le, and G.S. Giebink.** 1996. Roles of autolysin and pneumolysin in middle ear

moniae affect adherence to eucaryotic cells. Infect. Immun. **63:**2493–2498.

inflammation caused by a type 3 *Streptococcus pneumoniae* strain in the chinchilla otitis media model. Infect. Immun. **64:**1140–1145.

27. **Spellerberg, B., D.R. Cundell, J. Sandros, B.J. Pearce, I. Idän-pään-Heikkilä, C. Rosenow, and H.R. Masure.** 1996. Pyruvate oxidase, as a determinant of virulence in *Streptococcus pneumoniae*. Mol. Microbiol. **19:**803–813.

28. **Talkington, D.F., B.G. Brown, J.A. Tharpe, A. Koenig, and H. Russell.** 1996. Protection of mice against fatal pneumococcal challenge by immunization with pneumococcal surface adhesin A (PsaA). Microb. Pathogen. **21:**17–22.

29. **Talkington, D.F., D.L. Crimmins, D.C. Voellinger, J. Yother, and D.E. Briles.** 1991. A 43-kilodalton pneumococcal surface protein, PspA: Isolation, protective abilities and structural analysis of the amino terminal sequence. Infect. Immun. **59:**1285–1289.

30. **Tart, R.C., L.S. McDaniel, B.A. Ralph, and D.E. Briles.** 1995. Truncated *Streptococcus pneumoniae* PspA molecules elicit pro-tective immunity against fatal pneumococcal challenge in mice, abstr. B65. *In* Abstracts of the 35th Interscience Conference on Antimicrobial Agents and Chemotherapy. American Society for Microbiology, Washington, D.C.

31. **Yother, J., G.L. Handsome, and D.E. Briles.** 1992. Truncated forms of PspA that are secreted from *Streptococcus pneumoniae* and their use in functional studies and cloning of the *pspA* gene. J. Bacteriol. **174:**610–618.

Address reprint requests to:
James C. Paton
Molecular Microbiology Unit
Women's and Children's Hospital
North Adelaide, S.A., 5006, Australia

Relationship of Structure to Function in Pneumolysin

PETER W. ANDREW, TIMOTHY J. MITCHELL, PETE MORGAN, and ROBERT J.C. GILBERT

INTRODUCTION

PORE-FORMING TOXINS probably represent the largest group of bacterial toxins. Within this group of toxins there is a family that requires activation by the addition of thiol-reducing agents when they are present in crude preparations. These thiol-activated toxins (TATs) are produced by four genera of Gram-positive bacteria, *Streptococcus*, *Listeria*, *Clostridium*, and *Bacillus*. Pneumolysin is the TAT produced by *Streptococcus pneumoniae.*

Pneumolysin in a purified form is extremely lethal to animals and doubtless to humans also. *In vitro*, it lyses all eukaryotic cells tested, but for reasons of convenience most work is done with erythrocytes as the target cells, and hence the toxin is often referred to as a hemolysin. At sublytic concentrations pneumolysin modulates the activity of various mammalian tissues and isolated cells, inhibiting some cellular activities[7,33,39,46] but also activating others.[13,45] In addition to these anticellular activities, the toxin can activate the classical complement pathway independently of antipneumolysin antibodies.[40] Activation is, however, dependent on the presence of immunoglobulin and is believed to be linked to the ability of pneumolysin to bind IgGFc.[26] Such interactions between pneumolysin and cells and soluble molecules of the immune system probably explain why pneumolysin has a prominent role in pneumococcal disease.[5,44] These *in vitro* and *in vivo* activities of pneumolysin are reviewed in fuller detail elsewhere in this volume. This review addresses the mode of action of pneumolysin and how the structure of the toxin has been related to its function.

GENERAL PROPERTIES OF PNEUMOLYSIN

In common with other TATs, pneumolysin is inactivated by exposure to oxygen in a manner reversible by thiol reducing agents. This property, however, is only apparent in crude preparations. When pure, the toxins are not oxygen labile and hence are no longer activated by thiol-reducing agents because they are fully active. Pneumolysin shares a further distinguishing feature with other members of the family, in that lytic and other anticellular activities are irreversibly inhibited by nanomolar quantities of cholesterol. The ability to activate complement is not inhibited by oxygen or cholesterol. Not surprisingly, pneu-molysin is antigenically related to the other TATs. Polyclonal antiserum against another member of the family will precipitate and neutralize pneumolysin. Unlike other members of the family, pneumolysin is synthesized without a signal peptide[52] and is intracytoplasm[17] only being released when the bacterium lyses under the influence of autolysin or lytic antibiotic.

MODE OF ACTION: WHAT IS KNOWN AND UNKNOWN

It is believed that pneumolysin, and other TATs, share a common mode of anticellular action involving two steps. In the first step monomeric, water-soluble toxin binds to the membrane of the target cell. It is presumed that the monomers then move laterally, self-associate and form oligomeric structures, seen as arcs and rings by electron microscopy (Fig. 1).[30] This series of events involves several poorly understood protein-protein and protein-lipid interactions. The details of several aspects of this hypothesis of pore formation remain to be determined for pneumolysin.

Two pieces of evidence favor the two-step hypothesis of pore formation. Firstly, binding of pneumolysin is apparently independent of temperature, whereas oligomerization is dependent on it. Secondly, some monoclonal antibodies block oligomerization but have no effect on binding,[6] indicating that binding precedes oligomerization. Similar observations have been seen with streptolysin, the TAT of *Streptococcus pyo-genes.*[14]

There are data, however, that oppose this simple view and suggest that oligomerization occurs in the absence of cells but probably with much reduced efficiency. Data from application of a combination of analytical ultracentrifugation techniques indicate that a dimeric toxin form of pneumolysin occurs even at low concentrations and that oligomerization occurs in a concentration-dependent manner.[9] The oligomers formed appear to have the same form as those previously associated exclusively with membrane interaction. The fact that oligomerization occurs spontaneously in solution may offer the opportunity of shedding light on the mechanism by which it occurs on the cell membrane.

The mechanism of binding of pneumolysin to mammalian cells is not understood. It is generally assumed that the cell receptor is cholesterol,[1] but definitive proof is lacking. Amongst

Department of Microbiology and Immunology, University of Leicester, Leicester, U.K.

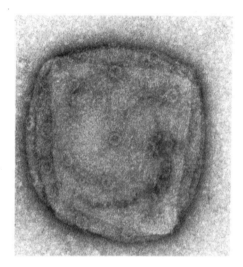

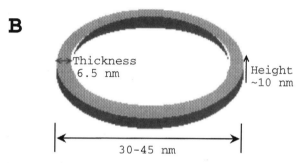

FIG. 1. (**A**) Electron micrograph of oligomeric pneumolysin pores formed in a red blood cell ghost visualized using negative staining. Bar = 100 nm. (**B**) Representation of ring showing dimensions. (Reprinted with permission from Morgan et al.[30])

the evidence supporting this conclusion is the observation that cells which do not contain cholesterol in their membranes are insensitive to lysis by TATs.[1] Also, cytolysis by pneumolysin, and other TATs is irreversibly inhibited by free cholesterol.[1] However, it is possible to obtain pneumolysin pores in planar lipid bilayers with ergosterol but not cholesterol.[20,21] An alternative hypothesis, although not mutually exclusive, is that cholesterol functions to stabilize oligomers in membranes. A recent report suggested that the role of cholesterol is more involved with pore formation than with binding.[16]

It is unclear if insertion of pneumolysin into the target membrane precedes oligomerization, in which case it is monomers that insert, or if oligomerization occurs on the membrane surface before insertion. Indeed what is the mechanism that takes pneumolysin into the membrane? The pattern of assembly of pneumolysin oligomers and the relation of arcs to rings also is unknown. A recent analysis of the kinetics of self-assembly of streptolysin concluded that oligomerization begins with association of two membrane-bound monomers and then continues with the sequential addition of further subunits.[37] A detailed analysis of the kinetics of binding and oligomerization of pneumolysin remains to be determined.

The arc and ring structures are thought to be transmembrane pores, the presence of which results in cell lysis or modulation in cell activity. Pneumolysin is able to induce leakage of solutes from erythrocytes, nucleated cells, liposomes,[21] and conductance through planar lipid bilayers.[20] Leakage and conductance is inhibited by divalent cations and conductance is voltage-dependent. The divalent cations do not prevent formation of the pore or displace it from the membrane, rather they maintain the pores in a nonleaky state.[20,21]

Pneumolysin does not form uniform channels. Voltage-sensitive channels formed in planar lipid bilayers can be categorized as small (conductance <50 pSiemens), medium (50–1,000 pS), or large (>1 nS) on the basis of conductance.[20,21] It is the small and medium sized channels that are primarily closed by divalent cations but the biological significance of these observations is not clear. If the arcs and rings truly represent transmembrane channels, it is a conundrum how the bulk flow through such structures with apparently large apertures (30–40 nm) is inhibited by divalent cations and voltage changes. In considering the flow of solutes, the internal volume of the pores is important, but it is a parameter that is unknown.

It is presumed that the presence of pores allows an influx of water and this eventually leads to cell lysis; a process known as colloid-osmotic lysis.[47] It is noteworthy, however, that a related toxin, listeriolysin from *Listeria monocytogenes*, has been shown to bring about cell death by apoptosis in some cells.[10] Formation of pores by pneumolysin does not inevitably lead to lysis,[21] but the molecular events that link exposure to sublytic amounts of toxin to the changes in activity of cells are not known. There is some evidence that cells can recover from exposure to pneumolysin,[21] but the mechanism is unknown. Cells, other than erythrocytes, do recover from exposure to other cytolysins.[2,4] It may be significant that phagocytes become more resistant to pneumolysin after exposure to interferon-γ (our unpublished data).

We have sought to understand the mechanisms of toxicity of pneumolysin by the determination of the structure of the monomer, the use of mutagenetic and chemical strategies to probe the role of individual regions in the protein, and the determination of the structure of the oligomer.

RELATIONSHIP OF STRUCTURE TO FUNCTION

Structure of the monomer and relationship to anticellular activity

Pneumolysin is a polypeptide of 470 amino acids with a molecular weight of 52,800, calculated from the deduced amino acid sequence.[52] Comparison of amino acid sequences deduced from the gene sequence of two pneumococcal isolates, a type 1 and a type 2, revealed only a single amino acid difference.[28] The far-UV circular dichroism spectrum for pneumolysin predicts 36% β-sheet and 31% α-helix.[31] A similar picture is seen with perfringolysin.[32] Hydropathy plots from the primary amino acid sequence do not show any significant regions of hydrophobicity; rather a hydrophilic molecule. It appears that pneumolysin is an example of a growing number of bacterial toxins which share the properties of being a protein of hydrophilic character and lacking hydrophobic regions, being rich in β-sheet and needing to oligomerize to form channels. These toxins have been called hydrophilic channel-forming proteins and include aerolysin from *Aeromonas* spp. and hemolysins from *Vibrio* and *Pseudomonas* spp.[38]

The crystal structure of the closely related TAT, perfringolysin from *Clostridium perfringens*, has recently been solved.[42] Perfringolysin has 48% sequence identity and 60% sequence similarity to pneumolysin.[43] A homology model of pneumolysin based on perfringolysin has been constructed and a mechanistic model proposed.[43] Figure 2 shows this structure, with its four domains and N- and C-termini labeled. The structure predominately consists of β-sheet, as predicted from CD measurements, arranged in a complex fold. As described below, the fourth domain is expected to contain the site involved

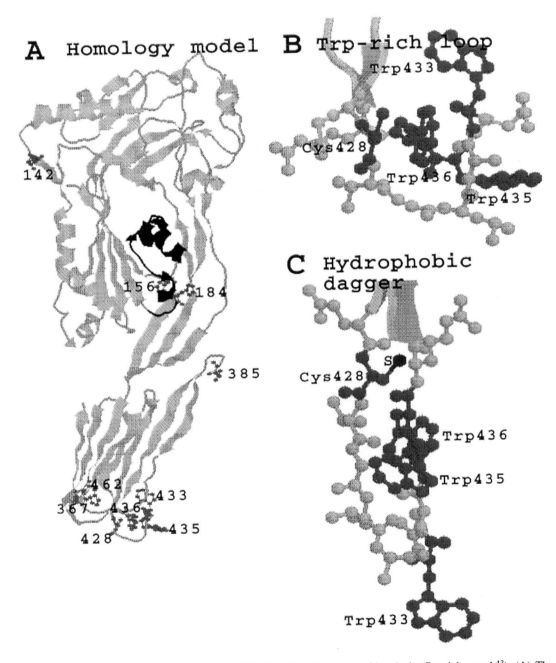

FIG. 2. Structure of the pneumolysin monomer modelled by homology to perfringolysin (Rossjohn et al.[43]). (**A**) The whole structure, with domains 1–4 and the N- and C-termini labeled. The secondary structure is shown in yellow as a ribbon representation. Residues known to be important from mutation, antibody, and proteolytic analyses are shown in red ball-and-stick representation. The region of domain 3 (residues 158–187) thought from spectroscopic assays to be involved in membrane penetration is shown as a white ribbon. (**B**) An expanded view of the Trp-rich loop in the region of which pneumolysin binds the membrane. (**C**) A view of the Trp-rich loop in its presumed conformation following binding to cholesterol.

in cell binding by pneumolysin, while the third domain is proposed to be involved in membrane insertion and pore formation. The second domain seems to act as a linker between the head and tail of the molecule, while the upper surface of the first domain consists entirely of negatively charged amino acids, which may have a role in the orientation of the molecule with respect to the membrane.

Pneumolysin only contains one cysteine residue, at position 428, which is labeled in Fig. 2. Analysis of the available sequences of other TATs showed that they too only possess one cysteine residue,[8,11,19,23,51,54] except for ivanolysin from Listeria ivanovi, which has two cysteines.[11] The presence of a single cysteine in TATs is inconsistent with the models for thiol activation involving reduction of intramolecular disulphide bonds, that had previously been expounded.[50] The single cysteine is within an eleven amino acid sequence, ECTGLAWEWWR, the Trp-rich motif, lying towards the C-terminus of the molecule. In addition to being rich in tryptophans, this region was likely to be significant because it is the largest region of identity between the TATs. Changes to various amino acids in this group of residues reduced hemolytic activity, but it was the conversion Trp433 > Phe that had the most dramatic effect, causing a greater than 99% loss of cytotoxicity.[25] Pneumolysin is thought to bind cholesterol at a site close to the Trp-rich motif, leading to the ejection of Trp433 from its hydrophobic pocket (Fig. 2B). The resulting refolding of the loop forms a hydrophobic dagger (Fig. 2C), which pierces the membrane and may associate its Trp residues with the cholesterol ring system. The main findings pointing to the role of this region in both binding and pore formation by pneumolysin are summarized below.

The substitution of the cysteine by alanine had no effect on the activity of pneumolysin and thus ruled out an essential role for its thiol group.[46] Similar experiments with other TATs resulted in the same conclusion.[24,41] Further mutagenesis experiments, however, showed that the amino acid at position 428 of pneumolysin is important. Substitution of the cysteine with serine or glycine substantially reduced cytolytic activity.[46] The derivatization of the cysteine with a benzyl moiety inhibits both cell-binding[15,53] and self-interaction of pneumolysin,[9] demonstrating that the fourth domain mediates binding and self-association of toxin and more specifically that this involves the region containing Cys-428. Interestingly, according to the homology model, this region adopts a β-sandwich fold highly reminiscent of both the Fc domain of IgG and the amyloidogenic human serum protein.[9]

Although a series of mutants in domain 4 display much-reduced activities, the pneumolysin toxoids are still capable of both cell-binding and oligomerization. Clearly, oligomer formation per se is not enough to bring about target cell lysis. Either the arrangement of toxin monomers within the oligomer, and/or the alignment of the oligomers in the membrane, may be crucial for lysis to occur. We have suggested before[3] that the cysteine region plays a role in orientation of pneumolysin, and other TATs, in cell membranes. This suggestion was based on a proposal by de Kruijff.[22] The antibiotic, gramicidin A, has four tryptophan residues towards the C-terminus of the molecule and, like the TATs, forms channels in membranes. De Kruijff[22] proposed that the tryptophan residues interact with the nucleus of cholesterol to correctly orientate gramicidin A in the

membrane. As mentioned above, we believe that pneumolysin may associate the Trp-rich motif with cholesterol in a comparable way.

Further evidence that the cysteine region is important for the functioning of the channels came when we found that channels, formed in cells and planar lipid bilayers by the TrP433 > Phe modified toxin were less sensitive to closure by divalent cations and that there was an increase in the proportion of large conductance channels in these bilayers.[21] Disruption of the entire fourth domain by deletion of the C-terminal 6 amino acids eradicated hemolytic activity and reduced binding by 98%.[35] Also a point mutation close to this region, Pro462 > Ser, caused a 90% decrease in cell binding.[35] Further evidence for the importance of this region in cell binding, came from the demonstration that a monoclonal antibody that neutralizes hemolytic activity and blocks binding, recognizes an epitope within the six C-terminal amino acids.[6] A second monoclonal antibody, which recognizes an epitope around residue 419, also blocked binding. Like the C-terminus, residue 419 resides in domain 4, and the effects of antibody binding at both of these sites are likely to be due to prevention of interaction by cell-binding regions of domain 4 with the membrane. The degree of insertion of domain 4 into the membrane is unknown, but is thought only to involve the Trp-rich motif in interaction with the hydrophobic interior of the bilayer.[32]

Mutants in other regions of the molecule also have reduced activities against cells. Histidines were shown to be important in anticellular activity when chemical modification of pneumolysin with diethyl pyrocarbonate resulted in abolition of hemolytic activity.[27] Pneumolysin contains eight histidines, one of which is conserved in the TATs: position 367 in pneumolysin. The modification His367 > Arg caused a >99% loss of activity. This mutant was able to bind cells but had vastly reduced ability to form oligomers.[25] Other histidines have also been shown to be important in pore formation by pneumolysin. Mutation of the residue His156 occurring within domain 3 severely reduces the activity of pneumolysin.[12] His156 along with His184 brackets a region of domain 3 predicted from experiments on perfringolysin to insert into the membrane during pore formation.[49] The membrane-inserted region of domain 3, stretching from residues 158–187 has a helical structure in the monomeric toxin (Fig. 2A), but undergoes a transition to an amphipathic β-sheet on membrane insertion.[49] This is the first helical-to-sheet transition observed for a pore-forming toxin. Domain 3 has also been implicated in membrane insertion by experiments on streptolysin.[36] Interestingly, a monoclonal antibody that recognizes an epitope close to this histidine, at around position 142, had no effect on binding but abolished oligomerization.[6] We believe that following cell binding via the fourth domain and the refolding and membrane insertion of the cysteine-containing region, domain 3 refolds to form a pore-forming structure within the bilayer. Spectroscopic studies of both perfringolysin and pneumolysin have suggested that membrane insertion by TATs is accompanied by only modest changes in secondary structure.[32,43] It may therefore be that rearrangements in secondary structure are limited to the three small helices in domain 3. Despite the identification of pneumolysin residues 158–187 as a membrane-insertion region, the identity of the residues lining the pore, that participate in flow through the pore, respond to voltage changes and to which divalent cations bind, is at best a matter of speculation and largely is unknown.

Relationship to complement activating activity

None of the mutations discussed above altered the ability of pneumolysin to activate the classical complement cascade. A clue to the identity of some of the amino acids involved came when we found that two distinct regions of pneumolysin had limited homology to two contiguous regions of the human acute phase molecule C-reactive protein, CRP. This was a significant observation because CRP also is able to activate the classical complement cascade independently of specific antibody.[18] Site-directed mutations within one of these regions of pneumolysin, residues 368–397 in domain 4, had marked effects on complement activation and on binding of IgGFc[26] and one change, Asp385 > Asn, completely abolished complement activation by pneumolysin. This change also resulted in a substantial, although not complete, reduction in binding of IgGFc in the absence of which activation of complement by pneumolysin does not occur.[26] The binding of Fc is fundamental to the way in which pneumolysin activates the complement system.[26] The structure of the fourth toxin domain is in fact very similar to that of Fc, as discussed above, and is associated with other proteins which undergo self-interaction.[9] As a result we have proposed that the mechanism of complement activation employed by pneumolysin may involve association between domain 4 and Fc based on their similar folds.

STRUCTURE OF THE OLIGOMER

Large arc and ring structures can be seen in cell membranes and liposomes treated with pneumolysin (Fig. 1).[29,30] These structures are approximately 30–40 nm in diameter, and the width of the rings is approximately 6.5 nm. The dimensions of the arc and rings are identical whether they are in liposomes or cells. Negative stain electron microscopy combined with image analysis has been used to investigate the organization of pneumolysin monomers within the ring structures. Analysis of the rotational symmetry gave a subunit number variable within the range of 40–50.[29] The negatively stained images were used to produce a protein density map in which the oligomers appear as two concentric rings of protein density, separated by a gap of lower protein density.[29] A similar picture was seen with the oligomers of perfringolysin.[34] Two concentric rings of protein density also were seen in the oligomers of streptolysin and this was interpreted as being due to two rings of protein subunits.[48] We disagree with this view and instead propose that the two rings of protein density represent a single ring of subunits.

It is possible to isolate the oligomers by exposure of pneumolysin-treated cells to deoxycholate. Metal shadowing of these isolated oligomers enable their height to be estimated as 9.3 nm.[30] Another measure of the height of the oligomers was obtained by happenstance. At high concentrations of pneumolysin in presence of liposome, stacks of toxin oligomers are formed. These stacks of oligomers lay on their sides on mica grids enabling direct measurement of the height, at approximately 10 nm.[29] Based on our analysis of the structure of the pneumolysin oligomers and monomers, our working model for pneumolysin

oligomers is that each subunit of the oligomer is made up of four domains packed in a square planar arrangement.

ACKNOWLEDGMENTS

We are grateful to the colleagues who have collaborated with us on this project, including C.L. Bashford, O. Byron, J.R. de los Toyos, F.J. Mendez, C.A. Pasternak, J.C. Paton, M.W. Parker, J. Rossjohn, A.J. Rowe, H.R. Saibil, R. Sowdhamini, and R.K. Tweten.

REFERENCES

1. **Alouf, J.E., and C. Geoffroy.** 1991. The family of the antigenically related cholesterol binding (sulphydryl activated) cytolytic toxins. *In* J.E. Alouf and J.H. Freer (eds.), Source of bacterial protein toxins. Academic Press, New York, pp. 147–186.

2. **Bashford, C.L., G. Menestrina, P.A. Henkart, and C.A. Pasternak.** 1988. Spontaneous recovery and reversible inhibition by divalent cations. J. Biol. Chem. **141:**3965–3974.

3. **Boulnois, G.J., T.J. Mitchell, F.K. Saunders, R.H.G. Owen, J.R. Canvin, R. Wilson, C. Feldman, L. Bashford, C. Pasternack, and P.W. Andrew.** 1990. The protein virulence factors of *Streptococcus pneumoniae. In* G.M. Dunny, P.P. Cleary, and L.L. McKay. Genetics and molecular biology of Streptococci, Lactococci and Enterococci. ASM, Washington, D.C., pp. 83–87.

4. **Campbell, A.K. and B.P. Morgan.** 1985. Monoclonal antibodies demonstrate protection of polymorphonuclear leukocytes against complement attack. Nature **317:**164–166.

5. **Canvin, J.R., A.P. Marvin, M. Sivakumaran, J.C. Paton, G.J. Boulnois, P.W. Andrew, and T.J. Mitchell.** 1995. The role of pneumolysin and autolysin in the pathology of pneumonia and septicaemia in mice infected with a type 2 pneumococcus. J. Infect. Dis. **172:**119–123.

6. **de los Toyas, J.R., F.J. Mendez, J.F. Aparico, F. Vazquez, M.M.G. Suarez, A. Fleites, C. Hardisson, P.J. Morgan, P.W. Andrew, and T.J. Mitchell.** 1996. Functional analysis of pneumolysin by use of monoclonal antibodies. Infect. Immunol. **64:**480–484.

7. **Feldman, C., T.J. Mitchell, P.W. Andrew, G.J. Boulnois, S.C. Reed, H.C. Todd, P.J. Cole, and R. Wilson.** 1990. The effect of *Streptococcus pneumoniae* pneumolysin on human respiratory epithelium *in vitro.* Microbial Pathog. **9:**275–284.

8. **Geoffroy, C., J. Mengaud, J.E. Alouf, and P. Cossart.** 1990. Alveolysin, the thiol-activated toxin of *Bacillus alvei* is homologous to listeriolysin O, perfringolysin O, pneumolysin and streptolysin O and contains a single cysteine. J. Bacteriol **172:**7301–7305.

9. **Gilbert, R., J. Rossjohn, M. Parker, R. Tweten, P. Morgan, T. Mitchell, N. Errington, A. Rowe, P. Andrew, and O. Byron.** 1990. Self-interaction of pneumolysin, the pore-forming protein toxin of *Streptococcus pneumoniae.* J. Mol. Biol. **284:**1223–1237.

10. **Guzman, C.A., E. Domann, M. Rohde, D. Bruder, A. Darji, S. Weiss, J. Wehland, T. Chakraborty, and K.N. Timmis.** 1996. Apoptosis of mouse dendritic cells is triggered by listeriolysin, the major virulence determinant of *Listeria monocytogenes.* Mol. Microbiol. **20:**119–126.

11. **Haas, A., M. Dumbsky, and J. Kreft.** 1992. Listeriolysin genes: complete sequence of ivanolysin from *Listeria ivanovii* and of listeriolysin from *Listeria seeligeri.* Biochim. Biophys. Acta **1130:**81–84.

12. **Hill, J., P.W. Andrew, and T.J. Mitchell.** 1994. Amino acids in

pneumolysin important for hemolytic activity identified by random mutagenesis. Infect. Immunol. **62:**757–758.

13. **Houldsworth, S., P.W. Andrew, and T.J. Mitchell.** 1994. Pneumolysin stimulates production of tumor necrosis factor alpha and interleukin-1β by human mononuclear phagocytes. Infect. Immunol. **62:**1501–1503.

14. **Hugo, F., J. Reichwein, M. Arvand, S. Kramer, and S. Bhakdi.** 1986. Use of a monoclonal antibody to determine the mode of transmembrane pore formation by streptolysin O. Infect. Immunol. **54:**641–645.

15. **Iwamoto, M., Y. Ohno-Iwashita, and S. Ando.** 1987. Role of the essential thiol group in the thiol-activated cytolysin from *Clostridium perfringens*. Eur. J. Biochem. **167:**425–430.

16. **Jacobs, T., A. Darji, M. Frahm, M. Rohde, J. Wehland, T. Chakraborty, and S. Weiss.** 1998. Listeriolysin O: cholesterol inhibits cytolysis but not binding to cellular membranes. Mol. Microbiol. **28:**1081–1089.

17. **Johnson, M.K.** 1977. Cellular location of pneumolysin. F.E.M.S. Microbiol. Lett. **2:**243–245.

18. **Kaplan, M.H., and J.E. Volankis.** 1974. Interaction of C reactive protein complexes with the complement system. J. Immunol. **112:**2135–2147.

19. **Kehoe, M.A., L. Miller, J.A. Walker, and G.J. Boulnois.** 1987. Nucleotide sequence of the streptolysin O (SLO) gene: structural homologies between SLO and other membrane-damaging, thiol-activated toxins. Infect. Immunol. **55:**3228–3232.

20. **Korchev, Y.E., C.L. Bashford, and C.A. Pasternak.** 1992. Differential sensitivity of pneumolysin-induced channels to gating by divalent cations. J. Memb. Biol. **127:**195–203.

21. **Korchev, Y.E., C.L. Bashford, C. Pederzolli, C.A. Pasternak, P.J. Morgan, P.W. Andrew, and T.J. Mitchell.** 1998. A conserved tryptophan in pneumolysin is a determinant of the characteristics of channels formed by pneumolysin in cells and planar lipid bilayers. **329:**571–577.

22. **Kruiff, B.D.** 1990. Cholesterol as a target for toxins. Biosci. Rep. **10:**127–130.

23. **Mengaud, J., M.F. Vicente, J. Chenevert, J.M. Pereira, C. Geoffroy, B. Gicquel-Sanzey, B. Baquero, J.C. Perez-Diaz, and P. Cossart.** 1988. Expression of *E. coli* and sequence analysis of the listeriolysin O determinant of *Listeria monocytogenes*. Infect. Immunol. **56:**766–772.

24. **Michel, E., K.A. Reich, R. Favier, P. Berche, and P. Cossart.** 1990. Attenuated mutants of the intracellular bacterium *Listeria monocytogenes* obtained by single amino acid substitutions in listeriolysin O. Mol. Microbiol. **4:**2167–2178.

25. **Mitchell, T.J., P.W. Andrew, G.J. Boulnois, C.-J. Lee, R.A. Lock, and J.C. Paton.** 1992. Molecular studies of pneumolysin as an aid to vaccine design. Zbl. Bakt. **23:**429–438.

26. **Mitchell, T.J., P.W. Andrew, F.K. Saunders, A.N. Smith, and G.J. Boulnois.** 1991. Complement activation and antibody binding by pneumolysin via a region homologous to a human acute phase protein. Mol. Microbiol. **5:**1883–1888.

27. **Mitchell, T.J., J. Hill, and P.W. Andrew.** 1994. The role of histidine residues in the cytolytic action of pneumolysin. Zent. Bakt. **S24:**335–336.

28. **Mitchell, T.J., F.J. Mendez, J.C. Paton, P.W. Andrew, and G.J. Boulnois.** 1990. Comparison of pneumolysin genes and proteins from *Streptococcus pneumoniae* types 1 and 2. Nucl. Acids Res. **18:**4010.

29. **Morgan, P.J., S.C. Hyman, A.J. Rowe, T.J. Mitchell, P.W. Andrew, and H.R. Saibil.** 1995. Subunit organisation and symmetry of pore-forming oligomeric pneumolysin. F.E.B.S. Lett. **371:**77–80.

30. **Morgan, P.J., P.G. Varley, S. Hyman, O. Byron, P.W. Andrew, T.J. Mitchell, and A.J. Rowe.** 1994. Modelling the bacterial toxin pneumolysin in its monomeric and oligomeric forms. J. Biol. Chem. **269:**25315–25320.

31. **Morgan, P.J., P.G. Varley, A.J. Rowe, P.W. Andrew, and T.J. Mitchell.** 1993. Characterization of the solution properties and conformation of pneumolysin, the membrane-damaging toxin of *Streptococcus pneumoniae*. Biochem. J. **296:**671–674.

32. **Nakamura, M., N. Sekino, M. Iwamoto, and Y. Ohno-Iwashita.** 1995. Interaction of theta toxin (perfingolysin O) a cholesterol binding cytolysin, with liposomal membranes: change in the aromatic side chains upon binding and insertion. Biochem. **34:**6513–6520.

33. **Nandoskar, M., A. Ferrante, E.J. Bates, N. Hurst, and J.C. Paton.** 1986. Inhibition of human monocyte respiratory burst, degranulation, phospholipid metabolism and bactericidal activity by pneumolysin. Immunology **59:**515–520.

34. **Olofsson, A., H. Herbert, and M. Thelestam.** 1993. The projection structure of perfringolysin O (*Clostridium perfringens* theta toxin). F.E.B.S. Lett. **319:**125–127.

35. **Owen, R.H.G., G.J. Boulnois, P.W. Andrew, and T.J. Mitchell.** 1994. A role in cell-binding for the C-terminus of pneumolysin, the thiol-activated toxin of *Streptococcus pneumoniae*. F.E.M.S. Microbiol. Lett. **121:**217–222.

36. **Palmer, M., P. Saweljew, I. Vulicevic, A. Valeva, M. Kehoe, and S. Bhakdi.** 1996. Membrane penetrating domain of streptolysin O identified by cysteine scanning mutagenesis. J. Biol. Chem. **271:**26664–26667.

37. **Palmer, M., A. Valeva, M. Kehoe, and S. Bhakdi.** 1995. Kinetics of streptolysin O self-assembly. Eur. J. Biochem. **231:**388–395.

38. **Parker, M.W., F.G. Goot, and J.T. Buckley.** 1996. Aerolysin—ins and outs of a model channel-forming toxin. Mol. Microbiol. **19:**205–212.

39. **Paton, J.C., and A. Ferrante.** 1983. Inhibition of human polymorphonuclear leukocyte respiratory burst, bactericidal activity and migration by pneumolysin. Infect. Immunol. **41:**1212–1216.

40. **Paton, J.C., K.B. Rowan, and A. Ferrante.** 1984. Activation of human complement by the pneumococcal toxin pneumolysin. Infect. Immunol. **43:**1085–1087.

41. **Pinkey, M., E. Beachey, and M. Kehoe.** 1989. The thiol-activated toxin streptolysin O does not require a thiol group for cytolytic activity. Infect. Immunol. **57:**2553–2558.

42. **Rossjohn, J., S.C. Feil, W.J. McKinstry, R.K. Tweten, and M.W. Parker.** 1997. Structure of a cholesterol-binding, thiol-activated cytolysin in water soluble and membrane forms. Cell **89:**685–692.

43. **Rossjohn, J., R.J.C. Gilbert, D. Crane, P.J. Morgan, T.J. Mitchell, A.J. Rowe, P.W. Andrew, R.K. Tweten, and M.W. Parker.** 1998. The molecular mechanism of pneumolysin, a virulence factor from *Streptococcus pneumoniae*. J. Mol. Biol. **284:**449–461.

44. **Rubins, J., D. Charboneau, C. Fashing, A.M. Berry, J.C. Paton, J.E. Alexander, P.W. Andrew, T.J. Mitchell, and E.N. Janoff.** 1996. Distinct roles for pneumolysin's cytotoxic and complement activities in the pathogenesis of pneumococcal pneumonia. Am. J. Respir. Crit. Care Med. **153:**1339–1346.

45. **Rubins, J.B., P.W. Andrew, T.J. Mitchell, and D.E. Niewoehner.** 1994. Pneumolysin activates phospholipase A_2 in pulmonary artery endothelial cells. Infect. Immunol. **62:**3829–3836.

46. **Saunders, F.K., T.J. Mitchell, J.A. Walker, P.W. Andrew, and G.J. Boulnois.** 1989. Pneumolysin, the thiol-activated toxin of *Streptococcus pneumoniae*, does not require a thiol group for *in vitro* activity. Infect. Immunol. **57:**2547–2452.

47. **Sears, D.A., R.I. Weed, and S.N. Swisher.** 1964. Differences in the mechanism of *in vitro* immune hemolysis related to antibody specificity. J. Clin. Invest. **43:**975–985.

48. **Sekiya, K., R. Satoh, H. Danbara, and Y. Futaesaku.** 1993. A ring-shaped structure with a crown formed by streptolysin O on the erythrocyte membrane. J. Bacteriol **175:**5953–5961.

49. **Shepard, L.A., A.P. Heuck, B.D. Hamman, J. Rossjohn, M.W. Parker, K.R. Ryan, A.E. Johnson, and R.K. Tweten.** 1998. Iden-

tification of a membrane spanning domain of the thiol-activated pore-forming toxin *Clostridium perfringens* perfringolysin O: an α helical to β sheet transition identified by fluorescence spectroscopy. Biochemistry 37:14563–14574.

50. **Smyth, C.J., and J.L. Duncan.** 1978. Thiol-activated (oxygen-labile) cytolysins. *In* J. Jeljaszewicz and T. Wadstrom (eds.), Bacterial toxins and cell membranes. Acdemic Press, New York, pp. 129–183.

51. **Tweten, R.K.** 1988. Nucleotide sequence of the gene for perfringolysin O (theta toxin) from *Clostridium perfringens:* significant homology with the genes for streptolysin O and pneumolysin. Infect. Immunol. **56:** 3235–3240.

52. **Walker, J.A., R.L. Allen, P. Falmalgne, and M.K. Johnson.** 1987. Molecular cloning, characterisation and complete nucleotide sequence of the gene for pneumolysin, the sulfhydryl-activated toxin of *Streptococcus pneumoniae.* Infect. Immunol. **55:**1184–1189.

53. **Yamakawa, Y., and A. Ohsaka.** 1986. Hydrophobic interaction between θ toxin of *Clostridium perfringens* and erythrocyte membrane. Jpn. J. Med. Sci. Biol. **39:**254–255.

54. **Yutsudo, T.** 1994. Genbank accession number D21270.

Address reprint requests to:
P.W. Andrew
Department of Microbiology and Immunology
University of Leicester
POB 138
University Road
Leicester LE1 9HN
U.K.

Biological Properties of Pneumolysin

TIMOTHY J. MITCHELL[1] and PETER W. ANDREW

ABSTRACT

Pneumolysin is a thiol-activated membrane-damaging toxin produced by *Streptococcus pneumoniae*. The toxin plays a role in virulence of the pneumococcus in animal models of infection. Pneumolysin has a range of biological activity including the ability to lyse eukaryotic cells and to interfere with the function of cells and soluble molecules of the immune system. The use of purified native and mutant toxin and of isogenic mutants of the pneumococcus expressing altered versions of the toxin has allowed the contribution of the various activities of this multifunctional toxin to virulence to be defined.

INTRODUCTION

THE FIRST REPORT that pneumococci make a hemolysin was made in 1905.[29] During the next 50 years studies were carried out on crude toxin preparations[13,14,22,34,35,42] and showed that the hemolysin was toxic, susceptible to oxidation, antigenic and irreversibly inactivated by treatment with cholesterol. A role was first suggested for the hemolysin in the pathogenesis of pneumococcal infections by Shumway[48] who noted spherocytosis and increased osmotic fragility of erythrocytes in rabbits with pneumococcal bacteremia. These effects could be reproduced by injection of a cell free pneumococcal extract.[50] This effect was shown to be due to a single protein species (pneumolysin) when purified material became available.[49] Pneumolysin is now known to have a range of effects in different biological systems and these effects will be the subject of this review.

BIOLOGICAL EFFECTS OF PURIFIED PNEUMOLYSIN

The biological activities of pneumolysin are summarized in Table 1 and discussed in detail below.

Isolated cells

Pneumolysin is known to be lytic for all eukaryotic cells that have cholesterol in their membrane. The toxin belongs to the family of thiol activated toxins whose mechanism of action is believed to follow a common pathway involving two steps. The first step involves binding to membrane cholesterol and insertion of the toxin into the lipid bilayer. The second stage involves lateral diffusion and assembly of a high molecular weight oligomeric structure that is believed to represent a transmembrane pore.[9] Pneumolysin is thus able to injure a range of eukaryotic cells including bronchial epithelial cells,[51] alveolar epithelial cells,[44] and pulmonary arterial endothelial cells.[43] As these cell types are involved in lung-capillary barrier, destruction by the toxin may account for much of the histopathology typical of early pneumococcal pneumonia such as alveolar flooding and hemorrhage.[56]

As well as being lytic for eukaryotic cells, pneumolysin can have a range of physiological effects on cells at sublytic concentrations. Low doses of the toxin (1 ng/ml) have been shown to inhibit the respiratory burst of human polymorphonuclear leukocytes (PMNL).[37] The reduction in respiratory burst activity of PMNL was also associated with reduced ability to take up and kill opsonized pneumococci. Chemotaxis and random migration of the PMNL was inhibited, indicating that pneumolysin has a dramatic effect on the function of these cells. The effect of the toxin could be blocked with cholesterol. It has been shown that a region of the toxin important in the lytic mechanism of the protein is also involved in the sublytic effects on PMNL.[47] Similar inhibitory effects of pneumolysin on the respiratory burst, degranulation, bactericidal activity and phospholipid methylation of human monocytes have also been reported.[33] At very low doses pneumolysin is also capable of stimulating human monocytes to produce the inflammatory cytokines TNF-α and IL1-β.[25] Pretreatment of human lymphocytes with sub-lytic concentrations of the toxin was shown to block proliferation in response to several mitogens.[20] Toxin

---

[1]Division of Infection and Immunity, University of Glasgow, Glasgow, G12 8QQ, Scotland.
Reprinted from *Microbial Drug Resistance*, Vol. 3, No. 1, 1997.

TABLE 1. BIOLOGICAL EFFECTS OF PURIFIED PNEUMOLYSIN

Activity	Reference
Lysis of red blood cells	31
Inhibition of respiratory cilial beat in organ culture	18
Inhibition of cilial beat of brain ependymal cells in organ culture	32
Increases alveolar permeability in rat isolated lungs	44
Toxic to bovine artery endothelial cells	43
Toxic to pulmonary alveolar epithelial cells	44
Inhibition of mitogen induced proliferation and antibody production by human lymphocytes	20
Inhibits PMNL respiratory burst, random migration and chemotaxis	37
Activates classical complement pathway by binding to the Fc portion of antibody	30, 39
Stimulates the production of TNFα and IL-1β from human monocytes	25
Activates phospholipase A$_2$	45
Induces inflammation in the rat lung	19
Induces CSF leukocytocyes and increased TNF in rabbit brain	21
Electrophysiological and histological damage when perfused into the cochlea of guinea pigs	15

treated, stimulated lymphocytes also showed a decreased ability to produce lymphokines and antibody.

A further possible mechanism of toxin mediated injury and inflammation is suggested by the finding that pneumolysin is a potent activator of phospholipase A in pulmonary artery endothelial cells.[45] The activation of phospholipase A by pneumolysin required the toxin to form functional transmembrane pores. Once activated the phospholipase showed broad substrate specificity for cellular membrane phospholipid. It was also shown that the toxin was capable of activating purified phospholipase A$_2$ to degrade phospholipids isolated from membrane and incubated in vitro. Such activation of phospholipase A during an infection could contribute both to direct lung injury and to the inflammatory response. Direct cytotoxity would result from the release of free fatty acids and lysophosphatides. Arachidonic acid released by phospholipase A is capable of evoking chemotaxis and a respiratory burst in neutrophils.[4,16] Released arachidonic acid could also be metabolized through the eicosanoid cascade with the production of leukotrienes and platelet activating factor precursor.[24] Products of the eicosanoid pathway are a major source of neutrophil chemotaxins.[11] Recruitment and activation of PMNL followed by release of toxic molecules could injure pulmonary tissue. The activation of phospholipase A therefore could underlie the connection between the lytic activity of pneumolysin and its ability to cause inflammation in models of pneumonitis.[19]

Studies of the effect of pneumolysin on a range of cell types have therefore shown that there is a complexity of effects that can lead to inhibition of some cellular functions such as bacterial killing while stimulating others such as cytokine production and phospholipase activity. The possible contribution of these effects to the disease process will be discussed below.

Interaction with the complement pathway

Pneumolysin, when added to normal human serum, can activate the classical complement pathway in the absence of specific antibody.[39] Activation of the pathway results in a reduction in serum opsonic activity. The ability of pneumolysin to activate the complement pathway is due, at least in part, to nonspecific binding of IgG Fc by the toxin.[30] Activation also occurs with membrane fixed toxin (our unpublished data) and this may lead to complement attack on host tissues and promote inflammation. Complement activation by pneumolysin, unlike the lytic activity, is not blocked by incubation with cholesterol[39] and mutations within the pneumolysin gene that reduce haemolytic activity have no effect on the ability of the toxin to activate complement,[30] indicating that the two effects are mediated by different parts of the molecule.

Effects on animal tissues

Introduction of pneumolysin into the ligated apical lobe of rat lung induces the salient histological features of pneumonia.[19] It was shown that the histological changes induced were less when altered forms of the pneumolysin protein that lacked either the lytic or complement-activation properties of the wildtype toxin were used. This was the first indication from in vivo studies that the cytotoxic and complement activating ability of the toxin both play a role in pathogenesis.

Pneumolysin has detrimental effects on ciliated epithelium. The toxin causes a slowing of cilial beat of human nasal epithelium maintained in organ culture and at higher toxin concentrations disrupts the cells of this tissue.[18] Such effects may reduce the ability of the mucociliary escalator to clear particles from the respiratory tract. Pneumolysin is also directly toxic to primary cultures of type II rat alveolar epithelial cells[44] and increases the alveolar permeability in isolated perfused rat lungs. The alveolar epithelium is important as the limiting membrane in alveolar water and solute transport and may also provide a barrier to tissue invasion by bacteria. Damage to this barrier by pneumolysin could therefore be involved in the pathogenesis of pneumococcal infections.

It has been shown that pneumolysin has dramatic effects on the ciliated ependymal cells from the brain of rats. Brain cilia were more sensitive to the toxin than respiratory cilia and as little as 100 ng/ml of the toxin caused ciliary stasis within 15 minutes (Mohammed, Mitchell, Andrew, O'Callaghan, manuscript in preparation). This concentration of toxin had no effect on respiratory cilia.[18] Ciliated ependymal cells line the ventricular surface of the brain and cerebral aqueducts and form a barrier between the cerebrospinal fluid which is infected during meningitis and neuronal tissue.[2] It has been suggested that these cilia may protect the neuronal tissue from damage during infection by allowing continual movement of the CSF and preventing margination of bacteria during meningitis. Perturbation of cilial function could play a role in the pathophysiology of pneumococcal meningitis and pneumolysin therefore has effects on host tissue that could compromise nonspecific host defence mechanisms.

A common complication of pneumococcal meningitis is sensorineural hearing loss. Studies in a guinea pig model of hearing loss suggest that pneumolysin plays a key role. When pneumolysin was perfused through the scala tympani widespread electrophysiological and histological damage resulted.[15] Subsequent studies suggest that the toxic effects in the guinea pig cochlea are mediated by nitric oxide.[3] The role of pneumolysin in hearing loss during meningitis has since been confirmed in an infection model of meningitis and this is discussed further below. Pneumolysin may also perturb the round-window membrane during pneumococcal otitis media and allow the toxin to diffuse from the middle ear to the cochlea.[17]

Studies involving ocular instillation of pneumolysin have shown that the toxin plays a role in inflammation at that site also.[26] In this study when the toxin was given by intracorneal injection it induced pathology similar to that observed in natural infections with the organism. The pathology induced by the toxin in this system was significantly diminished if the rabbits were made leukopenic prior to challenge, suggesting that leukocytes could be a source of cornea damaging enzymes such as collagenase.[23]

Using a variety of systems purified pneumolysin has been shown to compromise host defence mechanism, cause tissue damage and promote inflammation. The role played by pneumolysin during an infection with *Streptococcus pneumoniae* can only be inferred from studies with the purified protein. With the availability of defined isogenic mutants of the pneumococcus the exact role played by the toxin during experimental infections could be determined.

STUDIES WITH ISOGENIC MUTANTS OF THE PNEUMOCOCCUS

Pneumolysin-negative mutant

The first suggestion that pneumolysin plays a role in virulence in animal models of pneumococcal disease came from the finding in James Paton's laboratory that immunization of mice with pneumolysin could partially protect mice from subsequent challenge with virulent organisms.[38] The gene for the toxin was subsequently cloned and sequenced[36,52] and the sequence used to construct isogenic mutants of type 2 and type 3 pneumococci in which the gene for pneumolysin had been disrupted by insertion duplication mutagenesis.[7,8] The loss of ability to synthesize pneumolysin reduced the virulence of the organism. In the case of the type 2 pneumolysin negative mutant (termed PLN-A) virulence was reduced by 10-fold and 100-fold when the organisms were administered via the intranasal and intraperitoneal routes respectively.[8] These workers also showed that PLN-A survived less well than the wild-type when injected intravenously. The PLN-A mutant has been pivotal in defining the biological role of pneumolysin in several systems. Canvin et al.[12] used an intranasal challenge of mice to investigate the role of pneumolysin in pneumonia and bacteremia. When compared to wild-type, PLN-A was shown to induce much less inflammation in the lung. PLN-A also showed reduced ability to replicate in the lung and a delayed invasion of the bloodstream. It has also been shown that if the pneumolysin-negative mutant is coinfected with the wild-type parent the mutant exhibits wild-type growth kinetics in the blood suggesting that pneumolysin exerts its effects at a distance.[5] It was also shown in this study that the pneumolysin-negative mutant causes a chronic bacteremia in mice. After intraperitoneal injection of wild-type

pneumococci into mice a bacteremia ensues and continues to increase until the animals die. Those animals inoculated with PLN-A initially develop a similar bacteremia until a level of about 1×10^6 CFU/ml of blood is reached at which point the number plateaued. Once this chronic bacteremia was established the mice were resistant to wild-type pneumococci. These workers concluded that pneumolysin plays an important role early in infection in preventing the generation of inflammation based immunity and allowing maximal growth of pneumococci.

PLN-A has also been used in a pneumonia model based on intratracheal inoculation into mice.[42] The use of this model established a lobar pneumonia rather than the bronchopneumonia seen with intranasal inoculation.[12] When PLN-A was used in this system it was less virulent than wild-type (LD_{50} of wild-type 10 times lower than PLN-A). Infection with wild-type pneumococci was found to cause an increase in the permeability of the alveolar capillary barrier as measured by the leakage of serum albumin into the alveolar air space. PLN-A had a reduced ability to multiply within the lungs and did not cause permeability changes in the alveolar capillary barrier. The toxin-negative mutant also had decreased ability to grow within the tissue of the lung and to invade the bloodstream. If the inoculum of PLN-A was augmented with a bolus of purified pneumolysin the pattern of growth in the lung was similar to that seen with wild-type organisms. A mechanism by which pneumolysin may mediate the permeability change and promote invasion of organs in the lung was suggested by studies with human respiratory mucosa grown in organ culture and infected with PLN-A.[40] PLN-A caused significantly less damage to human mucosa than the wild-type parent. Wild-type pneumococci induced separation of the tight junctions of the epithelial cells and pneumococci could be seen adhering to the separated edges of the cells. It was proposed that this mechanism may be important in the invasion process. PLN-A did not induce the same separation of tight junctions or adherence of pneumococci.

The role of pneumolysin in infection has also been studied using genetically complement-deficient mice.[42] Intratracheal infection of these mice with wild-type pneumococci or PLN-A showed several differences to the infection in complement-sufficient mice. The total number of bacteria in lungs were 2-fold greater at all times post-infection and an earlier and greater bacteremia occurred in the complement deficient mice. The net clearance of PLN-A and especially wild-type organisms from the lung was substantially reduced in C5 deficient mice. The total number of PLN-A bacteria increased in the lungs of C5 deficient mice in contrast to net clearance in C5 sufficient mice. The effect of deletion of pneumolysin expression can to some extent be reversed by use of complement deficient mice, indicating the interaction of pneumolysin with the complement pathway is important in the course of infection.

The contribution of pneumolysin to meningitis-associated sensorineural deafness has been studied using PLN-A. As already discussed, purified pneumolysin perfused through the guinea pig cochlea causes substantial electrophysiological and ultrastructural damage.[15] When experimental meningitis was established in a guinea pig model by subarachnoid inoculation of virulent type 2 organisms there was bacterial invasion of the scala tympani and ultrastructural damage to the organ of Corti.[54] The role of pneumolysin was investigated with PLN-A in this model.[55] The CSF inflammatory response was similar in the

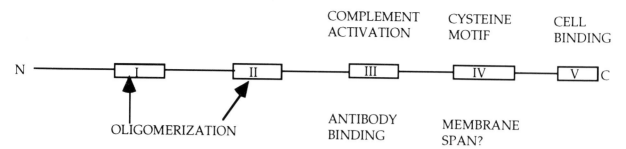

FIG. 1. Schematic representation of functional regions of pneumolysin within the primary amino sequence. Roman numerals indicate regions identified for function by site-directed mutagenesis of the primary sequence.

wild-type and PLN-A infection. Infection with the wild-type also caused a progressive hearing loss at all frequencies tested. There was a significant difference both in the degree and rate of hearing loss when animals were infected with PLN-A. All animals developed labyrinthitis but only infection with the wild-type (and not PLN-A) caused damage to the reticular lamina of the organ of Corti. Therefore in this acute model of meningogenic deafness there was clear structural and physiological evidence of local cochlear damage and this damage was mediated largely by pneumolysin.

Johnson et al.[28] also constructed a pneumolysin negative mutants of the pneumococcus. When a deletion mutant was used in a rabbit model of ocular infection it showed greatly reduced virulence. However, a nonhemolytic strain produced by chemical mutagenesis (probably a point mutation) was found to be no less virulent than the parent strain. These workers suggested that a property of the pneumolysin molecule other than its cytolytic activity may be important in its pathogenic mechanism of action. This proved to be the case in the studies done to determine the contribution of the various activities to virulence of whole pneumococci described below.

Although pneumolysin clearly plays a role in the pathogenesis of pulmonary, ocular, and systemic infections by the pneumococcus its role in other diseases is less clear. Use of a pneumolysin negative mutant of the pneumococcus in a rabbit model of meningitis[21] suggests that the toxin does not play a major role in the generation of inflammation in this system. However, although pneumolysin does not play a role in the gross inflammation seen in meningitis it does play a role in the hearing loss associated with this infection.[55] Examination of middle ear inflammation in the chinchilla otitis media model caused by infection with wild-type and a pneumolysin-negative mutant of the pneumococcus showed that the contribution of pneumolysin to inflammation was minimal.[46]

Isogenic mutants expressing altered versions of the toxin

Pneumolysin is a multifunctional molecule and various activities can be ascribed to various regions of the protein (see the contribution of Andrew et al.). A summary of the structure/function relationships determined for the protein is shown in Figure 1. This knowledge has enabled several series of experiments to be done to determine the relative contribution of lytic activity and complement activation by the toxin to the virulence of pneumococci. These studies are reviewed here. The first evidence that both lytic and complement activating activities of pneumolysin are important came from the studies of Feldman et al.[19] who showed that instillation of purified toxin into the rat lung caused inflammation. The use of mutant forms of the toxin in this system indicated that both activities of pneumolysin contributed to this inflammation. The contribution of the two activities to virulence was studied in more detail in a mouse model of lobar pneumonia.[42] In these studies (as discussed above) it was shown that a pneumolysin negative mutant (PLN-A) was less virulent and that wild-type behavior could be conferred by the addition of purified toxin to the in-

TABLE 2. ALLELIC REPLACEMENT MUTANTS OF *S. Pneumoniae* USED IN ANIMAL CHALLENGE EXPERIMENTS AND THE RELATIVE ACTIVITIES OF THE PNEUMOLYSIN PROTEINS EXPRESSED[1,6]

Strain designation	Point mutation(s) in pneumolysin	Region of protein (FIG. 1)	Hemolytic activity (%)	Complement activity (%)
H+/C+	Wild-type		100	100
H1−/C+	W433>F	IV	0.1	100
H2−/C+	H367>R	II	0.02	100
H3−/C+	C428>G	IV	0.001	100
	W433>F	IV		
H+/C−	D385>N	III	100	0
H3−/C−	D385>N	III	0.001	0
	C428>G	IV		
	W433>F	IV		
PLY-(PLN-A)	Inactivation		0	0

oculum of PLN-A. Experiments using coinstillation of mutated forms of the toxin lacking either cytotoxic activity or complement activation showed that lytic activity was important for allowing growth of the bacteria in the lung and invasion into lung tissue during the early period of the infection. Complement activation by pneumolysin appeared to be important for survival of the organisms in the lung at later times. The role of complement activation by pneumolysin has also been confirmed in the rabbit intracorneal model of infection.[27] In this study a strain was constructed that produced pneumolysin that was hemolytic but carried a point mutation that reduced the ability of the toxin to activate complement. This strain was less virulent than the wild-type parent showing that complement activation by pneumolysin plays a significant role in the pathology observed in the model of corneal infection.

To understand in detail how the lytic and complement activating activities of pneumolysin are involved in the pathogenesis of disease a series of derivatives of type 2 *S. pneumoniae* strain D39 have been constructed in which the wild type pneumolysin gene has been replaced by genes encoding toxins with one or more of a series of defined point mutations that alter the cytolytic or complement activation properties.[6] This panel of mutants has been used in several models of pneumococcal in-

fection. A summary of the location of these mutations and their activities is given in Table 2 (strain designations are based on).[1]

Use of isogenic mutants that differ in the ability of the pneumolysin they produce to activate complement or cause cytotoxicity (Table 2: H3−/C+, H+/C− and H3−/C−) *in vitro* in an assay for complement mediating killing of pneumococci by human phagocytes showed complement activation by pneumolysin to interfere with this process. The complement system is essential for opsonophagocytosis and clearance of pneumococci from the lung.[53] The alternative complement pathway can be activated by pneumococcal cell wall, but the polysaccharide capsule of the pneumococcus is thought to act as a barrier to the recognition of cell wall bound opsonins by phagocytes.[53] It has therefore been proposed that activation of the classical complement pathway is essential for effective opsonisation of pneumococci by deposition of complement C3b on the capsule.[10] Using isogenic mutants of the pneumococcus expressing pneumolysin with reduced ability to activate complement suggests that this activity may allow pneumococci to evade classic complement system-dependent opsonophagocytosis by consuming classical complement factors in solution. Evasion of the complement system in this way would produce increased bacterial growth especially when the concentrations of complement fac-

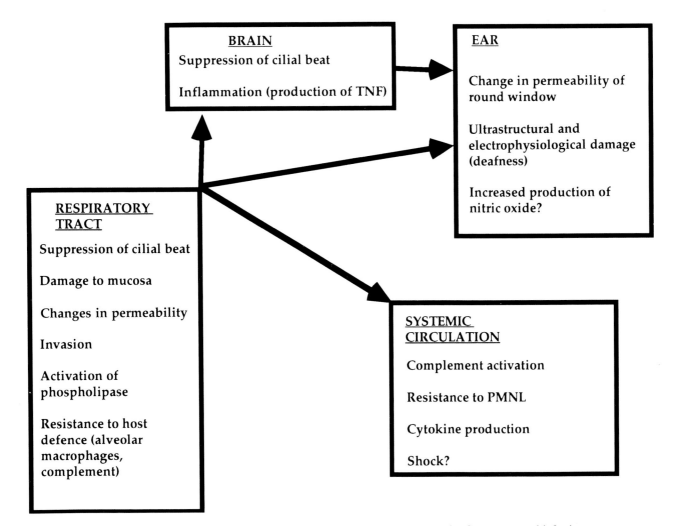

FIG. 2. Summary of the possible side effects of pneumolysin during the pathogenesis of pneumococcal infection.

tors are already limiting such as in the alveoli of the infected lung.

The contribution of the various biological activities of pneumolysin has been investigated in a range of animal models. Interestingly, the contribution of the activities of pneumolysin varies according to the model used. When the mutants were used in a model of systemic infection (intraperitoneal challenge) the cytotoxic property of the toxin was important while complement activating ability was irrelevant.[6] The evasion of opsonophagocytosis by consumption of classical complement components by pneumolysin would allow increased bacterial growth especially where the concentrations of the components are limited to begin with. Activation of complement by pneumolysin may not affect growth if the complement components are present in excess. This reasoning may explain why complement activation by pneumolysin has no effect on virulence when organisms are given via the systemic route. Mutants in which the lytic activity of the toxin was reduced to 0.02 and 0.0001% (Table 2 H2−/C+ and H3−/C+) of wild-type levels were less virulent than D39. The amount of pneumolysin required for full virulence may be very small as D39 derivatives carrying a mutation that reduces the lytic activity of the toxin to 0.1% of wild-type level showed intermediate virulence.

When mutant pneumococci were given to mice via the intranasal route of challenge both activities of pneumolysin were shown to be important but it was the ability of pneumolysin to activate complement that had most effect on the behavior of pneumococci in the lungs and associated bacteremia in the first 24 hours following infection.[1] Reduction in hemolytic activity was only influential 6h post infection. The level of bacteremia mirrored the number of bacteria present in the lung and therefore in the absence of complement activation by pneumolysin there was a lower level of bacteremia. Intriguingly, pneumococci carrying three point mutations in the pneumolysin gene were more virulent than the PLN-A gene disruption mutant. This indicates that some unidentified activity of pneumolysin also has a role in bronchopneumonia. This could be related to the residual ability of pneumolysin from strain H3−/C− to bind the Fc portion of antibody.[30] Alternatively, the activity could be related to the anticellular activity seen at sublytic concentrations of the toxin. To date mutations affecting the lytic activity of the toxin have been shown to reduce the sublytic anticellular activity to the same extent, although these studies have been limited to effects on neurophils and monocytes.[25,47]

Perhaps the most definitive analysis of the role of pneumolysin has also been done using the intratracheal route of inoculation into mice.[41] Using the H3−/C+, H+/C− and H3−/C− mutants described in Table 2 it was shown that absence of either lytic or complement activating ability from pneumolysin rendered mutant strains less virulent than the parent strain in this model of pulmonary infection. In contrast to inoculation by the intranasal route the combined mutations were not additive in their effect. The lack of additive effect was proposed to show that the lytic effect of pneumolysin is involved in several steps during pathogenesis whereas complement activation by the toxin has a more limited role in reducing bacterial clearance in the lung. The lytic activity of the toxin correlated with acute lung injury and bacterial growth for up to six hours after inoculation. The complement activating activity of the toxin correlated with bacterial growth and bacteremia at 24

hours post inoculation. It was proposed in this study that complement activation by the toxin has a singular role in pulmonary infection by promoting bacterial survival in the lung tissues and facilitating invasion into the blood.

CONCLUSION

Pneumolysin is an important virulence factor of the pneumococcus. Immunization with the toxin can protect against infection with the organism. Isogenic mutants of the pneumococcus in which the gene encoding pneumolysin has been disrupted are less virulent in animal models of infection. The toxin is multi-functional and has a range of effects on cells and soluble molecules of the immune system. A detailed structure/function study of the toxin allowed the definition of the areas of the protein involved in several of these activities. Use of isogenic mutants of the pneumococcus in which the pneumolysin gene has either been disrupted or replaced to allow expression of altered versions of the toxin has allowed the definition of the role played by various activities of the toxin in the infection process. The toxin mediates its effects on virulence both by its lytic properties and its ability to activate the classical complement pathway. The studies reviewed here show how it is now possible to define the role played by individual proteins, protein domains or even individual amino acids of virulence factors in the pathogenesis of infection. It is also clear that the role played by the virulence factors and their activity can differ dramatically according to the system chosen for their evaluation. For example, pneumolysin appears to play no role in the inflammation associated with meningitis but plays a key role in the hearing loss associated with this infection. Studies of pneumolysin therefore demonstrate how a combination of genetics, microbiology, and animal infection studies can define the role played by bacterial virulence factors in a range of infections. Such studies of virulence factors are key to the understanding of the pathogenesis of infectious disease and to the design of new treatments and vaccines.

ACKNOWLEDGMENTS

Work in the authors laboratories is supported by the Medical Research Council, The Royal Society and RIVM. We would like to thank our many collaborators who have contributed to this work, but in particular James Paton and Jeff Rubins for their contribution to this work.

REFERENCES

1. **Alexander, J.E., A.M. Berry, J.C. Paton, J.B. Rubins, P.W. Andrew, and T.J. Mitchell.** 1996. The course of pneumococcal pneumonia is altered by amino acid changes affecting the activity of pneumolysin. In Preparation.

2. **Alfzelius, B.A.** 1979. The immotile-cilia syndrome and other ciliary diseases. Int. Rev. Exp. Pathol. **19**:1–43.

3. **Amee, F.Z., S.D. Comis, and M.P. Osbourne.** 1995. N^G-methyl-L-arginine protects the guinea pig cochlea from the cytotoxic effects of pneumolysin. Acta Otolaryngol. **115**:386–391.

4. **Badwey, J.A., J.T. Curnutte, J.M. Robinson, C.B. Berde, M.J. Karnovsky, and M.L. Karnovsky.** 1984. Effects of free fatty acids on release of superoxide and on change of shape by human neutrophils. Reversibility by albumin. J. Biol. Chem. **259:**7870–7877.

5. **Benton, K.A., M.P. Everson, and D.E. Briles.** 1995. A pneumolysin-negative mutant of Streptococcus pneumoniae causes chronic bacteremia rather than acute sepsis in mice. Infection and Immunity **63:**448–455.

6. **Berry, A.M., J.E. Alexander, T.J. Mitchell, P.W. Andrew, D. Hansman, and J.C. Paton.** 1995. Effect of defined point mutations in the pneumolysin gene on the virulence of *Streptococcus pneumoniae.* Infect. Immun. **63:**1969–1974.

7. **Berry, A.M., J.C. Paton, and D. Hansman.** 1992. Effect of insertional inactivation of the genes encoding pneumolysin and autolysin on the virulence of *Streptococcus pneumoniae* type 3. Microbial Pathogen. **12:**87–93.

8. **Berry, A.M., J. Yother, D.E. Briles, D. Hansman, and J.C. Paton.** 1989. Reduced virulence of a defined pneumolysin-negative mutant of *Streptococcus pneumoniae.* Infect. Immun. **57:**2037–2042.

9. **Bhakdi, S., and J. Tranum-Jensen.** 1986. Membrane damage by pore-forming bacterial cytolysins. Microb. Pathogen. **1:**5–14.

10. **Brown, E.J., K.A. Joiner, R.M. Cole, and M. Berger.** 1983. Localization of complement component 3 on *Streptococcus pneumoniae:* anti-capsular antibody causes complement deposition on the pneumococcal capsule. Infect. Immun. **39:**403–409.

11. **Cabellos, C., D.E. MacIntyre, M. Forrest, M. Burroughs, S. Prasad, and E. Tuomanen.** 1992. Differing roles for platelet-activating factor during inflammation of the lung and sub-arachnoid space: the special case of *Streptococcus pneumoniae.* J. Clin. Invest. **90:**612–618.

12. **Canvin, J.R., A.P. Marvin, M. Sivakumaran, J.C. Paton, G.J. Boulnois, P.W. Andrew, and T.J. Mitchell.** 1995. The role of pneumolysin and autolysin in the pathology of pneumonia and septicemia in mice infected with a type 2 pneumococcus. J. Infect. Dis. **172:**119–123.

13. **Cohen, B., M.E. Perkins, and S. Putterman.** 1940. The Reaction between Hemolysin and Cholesterol. J. Bacteriol. **39:**59–60.

14. **Cole, R.** 1914. Pneumococcus hemotoxin. J. Exp. Med. **20:**346–362.

15. **Comis, S.D., M.P. Osborne, J. Stephen, M.J. Tarlow, T.L. Hayward, T.J. Mitchell, P.W. Andrew, and G.J. Boulnois.** 1993. Cytotoxic effects on hair cells of guinea pig cochlea produced by pneumolysin, the thiol activated toxin of Streptococcus pneumoniae. Acta Otolaryngol. **113:**152–159.

16. **Curnutte, J.T., J.M. Badwey, J.M. Robinson, M.J. Karnovsky, and M.L. Karnovsky.** 1984. Studies on the mechanism of superoxide release from human neutrophils stimulated with arachidonate. J. Biol. Chem. **259:**11851–11857.

17. **Engel, F., R. Blatz, J. Kellner, M. Palmer, U. Weller, and S. Bhakdi.** 1995. Breakdown of the round window permeability barrier evoked by streptolysin O: Possible etiologic role in the development of sensorineural hearing loss in acute otitis media. Infect. Immun. **63:**1305–1310.

18. **Feldman, C., T.J. Mitchell, P.W. Andrew, G.J. Boulnois, R.C. Read, H.C. Todd, P.J. Cole, and R. Wilson.** 1990. The effect of Streptococcus pneumoniae pneumolysin on human respiratory epithelium *in vitro.* Microbial Pathogenesis. **9:**275–284.

19. **Feldman, C., N.C. Munro, D.K. Jeffrey, T.J. Mitchell, P.W. Andrew, G.J. Boulnois, D. Gueirreiro, J.A.L. Rohde, H.C. Todd, P.J. Cole, and R. Wilson.** 1991. Pneumolysin induces the salient features of pneumococcal infection in the rat lung *in vivo.* Am. J. Resp. Cell. Mol. Biol. **5:**416–423.

20. **Ferrante, A., B. Rowan-Kelly, and J.C. Paton.** 1984. Inhibition of in vitro human lymphocyte response by the pneumococcal toxin pneumolysin. Infect. Immun. **46:**585–589.

21. **Friedland, I.R., M.M. Paris, S. Hickey, S. Shelton, K. Olsen, J.C. Paton, and G.H. McCracken.** 1995. The limited role of pneumolysin in the pathogenesis of pneumococcal meningitis. J. Infect. Dis. **172:**805–809.

22. **Halbert, S.P., B. Cohen, and M.E. Perkins.** 1946. Toxic and immunological properties of pneumococcal hemolysin. Bull. Johns Hopkins Hosp. **78:**340–359.

23. **Harrison, J.C., Z.A. Karcioglu, and M.K. Johnson.** 1993. Response of leukopenic rabbits to pneumococcal toxin. Curr. Eye Res. **2:**705–710.

24. **Holtzman, M.J.** 1991. Arachidonic acid metabolism. Implications of biological chemistry for lung function and disease. Am. Rev. Resp. Dis. **143:**188–203.

25. **Houldsworth, S., P.W. Andrew, and T.J. Mitchell.** 1994. Pneumolysin stimulates production of tumor necrosis factor alpha and interleukin-1beta by human mononuclear phagocytes. Infection and Immunity **62:**1501–1503.

26. **Johnson, M.K., and J.H. Allen.** 1975. The role of cytolysin in pneumococcal ocular infection. Am. J. Opthalm. **80:**518–520.

27. **Johnson, M.K., M.C. Callegan, L.S. Engel, R.J. O'Callaghan, J.M. Hill, J.A. Hobden, G.J. Boulnois, P.W. Andrew, and T.J. Mitchell.** 1995. Growth and virulence of a complement-activation-negative mutant of *Streptococcus pneumoniae* in the rabbit cornea. Curr. Eye Res. **14:**281–285.

28. **Johnson, M.K., J.A. Hobden, M. Hagenah, R.J. O'Callaghan, J.M. Hill, and S. Chen.** 1990. The role of pneumolysin in ocular infections with *Streptococcus pneumoniae.* Current Eye Res. **9:**1107–1114.

29. **Libman, E.** 1905. A pneumococcus producing a peculiar form of hemolysis. Proc. N.Y. Pathol. Soc. **5:**168.

30. **Mitchell, T.J., P.W. Andrew, F.K. Saunders, A.N. Smith, and G.J. Boulnois.** 1991. Complement activation and antibody binding by pneumolysin via a region of the toxin homologous to a human acute-phase protein. Molecular Microbiol. **5:**1883–1888.

31. **Mitchell, T.J., J.A. Walker, F.K. Saunders, P.A. Andrew, and G.J. Boulnois.** 1989. Expression of the pneumolysin gene in *Escherichia coli:* Rapid purification and biological properties. Biochim. et Biophys. Acta. **1007:**67–72.

32. **Mohammed, B.J., T.J. Mitchell, P.W. Andrew, and C. O'Callaghan.** 1996. Pneumolysin inhibits cilial beat in rat brain ependymal cells. Manuscript in preparation.

33. **Nandoskar, N., A. Ferrante, E.J. Bates, N. Hurst, and J.C. Paton.** 1986. Inhibition of human monocyte respiratory burst, degranulation, phospholipid methylation and bactericidal activity by pneumolysin. Immunology. **59:**515–520.

34. **Neill, J.M.** 1926. Studies on the oxidation and reduction of immunological substances. I. Pneumococcus hemotoxin. J. Exp. Med. **44:**199–213.

35. **Neill, J.M.** 1927. Studies on the oxidation and reduction of immunological substances. V. Production of anti-hemotoxin by immunization with oxidized pneumococcus hemotoxin. J. Exp. Med. **45:**105–113.

36. **Paton, J.C., A.M. Berry, R.A. Lock, D. Hansman, and P.A. Manning.** 1986. Cloning and expression in *Escherichia coli* of the *Streptococcus pneumoniae* gene encoding pneumolysin. Infect. Immun. **54:**50–55.

37. **Paton, J.C., and A. Ferrante.** 1983. Inhibition of human polymorphonuclear leukocyte respiratory burst, bactericidal activity, and migration by pneumolysin. Infect. Immun. **41:**1212–1216.

38. **Paton, J.C., R.A. Lock, and D.J. Hansman.** 1983. Effect of immunization with pneumolysin on survival time of mice challenged with *Streptococcus pneumoniae.* Infect Immun. **40:**548–552.

39. **Paton, J.C., B. Rowan-Kelly, and A. Ferrante.** 1984. Activation of human complement by the pneumococcal toxin pneumolysin. Infect. Immun. **43:**1085–1087.

40. **Rayner, C., A.D. Jackson, A. Rutman, A. Dewar, T.J. Mitchell,**

P.W. Andrew, P.J. Cole, and R. Wilson. 1995. Interaction of pneumolysin-sufficient and -deficient isogenic variants of *Streptococcus pneumoniae* with human respiratory mucosa. Infection and Immunity **63**:442–447.

41. **Rubins, J.B., D. Charboneau, C. Fasching, A.M. Berry, J.C. Paton, J.E. Alexander, P.W. Andrew, T.J. Mitchell, and E.N. Janoff.** 1996. Distinct role for pneumolysin's cytotoxic and complement activities in the pathogenesis of pneumococcal pneumonia. Am. J. Respir. and Critical Care Medicine. **153**:1339–1346.

42. **Rubins, J.B., D. Charboneau, J.C. Paton, T.J. Mitchell, P.W. Andrew, and E.N. Janoff.** 1995. Dual function of pneumolysin in the early pathogenesis of murine pneumococcal pneumonia. J. Clin. Invest. **95**:142–150.

43. **Rubins, J.B., P.G. Duane, D. Charboneau, and E.N. Janoff.** 1992. Toxicity of pneumolysin to pulmonary endothelial cells in vitro. Infection and Immunity **60**:1740–1746.

44. **Rubins, J.B., P.G. Duane, D. Clawson, D. Charboneau, J. Young, and D.E. Niewoehner.** 1993. Toxicity of pneumolysin to pulmonary alveolar epithelial cells. Infection and Immunity **61**:1352–1358.

45. **Rubins, J.B., T.J. Mitchell, P.W. Andrew, and D.E. Niewoehner.** 1994. Pneumolysin activates phospholipase A in pulmonary artery endothelial cells. Infection and Immunity **62**:3829–3836.

46. **Sato, K., M.K. Quartey, C.L. Liebeler, C.T. Le, and G.S. Giebink.** 1996. Roles of autolysin and pneumolysin in middle ear inflammation caused by a type 3 *Streptococcus pneumoniae* strain in the chinchilla otitis media model. Infect. Immun. **64**:1140–1145.

47. **Saunders, F.K., T.J. Mitchell, J.A. Walker, P.W. Andrew, and G.J. Boulnois.** 1989. Pneumolysin, the thiol-activated toxin of *Streptococcus pneumoniae*, does not require a thiol group for in vitro activity. Infection and Immunity **57**:2547–2552.

48. **Shumway, C.N.** 1958. Spherocytic hemolytic anemia associated with acute pneumococcal infection in rabbits. J. Lab. Clin. Med. **51**:240–247.

49. **Shumway, C.N., and S.J. Klebanoff.** 1971. Purification of pneumolysin. Infect. Immun. **4**:388–392.

50. **Shumway, C.N., and D. Pollock.** 1965. The effect of a pneumococcal product upon rabbit erythrocytes in vitro and in vivo. J. Lab. Clin. Med. **65**:432–439.

51. **Steinfort, C., R. Wilson, T. Mitchell, C. Feldman, A. Rutman, H. Todd, D. Sykes, J. Walker, K. Saunders, P.W. Andrew, G.J. Boulnois, and P.J. Cole.** 1989. Effect of Streptococcus pneumoniae on human respiratory epithelium in vitro. Infection and Immunity **57**:2006–2013.

52. **Walker, J.A., R.L. Allen, P. Falmagne, M.K. Johnson, and G.J. Boulnois.** 1987. Molecular cloning, characterization, and complete nucleotide sequence of the gene for pneumolysin, the sulfhydryl-activated toxin of *Streptococcus pneumoniae*. Infect. Immun. **55**:1184–1189.

53. **Winkelstein, J.A.** 1981. Complement and the host's defence against the pneumococcus. CRC Crit. Rev. Microbiol. **11**:187–208.

54. **Winter, A., S. Marwick, M. Osborne, S. Comis, J. Stephen, and M. Tarlow.** 1996. Ultrastructural damage to the organ of Corti during acute experimental *Escherichia coli* and pneumococcal meningitis in guinea pigs. Acta Otolaryngol. **116**:401–407.

55. **Winter, A.J., S.D. Comis, M.P. Osbourne, M.J. Tarlow, J. Stephen, P.W. Andrew, and T.J. Mitchell.** 1996. Pneumolysin rather than neuraminidase is chiefly responsible for deafness during experimental pneumococcal meningitis in guinea pigs. 7th International Congress for Infectious Diseases, Hong Kong, June 1996. Abstract **73**:004.

56. **Wood, W.B.J.** 1941. Studies on the emchanism of recovery in pneumococcal pneumonia. I. The action of type specific antibody upon the pulmonary lesion of experimental pneumonia. J. Exp. Med. **73**:201–222.

Address reprint requests to:
T.J. Mitchell
Division of Infection and Immunity
Joseph Black Building
University of Glasgow
Glasgow, Scotland G12 8QQ

Calcium Signaling in *Streptococcus pneumoniae*: Implication of the Kinetics of Calcium Transport

MARIE-CLAUDE TROMBE

ABSTRACT

The kinetics and pharmacological characterization of a Na^+/Ca^{2+} exchange system, essential for the growth of the extracellular pathogen *Streptococcus pneumoniae* in high-calcium media, demonstrated that calcium transport, in addition to its role in calcium homeostasis, is involved in the induction of autolysis and competence for genetic transformation. These responses are expressed, respectively, in cultures entering the stationary phase and growing with exponential rates. Experimental virulence also appears to be modulated by the kinetics of calcium transport. Calcium transport in *S. pneumoniae* is electrogenic and shows sigmoidicity, indicating a cooperative mechanism, with an inflexion point at 1 mM Ca^{2+}. Mutant strains with Hill number values of 4 and 1, compared to 2 in the wild-type strain, were isolated. These changes were associated with altered regulation of competence and autolysis, and also with reduced experimental virulence. By contrast, they could not be related to specific calcium requirements for growth. This indicates that the cooperativity of Ca^{2+} transport is not involved in vegetative growth, but rather regulates competence and autolysis. Competence and autolysis represent two growth-phase-dependent responses to an oligopeptide-activator exported to the medium, the competence-stimulating peptide. Addition of this activator to noncompetent cells, triggers net and transient $^{45}Ca^{2+}$ influx. One effect of the activator might be to activate a calcium transporter by enhancing its cooperativity. In addition to an increase in intracellular calcium, a transient membrane depolarization induced by electrogenic calcium influx may be part of the signaling mechanism. The competence activator is a quorum-sensing molecule whose synthesis is autoregulated. This regulation might involve calcium-mediated signaling. As an extracellular pathogen, *S. pneumoniae* probably develops in niches with variable calcium concentrations. Interestingly, virulence depends strongly upon the kinetics of Ca^{2+} transport. Regulation of calcium influx may represent a common mechanism of sensing the environment, if the Na^+/Ca^{2+} exchanger is the target for external mediators, including the competence activator.

INTRODUCTION

THE EXTRACELLULAR PATHOGEN *Streptococus pneumoniae* is well known for its transformability by naked DNA. Another trait of these bacteria is their high suceptibility to autolysis catalyzed by an *N*-acetylmuramylalanine amidase encoded by *lytA*.[20,51] Tranformability, a property of competent bacteria, requires a single-strand DNA import machinery as well as functions involved in homologous recombination. Competence and autolysis constitute responses to the same stimulus, high calcium and alkaline pH. They are under the control of an autoregulated ring involving the competence-stimulating peptide (CSP) and its cognate two-component system COMD, COME (for a recent review, see ref. 16). These responses occur at different windows of the growth curve with competence in expo-

nential cultures and autolysis in early-stationary cultures.[53] The calcium concentration required for optimal competence induction and autolysis activation is in the range of 1 to 1.5 m*M*, values characteristic of body fluids. This raises the question of calcium handling in *S. pneumoniae*. Data supporting specific physiological roles for calcium in cell wall and cell membrane structures and in calcium signaling in prokaryotes, are rather disparate (for reviews, see ref. 34, 36, 37, 44). A putative role for calcium in signaling involves first, as a prerequisite, tight control of the Ca^{2+} level in the cytoplasm. This appears to be fulfilled in *Escherichia coli*. At external concentrations up to 10 m*M*, free cytoplasmic calcium levels are between 0.1 and 0.2 μM,[13,48,57] but little is known about the functions involved in calcium traffic. Brey and Rosen[5] established that calcium transport is electrogenic in *E. coli* cells and vesicles. Recently,

Universite Paul Sabatier, Laboratoire de Bactériologie, Centre Hospitalo Universitaire de Rangueil, 31403 Toulouse, France.

genetic characterization of a locus (*chaA*) encoding a Ca^{2+}/H^+ antiporter activity and showing protein sequence homologies with a eukaryotic Na^+/Ca^{2+} antiporter, was reported.[21,35] In addition to such apparently drug-sensitive Ca^{2+} channels, a P-type ATPase (blocked by orthovanadate) very likely exports calcium at the expense of ATP in streptococci.[17,18,19,42] It has been proposed also that calcium transport in *E. coli* might occur via voltage-dependent channels formed by the lipid polymer poly-β-hydroxybutyrate, incorporated into membranes[41] and via the constitutive phosphate transporter encoded by *pit*.[55]

However, apart from the demonstrated role for calcium transport in chemotaxis, both in *E. coli*[47–49] and in *Bacillus subtilis*,[29,30] little is known about the physiological function of intracellular calcium. The possible role of cytoplasmic calcium as a second messenger in prokaryotes is supported by the presence of proteins with calcium binding motif,[4,12,46,56] reminiscent of calmodulins and other calcium-binding proteins from eukaryotes.[24] Moreover, a direct and primary role for divalent cations, including Ca^{2+} and Mg^{2+}, in signal transduction has been reported in *Salmonella typhimurium*, where divalent cations regulate the expression of genes belonging to the *phoP/phoQ* regulon with clear evidence for sensing periplasmic levels of Ca^{2+} and Mg^{2+} via a two-component signal transducing system.[14]

In this review, we present pharmacological and kinetics data demonstrating that in *S. pneumoniae* an electrogenic Na^+/Ca^{2+} exchange is involved in calcium homeostasis, and also that the kinetics of Ca^{2+} transport represent a key point for regulating genetic exchanges, autolysis, and experimental virulence.

CALCIUM CIRCULATION IN *S. PNEUMONIAE*

Inhibitor definition

Calcium circulation involves, as in other streptococci, a vanadate-sensitive function that is probably an ATPase (P-type ATPase),[19] in addition to a function sensitive to an amiloride derivative, the 2'-4'-dimethylbenzamil (DMB).[22]

The involvement of a vanadate-sensitive function that exports calcium at the expense of ATP is suggested by three lines of evidence: (i) $^{45}Ca^{2+}$ uptake cannot be measured in fully energized bacteria; (ii) addition of 100 μM vanadate to the uptake medium permits measurements of $^{45}Ca^{2+}$ uptake; (iii)

$^{45}Ca^{2+}$ uptake in a vanadate-free medium can be measured if the ATP pool is depleted. In addition to this vanadate-sensitive function, a DMB-sensitive porter participates in calcium traffic. Indeed, $^{45}Ca^{2+}$ uptake is abolished by 15 μM DMB, in vanadate-treated as well as in energy-depleted bacteria. These data are summarized in Table 1.

Because of its implications for *S. pneumoniae* physiology (see next sections), we have characterized the kinetics of calcium transport via the DMB-sensitive porter in the wild-type strain Cp1015 and in two derivatives carrying DMB-resistant mutations. These mutant strains were from independent clones isolated on plates containing 15 μM DMB. Transfer of the mutations into the Cp1015 background was obtained by genetic transformation using DNA from the DMB-resistant clones at a concentration 10-fold lower than the saturation level. Selection of transformants was obtained on blood agar plates containing 15 μM DMB and 1 m*M* calcium. Two successive rounds of transformation were performed for each construction, giving rise to strains Cp2200 and Cp3300. Both strains resisted up to 30 μM DMB in calcium-rich medium compared to the wild-type parent, for which growth is totally inhibited by 10 μM DMB. In each case, the DMB^R trait was transferred as a single transformation event as compared with well-defined point mutations, suggesting that each mutant strain contains a single mutation (Salis and Trombe, 1998, unpublished).[52,54]

Pharmacological and kinetic definition of the DMB-sensitive component of calcium transport

The amiloride derivative DMB, already known to inhibit an eukaryotic Na^+/Ca^{2+} transporter,[22] also inhibits $^{45}Ca^{2+}$ transport in *S. pneumoniae*. This molecule made possible the characterization of an electrogenic $^{45}Ca^{2+}$ transport in exchange with Na^+ with kinetics that show sigmoidicity. The inflexion point occurs at 1 m*M* and the Hill number (nH) is 1.9 in the wild-type strain, suggesting a cooperative process; this was indicated by an abrupt increase in the initial rate of uptake when the calcium concentration progressively increased to 1 m*M*. Cooperativity of Ca^{2+} transport was changed by mutations selected by their ability to confer resistance to DMB. Strain Cp2200, carrying the *dmb1* mutation, shows an nH value of 1.3 whereas strain Cp3300 carrying the *dmb2* mutation shows an nH value of 4. These shifts in nH values are not associated with changes in the inflexion point, which remained at 1 m*M* Ca^{2+},

TABLE 1. INVOLVEMENT OF FUNCTIONS INHIBITED BY ORTHOVANADATE AND BY DMB IN $^{45}Ca^{2+}$ TRANSPORT

Experimental conditions	$ATP_i = 3$ m*M*	$ATP_i = 3$ m*M* $V_2O_5 = 100$ μM	$ATP_i < 3$ μM	$ATP_i = 3$ m*M* $V_2O_5 = 100$ μM $DMB = 15$ μM
$^{45}Ca^{2+}$ uptake (cpm/μl)				
Net uptake	a-0	4,700		
(-blank value)	b-0		3,384	
	c-0	3,288		0

The amount of radioactivity retained by the bacteria was measured by filtration assays after 7 min incubation at 20°C in a medium containing 1 mM, $^{45}Ca^{2+}$, 1.5×10^6 cpm/μmole. Blank values were obtained at time 0 at 4°C. V_2O_5 and DMB treatment of the bacteria were performed during 2 min at 20°C in CAT medium. For more details on transport methods, see ref 79. a, b, and c are independent representative experiments. Each experiment has been repeated three times to verify reproducibility.

as in the wild-type strain.[52,54] Thus, for extracellular Ca^{2+} concentrations above 1 mM, the rate of $^{45}Ca^{2+}$ uptake shifts abruptly and reaches 10, 27, and 6 nmoles/min per mg of proteins, respectively, for the wild type and the *dmb2* and *dmb1* mutant strains.

CALCIUM AND PHYSIOLOGY

Calcium transport and growth

The optimum calcium concentration for growth in rich medium is 0.15 mM. Growth inhibition by DMB is strongly dependent on the extracellular calcium concentration, suggesting that the DMB-sensitive function is likely to be involved in the regulation of calcium homeostasis. In low-calcim medium (0.15 mM), increasing the DMB concentration increased the lag period of growth without changing the growth rate. In calcium-rich medium (1.5 mM), a dose–response reduction of the growth rate was observed for DMB concentrations ranging from 2 to 10 μM. This indicates that the role of the DMB target depends on the Ca^{2+} concentrations of the growth medium. At low Ca^{2+} concentration, it is limited to growth initiation from a frozen culture, whereas in calcium-rich medium, the DMB target is involved throughout growth.[52,53] Mutations leading to DMB-resistance that change the cooperativity of calcium transport do not shift the calcium threshold requirement for growth (Trombe, unpublished).

Calcium transport and genetic exchanges

The role of divalent cations, including Ca^{2+}, on genetic transformation was described in early studies by Fox and Hotchkiss,[11] Lacks,[26] and Seto and Tomasz.[43] More precise evidence for the involvement of calcium in the complex process of transformation was obtained by checking the calcium requirement and the role of the DMB-sensitive function at competence induction and for DNA degradation, DNA uptake, and the isolation of transformed bacteria.[53]

Calcium transport and competence expression: The optimal calcium concentration for competence-specific DNA degradation and for DNA uptake is 0.4 mM.[6] However, addition of DMB to competent cultures did not interfere with competence expression, *i.e.*, DNA degradation, transport, and genetic transformation, suggesting that once competence is induced, within the 30 min following DNA addition, calcium traffic via the DMB-sensitive transporter is not essential for obtaining transformants.[53]

Calcium transport and competence induction: Competence induction requires a higher calcium concentration compared with competence expression. Optimum induction is obtained at 1 mM Ca^{2+}.[6] DMB at a concentration subinhibitory for growth (5 μM) reduces competence induction by 80%.[53] $^{45}Ca^{2+}$ transport measurements indeed show that CSP addition to a culture triggers a net $^{45}Ca^{2+}$ influx and a Na^+ efflux within 1 min. Both are blocked specifically by 5 μM DMB. A related amiloride derivative, hexamethylene amiloride (HMA), is an inhibitor of the Na^+/H^+ antiporter in eukaryotic cells[25] and is also active in *S. pneumoniae*[53] (Thomas and Trombe, 1997, unpublished); it showed a minor effect on competence induction and on calcium influx in response to CSP. This indicates

that Ca^{2+} influx in response to CSP triggers induction with a dominant role for Na^+/Ca^{2+} rather than Na^+/H^+ exchange.[8,53] Also, the addition of the Ca^{2+} ionophore A23187[40] to a culture containing calcium at concentration that is suboptimal for induction (0.4 mM) restores full competence in the wild-type strain Cp1015.[53] Moreover, DMB at a concentration that is subinhibitory for growth (5 μM) reduces competence induction by 80% and inhibits the initial rate of Ca^{2+} transport by 50%.

Interestingly, mutant Cp3300, which shows an increased cooperativity for calcium transport and therefore a higher uptake rate at 1 mM calcium than the wild-type strain, shows a similar resistance level to DMB for competence induction and for growth but expresses a higher competence level.[54] By contrast, strain Cp2200, in which cooperativity of calcium transport is reduced, and therefore shows a low uptake rate at 1 mM Ca^{2+}, requires 20-fold more CSP to be activated.[52]

Together these physiological, pharmacological, biochemical, and genetic data converge to show the involvement of the kinetics of calcium transport in competence regulation via its impact on the amplitude of calcium influx. The *dmb* mutations define new loci involved in the kinetics of calcium transport and in competence regulation. These loci map away from the *comAB* locus involved in the export of the activator[52,54] (Salis and Trombe, 1997, unpublished).

Calcium transport and autolysis

Autolysis mediated by the N-acetylmuramylalanine amidase,[20] the product of *lytA*,[51] is activated in early stationary phase, when cultures are grown in calcium-rich medium. Like competence induction, autolysis is under the control of CSP, as shown by the requirement for extra CSP to trigger autolysis in cultures of the *comO* mutant Cp1322.[33] These results are in line with recent findings showing that *lytA* belongs to a late-competence operon[28,39] and with the known influence of the kinetics of calcium transport on the autolysis susceptibility of cultures. Strain Cp3300, in which cooperativity is high (nH = 4), shows a greater susceptibility to autolysis than the wild-type strain (nH = 2), whereas strain Cp2200, whose cooperativity is reduced (nH = 1.3), is resistant to autolysis. Moreover, protection from autolysis by subinhibitory concentrations of DMB reinforces the conclusion that calcium circulation may be a major determinant in this process. It is worth noting that in fully competent cultures, DNA transport prevents autolysis.[53]

Calcium transport and virulence

Functions involved in host colonization and growth should be considered with regard to the ecological niche of *S. pneumoniae* (for review see ref. 58). Metabolic versatility and genetic control allow bacteria to respond rapidly to changing environmental conditions and to colonize a vast range of habitats.[31] Furthermore, expression of virulence factors in several pathogens is shown to be regulated by environmental conditions, including the concentrations of cations.[15,32,38] The correlation between the kinetics of calcium transport, the regulation of *lytA*-dependent autolysis, and the control of genetic exchange via competence regulation raises the question of the impact of the kinetics of calcium transport on experimental virulence. Indeed, on the one hand, $lytA_0$ mutants were constructed in different laboratories and checked for their experimental virulence. In all the systems tested, the $lytA_0$ strains exhibited an attenuated virulence, suggesting a role for autolysis in virulence.[2,3] Because autolysis susceptibility is influenced by the *dmb* mutations, virulence determination in a set of isogenic strains carrying either *dmb1* or *dmb2* and expressing the serotype3 capsule[1] has been investigated in mice. Both mutations reduce virulence but, in contrast to $lytA_0$ the *dmb* mutations do not lead to rapid clearance from the bloodstream. Moreover, both $lytA_0$ and *dmb1* mutation conferring decreased autolysis susceptibility show an additive effect, resulting in total avirulence. This result suggests that the kinetics of calcium transport impacts on virulence via its control of autolysis in addition to yet nondefined pathway(s).

CONCLUSIONS AND PERSPECTIVES

The data presented here provide evidence for Ca^{2+} regulation of experimental virulence, competence, and autolysis in *S. pneumoniae*. A transporter, the target for the amiloride derivative DMB that uses the electrochemical potential of ionic gradients and that shows cooperative kinetics, is involved in this regulation. This porter fulfills the conditions required for Ca^{2+} signaling by mediating Ca^{2+} influx or efflux in response to environmental stimuli.

In *S. pneumoniae*, P-type ATPase-mediated calcium export and the DMB-sensitive transport are both involved in calcium traffic. The high sensitivity to DMB points to the important role of the DMB target in the regulation of growth, competence, and autolysis. Calcium influx causes a transient increase in cytoplasmic concentration and membrane depolarization. Both may be involved in signaling via different routes: the membrane depolarization resulting from electrogenic Ca^{2+} influx and/or transient increase in intracellular Ca^{2+} and its recognition by target proteins. So far such proteins are not identified.

Interestingly, competence involves the expression of a set of specific operons as well as an increased energetic potential as a consequence of the elevated ATP pool, the accumulation of PHB, and the increased $\Delta\mu H^+$ due to cytoplasmic alkalinization.[27] These changes are relevant with regard to genetic transformation. An alkaline pH value associated with a high ATP level represents optimal conditions for DNA uptake by competent bacteria.[6,7,9] Moreover, metabolic stimulation should lead to the accumulation of phospho-donors in the form of acetyl-P and ATP. In exponential cultures, this may trigger signaling through phospho-transfer, resulting in the induction of proteins required for the competence program. Because the same parameters control both competence and autolysis, it is possible that the conditions required for competence induction impose a stress on the bacteria. Indeed, the fact that PHB accumulates in competent bacteria also suggests a metabolic stress.[10] In the pioneering work of Tomasz,[50] competence was shown to be triggered in vigorously and exponentially growing cultures. The stress associated with competence is not likely to be due to classical starvation but might result from a metabolic imbalance. PHB accumulation in bacteria is associated with imbalanced growth conditions, such as these that accompany spore formation in certain bacilli[23] and cyst formation in *Azotobacter*. PHB synthesis depends on the concentrations of the reducing equivalents NADH and NADPH, which participate in the autocondensation of acetyl coenzyme A (CoA) catalyzed by a PHB synthetase to give PHB and $NAD(P)^+$.[10]

In bacteria growing on glucose or on another carbohydrate, glycolysis is the main source of the reducing equivalents, whereas production of acetyl-CoA suggests an oxidative metabolism of pyruvate. The gene encoding pyruvate oxidase in *S. pneumoniae* was recently identified.[45] This enzyme could lead to production of acetyl-CoA via pyruvate oxidation. Activation of acetyl-CoA production might switch carbohydrate metabolism toward "rich-energy molecules" such as ATP, acetyl-P, and PHB, instead of pentose biosynthesis. This might lead to pentose "deprivation" in energy-rich bacteria. In natural populations of pneumococci, such an "imbalance" might trigger competence and autolysis according to the physiological status of different subpopulations and thus allow cross-feeding. DNA uptake at competence prevents autolysis, suggesting that both responses might allow cross-feeding among subpopulations in different physiological states.[53]

Mutations that change the cooperativity of Ca^{2+} transport, competence, and autolysis regulation attenuate virulence at high bacteremia levels, which is in contrast to the $lytA_0$ mutation.[2] It is likely that the mechanism leading to the attenuated virulence of strains carrying the *dmb* mutations is complex. The link, if any, between the increased susceptibility to autolysis in *in vitro* cultures and virulence attenuation in mice of the mutant strain carrying the *dmb2* mutation is not established. However, the additive effect of the *dmb1* and the $lytA_0$ mutations, both conferring reduced autolysis susceptibility, clearly points to different mechanisms leading to virulence attenuation. In *S. pneumoniae* virulence, regulation may be part of a more general regulatory network, controlled by Ca^{2+} influx, including competence and autolysis.

Modulation of Ca^{2+} influx either by changes in the environmental Ca^{2+} level or by effectors regulating the kinetics of Ca^{2+} transport might represent one mechanism that allows the bacteria to "sense" and respond to its environment, with the CSP as a quorum-sensing oligopeptide, thus mediating the communication between the bacterial population and its environment.

ACKNOWLEDGMENTS

The work was supported by Université Paul Sabatier, Equipe DRRE 1968, and the "Foundation pour la Recherche Médicale". I thank Professor Barry Holland and Professor Vic Norris for discussions during the preparation of the manuscript.

REFERENCES

1. **Arrecubetia, C., E. Garcia, and R. Lopez.** 1995. Sequence and transcription analysis of a DNA region involved in the production of capsular polysaccharide in *Streptococcus pneumoniae* type 3. Gene **167:**1–7.

2. **Azoulay-Dupuis, E., V. Rieux, C. Rivier, and M.C. Trombe.** 1998. Pleiotropic mutations alter the kinetics of calcium transport, competence regulation, autolysis and experimental virulence in *Streptococcus pneumoniae*. Res. Microbiol. **149:**5–13.

3. **Berry, A.M., R.A. Lock, D. Hausman, and J.C. Paton.** 1998. Contribution of autolysis to virulence of *Streptococcus pneumoniae*. Infect. Immun. **57:**2324–2330.

4. **Bouquin, N., M. Tempete, I.B. Holland, and S.J. Séror.** 1995. Resistance to trifluoroperazine, a calmodulin inhibitor, maps to the fabD locus in E. coli. Mol. Gen. Genet. **246:**628–637.

5. **Brey, R.N., and B.P. Rosen.** 1979. Properties of *Escherichia coli* mutants altered in calcium/proton antiport activity. J. Bacteriol. **139:**824–834.

6. **Clavé, C., and M.C. Trombe.** 1989. DNA uptake in competent *Streptococcus pneumoniae* requires ATP and is regulated by cytoplasmique pH. FEMS Microbiol. **65:**113–118.

7. **Clavé, C., D. Morrison, and M.C. Trombe.** 1987. Is DNA transport driven by the proton electrochemical potential difference in the naturally transformable bacteria *Streptococcus pneumoniae*. Bioelectrochem. Bioenerget **17:**269–276.

8. **Clavé, C., F. Ragueh, M-H. Lebas, and M.C. Trombe.** 1989. Competence induction in *Streptococcus pneumoniae*: a metabolic response to calcium influx involving Na$^+$/Ca^{++} antiport, pp. 13–26. *In* L.O. Butler, C. Harwood, and B.E.B. Moseley (ed.). Genetic Transformation and Expression. Intercept, Andover.

9. **Clavé, C., F. Martin, and M.C. Trombe.** 1989. DNA uptake in competent *Streptococcus pneumoniae*: an insight into energetics and mechanism, pp. 27–40. *In* L.O. Butler, C. Harwood, and B.E.B. Moseley (ed.). Genetic Transformation and Expression. Intercept Andover.

10. **Dawes, E.A., and P.J. Senior.** 1973. Energy reserve polymers in microorganisms. Adv. Microb. Physiol. **14:**203–266.

11. **Fox, H., and R. Hotchkiss.** 1957. Initiation of bacterial transformation. Nature **179:**1322–1325.

12. **Fry, I.J., M. Becker-Hapak, and J.H. Hageman.** 1991. Purification and properties of an intracellular calmodulin-like protein from *Bacillus subtilis* cells. J. Bacteriol. **173:**2506–2513.

13. **Gangola, P., and B.P. Rosen.** 1987. Maintenance of intracellular calcium in *Escherichia coli*. J. Biol. Chem. **262:**12570–12574.

14. **Garcia Vescovi, E., F.C. Soncini, and E.A. Groisman.** 1996. Mg^{2+} as an extracellular signal: Environmental regulation of salmonella virulence. Cell **84:**165–174.

15. **Griffiths, E.** 1987. The iron-uptake systems of pathogenic bacteria, pp. 69–137. *In* J.J. Bullen and E. Griffiths (ed.). Iron and Infection. John Wiley & Sons, New York.

16. **Havarstein, L.S.** 1998. Identification of a competence regulon in streptococcus pneumoniae by genomic analysis. Trends Microbiol. **6:**297–299.

17. **Harold, F.M.** 1982. Pumps and currents: a biological perspective. Curr. Top. Memb. Transp. **16:**485–516.

18. **Hefner, D.L.** 1982. Transport of H$^+$, K$^+$, Na$^+$, and Ca^{2+} in streptococcus. Mol. Cell. Biochem. **44:**81–106.

19. **Hefner, D.L., and F.M. Harold.** 1982. ATP-driven sodium pump in *Streptococcus faecalis*. Proc. Natl. Acad. Sci. USA **79:**2798–2802.

20. **Holtje, J.V., and A. Tomasz.** 1976. Purification of the pneumococcal N-acetyl-L-alanine amidase to biochemical homogeneity. J. Biol. Chem. **251:**4199–4207.

21. **Ivey, D.M., A.A. Guffanti, J. Zemski, E. Pinner, R. Karpel, E. Padan, S. Schuldiner, and T.A. Krulwich.** 1993. Cloning and characterization of a putative Ca^{2+}/H$^+$ antiporter gene from *E. coli* upon functional complementation of Na$^+$/H$^+$ antiporter deficient strains by overexpressed gene. J. Biol. Chem. **268:**11296–11303.

22. **Kaczorowski, G.J., F. Barros, J.K. Dethmers, and M.J. Trumble.** 1985. Inhibition of Na$^+$/Ca^{2+} exchange in pituitary plasma membrane vesicles by analogues of amilorides. Biochemistry **24:**1394–1403.

23. **Kominek, L.A. and H.O. Halvorson.** 1965. Metabolism of poly-β-hydroxybutyrate and acetoin in *Bacillus cereus*. J. Bacteriol. **90:**1251–1259.

24. **Kretzinger, R.H., D. Tolbert, S. Nakayama, and W. Pearson.** 1991. The EF-hand homologs and analogs, pp. 20–35. *In* C.W. Heizman (ed.). Novel Calcium Binding Proteins. Springer-Verlag.

25. **Krulwich, T.A.** 1983. Na$^+$/H$^+$ antiporters. Biochem. Biophys. Acta **726:**254–264.

26. **Lacks, S.** 1962. Molecular fate of DNA in genetic transformation of Pneumococcus. J. Mol. Biol. **5:**119–131.

27. **Lopez, A., C. Clavé, R. Capeyrou, V. Lafontan, and M.C. Trombe.** 1989. Ionic and energetic changes at competence in the naturally transformable bacteria *Streptococcus pneumoniae*. J. Gen. Microbiol. **135:**2189–2197.

28. **Martin, B., P. Garcia, M.P. Castanie, and J.P. Claverys.** 1995. The recA gene of *Streptococcus pneumoniae* is part of a competence-induced operon and controls lysogenic induction. Mol. Microbiol. **15:**367–379.

29. **Matsushita, T., T. Ueda, and I. Kusaka.** 1986. Purification and characterization of Ca^{2+}/H$^+$ antiporter from *Bacillus subtilis*. Eur. J. Biochem. **156:**95–100.

30. **Matsushita, T., H. Hirata, and I. Kusaka.** 1988. Calcium channel blockers inhibit bacterial chemotaxis. Febs. Lett. **236:**400–437.

31. **Mazodier, P., and J. Davies.** 1991. Gene transfer between distantly related bacteria. Annu. Rev. Genet. **25:**147–171.

32. **Mekalanos, J.J.** 1992. Environmental signals controlling expression of virulent determinant in bacteria. J. Bacteriol. **174:**1–7.

33. **Morrison, D., M-C. Trombe, G. Hayden, G. Waszack, and J-D. Chen.** 1984. Isolation of transformation deficient mutants of *Streptococcus pneumoniae* defective in control of competence, using insertion-duplication mutagenesis with EM determinant of pAMB1. J. Bacteriol. **159:**870–876.

34. **Norris, V., M. Chen, M. Goldberg, J. Voskuil, G. McGurk, and I.B. Holland.** 1991. Calcium in bacteria: a solution to which problem? Mol. Microbiol. **5:**775–778.

35. **Ohyama, T., K. Igarashi, and H. Kobayashi.** 1994. Physiological role of the chaA gene in sodium and calcium regulations at high pH in *Escherichia coli*. J. Bacteriol. **176:**4311–4315.

36. **Oneck, L.A., and R.J. Smith.** 1992. Calmodulin and calcium mediated regulation in procaryotes. J. Gen. Microbiol. **138:**1039–1049.

37. **Ordal, G.W.** 1977. Calcium ion regulates chemotactic behaviour in bacteria. Nature **270:**66–67.

38. **Paton, J.C., P.W. Andrew, G.J. Boulnois, and T.J. Mitchell.** 1993. Molecular analysis of the pathogenicity of *Streptococcus pneumoniae*: the role of pneumococcal proteins. Annu. Rev. Microbiol. **47:**89–115.

39. **Pearce, B.J., A.M. Baughton, E.A. Campbell, and H.R. Masure.** 1995. The rec locus, a competence-induced operon in *Streptococcus pneumoniae*. J. Bacteriol. **177:**86–93.

40. **Rensendez, E.J., J. Ting, K.S. Kim, S.K. Wooden, and A.S. Lee.** 1986. The calcium ionophore A23187 as a regulator of gene expression in mammalian cells. J. Cell. Biol. **103:**2145–2152.

41. **Reusch, R.N., R. Huang, and L.L. Bramble.** 1995. Poly-3-hydroxybutyrate/polyphosphate complexes form voltage activated Ca^{2+} channels in the plasma membranes of *Escherichia coli*. Biophys. J. **37:**754–766.

42. **Rosen, B.P.** 1987. Bacterial calcium transport. Biochem. Biophys. Acta **906:**101–110.

43. **Seto, H., and A. Tomasz.** 1976. Calcium-requiring step in the uptake of deoxyribonucleic acid molecules through the surface of competent pneumococci. J. Bacteriol. **126:**1113–1118.

44. **Smith, R.J.** 1995. Calcium and bacteria. Adv. Microbial Physiol. **37:**83–133.

45. **Spellberg, B., D.R. Cundell, J. Sandros, B.J. Pearce, I. Idanpaan-Heikkila, C. Rosenow, and H.R. Masure.** 1996. Pyruvate oxydase, as a determinant of virulence in *Streptococcus pneumoniae*. Mol. Microbiol. **19:**803–813.

46. **Swan, D.G., R.S. Hale, N. Dhillon, and P.F. Leadlay.** 1987. A bacterial calcium binding protein homologous to calmodulin. Nature **329:**84–85.

47. **Tisa, L.S., and J. Adler.** 1992. Calcium ions are involved in *Es-*

cherichia coli chemotaxis. Proc. Natl. Acad. Sci. USA **89:**11804–11808.

48. **Tisa, L.S., and J. Adler.** 1995. Cytoplasmic free-Ca^{++} level rises with repellents and falls with attractants in Escherichia coli chemotaxis. Proc. Natl. Acad. Sci. USA **92:**10777–10781.

49. **Tisa, L.S., B.M. Olivera, and J. Adler.** 1993. Inhibition of *Escherichia coli* chemotaxis by ω conotoxin, a calcium ion channel blocker. J. Bacteriol. **175:**1235–1238.

50. **Tomasz, A.** 1970. Cellular metabolism in genetic transformation of pneumonococci: requirement for protein synthesis during induction of competence. J. Bacteriol. **101:**860–871.

51. **Tomasz, A., P. Moreillon, and G. Pozzi.** 1988. Insertional inactivation of the major autolysin of *Streptococcus pneumoniae*. J. Bacteriol. **170:**5931–5934.

52. **Trombe, M-C.** 1993. Characterization of the calcium porter involved in regulation of growth and competence induction in *Streptococcus pneumoniae*. J. Gen. Microbiol. **139:**443–439.

53. **Trombe, M-C., C. Clavé, and J-M. Manias.** 1992. Calcium regulation of growth and of differentiation in *Streptococcus pneumoniae*. J. Gen. Microbiol. **138:**77–84.

54. **Trombe, M-C., V. Rieux, and F. Bailles.** 1994. Calcium regulation of growth, autolysis and competence induction in *Streptococcus pneumoniae*: effect of mutations which alter the cooperativity of ^{45}Ca^{2+} transport. J. Bacteriol. **176:**1992–1996.

55. **van Veen, H.W., T. Abee, G.J. Kortstee, W.N. Konings, and A.J. Zehnder.** 1994. Translocation of metal phosphate via the phosphate inorganic transport system of *Escherichia coli*. Biochemistry **33:**1766–1770.

56. **Vyas, N.K., M.N. Vyas, and F.A. Quiocho.** 1987. A novel calcium binding site in the galactose-binding protein of bacterial transport and chemotaxis. Nature **327:**635–638.

57. **Watkins, N.J., M.R. Knight, A.J. Trewavas, and A.K. Campbell.** 1995. Free calcium transients in chemotactic and non chemotactic strains of E. coli determined by using recombinant aequorin. Biochem. J. **306:**865–869.

58. **Watson, D.A., D.M. Musher, and J. Verhoef.** 1995. Pneumococcal virulence factors and host immune response to them. Eur. J. Clin. Microbiol. Infect. Dis. **14:**479–490.

Address reprint requests to:
Dr. Marie-Claude Trombe
Universite Paul Sabatier
Laboratoire de Bactériologie
Centre Hospitalo Universitaire de Rangueil
Avenue J. Poullhès
31403 Toulouse, France

Part 4

Pneumococcal Disease and Animal Models

Molecular and Cellular Biology of Pneumococcal Infection

ELAINE I. TUOMANEN and H. ROBERT MASURE

INTRODUCTION

THE THREE MAJOR INVASIVE PATHOGENS OF CHILDREN, including *Streptococcus pneumoniae*, *Neisseria meningitidis*, and *Haemophilus influenzae*, are carried in the nasopharynx by a significant proportion of healthy individuals. For the pneumococcus, an asymptomatic carrier state persists for several weeks at a time in as many as 40% of the general population. During a small fraction of these encounters, pneumococci spread and gain access to the ear, lung or blood stream but do not necessarily evoke symptoms. In only a few, does symptomatic otitis media, pneumonia, bacteremia or meningitis develop. These epidemiological observations imply that there exists three levels of encounter between the human host and this pathogen. In the first, recognition of and attachment to human nasopharyngeal cells, all pneumococci appear to be able to establish a carrier state since the human is the only known host. Some variability in the efficiency of this property may exist since some strains are found more frequently than others. The second level of encounter in which pneumococci move to another body site may arise from a less widely distributed set of capabilities since most disease is limited to ~20 of the 90 serotypes. Finally, still other events, often derived from the host, contribute to development of symptoms referrable to the infected site.

This review will evaluate current understanding of the molecular events contributing to targeting pneumococci to various sites of infection and then examine additional steps that promote development of symptomatic pneumococcal disease. This information has been assembled by first identifying the receptors for pneumococci on various human cells and then searching libraries of mutants for nonadherent clones indicative of potential bacterial adhesins. Similarly, for the dissection of disease, the pneumococcal components responsible for initiating inflammation have been identified by a systematic analysis of the bioactivities of several classes of surface molecules.

ADHERENCE, INVASION, AND VIRULENCE

Pneumococci bind avidly to cells of the upper and lower respiratory tract and endovasculature (Fig. 1). The attachment interface is characterized by a broad area of contact between the bacterial surface and host cell suggesting multiple receptor interactions. No structures reminiscent of fimbriae have been detected at the attachment site despite significant search efforts using multiple techniques to prepare the cells. Rather, there is a uniform, electron dense haze that fills the space between the apposed membranes. Attachment does not invoke actin polymerization or formation of unusual human cellular protrusions as has been seen for other invasive bacteria. Yet, adherence appears to proceed to internalization into a vacuole that is formed by invagination of the cell surface membrane compatible with receptor-mediated endocytosis. This physiological event is somehow corrupted by the pneumococcus such that the bacteria-vacuole complex transits the cytoplasm and extrudes the bacteria on the opposite side of mammalian cells. This trafficking pattern has been demonstrated in *in vitro* systems for both the lung and the blood brain barrier.[1]

Receptors tethering pneumococci to human cells

For most bacteria, adherence to human cells is achieved by presentation of surface proteins that bind to eukaryotic carbohydrates in a lectin-like fashion. Pneumococci display at least five lectin specificities depending on the target cell (Table 1). The carriage interaction is sustained for several weeks and several serotypes can coexist at one time. The event is not associated with an overt inflammatory response yet it leads to serotype specific immunity based on the structure of the capsular polysaccharide of the infecting strain.

Nasopharynx

Early studies using buccal epithelial cells and hapten inhibition assays identified GlcNAc (β1-3) Gal as capable of blocking pneumococcal attachment.[2] More recent studies confirm that pneumococci can bind this determinant but how this relates to binding to *in vivo* niches is less clear. This sugar does not affect pneumococcal binding to upper respiratory tract cells, represented by either Chang conjunctival cells or primary bronchial epithelial cells.[3] Effective inhibition of adherence is seen by glycoconjugates of Gal (β1,4) GlcNAc, particularly if the sugar is sialylated. These sialylated lactosamines are likely to be present on many different human cell surface glycoconjugates and it is not known if a particular receptor is preferred. If so, then the receptor is universally distributed since there is no known example of resistance to pneumococcal carriage. Pneumococcal neuraminidase activity has been detected during

Department of Infectious Diseases, St. Jude Children's Research Hospital, Memphis, Tennessee.

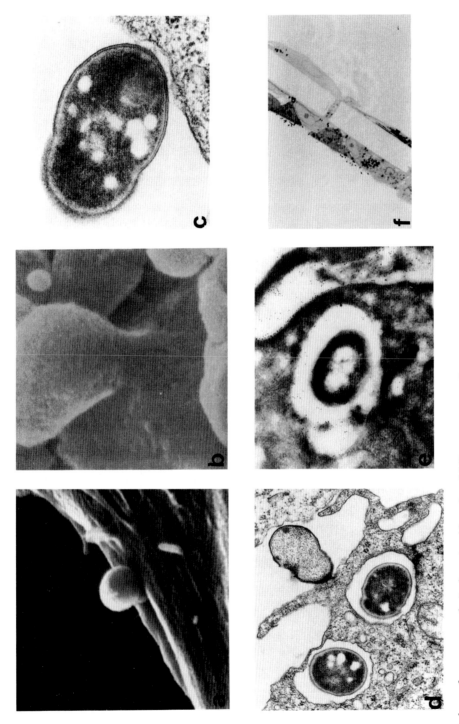

FIG. 1. Morphology of pneumococcal attachment and invasion. (**a**) Pneumococcus adherent to A549 lung epithelial cell. (**b**) Higher magnification view of (a) demonstrating that the zone of adherence between the bacteria and cell is broad and sufficiently strong so as to tent the human cell membrane. (**c**) Pneumococcus adherent to human vascular endothelial cell. Zone of contact is broad with fine, fibrillar mesh localized to and filling space between the cells. (**d**) Pneumococci adherent to and inside vacuoles of endothelial cell. (**e**) Pneumococcus within a vacuole of an endothelial cell. Surface of the cell was labeled with biotin and internalization was allowed for 30 min. Distribution of biotin is indicated by streptavidin conjugated gold particles. Vacuolar membrane maintains biotin labeling indicating it is derived from the cell surface. (**f**) Pneumococcal transmigration through a bilayer consisting of A549 cells on top and umbilical vein endothelial cells on the bottom. Bacteria, visualized as dark spheres by gram stain 10 h after inoculation of the upper chamber, are seen adherent to and within the upper A549 cells and within the lower endothelial cells. No intercellular bacteria were detected indicating that transmigration follows a transcellular route. (a,b) Scanning electron micrographs made by K. McDonough and M. Florczyk, N.Y. State Department of Health, Albany, NY, with technical advice of C. Rosenow, Rockefeller University. (c–e) Transmission electron micrographs made by U. Kavita and H. Chiao, Rockefeller University. (f) Light micrograph made by C. Rosenow, Rockefeller University.

TABLE 1. PNEUMOCOCCAL BINDING TO CARBOHYDRATES

Carbohydrate specificity	Proposed target cell	Reference
GlcNAc (β1-3) Gal	Buccal epithelium	2,6
NANA[a] Gal (β1-4) GlcNAc	Conjunctival epithelium	3
	Bronchial epithelium	3
GalNAc (β1-4) Gal	Alveolar epithelium	5,6
	Vascular endothelium	6
GalNAc (β1-3) Gal	Alveolar epithelium	6
	Vascular endothelium	6
GlcNAc	Activated alveolar epithelium	8
	Activated vascular endothelium	8

[a]A wide range of sialylated compounds are effective, particularly with the lactosamine core.

the advance of pneumococci up the eustachian tube suggesting that adherence to sialic acid may be a prelude to attachment via other masked specificities.[4]

Pulmonary epithelial cells and vascular endothelial cells

Pneumococci bind to at least two different ligands on non-inflamed pulmonary epithelium and vascular endothelium. No differences in these two sites have been found as yet. Attachment to resting cells occurs via two classes of glycoconjugates. The disaccharide GalNAc (β1-4) Gal was first described by Krivan et al.[5] as a specificity shared between several respiratory pathogens. Subsequent studies confirmed these results and added an additional capability to bind to GalNAc (β1-3) Gal on resting cells.[6] Soluble versions of both carbohydrates block pneumococcal adherence to human cells and immobilized carbohydrates support pneumococcal binding directly. A combination of the two sugars, as represented by asialo-GM2 and globoside, virtually eliminates adherent bacteria *in vitro*. This additive effect suggests that these glycoconjugates define independent receptors and that there are no other significant receptors on these cells in the resting state. In an extension of the *in vitro* data, mixture of the same combination of glycoconjugates with pneumococci prior to intratracheal challenge of rabbits results in rapid clearance of the pneumococcal load from the lung as compared to challenge with bacteria alone. These two resting cell surface sugar specificities can be viewed as the molecular targets involved in the asymptomatic presence of pneumococci in the lung and vascular space. In experimental models, low levels of pneumococci have been shown to persist on the mucosa of the alveolar space without overt disease.[7] Transient pneumococcal bacteremia, which is either asymptomatic or accompanied by a brief episode of fever, is a well-documented clinical phenomenon, particularly in children.

PAF receptor on activated human cells

The incidence of bacteremia resulting from pneumococcal pneumonia is less than 1 in 100. Similarly, the incidence of invasion of the meningeal space, even in the face of high grade bacteremia, is rare. These clinical observations suggest that invasive disease requires more than simple adherence capabilities. A molecular mechanism for a transition from a state of pneumococcal binding to a state promoting cellular transloca-

tion and invasion has been proposed and involves proinflammatory activation of the target human cell (Table 2).[8] By analogy with other human cell migration systems, the local generation of inflammatory factors can cause profound changes in the number and type of receptors available on activated cells. For example, activation of vascular endothelial cells by thrombin, tumor necrosis factor (TNF) or interleukin-1 (IL-1) increases expression of cell adhesion molecules important for leukocyte trafficking.[9,10] Pneumococci appear to take advantage of this scenario and engage one of these upregulated receptors, the platelet-activating factor (PAF) receptor.[8] Coincident with the appearance of the PAF receptor following an inflammatory stimulus, pneumococci undergo waves of enhanced adherence. In the case of thrombin, binding occurs in minutes, while for IL-1 and TNF, it occurs over hours. COS cells acquire the ability to bind pneumococci upon transfection with PAF receptor cDNA. The binding to activated cells is inhibitable by PAF receptor antagonists and by sugars, GlcNAc or lacto-N-neotetraose, which show no activity in blocking adherence to resting cells. The potency of these two distinct inhibitors suggests that pneumococci may bind to the PAF receptor at two sites: one shared with PAF and the other at a site

TABLE 2. PROPOSED STEPS IN PNEUMOCOCAL ADHERENCE AND TRANSMIGRATION

Targeting to nasopharynx or lung
  Adherence to nasopharyngeal cells bearing sialylated GlcNAc (β1-4) GalNAc glycoconjugates by transparent pneumococci
  Adherence to resting lung cells bearing GalNAc β1-4 Gal or GalNac (β1-3) Gal glycoconjugates by transparent pneumococci
Transmigration
  Activation of eukaryotic cells by thrombin or cytokines with resultant expression of PAF receptor
  Shift in pneumococcal binding by transparent variants only to the PAF receptor involving the cell wall phosphorylcholine
  Internalization of pneumococci by PAF receptor recycling without G-protein signalling
  Transcytosis of pneumococci in vesicles and extrusion on ablumenal surface
  Strong binding to fibronectin of extracellular matrix

of glycosylation of the receptor (Fig. 2). It is also possible that the glycosyl determinant is on a co-receptor that caps with the PAF receptor. This latter possibility is of interest in the search for alternative downstream signals generated after pneumococcal attachment.

PAF is a powerful lipid chemokine and upon binding to the PAF receptor induces endothelial permeability and leukocyte extravasation.[11] The PAF receptor is a G-protein coupled, serpentine receptor.[12,13] Although binding to the receptor in a manner inhibited by PAF, pneumococci do not induce G-protein–mediated signal transduction or interfere with PAF-induced signalling.[8] Rather, it appears that the PAF receptor facilitates internalization of pneumococci into endothelial cells, a process that may promote invasion. Pneumococci fail to invade resting cells (0.1%). However, 2–3% of the inoculum moves to an intracellular vacuole in activated cells as demonstrated by gentamicin protection studies[8] as well as electron microscopy (Fig. 1).[14] The PAF receptor is known to be rapidly internalized after interaction with the ligand.[15] Such receptor-mediated endocytosis is consistent with the demonstration that the membrane of the pneumococcal vacuole retains cell surface markers (U. Kavita and E. Tuomanen, unpublished data) (Fig. 1d) and that PAF receptor antagonists inhibit pneumococcal uptake.[8]

That the PAF receptor–dependent uptake of pneumococci leads to transcellular migration and exit of living bacteria at the ablumenal surface remains to be studied in detail. Three pieces of evidence suggest this is the case. In a rabbit model of pneumonia, the development of bacteremia following intratracheal challenge with pneumococci is attenuated upon treatment with the PAF receptor antagonist.[8] Increased pinocytotic vesicle traffic across the blood brain barrier endothelium follows intravenous application of pneumococcal cell wall components.[16] Finally, preliminary studies using an *in vitro* bilayer model system developed by Birkness and Quinn[17] indicate that pneumococcal translocation is PAF receptor dependent. Pneumococci can transit from the upper to the lower chamber across a bilayer consisting of type 2 pulmonary epithelial cells and umbilical vein endothelial cells. The process takes 9–11 h to complete and is attenuated in the presence of the PAF receptor antagonist (C. Rosenow and Tuomanen, unpublished data; Fig. 1e). Histologic examination indicates pneumococci accumulate within both epithelial and endothelial cells and are not seen in between cells. Results in the rabbit pneumonia model suggest this transmigration, at least in part PAF receptor dependent, is a critical step in advancing disease. Thus, the participation of the host in an inflammatory response, in this case upregulating the presentation of the PAF receptor, is an important element contributing to development of symptomatic, invasive infection. It also suggests that pneumococcal elements required to negotiate this step will be key virulence determinants operative more frequently in virulent strains and likely to be subject to regulated expression.

Crossing the blood-brain barrier: pneumococcal recycling

Meningitis due to *S. pneumoniae* develops during high-grade bacteremia in relatively few individuals. Using an *in vitro* human blood-brain barrier (BBB) system, a specific mechanism for pneumococcal targeting of the BBB has been characterized.[1] Invasion requires prior adherence of the bacteria to the surface

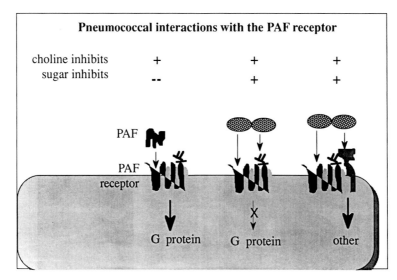

FIG. 2. Pneumococcal interactions with the PAF receptor. Left diagram: PAF binds to the PAF receptor in a choline-dependent fashion and elicits a G protein mediated signal. Middle and right diagram: Pneumococci also interact with the PAF receptor in a choline-dependent fashion, but there is no G protein elicited signal. Furthermore, pneumococcal binding, but not PAF binding, is inhibited by exogenous carbohydrate suggesting that pneumococcal attachment is qualitatively different than that of the native ligand PAF. There are two models to explain this difference: as shown in the middle diagram, pneumococci may engage both the PAF binding site and a carbohydrate on the PAF receptor. Alternatively, as shown on the right diagram, pneumococci might bind the PAF binding site on PAF receptor and a carbohydrate on an unidentified receptor which co-caps with the PAF receptor. This second co-receptor may produce an as yet unknown signal not shared by the G-protein pathway. (Analysis based on Cundell *et al.*[8])

of BBB, a step requiring the pneumococcal adhesin CbpA. Internalization lags behind adherence temporally, and a maximum of ~10% of the adherent bacterial population becomes intracellular. Pneumococci are approximately 10-fold more efficient at invasion of cerebral as compared to peripheral endothelial cells. However, this capability is widely variable depending in part on the amount of bacterial capsule (not on serotype). Spontaneous nonencapsulated variants of clinical isolates and nonencapsulated laboratory strains demonstrated up to 200 fold greater invasion of BBB than isogenic encapsulated strains. Transparent colony variants have a 3–5-fold selective advantage over opaque variants for BBB transmigration.

The PAF receptor appears to play a role in pneumococcal trafficking across the BBB and activated BBB cells support greater transmigration, as has been found in the periphery. Once inside BBB cells, the bacteria appear to undergo one of three fates: death within the vacuole, transit through the cells to exit the basolateral surface, or recycling of bacteria back to the apical surface. Ten percent of internalized bacteria recycle to the surface within 30 min. Transmigration of similar numbers of bacteria to the lower chamber requires 120 min. Only transparent bacteria can travel either of these routes; opaque bacteria are killed intracellularly. A circular recycling pathway in which bacteria enter and exit the same cellular surface could enhance the total number of bacteria positioned to cross a substantial barrier such as the BBB. The details of this process remain to be established, but this behavior represents an important potential tool to investigate vectorial vesical transport across mammalian cells.

Extracellular matrix

Upon exit at the basolateral surface of a human cell, pneumococci would encounter extracellular matrix components such as fibronectin. Pneumococci adhere avidly to immobilized but not soluble fibronectin.[18] Most other bacteria bind to the amino terminus of fibronectin. Pneumococci, however, preferentially bind the carboxy-terminal heparin binding domain within a region that shares sequence similarity to vascular cell adhesion molecule–1 (VCAM-1).[19] Pneumococci also bind recombinant VCAM-1.

Pneumococcal components contributing to adherence

To identify the important adhesive ligands of pneumococcus, several new genetic strategies were developed and then coupled to an array of in vitro assays based on the biology of pneumococcal interactions with human cells as described above (Table 3). Several genetic loci which affected adherence were rapidly identified from a library of phoA fusion mutants in which targeted insertion duplication mutagenesis yielded loss of function in an array of pneumococcal surface molecules.[20–23] The nature and multiplicity of the adhesive determinants identified indicated that pneumococcal attachment is complex (Table 4). Structural, regulatory and accessory components were identified (Table 5).

Interpretation of these results led to a number of conclusions: (1) Of the five sugars recognized by pneumococci, mutants were found that were defective in binding each individual sugar. This provided genetic evidence to support the biochemical data that each adhesive specificity is distinct from the others and suggested that there may be as many as five specific adhesins. (2)

TABLE 3. GENETIC AND *in Vitro* ANALYSIS OF PNEUMOCOCCAL VIRULENCE

Libraries of pneumococcal mutants
   phoA fusion for identification of surface proteins
   lacZ fusion for promoter probes
   Gain of function in *B. subtilis*
   Saturated mutagenesis of entire chromosome
Assays of steps in pneumococcal disease
   Adherence/internalization into resting and activated cells
      Nasopharynx
      Lung
      Peripheral and brain vascular endothelium
      PAF receptor transfectants
   Adherence to extracellular matrix
   Transmigration through lung-blood and blood-brain bilayer models
   DNA transformation
   Autolysis

Several mutants were found that failed to adhere to all carbohydrates, indicating that global down regulation of adherence was possible. (3) Some mutants defective in autolysis or transformation were also deficient in adherence, suggesting that there may be cross-regulation of important events in pneumococcal physiology.

A model of pneumococcal adherence

Appreciation that important events in pneumococcal physiology were interrelated provided the key to the development of a model of pneumococcal adherence and virulence consistent with the surprisingly large number of potential participating elements. Reexamination of adherence as a function of cell density revealed changes over time, a feature also characteristic of transformation and autolysis (A. Cauwels and E. Tuomanen, unpublished data). Temporal analysis of the wild-type pneumococcal life cycle is shown in Fig. 3. Major events appear to be regulated with time in accordance with a quorum sensing paradigm. Transformation occurs in a brief window during early log phase coincident with the extracellular appearance and disappearance of the 17–amino acid activator substance (competence stimulating peptide).[24] Transformation is followed by a transient ability to adhere to the PAF receptor and subsequently to sialic acid. These transient binding capacities are distinct from the constitutive ability to bind to resting cell receptors of the lung and vascular endothelium. Finally, in stationary phase, autolysis is triggered. Supernatant fluids collected at the peak of each activity can confer that activity on cells from other points in the life cycle consistent with cell signalling triggered by autoinducers produced at discrete cell densities. This model suggests that for transformation, autolysis and two types of adhesion there exist extracellular autoinducers that indicate four different cell densities. For each of these four checkpoints, a signalling cascade exists that triggers expression of a regulon resulting in the coordinate appearance of many gene products required to enact each physiological event.

Regulation of adherence

Class 1: Regulatory elements affecting adherence, transformation, and autolysis. (A) The opacity locus: Pneumococci

TABLE 4. PNEUMOCOCCAL MUTANTS IDENTIFIED AS DEFICIENT IN ADHERENCE FROM A
LIBRARY OF 300 *phoA* MUTANTS SCREENED AGAINST EUKARYOTIC SUGAR RECEPTORS

| | Resting receptor/Activated receptor | | | |
Mutant	β(1-3)Gal	β(1-4)Gal	GlcNac	Gene
4	+		+	Pyrrolidine 5 carboxylate reductase
5			+	PTS family of permeases
11	+	+		*amiD*, peptide permease
14	+			Amylopullulanase receptor
16	+	+	+	Pyruvate oxidase
19			+	PTS family of permeases
25	+	+	+	Spore coat protein
30			+	Glycerol 3 phosphate dehydrogenase
31			+	tRNA synthetase
40		+		Methionine sulfoxide reductase
72	+			Pyruvate formate lyase
77		+	+	Ornithine carbamoyl transferase
87			+	PTS family of permeases
98	+			*plpA*, peptide permease
101	+			*lacX* glucose metabolism
104	+			Proline-rich protein
121		+		*amiA*, peptide permease

+Mutant is defective in adherence to this sugar.

Resting, human cell (lung or endothelial cell) not stimulated with cytokines; activated, human cell (lung or endothelial cell) stimulated with IL-1β or TNF; β13 Gal, GlcNAc β(1-3)Gal; β14 Gal, GlcNAc β(1-4)Gal; GlcNAc, Lacto-*N*-neotetraose.

Analysis performed by Dr. D. Cundell; library created by Drs. B. Pearce and P. Sreenivasan.

spontaneously vary colonial morphology at high frequency between opaque and transparent colony variants.[25] Opaque colonies fail to cause disease in a rat intranasal challenge model, while transparent variants that colonize the nasopharynx cause bacteremia. A genetic locus conferring opacity has been identified although its function has not been clarified.[26] Although opaque and transparent pneumococcal variants adhere to a sim-

TABLE 5. CLASSIFICATION OF LOSS OF FUNCTION
MUTATIONS THAT CAUSE DEFECTIVE ADHERENCE

Peptide permeases
  Exp 5, PTS family
  Exp 19, PTS family
  AmiD
  AmiA
  PlpA[a]
Signal transduction
  Pyruvate oxidase
  Pyruvate formate lyase
Amino acid biosynthesis
  Pyrolidine 5 carboxylate reductase
  Ornithine carbamoyl transferase
  tRNA synthetase
Glucose metabolism
  Glycerol 3 phosphate dehydrogenase
  lacX
Other
  Amylo pullulanase receptor precursor
  Spore coat protein
  Methionine sulfoxide reductase
  Proline-rich protein

[a]As described by Paton.

ilar degree to nonactivated epithelial and endothelial cells, enhanced adherence to cytokine stimulated cells or PAF receptor transfected COS cells is limited to transparent variants (Fig. 4).[27] This is consistent with the advantage shown by the transparent pneumococci in producing invasive disease *in vivo* and in enhanced transmigration across the blood brain barrier *in vitro*.[1] Transparent pneumococci are also transformation deficient and exhibit reduced autolytic properties. Recent studies indicate that the pattern of surface proteins on the two phenotypes differs, suggesting a class of proteins are regulated together with phase variation. Of particular note is the increased expression of the adhesin, choline binding protein A, consistent with the enhanced adherence capabilities of the transparent variants. *(B) Bacterial permeases:* Peptide permeases capture and transport small peptides or amino acids from the environment into the cell. They are excellent candidates for the transport of quorum sensing molecules, and genetic experiments suggest this is the case for pneumococci. Mutants with defects in either of two peptide permeases, PlpA and AmiA, show differences in the cell density dependent initiation of transformation and changes in adherence.[21] Loss of function of PlpA eliminates adherence to GalNac (β1-3) Gal and shifts the onset of transformation to very low cell densities. Mutations in AmiA result in loss of binding to GalNac (β1-4) Gal and shifts the onset of transformation to higher cell densities. Both mutants adhere normally to the PAF receptor. Recently, a protein, PsaA, was implicated in adherence[28] but subsequently was shown by sequence similarity and functional studies to be another permease.[29] Mutants with defects in PsaA are deficient in adherence to alveolar cells.[30] Further analysis of this phenotype indicates that mutants defective in this permease do not carry several proteins on the bacterial surface, including a major

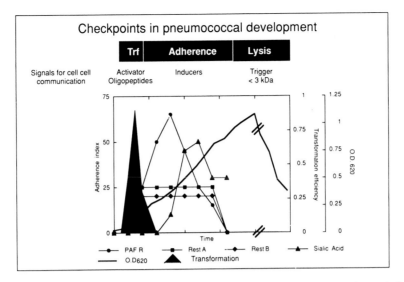

FIG. 3. A program for pneumococcal development. Pneumococci pass through three distinct phases during logarithmic growth *in vitro*. Each is triggered at a specific cell density consistent with a quorum sensing event although the molecules involved are unknown. Phase 1 involves competence for natural DNA transformation. At low bacterial cell density, production of the 17-mer activator peptide is triggered and induces expression of over a dozen genes required from the binding, uptake and incorporation of exogenous DNA. Phase II is characterized by adherence. While adherence to resting human cells is expressed throughout the growth cycle at the same intensity, adherence to the PAF receptor and subsequently to sialic acid occurs in transient peaks. The extracellular signals for these events are unknown. Phase III is stationary phase in which pneumococci autolyse through the activity of the endogenous murein hydrolase, the N-acetylmuramyl-L-alanine amidase. The enzyme is triggered by an unknown extracellular product of <3 kDa size.

structural adhesion, CbpA.[31] *(C) Two component signal transduction systems:* Three two component systems have been characterized in pneumococcus and they appear to link regulation of transformation to cell wall metabolism without changing adherence (Figs. 5 and 6). The first such example *ciaH/ciaR* was described by Hackenbeck, and the characteristics associated with this element are reviewed by her.[73] Mutations of

CiaH/CiaR down regulate transformation and result in enhanced resistance to penicillin. A second two component system is within the *com* locus. This locus consists of three genes, *comC, D,* and *E*, which encode the pheromone competence stimulating peptide and a sensor kinase and response regulator.[32,33] Genetic and biochemical analysis show that these elements are required for the induction of transformation but not appear to alter

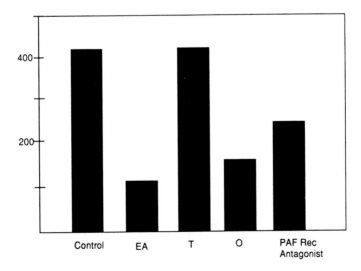

FIG. 4. Modulation of pneumococcal adherence to activated cells. Pneumococci adhere strongly to human endothelial cells activated by cytokines. Replacement of cell wall choline by ethanolamine (EA) substantially reduces adherence as does the PAF receptor antagonist suggesting that pneumococci bind to the PAF receptor in a choline dependent fashion similar to the endogenous mediator PAF. Transparent (T) but not opaque (O) pneumococci exhibit enhanced binding to cells in a PAF dependent fashion consistent with the enhanced virulence of transparent colony forms. (Summarized from other sources.[8,27])

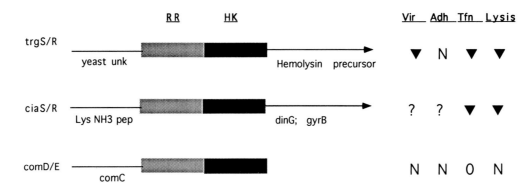

N = normal; ▼ = decreased
0 = absent; ? = not tested

FIG. 5.   Three two-component systems described in pneumococci. In each case, the response regulator precedes the coupled histidine kinase. Genes contiguous with these systems are indicated. TrgS/R is the only system described that affects virulence. All three affect transformation and TrgS/R and ComD/E are also involved in transformation. (Compiled from Cheng et al.[33]; Havarstein et al.[24]; Hackenbeck, this volume; Couwels and Tuomanen, unpublished data.)

adherence, autolysis or virulence. We have identified a third two component sensor-regulator pair, TrgH/TrgR. Mutants with defects in this locus display a decrease in transformation efficiency of >98% and dramatic loss of autolysis in stationary phase and in response to penicillin.[34] Radical changes in the surface protein profile of this mutant suggests that it might be a global regulator of choline binding proteins.

Class 2: Regulation affecting only adherence. (A) The second messenger, acetyl phosphate: Acetyl phosphate is generated by pyruvate oxidase (SpxB) and is the preferred substrate for phosphorylation of response regulators of two component signal transduction systems. In pneumococci, mutation of *spxB* eliminates all adherence to resting and activated cells indicating that multiple adherence specificities can be co-regulated.[22] The link between acetyl phosphate and signal transduction suggests that as yet unidentified two component systems may coordinately regulate the adherence phenotype. *(B) Repair of extracellular oxidative damage by peptide methionine sulfoxide reductase:* Loss of pneumococcal adherence to all cell types was observed for mutants with defects in *msrA*, which encodes a peptide methionine sulfoxide reductase.[23] This enzyme is responsible for the maintenance of methionine residues in a re-

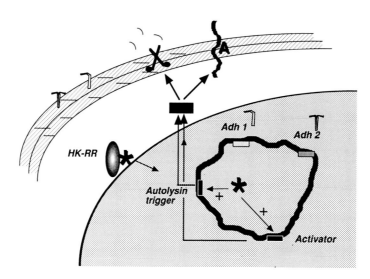

FIG. 6.   A model for two-component regulatory systems in pneumococci. The histidine kinase (HK) becomes phosphorylated upon binding ligand. The phosphate is transferred to the cognate response regulator (RR) which then acts as a DNA binding protein changing gene expression. In the three cases of HK/RR pairs known for pneumococci, the regulation has affected transformation ± autolysis. No system affecting adherence has yet been described. The activator substance, the autolysin and the adhesins are extracellular products which may be subject to regulation at the level of gene expression, transport of the gene products and extracellular proteolysis.

duced state in the face of oxidative stress. Clearly, surface adhesive determinants would be exposed to environmental oxidation and this enzyme appears to be critical to sustaining biological activity of a number of pneumococcal adherence proteins. The phenotype of the homologous mutation in *E. coli* and *Neisseria* also revealed changes in adherence and demonstrated distortion of adhesive pilus structures presumably resulting from the cumulative effects of unrepaired oxidative damage.

Choline-binding proteins: candidate structural genes

Several laboratories have described a family of surface proteins bound to the choline component of the cell wall teichoic acid or lipoteichoic acid of pneumococci. A signature choline-binding domain was discovered and fully characterized by Lopez et al.[35] in his studies of the autolytic enzyme. Other proteins containing this domain include the autolysin of the pneumococcal phage and the protective antigen pneumococcal surface protein A (PspA).[35,36] Some choline-binding proteins are released from the bacteria by exogenous choline, while others are not, suggesting there exist functional subgroups within this family.[37]

A total of 12 choline-binding proteins have been identified in our laboratory by virtue of genomic analysis. Studied as a family,[38] these proteins are surface exposed and react with convalescent human antisera. When co-purified, these proteins can inhibit pneumococcal adherence to endothelial and epithelial cells suggesting that several may contribute to adherence. Antiserum to the mixture of proteins is protective against pneumococcal challenge in rats. A mutant defective in one choline-binding protein, CbpA, fails to colonize the rat nasopharynx. Thus, the choline-binding protein family of surface elements contains the structural gene for autolysis (amidase), at least one candidate adhesin (CbpA), and the protective antigen, PspA. Recent evidence suggests that a choline-binding protein may also stabilize the activity of the activator substance for transformation.[39] Variation in the expression of choline binding proteins during opaque and transparent phase switching is consistent with the multiple changes that occur in bacterial physiology with this transition.[25] Choline-binding proteins may serve as a family of structural genes for much of the important cellular physiology of the pneumococcus.

CbpA has been studied in more detail than many of the other newly found choline-binding proteins.[38] Mature CbpA is a protein of 663 amino acids with two distinct domains. Like all other choline-binding proteins, the C-terminus consists of a choline binding domain, in this case formed by ten tandem repeats. The N-terminal domain (amino acids 1–433) is different from all other choline binding proteins. It contains two large repeat regions, each containing three alpha helices. Repeat 1 spans residues 153–321, and repeat 2 spans 327–433. Recombinant CbpA blocks pneumococcal binding to lacto-N-neotraose, sialic acid, lung cells and nasopharyngeal cells. Similarly recombinant forms of the repeats fulfill the same functions with two repeats being of greater potency than one. These data suggest that the repeats constitute lectin domains. It is of interest that recent data suggest that a variant of CbpA containing only one repeat and the choline binding domain (which arose during cloning in *E. coli*) was reported to bind IgA and secretory component.[40]

Whether this represents a lectin type of interaction remains to be determined. Of further interest, Hostetter and colleagues also identified a protein, named PbcA, with sequence identical to CbpA which binds but does not cleave C3.[41] While the functions of CbpA may be multiple, it is encouraging that, in passive and active protection studies, CbpA is protective in several animal models across heterologous serotypes (42). A conserved, multifunctional pneumococcal surface protein would logically be an excellent vaccine candidate.

Cell wall choline as an adhesive ligand

An unusual feature of the pneumococcal cell wall structure is the presence of phosphorylcholine in the teichoic acid and lipoteichoic acid.[43] Treatment of pneumococci with trypsin eliminates approximately half of the adherence capacity of wild type bacteria for endothelial cells, suggesting that components other than proteins mediate some adherence.[14] The remaining adherence is eliminated by competition with soluble, purified cell wall or when the choline is replaced by ethanolamine suggesting that choline on the cell wall itself may directly participate in adherence. This choline-dependent binding was demonstrated to involve the PAF receptor on host cells.[8]

Pneumococcal choline-bearing cell wall structures appear to serve several functions. First, they are a platform for docking of a family of choline binding proteins on the bacterial surface, some of which bind to carbohydrates on human cells during bacterial adherence. Secondly, choline potentially interacts directly with the PAF receptor during bacterial adherence. Finally, choline-mediated binding of some soluble cell wall fragments to human cells induces signalling in the host cell resulting in generation of some elements of the acute phase response. This represents substantial evidence that a significant amount of pneumococcal pathophysiology is focused on the cell wall choline (at least as a determinant of bacterial binding and migration across cells and as a key inflammatory mediator; Fig. 7). Differences in the amount of choline on the cell wall correlates with pneumococcal virulence.[44] That such choline-related biology might extend to other respiratory pathogens is an exciting possibility that has been suggested by two findings: choline decorates the surface polar lipid of Mycoplasma[45] and phase variable, serum sensitivity of *Haemophilus influenzae* correlates with the presence of a choline adduct on endotoxin[46,47]. These similarities raise the possibility of similarities in gene products involved in placement of choline on the surface of these pathogens. The *lic* locus performs this function in *Haemophilus*, and a related *lic* locus has been found and characterized in pneumococcus.[48] These findings imply convergent evolution of pathogens capable of targeting the choline-rich environment of the human lung.

MECHANISMS OF PNEUMOCOCCAL INFLAMMATION

Cell wall as a library of inflammatory fragments

When cell wall, cytoplasm, and capsule are compared for inflammatory capacity, cell wall has the highest specific activity

Pneumococcal transmigration   Cell wall entry and signalling

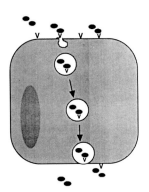   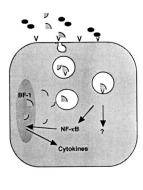

FIG. 7. Common features of pneumococcal transmigration and cell signalling. Left: Pneumococcal transmigration involves internalization into a vacuole, at least in part involving the PAF receptor and its natural recycling pathway. The events which direct the bacteria laden vacuole across the cell to the basolateral surface are unknown. Right: In addition to pneumococci, pneumococcal cell wall pieces, particularly those bearing choline, can be bound and internalized into human cells. Signalling can be initiated by wall bound at the cell surface by CD14 or PAF receptor. These receptors engender as yet uncharacterized signals which lead to activation of NF-kB, its translocation to the nucleus and induction of cytokine production. Events associated with cell wall internalized into vacuoles remain to be studied. (Compiled from other sources.[8,14,60,62,72])

(Table 6).[49,50] This activity is not shielded by overlying capsule on the native bacteria. The signs and symptoms of infection induced by cell wall mimic that of living bacteria in animal models of meningitis, pneumonia and otitis media.[49,51,52] In addition, clinical strains and their isogenic lab derivatives, which have defects in release of cell wall fragments, induce an attenuated pattern of disease.[53]

The teichoic acid and lipteichoic acid contribute strongly to host defense responses associated with acute inflammation. They activate the alternative pathway of the complement cascade, bind the acute phase reactant C-reactive protein, activate procoagulant activity on the surface of endothelial cells, induce

TABLE 6.   BIOACTIVITIES OF PNEUMOCOCCAL
CELL WALL COMPONENTS

Teichoicated cell wall
  Fix complement
  Induce procoagulant activity on endothelial cells
  Activate endothelia, epithelia and leukocytes to produce
    IL-1 and TNF
  Chemotactic for leukocytes
Peptidoglycan
  Induction of NF-kB
  Induction of BBB permeability by increased vesicle
    transport
  Cytotoxic to ciliated cells of the choroid plexus
  Cytotoxic to neurons
  Induce sleep

cytokines and PAF upon binding to epithelia, endothelia, and macrophages, and initiate the influx of leukocytes.[14,54–60] The IL-1 response is particularly strong, exceeding that for endotoxin at least 10-fold on a bacterial cfu basis. In contrast, induction of TNF requires >100 times more cell wall than the induction of IL-1, even in the presence of putative serum binding components.[55,60] New evidence indicates that IL-12, an important component inducing cell mediated immunity, is induced by pneumococcal cell wall (Fig. 8).[61] Some of these effects arise through the interaction of cell walls with CD14, a cell surface receptor known to initiate the inflammatory cascade for endotoxin.[60,62] Other receptors are suspected also to participate in cell wall–induced events since mice resistant to endotoxin/CD14 effects by virtue of knockout mutations in the TNF receptor or p50 of NF-kB still die of pneumococcal infection.[63,64] Conversely, mice deficient in ICAM-1 have a poorer prognosis for gram negative than for gram positive meningitis.[65]

The bioactivities of bacterial glycopeptides lacking teichoic acid are numerous and depend on the structure of the glycopeptide and the nature of the target eukaryotic cell (Table 6). For instance, modification of the disaccharide moiety to a 1,6 anhydro linkage defines the sleep peptide known to induce slow wave sleep in rabbits,[66] while a lactyl-tetrapeptide derivative is toxic to respiratory ciliated cells.[67] The peptidoglycan portion of the pneumococcal cell wall is a potent stimulus of blood brain barrier permeability. The activation of cerebral endothelia by disaccharides linked to two or three amino acids results in increased vesicle translocation and enhanced barrier permeability.[16] The accumulation of penicillin in brain increases up to 250%.

Attenuation of disease

Intervention at the level of adherence. It has long been suggested that understanding bacterial adherence would generate excellent vaccine candidates and novel therapeutics. Clearly, many of the proteins described above will be analyzed as potential vaccine candidates. To examine possible therapeutics based on antiadherence strategies, both the PAF receptor antagonist and a series of antiadhesive oligosaccharides were tested for the ability to attenuate the course of pneumococcal disease, i.e., pneumonia in a rabbit model and colonization of the nasopharynx in a rat model.[8,68] Intratracheal administration of either the PAF receptor antagonist or lacto-*N*-neotetraose or its alpha 2,3 and alpha 2,6 sialylated derivatives eliminated pneumococci from the lungs of rabbits over a period of 48 h (Fig. 9). This activity was accompanied by protection from bacteremia. The activity of these compounds extended to the prevention of colonization of the nasopharynx of infant rats. Further, these agents were capable of eliminating pneumonia and bacteremia when given 24 h *after* infection was established. Although *in vitro* studies suggested that the effects of the oligosaccharides *in vivo* correlated with the capacity to block adherence *in vitro*, another possible mechanism of action includes direct effects of the oligosaccharide on human cells resulting in down modulation of the ability of the cell to support adherence. The PAF receptor antagonist and the antiadhesive oligosaccharides are promising agents for interrupting carriage and transmission

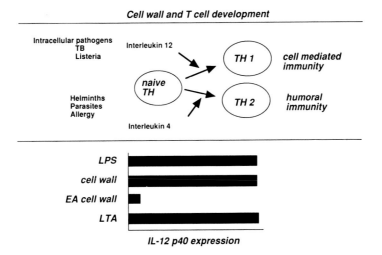

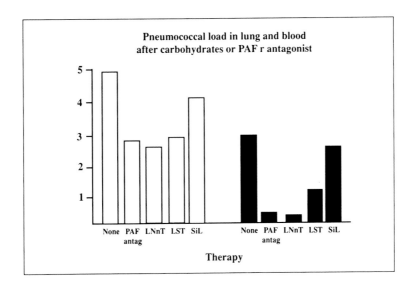

FIG. 8. Cell wall–induced production of interleukin-12. Cell walls can induce production of a large variety of cytokines from human cells. TNF and IL-1 are expected products of a challenge with a bacterial component which elicits an acute phase response. However, it was unanticipated that these same cell wall pieces would also enhance IL-12 production, a feature associated with intracellular bacteria cleared by cell mediated immunity. The activities of cell wall and lipoteichoic acid were similar to each other and to endotoxin (LPS). Choline was critical to the response since ethanolamine (EA)–grown bacteria failed to induce IL-12. (Adapted from Cleveland et al.[16])

of pneumococci particularly in view of the current interest in limiting the use of antibiotics in the absence of overt disease so as to decrease the emergence of resistance.

Intervention at the level of cell wall–induced inflammation. Given the complex relationships between the participants in the acute inflammatory response to pneumococci, it is not surprising that a single critical agent has not been identified. Attenuating the acute host response, however, has direct clinical application to improving the outcome of disease.

A major change in the therapy of meningitis arose from the observation that pneumococcal cell wall pieces are bioactive from intact bacteria and, even more so, from bacteria undergoing antibiotic induced lysis. This provided an opportunity to mitigate cell wall associated damage by down modulating the host response during antibiotic therapy. Over the first few hours of antibiotic therapy, the leukocyte density in cerebrospinal fluid can increase one to two orders of magnitude.[69] This burst is sufficient to injure host tissues as evidenced by

FIG. 9. Effect of antiadhesive carbohydrates and PAF receptor antagonist on the progression of pneumococcal disease. The log of bacterial counts in lung lavage fluid (open bars) and blood (closed bars) was determined at 48 h in animals receiving the indicated therapy 24 h after type 2 pneumococcal challenge intratracheally. LNnT, lacto-*N*-neotetraose; LST, Sialylated LNnT; SiL, sialyl α2,3 lactose; PAF antag, PAF receptor antagonist. (Adapted from elsewhere.[8,68])

the significant attenuation of damage upon the inhibition of leukocyte recruitment.[70,71] The use of steroids during the early phase of antibiotic therapy to inhibit this response has recently become accepted in the clinical setting of childhood meningitis.[69]

REFERENCES

1. Ring, A., J. Weiser, and E. Tuomanen. 1998. Pneumococcal trafficking across the blood brain barrier. J. Clin. Invest. **102**:1–14.

2. Andersson, B., J. Dahmen, T. Frejg, H. Leffler, G. Magnusson, and C. Svanborg Eden. 1983. Identification of an active disaccharide unit of a glycoconjugate receptor for pneumococci attaching to human pharyngeal epithelial cells. J. Exp. Med. **158**:559–570.

3. Barthelson, R., A. Mobasseri, D. Zopf, and P. Simon. 1998. Adherence of *Streptococcus pneumoniae* to respiratory epithelial cells is inhibited by sialylated oligosaccharides. Infect. Immunol. **66**:1439–1444.

4. Linder, T., R. Dandiles, D. Lime, and T. DeMaria. 1994. Effect of intranasal inoculation of *Streptococcus pneumoniae* on the structure of the surface carbohydrates of the chinchilla eustachian tube and middle ear mucosa. Microb. Pathog. **16**:435–441.

5. Krivan, H.C., D.D. Roberts, and V. Ginsburg. 1988. Many pulmonary pathogenic bacteria bind specifically to the carbohydrate sequence GalNacβ1-4Gal found in some glycolipids. Proc. Natl. Acad. Sci. U.S.A. **85**:6157–6161.

6. Cundell, D., and E. Tuomanen. 1994. Receptor specificity of adherence of *Streptococcus pneumoniae* to human type II pneumocytes and vascular endothelial cells *in vitro*. Microb. Pathog. **17**:361–374.

7. Hamburger, M., and O. Robertson. 1940. Studies of the pathogenesis of experimental pneumococcus pneumonia in the dog. J. Exp. Med. **72**:261–274.

8. Cundell, D., N. Gerard, C. Gerard, I. Idanpaan-Heikkila, and E. Tuomanen. 1995. *Streptococcus pneumoniae* anchors to activated eukaryotic cells by the receptor for platelet-activating factor. Nature **377**:435–438.

9. Lasky, L.A. 1992. Selectins: interpreters of cell-specific carbohydrate information. Science **258**:964–969.

10. Zimmerman, G., S. Prescott, and T. McIntyre. 1992. Endothelial cell interactions with granulocytes: tethering and signaling molecules. Immunol. Today **13**:93–100.

11. Geng, J., K. Moore, A. Johnson, and R. McEver. 1991. Neutrophil recognition requires a Ca-induced conformational change in the lectin domain of GMP-140. J. Biol. Chem. **266**:22313–22318.

12. Honda, Z.-I., M. Nakamura, I. Miki, M. Minami, T. Watanabe, Y. Seyama, H. Okado, H. Toh, K. Iot, T. Miyamoto, and T. Shimizu. 1991. Cloning by functional expression of platelet-activating factor receptor from guinea pig lung. Nature **349**:342–346.

13. Kunz, D., N. Gerard, and C. Gerard. 1992. The human leukocyte platelet activating factor receptor. J. Biol. Chem. **267**:9101–9106.

14. Geelen, S., C. Battacharyya, and E. Tuomanen. 1993. Cell wall mediates pneumococcal attachment and cytopathology to human endothelial cells. Infect. Immunol. **61**:1538–1543.

15. Gerard, N., and C. Gerard. 1994. Receptor-dependent internalization of platelet-activating factor. J. Immunol. **152**:793–800.

16. Spellerberg, B., S. Prasad, C. Cabellos, M. Burroughs, P. Cahill, and E. Tuomanen. 1995. Penetration of the blood-brain barrier: enhancement of drug delivery and imaging by bacterial glycopeptides. J. Exp. Med. **182**:1037–1044.

17. Birkness, K., B. Swisher, E. White, E. Long, E. Ewing, and F.

Quinn. 1995. A tissue culture bilayer model to study the passage of *Neisseria meningitidis*. Infect. Immunol. **63**:402–409.

18. van der Flier, M., N. Chhun, T. Wizemann, J. Min, J. McCarthy, and E. Tuomanen. 1995. Adherence of *Streptococcus pneumoniae* to immobilized fibronectin. Infect. Immunol. **63**:4317–4322.

19. Wizemann, T., J. Min, J. McCarthy, and E. Tuomanen. 1996. Adherence of *Streptococcus pneumoniae* to VCAM-1 and the HepII region of fibronectin [Abstract B358]. Proceedings of American Society of Microbiology. p. 216.

20. Pearce, B., Y. Yin, and H. Masure. 1993. Genetic identification of exported proteins in *Streptococcus pneumoniae*. Mol. Microbiol. **9**:1037–1050.

21. Cundell, D., B. Pearce, J. Sandros, A. Naughton, and H. Masure. 1995. Peptide permeases from *Streptococcus pneumoniae* affect adherence to eucaryotic cells. Infect. Immunol. **63**:2493–2498.

22. Spellerberg, B., D. Cundell, J. Sandros, B. Pearce, I. Idänpään-Heikkilä, C. Rosenow, and H. Masure. 1996. Pyruvate oxidase as a determinant of virulence in *Streptococcus pneumoniae*. Mol. Microbiol. **19**:803–813.

23. Wizemann, T., J. Moskovitz, B. Pearce, D. Cundell, H. Weissbach, N. Brot, and H. Masure. 1996. Peptide methionine sulfoxide reductase contributes to the maintenance of adhesins for three major pathogens. Proc. Natl. Acad. Sci. U.S.A. **93**:7985–7990.

24. Havarstein, L., G. Coomaraswamy, and D. Morrison. 1995. An unmodified heptadecapeptide pheromone induces competence for genetic transformation in *Streptococcus pneumoniae*. Proc. Natl. Acad. Sci. U.S.A. **92**:11140–11144.

25. Weiser, J., R. Austrian, P. Sreenivasan, and H. Masure. 1994. Phase variation in pneumococcal opacity: relationship between colonial morphology and nasopharyngeal colonization. Infect. Immunol. **62**:2582–2589.

26. Saluga, S., and J. Weiser. 1995. The genetic basis of colonial opacity in *Streptococcus pneumoniae*: evidence for the effect of box elements on phenotypic variation. Mol. Microbiol. **2**:215–227.

27. Cundell, D., J. Weiser, J. Shen, A. Young, and E. Tuomanen. 1995. Relationship between colonial morphology and adherence of *Streptococcus pneumoniae*. Infect. Immunol. **63**:757–761.

28. Sampson, J., R. O'Connor, A. Stinson, J. Tharpe, and H. Russell. 1994. Cloning and nucleotide sequence analysis of psaA, the *Streptococcus pneumoniae* gene encoding a 37-kilodalton protein homologous to previously reported *Streptococcus* sp. adhesins. Infect. Immunol. **62**:319–324.

29. Dintilhac, A., G. Alloing, C. Granadel, and J.P. Claverys. 1997. Competence and virulence of *Streptococcus pneumoniae*: Adc and PsaA mutants exhibit a requirement for An and Mn resulting from inactivation of putative ABC metal permeases. Mol. Microbiol. **25**:727–739.

30. Talbot, U., A. Paton, and J. Paton. 1996. Uptake of *Streptococcus pneumoniae* by respiratory epithelial cells. Infect. Immunol. **64**:3772–3777.

31. Novak, R., J. Braun, E. Charpentier, and E. Tuomanen. 1998. Penicillin tolerance genes of *Streptococcus pneumoniae*: the ABC-type manganese permease complex PsaA. Mol. Microbiol. **29**:1285–1294.

32. Pestova, E., L. Havarstein, and D. Morrison. 1996. Regulation of competence for genetic transformation in *Streptococcus pneumoniae* by an auto-induced peptide pheromone and a two-component regulatory system. Mol. Microbiol. **21**:853–862.

33. Cheng, Q., E. Campbell, A. Naughton, S. Johnson, and H. Masure. 1997. The *com* locus controls genetic transformation in *Streptococcus pneumoniae*. Mol. Microbiol. **23**:683–692.

34. Novak, R., B. Henriques, S. Normark, and E. Tuomanen. Vancomycin tolerance in *Streptococcus pneumoniae*. Proceedings of the International Congress of Antimicrobial Agents and Chemotherapy (in press).

35. **Ronda, C., J. Garcia, E. Garcia, J. Sanchez-Puelles, and R. Lopez.** 1987. Biological role of the pneumococcal amidase: cloning of the lytA gene. Eur. J. Biochem. **164:**621–624.

36. **McDaniel, L.S., J.S. Sheffield, E. Swiatlo, J. Yother, M.J. Crain, and D.E. Briles.** 1992. Molecular localization of variable and conserved regions of *pspA* and identification of additional *pspA* homologous sequences in *Streptococcus pneumoniae*. Microb. Pathog. **13:**261–269.

37. **Yother, J., G.L. Handsome, and D.E. Briles.** 1992. Truncated forms of PspA that are secreted from *Streptococcus pneumoniae* and their use in functional studies and cloning of the *pspA* gene. J. Bacteriol. **174:**610–618.

38. **Rosenow, C., P. Ryan, J. Weiser, S. Johnson, P. Fontan, A. Ortqvist, and H. Masure.** 1997. Contribution of a novel choline binding protein to adherence, colonization, and immunogenicity of *Streptococcus pneumoniae*. Mol. Microbiol. **25:**819–829.

39. **Zaitseva, F., E. Campbell, and H. Masure.** 1996. Surface localization and cell signalling by activator, the competence inducing protein of *Streptococcus pneumoniae* is dependent on phosphorylcholine, a component of the cell wall [Abstract H108]. Proceedings of the American Society of Microbiology, p. 502.

40. **Hammerschmidt, S., S. Talay, P. Brandtzaeg, and G. Chhatwal.** 1997. SpsA, a novel pneumococcal surface protein with specific binding to secretory immunoglobulin A and secretory component. Mol. Microbiol. **25:**1113–1124.

41. **Smith, B., Q. Cheng, and M. Hostetter.** 1998. Characterization of a pneumococcal surface protein that binds complement protein C3 and its role in adhesion [Abstract D-122]. Proceedings of the Meeting of the American Society of Microbiology, p. 233.

42. **Dormitzer, M., T. Wizemann, J. Adamou, B. Walsh, T. Gayle, S. Koenig, S. Lanermann, and S. Johnson.** 1998. Sequence and structural analysis of CbpA, a novel choline binding protein of *Streptococcus pneumoniae* [Abstract B3]. Proceedings of the American Society of Microbiology, p. 56.

43. **Tomasz, A.** 1967. Choline in the cell wall of a bacterium: novel type of polymer-linked choline in pneumococcus. Science **157:**694–697.

44. **Kim, J., and J. Weiser.** 1998. Association of intrastrain phase variation in quantity of capsular polysaccharide and teichoic acid with the virulence of *Streptococcus pneumoniae*. J. Infect. Dis. **177:**368–377.

45. **Deutsch, J., M. Salman, and S. Rottem.** 1995. An unusual polar lipid from the cell membrane of *Mycoplasma fermentans*. Eur. J. Biochem. **227:**897–902.

46. **Weiser, J., M. Shchepetov, and S. Chong.** 1997. Decoration of lipopolysaccharide with phosphorylcholine: a phase-variable characteristic of *Haemophilus influenzae*. Infect. Immunol. **65:**943–950.

47. **Weiser, J., N. Pan, K. McGowan, D. Musher, A. Martin, and J. Richards.** 1998. Phosphorylcholine on the lipopolysaccharide of *Haemophilus influenzae* contributes to persistence in the respiratory tract and sensitivity to serum killing mediated by C-reactive protein. J. Exp. Med. **187:**631–640.

48. **Zhang, J., I. Idanpaan-Heikkila, and E. Tuomanen.** 1999. The pneumococcal *lic* locus: involvement in choline metabolism and virulence. Molec. Microb. **31:**1477–1488.

49. **Tuomanen, E., H. Liu, B. Hengstler, O. Zak, and A. Tomasz.** 1985. The induction of meningeal inflammation by components of the pneumococcal cell wall. J. Infect. Dis. **151:**859–868.

50. **Tuomanen, E.I., A. Tomasz, B. Hengstler, and O. Zak.** 1985. The relative role of bacterial cell wall and capsule in the induction of inflammation in pneumococcal meningitis. J. Infect. Dis. **151:**535–540.

51. **Tuomanen, E., R. Rich, and O. Zak.** 1987. Induction of pulmonary inflammation by components of the pneumococcal cell surface. Am. Rev. Respir. Dis. **135:**869–874.

52. **Ripley-Petzoldt, M.L., G.S. Giebink, S.K. Juhn, D. Aeppli, A. Tomasz, and E. Tuomanen.** 1988. The contribution of pneumococcal cell wall to the pathogenesis of experimental otitis media. J. Infect. Dis. **157:**245–255.

53. **Tuomanen, E., H. Pollack, A. Parkinson, M. Davidson, R. Facklam, R. Rich, and O. Zak.** 1988. Microbiological and clinical significance of a new property of defective lysis in clinical strains of pneumococci. J. Infect. Dis. **158:**36–43.

54. **Winkelstein, J., and A. Tomasz.** 1978. Activation of the alternative complement pathway by pneumococcal cell wall teichoic acid. J. Immunol. **120:**174–178.

55. **Riesenfeld-Orn, I., S. Wolpe, J.F. Garcia-Bustos, M.K. Hoffman, and E. Tuomanen.** 1989. Production of interleukin-1 but not tumor necrosis factor by human monocytes stimulated with pneumococcal cell surface components. Infect. Immunol. **57:**1890–1893.

56. **Tomasz, A., and K. Saukkonen.** 1989. The nature of cell wall–derived inflammatory components of the pneumococci. Pediatr. Infect. Dis. J. **8:**902–903.

57. **Tuomanen, E., and S. Sande.** 1989. Inhibition of the binding of penicillin to the pneumococcal penicillin binding proteins (PBPs) by exogenous cell wall peptides. J. Gen. Microbiol. **135:**639–642.

58. **Cabellos, C., D.E. MacIntyre, M. Forrest, M. Burroughs, S. Prasad, and E. Tuomanen.** 1992. Differing roles of platelet-activating factor during inflammation of the lung and subarachnoid space. J. Clin. Invest. **90:**612–618.

59. **Geelen, S., C. Bhattacharyya, and E. Tuomanen.** 1992. Induction of procoagulant activity on human endothelial cells by *Streptococcus pneumoniae*. Infect. Immunol. **60:**4179–4183.

60. **Heumann, D., C. Barras, A. Severin, M. Glauser, and A. Tomasz.** 1994. Gram-positive cell walls stimulate synthesis of tumor necrosis factor alpha and interleukin-6 by human monocytes. Infect. Immunol. **62:**2715–2721.

61. **Cleveland, M., J. Gorham, T. Murphy, E. Tuomanen, and K. Murphy.** 1996. Lipoteichoic acids of gram-positive bacteria induce interleukin 12 through CD-14–dependent pathway. Infect. Immunol. **64:**1906–1912.

62. **Pugin, J., D. Heumann, A. Tomasz, V. Kravchenki, Y. Akamatsu, M. Nishijima, M. Lauser, P. Tobias, and R. Ulevitch.** 1994. CD14 is a pattern recognition receptor. Immunity **1:**509–516.

63. **Pfeffer, K., T. Matsuyama, T. Kundig, and T. Mak.** 1993. Mice deficient for the 55-kD tumor necrosis factor receptor are resistant to endotoxic shock, yet succumb to *L. monocytogenese* infection. Cell **73:**457–467.

64. **Sha, W., H. Liou, E. Tuomanen, and D. Baltimore.** 1995. Targeted disruption of the p50 subunit of NF-kB leads to multifocal defects in immune responses. Cell **80:**321–330.

65. **Tan, T., C. Smith, E. Hawkins, E. Mason, and S. Kaplan.** 1995. Hematogenous bacterial meningitis in an ICAM-1–deficient infant mouse model. J. Infect. Dis. **171:**342–349.

66. **Krueger, J., D. Davenne, J. Walter, S. Shoham, S. Kubillus, R. Rosenthal, S. Martin, and K. Biemann.** 1987. Bacterial peptidoglycans as modulators of sleep. Brain Res. **403:**258–266.

67. **Heiss, L., J. Lancaster, J. Corbett, and W. Goldman.** 1994. Epithelial autotoxicity of nitric oxide: role in the respiratory cytopathology of pertussis. Proc. Natl. Acad. Sci. U.S.A. **91:**267–270.

68. **Idanpaan-Heikkila, I., P. Simon, C. Cahill, K. Sokol, and E. Tuomanen.** 1997. Oligosaccharides interfere with the establishment and progression of experimental pneumococcal pneumonia. J. Infect. Dis. **176:**704–712.

69. **Lebel, M.H., B.J. Freij, G.A. Syrogiannopoulos, D.F. Chrane, M.J. Hoyt, S.M. Stewart, B.D. Kennard, K.D. Olsen, and G.H. McCracken, Jr.** 1988. Dexamethasone therapy for bacterial meningitis. N. Engl. J. Med. **15:**964–971.

70. **Tuomanen, E., B. Hengstler, R. Rich, M. Bray, O. Zak, and A. Tomasz.** 1987. Nonsteroidal anti-inflammatory agents in the therapy of experimental pneumococcal meningitis. J. Infect. Dis. **155:**985–990.

71. **Tuomanen, E., K. Saukkonen, S. Sande, C. Cioffe, and S.D. Wright.** 1989. Reduction of inflammation, tissue damage, and mortality in bacterial meningitis in rabbits treated with monoclonal antibodies against adhesion-promoting receptors of leukocytes. J. Exp. Med. **170:**959–969.

72. **Spellerberg, B., C. Rosenow, W. Sha, and E. Tuomanen.** 1996. Pneumococcal cell wall activates NF-kB in human monocytes. Microb. Pathog. **20:**309–317.

73. **Guenzi, E., and R. Hackenbeck.** 1996. Cia S/R: A two component regualatory system in Pneumococci. Molec. Micro. **12:**505–515.

Address reprint requests to:
Elaine I. Tuomanen
Department of Infectious Diseases
St. Jude Children's Research Hospital
332 North Lauderdale St.
Memphis, TN 38105

Opsonic and Nonopsonic Interactions of C3 with *Streptococcus pneumoniae*

MARGARET K. HOSTETTER

INTRODUCTION

BECAUSE COMPLEMENT PROTEINS cannot lyse the rigid cell wall of *Streptococcus pneumoniae*, deposition of opsonic C3b on the pneumococcal surface is the principal mediator of pneumococcal clearance in the nonimmune host. In the past, efforts to understand the interactions between C3 and the pneumococcus have focused primarily on the opsonic interactions that occur in the bloodstream.

Although Wright and Douglas were the first to show that serum elements were required for phagocytosis of *S. pneumoniae*,[1] 30 years elapsed before Ward and Enders dissected the opsonic capacities of anticapsular antibody alone versus antibody plus serum factors in the phagocytosis of serotype 3 pneumococci.[2] In the presence of anticapsular antibody alone, phagocytosis of type 3 pneumococci *in vitro* was an extraordinarily slow process and was not complete until approximately 8 h. Adding normal serum as complement source completed the process within 2 h.

Definitive proof that these "serum factors" were indeed complement proteins required another 30 years and the demonstration that depletion of the third component of complement (C3) in rat serum with zymosan or cobra venom factor suppressed phagocytosis of encapsulated *S. pneumoniae*.[3] Simultaneous proof arose from experiments depleting human C3 *in vitro* and from case histories of patients genetically deficient in C3.[4,5] Later models of pneumococcal sepsis in mice, guinea pigs, and dogs[6–8] have fortified these conclusions: C3 is the primary opsonin for *Streptococcus pneumoniae*. This contribution will summarize some of the salient features of the biochemistry of pneumococcal opsonization and will highlight novel mechanisms by which pneumococci are able to elude complement-mediated host defense.

BIOCHEMISTRY OF OPSONIZATION

Structurally, C3 is composed of an α-chain of 115 kDa connected by a single disulfide bond to the β chain of 75 kDa.[9] When the classical, alternative, or lectin pathways are activated, a small 10-kDa fragment of the C3 molecule, C3a, is cleaved from the amino terminus of the α-chain. This cleavage reaction engenders a conformational change that culminates in the exposure of an internal thioester bond, a labile binding site in the C3d subdomain that links a cysteinyl residue with a glutamyl residue just three amino acids downstream.[10] In native C3, the form of the protein that circulates in plasma, the thioester bond is protected within a hydrophobic pocket. When C3 is cleaved to C3b as a consequence of activation of either the classical or the alternative pathway, the thioester site is exposed and the bond itself is disrupted. The biochemical consequences of this reaction are two-fold: (a) the appearance of a titrable sulfhydryl group at the cysteinyl residue and (b) the potential for the reactive carbonyl group of the glutamyl residue to participate in a transacylation reaction with hydroxyl or amino groups, either soluble or surface-borne, during the 60 μs of its half-life. A detailed review of the biochemistry of this reaction can be found elsewhere.[11]

The thioester bond is the functional "cockpit" of the entire molecule, and the reactive carbonyl group is the means by which C3 binds covalently in ester linkage to free hydroxyl groups on simple sugars or complex polysaccharides or in amide linkage to free amino groups on amino sugars or amino acids.[12] Covalent binding of C3 to simple sugars *in vitro* is a paradigm for opsonic deposition of C3b on pneumococcal capsular polysaccharides *in vivo*.[12–14] That C3b does indeed deposit opsonically on the pneumococcal capsule, as well as on proteins of the teichoic acid fraction of the cell wall,[15–18] can be confirmed by methylamine release of ester-linked C3 fragments, by removal of capsule with attached radiolabeled C3,[19] or by electron microscopy (Fig. 1). Using biochemically modified forms of C3 in which the reactive carbonyl group was replaced with hydroxyl or methylamine substitutions, studies from our laboratory have demonstrated that the biochemical integrity of the C3 thioester bond is an absolute requirement for efficient opsonization.[21] Phagocytosis ensues when carboxy-terminal sequences of opsonically deposited C3b are recognized by complement receptors on phagocytic cells; the opsonized organism is brought into close approximation with the neutrophil and ingested. A graphic representation of the biochemistry of opsonization and phagocytosis is shown in Fig. 2.

After covalent deposition on the surface of the pneumococcus, C3b is cleaved by serum proteases to smaller fragments such as iC3b and C3d (Fig. 3), which in turn determine subse-

Formerly American Legion and Women's Auxiliary Heart Research Chair in Pediatrics, University of Minnesota, Minneapolis, Minnesota. Current Address: Professor of Pediatrics and Director, Child Health Research Center, Yale University School of Medicine, New Haven, Connecticut.

Reprinted from *Microbial Drug Resistance*, Vol. 5, No. 2, 1999.

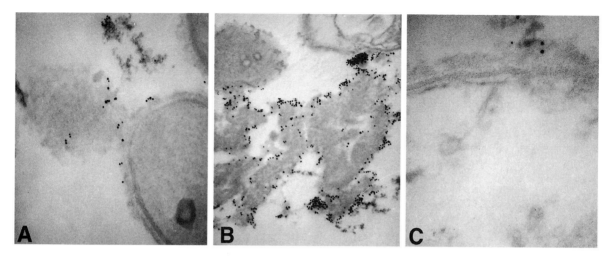

FIG. 1. Deposition of purified human C3 on *Streptococcus pneumoniae*, serotype 3, after exposure of the thiolester bond with trypsin. No other serum components are present. Twelve nanometer colloidal gold particles coupled to goat anti–human C3 are used to localize the site of deposition. (A) Section through intact organism and extruded capsule (×80,000). (B) Section through capsular polysaccharide (×60,000). (C) Section showing inner plasma membrane, cell wall, and capsule, the latter with bound C3 (×105,000). Electron micrographs courtesy of Elena M. Retsinas and Margaret K. Hostetter. (From Hostetter et al.,[21] with permission.)

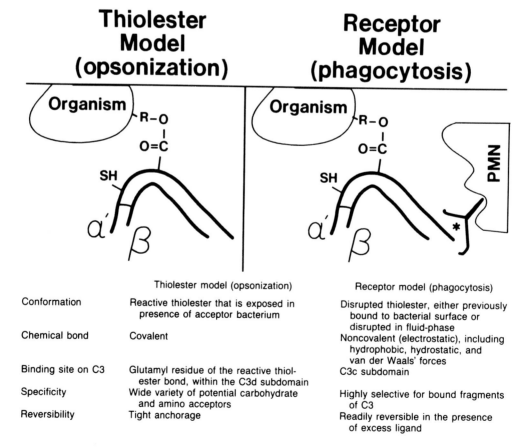

	Thiolester model (opsonization)	Receptor model (phagocytosis)
Conformation	Reactive thiolester that is exposed in presence of acceptor bacterium	Disrupted thiolester, either previously bound to bacterial surface or disrupted in fluid-phase
Chemical bond	Covalent	Noncovalent (electrostatic), including hydrophobic, hydrostatic, and van der Waals' forces
Binding site on C3	Glutamyl residue of the reactive thiolester bond, within the C3d subdomain	C3c subdomain
Specificity	Wide variety of potential carbohydrate and amino acceptors	Highly selective for bound fragments of C3
Reversibility	Tight anchorage	Readily reversible in the presence of excess ligand

FIG. 2. Comparison of the biochemical mechanisms of opsonization and phagocytosis. In opsonization (left), the glutamyl carbonyl of C3 may attach covalently in either ester (as shown) or amide linkage.

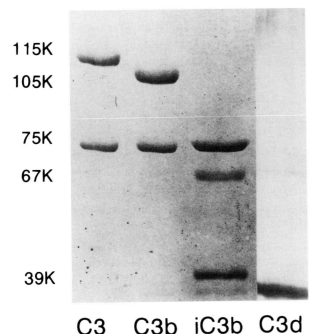

FIG. 3. Native C3 and its cleavage fragments—C3b, iC3b, C3d—after purification to homogeneity and electrophoresis on 10% SDS-PAGE gels under reducing conditions.

quent interactions with complement receptors on leukocytes. Differing C3b cleavage patterns among representative pneumococcal serotypes help to explain serotype-specific differences in susceptibility to phagocytosis and in capsular antigenicity.[19] For example, serotypes 3 and 4, most often found in adult infections, are highly resistant to phagocytosis and yet potent immunogens. Serotypes 6A and 14, most commonly found in childhood otitis, bacteremia, or meningitis, are readily phagocytized but poorly immunogenic. When surface-bound C3 fragments are compared after opsonization in non-immune serum, the predominant C3 fragment on serotypes 3 and 4 was C3d.[19] In contrast, serotypes 6A and 14 displayed only the cleavage fragment iC3b. These distinctions are critical because C3d is recognized by receptors on the B lymphocyte, but not by those on the phagocyte, while iC3b readily serves as a ligand for complement receptor type 3 on the neutrophil, thereby enhancing phagocytosis and clearance. Pneumococcal surfaces that halt C3 cleavage at iC3b will not generate C3d; at a cellular level, communication with the phagocyte will be enhanced, but interaction with the B lymphocyte will be retarded,

if not abolished. Thus, the absence of C3d on the pneumococcal surface protects serotypes 6A and 14 from interaction with B lymphocytes but allows these serotypes to be easily phagocytized. The converse is true for serotypes 3 and 4: the predominance of C3d facilitates interaction with B lymphocytes but retards phagocytosis; thus, serotypes 3 and 4 are potent immunogens but markedly resistant to phagocytosis. These interactions are summarized in Table 1.

ROLE OF C3D AND COMPLEMENT RECEPTOR TYPE 2 IN THE ANTIBODY RESPONSE TO PNEUMOCOCCAL POLYSACCHARIDES

Pneumococcal polysaccharides have long been known to induce antibody formation by human B lymphocytes *in vitro*. Pneumovax@-polysaccharides cultured with B lymphocytes from nonimmunized adults and serotype 4 or serotype 19F polysaccharide used singly in B lymphocytes from immunized adults were able to induce antigen-specific plaque-forming cells, as identified by polysaccharide-coated sheep erythrocytes.[23] The hypothesis that pneumococcal polysaccharides bearing C3d could interact directly with B lymphocytes was confirmed in two separate studies.[24,25] Incubation of pneumococcal polysaccharide (PS) from serotype 1, 3, 4, and 14 in serum supporting only alternative pathway activation led to the generation of C3d and the binding of this fragment to Ps, as measured by ELISA.[25] Most active in this regard were polysaccharides from serotypes 3 and 4. Binding of the PS-C3d complex to complement receptor type 2 (CR2) on B lymphocytes was blocked by an anti-CR2-monoclonal antibody.[24] Pneumococcal polysaccharide type 4 (PS4) was able to stimulate adult B lymphocytes, and neonatal B lymphocytes to a lesser extent, when coincubated with antibodies to CR2 on B lymphocytes.[25] Immunogenicity of PS4 complexed to C3d after incubation in serum from a patient with severe combined immunodeficiency showed an enhanced immunogenicity in adult B lymphocytes.[25] The potency of C3d as an adjuvant for proteins has been demonstrated in recent studies by Fearon's group. When hen egg lysozyme was coupled to a C3d trimer, the immune response was increased 10,000-fold.[26] The potency of a C3d trimer outdistanced complete Freund's adjuvant by approximately 100-fold. These studies did not assess whether C3d itself is able to induce an autoantibody response—a critical consideration. However, these "lessons of nature" indicate that surface-bound C3d is a highly potent molecular adjuvant

TABLE 1. SEROTYPE-SPECIFIC DIFFERENCES IN C3 DEGRADATION FRAGMENTS AFTER OPSONIZATION

Pneumococcal serotype	Resistance to phagocytosis	Capsular antigenicity	C3 cleavage fragments	Leukocyte receptors
3	++++	++++	Predom. C3d	CR2 on B cells
4	++++	++++	Predom. C3d	CR2 on B cells
6A	++	+	iC3b only	CR3 on PMN
14	++	+	iC3b only	CR3 on PMN

CR2, complement receptor type 2; CD21. CR3, complement receptor type 3; CD11b/CD18. B cells, B lymphocytes.

for both proteins and polysaccharides. Coupling C3d to pneumococcal polysaccharides may enhance immunogenicity and improve the formulation of pneumococcal vaccines.

ROLE OF iC3B AND COMPLEMENT RECEPTOR TYPE 3 IN PNEUMOCOCCAL PHAGOCYTOSIS

Experiments utilizing differential blockade of CR1 (C3b receptor) or CR3 (iC3b receptor) with monoclonal and polyclonal antibodies have confirmed that iC3b-bearing pneumococci (serotypes 6A and 14) are phagocytized through CR3; phagocytosis is inhibited by more than 90% when the ligand-binding site on CR3 is blocked with the monoclonal antibody OKM10.[27] Moreover, when covalently bound to prototypic surfaces such as inert 1-μm microspheres, iC3b consistently surpasses C3b in the elicitation of superoxide, myeloperoxidase, and lactoferrin from normal adult neutrophils.[28] These experiments confirm that iC3b-bearing microorganisms are readily phagocytized via CR3 and are able to elicit the release of potent microbicidal mediators. In contrast, C3b- or C3d-bearing organisms are ineffective in both regards. Thus, the serotype-specific pattern of C3 fragmentation (iC3b or C3d) determines the subsequent disposition of opsonized pneumococci through their interaction with complement receptors on phagocytes or B lymphocytes.

Recently, novel proteins that permit the pneumococcus to elude these well-defined mechanisms of host defense have come to light. As we have previously described, clinical and laboratory isolates of encapsulated and unencapsulated pneumococci are able to degrade C3; this activity is most prominent during exponential growth and results in attack at the C3 β-chain, thereby destabilizing the C3 molecule.[29] *In vitro*, approximately half of available C3 molecules are inactivated by this mechanism. Two pneumococcal surface proteins of 29 and 20 kDa, identified in our laboratory, have been shown to be responsible for this activity. A gene presumptively encoding the 20-kDa proteinase has now been completely sequenced and is unrelated to all previously characterized pneumococcal proteins including pneumolysin, autolysin, PspA, or PsaA.

Our laboratory has also identified a third pneumococcal protein of 90 kDa that interacts with C3 molecules independently of thioester conformation. This protein has been purified, and studies to isolate the gene are underway. Thus in pneumococcal biology, traditional mechanisms of C3-mediated opsonization and phagocytosis are combated by pneumococcal surface proteins that interact non-opsonically with C3. The pneumococcus is indeed a wily pathogen.

ACKNOWLEDGMENTS

This work was supported by NIH grant AI24162 and by funds from the American Legion Heart Research Chair.

NOTE ADDED IN PROOF

Genes encoding all three proteins have now been isolated; the sequence of the 90 kDa C3-binding protein can be found at accession #AF067128.

REFERENCES

1. **Wright, A.E., and S.R. Douglas.** 1903. An experimental investigation of blood fluids in connection with phagocytosis. Proc. R. Soc. Lond. B. Biol. Sci. **72**:357–370.
2. **Ward, H.K., and J.F. Enders.** 1933. An analysis of the opsonic and tropic action of normal and immune sera based on experiments with the pneumococcus. J. Exp. Med. **57**:527–547.
3. **Smith, M.R., and W.B. Wood, Jr.** 1969. Heat labile opsonins to pneumococcus. I. Participation of complement. J. Exp. Med. **129**:1209–1225.
4. **Johnston, R.B., M.R. Klemperer, C.A. Alper, and F.S. Rosen.** 1969. The enhancement of bacterial phagocytosis by serum. J. Exp. Med. **129**:1275–1290.
5. **Alper, C.A., H.R. Colten, F.S. Rosen, A.R. Rabson, G.M. MacNab, and J.S.S. Gear.** 1972. Homozygous deficiency of C3 in a patient with repeated infections. Lancet **2**:1179–1181.
6. **Hosea, S.W., E.J. Brown, and M.M. Frank.** 1980. The critical role of complement in experimental pneumococcal sepsis. J. Infect. Dis. **42**:903–909.
7. **Auerbach, H.S., R. Burger, A. Dodds, and H.R. Colten.** 1990. Molecular basis of complement C3 deficiency in guinea pigs. J. Clin. Invest. **86**:96–106.
8. **Winkelstein, J.A., L.C. Cork, D.E. Griffin, R.J. Adams, and D.L. Price.** 1981. Genetically determined efficiency of the third component of complement in the dog. Science. **212**:1169–1173.
9. **Tack, B.F., and J.W. Prahl.** 1976. Third component of human complement: purification from plasma and physiochemical characterization. Biochemistry **15**:4513–4521.
10. **Tack, B.F., R.A. Harrison, J. Janatova, M.L. Thomas, and J.W. Prahl.** 1980. Evidence for presence of an internal thiolester bond in third component of human complement. Proc. Natl. Acad. Sci. U.S.A. **77**:5764–5768.
11. **Tack, B.F.** 1983. The b-CYS-g-GLU thiolester bond in human C3, C4, and a2-macroglobulin. Springer Sermin. Immunopathol. **6**:259–282.
12. **Hostetter, M.K., M.L. Thomas, F.S. Rosen, and B.F. Tack.** 1982. Binding of C3b proceeds by a transesterification reaction at the thiolester site. Nature **298**:72–75.
13. **Capel, P.J.A., R.O. Groeneboe, G. Grosveld, and K.W. Pondman.** 1978. The binding of activated C3 to polysaccharides and immunoglobulins. J. Immunol. **121**:2566–2572.
14. **Mann, J., R. O'Brien, M.K. Hostetter, C.A. Alper, S.R. Rosen, and B.M. Babior.** 1981. The third component of complement: covalent attachment of a radioactive sugar to the labile binding site of C3 via the alternative pathway. J. Immunol. **236**:2370–2372.
15. **Winkelstein, J.A., and A. Tomasz.** 1977. Activation of the alternative pathway by pneumococcal cell walls. J. Immunol. **118**:451–454.
16. **Winkelstein, J.A., and A. Tomasz.** 1978. Activation of the alternative complement pathway by pneumococcal cell wall teichoic acid. J. Immunol. **120**:174–178.
17. **Winkelstein, J.A., A.S. Abramovitz, and A. Tomasz.** 1980. Activation of C3 via the alternative complement pathway results in fixation of C3b to the pneumococcal cell wall. J. Immunol. **124**:2502–2506.
18. **Hummell, D.S., R.W. Berninger, A. Tomasz, and J.A. Winkelstein.** 1981. The fixation of C3b to pneumococcal cell wall polymers as a result of activation of the alternative complement pathway. J. Immunol. **127**:1287–1289.
19. **Hostetter, M.K.** 1986. Serotypic variations among virulent pneumococci in deposition and degradation of covalently bound C3b. Implications for phagocytosis and antibody production. J. Infect. Dis. **153**:682–693.
20. **Hostetter, M.K.** 1993. C3 and C4 as opsonins in natural immunity. *In* E. Sim (ed.), Humoral factors. Oxford University Press, Oxford, pp. 176–208.

21. **Hostetter, M.K., R.A. Krueger, and D.J. Schmeling.** 1984. The biochemistry of opsonization: central role of the reactive thiolester of the third component of complement. J. Infect. Dis. **150:**653–661.

22. **Hostetter, M.K., and D.L. Gordon.** 1987. Biochemistry of C3 and related thiolester proteins in infection and inflammation. Rev. Infect. Dis. **9:**97–109.

23. **Rijkers, G.T., and D.E. Mosier.** 1985. Pneumococcal polysaccharides induce antibody formation by human B lymphocytes *in vitro.* J. Immunol. **135:**1–4.

24. **Griffioen, A.W., G.T. Rijkers, P. Janssens-Korpela, and B.J.M. Zegers.** 1991. Pneumococcal polysaccharides complexed with C3d bind to human B lymphocytes via complement receptor type 2. Infect. Immunol. **59:**1839–1845.

25. **Griffioen, A.W., E.A.H. Toebes, B.J.M. Zegers, and G.T. Rijkers.** 1992. Role of CR2 in the human adult and neonatal in vitro antibody response to type 4 pneumococcal polysaccharide. Cell. Immunol. **143:**11–22.

26. **Dempsey, P.W., M.E. Allison, S. Akkaraju, C.C. Goodnow, and D.T. Fearon.** 1996. C3d of complement as a molecular adjuvant: bridging innate and acquired immunity. Science **271:** 348–350.

27. **Gordon, D.L., G.M. Johnson, and M.K. Hostetter.** 1986. Ligand-receptor interactions in the phagocytosis of virulent *Streptococcus pneumoniae* by polymorphonuclear leukocytes. J. Infect. Dis. **154:**619–626.

28. **Hostetter, M.K., and G.M. Johnson.** 1989. The erythrocyte as instigator of inflammation. J. Clin. Invest. **84:**665–671.

29. **Angel, C.M., M. Ruzek, and M.K. Hostetter.** 1994. Degradation of C3 by *Streptococcus pneumoniae.* J. Infect. Dis. **170:**600–608.

Address reprint requests to:
Margaret K. Hostetter
Section of Immunology
Department of Pediatrics
Yale Child Health Research Center
464 Congress Ave.
New Haven, CT 06519-1313

Streptococcus pneumoniae
Copyright © 2000 Mary Ann Liebert, Inc., 2 Madison Avenue, Larchmont, NY 10538

Pneumococcal Meningitis: Current Pathophysiologic Concepts

MERLE A. SANDE[1] and MARTIN G. TÄUBER[2]

INTRODUCTION

MENINGITIS CAUSED BY *Streptococcus pneumoniae* has become the most common bacterial infection of the central nervous system.[1] It is rapidly fatal if not treated early and effectively with antibiotics that achieve bactericidal activity at the site of infection which is in the subarachnoid space filled with cerebrospinal fluid (CSF).[2] For the last 40–50 years, the β-lactam antibiotics have fulfilled this function. However, with the emergence of resistance to these and other antibiotics, the future approach to treatment of this infection could be problematic. This renewed interest in pneumococcal disease stimulates us to review what we have learned about the pathophysiology of this disease since the development of the Dacey/Sande meningitis model in the early 1970s.[3] It has always been our hope that an in-depth understanding of the mediators that lead to abnormalities in brain function and eventual neuronal death would lead to therapeutic interventions that would reduce these destructive consequences. Today, these goals are more important that ever.

THE MODEL

The model was first described by Dacey and Sande in 1974, when it was used to demonstrate that probenecid increased the concentration of penicillin in the CSF fluid by blocking the organic acid exit pump located in the choroid plexus.[3] The model consisted of a rabbit suspended in a stereotactic frame that allowed instillation of microorganisms (usually the pneumococcus) directly into the cisterna magna of the animal and then, with the needle left in place, continuous sampling of CSF as the infection developed. CSF could be analyzed for viable bacteria, various mediators and indicators of inflammation, drug concentrations as a function of simultaneous serum concentrations, and CSF pressure. Brain histology and brain water content could be measured at the conclusion of the experiment.[4] The unique ability to monitor the infection over time allowed for a real-time assessment of the importance of the various components of the inflammatory process and allowed a direct measure of their contribution to the pathophysiology of the disease by the use of selective inhibitors. While the experimental work has expanded into various other *in vivo* and *in vitro* models over

the past 30 years by numerous investigators, most of the initial observations were made using this rabbit model.

THE INFECTION

It was found that a very low inoculum of encapsulated pneumococci could produce a progressive infection in the rabbit,[5] an observation confirmed by Moxon in the infant rat model of *Haemophilus influenza* type b meningitis, who found that it only took a single organism in the CSF to produce meningitis.[6] Unencapsulated mutants were nonpathogenic. Each bacterial strain had its own unique infectious dose 50 (ID50), which is the number of organisms necessary to produce progressive infection in 50% of the animals when directly injected into the CSF. This proved to be a measure of virulence for the meningitis potential of the various bacteria. With a well-characterized type 3 *S. pneumoniae*, the ID50 was less than 100 organisms. After injection, a lag phase with stationary growth lasted for approximately 2 h, and then the bacteria grew with a generation (or doubling) time of approximately 60 min (compared to 20 min in broth) until they reached "maximum population densities" of 10^6 to 10^8 cfu/ml after 18–36 h. Adapting the model to the dog, we found that shortly after initiation of log phase growth in CSF, the pneumococcus appeared in the sagittal sinus, followed 2 h later by appearance in the arterial circulation, thus demonstrating a unique clearance mechanism for bacteria from the central nervous system.[7]

THE HOST'S RESPONSE

Within 8–12 h after inoculation of the pneumococcus, white blood cells (WBC) of the polymorphonuclear type appear in the CSF. Just preceding this is an opening of the blood brain barrier extensively characterized by Scheld as an opening of the tight junctions between brain capillary endothelial cells associated with enhanced pinocytotic activity.[8] This results in the influx of serum components, including chemotactic components of the complement system, especially C5a, which is in part responsible for the PMN migration.[9] It is significant that the appearance of WBC has no effect on the rate of proliferation of the bacteria and neutropenic animals showed the same bacter-

---

[1]Department of Medicine, School of Medicine, University of Utah, Salt Lake City, Utah.
[2]Institute for Medical Microbiology, University of Berne, Berne, Switzerland.

ial growth characteristics as normal animals.[10] This lack of effect of granulocytes in the CSF against the encapsulated pathogen is a reflection of the low concentrations of opsonins (anticapsular antibodies, complement) in this compartment of relative host defense deficiency.[11,12] Consequently, when serum or anticapsular antibody was injected directly into the CSF prior to inoculation of the *S. pneumoniae*, the WBCs effectively killed the bacteria (W.M. Scheld, B. Perkins, and M.A. Sande, unpublished observations). Conversely, complement depletion of animals increases the virulence of pneumococci during experimental meningitis.[13] One apparently effective host response in the CSF is the generation of fever in the rabbit. Bacterial growth is significantly reduced and the ID50 significantly increased in animals that were allowed to develop high temperatures compared to those in which the febrile response was suppressed.[5,14]

Another consistent pathophysiological alteration that developed during the first phase of infection in parallel with the opening of the blood brain barrier was the decline of CSF glucose concentration (hypoglycorrhachia) and the increase in lactic acid concentration.[15,16] Both changes were felt to represent increased utilization of glucose in response to relative cerebral ischemia caused by a reduction or mismatch of cerebral blood flow and a subsequent switch to the glycolytic cycle and away from the Krebs cycle of metabolism.[17] This metabolic switch utilizes more glucose and produces lactate. It has been shown that tumor necrosis factor–alpha (TNF-α), when injected directly into the CSF, can induce this switch to anaerobic glycolysis with a subsequent increase in CSF lactate concentrations.[18] Other studies have implicated reduced glucose transport as another potential cause of a low CSF glucose concentration.[19]

MOLECULAR MEDIATORS OF INFLAMMATION IN MENINGITIS

One of the most fruitful areas of research in bacterial meningitis was the exploration of the molecular mediators of inflammation. The question, how the host recognizes the presence of the pneumococcus in the subarachnoid space, and how it responds to this invasion could be addressed almost ideally in the Dacey/Sande rabbit model, in which substances can be directly injected into the CSF space and CSF can then be sampled almost continuously to monitor the response of the host. Work by several groups, notably Alex Tomasz and Elaine Tuomanen and their colleagues at Rockefeller University, has documented that fragments of the bacterial cell, not the bacterial polysaccharide capsule, are critical stimuli for the host's own inflammatory response.[20,21] The pneumococcal cell wall is composed of a sugar back bone consisting of alternating molecules of *N*-acetyl-muramic acid and *N*-acetyl-glucosamine, which are connected to a three dimensional network by pentapeptide side chains. In addition, the cell wall contains teichoic acid and lipoteichoic acids. All of these components of the cell wall are released as fragments from dying organisms undergoing autolysis and are able to induce mononuclear macrophages to express and release proinflammatory cytokines, such as TNF-α, interleukin-1 (IL-1), IL-6, and many others.[22] Release of cell wall fragments is dramatically increased immediately after initiation of antibiotic therapy, when large numbers of bacteria are killed, and the increased liberation of cell wall fragments leads to a heightened inflammatory response of the host.[23,24] The exact potency of various cell wall fragments of the pneumococcus in inducing cytokines seems to vary, but small muramic acid-dipeptides are thought to represent the minimal proinflammatory unit. The composition and amount of cell wall fragments released spontaneously or after initiation of antibiotic therapy can vary substantially from one pneumococcal strain to another. This variability may be one factor explaining the dramatic differences in the evolution of pathophysiologic changes, when different pneumococcal strains are injected into the CSF of rabbits.[25]

Induction of proinflammatory cytokines (TNF-α, IL-1, IL-6) triggers a complex network of additional inflammatory mediators that in concert regulate the humoral and cellular inflammation during meningitis. Other proinflammatory cytokines, antiinflammatory cytokines (IL-10, TGF-β), soluble cytokine receptors and receptor antagonists, several members of the more recently discovered class of chemokines, and lipid mediators such as platelet activating factor (PAF) all appear to be involved in the meningeal inflammation and the subsequent pathophysiologic changes (for a recent review, see Täuber and Moser[26]). The complexity of the inflammatory mediator network, and limitations of the currently used experimental systems rarely allow a conclusive determination as to what extent bacterial components or host-derived mediators are responsible for the changes observed during bacterial meningitis. It is possible that the only role of bacterial products is to start and maintain the inflammatory response of the host. Accordingly, inhibition of inflammatory mediators by administration of corticosteroids or nonsteroidal antiinflammatory drugs is effective in preventing the pathophysiologic changes in models of meningitis, particularly when the substances are given prior to the development of meningitis.[4,23,27] Corticosteroids, with their broad mode of action which includes potent inhibition of cytokines, seem more effective in downmodulating inflammation and pathophysiologic changes in meningitis than nonsteroidal antiinflammatory drugs. The latter class of drugs, represented for example by indomethacin, primarily influences the generation of some lipid mediators and has shown limited effects on the pathophysiology of meningitis.[27]

ADVANCED PATHOPHYSIOLOGY OF MENINGITIS

As a consequence of the increasing inflammatory reaction in the subarachnoid and ventricular space, meningitis leads to multiple, well-defined alterations of the intracranial physiology. These include brain edema, increased intracranial pressure, reduction in cerebral blood flow, and increased resistance to CSF resorption.[4,28-30] Increased intracranial pressure represents probably the most critical single alteration that is both the result of other changes and contributes critically to cerebral ischemia with its devastating effect on the brain.[29] Three factors can contribute to increased intracranial pressure during meningitis: brain edema, increased cerebral blood volume, and alterations of CSF hydrodynamics, in particular disturbed CSF resorption.[30–32] Brain edema in meningitis appears to be a combination of vasogenic edema, resulting from the disruption of the blood-brain barrier, cytotoxic edema, resulting from cytotoxic mediators such as excitatory amino acids (EAA), and interstitial edema.[31] The latter is the consequence of a mechanical plugging of the CSF clearance system across the arachnoid villi in the superior sagittal sinus by the inflammation in the subarachnoid space.[30] White blood cells, fibrin, and bacteria collect in the villi, thus obstructing the CSF outflow and leading to increased CSF pressure, increased intracranial pressure, and possibly hydrocephalus. Downmodulation of inflammation with corticosteroids improves, as one would expect, the function of the CSF clearance system across the arachnoid villi.[30] Finally, intracranial blood volume can also contribute to increased intracranial pressure. Early in the disease, increased blood flow to the brain (hyperemia) may be the most important contributing factor to increased intracranial blood volume and increased intracranial pressure.[33] As the disease progresses, blood flow is overall reduced, but the venous blood volume may nevertheless be increased, leading to an increase of total intracerebral blood volume.[32]

The most significant consequence of increased intracranial pressure is its effect on cerebral blood flow. At least in severe cases of meningitis, typically caused by pneumococci, cerebral blood flow autoregulation is impaired and cerebral blood flow is directly dependent on cerebral perfusion pressure, which results from arterial pressure minus intracranial pressure.[28,29] Thus, high intracranial pressure directly reduces cerebral perfusion pressure (particularly when the patient at the same time has a low systemic blood pressure because of dehydration or sepsis) and thus leads to reduced cerebral blood flow and subsequent cerebral ischemia.[29,34] In practical terms, correction of cerebral perfusion pressure by normalizing arterial blood pressure and reducing intracranial hypertension is one of the most critical goals of the supportive management of patients with severe meningitis.

MECHANISMS OF BRAIN DAMAGE

The net result of the many changes occurring in the brain during meningitis is the development of brain damage, characterized by neuronal drop out and other, less well defined cellular changes in the brain. As a clinical result, patients who survive the disease with neuronal damage show neurologic sequelae, such as learning deficits, mental retardation, sensory-motor deficits, and seizure disorders.[35] The most common neurologic sequelae is hearing loss, which appears to result from inflammation affecting the inner ear after direct extension from the subarachnoid space along the cochlear aqueduct into the perilymphatic space of the cochlea.[36,37] Molecular mediators of the processes that lead to the destruction of the hair cells of the inner ear are incompletely characterized, but may involve cytokines, oxygen-derived radicals, and in the case of the pneumococcus, the bacteria-derived, highly potent cytotoxin pneumolysin.[38]

The molecular mechanisms that lead to neuronal damage during meningitis have started more recently to emerge from work in infant rats with experimental meningitis. Initial studies in this model were performed using group B streptococci as the infecting organism, but more recent experiments have shown that the pneumococcus produces very similar alterations as the group B streptococcus. The advantage of this model is the fact that substantial neuronal injury occurs as a result of the disease.[39] This is in contrast to most other models of meningitis previously employed, particularly the rabbit model, where very little neuropathologic changes can be identified even in advanced meningitis. The new model has thus opened the door to investigate directly the role of various mediators in causing neuronal injury. The most important form of neuronal injury in this model involves focal cortical injury that resembles very much the focal damage seen in neonates and young children suffering from meningitis.[39] The morphology of these changes shows all the features of ischemic cortical damage; that is, it is wedge shaped and most severe in watershed areas of the cerebral circulation. Indeed, blood flow studies have documented severe focal ischemia in the model, in a pattern that was identical to the histopathologic changes observed. Further supporting the ischemic nature of the cortical injury were studies that showed improved neurologic outcome in animals, in which the extent of blood flow changes was reduced, and worsened neurologic outcome, when blood flow changes were aggravated. Thus, molecular mediators of blood flow alterations during meningitis became an important area of investigation in this model.

Early in experimental meningitis, cerebral blood flow increases as a result of vasodilation. Work in an adult rat model of pneumococcal meningitis by Walter Pfister's group in Munich has documented that this early vasodilation is mediated by nitric oxide (NO).[40] We have found subsequently that NO continues to play an important role as regulator of cerebral blood flow far into the course of the disease.[41] We observed that inhibition of the inducible nitric oxide synthase (NOS), which is upregulated during meningitis in the subarachnoid space inflammation and vasculature and which is responsible at least for part of the NO produced during meningitis, led to a harmful increase in cerebral ischemia in animals with advanced meningitis. This increased ischemia was associated with an increase in neuronal damage. Thus, NO produced by the inducible NOS in or close to the cerebral vasculature has a beneficial effect, because its vasodilative effect counteracts other processes that tend to lead to vasoconstriction and subsequent ischemia.

Some of the vasoconstrictive mediators have also been identified. Most notably are oxygen-derived radicals, such as superoxide, hydrogen peroxide, and others. These metabolic products of essential biologic processes, such as mitochondrial respiratory chain and activation of macrophages, have multiple harmful effects on cells and macromolecules, including lipid peroxidation, DNA damage, and protein oxidation. In the infant rat model of meningitis, lipid peroxidation is strongly increased in advanced disease, and histochemical methods have allowed to directly localize the production of superoxide to the subarachnoid space and the cerebral vasculature.[42] Importantly, scavenging of these radicals by so-called spin-trapping agents, which can bind and detoxify radicals, led to a reduction of lipid peroxidation, but also to an improvement of cerebral blood flow with associated reduction of ischemic neuronal damage.[42] Thus, oxidative radicals, by mechanisms that are currently not completely understood, are important mediators of vasoconstriction during meningitis, and their inhibition is beneficial by improving cerebral blood flow. Another molecule with vasoconstrictive properties that has recently been implicated in the ischemia developing during meningitis is endothelin. This vasoactive peptide is increased in the CSF of patients with meningitis, and we found that an endothelin-receptor antagonist, bosentan, dramatically improved the neurologic outcome of meningitis in the infant rat model, apparently at least in part by improving cerebral blood flow (L.A. Pfister, manuscript in preparation). Other mediators of vasoconstriction likely play also a role in meningitis and will need to be identified in future studies. Importantly, it is likely that increased local coagulation leads to thrombosis with associated disturbances of cerebral blood flow, but this has not been investigated in any of the available models of meningitis.

Some of the molecules that are directly neurotoxic during meningitis have also been identified. Since ischemia appears to play a critical role in causing brain injury, studies have focused on the role of EAA in causing neuronal cell death. EAA (e.g., glutamate) are physiologic neurotransmitters that are released at increased concentrations from neurons subjected to stress, such as ischemia or hypoglycemia. Their increased concentrations in the extracellular fluid leads to overstimulation of postsynaptic EAA receptors, in particular the NMDA receptor, with subsequent increased influx of calcium through the receptor channel, activation of various cellular pathways, including production of NO by neuronal NOS and generation of oxidative radicals. All these processes ultimately lead to cellular death. This appears to be an important mechanism of cell death in stroke. In models of meningitis, we and others have documented an increase in glutamate concentrations both in the CSF and, more importantly, in the intercellular fluid, and have shown that an antogonist of the NMDA receptor, kynurenic acids, is neuroprotective.[43–45] Thus, EAA represent the first neurotoxic molecules shown directly to play a role in bacterial meningitis.

One consequence of overstimulation of NMDA receptors is the generation of NO by neurons containing neuronal NOS. NO can potentially be neurotoxic directly, as shown in brain cell culture systems stimulated with pneumococcal cell walls,[46] or it can combine with superoxide to form the highly cytotoxic molecule peroxynitrite (ONOO). Superoxide is likely to be formed during meningitis in the brain, either as a result of ischemic insult and associated activation of the glycolytic pathway, or as a result of activation of microglia and other phagocytic cells by cytokines and bacterial products. Preliminary evidence suggests that peroxynitrite is indeed formed in the brain during experimental meningitis, and that it contributes to the development of neuronal injury. In the infant rat model, we found evidence for increased production of nitrotyrosine, the chemical hallmark of the presence of peroxynitrite, by immunocytochemistry and HPLC (unpublished observations). A role of peroxynitrite, in meningitis was further supported by treatment studies. Both scavengers of peroxynitrite (uric acid), and an inhibitor (3-aminobenzamine) of the enzyme poly-(ADP-ribose) polymerase (PARP), which is activated by the action of peroxynitrite on mitochondria, significantly reduced neuronal injury in the treated compared to the untreated animals.[47]

Thus, molecules that contribute to the demise of neurons during meningitis may emerge as targets for adjunctive therapy. It would appear that a combined inhibition of oxidative radicals, EAA, and peroxynitrite should have profound effects on the development of neuronal injury. Such therapies could be effective even when instituted in relatively advanced stages of the disease, since the interrupted pathways are late events in the sequence leading from subarachnoid space inflammation to neuronal injury. Specific neuroprotective therapies could represent a potential advantage over the use of corticosteroids, which act primarily by downmodulating inflammation and thus at a relatively early stage in the pathophysiologic cascade of meningitis. This effect primarily on early events in meningitis may, at least in part, be a reason why corticosteroids, while clearly beneficial in several clinical studies, have shown overall modest benefits. This has led to a continued controversy regarding their usefulness in meningitis.[48,49] We hope that the lessons that have been and will be learned from the use of models such as the Dacey/Sande rabbit model will lead to new therapies that can improve the outcome of bacterial meningitis.

REFERENCES

1. **Schuchat, A., K. Robinson, J.D. Wenger, L.H. Harrison, M. Farley, A.L. Reingold, L. Lefkowitz, and B.A. Perkins.** 1997. Bacterial meningitis in the United States in 1995. N. Engl. J. Med. **337:**970–976.

2. **Scheld, W.M., and M.A. Sande.** 1983. Bactericidal versus bacteriostatic antibiotic therapy of experimental pneumococcal meningitis in rabbits. J. Clin. Invest. **71:**411–419.

3. **Dacey, R.G., and M.A. Sande.** 1974. Effect of probenecid on cerebrospinal fluid concentrations of penicillin and cephalosporin derivatives. Antimicrob. Agents Chemother. **6:**437–441.

4. **Täuber, M.G., H. Khayam-Bashi, and M.A. Sande.** 1985. Effects of ampicillin and corticosteroids on brain water content, CSF pressure and CSF lactate in experimental pneumococcal meningitis. J. Infect. Dis. **151:**528–534.

5. **Sande, M.A., E.R. Sande, J.D. Woolwine, C.J. Hackbarth, and P.M. Small.** 1987. The influence of fever on the development of experimental *Streptococcus pneumoniae* meningitis. J. Infect. Dis. **156:**849–850.

6. **Moxon, E.R., and P.A. Murphy.** 1978. *Haemophilus influenzae* bacteremia and meningitis resulting from the survival of a single organism. Proc. Natl. Acad. Sci. U.S.A. **75:**1534–1536.

7. **Scheld, W.M., T. Park, R.G. Dacey, H.R. Winn, J.A. Jane, and M.A. Sande.** 1979. Clearance of bacteria from cerebrospinal fluid to blood in experimental meningitis. Infect. Immunol. **24:**102–105.

8. **Quagliarello, V.J., W.J. Long, and W.M. Scheld.** 1986. Morphologic alterations of the blood-brain barrier with experimental meningitis in the rat. J. Clin. Invest. **77:**1085–1095.

9. **Ernst, J.D., K. Hartiala, I.M. Goldstein, and M.A. Sande.** 1984. Complement (C5)–derived chemotactic activity accounts for accumulation of polymorphonuclear leukocytes in cerebrospinal fluid of rabbits with pneumococcal meningitis. Infect. Immunol. **46:**81–86.

10. **Ernst, J.D., J.M. Decazes, and M.A. Sande.** 1983. Experimental pneumococcal meningitis: role of leukocytes in pathogenesis. Infect. Immunol. **41:**275–279.

11. **Propp, R.P., B. Jannari, and K. Barron.** 1977. Measurement of the third component of complement in cerebrospinal fluid by modified electroimmunodiffusion. Scand. J. Clin. Lab. Invest. **37:**385–390.

12. **Smith, H., B. Bannister, and M.J. O'Shea.** 1973. Cerebrospinal fluid immunoglobulins in meningitis. Lancet **1**:591–593.

13. **Tuomanen, E., B. Hengstler, O. Zak, and A. Tomasz.** 1986. The role of complement in inflammation during experimental pneumococcal meningitis. Microb. Pathog. **1**:15–32.

14. **Small, P.M., M.G. Täuber, C.J. Hackbarth, and M.A. Sande.** 1986. Influence of body temperature on bacterial growth rates in experimental pneumococcal meningitis in rabbits. Infect. Immunol. **52**:484–487.

15. **Cooper, A., H. Beaty, S. Oppenheimer, R. Goodner, and R. Petersdorf.** 1968. Studies on the pathogenesis of meningitis. Glucose transport and spinal fluid production in experimental pneumoccocal meningitis. J. Lab. Clin. Med. **71**:473–483.

16. **Hochwald, G., S. Nakamura, R. Chase, and J. Gorelick.** 1984. Cerebrospinal fluid glucose and leukocyte responses in experimental meningitis. J. Neurol. Sci. **63**:381–391.

17. **Guerra-Romero, L., M.G. Täuber, M.A. Fournier, and J.H. Tureen.** 1992. Lactate and glucose concentrations in brain interstitial fluid, cerebrospinal fluid, and serum during experimental pneumococcal meningitis. J. Infect. Dis. **166**:546–550.

18. **Tureen, J.** 1995. Effect of recombinant human tumor necrosis factor-alpha on cerebral oxygen uptake, cerebrospinal fluid lactate, and cerebral blood flow in the rabbit: role of nitric oxide. J. Clin. Invest. **95**:1086–1091.

19. **Brooke-Williams, R.** 1964. Alterations in the glucose transport mechanism in patients with complications of bacterial meningitis. Pediatrics **34**:491–502.

20. **Tuomanen, E., H. Liu, B. Hengstler, O. Zak, and A. Tomasz.** 1985. The induction of meningeal inflammation by components of the pneumococcal cell wall. J. Infect. Dis. **152**:859–868.

21. **Tuomanen, E., A. Tomasz, B. Hengstler, and O. Zak.** 1985. The relative role of bacterial cell wall and capsule in the induction of inflammation in pneumococcal meningitis. J. Infect. Dis. **151**:535–540.

22. **Tuomanen, E., B. Hengstler, O. Zak, and A. Tomasz.** 1986. Induction of meningeal inflammation by diverse bacterial cell walls. Eur. J. Clin. Microbiol. **5**:682–684.

23. **Tuomanen, E., B. Hengstler, R. Rich, M.A. Bray, O. Zak, and A. Tomasz.** 1987. Nonsteroidal anti-inflammatory agents in the therapy for experimental pneumococcal meningitis. J. Infect. Dis. **155**:985–990.

24. **Täuber, M.G., A.M. Shibl, C.J. Hackbarth, J.W. Larrick, and M.A. Sande.** 1987. Antibiotic therapy, endotoxin concentration in cerebrospinal fluid, and brain edema in experimental *Escherichia coli* meningitis in rabbits. J. Infect. Dis. **156**:456–462.

25. **Täuber, M.G., M. Burroughs, U.M. Niemöller, H. Kuster, U. Borschberg, and E. Tuomanen.** 1991. Differences of pathophysiology in experimental meningitis caused by three strains of *Streptococcus pneumoniae*. J. Infect. Dis. **163**:806–811.

26. **Täuber, M.G., and B. Moser.** 1999. Cytokines and chemokines in meningeal inflammation: biology and clinical implications. Clin. Infect. Dis. **28**:1–11.

27. **Tureen, J.H., M.G. Täuber, and M.A. Sande.** 1991. Effect of indomethacin on the pathophysiology of experimental meningitis in rabbits. J. Infect. Dis. **163**:647–649.

28. **Tureen, J.H., R.J. Dworkin, S.L. Kennedy, M. Sachdeva, and M.A. Sande.** 1990. Loss of cerebrovascular autoregulation in experimental meningitis in rabbits. J. Clin. Invest. **85**:577–581.

29. **Tureen, J.H., M.G. Täuber, and M.A. Sande.** 1992. Effect of hydration status on cerebral blood flow and cerebrospinal fluid lactic acidosis in rabbits with experimental meningitis. J. Clin. Invest. **89**:947–953.

30. **Scheld, W.M., R.G. Dacey, H.R. Winn, J.E. Welsh, J.A. Jane, and M.A. Sande.** 1980. Cerebrospinal fluid outflow resistance in rabbits with experimental meningitis. J. Clin. Invest. **66**:243–253.

31. **Täuber, M.G.** 1989. Brain edema, intracranial pressure and cerebral blood flow in bacterial meningitis. Pediatr. Infect. Dis. J. **8**:915–917.

32. **Tureen, J., Q. Liu, and L. Chow.** 1996. Near-infrared spectroscopy in experimental pneumococcal meningitis in the rabbit: cerebral hemodynamics and metabolism. Pediatr. Res. **40**:759–763.

33. **Pfister, H.W., U. Koedel, R.L. Haberl, U. Dirnagl, W. Feiden, L.G. Kuckdesche, and K.M. Einhaupl.** 1990. Microvascular changes during the early phase of experimental bacterial meningitis. J. Cereb. Blood Flow Metab. **10**:914–922.

34. **Täuber, M.G., E. Sande, M.A. Fournier, J.H. Tureen, and M.A. Sande.** 1993. Fluid administration, brain edema, and cerebrospinal fluid lactate and glucose concentrations in experimental *Escherichia coli* meningitis. J. Infect. Dis. **168**:473–476.

35. **Grimwood, K., V.A. Anderson, L. Bond, C. Catroppa, R.L. Hore, E.H. Keir, T. Nolan, and D.M. Robertson.** 1995. Adverse outcome of bacterial meningitis in school-age survivors. Pediatrics **95**:646–656.

36. **Dodge, P.R., D. Hallowell, R.D. Feigin, S.J. Holmes, S.L. Kaplan, D.P. Jubelirer, B. Stechberg, and S.K. Hirsh.** 1984. Prospective evaluation of hearing impairment as a sequela of acute bacterial meningitis. N. Eng. J. Med. **311**:869–874.

37. **Bhatt, S.M., A. Lauretano, C. Cabellos, C. Halpin, R.A. Levine, W.Z. Xu, J.B.J. Nadol, and E. Tuomanen.** 1993. Progression of hearing loss in experimental pneumococcal meningitis: correlation with cerebrospinal fluid cytochemistry. J. Infect. Dis. **167**:675–683.

38. **Comis, S.D., M.P. Osborne, J. Stephen, M.J. Tarlow, T.L. Hayward, T.J. Mitchell, P.W. Andrew, and G.J. Boulnois.** 1993. Cytotoxic effect on hair cells of guinea pig cochlea produced by pneumolysin, the thiol activated toxin of *Streptococcus pneumoniae*. Acta Otolaryngol. **113**:152–159.

39. **Kim, Y.S., R.A. Sheldon, B.R. Elliot, Q. Liu, D.M. Ferriero, and M.G. Täuber.** 1995. Brain damage in neonatal meningitis caused by group B streptococci in rats. J. Neuropathol. Exp. Neurol. **54**:531–539.

40. **Koedel, U., A. Bernatowicz, R. Paul, K. Frei, A. Fontana, and H.-W. Pfister.** 1995. Experimental pneumococcal meningitis: cerebrovascular alterations, brain edema, and meningeal inflammation are linked to the production of nitric oxide. Ann. Neurol. **37**:313–323.

41. **Leib, S.L., Y.S. Kim, S.M. Black, J.H. Tureen, and M.G. Täuber.** 1998. Inducible nitric oxide synthase and the effect of aminoguanidine in experimental neonatal meningitis. J. Infect. Dis. **177**:692–700.

42. **Leib, S.L., Y.S. Kim, L.L. Chow, R.A. Sheldon, and M.G. Täuber.** 1996. Reactive oxygen intermediates contribute to necrotic and apoptotic neuronal injury in an infant rat model of bacterial meningitis due to group B streptococci. J. Clin. Invest. **98**:2632–2639.

43. **Guerra-Romero, L., J.H. Tureen, M.A. Fournier, V. Makrides, and M.G. Täuber.** 1993. Amino acids in cerebrospinal and brain interstitial fluid during experimental pneumococcal meningitis. Pediatr. Res. **33**::510–513.

44. **Perry, V., R.S.K. Young, W.J. Aquila, and M.J. During.** 1993. Effect of experimental *Escherichia coli* meningitis on concentrations of excitatory and inhibitory amino acids in the rabbit brain: *in vivo* microdialysis study. Pediatr. Res. **34**:187–191.

45. **Leib, S.L., S.Y. Kim, D.M. Ferriero, and M.G. Täuber.** 1996. Neuroprotective effect of excitatory amino acid antagonist kynurenic acid in experimental bacterial meningitis. J. Infect. Dis. **173**:166–171.

46. **Kim, Y.S., S. Kennedy, and M.G. Täuber.** 1995. Toxicity of *Streptococcus pneumoniae* in neurons, astrocytes, and microglia *in vitro*. J. Infect. Dis. **171**:1363–1369.

47. **Ho, T.C., L. Chow, D.M. Ferriero, M.G. Täuber, and J.H. Tureen.** 1998. Peroxynitrite-mediated brain injury in experimen-

tal group B streptococcal meningitis in the neonatal rat. J. Invest. Med. **46**:115.

48. **McIntyre, P.B., C.S. Berkey, S.M. King, U.B. Schaad, T. Kilpi, G.Y. Kanra, and C.M. Odio Perez.** 1997. Dexamethasone as adjunctive therapy in bacterial meningitis. A meta-analysis of randomized clinical trials since 1988. J.A.M.A. **278**:925–931.

49. **Quagliarello, V.J., and W.M. Scheld.** 1997. Treatment of bacterial meningitis. N. Engl. J. Med. **336**:708–716.

Address reprint requests to:
Merle A. Sande
Department of Internal Medicine
University of Utah
50 North Medical Drive
Salt Lake City, UT 84132

Invasive Pneumococcal Disease in the Immunocompromised Host

EDWARD N. JANOFF[1] and JEFFREY B. RUBINS[2]

ABSTRACT

A normal constituent of the human upper respiratory flora, *Streptococcus pneumoniae* also produces respiratory tract infections that progress to invasive disease at high rates in specific risk groups. The individual factors that contribute to the development of invasive pneumococcal disease in this distinct minority of persons, include immune (both specific and innate), genetic, and environmental elements. Specific defects in host responses may involve age, deficiencies in levels of and receptors for antibodies and complement factors, and splenic dysfunction. Combinations of these immune defects contribute to the increased rates of invasive pneumococcal disease in patients with sickle cell disease, nephrotic syndrome, neoplasms, and possibly those with underlying medical conditions such as diabetes and alcoholic liver disease. The numbers of risk factors are greatest and the rates of invasive disease are highest in patients with HIV-1 infection, which has emerged as a major risk factor for serious *S. pneumoniae* infection worldwide.

INTRODUCTION

STREPTOCOCCUS PNEUMONIAE commonly colonizes the nasopharynx asymptomatically in healthy children and adults. This encapsulated potential pathogen is considered a constituent of the normal upper respiratory flora in humans. Transient or mild-to-moderately severe mucosal infections of the auditory canal (otitis media), upper respiratory tract (sinusitis), large airways (bronchitis), or lower airways (pneumonia) comprise the vast majority of *S. pneumoniae*–associated illness and morbidity. However, a subset of these infections progress to cause severe pneumococcal disease with tissue invasion (e.g., necrotizing pneumonia, meningitis, bacteremia). These invasive syndromes cause the preponderance of *S. pneumoniae*–related mortality.

Invasive pneumococcal disease affects persons of selected races and ages, in certain social conditions, and with specific underlying diseases at rates that greatly exceed those of the general population. In the United States, rates of pneumococcal bacteremia, a reliable if insensitive marker of the burden of this bacterial infection, are remarkably consistent at approximately 19 per 100,000 per year in most heterogeneous populations (Table 1). However, even within these populations, rates vary by race, with a threefold higher incidence among black Americans than among Caucasians,[16] differences that have not been explained entirely by differences in socioeconomic factors. Similarly, Native American populations in geographically divergent areas from Alaska to Arizona have a five- to 10-fold higher annual incidence of pneumococcal bacteremia than that of most U.S. populations (74–207 per 100,000).[34,37,38] Independent of race, children under 2 years experience yet another 10-fold increased incidence of bacteremia compared with matched adult populations.[14,19,34,36,38,46] Thus, specific communities within the general population and those living with poverty, crowding, pollution, and extreme stress, are preferentially susceptible to invasive pneumococcal disease.[26,82,107,151,154]

In the following discussion, we will characterize groups with certain known immune defects and consider their rates of serious pneumococcal infections and attendant mortality. We will introduce the functional relationship of host defenses acting in concert to protect against pneumococcal disease. Other instructive articles in this series on *S. pneumoniae* highlight the pathogenic mechanisms utilized by the organism to evade these host defenses. We describe how individual host defects may each contribute independently to the increased risk of invasive disease, and observe that the potential number of immunologic risk factors is greatest and rates of invasive pneumococcal disease are highest among HIV-1–infected patients. In this context, the reader is encouraged to consider what factors convey natural immunity against initial pneumococcal infection, and

---

[1]Infectious Disease and [2]Pulmonary Sections, Department of Medicine, Veterans Affairs Medical Center, University of Minnesota School of Medicine, Minneapolis, Minnesota.

TABLE 1. INCIDENCE OF INVASIVE PNEUMOCOCCAL
DISEASE IN U.S. POPULATIONS

Group, location (reference)	Cases/100,000 persons/year	
	All ages	<2 years
General population, Charleston, SC[21]	18.7	162
General population, Monroe Co., NY[16]	18.8	175
White Mountain Apache, Arizona[34]	207	1820
Native Americans, Alaska[38]	108	1235

what are the critical components of protection against lethal invasive disease (e.g., immune versus nonimmune factors, anatomic defenses, inflammation, and systemic versus mucosal immunity). Identifying these factors may stimulate innovative approaches to prevent invasive pneumococcal disease in the immunocompromised host.

SPECIFIC POPULATIONS AT RISK

Children

Relative immune dysfunction may be a manifestation of an immature or inexperienced immune system. As highlighted in Table 1, rate of invasive pneumococcal disease are typically 10-fold higher in children under 2 years compared with those in adults in the same population. These high rates may be due to anatomic imbalances (e.g., alignment of the eustachian tube), humoral immune dysfunction, or high rates of preceding viral and allergic episodes. A prominent predisposing factor is the inability of young children to produce antibodies to polysaccharide antigens, such as those in the serotype-specific pneumococcal capsule. This humoral defect, likely under T cell control, may derive in part from compromised production of the IgG$_2$ subclass, which comprises an appreciable proportion of capsule-specific IgG.[4,32,177] The enhanced ability of capsular polysaccharides to stimulate specific IgG when conjugated to protein antigens was the basis for the outstanding clinical efficacy of newer vaccines directed to prevent invasive *Haemophilus influenzae* disease in children.[45] This success derived in part from the shift to production from IgG$_2$ to predominantly IgG$_1$ subclass anticapsular antibodies, which are readily produced by young children. Such conjugate vaccines using pneumococcal polysaccharide antigens are now in development.[104] Field trials will establish whether these multivalent pneumococcal conjugate vaccines can prevent invasive disease (e.g., bacteremia and meningitis) and colonization as effectively as the antecedent conjugate vaccine directed to *H. influenzae* type b. Whether newer vaccines can effectively prevent *S. pneumoniae*-related otitis media, the most common manifestation of pneumococcal disease in children (6 million cases per year in the United States),[29] is a crucial area of concern and investigation.

The risks for invasive pneumococcal disease in children may decline with age due to maturation of the immune system, to an expanded repertoire of immunologic memory, and, likely in the near future, to the use of a new generation of vaccines. Nevertheless, some patients with specific genetic immune defects

remain at risk for life, whereas other previously healthy persons develop into high risk patients due to the acquisition of hematologic, oncologic, or medical problems.

Antibody defects

Specific humoral responses to pneumococcal capsular polysaccharides are critical to effective opsonophagocytosis and killing of the organism.[24,68] Defective humoral responses to *S. pneumoniae* contribute to the increased rates of invasive infection not only in patients with primary antibody deficiencies but also in those with defects in complement and splenic function. Although specific rates are not available, patients with hypogammaglobulinemia are susceptible to invasive *S. pneumoniae* infection.[160] Specifically, IgG$_2$ appears to the critical antibody class for protective humoral responses to *S. pneumoniae*,[120,166] presumably because of the proposed unique ability of IgG$_2$ to support neutrophil phagocytosis of pneumococci in the absence of complement.[120] IgG$_2$ deficiency probably underlies, in part, the increased rates of pneumococcal bacteremia in hypogammaglobulinemia, and in some patients with IgA deficiency.[117] Although patients with selective IgA deficiency are not generally susceptible to higher rates of pneumococcal infection, the subset who have concomitantly impaired IgG$_2$ responses to pneumococcal capsular polysaccharides do appear to be at increased risk.[117]

Complement defects

Efficient opsonophagocytosis of *S. pneumoniae* also requires fixation of early complement components (especially C3b) to the bacterial surface. Complement can bind to *S. pneumoniae* and mediate phagocytosis by both antibody-dependent and antibody-independent mechanisms.[83] Accordingly, *S. pneumoniae* is the most common etiology of invasive bacterial infection among patients with congenital or acquired deficiencies of early components of the classical pathway (C1, C4, and C2) and the alternative pathway (factor I and factor H); C3 is common to both pathways. Factor C2 deficiency, one of the most common complement deficiencies, is associated with an increased incidence of invasive *S. pneumoniae* infection, particularly when additional defects in alternate pathway components are present.[135] However, even isolated C2 deficiency causes an increased incidence of *S. pneumoniae* infection, presumably because C3 is more rapidly fixed by the classical complement pathway.[83] Although less common, C3 deficiency is associated with increased rates of pyogenic infections with encapsulated organisms such as *S. pneumoniae*.[194] Unlike defects in other early components of complement, C3 deficiency is also reported with recurrent pneumococcal infections.[52] The distinct susceptibility of such patients to recurrent pneumococcal infection derives from defects in both complement and antibody functions. In addition to their inability to fix C3b to the bacterial surface for opsonophagocytosis, these patients have almost total deficiency of antibodies to pneumococcal capsular polysaccharides,[78] perhaps related in part to the requirement for C3 to induce humoral responses to polysaccharide antigens.[40,72,73,144]

Splenic dysfunction

Asplenia and splenic dysfunction are associated with higher rates of invasive *S. pneumoniae* infection both because of abnormal immune responses to *S. pneumoniae* antigens and loss of splenic clearance of intravascular bacteria. The annual incidence of *S. pneumoniae* bacteremia in splenectomized adults is estimated to be significantly increased at 92–210 per 100,000 patients.[137,170] At least half of the cases of overwhelming postsplenectomy sepsis are caused by *S. pneumoniae*.

Splenectomized patients may exhibit defective humoral responses to *S. pneumoniae* polysaccharides.[41,75,108,153] Optimal induction of primary immune responses to polysaccharide antigens likely involve a functionally intact spleen containing B cells expressing a high density of surface C3d-receptors (CD21).[144] However, not all patients with splenectomy have deficient antibody responses to pneumococcal vaccine,[110,138] suggesting that additional immune deficiencies contribute to their higher rates of invasive *S. pneumoniae* infection. Loss of splenic clearance of intravascular pneumococci, which is critical in patients with impaired complement-dependent opsonization, may also contribute to the higher frequency of *S. pneumoniae* bacteremia in these patients.[194]

Combined immune defects

Additional groups of immunocompromised patients who experience increased rates of invasive pneumococcal disease include those with combined, and, most often, acquired defects in humoral, complement, and splenic functions.

Sickle cell disease

Sickle cell anemia produces functional asplenia resulting in an extraordinary susceptibility to pneumococcal bacteremia. Prior to the introduction of the pneumococcal vaccine in 1978, the age-specific annual incidence of *S. pneumoniae* bacteremia in patients with sickle cell disease varied from 5,700 to 42,100 per 100,000 for children under 2 years old, and was approximately 1,100 per 100,000 for those over 4 years old, with a total case-fatality rate of 26.8%.[197,199] Children with sickle cell anemia may have reduced serum opsonization of *S. pneumoniae* via the classical complement pathway secondary to low levels of IgG and IgM antibodies to capsular polysaccharides.[18] B cell maturation appears to be arrested at a step dependent on the B cell-activating cytokine interleukin-4. An abnormality associated with decreased numbers of antibody producing cells in response to *S. pneumoniae* polysaccharides and mitogens.[149] Despite these humoral defects, older children with sickle cell disease can generate adequate antibody responses to pneumococcal vaccine, especially after a booster immunization.[102,148]

Use of the vaccine has decreased the overall incidence of *S. pneumoniae* infection in these children.[197] However, as noted, the pure polysaccharide vaccine is substantially less effective in all children under 2 years,[18] and has not reduced the high rates of invasive infection in this age range.[197] Additional defects in unidentified classical and alternative complement cofactors,[19] as well as in neutrophil oxidative activity,[85] which have not as yet been fully characterized, have been proposed in these children.

Nephrotic syndrome

Patients with nephrotic syndrome are particularly susceptible to peritonitis and bacteremia due to *S. pneumoniae*, particularly during periods of relapse of their renal disease. The marked decrease in serum opsonizing activity in these patients is likely related to decreased serum levels of complement factor B (MW 80,000) secondary to urinary losses.[194] In addition, serum IgG antibodies to *S. pneumoniae* polysaccharides are decreased, partly due to urinary losses but also due in part to decreased antibody production.[58,181]

Cancer

Hematologic malignancies, especially lymphomas, are associated with higher rates of *S. pneumoniae* infection. Splenectomy in Hodgkin's disease carries the risk of fulminant bacterial sepsis, usually caused by *S. pneumoniae*, at an adjusted annual rate of approximately 330 cases per 100,000 patients.[56] In addition to specific immune defects attributable to splenectomy, Hodgkin's lymphoma and acute lymphocytic lymphoma are associated with decreased responsiveness to *S. pneumoniae* capsular polysaccharides.[51,54] Furthermore, bone marrow transplant therapy for hematologic malignancies can cause increased rates of pneumococcal infection[195] and depressed specific antibody response to *S. pneumoniae* capsular polysaccharides, especially in the presence of chronic graft-versus-host reactions.[11,63,76] Historically, multiple myeloma has been associated with recurrent pneumococcal infections, which carry increased mortality.[158] Sera from myeloma patients with recurrent pneumococcal infections have significantly decreased C3b binding to *S. pneumoniae* despite normal levels of C3, total hemolytic complement and C-reactive protein, which may be related to inadequate C3 activation.[30] The predisposition for invasive pneumococcal disease among adults with chronic lymphocytic leukemia (CLL) likely derives from their arrested B cell development and associated hypogammaglobulinemia.[31,87,111,188]

Underlying medical conditions

In addition to these conditions where specific defects in humoral, complement, or splenic defense functions can be identified, a number of other potentially immunocompromising diseases have been associated with increased susceptibility to invasive *S. pneumoniae* infection.[26] Diseases such as diabetes mellitus, alcoholism, cirrhosis, and nonhematologic malignancies appear to confer a 2.5-fold increased risk of pneumococcal bacteremia in case-control series; true population-based incidences are not known.[16,23,26,71,99,112,116,122,123,141,143,192] The predisposition of such patients to pneumococcal bacteremia is often multifactorial, with defects in mechanical defenses (e.g., weakened gag reflex and cough) and suppression of neutrophil phagocytosis and killing activities contributing to potential deficiencies in humoral responses and reticuloendothelial clearance mechanisms.

HIV-1 infection and S. pneumoniae

In the early to mid 1980s, the presence of severe, persistent, or unusual opportunistic infections in previously healthy young adults characterized the syndrome of HIV-1/AIDS.[125] These infections included protozoal, fungal, and viral pathogens. As early HIV-1 infection was more readily detected with commercial immunoassay (beginning mid-1985) and as antiretroviral therapy and prophylactic antimicrobial regimens were introduced and widely used, the spectrum of HIV-1–associated illness changed.[103,171] Initially, P. carinii infections accounted for up to three quarters of primary diagnoses of AIDS and were by far the most commonly recognized cause of pulmonary disease. Now, bacterial pneumonias are among the leading indications for hospitalization among HIV-1–infected patients.[13,89,115,130,146,173]

Epidemiology of S. pneumoniae in HIV-1–infected patients

In the United States and Europe, bacterial infections, particularly bacterial pneumonia, comprise an increasing proportion of major clinical events as rates of P. carinii and Salmo-nella infections decrease with the use of prophylactic agents.[119,121,167] The incidence of bacterial pneumonia is increased 5–10 fold during HIV-1 infection (5.5 versus 0.9 per 100 person-years in seronegative persons),[80] particularly in drug users, whose incidence of bacterial pneumonia is almost 10% per year compared with 1–2% in HIV-1–seronegative current or former addicts.[20,173] The most common organisms identified in these patients are S. pneumoniae and Haemophilus influenzae.[80,115,130,146,173] However, whereas pneumonia with H. influenzae is uncommonly bacteremic, rates of bacteremic pneumococcal pneumonia are high. Pneumococcal pneumonia is complicated by bacteremia in the majority of cases in HIV-1–infected patients (60–80%, compared with 10–20% with typical community-acquired pneumococcal pneumonia).[10,17,21,89,91,113,115,146,150,156,168,172,173,196]

As a result of these high rates of invasion, S. pneumoniae is a leading cause of bacteremia during HIV-1 infection, accounting for 13–31% of all bacteremias in these patients.[89] Two population-based studies demonstrate that the incidence of pneumococcal bacteremia during HIV-1 infection is approximately 100-fold higher among 20–55-year-old patients with HIV/AIDS[150,168] compared with the age-matched population (9.4 cases versus 0.07 cases per 1,000 per year; Table 2).[21] Moreover, HIV-1 infection is a common coinfection among all adults with pneumococcal bacteremia (10–28%).[57,79,89,96,168]

Serious bacterial infections have also been recognized

TABLE 2. IMPACT OF HIV-1 INFECTION ON THE INCIDENCE OF PNEUMOCOCCAL DISEASE IN POPULATION-BASED STUDIES

Reference	Location (years)	Group (age)	Syndrome[a]	HIV-1 status	Incidence (cases/1,000 person-years)	Comments
150	San Francisco (1983–87)	Adults (20–55 years)	Invasive	+	9.4	Retrospective study
				−	0.08–0.16[b]	Recurrence: HIV-1+, 13% Seronegative, 7%
168	New Jersey (1986)	Adults (25–44 years)	Invasive	+ AIDS	10.7	Retrospective study
				+ pre-AIDS	5.3	
				−	0.03	
64	Nairobi (1989–92)	Adult female sex workers (mean 29 years)	Invasive	+	23.8	Prospective study
				−	0	Recurrent 19.1% per year in HIV-1+
3	Barcelona (1985–97)	Adults	Meningitis	+	0.4	Prospective study Estimated 150–400 times greater than general population Recurrences in 2/9 patients (22%)
173	New York City (1985–86)	Adult IVDU (mean 34 years)	Pneumonia	+ non-AIDS	34.6	Prospective study
				−	3.5	
20	Rome (1991–94)	Adult IVDU	Pneumonia	+	18.6	Prospective study
				−	1.2	
50	Baltimore, MD (1986–92)	Children (6–36 months)	Invasive	+	113	Prospective study
				− (exposed)	11	Some HIV-1+ children receiving intravenous immunoglobulin
				−	5	
7	New Haven, CT (1985–91)	Children	Invasive	+	124	Prospective study
				−	13	

[a]Invasive indicates bacteremia, meningitis, or isolation of S. pneumoniae from other sterile sites.
[b]Historical age-matched controls.
IVDU, intravenous drug user.

as a prominent problem in children with HIV-1/AIDS.[8,49,61,113,165,169] As described in other populations earlier, the incidence of pneumococcal bacteremia in young children is approximately 10-fold higher than in geographically and ethnically matched adults (Table 1). Consistent with this pattern, invasive pneumococcal disease (bacteremia or meningitis) affects 10–12% of HIV-1–infected children per year in the United States[7,50] compared with approximately 1% of seropositive adults (Table 2). Although well-recognized in HIV-1–infected children in Africa as well,[118] no data on the rates of pneumococcal infections are available, and little is known about the clinical manifestations or outcome of HIV-1–associated pediatric pneumococcal infections in this part of the world.

Although the incidence of invasive pneumococcal disease is quite high in HIV-1–infected adults in the United States, rates in African adults are higher still. The World Health Organization estimates that over 3 million cases of AIDS, representing two thirds of all cases worldwide, have occurred in sub-Saharan Africa, and that 9 million people in this area have been infected with HIV.[39] The epidemiology of HIV-1 disease in sub-Saharan Africa is quite different than in the United States, with a much higher proportion of the total population infected, with women and children comprising a higher proportion of cases, and with death occurring earlier in the course of infection. Moreover, the natural distribution of infections which complicate HIV-1 disease in Africa are quite different. In the absence of prophylaxis, pneumococcus, rather than pneumocystis, is prominent among the infections which complicate HIV-1 disease in Africa.[65,66] In Nairobi, Kenya, S. pneumoniae is the second most common cause of community-acquired bacteremia (after non–typhi Salmonellae). The only population-based data from Africa reveal that invasive pneumococcal disease affects 2–4% of HIV-1–infected women per year, rates two- to fourfold higher than those in HIV-1–infected adults in the United States (Table 2).[66] Thus, with higher numbers of persons infected with HIV-1 and higher rates of this bacterial infection, the impact of HIV-1–associated pneumococcal disease in Africa is far greater than in industrialized nations.

Clinical manifestations

Pneumonia is the most common source of pneumococcal bacteremias (up to 80–90%) in HIV-1–infected adults in the United States, Europe, and Africa.[60,101,115,131,150,156] Other sites include meningitis, sinusitis, or endocarditis. Among U.S. children and African adults, approximately 50% of pneumococcal bacteremias begin with pneumonia, but primary bacteremias without definable source and sinusitis are more common.[7,50,61,66,113] Despite the high rates of pneumococcal pneumonia and the striking predisposition to invasive infection among HIV-1–infected patients, the clinical manifestations of S. pneumoniae infections are similar to those in age-matched seronegative patients.[57,89,150] HIV-1–infected patients with community-acquired pneumonia usually present with typical symptoms of fever, shortness of breath, cough, and sputum, often in association with pleuritic chest pain.[57,60,89,91,96,150] Most patients respond quickly to antimicrobial agents; failure to improve over 48–72 h of therapy suggests the presence of a second coinfection, for example, P. carinii, empyema or abscess. Chest radiographs may show uni- or multilobar infiltrates, with or without effusion, and peripheral leukocyte counts are most often elevated.

A striking characteristic of pneumococcal disease during HIV-1 infection is the high rate of recurrence. Recurrences, defined as a second episode of pneumococcal disease within 6 months of the initial episode, follow 10–25% of adult cases[53,60,89,150] compared with 0–8% of episodes in seronegative adults. Indeed, the presence of recurrent bacterial infections is now sufficient criteria to establish a diagnosis of AIDS. Recurrent pneumococcal disease is particularly common among HIV-1–infected children; up to six episodes have been reported in a single child.[61] That recurrent infections may be due to the same or different serotypes suggests that a subset of HIV-1–infected patients are at particular risk for these infections.

Mortality with invasive pneumococcal infections

The development of an acute, rapidly invasive systemic bacterial infection in an immunocompromised host prompts concern about the potential for high rates of mortality. Mortality with overwhelming postsplenectomy sepsis, a syndrome most often caused by S. pneumoniae, approaches 40% in young adults, and HIV-1–infected patients often show splenic dysfunction. Nevertheless, most studies support the concept that death from HIV-1–associated pneumococcal bacteremia is no more common than that among age-matched seronegative bacteremic patients (Tables 3 and 4). Differences in mortality ascribed to coinfection with HIV-1 have been more likely related to differences in rates of bacteremia, age, and pneumococcal syndrome among patient groups studied.[47,57,150,168]

Therefore, despite the high incidence of infection, careful matching of patients by age and clinical syndrome revealed that mortality was appreciable but similar among HIV-1–infected and control subjects with bacteremia and meningitis.[53,79,89,90,145] Of note, the absence of deaths in 42 seropositive patients with pneumococcal disease in Nairobi under study conditions[66] highlights the value of rapid diagnosis and treatment of these serious infections. Efforts to prevent these infections depend on our understanding the risk factors involved in causing them.

Risk factors for pneumococcal disease during HIV-1 infection

The accumulated epidemiological and clinical evidence suggests that the predominant predisposing risk factor for invasive pneumococcal disease in this population is not behavioral, medical, environmental, or bacteriologic, but rather HIV-1–associated immunodeficiency.[91,150] The seasonal incidence of disease (peaking in November to April), frequency and severity of preceding viral infections, and rates of smoking and alcohol use all appear to be similar or lower in HIV-1–infected patients compared with control subjects with pneumococcal disease.[79,96,101,173] Underlying medical illness, including asplenia, are no more common in bacteremic patients with HIV-1 disease; rather, liver disease, chronic lung disease, and other forms of immunosuppression may be identified more frequently in seronegative patients with pneumococcal bacteremia.[57,101,150,168]

Intravenous drug use is a consistent risk factor for increased rates of bacterial pneumonia, but this predilection is independent of HIV-1 infection.[20,80,172,173] Although high rates of pharyngeal colonization may be associated with an increased inci-

TABLE 3. MORTALITY WITH INVASIVE PNEUMOCOCCAL DISEASE DURING HIV-1 INFECTION IN ADULTS

Reference	Location (years)	Group	Syndrome	HIV-1 status	Mortality/ no. studied	(%)	Comments
60	San Francisco	Adults	Bacteremia	+	3/29	(8)	
168	New Jersey (1986)	Adults	Bacteremia	+	1/17	(6)	
				−	NR	(11)	
150	San Francisco (1983–87)	Adults	Bacteremia	+	6/75	(8)	Seronegative patients older than HIV-1+
				−	39/219	(18)	
79	Denver (1985–94)	Adults (15–44 years)	Bacteremia	+	3/40	(8)	
				−	4/74	(5)	
65	Nairobi (1988–89)	Adults	Bacteremia	+	2/7	(29)	
				−	3/7	(43)	
66	Nairobi (1989–92)	Adults	Bacteremia	+	0/42		Ready access to care provided in study
145	New York City (1989–90)	Adults	Bacteremia, pneumonia	+	8/26	(31)	8/14 (57%) AIDS patients and 0/12 non-AIDS HIV-1+ died
				−	6/24	(25)	
57	Madrid (1988–90)	Adults	Pneumonia	+	1/21	(5)	Seronegative patients older than HIV-1+
				−	10/54	(19)	
47	Barcelona (1988–90)	Adults	Pneumonia	+	4/21	(19)	Bacteremia in 71% HIV-1+ and 41% of seronegative patients
				−	3/69	(4)	
94	10 cities, U.S. (1986–91)	Adults (16–55 years)	Meningitis	+	8/22	(36)	
				−	19/81	(24)	
53	New Haven, CT (1992–93)	Adults	Bacteremia, meningitis	+	3/25	(12)	
				−	11/81	(14)	
101	Johannesburg (1996)	Adults	Bacteremia	+	7/58	(12)	Seronegative patients older than HIV-1+
				−	15/71	(21)	
3	Barcelona (1985–97)	Adults	Meningitis	+	1/9	(11)	
				−	18/81	(22)	

NR, not reported.

dence of pneumococcal disease,[81,134] rates of colonization in the United States and Spain are quite comparable in HIV-1–infected patients and seronegative subjects without clinical signs of pneumococcal infection (9–14% versus 9–10%, respectively).[48,96,157] In East Africa, however, rates of colonization may be increased among seropositive patients (C.F. Gilks, personal communication). Although limited data are available characterizing the virulence factors in pneumococcal strains isolated from HIV-1–infected patients, the distribution of capsular serotypes identified in these patients (more than 85% in the 23-valent vaccine) shows no appreciable differences from that in control patients.[66,89,150] In the absence of other identifiable risk factors, the presence of immunologic compromise most plausibly underlies the high rates of pneumococcal disease during HIV-1 infection.

Immune status of HIV-1–infected patients with S. pneumoniae

Pneumococcal infections occur at all stages of HIV-1 infection. Studies from Kenya suggest that pneumococcal infections occur at CD4+ T cell counts in the range of 300 cells/μL, before most patients have shown clinical manifestations of AIDS.[64,67,178] In San Francisco, half of the HIV-1–infected patients with invasive pneumococcal disease had CD4+ T cell counts above 200 cells/μL (Fig. 1), and in New Haven, 23 such patients showed mean counts of 185 cells/μL (range 0–700).[53] Among 16 patients reported from Denver, eight of nine tested showed counts below 200 cells/μL,[92] and of all 16 patients, eight had a previous diagnosis of AIDS, four had AIDS-related complex, and four were asymptomatic.[96] Several studies suggest an association between invasive pneumococcal disease, particularly bacteremia, and advanced HIV-1 disease and AIDS. In New Jersey, the diagnosis of AIDS was temporally correlated with an increased risk of preceding pneumococcal bacteremia (Fig. 2).[168] In New York, major clinical events among drug users, for example, development of bacterial pneumonia and sepsis, independently predicted HIV-1 disease progression.[172] However, that these infections occurred at several levels of CD4+ T cell counts from <200/μL[96] to 300–400 μL,[136,172] suggested that many patients were not at a very advanced stage of HIV-1 disease at the onset of bacterial infection. Thus, pneumococcal infections may affect patients with HIV-1 at all clinical stages of the disease, although the rates appear to be highest later in the course. However, numbers of CD4+ T cells are at best only markers of immune status. More relevant are the specific mechanisms of host defense against S. pneumoniae.

TABLE 4. MORTALITY WITH INVASIVE PNEUMOCOCCAL DISEASE DURING HIV-1 INFECTION IN CHILDREN

Reference	Location (years)	Group	Syndrome	HIV-1 status	Mortality/ no. studied	(%)	Comments
94	10 cities, U.S. (1986–91)	Children	Meningitis	+	2/15	(15)	
				–	5/90	(6)	
53	New Haven, CT (1992–93)	Children	Bacteremia, meningitis	+	1/8	(13)	
				–	4/33	(12)	
8	New York City (1982–89)	Children <5 years old	Bacteremia	+	0/5		
165	Madrid (1984–94)	Children	Bacteremia	+	0/9		3/9 recurrences
61	New York City (1978–93)	Children	Bacteremia, meningitis	+	2/31	(6)	31 episodes in 19 children; 4/19 with 2–6 recurrences
113	New York City (1983–87)	Children	Bacteremia	+	0/11		
101	Johannesburg (1996)	Children	Bacteremia	+	2/25	(8)	
				–	1/24	(4)	

Mucosal defense

Because *S. pneumoniae* is a mucosal pathogen which typically colonizes the nasopharynx asymptomatically, mucosal immune defects may contribute to the high rates of pneumonia and associated bacteremia caused by this pathogen.[89] Secretory IgA, the predominant antibody at mucosal surfaces, comprises two subclasses (IgA1 and IgA2) which may prevent the adherence of pathogenic organisms and neutralize their toxins.[35,106] Functional activity of IgA1 against *S. pneumoniae* may be compromised by pneumococcal IgA1 protease, an enzyme which cleaves the functional constant portion (Fc) from the antigen-binding variable fragment (F[ab]′2) of IgA1.[106] However, levels and proportions of the protease-resistant subclass, IgA2, in upper respiratory secretions (saliva), were similar among patients with and without HIV-1 and with and without pneumococcal bacteremia. Moreover, levels of innate or nonspecific factors (lactoferrin, lysozyme, and lactoperoxidase), each of which may also contribute to mucosal defense against *S. pneumoniae*, were also comparable in these groups.[140] Finally, serotype-specific capsular salivary IgA has been detected in only a minority of bacteremic patients, independent of HIV-1 infection. Thus, neither selective mucosal IgA2 deficiency nor impaired nonspecific upper respiratory mucosal responses were associated with invasive pneumococcal disease during HIV-1 infection. Therefore, other defects in mucosal cellular responses or systemic immunity may predispose HIV-1–infected patients to invasive pneumococcal disease.

Natural humoral immunity to *S. pneumoniae*

Adequate host defense against *S. pneumoniae* is in large part dependent upon the presence of natural antibodies reactive with the polysaccharide capsule.[10,24,68] Natural antibodies are those found in sera of healthy persons in the absence of overt previous infection or immunization. They may result from asymptomatic colonization,[133] exposure to cross-reactive antigens, or the presence of polyreactive low-affinity antibodies.[28] Capsule-specific antibodies are critical in defense against *S. pneumoniae* as they mediate opsonization, efficient complement activation, and killing of the organism by phagocytic cells.[68] Several studies suggest that baseline levels of IgG to pneumococcal polysaccharides are significantly lower in both asymptomatic HIV-1–infected patients and AIDS patients compared with those in seronegative homosexual and heterosexual subjects (Fig. 3).[6,93,94] Other reports demonstrated similar levels by ELISA in asymptomatic HIV-1–infected patients and seronegative subjects.[27,193]

Among HIV-1–infected patients with acute pneumococcal bacteremia, levels of capsule-specific IgG are significantly lower than those in healthy seronegative control subjects.[91] Moreover, these levels were also lower than those in control

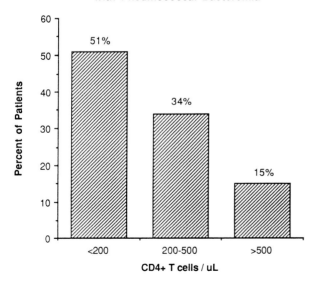

CD4+ T Cells in 41 HIV-Infected Patients with Pneumococcal Bacteremia

FIG. 1. Distribution of CD4$^+$ T cell counts in 41 HIV-1-infected patients with pneumococcal bacteremia at San Francisco General Hospital, 1991–92.[140]

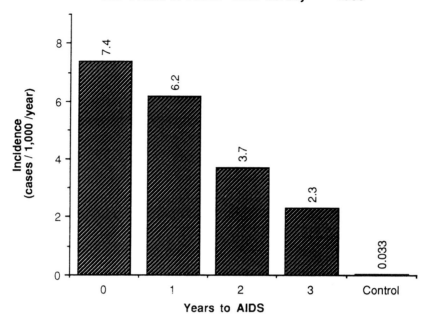

FIG. 2. Incidence of pneumococcal bacteremia based on the interval between the occurence of the bacteremic episode and the subsequent diagnosis of advanced HIV-1 disease (AIDS). Rates are compared with those in age-matched HIV-1-seronegative control subjects. Adapted with permission from Schuchat et al.[168]

subjects in otherwise asymptomatic HIV-1–infected subjects for three of four serotypes that commonly cause disease in HIV-1–infected patients (serotypes 4, 8, and 12F but not 14).[91,96,150] These results in U.S. patients were confirmed in East Africa.

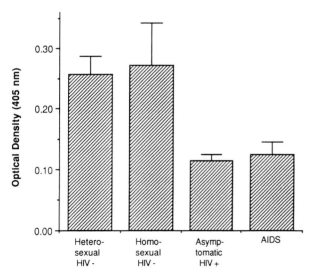

FIG. 3. Baseline pre-immunization levels of IgG to pneumococcal polysaccharides (23-valent vaccine) by ELISA in 53 HIV-1-seronegative adults (28 heterosexual and 25 homosexual), 27 asymptomatic HIV-1-infected men, and 21 patients with AIDS. Adapted with permission from Janoff et al.[93]

In Africa, baseline levels of capsule-specific IgG were decreased for two of four common serotypes (14 and 19F) among HIV-1–infected women compared with HIV-1–seronegative women ($p < 0.05$),[94] but similar in Ugandan adults with and without HIV-1 infection.[55]

Although the majority of IgG in serum is of the IgG$_1$ subclass, an appreciable proportion of pneumococcal capsule-specific IgG is of the IgG$_2$ subclass,[32,177] and IgG$_2$ levels may be decreased during HIV-1 infection.[129,152] Indeed, baseline levels of IgG$_2$ to two serotypes tested (types 8 and 14) were lower among asymptomatic HIV-1–infected patients in the United States,[27] and preliminary data indicate that both the levels and proportions of total IgG$_2$ in serum are decreased in HIV-1–infected patients with acute bacteremia (E.N. Janoff and R. Hamilton, unpublished data). However, more important than the levels or structure of antibodies to *S. pneumoniae* is their ability to mediate clearance of the organism.

Functional activity of S. pneumoniae–*specific antibodies*

Levels of capsule-specific antibodies are directly related to the functional ability of serum to support phagocytic killing of the organism.[68,89] In sera from HIV-1–infected men with pneumococcal bacteremia, the ability of their sera to kill the organism in the presence of exogenous complement and PMNs from healthy donors was lower in four of six acute sera compared with that of baseline sera from seven HIV-1–seronegative healthy subjects.[96] Moreover, despite rises in bactericidal activity after infection, the killing activity of convalescent sera was still below that of sera from unvaccinated seronegative subjects.

Consistent with these results, killing of type 14 *S. pneumoniae* by serum in the presence of complement and phagocytic cells was significantly lower among HIV-1–infected women in Kenya than with sera from seronegative subjects. In addition, serum killing titers were proportional to the amount of capsule-specific antibody present by ELISA.[94] Thus, for selected serotypes, levels of functionally active antibody to the pneumococcal capsule, a critical virulence factor, may be decreased in association with high rates of invasive disease during HIV-1 infection. That levels are not low in all patients to all serotypes may explain why only certain patients become infected. Alternatively, antibody avidity, a measure of the strength of antibody-antigen binding and, often, functional activity, may be decreased during HIV-1 infections. Finally, impairment of other mechanisms of defense may participate, such as antibodies to pneumococcal toxins.

Inhibition of pneumolysin

Studies have examined whether the decreased protective function of serum antibodies to *S. pneumoniae* in HIV-1–infected patients extend to their ability to protect against the effects of pneumococcal toxins. Pneumolysin, the major cytotoxin produced by *S. pneumoniae*,[25] damages both pulmonary endothelial cells[164] and epithelial cells[42] *in vitro*. Pneumolysin may act at several sites to promote the course of infection, inducing both tissue injury, invasion, and impairment of host defense.[25,140,162,163] Moreover, pneumolysin may inhibit both proliferation and antibody production by human lymphocytes, while cell viability remains intact. To determine whether the predisposition of HIV-1–infected patients to invasive pneumococcal infection may be related, in part, to an impaired natural immunity to pneumolysin, serum antipneumolysin antibodies were measured in two separate populations of HIV-1–infected and seronegative controls. Both by ELISA and by a functional assay in which antibody inhibited pneumolysin-induced hemolysis and cytotoxicity, HIV-1–infected patients in the United States had significantly lower titers of antipneumolysin antibodies than did seronegative control subjects (Fig. 4).[5] Similarly, HIV-1–infected patients in Kenya who later developed pneumococcal bacteremia also had significantly lower levels of antipneumolysin antibody levels at baseline compared with those in seronegative control subjects. Thus, lower levels of antibodies to pneumolysin, a toxin that promotes tissue invasion, were associated with the higher incidence of bacteremic pneumococcal infections among HIV-1–infected patients.

Complement and phagocytes

Although humoral defects are prominent, the immunologic predisposition to invasive pneumococcal disease during HIV-1 infection also may involve defects in complement and PMN function. Because gram-positive bacteria resist the direct bactericidal activity of the terminal membrane attack complex (C5–C9), the early complement components, particularly C3, figure prominently in control of pneumococcal disease.[161] In patients with HIV-1 infection, complement activity (CH_{50}, C3, C4) may be normal or low,[14,184] and products of abnormal complement activation, which may inhibit clearance of opsonized particles, are increased.[147] Nevertheless, pneumococcal infections have not been ascribed specifically to complement-related defects in HIV-1–infected patients.

Similarly, PMN-mediated, antibody-dependent cellular cytotoxicity may be normal[174] or depressed[132] and chemotaxis may be impaired[44] in HIV-1–infected patients. Recently, an expressed polymorphism in the gene for the phagocyte IgG receptor FcγRIIa (CD32) has been characterized. Although the alleles code for receptors with high, intermediate, or low affinity for IgG_2, to date no association has been found between FcγRIIa allotype and pneumococcal disease during HIV-1 infection.[1,155,191] Nevertheless, PMN dysfunction and other defects in phagocyte function, such as delayed and decreased clearance of opsonized particles by macrophages in the liver and spleen,[14,15,68] may contribute to the high rates of pneumococcal infection in these patients. The defects may not be severe enough to increase the mortality associated with HIV-1–related pneumococcal disease, and other host factors may also contribute to the outcome of this infection.

Inflammatory response to S. pneumoniae infection in HIV-1–infected patients

Mortality related to invasive pneumococcal disease occurs very early in the course of infection (80% of deaths occur within 5–7 days of admission),[10] and mortality has been associated with the acute inflammatory response to pneumococcal infection.[69,187] As discussed previously, despite a high incidence of pneumococcal infection and a high rate of invasive disease in these patients, mortality is similar among HIV-1–infected and seronegative patients. Consistent with this hypothesis, the acute clinical inflammatory responses in patients with and without HIV-1 disease who had pneumococcal disease appear to be quite similar. In adults with bacteremia, the days of symptoms, the presence and height of fever, and the manifestations of pneu-

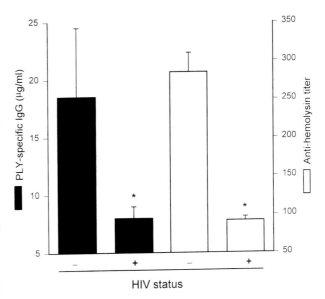

FIG. 4. Levels of IgG to pneumolysin, the major pneumococcal toxin, in sera from HIV-1-infected (+) and seronegative (−) adults without known prior pneumococcal disease by ELISA (black bars) and by functional assay for neutralization of the hemolytic/cytotoxic activity of pneumolysin (white bars). Results are shown as mean ± SD. *p < 0.05 compared with values in HIV-1-seronegative adults. Adapted with permission from Amdahl et al.[5]

monia by history, examination, and chest x-ray were comparable in the two groups.[92] In addition, among age-matched patients with meningitis, the mean duration of symptoms, the proportion with and magnitude of fever, meningismus, coma, all reflecting the clinical inflammatory response, were comparable in those with and without known HIV-1 infection.[90] Similarly, although laboratory results showed greater signs of inflammation in adults (higher protein and lower glucose in association with greater mortality) than in children, mortality were similar in age-matched HIV-1–infected and control patients.

Among asymptomatic control subjects, levels of C-reactive protein (CRP), a prototypic hepatic acute phase reactant, were normal in sera and commensurate in those with and without HIV-1 infection.[92] Among bacteremic patients, levels were well over 25 times higher in acute sera, independent of HIV-1 status. These data suggest that, although immunologic defects may predispose patients with HIV-1 disease to a high incidence of pneumococcal disease, they can generate a vigorous acute inflammatory response to acute bacterial infection, independent of immunologic status. These non-immune responses may be important in the initial defense to contain invasive pathogens and result in the relatively normal mortality observed with invasive pneumococcal infections during HIV-1 disease. Although mortality is "normal" in patients coinfected with HIV-1 and *S. pneumoniae*, death rates are still high (approximately 10% in adults) and, much too high, for a disease that can be prevented.

Prevention of invasive pneumococcal disease during HIV-1 infection

When a disease is so prevalent and serious, prevention is the most cost-effective strategy. Limiting exposure requires substantial changes in population density, socioeconomic status, and behavior, for example, smoking. In the absence of such changes, prevention is particularly important where rates are highest, resources are few, and access to care may be limited, as in Africa. Several prophylactic approaches have been considered and, to a limited extent, analyzed.

Chemoprophylaxis. Chronic daily use of penicillin has been very effective in preventing invasive pneumococcal disease in children with sickle-cell disease,[59,197,199] is often recommended for asplenic patients, particularly following an initial episode of pneumococcal disease. The effectiveness of chronic antimicrobial agents (particularly trimethoprim-sulfamethoxazole [TMP-SMX]) in HIV-1–infected patients has been evaluated in several epidemiologic studies. Use of TMP-SMX has also been associated with lower rates of bacteremia and bacterial pneumonia, including those due to *S. pneumoniae*, in studies in related areas of HIV-1 disease.[43,77] Moreover, only a minority of HIV-1–infected patients are taking TMP-SMX at the time of pneumococcal infection.[53,96,130] In a prospective observational cohort study in San Francisco, use of TMP-SMX, typically taken three times weekly, was associated with a 32–67% reduction in rates of bacterial pneumonia in HIV-1–infected adults with fewer than 200 CD4$^+$ T cells/μL.[80] However, in Spain, six of 12 episodes of pneumococcal meningitis occurred in patients of active TMP-SMX prophylaxis.[3] Randomized, double-blind, placebo-controlled intervention studies with prophylactic antimicrobial agents have not been done.

In addition to considerations of the efficacy of prophylaxis among HIV-1–infected patients, issues of cost, compliance, and complications emerge. The cost of penicillin and TMP-SMX is low, but relatively less so in Africa. Compliance is likely variable. Complications of drug-reactions, especially with TMP-SMX, are an issue, as is emergence of resistance. In some areas, multidrug resistance is common among *S. pneumoniae* isolates identified from patients with HIV-1 infection, particularly those with low CD4$^+$ T cell numbers (Table 5).[53,157] Antimicrobial prophylaxis used specifically to prevent *S. pneumoniae* infections is likely best employed for HIV-1–infected patients, particularly children, who are asplenic, have had one or more prior pneumococcal infections, and have low numbers of leukocytes or CD4$^+$ T cells.

Intravenous immunoglobulins. Replacement of low levels of *S. pneumoniae*–specific antibodies, particularly those to the polysaccharide capsule, seems a logical prophylactic strategy for HIV-1–infected patients. Such antibodies are routinely present in commercial immunoglobulin preparation and replacement has successfully decreased infections with encapsulated pathogens in hypogammaglobulinemic patients.[33,86] The first randomized placebo-controlled trial of intravenous immunoglobulin showed a significant decrease in the rate of serious bacterial infections, including *S. pneumoniae*, in symptomatic HIV-1–infected children with low CD4$^+$ T cell counts.[186] Complications of this therapy were few. Subsequent studies confirmed and extended these promising results,[127,180] but one subgroup analysis suggested that concomitant use of TMP-SMX in children receiving immunoglobulin was associated with an increase in streptococcal infections.[180] However, this latter study was not designed to test the potential interaction between immunoglobulin and TMP-SMX, and other results have not noted such increased rates with combined prophylactic regimens.[127,128] It should also be noted that the effects of immunoglobulin on survival have been minimal, despite the decreased and delayed incidence of bacterial infections. In the absence of data from a randomized, controlled trial in adults, children with HIV-1 disease, rather than adults, particularly after an initial pneumococcal infection,[198] appear to be the most appropriate beneficiaries of such treatment, as long as safety is assured.

Immunization. No proposed prophylactic approach is as safe and inexpensive as immunization. The currently available 23-valent vaccine contains the capsular polysaccharides from serotypes associated with more than 90% of cases of invasive pneumococcal disease in HIV-1–infected and seronegative adults in the United States.[53,78,89] The ability to generate antibody responses to pneumococcal vaccine polysaccharides was of both theoretical and clinical significance because these capsular polysaccharides are considered T cell-independent antigens,[12,105] and because of the clinical frequency of *S. pneumoniae* in patients with HIV-1 infection.[146,150,179] Antibodies of the IgM class are prominent in responses to T-independent antigens,[74] and capsule-specific antibodies, particularly IgM, activate complement binding and opsonize the organisms to facilitate killing by phagocytic cells.[68,89,100,176] Following immunization, significantly impaired responses to pneumococcal polysaccharides, including specific IgM, have been reported both in patients with AIDS and in asymptomatic HIV-infected men compared with those in control subjects.[6,97] Impairment of

TABLE 5. PENICILLIN-RESISTANT *S. pneumoniae* IN PERSONS WITH HIV-1 INFECTION

Reference	Location (years)	Group	Source	HIV status	PCN-resistant/ no. tested	(%)	Comments
79	Denver (1985–94)	Adults	Blood	+	2/47	(4)	Resistance predom-
				−	3/144	(2)	inantly serogroups 14 and 6
142	Nairobi (1992)	Adults	Pneumonia (sterile sites)	+	12/45	(27)	50% of resistant
				−	3/42	(7)	isolates = serotype 1
126	Paris (1992–94)	Adults	Respiratory	+	14/45	(31)	8/10 resistant isolates = serogroup 23
96	Denver (1989–90)	Adults	Colonization	+	0/8		
				−	0/9		
53	New Haven, CT (1992–93)	Adults	Blood; CSF	+	0/25		5/10 resistant isolates = serogroup 9v
				−	7/81	(9)	
		Children		+	1/8	(13)	
				−	2/33	(6)	
61	New York City (1978–93)	Children	Blood; CSF	+	0/26		
3	Barcelona (1985–97)	Adults	CSF	+	5/9	(56)	4 intermediate and 1 high-level resistance
101	Johannesburg (1996)	Adults	Blood	+	15/57	(26)	7/173 isolates (4%)
				−	3/69	(4)	high-level resistance
		Children		+	9/24	(38)	
				−	7/23	(30)	

IgM responses *in vivo* following immunization with pneumococcal vaccine was confirmed in HIV-1–infected patients with varied CD4+ T cell counts compared with those in 18 healthy seronegative control subjects.[27] Although the numbers of vaccine-specific IgG and IgA antibody-secreting B cells (ASC) in blood 1 week after immunization were not significantly different among the groups (Fig. 5a), specific IgM ASC were pro-foundly and consistently depressed in all HIV-1–infected patients, independent of T cell number (Fig. 5b).

Thus, humoral immune defects among HIV-1–infected patients include a consistently impaired ability to produce IgM to pneumococcal polysaccharides,[93,97] which occurs early in the course of HIV-1 infection.[88,185] Ultimately, however, primary IgM responses should switch to IgG responses, which comprise

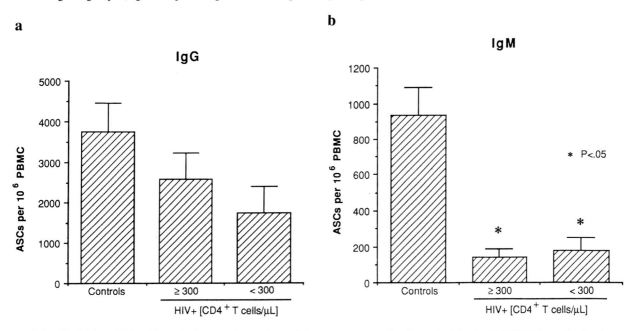

FIG. 5. IgG (**a**) and IgM (**b**) antibody-secreting cells (ASC) to pneumococcal polysaccharides by ELISPOT 1 week after immunization with 23-valent pneumococcal capsular polysaccharide vaccine in 18 healthy HIV-1-seronegative control subjects and 18 HIV-1-infected patients (10 with ≥300 CD4+ T cells/μL [mean ± SD, 519 ± 68] and 8 with <300 CD4+ T cells/μL [mean ± SD, 166 ± 40]). Results are shown as mean ± SEM of ASC/10^6 peripheral blood mononuclear cells (PBMC). *p < 0.01. Adapted with permission from Carson et al.[27]

Table 6. IgG Responses to Immunization With Pneumococcal Capsular Polysaccharides in Persons with HIV-1 Infection[a]

Reference	Assay	Serotypes tested	Group	HIV-1	No.	Specific IgG levels[b]		Comments
						Baseline	Postvaccine	
6	RIA	12 individually	AIDS	+	18	Lower (5 of 6)	Lower (5 of 6)	
			Controls	−	20			
84	ELISA	12 individually	Non-AIDS	+	35	Similar	Similar	
			Controls	−	39			
93	ELISA	23 together (vaccine)	AIDS	+	21	Lower	Lower	
			Asymptomatic	+	21	Lower	Lower	
			Controls	−	53			
109	RIA	12 individually	IVDU/partners	+	21	Variable	Lower (9 of 12)	
			IVDU/partners	−	23			
139	Nitrocellulose binding	23 together (vaccine)	Symptomatic	+	10	Higher	Lower	
			Control pool	−				
156	ELISA[c]	3, 4, 6A, 8, 23	CD4 ≤500	+	39	ND	Lower (5 of 5)	
			CD4 >500	+	12	ND	Lower (2 of 5)	
			Controls	−	25			
114	ELISA	23 together (vaccine)	Infected	+	51	Similar	Similar	
			Controls	−	10			
193	ELISA[c]	4, 6B, 12F, 14	Recent seroconverters	+	20	Similar	Similar (3 of 4)	
			Controls	−	15			
27	ELISA[c]	23 together; 8, 14	Infected	+	18	Similar	Lower or similar	
189	ELISA[c]	23 together (vaccine)	Controls	−	18			
			Infected	+	98			>4 fold rise in 83%; no differences by stage or CD4 count
124	ELISA[c]	23 together (vaccine)	Non-AIDS	+	35	Lower ≥200 CD4 Similar <200 CD4		
			Controls	−	12			

Reference	Assay	Serotypes	Subjects	HIV-1	No.			
2	ELISA[c]	6B, 14, 18c, 19F, 23F	*Conjugate* Infected	+	92	Similar[d]	Lower (5 of 5)	Conjugate more immunogenic among controls (3 of 5 types)
			Controls	−	48			
			Polysaccharide Infected	+	86	Similar[d]	Lower <500 CD4 (4 of 5)	
			Controls	−	48			
22	ELISA[c]	23 together (vaccine)	Asymptomatic	+	12	Similar	Lower	
			Control	−	18			
94	ELISA[c]	1, 6B, 14, 19F	African women	+	33	Similar	Lower (2 of 4)	
			Prior pneumococcal disease	+	21	Lower (2 of 4)	Lower (3 of 4)	
			Controls	−				
55	ELISA[c]	1, 6B, 14, 19F	Ugandan adults	+	15	Similar	Lower (3 of 4)	

[a]Although postvaccination levels were often lower among groups of HIV-1–infected patients compared with those in matched seronegative control subjects, both groups showed a significant rise in type-specific antibody after vaccination compared with baseline levels for most serotypes tested.
[b]"Similar," "variable," and "lower" refer to comparison with values in HIV-1–seronegative control subjects at the same time. Numbers in parentheses refer to numbers of serotypes.
[c]Sera preadsorbed with pneumococcal cell-wall polysaccharide.
[d]Preimmunization levels were lower for two of five serotypes (18C and 19F) among patients with <200 CD4+ T cells/μL.
ND, not done.

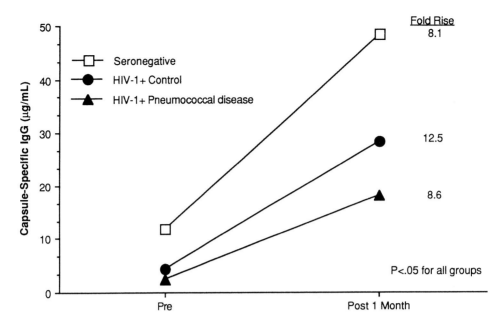

FIG. 6. Mean *S. pneumoniae* type 14 capsule-specific IgG in serum prior to and one month after immunization of 15 HIV-1-seronegative women, and HIV-1-infected women who did (*n* = 21) and did not (HIV-1 + controls; *n* = 33) previously develop pneumococcal disease, Nairobi, Kenya. Adapted with permission from Janoff et al.[94]

the majority of polysaccharide-specific antibodies in blood. Most studies in the United States and Europe show that HIV-1-infected adults do indeed show a significant IgG response to pneumococcal capsular polysaccharides in the vaccine following immunization (Table 6). Despite these responses, the magnitude of these responses to many individual capsular serotypes is most often lower than that among seronegative subjects.

These results in the United States and Europe are similar to those in East Africa. In Nairobi, Kenya, where serotype 1 commonly causes invasive pneumococcal disease,[66] immunized commercial sex workers (15 HIV-1-seronegative, 33 HIV-1-infected controls, and 21 HIV-1-infected women who had recovered from invasive pneumococcal disease) all showed significant increases in levels of capsule-specific IgG in serum in all serotypes tested one month after immunization (*p* < 0.05; Fig. 6).[94] These levels were greater in HIV-1-negative compared with both HIV-1-infected groups for three or four serotypes (1, 6B, and 14) (*p* < 0.05). Despite significant differences in CD4+ T cell counts between HIV-1-infected controls and previously bacteremic patients (330 ± 37 versus 189 ± 37 cells/mL; *p* < 0.05), levels of specific IgG were similar both prior to and following immunization for each serotype. Therefore, as in the United States, HIV-1 infection in Kenyan women is associated with decreased levels of natural antibody to selected pneumococcal capsular serotypes, but the development of invasive pneumococcal disease prior to immunization does not predict a generalized inability to respond to the common local capsular polysaccharides that is independent of HIV-1 infection. Despite the ability to respond, levels of capsule-specific antibodies are not optimal in Kenya, Uganda,[55] or more developed nations among HIV-1-infected patients, who often have other immunologic defects which may limit their ability to prevent or control pneumococcal infections.

Strategies to enhance the effects of pneumococcal vaccine in the HIV-1-infected patients have included the use of protein-polysaccharide conjugate vaccines. Antibody responses to recall antigens, such as tetanus and diphtheria toxoids, which are used as protein conjugates and to which patients were exposed prior to HIV-1 infection, may be relatively spared in these patients.[95] Although humoral responses to *H. influenzae* capsular polysaccharide antigen could be enhanced by linkage to recall protein antigens,[98,182] a conjugate pneumococcal vaccine was no more immunogenic than unconjugated capsular polysaccharides among HIV-1-infected adults.[2] Conjugate vaccines do hold promise for inducing protective immunity in children with HIV-1 disease, who experience the highest rates of invasive disease but poor responses to the current vaccine.[9,62]

For adults, other options for eliciting adequate capsule-specific immunity with vaccine include immunizing early in the course of HIV-1 infection. Indeed, recent seroconverters immunized within one year of primary HIV-1 infection showed specific antibody levels comparable to those of seronegative control subjects for most serotypes tested.[193] Reversing immunosuppression with anti-retroviral therapy may also promote maximal response. In this regard, the modestly increased titers of capsule-specific IgG measured in patients upon initiation of zidovudine therapy compared with untreated patients[70] may be further amplified with more effective anti-retroviral therapy currently available. Finally, elucidating the mechanisms of impaired B cell function and trials with alternative conjugate vaccines may help bolster responses to prevent the morbidity and mortality associated with *S. pneumoniae* infections.

For a vaccine to be truly effective, its use must be promoted and accepted by caregivers and patients. Currently, approximately 25–35% of HIV-1-infected patients in the United States receive pneumococcal vaccine and estimates suggest that its use is cost-effective.[159] However, the most important issue is whether the vaccine is effective in preventing pneumococcal disease. Preliminary results of a case-control study suggest a 40% efficacy in preventing pneumococcal pneumonia during HIV-1 infection,[190] a rate comparable to the efficacy of prevention of bacteremia in older adults ($\cong 60\%$).[175] A prospective, randomized, placebo-controlled efficacy trial is on-going in Uganda to determine the impact of pneumococcal vaccine on the incidence of *S. pneumoniae* infection in patients with HIV-1 disease, on rates of disease progression, and on overall mortality.

Therapy of HIV-1. Perhaps the most striking recent advance in the care of patients with HIV-1 has been the development and efficacy of highly active antiretroviral therapy (HAART). These multidrug regimens have dramatically lowered the rates of death and opportunistic infections in this group. Preliminary data suggest that rates of invasive bacterial infections may be reduced as well.[183] Unfortunately, this therapy has not reduced the cost of care. As a result, patients with limited access to care and to the tremendous financial resources required to initiate and sustain HAART, such as patients in developing countries, will not share this potential benefit.

CONCLUSION

Specific immune defects can be identified for particular groups at higher risk of invasive pneumococcal infection, whereas more generalized deficiencies in immune and nonimmune defenses underlie bacteremia in others. The most prominent identified defect underlying the dramatic susceptibility of HIV-1–infected persons to invasive pneumococcal disease is deficient systemic humoral responses to pneumococcal virulence factors, capsular polysaccharides, and pneumolysin. Prevention of invasive pneumococcal disease during HIV-1 infection, which has emerged as a major risk for pneumococcal bacteremia worldwide, will require improved vaccination strategies and consideration of alternative prophylactic approaches, including chemoprophylaxis and passive immunization, in selected patients.

ACKNOWLEDGMENTS

We thank Claudine Fasching, Charles F. Gilks, James O'Brien, Charles Daly, Paul Carson, and John M. Douglas, Jr., for providing much of the data presented, and Ann Emery for excellent secretarial assistance. This work was supported by NIH grants AI 39445, DE 42600, HL 96-008, and AI 34051, and the Veterans Affairs Research Service.

REFERENCES

1. **Abadi, J., Z. Zhong, J. Dobroszycki, and L.-A. Pirofski.** 1997. FcγRIIa polymorphism in human immunodeficiency virus–infected children with invasive pneumococcal disease. Pediatr. Res. **42:**259–262.

2. **Ahmed, F., M.C. Steinhoff, M.C. Rodriguez-Barradas, R.G. Hamilton, D.M. Musher, and K.E. Nelson.** 1996. Effect of human immunodeficiency virus type 1 infection on the antibody response to a glycoprotein conjugate pneumococcal vaccine: results from a randomized trial. J. Infect. Dis. **173:**83–90.

3. **Almirante, B., M. Saballs, E. Ribera, C. Pigrau, J. Gavalda, I. Gasser, and A. Pahissa.** 1998. Favorable prognosis of purulent meningitis in patients infected with human immunodeficiency virus. Clin. Infect. Dis. **27:**176–180.

4. **Ambrosino, D.M., G. Schiffman, E.C. Gotschlich, P.H. Schur, G.A. Rosenberg, G.G. DeLange, E. vanLoghem, and G.R. Siber.** 1985. Correlation between G2M(n) immunoglobulin allotype and human antibody response and susceptibility to polysaccharide encapsulated bacteria. J. Clin. Invest. **75:**1935–1942.

5. **Amdahl, B.D., J.B. Rubins, C.L. Daley, C.F. Gilks, P.C. Hopewell, and E.N. Janoff.** 1995. Impaired natural immunity to pneumolysin during human immunodeficiency virus infection in the United States and Africa. Am. J. Respir. Crit. Care Med. **152:**2000–2004.

6. **Amman, A.J., G. Schiffman, D. Abrams, P. Volberding, J. Ziegler, and M. Conant.** 1984. B-cell immunodeficiency in acquired immune deficiency syndrome. J.A.M.A. **251:**1447–1449.

7. **Andiman, W.A., J. Mezger, and E. Shapiro.** 1994. Invasive bacterial infections in children born to women infected with human immunodeficiency virus type 1. J. Pediatr. **124:**846–852.

8. **Arpadi, S., and S.B. Hauger.** 1992. Causes of fever and predictors of pneumococcal bacteremia in HIV-infected children. Pediatr. AIDS HIV **4:**187–192.

9. **Arpadi, S.M., S. Back, J. O'Brien, and E.N. Janoff.** 1994. Antibodies to pneumococcal capsular polysaccharides in HIV-infected children given polyvalent pneumococcal vaccine. J. Pediatr. **125:**77–79.

10. **Austrian, R., and J. Gold.** 1964. Pneumococcal bacteremia with especial reference to bacteremic pneumococcal pneumonia. Ann. Intern. Med. **60:**759–776.

11. **Avanzini, M.A., A.M. Carra, R. Maccario, M. Zecca, P. Pignatti, M. Marconi, P. Comoli, F. Bonetti, P. DeStefano, and F. Locatelli.** 1995. Antibody response to pneumococcal vaccine in children receiving bone marrow transplantation. J. Clin. Immunol. **15:**137–144.

12. **Baker, P.J., D.F. Amsbaugh, P.W. Stashak, G. Caldes, and B. Prescott.** 1981. Regulation of the antibody response to pneumococcal polysaccharide by thymus-derived cells. Rev. Infect. Dis. **3:**332–341.

13. **Barat, L.M., J.E. Gunn, K.A. Steger, C.J. Perkins, and D.E. Craven.** 1996. Causes of fever in patients infected with human immunodeficiency virus who were admitted to Boston City Hospital. Clin. Infect. Dis. **23:**320–328.

14. **Bender, B.S., J.F. Bohnsack, S.H. Sourlis, M.M. Frank, and T.C. Quinn.** 1987. Demonstration of defective C3-receptor–mediated clearance by the reticuloendothelial system in patients with acquired immunodeficiency syndrome. J. Clin. Invest. **79:**715–720.

15. **Bender, B.S., M.M. Frank, et al.** 1985. Defective reticuloendothelial system Fc-receptor function in patients with the acquired immunodeficiency syndrome. J. Infect. Dis. **152:**409–412.

16. **Bennett, N.M., J. Buffington, and F.M. La Force.** 1992. Pneumococcal bacteremia in Monroe County, New York. Am. J. Public Health **82:**1513–1516.

17. **Bernstein, L.J., B.Z. Krieger, B. Novick, M.J. Sicklick, and A. Rubinstein.** 1985. Bacterial infection in the acquired immunodeficiency syndrome of children. Pediatr. Infect. Dis. **4:**472–475.

18. **Bjornson, A.B., and J.S. Lobel.** 1987. Direct evidence that decreased serum opsonization of *Streptococcus pneumoniae* via the alternative complement pathway in sickle cell disease is related to antibody deficiency. J. Clin. Invest. **79:**388–398.

19. **Bjornson, A.B., J.S. Lobel, and K.S. Harr.** 1985. Relation between serum opsonic activity for *Streptococcus pneumoniae* and complement function in sickle cell disease. J. Infect. Dis. **152:**701–709.

20. **Boschini, A., C. Smacchia, M. Di Fine, A. Schiesari, P. Bal-larini, M. Arlotti, C. Gabrielli, G. Castellani, M. Genova, P. Pantani, A. Cozzi Lepri, and G. Rezza.** 1996. Community-ac-quired pneumonia in a cohort of former injection drug users with and without human immunodeficiency virus infection: incidence, etiologies, and clinical aspects. Clin. Infect. Dis. **23:**107–113.

21. **Breiman, R.F., J.S. Spika, V.J. Navarro, P.M. Darden, and C.P. Darby.** 1990. Pneumococcal bacteremia in Charleston County, South Carolina: a decade later. Arch. Intern. Med. **150:** 1401–1405.

22. **Brichacek, B., S. Swindells, E.N. Janoff, S. Pirrucello, and M. Stevenson.** 1996. Increased plasma HIV-1 burden following anti-genic challenge. J. Infect. Dis. **174:**1191–1199.

23. **Bruyn, G.A.W., J.W.M. van der Meer, J. Hermans, and W. Knoppert.** 1988. Pneumococcal bacteremia in adults over a 10-year period at University Hospital, Leiden. Rev. Infect. Dis. **10:**446–450.

24. **Bruyn, G.A.W., B.J.M. Zegers, and R. van Furth.** 1992. Mech-anisms of host defense against infection with *Streptococcus pneu-moniae.* Clin. Infect. Dis. **14:**251–262.

25. **Bulnois, G.J., J.C. Paton, T.J. Mitchell, and P.W. Andrew.** 1991. Structure and function of pneumolysin, the multifunctional thiol-activated toxin of *Streptococcus pneumoniae.* Mol. Micro-biol. **5:**2611–2616.

26. **Burman, L.Å., R. Norrby, and B. Trollfors.** 1985. Invasive pneumococcal infections: incidence, predisposing factors, and prognosis. Rev. Infect. Dis. **7:**133–142.

27. **Carson, P.J., R.L. Schut, M.L. Simpson, J. O'Brien, and E.N. Janoff.** 1995. Antibody class and subclass responses to pneumo-coccal polysaccharides following immunization of human im-munodeficiency virus-infected patients. J. Infect. Dis. **172:** 340–345.

28. **Casali, P., and A.L. Notkins.** 1989. CD5$^+$ lymphocytes and the human B cell repertoire. Immunol. Today **10:**364–368.

29. **Centers for Disease Control.** 1984. Update: Pneumococcal poly-saccharide vaccine usage—United States. Ann. Intern. Med. **101:**348–350.

30. **Cheson, B.D., H.S. Walker, M.E. Health, R. J. Gobel, and J. Janatova.** 1984. Defective binding of the third component of complement (C3) to *Streptococcus pneumoniae* in multiple myeloma. Blood **63:**949–957.

31. **Chou, M., A.E. Brown, A. Blevins, and D. Armstrong.** 1983. Severe pneumococcal infection in patients with neoplastic dis-ease. Cancer **51:**1546–1550.

32. **Chudwin, D.S., S.G. Artrip, and G. Schiffman.** 1987. Im-munoglobulin G class and subclass antibodies to pneumococcal capsular polysaccharides. Clin. Immunol. Immunopathol. **44:** 114–121.

33. **Cooperative Group for the Study of Immunoglobulin in Chronic Lymphocytic Leukemia.** 1988. Intravenous Im-munoglobulin for the prevention of infection in chronic lympho-cytic leukemia: a randomized, controlled trial. N. Engl. J. Med. **319:**902–907.

34. **Cortese, M.M., M. Wolff, J. Almeido-Hill, R. Reid, J. Ketcham, and M. Santosham.** 1992. High incidence rates of invasive pneumococcal disease in the White Mountain Apache population. Arch. Intern. Med. **152:**2277–2282.

35. **Crago, S.S., W.H. Kutteh, I. Moror, M.R. Allansmith, J. Radl, J.J. Haaijman, and J. Mestecky.** 1984. Distribution of IgA1, IgA2, and J-chain containing cells in human tissues. J. Immunol. **132:**16–18.

36. **Dagan, R., D. Engelhard, and E. Piccard.** 1992. Epidemiology of invasive childhood pneumococcal infections in Israel: the Is-raeli Pediatric Bacteremia and Meningitis Group. J.A.M.A. **268:**3328–3332.

37. **Davidson, M., A.J. Parkinson, L.R. Bulkow, M.A. Fitzgerald, H.V. Peters, and D.J. Parks.** 1994. The epidemiology of inva-sive pneumococcal disease in Alaska, 1986–90: ethnic differences and opportunities for prevention. J. Infect. Dis. **170:**368–376.

38. **Davidson, M., C.D. Schraer, A.J. Parkinson, J.F. Campbell, R.R. Facklam, R.B. Wainwright, A.P. Lanier, and W.L. Hey-ward.** 1989. Invasive pneumococcal disease in an Alaska native population, 1980 through 1986. J.A.M.A. **261:**715–718.

39. **De Cock, K.M., E. Ekpini, E. Gnaore, A. Kadio, and H.D. Gayle.** 1994. The public health implications of AIDS research in Africa. J.A.M.A. **272:**481–486.

40. **Dempsey, P.W., M.E. Allison, S. Akkaraju, C.C. Goodnow, and D.T. Fearon.** 1996. C3d of complement as a molecular ad-juvant: bridging innate and acquired immunity. Science **271:**348–350.

41. **DiPadova, F., M. Durig, F. Harder, C. DiPadova, and C. Zanussi.** 1985. Impaired antipneumococcal antibody production in patients without spleens. B.M.J. **290:**14–16.

42. **Duane, P., J.R. Rubins, H. Weisel, and E.N. Janoff.** 1993. Iden-tification of hydrogen peroxide as a *Streptococcus pneumoniae* toxin for rat alveolar epithelial cells. Infect. Immunol. **61:**4392–4397.

43. **Edge, M.D., and D. Rimland.** 1996. Community-acquired bac-teremia in HIV-positive patients: protective benefit of co-trimox-azole. A.I.D.S. **10:**1635–1639.

44. **Ellis, M., S. Gupta, S. Galant, S. Hakim, C. VandeVen, C. Toy, and M.S. Cairo.** 1988. Impaired neutrophil function in patients with AIDS or AIDS-related complex: a comprehensive evalua-tion. J. Infect. Dis. **158:**1268–1276.

45. **Eskola, J., H. Käyhty, A.K. Takala, H. Peltola, P.-R. Rönnberg, E. Kela, E. Pekkanen, P.H. McVerry, and P.H. Mäkelä.** 1990. A randomized, prospective field trial of a conju-gate vaccine in the protection of infants and young children against invasive *Haemophilus influenzae* type b disease. N. Engl. J. Med. **323:**1381–1387.

46. **Eskola, J., A.K. Takala, E. Kela, E. Pekkanen, R. Kalliokoski, and M. Leinonen.** 1992. Epidemiology of invasive pneumococ-cal infections in children in Finland. J.A.M.A. **268:**3323–3327.

47. **Falcó, V., T. de Sevilla, J. Alegre, J. Barbé, A. Ferrer, I. Ocaña, E. Ribera, and J.M. Martínez-Vázquez.** 1994. Bacterial pneu-monia in HIV-infected patients: a prospective study of 68 episodes. Eur. Respir. J. **7:**235–239.

48. **Falguera, M., J. Perez-Mur, C. Galindo, and M. Garcia.** 1993. Prevalence and outcome of pneumococcal carrier human immu-nodeficiency virus-infected patients [Letter]. J. Infect. Dis. **168:**511.

49. **Falloon, J., J. Eddy, L. Wiener, and P.A. Pizzo.** 1989. Human immunodeficiency virus infection in children. J. Pediatr. **114:**1–30.

50. **Farley, J.J., J.C. King, Jr., P. Nair, S.E. Hines, R.L. Tressler, and P.E. Vink.** 1994. Invasive pneumococcal disease among in-fected and uninfected children of mothers with human immuno-deficiency virus infection. J. Pediatr. **124:**853–858.

51. **Feldman, S., W. Malone, R. Wilbur, and G. Schiffman.** 1985. Pneumococcal vaccination in children with acute lymphocytic leukemia. Med. Pediatr. Oncol. **13:**69–72.

52. **Figueroa, J.E., and P. Densen.** 1991. Infectious diseases asso-ciated with complement deficiencies. Clin. Microbiol. Rev. **4:**359–395.

53. **Frankel, R.E., M. Virata, C. Hardalo, F.L. Altice, and G. Friedland.** 1996. Invasive pneumococcal disease: clinical fea-tures, serotypes, and antimicrobial resistance patterns in cases in-volving patients with and without human immunodeficiency virus infection. Clin. Infect. Dis. **23:**577–584.

54. **Frederiksen, B., L. Specht, J. Henrichsen, F.K. Pedersen, and J. Pedersen-Bjergaard.** 1989. Antibody response to pneumo-coccal vaccine in patients with early stage Hodgkin's disease. Eur. J. Haematol. **43:**45–49.

55. **French, N., C.F. Gilks, A. Mujugira, C. Fasching, J. O'Brien, and E.N. Janoff.** 1998. Pneumococcal vaccination in HIV-1–in-

fected adults in Uganda: humoral response and two vaccine failures. A.I.D.S. **12**:1683–1689.

56. **Frezzato, M., G. Castaman, and F. Rodeghiero.** 1993. Fulminant sepsis in adults splenectomized for Hodgkin's disease. Haematologica **78**:73–77.

57. **García-Leoni, M.E., S. Moreno, P. Rodeñó, E. Cercenado, T. Vicente, and E. Bouza.** 1992. Pneumococcal pneumonia in adult hospitalized patients infected with the human immunodeficiency virus. Arch. Intern. Med. **152**:1808–1812.

58. **Garin, E.H., and D.J. Barrett.** 1988. Pneumococcal polysaccharide immunization in patients with active nephrotic syndrome. Nephron **50**:383–388.

59. **Gaston, M.H., J.I. Verter, G. Woods, C. Pegelow, J. Kelleher, G. Presbury, H. Zarkowsky, E. Vichinsky, R. Iyer, J.S. Lobel, S. Diamond, C.T. Holbrook, F.M. Gill, K. Ritchey, and J.M. Falletta.** 1986. Prophylaxis with oral penicillin in children with sickle cell anemia: a randomized trial. N. Engl. J. Med. **314**:1593–1599.

60. **Gerberding, J.L., J. Krieger, and M.A. Sande.** 1986. Recurrent bacteremia infection with *S. pneumoniae* in patients with AIDS virus [Abstract]. *In* Proceedings of the 26th Interscience Conference on Antimicrobial Agents and Chemotherapy, New Orleans.

61. **Gesner, M., D. Desiderio, M. Kim, A. Kaul, R. Lawrence, S. Chandwani, H. Pollack, M. Rigaud, K. Krasinski, and W. Borkowsky.** 1994. *Streptococcus pneumoniae* in human immunodeficiency virus type 1–infected children. Pediatr. Infect. Dis. J. **13**:697–703.

62. **Gibb, D., V. Spoülou, A. Giacomelli, H. Griffiths, J. Masters, S. Misbah, L. Nokes, A. Pagliaro, C. Giaquinto, S. Kroll, and D. Goldblatt.** 1995. Antibody responses to *Haemophilus influenzae* type b and *Streptococcus pneumoniae* vaccines in children with human immunodeficiency virus infection. Pediatr. Infect. Dis. J. **14**:129–135.

63. **Giebink, G.S., P.I. Warkentin, N.K. Ramsay, and J.H. Kersey.** 1986. Titers of antibody to pneumococci in allogeneic bone marrow transplant recipients before and after vaccination with pneumococcal vaccine. J. Infect. Dis. **154**:590–596.

64. **Gilks, C., A. Adam, L. Otieno, F. Mwongera, M. Amir, and J. Paul.** 1993. HIV infection in acute medical admissions to Kenyatta Hospital: 1988/89 compared to 1992 [Abstract]. *In* Proceedings of the IX International Conference on AIDS, Berlin.

65. **Gilks, C.F., R.J. Brindle, L.S. Otieno, P.M. Simani, R.S. Newnham, S.M. Bhatt, G.N. Lule, G.B.A. Okelo, W.M. Watkins, P.G. Waiyaki, J.B.O. Were, and D.A. Warrell.** 1990. Life-threatening bacteraemia in HIV-1 seropositive adults admitted to hospital in Nairobi, Kenya. Lancet **336**:545–549.

66. **Bilks, C.F., S.A. Ojoo, J.C. Ojoo, R.J. Brindle, J. Paul, B.I.F. Batchelor, J.N. Kimari, R. Newnham, J. Bwayo, F.A. Plummer, and D.A. Warrell.** 1996. Invasive pneumococcal disease in a cohort of predominantly HIV-1–infected female sex-workers in Nairobi, Kenya. Lancet **347**:718–723.

67. **Gilks, C.F., L.S. Otieno, R.J. Brindle, R.S. Newnham, G.N. Lule, J.B.O. Were, P.M. Simani, S.M. Bhatt, G.B.A. Okelo, P.G. Waiyaki, and D.A. Warrell.** 1992. The presentation and outcome of HIV-related disease in Nairobi. Q. J. Med. **297**:25–32.

68. **Gillespie, S.H.** 1989. Aspects of pneumococcal infection including bacterial virulence, host response and vaccination. J. Med. Microbiol. **28**:237–248.

69. **Girgis, N.I., Z. Farid, I.A. Mikhail, I. Farrag, Y. Sultan, and M.E. Kilpatrick.** 1989. Dexamethasone treatment for bacterial meningitis in children and adults. Pediatr. Infect. Dis. J. **8**:848–851.

70. **Glaser, J.B., S. Volpe, A. Aguirre, H. Simpkins, and G. Schiffman.** 1991. Zidovudine improves response to pneumococcal vaccine among persons with AIDS and AIDS-related complex. J. Infect. Dis. **164**:761–764.

71. **Gransden, W.R., S.J. Eykyn, and I. Phillips.** 1985. Pneumococcal bacteremia: 325 episodes at St. Thomas's hospital. B.M.J. **290**:505–508.

72. **Griffioen, A.W., G.T. Rijkers, P. Janssens-Korpela, and B.J.M. Zegers.** 1991. Pneumococcal polysaccharides complexed with C3d bind to human B lymphocytes via complement receptor type 2. Infect. Immunity **59**:1839–1845.

73. **Griffioen, A.W., E.A. Toebes, B.J. Zeges, and G.T. Rijkers.** 1992. Role of CR2 in the human adult and neonatal *in vitro* antibody response to type 4 pneumococcal polysaccharide. Cell. Immunol. **143**:11–22.

74. **Griffioen, A.W., E.A.H. Toebes, G.T. Rijkers, F.H.J. Claas, G. Datema, and B.J.M. Zegers.** 1992. The amplifier role of T cells in the human in vitro B cell response to type 4 pneumococcal polysaccharide. Immunol. Lett. **32**:265–272.

75. **Grimfors, G., M. Bjorkholm, L. Hammarstrom, J. Askergren, C.I. Smith, and G. Holm.** 1989. Type-specific anti-pneumococcal antibody subclass response to vaccination after splenectomy with special reference to lymphoma patients. Eur. J. Haematol. **43**:404–410.

76. **Hammarström, V., K. Pauksen, J. Azinge, G. Oberg, and P. Ljungman.** 1993. Pneumococcal immunity and response to immunization with pneumococcal vaccine in bone marrow transplant patients: the influence of graft versus host reaction. Support Care Cancer **1**:195–199.

77. **Hardy, W.D., J. Feinberg, D.M. Finkelstein, M.E. Power, W. He, C. Kaczka, P.T. Frame, M. Holmes, H. Waskin, R.J. Fass, et al.** 1992. A controlled trial of trimethoprim-sulfamethoxazole or aerosolized pentamidine for secondary prophylaxis of *Pneumocystis carinii* pneumonia in patients with the acquired immunodeficiency syndrome. N. Engl. J. Med. **327**:1482–1488.

78. **Hazelwood, M.A., D.S. Kumararatne, A.D. Webster, M. Goodall, P. Bird, and M. Daha.** 1992. An association between homozygous C3 deficiency and low levels of anti-pneumococcal capsular polysaccharide antibodies. Clin. Exp. Immunol. **87**:404–409.

79. **Hibbs, J.R., J.M. Douglas, Jr., F.N. Judson, W.L. McGill, C.A.M. Rietmeijer, and E.N. Janoff.** 1997. HIV infection, mortality, and serogroup distribution among patients with pneumococcal bacteremia at Denver General Hospital, 1984–94. Clin. Infect. Dis. **25**:195–199.

80. **Hirschtick, R.E., J. Glassroth, M.C. Jordan, T.C. Wilcosky, J.M. Wallace, P.A. Kvale, N. Markowitz, M.J. Rosen, B.T. Mangura, and P.C. Hopewell.** 1995. Bacterial pneumonia in persons infected with the human immunodeficiency virus. N. Engl. J. Med. **333**:845–851.

81. **Hodges, R.G., C.M. MacLeod, and W.G. Bernhard.** 1946. Epidemic pneumococcal pneumonia. III. Pneumococcal carrier studies. Am. J. Hyg. **44**:207–230.

82. **Hoge, C.W., M.R. Reichler, E.A. Dominguez, J.C. Bremer, T.D. Mastro, K.A. Hendricks, D.M. Musher, J.A. Elliott, R.R. Facklam, and R.F. Breiman.** 1994. An epidemic of pneumococcal disease in an overcrowded, inadequately ventilated jail. N. Engl. J. Med. **331**:643–648.

83. **Hostetter, M.K.** 1986. Serotypic variations among virulent pneumococci in deposition and degradation of covalently bound C3b: implications for phagocytosis and antibody production. J. Infect. Dis. **153**:682–693.

84. **Huang, K.-L., F.L. Ruben, C.R. Rinaldo, Jr., L. Kingsley, D.W. Lyter, and M. Ho.** 1987. Antibody responses after influenza and pneumococcal immunization in HIV-infected homosexual men. J.A.M.A. **257**:2047–2050.

85. **Humbert, J.R., E.L. Winsor, J.M. Githens, and J.B. Schmitz.** 1990. Neutrophil dysfunctions in sickle cell disease. Biomed. Pharmacother. **44**:153–158.

86. **Hypogammaglobulinaemia in the United Kingdom.** 1969. Summary report of a Medical Research Council working-party. Lancet **1**:163–168.

87. **Itala, M., H. Helenius, J. Nikoskelainen, and K. Remes.** 1992. Infections and serum IgG levels in patients with chronic lymphocytic leukemia. Eur. J. Haematol. **48**:266–270.

88. Jacobson, D.L., J.A. McCutchan, P.L. Spechko, I. Abramson, R.S. Smith, A. Bartok, G.R. Boss, D. Durand, S.A. Bozzette, S.A. Spector, and D.D. Richman. 1991. The evolution of lymphadenopathy and hypergammaglobulinemia are evidence for early and sustained polyclonal B lymphocyte activation during human immunodeficiency virus infection. J. Infect. Dis. 163:240–246.

89. Janoff, E.N., R.F. Breiman, C.L. Daley, and P.C. Hopewell. 1992. Pneumococcal disease during HIV infection. Epidemiologic, clinical, and immunologic perspectives. Ann. Intern. Med. 117:314–324.

90. Janoff, E.N., C.L. Daley, F. Indacochea, C. Miller, B. Viner, K. Jobe, J.M. Douglas, Jr., P. Weiss, and C.R. Horsburgh, Jr. 1992. Streptococcus pneumoniae (SP) meningitis in the modern era: impact of HIV disease [Abstract]. In Proceedings of the 32nd Interscience Conference on Antimicrobial Agents and Chemotherapy, Anaheim, CA.

91. Janoff, E.N., C.L. Daley, C. Merrifield, J. O'Brien, and P.C. Hopewell. 1992. Natural immunity to Streptococcus pneumoniae in patients with HIV disease [Abstract]. In Proceedings of the 30th Infectious Diseases Society of America Meeting, Anaheim, CA.

92. Janoff, E.N., C.L. Daley, Y. Zhai, J.R. Thurn, and P. Hopewell. 1993. Acute inflammatory responses to Streptococcus pneumoniae are preserved in HIV-infected patients [Abstract]. In Proceedings of the 33rd Interscience Conference on Antimicrobial Agents and Chemotherapy, New Orleans.

93. Janoff, E.N., J.M. Douglas, M. Gabriel, M.J. Blaser, A.J. Davidson, D.L. Cohn, and F.N. Judson. 1988. Class-specific antibody response to pneumococcal capsular polysaccharides in men infected with human immunodeficiency virus type 1. J. Infect. Dis. 158:983–990.

94. Janoff, E.N., C. Fasching, J.C. Ojoo, J. O'Brien, and C.F. Gilks. 1997. Responsiveness of human immunodeficiency virus type 1–infected Kenyan women with and without prior pneumococcal disease to pneumococcal vaccine. J. Infect. Dis. 175:975–978.

95. Janoff, E.N., W.D. Hardy, P.D. Smith, and S.M. Wahl. 1991. Levels, specificity, and affinity of IgG specific for recall antigens in patients with HIV. J. Immunol. 147:2130–2135.

96. Janoff, E.N., J. O'Brien, P. Thompson, J. Ehret, G. Meiklejohn, G. Duvall, and J.M. Douglas, Jr. 1993. Streptococcus pneumoniae colonization, bacteremia, and immune response among persons with human immunodeficiency virus infection. J. Infect. Dis. 167:49–56.

97. Janoff, E.N., P.D. Smith, and M.J. Blaser. 1988. Acute antibody responses to Giardia lamblia are depressed in patients with AIDS. J. Infect. Dis. 157:798–804.

98. Janoff, E.N., S. Worel, and J.M. Douglas, Jr. 1990. Natural immunity and response to conjugate vaccine for Haemophilus influenzae type B in men with HIV [Abstract]. In Proceedings of the 30th Interscience Conference on Antimicrobial Agents and Chemotherapy, Atlanta.

99. Jetté, L.P., and F. Lamothe. 1989. Surveillance of invasive Streptococcus pneumoniae infection in Quebec, Canada, from 1984 to 1986: serotype distribution, antimicrobial susceptibility, and clinical characteristics. J. Clin. Microbiol. 27:1–5.

100. Johnston, R.R., Jr. 1991. Pathogenesis of pneumococcal pneumonia. Rev. Infect. Dis. 13:S509–S519.

101. Jones, N., R. Huebner, M. Khoosal, H. Crewe-Brown, and K. Klugman. 1998. The impact of HIV on Streptococcus pneumoniae bacteraemia in a South African population. A.I.D.S. 12:2177–2184.

102. Kaplan, J., S. Sarnaik, and G. Schiffman. 1986. Revaccination with polyvalent pneumococcal vaccine in children with sickle cell anemia. Am. J. Pediatr. 8:80–82.

103. Kaplan, J.E., H. Masur, H.W. Jaffe, and K.K. Holmes. 1995. Reducing the impact of opportunistic infections in patients with HIV infection. J.A.M.A. 274:347–348.

104. Käyhty, H., and J. Eskola. 1996. New vaccines for the prevention of pneumococcal infections. Emerg. Infect. Dis. 2:289–298.

105. Kehrl, J.H., and A.S. Fauci. 1983. Activation of human B lymphocytes after immunization with pneumococcal polysaccharides. J. Clin. Invest. 71:1032–1040.

106. Kilian, M., J. Mestecky, and M.W. Russell. 1988. Defense mechanisms involving Fc-dependent functions of immunoglobulin A and their subversion by bacterial immunoglobulin A proteases. Microbiol. Rev. 52:296–303.

107. Kim, P.E., D.M. Musher, W.P. Glezen, M.C. Rodriguez-Barradas, W.K. Nahm, and C.E. Wright. 1996. Association of invasive pneumococcal disease with season, atmospheric conditions, air pollution, and the isolation of respiratory viruses. Clin. Infect. Dis. 22:100–106.

108. Kiroff, G.K., A.N. Hodgen, P.A. Drew, and G.G. Jamieson. 1985. Lack of effect of splenic regrowth on the reduced antibody responses to pneumococcal polysaccharides in splenectomized patients. Clin. Exp. Immunol. 62:48–56.

109. Klein, R.S., P.A. Selwyn, D. Maude, C. Pollard, K. Freeman, and G. Schiffman. 1989. Response to pneumococcal vaccine among asymptomatic heterosexual partners of persons with AIDS and intravenous drug users infected with human immunodeficiency virus. J. Infect. Dis. 160:826–831.

110. Konradsen, H.B., and J. Henrichsen. 1991. Pneumococcal infections in splenectomized children are preventable. Acta Paediatr. Scand. 80:423–427.

111. Kontoyianis, D.P., E.J. Anaissie, and G.P. Bodey. 1993. Infection in chronic lymphocytic leukemia: a reappraisal in chronic lymphocytic leukemia scientific advances and clinical developments. In B.D. Cheson (ed.), Chronic lymphocytic leukemia. Marcel Dekker, New York, pp. 399–417.

112. Koziel, H., and M.J. Koziel. 1995. Pulmonary complications of diabetes mellitus: pneumonia. Infect. Dis. Clin. North Am. 9:65–96.

113. Krasinski, K., W. Borkowsky, S. Bonk, R. Lawrence, and S. Chandwani. 1988. Bacterial infections in human immunodeficiency virus–infected children. Pediatr. Infect. Dis. J. 7:323–328.

114. Kroon, F.P., J.T. van Dissel, J.C. de Jong, and R. Furth. 1994. Antibody response to influenza, tetanus and pneumococcal vaccines in HIV-1 seropositive individuals in relation to the number of CD4$^+$ lymphocytes. A.I.D.S. 8:469–476.

115. Krumholz, H.M., M.A. Sande, and B. Lo. 1989. Community-acquired bacteremia in patients with acquired immunodeficiency syndrome: clinical presentation, bacteriology and outcome. Am. J. Med. 86:776–779.

116. Kuikka, A., J. Syrjanen, O.V. Renkonen, and V.V. Valtonen. 1992. Pneumococcal bacteremia during a recent decade. J. Infect. 24:157–168.

117. Lane, P.J.L., and I.C.M. Maclennan. 1986. Impaired IgG2 antipneumococcal antibody responses in patients with recurrent infection and normal IgG2 levels but no IgA. Clin. Exp. Immunol. 65:427–433.

118. Lepage, P., P. Van de Perre, F. Nsengumuremyi, C. Van Goethem, J. Bogaerts, and D.G. Hitimana. 1989. Bacteraemia as predictor of HIV infection in African children. Acta Pediatr. Scand. 78:763–766.

119. Levine, W.C., J.W. Buehler, N.H. Bean, and R.V. Tauxe. 1991. Epidemiology of nontyphoidal Salmonella bacteremia during the human immunodeficiency virus epidemic. J. Infect. Dis. 164:81–87.

120. Lortan, J.E., A.S. Kaniuk, and M.A. Monteil. 1993. Relationship of in vitro phagocytosis of serotype 14 Streptococcus pneumoniae to specific class and IgG subclass antibody levels in healthy adults. Clin. Exp. Immunol. 91:54–57.

121. Magnenat, J.-L., L.P. Nicod, R. Auckenthaler, and A.F. Junod. 1991. Mode of presentation and diagnosis of bacterial

pneumonia in human immunodeficiency virus-infected patients. Am. Rev. Respir. Dis. **144:**917–922.

122. **Marfin, A.A., J. Sporrer, P.S. Moore, and A.D. Siefkin.** 1995. Risk factors for adverse outcome in persons with pneumococcal pneumonia. Chest **107:**457–462.

123. **Marrie, T.J.** 1994. Pneumonia and carcinoma of the lung. J. Infect. **29:**45–52.

124. **Mascart-Lemone, F., M. Gérard, M. Libin, A. Crusiaux, P. Franchioly, A. Lambrechts, M. Goldman, and N. Clumeck.** 1995. Differential effect of human immunodeficiency virus infection on the IgA and IgG antibody responses to pneumococcal vaccine. J. Infect. Dis. **172:**1253–1260.

125. **Masur, H., M.A. Michelis, J.B. Greene, I. Onorato, R.A. Vande Stouwe, R.A. Holzman, G. Wormser, L. Brettman, M. Lange, H.W. Murray, S. Cunningham-Rundles, and D. Armstrong.** 1981. An outbreak of community-acquired *Pneumocystis carinii* pneumonia: initial manifestation of cellular immune dysfunction. N. Engl. J. Med. **305:**1431–1438.

126. **Meynard, J.L., F. Barbut, L. Blum, M. Guiguet, C. Chouaid, M.C. Meyohas, O. Picard, J.C. Petit, and J. Frottier.** 1996. Risk factors for isolation of *Streptococcus pneumoniae* with decreased susceptibility to penicillin G from patients infected with human immunodeficiency virus. Clin. Infect. Dis. **22:**437–440.

127. **Mofenson, L.M., J. Moye, Jr., J. Bethel, R. Hirschhorn, C. Jordan, and R. Nugent.** 1992. Prophylactic intravenous immunoglobulin in HIV-infected children with CD4+ counts of 0.20×10^9/L or more; effect on viral, opportunistic, and bacterial infections. J.A.M.A. **268:**483–488.

128. **Mofenson, L.M., J. Moye, Jr., J. Korelitz, J. Bethel, R. Hirschhorn, and R. Nugent.** 1994. Cross-over of placebo patients to intravenous immunoglobulin confirms efficacy for prophylaxis of bacterial infections and reduction of hospitalizations in human immunodeficiency virus-infected children. Pediatr. Infect. Dis. J. **13:**477–484.

129. **Muller, F., S.S. Froland, and P. Brandtzaeg.** 1989. Altered IgG-subclass distribution in lymph node cells and serum of adults infected with human immunodeficiency virus (HIV). Clin. Exp. Immunol. **78:**153–158.

130. **Mundy, L.M., P.G. Auwaerter, D. Oldach, M.L. Warner, A. Burton, E. Vance, C.A. Gaydos, J.M. Joseph, R. Gopalan, R.D. Moore, T.C. Quinn, P. Charache, and J.G. Bartlett.** 1995. Community-acquired pneumonia: impact of immune status. Am. J. Respir. Crit. Care Med. **152:**1309–1315.

131. **Murata, G.H., M.J. Ault, and R.D. Meyer.** 1984/5. Community-acquired bacterial pneumonias in homosexual men: presumptive evidence for a defect in host resistance. A.I.D.S. Res. **1:**379–393.

132. **Murphy, P.M., H.C. Lane, A.S. Fauci, and J.I. Gallin.** 1988. Impairment of neutrophil bactericidal capacity in patients with AIDS. J. Infect. Dis. **158:**627–630.

133. **Musher, D.M., J.E. Groover, M.R. Reichler, F.X. Riedo, B. Schwartz, D.A. Watson, R.E. Baughn, and R.F. Breiman.** 1997. Emergence of antibody to capsular polysaccharides of *Streptococcus pneumoniae* during outbreaks of pneumonia: association with nasopharyngeal colonization. Clin. Infect. Dis. **24:**441–446.

134. **Musher, D.M., J.E. Groover, J.M. Rowland, D.A. Watson, J.B. Struewing, R.E. Baughn, and M.A. Mufson.** 1992. Antibody to capsular polysaccharides of *Streptococcus pneumoniae*: prevalence, persistence, and response to revaccination. Clin. Infect. Dis. **17:**66–73.

135. **Newman, S.L., L.B. Vogler, R.D. Feigin, and R.B. Johnston, Jr.** 1979. Recurrent septicemia associated with congenital deficiency of C2 and partial deficiency of factor B and the alternate complement pathway. N. Engl. J. Med. **299:**290–292.

136. **O'Connor, P.G., P.A. Selwyn, and R.S. Schottenfeld.** 1994.

Medical care for injection-drug users with human immunodeficiency virus infection. N. Engl. J. Med. **331:**450–459.

137. **O'Neal, B.J., and J.C. McDonald.** 1981. The risk of sepsis in the asplenic adult. Ann. Surg. **194:**775–778.

138. **Oldfield, S., S. Jenkins, H. Yeoman, D. Gray, and I.C.M. MacLennan.** 1985. Class and subclass anti-pneumococcal antibody responses in splenectomized patients. Clin. Exp. Immunol. **61:**664–673.

139. **Opravil, M., W. Fierz, L. Matter, J. Blaser, and R. Lüthy.** 1991. Poor antibody response after tetanus and pneumococcal vaccination in immunocompromised, HIV-infected patients. Clin. Exp. Immunol. **84:**185–189.

140. **Opstad, N.L., C.L. Daley, J.R. Thurn, J.B. Rubins, C. Merrifield, P.C. Hopewell, and E.N. Janoff.** 1995. Impact of *Streptococcus pneumoniae* bacteremia and human immunodeficiency virus type 1 on oral mucosal immunity. J. Infect. Dis. **172:**567–571.

141. **Ortqvist, A., M. Kalin, I. Julander, and M.A. Mufson.** 1993. Deaths in bacteremic pneumococcal pneumonia. A comparison of two populations—Huntington, WV and Stockholm, Sweden. Chest **103:**710–716.

142. **Paul, J., J. Kimari, and C.F. Gilks.** 1994. *Streptococcus pneumoniae* resistant to penicillin and tetracycline associated with HIV seropositivity [Letter]. Lancet **346:**1034–1035.

143. **Perlino, C.A., and D. Rimland.** 1985. Alcoholism, leukopenia, and pneumococcal sepsis. Am. Rev. Respir. Dis. **132:**757–760.

144. **Peset-Llopis, M.J., G. Harms, M.J. Hardonk, and W. Timens.** 1996. Human immune response to pneumococcal polysaccharides: complement-mediated localization preferentially on CD21-positive splenic marginal zone B cells and follicular dendritic cells. J. Allergy Clin. Immunol. **97:**1015–1024.

145. **Pesola, G.R., and A. Charles.** 1992. Pneumococcal bacteremia with pneumonia. Chest **101:**150–155.

146. **Polsky, B., J.W.M. Gold, E. Wimbey, J. Dryjansky, A.E. Brown, G. Schiffman, D. Armstrong, and T.C. Quinn.** 1986. Bacterial pneumonia in patients with the acquired immune deficiency syndrome. Ann. Intern. Med. **104:**38–41.

147. **Puppo, F., R. Ruzzenenti, S. Brenci, L. Lanza, M. Scudeletti, and F. Indiveri.** 1991. Major histocompatibility gene products and human immunodeficiency virus infection. J. Lab. Clin. Med. **117:**91–100.

148. **Rao, S.P., K. Rajkumar, G. Schiffman, N. Desai, C. Unger, and S.T. Miller.** 1995. Anti-pneumococcal antibody levels three to seven years after first booster immunization in children with sickle cell disease, and after a second booster. J. Pediatr. **127:**590–592.

149. **Rautonen, N., N.L. Martin, J. Rautonen, Y. Rooks, W.C. Mentzer, and D.W. Wara.** 1992. Low number of antibody producing cells in patients with sickle cell anemia. Immunol. Lett. **34:**201–211.

150. **Redd, S.C., G.W. Rutherford, M.A. Sande, A.R. Lifson, W.K. Hadley, R.R. Facklam, and J.S. Spika.** 1990. The role of human immunodeficiency virus in pneumococcal bacteremia in San Francisco residents. J. Infect. Dis. **162:**1012–1017.

151. **Reichler, M., R. Reynolds, B. Schwartz, D. Musher, D. Pratt, G. Hohenhaus, J. Struewing, B. Plikaytis, J. Elliot, and R. Breiman.** 1991. Epidemic of pneumococcal pneumonia at a military training camp [Abstract 49]. *In* Proceedings of the 31st Interscience Conference on Antimicrobial Agents and Chemotherapy, Chicago.

152. **Reimer, C.B., C.M. Black, R.C. Holman, T.W. Wells, R.M. Ramirez, J.A. Sa-Ferreira, J.K.A. Nicholson, and J.S. McDougal.** 1988. Hypergammaglobulinemia associated with human immunodeficiency virus infection (HIV). Monogr. Allergy **23:**83–96.

153. **Reinert, R.R., A. Kaufhold, O. Kuhnemund, and R. Lutticken.** 1994. Serum antibody responses to vaccination with 23-valent

pneumococcal vaccine in splenectomized patients. Int. J. Med. Microbiol. Virol. Parasitol. Infect. Dis. **281**:481–490.

154. **Riedo, F., B. Schwartz, S. Giono, J. Hierholzer, S. Ostroff, J. Groover, D. Musher, L. Martinez, R. Breiman, and The Pneumonia Study Group.** 1991. Pneumococcal pneumonia outbreak in a ranger training battalion, Georgia [Abstract 48]. *In* Proceedings of the 31st Interscience Conference on Antimicrobial Agents and Chemotherapy, Chicago.

155. **Rodriguez, M.E., W.-L. van der Pol, L.A.M. Sanders, and J.G.J. van de Winkel.** 1999. Crucial role of FcγRIIa (CD32) in assessment of functional anti-*Streptococcus pneumoniae* antibody activity in human sera. J. Infect. Dis. **179**:423–433.

156. **Rodriguez-Barradas, M.C., D.M. Musher, R.J. Hamill, M. Dowell, J.T. Bagwell, and C.V. Sanders.** 1992. Unusual manifestations of pneumococcal infection in human immunodeficiency virus-infected individuals: the past revisited. Clin. Infect. Dis. **14**:192–199.

157. **Rodriguez-Barradas, M.C., R.A. Tharapel, J.E. Groover, K.P. Giron, C.E. Lacke, E.D. Houston, R.J. Hamill, M.C. Steinhoff, and D.M. Musher.** 1997. Colonization by *Streptococcus pneumoniae* among human immunodeficiency virus–infected adults: prevalence of antibiotic resistance, impact of immunization, and characterization by polymerase chain reaction with BOX primers of isolates from persistent *S. pneumoniae* carriers. J. Infect. Dis. **175**:590–597.

158. **Rodriguez-Creixems, M., P. Munoz, E. Miranda, T. Pelaez, and R. Alonso.** 1996. Recurrent pneumococcal bacteremia. A warning of immunodeficiency. Arch. Intern. Med. **156**:1429–1434.

159. **Rose, D.N., C.B. Schechter, and H.S. Sacks.** 1993. Influenza and pneumococcal vaccination of HIV-infected patients: a policy analysis. Am. J. Med. **94**:160–168.

160. **Rosen, F.S., and C.A. Janeway.** 1966. The gamma globulins. III. The antibody deficiency syndromes. N. Engl. J. Med. **275**: 709–715.

161. **Ross, S.C., and P. Densen.** 1984. Complement deficiency states and infection: epidemiology, pathogenesis and consequences of neisserial and other infections in an immune deficiency. Medicine **63**:243–273.

122. **Rubins, J.B., D. Charboneau, J.C. Paton, T.J. Mitchell, P.W. Andrew, and E.N. Janoff.** 1995. Dual function of pneumolysin in the early pathogenesis of murine pneumococcal pneumonia. J. Clin. Invest. **95**:142–150.

163. **Rubins, J.B., P.G. Duane, D. Charboneau, and E.N. Janoff.** 1992. Toxicity of pneumolysin to pulmonary endothelial cells *in vitro*. Infect. Immunol. **60**:1740–1746.

164. **Rubins, J.B., T.J. Mitchell, P.W. Andrew, and D.E. Niewoehner.** 1994. Pneumolysin activates phospholipase A in pulmonary artery endothelial cells. Infect. Immunol. **62**:3829–3836.

165. **Ruiz-Contreras, J., J.T. Ramos, T. Hernandez-Sampelayo, M.D. Gurbindo, M. de José, M.J.G. de Miguel, M.J. Cilleruelo, M.J. Mellado, and the Madrid HIV Pediatric Infection Collaborative Study Group.** 1995. Sepsis in children with human immunodeficiency virus infection. Pediatr. Infect. Dis. J. **14**:522–526.

166. **Rynnel-Dagoo, B., A. Freijd, L. Hammarström, V. Oxelius, and M.A. Persson.** 1986. Pneumococcal antibodies of different immunoglobulin subclasses in normal and IgG subclass deficient individuals of various ages. Acta Otolaryngol. (Stockh.) **101**:146–151.

167. **Salmon, D., P. Detruchis, C. Leport, E. Bouvet, D. Karam, M.C. Meyohas, J.P. Couland, and J.L. Vildé.** 1991. Efficacy of zidovudine in preventing relapses of salmonella bacteremia in AIDS. J. Infect. Dis. **163**:415–416.

168. **Schuchat, A., C.V. Broome, A. Hightower, S.J. Costa, and W. Parkin.** 1991. Use of surveillance for invasive pneumococcal disease to estimate the size of the immunosuppressed HIV-infected population. J.A.M.A. **265**:3275–3279.

169. **Scott, G.B., B.E. Buck, J.G. Leterman, F.L. Bloom, and W.P. Parks.** 1984. Acquired immunodeficiency syndrome in infants. N. Engl. J. Med. **310**:76–81.

170. **Selby, C., S. Hart, P. Ispahani, and P.J. Toghill.** 1987. Bacteremia in adults after splenectomy or splenic irradiation. Q. J. Med. **63**:523–530.

171. **Selik, R.M., E.T. Starcher, and J.W. Curran.** 1987. Opportunistic diseases reported in AIDS patients: frequencies, associations, and trends. A.I.D.S. **1987**:175–182.

172. **Selwyn, P.A., P. Alcabes, D. Hartel, D. Buono, E.E. Schoenbaum, R.S. Klein, K. Davenny, and G.H. Friedland.** 1992. Clinical manifestations and predictors of disease progression in drug users with human immunodeficiency virus infection. N. Engl. J. Med. **327**:1697–1703.

173. **Selwyn, P.A., A.R. Feingold, D. Hartel, E.E. Schoenbaum, M.H. Alderman, R.S. Klein, and G.H. Friedland.** 1988. Increased risk of bacterial pneumonia in HIV-infected intravenous drug users without AIDS. AIDS **2**:267–272.

174. **Shah, T.P., and F.R. Sattler.** 1987. Polymorphonuclear leukocyte-mediated, antibody-dependent cellular cytotoxicity in patients with AIDS (letter). J. Infect. Dis. **155**:594–595.

175. **Shapiro, E.D., A.T. Berg, R. Austrian, D. Schroeder, V. Parcells, A. Margolis, R.K. Adair, and J.D. Clemens.** 1991. The protective efficacy of polyvalent pneumococcal polysaccharide vaccine. N. Engl. J. Med. **325**:1453–1460.

176. **Shyur, S.-D., H.V. Raff, J.F. Bohnsack, D.K. Kelsey, and H.R. Hill.** 1992. Comparison of the opsonic and complement triggering activity of human monoclonal IgG1 and IgM antibody against group B streptococci. J. Immunol. **148**:1879–1884.

177. **Siber, G.R., P.H. Schur, A.C. Aisenberg, S.A. Weitzman, and G. Schiffman.** 1980. Correlation between serum IgG2 concentrations and the antibody response to bacterial polysaccharide antigens. N. Engl. J. Med. **303**:178–182.

178. **Simani, P., C. Gilks, R. Brindle, Otieno, G.B. Okello, J. Ndinya-la, and J. Kreiss.** 1992. The role of pneumococcal disease among HIV seropositive and seronegative patients with acute pneumonia in Nairobi, Kenya [Abstract]. *In* Proceedings of the VIII International Conference on AIDS, Amsterdam.

179. **Simberkoff, M.S., W. El Sadr, G. Schiffman, and J.J. Rahal, Jr.** 1984. *Streptococcus pneumonia* infections and bacteremia in patients with acquired immune deficiency syndrome, with a report of pneumococcal vaccine failure. Am. Rev. Respir. Dis. **130**:1174–1176.

180. **Spector, S.A., R.D. Gelber, N. McGrath, D. Wara, A. Barzilai, E. Abrams, Y.I. Bryson, W.M. Danker, R.A. Livingston, E.M. Connor, *et al.*** 1994. A controlled trail of intravenous immune globulin for the prevention of serious bacterial infections in children receiving zidovudine for advanced human immunodeficiency virus infection. N. Engl. J. Med. **331**:1181–1187.

181. **Spika, J.S., N.A. Halsey, C.T. Le, A.J. Fish, G.M. Lum, B.A. Lauer, G. Schiffman, and G.S. Giebink.** 1986. Decline of vaccine-induced antipneumococcal antibody in children with nephrotic syndrome. Am. J. Kidney Dis. **7**:466–470.

182. **Steinhoff, M.C., B.S. Auerbach, K. Nelson, D. Vlahov, R.L. Becker, N.M. Graham, D.H. Schwartz, A.H. Lucas, and R.E. Chaisson.** 1991. Antibody responses to *Haemophilus influenzae* type b vaccines in men with human immunodeficiency virus infection. N. Engl. J. Med. **325**:1837–1842.

183. **Tacconelli, E., M. Tumbarello, K. de Gaetano, R. Cauda, and L. Ortona.** 1998. Highly active antiretroviral therapy decreases the incidence of bacteremia in human immunodeficiency virus-infected individuals [Brief Report]. Clin. Infect. Dis. **27**:901–902.

184. **Tausk, F.A., A. McCutchan, P. Spechko, R.D. Schreiber, and I. Gigli.** 1986. Altered erythrocyte C3b receptor expression, im-

mune complexes, and complement activation in homosexual men in varying risk groups for acquired immune deficiency syndrome. J. Clin. Invest. **78**:977–982.

185. **Terpstra, F.G., B.J.M. Al, M.T.L. Roos, F. De Wolf, J. Goudsmit, P.H.A. Schellekens, and F. Miedema.** 1989. Longitudinal study of leukocyte functions in homosexual men seroconverted for HIV: rapid and persistent loss of B cell function after HIV infection. Eur. J. Immunol. **19**:667–673.

186. **National Institute of Child Health and Human Development Intravenous Immunoglobulin Study Group.** 1991. Intravenous immune globulin for the prevention of bacterial infections in children with symptomatic human immunodeficiency virus infection. N. Engl. J. Med. **325**:73–80.

187. **Tuomanen, E.I., K. Saukkonen, S. Sande, C. Cioffe, and S.D. Wright.** 1989. Reduction of inflammation, tissue damage, and mortality in bacterial meningitis in rabbits treated with monoclonal antibodies against adhesion-promoting receptors of leukocytes. J. Exp. Med. **170**:959–968.

188. **Twomey, J.T.** 1973. Infections complicating multiple myeloma and chronic lymphocytic leukemia. Arch. Intern. Med. **132**:562–565.

189. **Vandenbruaene, M., R. Colebunders, F. Mascart-Lemone, Y. Haerden, D. Van Hove, M. Peeters, J. Goeman, P. Van Royen, and D. Avonts.** 1995. Equal IgG antibody response to pneumococcal vaccination in all stages of human immunodeficiency virus disease. J. Infect. Dis. **172**:551–553.

190. **Ward, J.W., D.L. Hanson, J. Jones, and J.O.N. Kaplan.** 1996. Pneumococcal vaccination and the incidence of pneumonia among HIV-1–infected persons [Abstract 245]. *In* Proceedings of the 34th Annual Meeting of the Infectious Diseases Society of America, New Orleans.

191. **Warmerdam, P.A.M., J.G.J. van de Winkel, A. Vlug, N.A.C. Westerdaal, and P.J.A. Capel.** 1991. A single amino acid in the second Ig-like domain of the human Fcγ receptor II is critical for human IgG2 binding. J. Immunol. **147**:1338–1343.

192. **Watanakunakorn, C., A. Greifenstein, K. Stroh, D.G. Jarjoura, D. Blend, A. Cugino, and A.J. Ognibene.** 1993. Pneu-

mococcal bacteremia in three community teaching hospitals from 1980 to 1989. Chest **103**:1152–1156.

193. **Weiss, P.J., M.R. Wallace, E.C. Oldfield III., J. O'Brien, and E.N. Janoff.** 1995. Response of recent human immunodeficiency virus seroconverters to the pneumococcal polysaccharide vaccine and *Haemophilus influenzae* type b conjugate vaccine. J. Infect. Dis. **171**:1217–1222.

194. **Winkelstein, J.A.** 1984. Complement and the host's defense against the pneumococcus. Crit. Rev. Microbiol. **11**:187–208.

195. **Winston, D.J., G. Schiffman, D.C. Wang, S.A. Feig, C.-H. Lin, E.L. Marso, W.G. Ho, L.S. Young, and R.P. Gale.** 1979. Pneumococcal infections after human bone-marrow transplantation. Ann. Intern. Med. **91**:835–841.

196. **Witt, D.J., D.E. Craven, and W.R. McCabe.** 1987. Bacterial infections in adult patients with the acquired immune deficiency syndrome (AIDS) and AIDS-related complex. Am. J. Med. **82**:900–906.

197. **Wong, W.Y., D.R. Powars, L. Chan, A. Hiti, C. Johnson, and G. Overturf.** 1991. Polysaccharide encapsulated bacterial infection in sickle cell anemia: a thirty-year epidemiologic experience. Am. J. Hematol. **39**:176–182.

198. **Wood, C.C., J.G. McNamara, D.F. Schwarz, W.W. Merrill, and E.D. Shapiro.** 1987. Prevention of pneumococcal bacteremia in a child with acquired immunodeficiency syndrome-related complex. Pediatr. Infect. Dis. J. **6**:564–566.

199. **Zarkowsky, H.S., D. Gallagher, F.M. Gill, W.C. Wang, J.M. Falletta, W.M. Lande, P.S. Levy, J.I. Verter, and D. Wethers.** 1986. Bacteremia in sickle hemoglobinopathies. J. Pediatr. **109**:579–585.

Address reprint requests to:
Edward N. Janoff
VA Medical Center
Infectious Disease Section (111F)
One Veterans Dr.
Minneapolis, MN 55417

Otitis Media: The Chinchilla Model[1]

G. SCOTT GIEBINK

ABSTRACT

Streptococcus pneumoniae infection and disease have been modeled in several animal species including infant and adult mice, infant and adult rats, infant Rhesus monkeys, and adolescent and adult chinchillas. Most are models of sepsis arising from intravenous or intraperitoneal inoculation of bacteria, and a few were designed to study disease arising from intranasal infection. Chinchillas provide the only animal model of middle ear pneumococcal infection in which the disease can be produced by very small inocula injected into the middle ear (ME) or intranasally, and in which the disease remains localized to the ME in most cases. This model, developed at the University of Minnesota in 1975, has been used to study pneumococcal pathogenesis at a mucosal site, immunogenicity and efficacy of pneumococcal capsular polysaccharide (PS) vaccine antigens, and the kinetics and efficacy of antimicrobial drugs.

Pathogenesis experiments in the chinchilla model have revealed variation in ME virulence among different pneumococcal serotypes, enhancement of ME infection during concurrent intranasal influenza A virus infections, and natural resolution of pneumococcal otitis media (OM) without intervention. Research has explored the relative contribution of pneumococcal and host products to ME inflammation. Pneumococcal cell wall components and pneumolysin have been studied in the model. Host inflammatory responses studied in the chinchilla ME include polymorphonuclear leukocyte oxidative products, hydrolytic enzymes, cytokine and eicosanoid metabolites, and ME epithelial cell adhesion and mucous glycoprotein production. Both clinical (tympanic membrane appearance) and histopathology (ME, Eustachian tube, inner ear) endpoints can be quantified.

Immunologic and inflammatory studies have been facilitated by the production of affinity-purified anti-chinchilla immunoglobulin G (IgG), IgM, and secretory IgA polyclonal antibody reagents, and the identification of cross-reactivity between human and chinchilla cytokines, and between guinea pig and chinchilla C3. Alteration of ME mucosa by pneumococcal neuraminidase and alteration of ME epithelial cell (MEEC) surface carbohydrates during intranasal pneumococcal infection have been demonstrated. Pathogenesis studies have been aided by cultured chinchilla MEEC systems, in which the ability of platelet activating factor and interleukin (IL)-1β to stimulate epithelial mucous glycoprotein synthesis has recently been demonstrated. Because chronic OM with effusion is characterized by presence of large amounts of mucous glycoprotein in the ME, pneumococcus may have an important role in both acute and chronic ME disease.

Both unconjugated PS and PS-protein-conjugated vaccines are immunogenic after intramuscular administration without adjuvant in chinchillas. Passive protection studies with human hyperimmune immunoglobulin demonstrated that anti-PS IgG alone is capable of protecting the chinchilla ME from direct ME challenge with pneumococci. Active PS immunization studies demonstrated protection following direct ME and intranasal pneumococcal challenge with and without concurrent influenza A virus infection. An attenuated influenza A virus vaccine also showed protection for pneumococcal OM.

Antimicrobial treatment of acute OM has been based almost exclusively on empirical drug use and clini-

Professor of Pediatrics and Otolaryngology, Director, Otitis Media Research Center, University of Minnesota School of Medicine, Minneapolis, MN 55455.

[1]Presented at the Workshop, "*Streptococcus pneumoniae:* Molecular Biology and Mechanisms of Disease—Update for the 1990s," Oeiras, Portugal, September 24–29, 1996.

Reprinted from *Microbial Drug Resistance*, Vol. 5, No. 1, 1999.

cal trials without a foundation of ME pharmacokinetics. Studies in the chinchilla model have started to bring a rational basis to drug selection and dosing. Microassays have been developed using high-pressure liquid chromatography for many relevant drugs. Studies have explored the *in vivo* ME response in pneumococcal OM to antimicrobial drugs at supra- and sub-minimum inhibitory concentration (MIC), the effect of concurrent influenza A virus infection on ME drug penetration, and the effect of treatment on sensorineural hearing loss produced by pneumococcal OM.

THE OTITIS MEDIA SPECTRUM IN HUMANS

OTITIS MEDIA (OM) is one of the most common diseases of infants and young children, with an estimated 6 million cases of OM annually in the United States.[15] The disease affects at least 7 out of every 10 children; one-third have repeated episodes and 5–10% develop chronic OM with effusion (OME). Acute OM initiates the continuum of OM, leading in many children to chronic OME and in some to chronic tissue sequelae such as mucosal granulation, mastoiditis, ossicular erosion and fixation, and cholesteatoma.

Streptococcus pneumoniae is the most frequent bacterium causing OM in infants and children.[23,53,104] There has been surprisingly little change in middle ear (ME) bacteriology reported during the past 18 years. Thirteen publications have enumerated the ME bacteriology of 4,157 cases of acute OM. Pneumococci were cultured from about one-third (20–37%) of acute ME effusions. About 20% (6–31%) yielded *Haemophilus influenzae*, most of which were nontypable strains, and smaller percentages yielded *Moraxella catarrhalis* (6%), *Streptococcus pyogenes* (2%), *Staphylococcus aureus* (2%), and others (6%). Antigen and DNA detection methods have revealed pneumococci in 30% to 60% of cases with sterile ME fluid (MEF).[104,120]

Otitis media is a disease manifest both in fluid that accumulates in the ME space and in the surrounding ME mucosa. The fluid may be serous, purulent, or mucoid. The relative frequency of effusion types differs in acute and chronic disease. In acute OM, purulent effusion is found in two-thirds of cases. In chronic OME, nearly one-half of the effusions are mucoid, only 10% are serous, and fewer than 10% are purulent.

Normal ME mucosa is composed of a single layer of squamous and cuboidal epithelial cells overlaying a thin subepithelial space and bone. Serous OM is associated with subepithelial edema but no change in the epithelium. Purulent OM is characterized by acute inflammatory cells in the submucosa and ME space and subepithelial edema; there is no epithelial metaplasia. In mucoid OM, epithelial metaplasia to tall columnar secreting goblet cells predominate with subepithelial edema and vascular dilatation; fluid with mucous strands but few inflammatory cells fills the ME space. Recently, a rat model of mucoid OM has been described; mucoid effusion was produced by pneumococcal ME infection followed by Eustachian tube obstruction.[67] Rat and human mucous glycoprotein cDNA probes have been used to explore factors that regulate the synthesis of mucous glycoprotein.[63,116]

Etiologic factors for OM have been investigated by several laboratories in the past two decades. Evidence indicates that OM occurs only in the presence of Eustachian tube dysfunction, and this dysfunction is caused principally by selected respiratory viruses (respiratory syncytial virus, adenovirus, influenza) and by anatomic abnormalities of the cartilaginous Eustachian tube and surrounding muscular structures in children with craniofacial dysmorphism. Bacterial replication in the obstructed ME leads to the release of bacterial and host inflammatory products and to clinical acute OM.

These events occur in the milieu of local and systemic host response to bacterial invasion. Potent biochemical mediators present in ME fluid and tissues during OM include arachidonic acid metabolites, which cause vascular leakage and edema, stimulation of mucous secretion, and bone resorption. Anti-proteases, such as α-2 macroglobulin, diffuse into the inflamed ME and neutralize microbial proteases, thereby protecting the host. Lysosomal enzymes, released by host epithelial, inflammatory, and bacterial cells, may have direct toxic effects on ME tissues. In defense of the host, complement proteins derived from serum, and perhaps synthesized by ME epithelium, attract leukocytes and facilitate bacterial killing. Host cellular elements, such as leukocytes, lymphocytes, and macrophages, aid in antibody production and eradication of microbes. Studies indicate that passively administered antibody or antibody induced by active immunization clear pneumococci and *H. influenzae* from the ME. Children lacking the ability to produce these antibodies after natural disease seem more susceptible to subsequent recurrent episodes of OM.

PATHOGENESIS

Chinchilla modeling of pneumococcal OM

We developed the chinchilla model of OM in 1975 to understand the pathophysiology of OM and to explore the efficacy of immunoprophylactic and therapeutic interventions.[48] This model closely parallels the continuum of human OM. Middle ear inoculation of living, encapsulated pneumococci causes a replicating local infection with polymorphonuclear leukocytes (PMNL) infiltration into the subepithelial space of the ME mucosa. Epithelial metaplasia, subepithelial edema, and MEF volume increase during the first week after inoculation, followed by gradual resolution of inflammation over the succeeding 8–10 weeks. Virulence of pneumococci for the chinchilla ME varies among some serotypes. For example, a type 3 strain produced more attenuated ME disease than a type 23B strain.[49] In untreated animals, the process ends with mucoperiosteal granulation tissue and osteoneogenesis, which is pathognomonic of chronic OM in humans.

Respiratory virus infection

The pathophysiology of acute OM caused by respiratory viruses has been investigated in the chinchilla model using influenza A virus strains and adenovirus. Intranasal influenza virus inoculation led to a profound drop in ME pressure, and negative pressure persisted for about 10 days.[51] Pressure returned to normal as the virus was cleared from the respiratory tract. In contrast, animals inoculated intranasally with saline or pneumococci alone showed no change in ME pressure. Influenza virus infection produced by intranasal inoculation caused marked metaplasia of the Eustachian tube epithelium, increased secretions, and obstruction of the tubal lumen.[57] Middle ear inoculation of influenza virus caused subepithelial hemorrhage, tissue edema, and acute inflammatory cell infiltration; ciliated cells were the primary target.[35] Ciliated epithelium of the tubotympanum was not restored to normal for 3 weeks. The chinchilla also readily supported adenovirus type 1 infection after intranasal or ME inoculation and responded serologically.[16]

Respiratory virus infection in children is frequently complicated by acute OM,[66] and influenza A viruses are commonly implicated.[68] We adapted the chinchilla OM model to study the interaction between pneumococci and influenza A viruses. Synergy between type 7F pneumococci and a wild-type influenza A H3N2 strain, both injected intranasally, caused a high incidence of pneumococcal OM.[51,55] Influenza infection in chinchillas followed a typical course of viral shedding from the nasopharynx for about 10 days and an increase in serum hemagglutinating antibody. Pneumococci colonized the nasopharynx for several weeks after injection. Most chinchillas survived intranasal inoculation with influenza and pneumococci without bacteremia.

In the animal model, influenza A virus strains varied in their ability to induce purulent OM.[55] When pneumococci were present in the nasopharynx during infection with an H3N2 influenza strain, purulent pneumococcal OM resulted in nearly every animal. However, an H1N1 influenza strain did not enhance the development of pneumococcal otitis, indicating that influenza viruses vary in their ability to cause acute OM. These observations in an animal model parallel clinical experience in children infected with the two virus strains and suggest that vaccines targeted against specific serotypes of influenza virus would impact the overall incidence of OM. This also may be true with other respiratory viruses.

The pathogenesis of influenza virus infection was further described by Abramson et al. Peak pneumococcal susceptibility occurred 4 days after influenza inoculation,[2] coinciding with a transient intracellular microbicidal and chemotactic defect in peripheral blood PMNL.[1] This defect appears to be caused by viral inhibition of early cell signaling, perhaps by altering binding of trimeric and monomeric G-proteins to leukocyte plasma membranes.[3]

Host inflammatory and tissue responses to nonreplicating pneumococci

Accumulating evidence from our laboratory and others suggests that pneumococcal tissue injury is triggered by cell envelope components. Thus, while many antimicrobial drugs effectively inhibit pneumococcal growth, the ensuing bacterial lysis generates pneumococcal cellular components presented to sensitive host defenses.

Pneumococcal replication in the ME is not required for development of inflammation and tissue injury.[111,123] We first reported in 1980 that nonviable pneumococci inoculated into the ME produced acute ME inflammation.[103] Tuomanen et al. demonstrated that the inflammatory response to pneumococci is triggered by the pneumococcal cell surface, particularly the cell wall.[145,146,148] We demonstrated by transmission electron micrographs that rapid heat killing (100°C for 10 min) leaves the pneumococcal capsule, cell wall, and cell membrane intact.[111] Therefore, we used heat-killed encapsulated and unencapsulated pneumococci as well as isolated native pneumococcal cell wall and cell wall digests to study local inflammatory responses in the ME of chinchillas.

Early triggering events in ME inflammation

Nonreplicating pneumococci induced an early, brief vascular response with leakage of albumin followed by α-2-macroglublin.[111] Sustained influx of acute inflammatory cells and lysozyme release into MEF began after onset of the vascular response. Killed unencapsulated pneumococci inoculated into the chinchilla ME space produced at least as much and possibly more ME inflammation than killed encapsulated pneumococci.[111] At least 10^6 pneumococcal cells (encapsulated and unencapsulated) were required to trigger the inflammatory cell influx. However, as few as 10^4 pneumococci caused an early unsustained release of lysozyme, probably from ME epithelial cells. The strong correlation between PMNL number and lysozyme concentration after 6 hr indicated that the later accumulation of lysozyme was derived predominantly from PMNL.[113] Threshold for a sustained lysozyme response was 1,000 times lower for unencapsulated than encapsulated pneumococci. Therefore, the pneumococcal cell wall initiated the early events of ME inflammation, and this response was attenuated by the organism's capsular polysaccharide. These events during the early stage of ME inflammation were not related to bacterial variability or encapsulation and most likely preceded specific humoral immune defenses.

Biochemical studies were performed to examine pathways of arachidonic acid metabolism.[112] Compared with saline-inoculated ears, significant increases in the mean concentrations of prostaglandin (PG) E_2, 6-keto-PGF$_{1a}$, leukotriene (LT) B$_4$, and LTC$_4$ were observed in pneumococcal-inoculated ears 24 hr after inoculation, but not at 6, 48, or 72 hr. Because pneumococcal inoculation caused an influx of inflammatory cells as early as 6 hr after inoculation, before the increase in eicosanoids, the initial stimulus for inflammatory cell chemotaxis is probably not eicosanoids, such as LTB$_4$; leukotrienes may, however, amplify the subsequent inflammatory response.

To determine the source of lysozyme early in the ME inflammatory response, chinchillas were irradiated to induce neutropenia, and their MEs were inoculated with heat-killed, encapsulated pneumococci.[113] In pneumococcal-inoculated ears, the mean number of inflammatory cells at 6 hr was significantly lower in irradiated than in nonirradiated animals. Mean concentrations of lysozyme, however, were similar in irradiated and nonirradiated animals at all sampling times, suggesting that ME epithelial cells were the initial source of MEF lysozyme. These results suggest that future therapeutic interventions to limit ME inflammation in acute OM will need to recognize the direct action of pneumococcal cell wall components on ME epithelium.

Capsular polysaccharide

The importance of capsular polysaccharide as a virulence factor in pneumococcal OM was demonstrated in a series of experiments using mid-log-phase, live encapsulated (type 7F) and unencapsulated (R6) pneumococci. One hundred times as many unencapsulated as encapsulated pneumococci were required to induce purulent OM. While the MEF lysozyme concentration increased significantly in ear inoculated with the unencapsulated strain (mean, 32 μg/mL) compared with saline-inoculated control ears (<1 mg/mL), lysozyme was even higher in ears inoculated with the encapsulated strain (50–100 μg/mL). Therefore, the pneumococcal capsule conferred the organism with partial resistance to host defense mechanisms. Encapsulation, however, was not required for pneumococcal-induced ME injury. Ears inoculated with the unencapsulated strain showed at least as much pathology as ears inoculated with the encapsulated strain.[123]

Cell wall

Because intact unencapsulated pneumococcal cells induced ME inflammation, an experiment was performed to measure ME responses to isolated native pneumococcal cell wall extracted from the unencapsulated R6 strain. Others have shown that pneumococcal cell walls contribute very significantly to the course of acute meningitis,[145,146,148] pneumonia,[149] and vasculitis (purpura) associated with sepsis.[33] Both acute and chronic ME mucoperiosteal histopathology were observed in ears inoculated with 10 μg of purified cell wall, an amount equivalent to approximately 10^8 bacterial cells.[123] We observed a dose-dependent increase in MEF inflammatory cells as the cell wall dose was increased from 0.7 ng to 10 μg; the threshold for inflammatory cell influx was 10 ng, which is equivalent to 10^5 pneumococci.

Different pneumococcal cell wall preparations were used to explore relationships between cell wall molecular structure and ME inflammation.[30] Native cell wall, muramidase cell wall digest, and amidase cell wall digest caused significantly more inflammatory cell influx and lysozyme accumulation in MEF than saline. Muramidase peptidoglycan digest free of teichoic acid also caused more inflammatory cell influx and lysozyme accumulation in MEF than saline, but caused less inflammation than native cell wall or either cell wall digest containing teichoic acid. Epithelial metaplasia was significantly greater in ears inoculated with native cell wall than in ears inoculated with the cell wall or peptidogylcan digests or with saline. Pneumococcal cell wall is, therefore, the principal factor that initiates ME inflammation in acute pneumococcal OM, and cell wall teichoication seems to be important in initiating this response. Middle ear mucoperiosteal granulation tissue and extensive osteoneogenesis observed in these chinchillas illustrated the chronicity of inflammation induced by pneumococcal cell wall and suggested that cell envelope components released during bacterial lysis may contribute to chronic OM in humans.[123]

Toxic oxygen species in ME injury

While PMNL contribute to ME defense during bacterial infection of the ME, the metabolic products of PMNL, which have profound cytotoxicity in other organ systems, have only recently been investigated in OM. We observed that free myeloperoxidase (MPO) in MEF was significantly increased 24 and 48 hr after either viable or nonviable pneumococci were inoculated into the ME.[83] In vitro-stimulated production of MPO and superoxide anion from MEF neutrophils was significantly less than from peripheral blood neutrophils 24 hr after pneumococcal inoculation, suggesting that oxidase metabolic products are released from phagocytic cells into the MEF during pneumococcal OM.

Chinchilla primary ME epithelial cell (MEEC) cultures were developed to study a variety of biochemical effects on MEEC function and structure.[5] Primary MEEC cultures were incubated with activated human neutrophils or with H_2O_2 to study the effect of reactive oxygen species on ME tissues. Epithelial cell viability, measured by [^{3}H]thymidine incorporation, was adversely affected by activated neutrophils and by 10^{-4} M H_2O_2, a concentration that did not affect viability of pneumococci.[85] Unstimulated neutrophils, the stimulant phorbol myristate acetate alone, and catalase alone did not affect cell viability. Catalase partially blocked the inhibitory effect of stimulated neutrophils and completely blocked the inhibitory effect of H_2O_2, indicating that H_2O_2 released from stimulated neutrophils accounted for some but not all the epithelial cell injury. These experiments revealed that inhibition of epithelial cell metabolism by neutrophil reactive oxygen species during OM may contribute to epithelial metaplasia and secretory cell transformation observed in the middle ear in chronic OM.

Lytic and nonlytic antibiotic effect on pneumococcal-induced ME inflammation

Procaine penicillin G given intramuscularly 12 hr after inoculation of pneumococci into chinchilla MEs caused a significant acceleration in MEF inflammatory cell influx and rise in lysosyzme concentrations compared with untreated controls.[84] Penicillin treatment of experimental pneumococcal OM accelerated inflammatory cell influx and lysozyme release, probably via lytic cell wall fragments and pneumolysin.[55,84] Viable pneumococci were not detected in MEF after the second penicillin dose, but pneumococcal wall was detected microscopically for 45 days. Therefore, penicillin treatment accelerated ME inflammation while killing pneumococci, but treatment did not accelerate clearance of the nonviable pneumococcal cells from MEF, perhaps contributing to chronic ME tissue injury.

The inflammatory effect of penicillin depended on the timing of penicillin administration and the concentration of pneumococci in MEF. Penicillin administered 12 hr after ME inoculation of type 3 pneumococcus, when there were approximately 10^3 pneumococcal colony forming units (CFU) per mL in MEF, produced accelerated MEF inflammatory cell influx, as seen using similar conditions with type 7F pneumococcus.[131] Penicillin did not produce this effect when administered 24 hr after pneumococcal inoculation, when there were approximately 10^7 CFU/mL in MEF. This is not surprising because the inflammatory cell threshold in the chinchilla middle ear is 10^5–10^6 pneumococci, a level surpassed at 24 hr. These results suggest that effective clinical antiinflammatory interventions will need to be applied very early in the course of ME inflammation.

Effects of the nonlytic antibiotic ciprofloxacin on pneumococcal-induced ME inflammation were studied in chinchillas sacrificed for temporal bone histopathology after 5 days of treatment (D. Canafax, unpublished observation). Middle ear mucosal histopathology included subepithelial edema, goblet cell hyperplasia, PMNL, and mononuclear infiltration. Pathology was significantly less in chinchillas treated with a ciprofloxacin dose that achieved MEF concentrations in excess of the pneumococcal ciprofloxacin minimum inhibitory concentration (MIC) compared to untreated chinchillas and those treated with a dose that achieved MEF concentrations slightly less than MIC.

Pneumolysin

Pneumolysin, the intracellular cytolysin of *S. pneumoniae* released on autolysin-induced cell lysis, appears to contribute to the inflammatory response caused by this organism in murine and rabbit models. Pneumolysin is produced during pneumococcal infection *in vivo* as evidenced by its detection in lung, spleen, and liver from mice challenged with virulent pneumococci,[118] and by presence of anti-pneumolysin antibody and circulating pneumolysin immune complexes in serum from patients with pneumococcal pneumonia.[78,81,95] Pneumolysin produced lung inflammation as demonstrated by intrapulmonary injection of pathogen-free Wistar rats with recombinant pneumolysin (rPL).[45] Tissue histopathology was identical to that induced by a living pneumolysin-producing pneumococcus. Heat-inactivation of rPL neutralized the injury. Reducing either the hemolytic activity or complement-activating property of rPL by isogenic mutation also reduced lung injury. Pneumolysin slowed ciliary beating and disrupted the surface integrity of human respiratory epithelium in organ culture,[44,46,121,141] and was cytotoxic for pulmonary endothelial[126] and epithelial cells.[127] Pneumolysin also caused toxic effects in rabbit cornea.[74]

Pertinent to pneumococcal OM, pneumolysin was found to cause disorganization and loss of cochlear cilia and damage to hair cell bundles in guinea pigs.[36] Guinea pig round window membranes treated *ex vivo* with streptolysin O, a pneumolysin-related cytolysin, showed permeability defects and marked epithelial cell pathology with defects in the cell membranes, detached cells, and denuded basal membrane.[40] These observations suggest a mechanism for sensorineural hearing loss in acute OM.

We used a type 3 pneumococcal strain (WT3) and its isogenic mutants to explore further the contribution of pneumolysin and autolysin-released cell wall products in OM pathogenesis.[132] Insertion-inactivation mutants lacking pneumolysin synthesis (P-1) and autolysin synthesis (A-1) were employed. Log-phase pneumococci were inoculated into the ME of chinchillas followed by procaine penicillin treatment 12 hr after pneumococcal inoculation. Penicillin significantly accelerated MEF inflammatory cell influx in WT3- and P-1-inoculated ears compared with respective untreated controls. Penicillin did not accelerate inflammatory cell influx in the A-1-infected group. Therefore, ME inflammation induced by a lytic antibiotic appears to be caused by release of lytic cell wall products and not pneumolysin.

Middle ear cytokine responses

Several cytokines—interleukin-1α (IL-1α), IL-1β, IL-2, IL-6, tumor necrosis factor-α (TNF-α), interferon-γ (IFN-γ) gran-ulocyte-macrophage colony-stimulating factor (GM-CSF)—have been demonstrated in MEF from children with chronic OME.[69,153,154] Compared to older children, younger children had higher IL-1 concentrations and lower TNF-α concentrations in MEF.[153] The number of cytokines present implies a "cytokine network."

We assayed 70 MEF samples from 56 children with chronic OME for several cytokines; highest concentrations of IL-1β and TNF-α were found in purulent MEF samples, and concentrations were higher in younger than older patients.[80] These observations suggest a linkage between acute OM and chronic OM because IL-1β and TNF-α have been shown to play a central role in regulating immune and inflammatory responses, including the stimulation of additional cytokines, fibroblast proliferation, osteoclast activation, endothelial leakage, intravascular thrombosis, vasodilation, and inflammatory cell activation.[142]

IL-8, a monocyte- and macrophage-derived cytokine with potent chemotactic-activating properties, contributes to OM pathogenesis as evidenced by detection of IL-8 mRNA in 75% of human MEF samples.[143] Another study found soluble IL-8 in 92% of MEF samples.[109] mRNAs for IL-1β, IL-6, and TNF-α were detected in 100% of OME samples, but IL-3, IL-5, and IFN-γ were present in only about 50% and mRNAs for IL-2 and IL-4 were present in none.[117] After *in vitro* infection of ME mucosal cultures with RSV, mRNA for IL-1β, IL-6, and TNF-α increased within 3 hr.[117] Cell adhesion molecule (CAM) expression (ICAM-1, VCAM-1, ELAM-1) increased over 12 hr. Kinetics of these responses suggest cytokines stimulate synthesis of CAMs in ME mucosa.

Johnson et al.[73] reported that chinchilla and human cytokines cross-reacted, and we have made similar observations.[132] Serous OM produced by Eustachian tube obstruction in chinchillas caused an increase in IL-1β and TNF-α in MEF. Presence of pneumococci in the ME further increased TNF-α but not IL-1β.[73] Recombinant IL-2 injected into the guinea pig ME produced a cellular MEF with predominant PMNLs, which cleared by 72 hr; recombinant TNF produced a MEF with lymphocytes that cleared by 48 hr; and recombinant IL-1 did not produce MEF.[31]

Recently, we assayed chinchilla MEF samples obtained 1–72 hr after ME inoculation of type 3 pneumococcus for IL-1β, TNF-α, and IL-6 using high-sensitivity enzyme-linked immunosorbent assay (ELISA) kits that employed human monoclonal antibodies (respective sensitivities: IL-1β = 0.125, TNF-α = 0.5, and IL-6 = 1.56 pg/mL) (G.S. Giebink, unpublished observation). IL-1β concentration peaked 6 hr after inoculating pneumococci, and TNF-α and IL-6 concentrations did not start to increase significantly until 72 hr.

Using radioimmunoassay, we reported detection of IL-6 activity in 100% of chinchilla purulent and 53% of serous MEF samples.[20] Both IL-1 and TNF have been shown to induce IL-6 production, the activity of which includes activation of cytotoxic cells and stimulation of T- and B-lymphocyte proliferation.

We have shown that TNF-α stimulates mucous glycoprotein (MGP) secretion in primary chinchilla MEEC cultures (J. Lin, unpublished observation). Others have demonstrated IL-1 stimulated mucus secretion from lung explants[108] and from intestinal explants.[64] TNF-α has been shown to regulate intestinal mucin production and changes in goblet cells in a murine *Salmonella typhimurium* model.[11] Thus, cytokine stimulation of MEEC is a likely trigger of chronic mucoid OM in children.

Platelet-activating factor

Platelet-activating factor (PAF) has been identified in human MEF, and a report suggested that PAF may develop and maintain OME by stimulating vascular permeability and chemotaxis.[32] PAF is an inflammatory mediator produced by macrophages, neutrophils, platelets, and endothelial cells in response to injury.[71,152] PAF activates cells by binding to a member of the superfamily of G-protein receptors.[70] PAF induces increased vascular permeability with protein exudation, accumulation of platelets and leukocytes, blood–brain barrier permeability and brain edema.[24,71]

Rhee et al. induced OME in chinchillas by injecting ME bullae with PAF; the PAF receptor antagonist WEB 2170 injected intraperitoneally prevented PAF-induced OME.[122] PAF is a strong secretagogue of MGP in the lower respiratory tract,[4] and we demonstrated that PAF stimulated MGP secretion from primary chinchilla MEEC cultures *in vitro*.[97] MGP secretion was inhibited by cycloheximide, a protein synthesis inhibitor, and it was also significantly, although not completely, inhibited by WEB 2170, suggesting that the inhibitor competitively bound to PAF receptors on MEEC but at lower affinity than PAF.[97]

PAF-stimulated MGP secretion by MEEC is also mediated by lipoxygenase metabolites of arachidonic acid, as demonstrated by our experiment in which nordihydroguaretic acid (an inhibitor of both cyclooxygenase and lipoxygenase metabolites) and A63162 (a lipoxygenase inhibitor) inhibited MGP secretion, but indomethacin (a cyclooxygenase inhibitor) did not.[98] PAF-stimulated MGP secretion was decreased by dexamethasone, and this effect was reversed by PLA_2, indicating that dexamethasone acted through the arachidonic acid pathway (J. Lin, unpublished observation).

We have also used primary chinchilla MEEC cultures to study the effects of arachidonic acid metabolites on MGP secretion. Each of three metabolites (PGD_2, PGE_2, and LTC_4) added in concentrations of 1–100 μM caused a dose-dependent increase in MGP secretion by MEEC cultures, which was inhibited by cycloheximide.[6]

Neuraminidase

Pneumococci are a rich source of several extracellular glycosidases. One of these, neuraminidase, has been demonstrated in ME effusions from patients with acute OM and chronic OME; and neuraminidase activity was highly correlated with the presence of pneumococci in MEF.[38,93] Because pneumococcal neuraminidase removed sialic acid residues from chinchilla ME mucosa, LaMarco et al. speculated that pneumococcal infection of the ME may increase mucosal susceptibility to attack by other bacterial and host hydrolases.[94]

Recent molecular evidence suggests that neuraminidase is a surface protein, or that it is released to the extracellular environment.[25] In patients with pneumococcal meningitis, there is a direct relationship between neuraminidase concentration in CSF and adverse outcome.[114] Moreover, death was caused by intracerebral inoculation of neuraminidase in mice.[86] Mice immunized with purified neuraminidase were partially protected against pneumococcal infection.[100] After pneumococcal inoculation of the ME in the chinchilla OM model, neuraminidase persisted in MEF for extended periods of time, and its persistence was independent of antibiotic treatment.[93] Its ability to decrease the viscosity of mucus[133] could also enhance pneumococcal colonization of underlying tissues. Linder et al. demonstrated exposure of *N*-acetylglucosamine in chinchilla ME and Eustachian tube epithelium during pneumococcal OM and after intranasal inoculation of pneumococci, respectively.[57,99] This observation suggests that pneumococcal enzymes facilitate colonization and middle ear invasion.

Semiquantitative ME histomorphometry

In the course of examining temporal bones from chinchillas with various forms of OM, we developed a semiquantitative scoring system.[123] The inferior bulla is examined and scored at three distinct anatomical levels. For statistical analyses, composite scores for similar histopathological parameters in the subepithelial space and middle ear space are used.

Rate of bacterial growth in chinchilla MEF

An experiment was conducted to determine whether soluble products of ME host defense affect the rate of pneumococcal growth. Encapsulated pneumococci were grown to mid-log phase in Todd-Hewitt broth supplemented with bovine albumin, centrifuged, and resuspended in one of three vehicles: sterile MEF (from chinchillas with serous MEF), normal chinchilla serum, and fresh Todd-Hewitt broth (control). Continued log-phase growth was observed in all three fluids during the succeeding 4-hr incubation at 37°C. Therefore, neither serous chinchilla MEF nor serum contain substances inhibitory to pneumococcal growth.

Pneumococcal adherence

Principal in the relationship of pneumococci with mammalian hosts is the initial attachment of pneumococci to respiratory tract epithelial cells.[47] During adherence, incompletely described pneumococcal adhesin(s)[19] interact with epithelial glycoconjugate receptors—a glycoconjugate with β1-3 linkage to GlcNAc[10] or β1-4 linkage to GalNAc.[91] Several methods for measuring pneumococcal adherence to nonciliated squamous cells have been described,[8,9,92,106,136] and pneumococci adhere to isolated oropharyngeal cells,[8,9,10,106,110] but these methods have questionable relevance to OM pathogenesis.

Major carbohydrate moieties expressed in the Eustachian tube epithelial glycocalyx have been identified by Lim et al.,[96] and many are known components of bacterial receptors.[135] A decreased incidence of infection by certain pathogens has been demonstrated after blocking specific carbohydrate moieties located in the glycocalyx of epithelial cells.[13]

Because ME infection most likely requires bacterial pathogens to adhere to cuboidal and columnar ciliated and nonciliated cells in the nasopharynx, Eustachian tube, and ME, we developed an assay employing isolated ciliated and nonciliated cells from the chinchilla ME.[65] Isolated epithelial cells had cilia beat frequency similar to nondissociated cells, and lectin binding indicated that terminal saccharide residues were intact. Pneumococcal adherence was proportional to the number of pneumococci adherent to human buccal epithelial cells reported by Andersson et al.[9]

We studied adherence of five pneumococcal serotypes.[65] All five strains adhered in greater numbers to ciliated than to non-ciliated MEEC and tracheal epithelial cells (TEC), and adherence of all five strains was greater to ciliated TEC than to ciliated MEEC. Type 18C was significantly less adherent than types 6B, 7F, and 23F, and type 14 adherence was intermediate. Wheat germ agglutinin (WGA) bound strongly to cilia of MEEC and TEC. Preincubation of ciliated TEC with WGA significantly reduced type 6B pneumococcal adhesion suggesting that the terminal GlcNAcβ1-4 sequence is specific for pneumococcal adherence to chinchilla respiratory epithelial cilia.[65]

Tuomanen also reported that unencapsulated pneumococci adhered *in vitro* to cilia of isolated rabbit tracheal ciliated cells, and adherence was greatly enhanced after pretreatment of ciliated cells with *B. pertussis* adhesins.[147] The exogenous adhesins had no effect, however, on adhesion of an encapsulated type 3 strain and only a modest effect on an encapsulated type 2 strain.

We found no consistent relationship between ME virulence in the chinchilla model and pneumococcal adherence to chinchilla MEEC.[65] Andersson et al.[8,9] also found no relationship between capsular serotype and adherence to human oropharyngeal epithelial cells. The discordance between adherence *in vitro* and virulence may reflect bacterial interaction with the mucous blanket *in vivo*, since some pneumococci may adhere to glycoconjugates in mucus secreted by underlying epithelial cells before they can interact with cilia.

Adherence of pneumococci to isolated chinchilla MEEC and TEC was also studied during influenza A virus (H$_3$N$_2$) infection in chinchillas. Adherence of type 6B and 7F strains was significantly increased in infected compared to control chinchillas (S. Hando and G.S. Giebink, unpublished observations). These observations suggest that pneumococcal OM susceptibility is influenced by the ability of influenza A virus to unmask or upregulate epithelial cell receptors for pneumococci.

OTITIS MEDIA IMMUNOLOGY

Affinity-purified chinchilla immunoglobulin reagents

Because immunologic studies in the chinchilla have been limited by the lack of antibodies against specific immunoglobulin isotypes, we prepared isotype-specific rabbit antibodies against the heavy-chain components of chinchilla immunoglobulins G, M, and A.[87] Chromatographic techniques were used to isolate chinchilla immunoglobulins from serum and breast milk; heavy-chain fractions were isolated and used as antigens to produce isotype-specific antibodies in rabbits, and anti-light chain cross-reactivity was removed by affinity chromatography. Using the affinity-purified antibodies, we developed a sensitive ELISA that is highly specific for IgG, IgM, and IgA antibodies against pneumococcal capsular polysaccharide (PS) types 6A, 6B, 14, 18C, 19A, and 19F and against C polysaccharide (C-Ps) in chinchilla serum and MEF.[89] Sensitivity of the type 14 antibody assay was enhanced using an avidin–biotin complex detection system to measure low concentrations of type 14 antibody produced during experimental OM. Using a modification of antibody quantitation described by Zollinger and Boslego,[157] microgram antibody values were assigned to reference chinchilla serum pools.

Pneumococcal antibody and susceptibility to homologous reinfection

We studied the hypothesis that early antibiotic treatment of POM suppresses the immune response during ME infection and predisposes to POM reinfections.[82] Acute, unilateral, type-14 pneumococcal OM was produced by direct ME inoculation, followed by prompt or delayed procaine penicillin G treatment. After full recovery 4 weeks later, animals were rechallenged bilaterally with the same type 14 strain. Susceptibility to pneumococcal OM was reduced from 88% in the initially inoculated right ear to 38% when this ear was reinoculated ($p < 0.001$); only 46% of previously uninoculated left ears became infected ($p < 0.001$). Thus, previous unilateral infection provided contralateral ME protection, suggesting that unilateral pneumococcal OM induced systemic immune defenses. Susceptibility of previously infected right ears to repeat OM was significantly greater in the prompt treatment group (64%) than in the delayed treatment group (35%), suggesting that early penicillin treatment interfered with local or systemic immune response. Type 14 anti-PCP IgG serum antibodies were similar, however, in the prompt and delayed treatment groups after initial infection. Moreover, there was not a significant correlation between serum antibody immediately preceding repeat pneumococcal inoculation and ME response to the second inoculation. Thus, the clinical response of the middle ear to rechallenge may be mediated by local IgA antibody.

Lymphoproliferative inhibitor

Middle ear fluid from chinchillas with pneumococcal OM inhibited the lymphoproliferative response of chinchilla peripheral blood lymphocytes to stimulation with phytohemagglutinin.[39] Inhibitor was absent in plasma suggesting local production of the inhibitor.

Pneumococcal immune complexes in MEF

We developed a sensitive ELISA method for measuring immune complexes carrying pneumococcal type 6B-PS and cell wall polysaccharide (C-Ps) as antigens.[88] The antigen portion was captured by anti-6B-PS or anti-C-Ps antibody-coated plates, and the antibody portion was detected using biotin-labeled rabbit IgG anti-chinchilla IgG, IgM, or IgA. MEF was obtained from 44 chinchillas with type 6B pneumococcal OM on days 3–9 after pneumococcal inoculation. Types 6B-PS IgG immune complexes were present in 10–32% of samples, and C-PS immune complexes were present in 23–56% of samples. IgM immune complexes were present in only one sample, and IgA immune complexes in none. There was no correlation between 6B-PS IgG and C-Ps IgG immune complexes. These results suggest that IgG immune complexes are formed during pneumococcal OM in humans and may contribute to the pathogenesis of pneumococcal OM.

Immunoprophylaxis

Development of vaccines to prevent pneumococcal AOM early in life is a major child health goal. Observations more than a decade ago revealed accelerated clearing of ME infection in children[140] and in the chinchilla model[52] when high type-specific anti-PS antibody concentrations were present in MEF. Clinical trials also showed that immunization with polyvalent PS vaccine gave serotype-specific protection in children[107] and the chinchilla model[50]; however, protection was limited to the most immunogenic types. In one trial, an octavalent vaccine prevented 67% of vaccine-type pneumococcal AOM episodes in 7- to 24-month-old children after excluding infections caused by the poorly immunogenic serogroup 6.[107] Enhanced immunogenicity of PS vaccines in infants, therefore, would be expected to have a major impact on the incidence of AOM disease.

Local secretion of IgA, IgG, and IgM by the ME mucosa has been considered to be important in preventing ME infection.[115,139] However, the proportionate contribution of local and systemic antibodies has been difficult to discern in vaccine studies because active immunization may stimulate both systemic and local antibody production.[119] Passive immunization studies in chinchillas demonstrated that intravenously-administered immune serum prevented middle ear infection with *H. influenzae* type b (Hib),[17] and systemically administered IgG anti-PS antibody prevented pneumococcal OM.[137] Similarly, IgG antibody against Hib enhanced bacterial clearance in the murine lower respiratory tract.[144] A clinical trial revealed that immune serum globulin-treated children had a 57% reduction of OM incidence compared to control subjects.[37] Thus, it seems reasonable to expect that vaccines designed to protect the ME should induce specific IgG antibodies.

Capsular polysaccharide vaccines

The chinchilla model has been useful in studying ME protection against pneumococci after systemic immunization. Systemically administered PS vaccines were modestly immunogenic in chinchillas, and subcutaneous immunization elicited at least a 10-fold increase in serum antibody in approximately two-thirds of immunized chinchillas.[54] Chinchillas with at least a two-fold serum antibody increase after immunization showed an 87% reduction in vaccine-type pneumococcal OM, compared to a 28% reduction in immunized nonresponding animals.[50] Animals with higher antibody titers in MEF showed more rapid clearing of viable pneumococci from MEF.[52]

Fortunately, only a few of the 90 pneumococcal serotypes—types 6A, 6B, 14, 19F, and 23F—account for nearly 60% of childhood pneumococcal AOM and other invasive diseases.[14] It is probably not coincidental that these are also the types against which antibody responsiveness appears later in childhood. Evidence that maturation of the pneumococcal antibody response leads to greater ME resistance against the pneumococci comes from an analysis of 704 first attacks of pneumococcal AOM; 61% occurred during the first year of life, 18% in the second, and 7% in the third year.[14]

Conjugate vaccines

Invasive disease caused by Hib, another polysaccharide encapsulated bacteria, now can be prevented in infants by systemic immunization with vaccines consisting of the capsular polysaccharide antigen, both high-molecular-weight polysaccharide and derived oligosaccharides, coupled to carrier proteins.[22,43,130] These conjugate vaccines produce an enhanced serum antibody response, which has been attributed to protein-elicited T lymphocyte helper effects.[124]

Similar approaches have been tried using PS. Schneerson et al.[134] first reported the immunogenicity of PS-protein conjugate vaccines: A tetanus toxoid conjugate of type 6A PS raised both 6A and tetanus antibodies in adults. Anderson and Betts[7] studied in adult volunteers the immunogenicity of types 6A, 14, 18C, 19F, and 23F saccharides of varying length and composition coupled by reductive amination to diphtheria toxoid. Immunogenicity of the type 6A conjugate was associated with higher overall saccharide content rather than chain length. Parallel changes in total anti-capsular and IgG-specific antibodies were noted. Eleven of 19 subjects who demonstrated significant antibody responses to one of the several conjugate preparations also had a significant rise in type-specific opsonic activity, and eight subjects did not.

We studied the immunogenicity and efficacy of PS conjugates composed of hydrolyzed PS conjugated to outer membrane protein complex (OMPC) from *Neisseria meningitidis* group B bacteria in the chinchilla model.[59] Type 6B monovalent, type 23F monovalent, type 6B + 23F bivalent, and type 6B + 14 + 19F + 23F tetravalent PS-OMPC conjugate vaccines were very immunogenic in chinchillas, producing 100–1,000 times more anti-PS antibody in serum than plain PS vaccines. These serum responses are relevant because both an earlier study[52] and this study showed strong relationships between serum antibody and type-specific ME protection. IgG, IgM, and some IgA type-6B antibodies were produced, and animals boosted 28 days after priming showed an anamnestic increase in IgG antibodies. Shorter intervals between priming and booster (7 and 14 days) did not accelerate type 6B antibody responses as has been observed in mice (P. Vella, unpublished observation).

Interactions between PS antigens in the vaccines were examined in bivalent and tetravalent preparations.[59] There was no interference of types 6B, 14, or 19F PS on the antibody response to type 23F PS, nor was there interference of type 23F PS on the antibody response to type 6B PS. However, the type 6B anti-PS antibody response to a booster dose of tetravalent vaccines was lower than the response to a booster dose of monovalent type 6B vaccine. Whether this represents antigen interference will require additional study. Such interference has not been observed with the tetravalent vaccine in infant Rhesus monkeys (P. Vella, unpublished observation). To our knowledge, this issue has not been addressed in previous studies with multivalent plain PS vaccines.

Type 6B containing conjugate vaccines prevented or greatly attenuated pneumococcal AOM in 63% of immunized animals.[59] Middle ear protection tended to be better in animals given one or two vaccine doses and challenged after 42–56 days. Protection was not significantly different among animals given one or two doses of monovalent vaccine, one dose of bivalent vaccine, or two doses of tetravalent vaccine, although the 28-day challenge protocol yielded significantly greater protection with bivalent than monovalent vaccine.

Type 19F conjugate in the tetravalent mixture elicited a highly protective ME response, but type 14 conjugate in the same mixture failed to protect.[59] Because type 14 conjugate elicited a slightly higher total mean serum antibody concentration before challenge (2.07 mg/mL) than either type 19F conjugate (1.85 mg/mL) or type 6B conjugate (0.82 mg/mL), differences in ME outcome among the three serotypes could be explained by a different isotype antibody response to type 14 conjugate or by an enhanced host inflammatory response to type 14 pneumococci.

Serum antibody correlates of ME protection

The concentrations of serum antibodies against 6B-PS and 19F-PS measured by radioimmunoassay (RIA) immediately before challenge were strongly associated with protection.[59] Correlation coefficients between antibody concentration and ME severity score were highly significant for both types. Type 6B pneumococcal OM developed in 72% of animals with anti-6B-PS serum antibody concentrations less than 1.0 mg/mL, and in only 13% with higher antibody concentrations. Type 19F pneumococcal OM developed in 75% of animals with anti-19F-PS serum antibody concentrations less than 1.0 mg/mL, and in none of seven with higher antibody concentrations.

Cross-protection between serotypes

Type 6B and 23F vaccines did not elicit heterologous antibodies (i.e., anti-23F and anti-6B, respectively), and immunization with type 23F vaccine did not protect against type 6B infection.[59] Cross-protection among pneumococcal subtypes within serogroups was reported.[60] Chinchillas were given two doses of a tetravalent vaccine composed of four pneumococcal PS (types 6B, 14, 19F, 23F) conjugated to OMPC. Vaccination induced at least a two-fold anti-PS IgG serum antibody rise against types 6A, 6B, 19A, and 19F PS in 71%, 89%, 94%, and 96% of chinchillas, respectively. Geometric mean post-vaccination antibody titers tended to be higher for subtypes contained in the vaccine (6B, 19F) than for related subtypes (6A, 19A).

Middle ear outcomes were not significantly different in ears of vaccinated chinchillas challenged with types 6B and 6A strains, and both groups had significantly better outcomes than the respective placebo vaccine groups. The vaccine was significantly more protective for type 19F OM than type 19A disease. Post-challenge OM severity for individual chinchillas was inversely correlated with serum anti-PS IgG antibody concentration at the time of challenge. Therefore, 6B-OMPC elicited type-specific antibody and protection for both subtypes within group 6. Type 19F-OMPC stimulated type specific antibody for both 19F and 19A PS, but it did not cross-protect against 19A disease.

Vaccine polyvalency

Clinically effective pneumococcal vaccines must be able to protect against several pneumococcal serotypes. Vaccine polyvalency may be a concern with PS conjugate vaccines because the conjugated protein antigens could adversely interact to reduce vaccine immunogenicity and efficacy. We studied this interaction in the chinchilla model using monovalent (types 6B and 14), tetravalent (types 6B, 14, 19F, 23F), and heptavalent (types 4, 6B, 9V, 14, 18C, 19F, 23F) PS-OMPC conjugate vaccines.[61] Types 6B and 14 IgG antibody distributions in serum were not significantly different in the respective monovalent and polyvalent vaccine groups; type 19F IgG antibody distributions were similar in the two polyvalent vaccine groups.

Vaccine efficacy was tested by injecting both MEs of immunized and control chinchillas with type 6B, 14, or 19F pneumococci. Middle ear outcomes after types 6B and 19F challenge were significantly better for immunized chinchillas than controls. Disease was not modified in the tetravalent vaccine group challenged with type 14 pneumococci, perhaps due to lower type 14 antibody concentrations prechallenge than in the 6B and 19F vaccine groups. Monovalent, tetravalent, and heptavalent preparations of 6B-OMPC vaccine yielded similar efficacy, as did tetravalent and heptavalent preparations of 19F-OMPC vaccine. Thus, 6B and 19F PS-OMPC monovalent and polyvalent vaccine mixtures have similar type-specific immunogenicity and OM efficacy.

Vaccine efficacy during influenza infection

Direct ME inoculation of pneumococci is an extremely vigorous test of vaccine efficacy. It bypasses the natural nasopharyngeal acquisition of pneumococci, their adherence to nasopharyngeal epithelium, and ascent to the ME via the Eustachian tube. Mucosal defense mechanisms, therefore, are less likely to contribute to ME protection in the direct ME challenge model than after nasopharyngeal colonization. Although a conservative test of vaccine efficacy is an important step in the evaluation of a new vaccine, conditions associated with the natural history of an illness should also be tested to measure true vaccine effectiveness in the target population of children.

We tested the efficacy of monovalent types 6B and 14 PS-OMPC conjugate vaccines by injecting the anterior nares of chinchillas with wild influenza A (H3N2) virus, and 4 days later injected the vaccine-type pneumococcal strain intranasally.[62] Both vaccines administered intramuscularly in two doses produced significant serum IgG anti-PS antibody responses. Prechallenge serum anti-PS IgG antibody titers were at least 0.5 μg/mL in 93% of chinchillas given type 6B conjugate vaccine and 88% given type 14 conjugate vaccine; this serum titer was previously demonstrated to predict vaccine-type ME protection in the chinchilla model.[60]

After intranasal influenza-pneumococcal challenge, type 6B pneumococcal OM developed in 45% and type 14 pneumococcal OM developed in 75% of unvaccinated control chinchillas. Compared with controls, type 6B vaccine efficacy was 72% against type 6B pneumococcal OM; type 14 vaccine efficacy was 29% against type 14 pneumococcal OM. Previously reported efficacy rates using direct ME pneumococcal challenge without influenza virus infection were 64% and 17% for types 6B and 14 conjugate vaccines, respectively.[59,60] Thus, conjugate vaccine efficacy for type 14 pneumococcal OM was nearly two-fold better after intranasal influenza-pneumococcal challenge than after direct ME challenge with pneumococci alone. Efficacy of type 6B conjugate vaccine was similar using both challenge protocols. Greater virulence of type 14 than type 6B pneumococci in the chinchilla model probably accounted for lower vaccine efficacy with type 14 conjugate vaccine compared to 6B conjugate in both challenge models.

Influenza vaccine efficacy

The efficacy of an attenuated influenza A virus vaccine (CR29) administered intranasally and formalin-inactivated influenza A vaccine given intramuscularly in preventing pneumococcal OM after intranasal challenge with wild influenza A virus and type 7F pneumococcus has been reported by our laboratory.[58] Seroconversion rates in the attenuated and inactivated influenza vaccine groups were similar (62% and 57%, respectively). The attenuated viral vaccine but not the inactivated vaccine significantly reduced nasal titers of both the challenge wild virus strain and pneumococci. The incidence of OM was significantly lower in the attenuated vaccine group (18%) than in controls (41%), but was not lower in the inactivated vaccine group (39%). Thus, attenuated influenza virus immunization administered intranasally may be an effective pneumococcal OM prophylaxis strategy in children.

ANTIMICROBIAL PHARMACOLOGY

The study of antibiotic dose, blood concentration, and tissue concentration is central to understanding and improving OM treatment.[21] It is intuitive that if concentrations of antibiotics reaching the infected ME space are below the MIC for the infecting bacteria, treatment failure or chronic OME may result. Pharmacokinetic characteristics that dictate antibiotic diffusion into the ME have just begun to be evaluated in models of OM.[26,27,28,75,79]

Most reports on the penetration of antibiotics into the ME have evaluated only the relative amount of drug distributing into the ME at a single time point. A modest number of reports describe antibiotic pharmacokinetic studies in patients with AOM or chronic OME.[18,90,138] Most are single-dose studies in which an antibiotic is given orally or intramuscularly, and a single MEF sample is obtained several hours later. Concentration data are pooled to determine a mean peak drug concentration in the MEF.

The pharmacokinetic characteristics of antibiotics differ between acute OM and chronic OME; MEF concentrations are higher in acute OM than in chronic OME. We have seen similar effects of acute inflammation in the chinchilla OM model, where amoxicillin and trimethoprim-sulfamethoxazole (TMP/SMX) concentrations were higher in experimental purulent than in serous OM.[26,27,75,79] One important implication of these findings is that doses of antibiotics used to prevent AOM in children with chronic OME need to be at least as high as doses used to treated AOM.

Pharmacologic assay methods

To study OM treatment, it is necessary to develop sensitive high-performance liquid chromatographic (HPLC) methods that measure antibiotic concentrations in extremely small amounts of plasma and MEF. We developed assays in these matrices for measuring trimethoprim and sulfamethoxazole,[41] amoxicillin,[42] ciprofloxacin,[101] and cefpodoxime.[102] Recently, we improved the sensitivity for measuring amoxicillin in human plasma and MEF.[155,156]

Pharmacokinetic animal studies

Otitis media animal models provide well-controlled conditions for measuring antibiotic pharmacokinetics in OM. The disease can be reliably produced with reasonably homogeneous pathology among animals, MEF can be sampled repetitively,

and the baseline pathology and MEF biochemistry has been described in untreated animals, providing a reference for future studies.[56]

Our studies in chinchilla models revealed that antibiotic distribution from blood into the ME cavity depends on ME mucosa blood vessel permeability.[26,27,75,79] Because the degree of inflammatory changes differs among OM types, the severity and characteristics of ME inflammation will affect treatment of the disease.

Small MEF volumes limit this model when studying the effect of certain factors on antibiotic penetration. We circumvented this limitation by instilling antibiotic solutions directly into the ME space, and measured "reverse" distribution of the drug from the ME to plasma.[75]

We found that TMP penetrates the mucosal membrane faster than amoxicillin or sulfamethoxazole in both the normal and infected ME.[26] However, TMP penetration increased the least of these three antibiotics when comparing normal with infected ME mucosa. Amoxicillin penetrated the mucosal membrane at the slowest rate in both the normal and infected ME, but amoxicillin penetration increased the most from normal to infected ME. Our findings paralleled those of Vogelman et al.[151] and suggest that time over bacterial MIC is the most significant parameter determining β-lactam antibiotic efficacy. Thus, there may be a need to attain supra-MIC concentration in MEF to produce maximal OM treatment response.

A recent study in children demonstrated a 10-fold greater antibiotic treatment failure rate in children with acute OM where both a pathogenic bacteria and virus were isolated from MEF compared to cases where only a bacteria was isolated.[34] The authors suggested that drug penetration into the ME may be altered by concomitant viral infection, resulting in subtherapeutic MEF antibiotic levels.[12] We explored this relationship in the chinchilla model. Influenza virus infection significantly decreased MEF penetration of amoxicillin, TMP and SMX in ears with pneumococcal OM compared to noninfluenza-infected chinchillas with POM.[77]

Adjunctive OM treatment could include drugs that limit ME inflammation. We observed the opposite effect, however, in the chinchilla model using the nonsteroidal antiinflammatory drug ibuprofen.[78] Chinchillas with pneumococcal OM treated with ibuprofen and penicillin had more ME pathology than control animals treated with penicillin alone. In contrast, methylprednisolone- and penicillin-treated animals had less inflammation than controls. Given the frequent use of antipyretic drugs in acute OM, further studies should explore relationships between antimicrobial and antiinflammatory drugs on ME response.

Chinchilla ME surface area and volume

The surface area (SA) to volume (V) ratio of an extravascular space is an important determinant of drug concentration behavior in the space. Using quantitative histomorphometry, we measured the ME space in 10 healthy chinchillas without OM and found a mean V of 2.09 mL and SA of 14.41 cm^2.[75] The chinchilla ME SA/V of 6.93 compares with other species and humans; therefore, a significant change in elimination rate constant (K_e) should not occur with small changes in volume, a fact we have supported experimentally.[75] In the clinical situation, this indicates that the concentration of an antibiotic achieved in the MEF is the same for any given effusion volume, although this assumes that the effusion is homogeneous and mixed, an issue that needs further study.

Antibiotic treatment trials in chinchillas

A randomized trial showed that cefixime in single or split daily dose and ampicillin thrice daily were equally effective in sterilizing MEF after pneumococcal infection.[105] Ceftibuten was studied in a controlled trial of *H. influenza* OM and found to be superior to ampicillin but comparable to cefixime in time to MEF sterilization.[125]

In vitro *OM model*

We used an *in vitro* model of antibiotic membrane diffusion to study amoxicillin concentration and bacterial killing.[150] This model system mimics ME and plasma antibiotic concentrations using a semipermeable membrane. We studied type 7F pneumococcal killing (amoxicillin MIC = 0.002 μg/mL) over 4 hr following a single amoxicillin bolus dose to produce peak plasma concentrations seen in children, ranging from 0.26 to 14.6 μg/mL. Amoxicillin elimination from the ME compartment was slower than from the plasma (mean $T_{1/2}$ = 2.3 vs. 0.97 hr).[128] Peak ear compartment concentrations occurred at 2 hr and were 30% of plasma compartment concentrations. The time for 99% killing of the bacterial inoculum was 1.5 hr at all concentrations tested. At peak amoxicillin concentrations of less than 2 μg/mL, a lag in bacterial killing occurred. The similarity of these amoxicillin *in vitro* pharmacokinetic data to *in vivo* chinchilla modeling experience suggests that the *in vitro* system will be useful for studying both antibiotic pharmacokinetics and bacterial killing for various drugs and ME conditions.

Ciprofloxacin ME pharmacokinetics

Ciprofloxacin has inhibitory but nonlytic activity against most OM bacteria, although pneumococcal activity is modest, and it penetrates into tissues extremely well. Although the safety of ciprofloxacin in children is still being established, we studied the pharmacokinetic behavior of this antibiotic in the chinchilla model preparatory to study dose-effect on ME inflammation.[128] Type 7F pneumococcal OM (cipro MIC = 0.5 μg/mL) was induced in chinchillas, and ciprofloxacin (6 mg/kg i.m.) was administered 2 days later. Using fluorescence HPLC detection, a 50 μL sample produced a detection limit of 5 ng/mL. Log-linear plots suggested the post-absorptive/penetration phase into MEF started about 6 hr after the dose. The average plasma ciprofloxacin K_e value was 0.24 hr,$^{-1}$ and half-life was 3.02 hr. For MEF, the mean K_e value was 0.1 hr,$^{-1}$ and half-life was 12.32 hr. Therefore, ciprofloxacin penetrated into MEF extremely well and was eliminated slowly. This pharmacokinetic behavior may provide an antibiotic advantage over the β-lactam agents, which are rapidly cleared from the MEF and, thus, affected by low doses and noncompliance.

Antibiotic protein binding

Antibiotic protein binding in plasma and MEF is likely an important determinant of antibiotic penetration and treatment efficacy. We found that the binding of amoxicillin in the chinchilla model was 35% for plasma, 35% in serous ME effusion, and 45% in purulent effusion compared to human plasma binding of 20–30%.[76] TMP binding in the chinchilla was 45% for plasma, 40% in serous effusion, and 25% in purulent effusion compared to human plasma binding of 40–70%. SMX binding in the chinchilla was 50% for plasma, 55% is serous effusion, and 35% in purulent effusion compared to human plasma binding of 65%.

Supra- and subinhibitory ciprofloxacin concentrations

We measured the effects of supra- and subinhibitory ciprofloxacin concentrations on MEF culture, hearing loss (measured electrophysiologically), and semiquantitative ME histopathology in chinchillas with pneumococcal OM.[29] High-dose treatment (12 mg/kg) achieved MEF concentrations exceeding MIC of the pneumococcal inoculum (MIC = 0.5 μg/mL) for the entire 8-hr dosing interval; low dose (4 mg/kg) achieved MEF concentrations just below MIC for the entire dosing interval. All MEF samples from control and low-dose chinchillas were pneumococcus culture-positive on days 5 and 7; in the high-dose group, only 2 of 8 ears were culture positive on day 5, and all were negative on day 7. Histopathologic exam demonstrated severe inflammatory changes in the control group, less change in the low-dose group, and little change in the high-dose group. Low-dose ciprofloxacin failed to clear pneumococci, produced hearing loss similar to untreated controls, and histopathology was only slightly improved compared with control. This experiment suggests that antimicrobial dosing must produce MEF concentrations above MIC to treat pneumococcal OM effectively. Sub-MIC MEF levels may improve AOM symptoms but the viable organisms remaining may multiply and produce recurrent AOM.

FUTURE RESEARCH DIRECTIONS

Virtually all of the issues confronting students of pneumococcal pathogenesis, immunoprophylaxis, and antimicrobial intervention can be studied in the chinchilla OM model. In studies of respiratory mucosal inflammation, OM modeling provides the ability to sample mucosal secretions easily and subepithelial transudates not possible in the lower respiratory tract.

The synergistic effect of pneumococci and influenza A virus has been carefully studied in this model, but clinically relevant interactions between pneumococci and other respiratory viruses, notable respiratory syncytial virus and adenovirus, have not been explored. It is possible that respiratory syncytial virus and adenovirus vaccines might have an effect similar to attenuated influenza vaccine on pneumococcal OM susceptibility.

Molecular events linking pneumococcal replication and lysis in the ME to host inflammatory responses are just starting to be revealed. Knowledge of these events is central in developing anti-inflammatory protection strategies. To this end, high-sensitivity human monoclonal antibodies have been useful in studying cytokine kinetics in chinchilla ME fluid, but these reagents are available only for a few cytokines. Study of cytokine synthesis using mRNA probes has not been attempted in chinchilla ME cells, and existing murine and human probes may not be cross-reactive with chinchilla RNA.

Caution should be exercised in extrapolating lower respiratory tract inflammatory events to the ME because pneumococcal pneumolysin appears to have a more important role in the lower than upper respiratory tract. Likewise, host inflammatory responses may not be parallel. Further use of primary ME epithelial cell cultures may be very useful in isolating the effect of pneumococcal components and host inflammatory mediators on mucous glycoprotein secretion. These studies are quite important in understanding the pathological basis of chronic mucoid OM, which is a major child health problem.

The relative contribution of IgG and IgA anti-PS antibodies in ME protection against pneumococcal diseases has not been explored carefully. Our pneumococcal OM reinfection study suggests that both local and systemic antibodies are produced during natural ME infection. Future studies might use lymphocyte plaque-forming assays to study IgA synthesis in ME mucosa during and after ME infection, and systemic IgA synthesis after pneumococcal immunization.

The susceptibility of infant chinchillas to pneumococcal OM has not been explored, and a number of clinically relevant issues could be studied. Middle ear mesenchyme is known to persist in some human infants after birth; its presence has been hypothesized to increase ME susceptibility to bacterial infection. Because young age of OM onset in humans is a strong determinant of subsequent ME infections, studies in infant chinchillas might clarify the role of mesenchyme. Relationships between maternal and infant antibody can also be studied in the infant model. Pneumococcal immunization of pregnant chinchillas and ME challenge of their offspring could clarify the interesting observation in human infants that cord blood anti-PS antibody is directly related to age of OM onset.[129]

The chinchilla model was first developed to study pneumococcal vaccines, and it remains the only nonbacteremic animal model of pneumococcal disease. As such, it will be very useful in studying the efficacy of new pneumococcal conjugate and common protein vaccines and other prophylactic and therapeutic strategies such as antiadhesive compounds.

Chinchilla and human cochlear structure and function are quite similar. Thus, the demonstration that pneumococcal OM caused hearing loss in chinchillas has important implications for transient and sometimes permanent sensorineural hearing loss in humans following acute OM. Further study in the chinchilla model might reveal the pathogenesis of this relationship.

REFERENCES

1. **Abramson, J.S., G.S. Giebink, E.L. Mills, and P.G. Quie.** 1981. Polymorphonuclear leukocyte dysfunction during influenza virus infection in chinchillas. J. Infect. Dis. **143:**836–845.

2. **Abramson, J.S., G.S. Giebink, and P.G. Quie.** 1982. Influenza A virus-induced polymorphonuclear leukocyte dysfunction in the pathogenesis of experimental pneumococcal otitis media. Infect. Immun. **36:**289–296.

3. **Abramson, J.S., and H.R. Hudnor.** 1995. Decreased binding of specific monomeric and trimeric G-proteins with the plasma membrane of polymorphonuclear leukocytes exposed to influenza A virus. J. Immunol. **155:**2571–2578.

4. **Adler, K.B., J.E. Schwarz, W.H. Anderson, and A.F. Welton.** 1987. Platelet activating factor stimulates secretion of mucin by

5. **Amesara, R., Y. Kim, S. Sano, et al.** 1992. Primary cultures of middle ear epithelial cells from chinchillas. Eur. Arch. Otorhinolaryngol. **249:**164–167.

6. **Amesara, R., Y. Kim, and S.K. Juhn.** 1993. Effects of arachidonic acid metabolites on mucous glycoprotein production in middle ear epithelial cell culture, pp. 411–413. In D.J. Lim, C.D. Bluestone, J.O. Klein, J.D. Nelson, and P.L. Ogra (ed.). Recent Advances in Otitis Media, Decker Periodicals, Hamilton, Ontario.

7. **Anderson, P., and R. Betts.** 1989. Human adult immunogenicity of protein-coupled pneumococcal capsular antigens of serotypes prevalent in otitis media. Pediatr. Infect. Dis. J. **8:**S50–S53.

8. **Andersson, B., O. Nylen, C.M. Peterson, and E.C. Svanborg.** 1980. Attachment of *Streptococcus pneumoniae* to human pharyngeal epithelial cells in vitro. Ann. Otol. Rhinol. Laryngol. **89:**115–116.

9. **Andersson, B., B. Eriksson, E. Falsen, et al.** 1981. Adhesion of *Streptococcus pneumoniae* to human pharyngeal epithelial cells in vitro: Differences in adhesive capacity among strains isolated from subjects with otitis media, septicemia, or meningitis or from healthy carriers. Infect. Immun. **32:**311–317.

10. **Andersson, B., J. Dahmen, T. Frejd, et al.** 1983. Identification of an active disaccharide unit of a glycoconjugate receptor for pneumococci attaching to human pharyngeal epithelial cells. J. Exp. Med. **158:**559–570.

11. **Arnold, J.W., G.R. Klimpel, and D.W. Niesel.** 1993. Tumor necrosis factor (TNFα) regulated intestinal mucus production during Salmonellosis. Cell. Immunol. **151:**336–344.

12. **Arola, M., T. Ziegler, and O. Ruuskanen.** 1990. Respiratory virus infection as a cause of prolonged symptoms in acute otitis media. J. Pediatr. **116:**697–701.

13. **Aronson, M., O. Medalia, L. Schori, et al.** 1979. Prevention of colonization of the urinary tract of mice with Escherichia coli by blocking of bacterial adherence with methyl-D-manno pyranoside. J. Infect. Dis. **139:**329–332.

14. **Austrian, R., V.M. Howie, and J.H. Ploussard.** 1977. The bacteriology of pneumococcal otitis media. Johns Hopkins Med. J. **141:**104–111.

15. **Austrian, R.** 1981. Some observations on the pneumococcus and on the current status of pneumococcal disease and its prevention. Rev. Infect. Dis. 3 (Suppl. 1):S1–S17.

16. **Bakaletz, L.O., R.L. Daniels, and D.J. Lim.** 1993. Modeling adenovirus type 1-induced otitis media in the chinchilla: Effect on ciliary activity and fluid transport function of eustachian tube mucosal epithelium. J. Infect. Dis. **168:**865–872.

17. **Barenkamp, S.J.** 1986. Protection by serum antibodies in experimental nontypable *Haemophilus influenzae* otitis media. Infect. Immun. **52:**572–578.

18. **Barry, B., M. Muffat-Joly, P. Gehanno, and J.J. Pocidalo.** 1993. Effect of increased dosages of amoxicillin in treatment of experimental middle ear otitis due to penicillin-resistant *Streptococcus pneumoniae*. Antimicrob. Agents Chemother. **37:**1599–1603.

19. **Beachey, E.H.** 1981. Bacterial adherence: adhesin-receptor interactions mediating the attachment of bacteria to mucosal surface. J. Infect. Dis. **143:**325–345.

20. **Benfield, M., Y. Kim, G.S. Giebink, and S. Juhn.** 1990. Interleukin 6 activity in middle ear effusion, p. 28. In D. Lim (ed.) Abstracts of the 13th Midwinter Research Meeting, Association for Research in Otolaryngology, February 4–8, 1990, St. Petersburg Beach, FL.

21. **Bergan, T.** 1981. Pharmacokinetics of tissue penetration of antibiotics. Rev. Infec. Dis. **3:**45–66.

22. **Black, S.B., H.R. Shinefield, B. Fireman, et al.** 1991. Efficacy

explants of rodent airways in organ culture. Exp. Lung Res. **13:**25–43.

in infancy of oligosaccharide conjugate *Haemophilus influenzae* type b (HbOC) vaccine in a United States population of 61,080 children. Pediatr. Infect. Dis. J. **10**:97–104.

23. **Bluestone, C.D., J.S. Stephenson, and L.M. Martin.** 1992. Ten-year review of otitis media pathogens. Pediatr. Infect. Dis. J. **11** (Suppl. 8):S7–S11.

24. **Cabellos, C., E.D. MacIntyre, M. Forrest, et al.** 1992. Differing roles for platelet-activating factor during inflammation of the lung and subarachnoid space. J. Clin. Invest. **90**:612–618.

25. **Cámara, M., G.J. Boulnois, P.W. Andrew, and T.J. Mitchell.** 1994. A neuraminidase from *Streptococcus pneumoniae* has the features of a surface protein. Infect. Immun. **62**:3668–3695.

26. **Canafax, D.M., G.S. Giebink, G.R. Erdmann, R.J. Cipolle, and S.K. Juhn.** 1988. Penetration of trimethoprim and sulfamethoxazole into the middle ear in experimental otitis media, pp. 219–222. *In* D.J. Lim (ed.). Recent Advances in Otitis Media. B.C. Decker, Philadelphia.

27. **Canafax, D.M., N. Nonomura, G.R. Erdmann, C.T. Le, S.K. Juhn, and G.S. Giebink.** 1989. Experimental animal models for studying antimicrobial pharmacokinetics in otitis media. Pharmaceut. Res. **6**:279–285.

28. **Canafax, D.M., H.Q. Russlie, M.J. Lovdahl, G.R. Erdmann, C.T. Le, and G.S. Giebink.** 1994. Comparison of two otitis media models for the study of middle ear antimicrobial pharmacokinetics. Pharmaceut. Res. **11**:855–859.

29. **Canafax, D.M., H.Q. Russlie, M.J. Lovdahl, K.H. Reher, S.K. Juhn C.T. Le, P.A. Schachern, S.F. Fulton, N. Johnson, T. Morizono, R.H. Margolis, M.M. Paparella, and G.S. Giebink.** 1995. Effects of ciprofloxacin treamtent on bacterial, histopathologic and sensorineural hearing response in experimental AOM. *In* Midwinter Meeting of the Association for Research in Otolaryngology, St. Petersburg Beach, Florida, February, 1995.

30. **Carlsen, B.D., M. Kawana, C. Kawana, A. Tomasz, and G.S. Giebink.** 1992. Role of the bacterial cell wall in middle ear inflammation caused by *Streptococcus pneumoniae*. Infect. Immun. **60**:2850–2854.

31. **Catanzaro, A., A. Ryan, S. Batcher, and S.I. Wasserman.** 1991. The response to human rIL-1, rIL-2, and rTNF in the middle ear of guinea pigs. Laryngoscope **101**:271–275.

32. **Cauwenberge, P., and J. Bernstein.** 1987. Inflammatory mediators in middle ear disease, pp. 338–339. *In* J. Bernstein, and P. Ogra (eds.). Immunology of the Ear. Raven Press, New York.

33. **Chetty, C., and A. Kreger.** 1985. Generation of purpura-producing principle from pneumococcal cell walls. J. Bacteriol. **163**:389–391.

34. **Chonmaitree, T., M.J. Owen, and V.M. Howie.** 1990. Respiratory viruses interfere with bacteriologic responses to antibiotics in children with acute otitis media. J. Infect. Dis. **162**:546–549.

35. **Chung, M.H., S.R. Griffith, K.H. Park, D.J. Lim, and T.F. DeMaria.** 1993. Cytological and histological changes in the middle ear after inoculation of influenza A virus. Acta Oto-Laryngol. **113**:81–87.

36. **Commis, S.D., P.M. Osbourne, J. Stephen, et al.** 1993. Cytotoxic effect on hair cells of the guinea pig cochlea produced by pneumolysin, the thiol activated toxin of *Streptococcus pneumoniae*. Acta Otolaryngol. (Stockholm) **113**:152–159.

37. **Diamant, M., S. Ek, P. Kallos, and G. Rubensohn.** 1961. Gammaglobulin treatment and protection against infections. Acta Otolaryngol. **53**:317–327.

38. **Diven, W.F., R.H. Glew, and K.L. LaMarco.** 1985. Hydrolase activity in acute otitis media with effusion. Ann. Otol. Rhinol. Laryngol. **94**:415–418.

39. **Diven, W.F., A. Zeevi, and W.J. Doyle.** 1992. Inhibition of lymphoproliferation by middle ear effusion in experimental otitis media. Arch. Otolaryngol. Head & Neck Surg. **118**:749–752.

40. **Engel, F., R. Blatz, J. Kellner, et al.** 1995. Breakdown of the round window membrane permeability barrier evoked by streptolysin O: Possible etiologic role in development of sensorineural hearing loss in acute otitis media. Infect. Immun. **63**:1305–1310.

41. **Erdmann, G.R., D.M. Canafax, and G.S. Giebink.** 1988. High-performance liquid chromatographic analysis of trimethoprim and sulfamethoxazole in microliter volumes of chinchilla middle ear effusion and serum. J. Chromatogr. **433**:187–195.

42. **Erdmann, G.R., K. Walker, G.S. Giebink, and D.M. Canafax.** 1990. High performance liquid chromatographic analysis of amoxicillin in microliter volumes of chinchilla middle ear effusion and plasma. J. Liq. Chrom. **13**:3339–3350.

43. **Eskola, J., H. Käyhty, A.K. Takala, et al.** 1990. A randomized, prospective field trial of a conjugate vaccine in the protection of infants and young children against invasive *Haemophilus influenzae* type b disease. N. Engl. J. Med. **323**:1381–1387.

44. **Feldman, C., T.J. Mitchell, P.W. Andrew, et al.** 1990. The effect of *Streptococcus pneumoniae* pneumolysin on human respiratory epithelium in vitro. Microb. Pathog. **9**:275–284.

45. **Feldman, C., N.C. Munro, D.K. Jeffrey, et al.** 1991. Pneumolysin induces the salient features of pneumococcal infection in the rat lung in vivo. Am. J. Respir. Cell Mol. Biol. **5**:416–423.

46. **Feldman, C., R. Read, A. Rutman, et al.** 1992. The interaction of *Streptococcus pneumoniae* with intact human respiratory mucosa in vitro. Eur. Respir. J. **5**:576–585.

47. **Gibbons, R.J.** 1977. Adherence of bacteria to host tissue, pp. 395–406. *In* D. Schlessinger (ed.). Microbiology. American Society for Microbiology, Washington, D.C.

48. **Giebink, G.S., E.E. Payne, E.L. Mills, et al.** 1976. Experimental otitis media due to *Streptococcus pneumoniae*: immunopathogenic response in the chinchilla. J. Infect. Dis. **134**:595–604.

49. **Giebink, G.S., and P.G. Quie.** 1977. Comparison of otitis media due to *Streptococcus pneumoniae* types 3 and 23 in the chinchilla model. J. Infect. Dis. **136** (Suppl.):191–195.

50. **Giebink, G.S., I.K. Berzins, G. Schiffman, and P.G. Quie.** 1979. Experimental otitis media in chinchillas following nasal colonization with type 7F *Streptococcus pneumoniae*: Prevention after vaccination with pneumococcal capsular polysaccharide. J. Infect. Dis. **140**:716–723.

51. **Giebink, G.S., I.K. Berzins, S.C. Marker, and G. Schiffman.** 1980. Experimental otitis media after nasal inoculation of *Streptococcus pneumoniae* and influenza A virus in chinchillas. Infect. Immun. **30**:445–450.

52. **Giebink, G.S.** 1981. The pathogenesis of pneumococcal otitis media in chinchillas and the efficacy of vaccination in prophylaxis. Rev. Infect. Dis. **3**:342–352.

53. **Giebink, G.S., S.K. Juhn, M.L. Weber, and C.T. Le.** 1982. The bacteriology and cytology of chronic otitis media with effusion. Pediatr. Infect. Dis. **1**:98–103.

54. **Giebink, G.S., and G. Schiffman.** 1983. Humoral immune response in chinchillas to the capsular polysaccharides of *Streptococcus pneumoniae*. Infect. Immun. **39**:638–644.

55. **Giebink, G.S., and P.F. Wright.** 1983. Different virulence of influenza A virus strains and susceptibility to pneumococcal otitis media in chinchillas. Infect. Immun. **41**:913–920.

56. **Giebink, G.S., W.L. Meyerhoff, and E.I. Cantekin.** 1986. Animal models of otitis media, pp. 213–236. *In* M. Sande and O. Zak (eds.). Animal Models in the Evaluation of Chemotherapy of Infectious Diseases. Academic Press, London.

57. **Giebink, G.S., M.L. Ripley, and P.F. Wright.** 1987. Eustachian tube histopathology during experimental influenza A virus infection in the chinchilla. Ann. Otol. Rhinol. Laryngol. **96**:199–206.

58. **Giebink, G.S.** 1989. Studies of *Streptococcus pneumoniae* and influenza virus vaccines in the chinchilla otitis media model. Pediatr. Infect. Dis. J. **8**:S42–S44.

59. **Giebink, G.S., M. Koskela, P.P. Vella, M. Harris, and C.T. Le.** 1993. Pneumococcal capsular polysaccharide-meningococcal

outer membrane protein complex conjugate vaccines: immunogenicity and efficacy in experimental pneumococcal otitis media. J. Infect. Dis. **167**:347–355.

60. **Giebink, G.S., J.D. Meier, M.K. Quartey, C.L. Liebeler, and C.T. Le.** 1996. Immunogenicity and efficacy of *Streptococcus pneumoniae* polysaccharide-protein conjugate vaccines against homologous and heterologous serotypes in the chinchilla otitis media model. J. Infect. Dis. **173**:119–127.

61. **Giebink, G.S., J.D. Meier, and M.K. Quartey.** 1996. Comparative immunogenicity and efficacy of monovalent and polyvalent pneumococcal conjugate vaccines. (Submitted).

62. **Giebink, G.S., J.D. Meier, and M.K. Quartey.** 1996. Pneumococcal capsular polysaccharide-protein conjugate vaccine efficacy in preventing pneumococcal otitis media during experimental influenza A virus infection in chinchillas. (Submitted).

63. **Gum, J.R., J.C. Byrd, J.W. Hicks, N.W. Toribara, D.T.A. Lamport, and Y.S. Kim.** 1989. Molecular cloning of human intestinal mucin cDNAs. Sequence analysis and evidence for genetic polymorphism. J. Biol. Chem. **264**:6480–6487.

64. **Han, V., J. Resau, R. Prendergast, et al.** 1987. Interleukin-1 induces mucus secretion from mouse intestinal explants. Archs. Allergy Appl. Immun. **82**:364–365.

65. **Hando, S., and G.S. Giebink.** 1994. Adherence of different *Streptococcus pneumoniae* serotypes to chinchilla middle ear and tracheal epithelial cells, pp. 613–618. *In* G. Mogi (ed.). Recent Advances in Otitis Media, Kugler Publications, New York.

66. **Harsten, G., K. Prellner, B. Logren, and O. Kalm.** 1991. Serum antibodies against respiratory tract viruses in episodes of acute otitis media. J. Laryng. Otol. **105**:337–340.

67. **Hellstrom, S.O.M., A. Hermansson, U. Johansson, and K. Prellner.** 1987. Experimentally induced effusion in rat middle ear: A complete model for otitis media research? pp. 462–464. *In* D.J. Lim, C.D. Bluestone, J.O. Klein, and J.D. Nelson (eds.). Recent Advances in Otitis Media. B.C. Decker, Philadelphia.

68. **Henderson, F.W., A.M. Collier, M.A. Sanyal, et al.** 1982. A longitudinal study of respiratory viruses and bacteria in the etiology of acute otitis media with effusion. N. Engl. J. Med. **306**:1377–1383.

69. **Himi, T., T. Suzuki, H. Kodama, et al.** 1992. Immunologic characteristics of cytokines in otitis media with effusion. Ann. Otol. Rhinol. Laryngol. **101**:21–25.

70. **Honda, Z., M. Nakamura, I. Miki, et al.** 1991. Cloning by functional expression of platelet-activating factor receptor from guinea-pig lung. Nature **349**:342–346.

71. **Issekutz, A.C., and M. Szpejda.** 1986. Evidence that platelet activating factor may mediate some acute inflammatory responses. Lab. Invest. **54**:275–281.

72. **Jalonen, E., J.C. Paton, M. Koskela, et al.** 1989. Measurement of antibody responses to pneumolysin—a promising method for the presumptive aetiological diagnosis of pneumococcal pneumonia. J. Infect. **19**:127–134.

73. **Johnson, M.D., J.E. Fitzgerald, G. Leonard G, et al.** 1994. Cytokines in experimental otitis media with effusion. Laryngoscope **104**:191–196.

74. **Johnson, M.K., and J.H. Allen.** 1975. The role of cytolysin in pneumococcal ocular infection. Am. J. Ophthalmol. **80**:518–521.

75. **Jossart, G.H., G.R. Erdmann, D.G. Livett, P. Kucera, C.T. Le, S.K. Juhn, G.S. Giebink, and D.M. Canafax.** 1990. An experimental model for measuring middle ear antimicrobial drug penetration in otitis media. Pharmaceutical Res. **7**:1242–1247.

76. **Jossart, G.H., G.R. Erdmann, J.C. Steury, C.T. Le, S.K. Juhn, G.S. Giebink, and D.M. Canafax.** 1993. Effects of pH and protein binding on middle ear antimicrobial drug penetration may explain acute otitis media treatment failures, pp. 446–449. *In* D.J. Lim (ed.). Recent Advances in Otitis Media. B.C. Decker, Philadelphia.

77. **Jossart, G.H., D.M. Canafax, G.R. Erdmann, M.R. Lovdahl, H. Russlie, S.K. Juhn, and G.S. Giebink.** 1994. Effect of *Streptococcus pneumoniae* and Influenza A virus on middle ear antimicrobial pharmacokinetics in experimental otitis media. Pharmaceut. Res. **11**:860–864.

78. **Jung, T.T.K., G.S. Giebink, and S.K. Juhn.** 1984. Effects of ibuprofen, corticosteroid, penicillin on the pathogenesis of experimental pneumococcal otitis media, pp. 269–272. *In* D.J. Lim (ed.). Recent Advances in Otitis Media. B.C. Decker, Inc., Philadelphia.

79. **Juhn, S.K., J. Edlin, T.T.K. Jung, and G.S. Giebink.** 1986. Kinetics of penicillin in serum and middle ear effusion in experimental otitis media. Arch. Otorhinolaryngol. **243**:183–185.

80. **Juhn, S.K., W.J. Garvis, C.J. Lees, et al.** 1994. Determining otitis media severity from middle ear fluid analysis. Ann. Otol. Rhinol. Laryngol. **103** (Suppl. 163):43–45.

81. **Kanclerski, K., S. Blomquist, M. Granström, and R. Möllby.** 1988. Serum antibodies to pneumolysin in patients with pneumonia. J. Clin. Microbiol. **26**:96–100.

82. **Karjalainen, H.K., M.K. Quartey, S.K. Juhn, and G.S. Giebink.** 1993. Pneumococcal otitis media treatment timing and susceptibility to homologous reinfection in the chinchilla model. Association for Research in Otolaryngology Annual Meeting, St. Petersburg, Florida.

83. **Kawana, M., C. Kawana, T. Yokoo, P.G. Quie, and G.S. Giebink.** 1991. Oxidative metabolic products released from polymorphonuclear leukocytes in middle ear fluid during experimental pneumococcal otitis media. Infect. Immun. **59**:4084–4088.

84. **Kawana, M., C. Kawana, and G.S. Giebink.** 1992. Penicillin treatment accelerates middle ear inflammation in experimental pneumococcal otitis media. Infect. Immun. **60**:1908–1912.

85. **Kawana, M., C. Kawana, R. Amesara, S.K. Juhn, and G.S. Giebink.** 1994. Neutrophil oxygen metabolite inhibition of cultured chinchilla middle ear epithelial cell growth. Ann. Otol. Rhinol. Laryngol. **103**:812–816.

86. **Kelly, R., and D. Greiff.** 1970. Toxicity of pneumococcal neuraminidase. Infect. Immun. **2**:115–117.

87. **Konietzko, S., M. Koskela, G. Erdmann, G.S. Giebink.** 1992. Isotype-specific rabbit antibodies against chinchilla immunoglobulins G, M, and A. Lab. Animal Sci. **42**:302–306.

88. **Koskela, M., M. Harris, J. Henrichsen, F.K. Pedersen, and G.S. Giebink.** 1991. Middle ear fluid immune complexes in experimental pneumococcal otitis media. Abstracts of the 5th International Symposium on Recent Advances in Otitis Media, Ft. Lauderdale, FL. May 20–24, 1991.

89. **Koskela, M., M. Harris, and G.S. Giebink.** 1992. Enzyme immunoassay for detection of immunoglobulin G (IgG), IgM, and IgA antibodies against type 6B pneumococcal capsular polysaccharide and cell wall C polysaccharide in chinchilla serum. J. Clin. Microbiol. **30**:1485–1490.

90. **Krause, P.J., N.J. Owens, C.H. Nightingale, et al.** 1982. Penetration of amoxicillin, cefaclor, erythromycin-sulfisoxazole, and trimethoprim-sulfamethoxazole into the middle ear fluid of patients with chronic otitis media. J. Infect. Dis. **145**:815–821.

91. **Krivan, H.C., D.D. Roberts, and V. Ginsburg.** 1988. Many pulmonary pathogenic bacteria bind specifically to the carbohydrate sequence GalNAcβ1-4Gal found in some glycolipids. Proc. Natl. Acad. Sci. USA **85**:6157–6161.

92. **Kurono, Y., K. Shimamura, H. Shigemi, and G. Mogi.** 1991. Inhibition of bacterial adherence by nasopharyngeal secretions. Ann. Otol. Rhinol. Laryngol. **100**:455–458.

93. **LaMarco, K.L., W.F. Diven, R.H. Glew, et al.** 1984. Neuraminidase activity in middle ear effusions. Ann. Otol. Rhinol. Laryngol. **93**:76–84.

94. **LaMarco, K.L., W.F. Diven, and R.H. Glew.** 1986. Experi-

mental alteration of chinchilla middle ear mcosae by bacterial neu-raminidase. Ann. Otol. Rhinol. Laryngol. **95:**304–308.

95. **Leinonen, M., H. Syrjälä, E. Jalonen, et al.** 1990. Demonstration of pneumolysin antibodies in circulating immune complexes—a new diagnostic method for pneumococcal pneumonia. Serodiag. Immunother. Infect. Dis. **4:**451–458.

96. **Lim, D.J., J.M. Coticchia, K. Ueno, et al.** 1991. Glycoconjugates in the chinchilla tubotympanum. Ann. Otol. Rhinol. Laryngol. **100:**933–943.

97. **Lin, J., Y. Kim, C. Lees, and S.K. Juhn.** 1995. Effect of platelet-activating factor on secretion of mucous glycoprotein from chinchilla middle ear epithelial cells in vitro. Eur. Arch. Otorhinolaryngol. **252:**92–96.

98. **Lin, J., Y. Kim, C. Lees, et al.** 1996. Effect of lipoxygenase inhibition on mucous glycoprotein secretion from chinchilla middle ear epithelial cells in vitro. Ann. Otol. Rhinol. Laryngol. **105:**916–921.

99. **Linder, T.E., D.J. Lim, and T.F. DeMaria.** 1992. Changes in the structure of the cell surface carbohydrates of the chinchilla tubotympanum following *Streptococcus pneomoniae*-induced otitis media. Microbial. Pathogenesis. **13:**293–303.

100. **Lock, R.A., J.C. Paton, and D. Hansman.** 1988. Comparative efficacy of pneumococcal neuraminidase and pneumolysin as immunogens protective against *Streptococcus pneumoniae*. Microb. Pathogen. **5:**461–467.

101. **Lovdahl, M., J. Steury, H.Q. Russlie, and D.M. Canafax.** 1993. Determination of ciprofloxacin levels in chinchilla middle ear effusion and plasma by high-performance liquid chromatography with fluorescence detection. J. Chromatogr. **617:**329–333.

102. **Lovdahl, M., K.E. Reher, H.Q. Russlie, and D.M. Canafax.** 1994. Determination of cefpodoxime levels in chinchilla middle ear fluid and plasma by HPLC. J. Chromatogr. **653:**227–232.

103. **Lowell, S.H., S.K. Juhn, and G.S. Giebink.** 1980. Experimental otitis media following middle ear inoculation of nonviable *Streptococcus pneumoniae*. Ann. Otol. Rhinol. Laryngol. **89:**479–482.

104. **Luotonen, J., E. Herva, P. Karma, et al.** 1981. The bacteriology of acute otitis media in children with special reference to *Streptococcus pneumoniae* as studied by bacteriological and antigen detection methods. Scand. J. Infect. Dis. **13:**177–183.

105. **Magit, A.E., J.N. Dolitsky, W.J. Doyle, J.D. Swarts, J.T. Seroky, and R.M. Rosenfeld.** 1994. An experimental study of cefixime in the treatment of *Streptococcus pneumoniae* otitis media. Int. J. Pediatr. Otorhinolaryngol. **29:**1–9.

106. **Mahajan, B., and B.R. Panhotra.** 1989. Adherence of *Streptococcus pneumoniae* to buccal epithelial cells of smokers and nonsmokers. Ind. J. Med. Res. **89:**381–383.

107. **Mäkelä, P.H., M. Sibakov, E. Herva, et al.** 1980. Pneumococcal vaccine and otitis media. Lancet **2:**547–551.

108. **Marom, Z., J.H. Schelmeimer, and M. Kaliner.** 1985. Human monocyte-derived mucus secretagogue. J. Clin. Invest. **75:**191–198.

109. **Maxwell, K.S., J.E. Fitzgerald, J.A. Burleson, et al.** 1994. Interleukin-8 expression in otitis media. Laryngoscope **104:**989–995.

110. **Mbaki, N., N. Rikitomi, M. Akiyama, and K. Matsumoto.** 1989. In vitro adherence of *Streptococcus pneumoniae* to oropharyngeal cells: Enhanced activity and colonization of the upper respiratory tract in patients with recurrent respiratory infections. Tohoku J. Exp. Med. **157:**345–354.

111. **Nonomura, N., G.S. Giebink, S.K. Kuhn, T. Harada, and D. Aeppli.** 1991. Pathophysiology of *Streptococcus pneumoniae* otitis media: Kinetics of the middle ear biochemical and cytologic host responses. Ann. Otol. Rhinol. Laryngol. **100:**236–243.

112. **Nonomura, N., G.S. Giebink, D. Zelterman, T. Harada, and S.K. Juhn.** 1991. Early biochemical events in pneumococcal oti-

tis media: arachidonic acid metabolites in middle ear fluid. Ann. Otol. Rhinol. Laryngol. **100:**385–388.

113. **Nonomura, N., G.S. Giebink, D. Zelterman, T. Harada, and S.K. Juhn.** 1991. Middle ear fluid lysozyme source in experimental pneumococcal otitis media. Ann. Otol. Rhinol. Laryngol. **100:**593–596.

114. **O'Toole, R.D., L. Goode, and C. Howe C.** 1971. Neuraminidase activity in bacterial meningitis. J. Clin. Invest. **50:**979–985.

115. **Ogra, R.L., J.M. Bernstein, A.M. Yrchak, et al.** 1974. Characteristics of secretory immune system in human middle ear: Implications in otitis media. J. Immunol. **112:**488–495.

116. **Ohmori, H., A.F. Dohrman, M. Gallup, T. Tsuda, H. Kai, J.R. Gum, Y.S. Kim, and C.B. Basbaum.** 1994. Molecular cloning of the amino-terminal region of a rat MUC2 mucin gene homologue. J. Biol. Chem. **269:**17833–17840.

117. **Okamoto, Y., K. Kudo, K. Ishikawa, et al.** 1993. Presence of respiratory syncytial virus genomic sequences in middle ear fluid and its relationship to expression of cytokines and cell adhesion molecules. J. Infect. Dis. **168:**1277–1281.

118. **Paton, J.C., P.W. Andrew, G.J. Boulnois, and T.J. Mitchell.** 1993. Molecular analysis of the pathogenicity of *Streptococcus pneumoniae*. The role of pneumococcal proteins. Annu. Rev. Microbiol. **47:**89–115.

119. **Pichichero, M.E., and R.A. Insel.** 1983. Mucosal antibody response to parenteral vaccination with *Haemophilus influenzae* type b capsule. J. Allergy Clin. Immunol. **72:**481–486.

120. **Post, J.C. R.A. Preston, J.J. Aul, M. Larkins-Pettigrew, J. Rydquist-White, K.W. Anderson, R.M. Wadowsky, D.R. Reagan, E.S. Walker, L.A. Kingsley, et al.** 1995. Molecular analysis of bacterial pathogens in otitis media with effusion. J. Am. Med. Assn. **273:**1598–1604.

121. **Rayner, C.F.J., A.D. Jackson, A. Rutman, et al.** 1995. Interaction of pneumolysin-sufficient and -deficient isogenic variants of *Streptococcus pneumoniae* with human respiratory mucosa. Infect. Immun. **63:**442–447.

122. **Rhee, C.-K., T.T.K. Jung, S. Miller, and D. Weeks.** 1993. Experimental otitis media with effusion induced by platelet activating factor. Ann. Otol. Rhinol. Laryngol. **102:**600–605.

123. **Ripley-Petzoldt, M.L., G.S. Giebink, S.K. Juhn, D. Aeppli, A. Tomasz, and E. Tuomanen.** 1988. The contribution of pneumococcal cell wall to experimental otitis media pathogenesis. J. Infect. Dis. **157:**245–255.

124. **Robbins, J.B., R. Austrian, S.C. Rastogi, et al.** 1983. Considerations for formulating the second-generation pneumococcal capsular polysaccharide vaccine with emphasis on the cross-reactive types within groups. J. Infect. Dis. **148:**1136–1159.

125. **Rosenfeld, R.M., W.J. Doyle, J.D. Swarts, J. Seroky, and I. Greene.** 1993. Efficacy of ceftibuten for acute otitis media caused by Hemophilus influenzae: An animal study. Ann. Otol. Rhinol. Laryngol. **102:**222–226.

126. **Rubins, J.B. P.G. Duane, D. Charboneau, and E.N. Janoff.** 1992. Toxicity of pneumolysin to pulmonary endothelial cells in vitro. Infect. Immun. **60:**1740–1746.

127. **Rubins, J.B., P.G. Duane, D. Clawson, et al.** 1993. Toxicity of pneumolysin to pulmonary alveolar epithelial cells. Infect. Immun. **61:**1352–1358.

128. **Russlie, H.Q., M.J. Lovdahl, G.S. Giebink, and D.M. Canafax.** 1996. Ciprofloxacin middle ear and plasma pharmacokinetics in experimental acute otitis media. *In* Proceedings of the 6th International Symposium on Recent Advances in Otitis Media, June 4–8, 1995, Ft. Lauderdale, FL. (in press).

129. **Salazar, J.C., K.A. Daly, G.S. Giebink, B.R. Lindgren, C.L. Liebeler, M. Meland, and C.T. Le.** 1997. Low cord blood pneumococcal IgG antibodies predict early onset acute otitis media in infancy. Am. J. Epidemiol. **145:**1048–1056.

130. **Santosham, M., M. Wolff, R. Reid, et al.** 1991. The efficacy in

Navajo infants of a conjugate vaccine consisting of *Haemophilus influenzae* type b polysaccharide and Neisseria meningitidis outer-membrane protein complex. N. Engl. J. Med. **324:**1767–1772.

131. **Sato, K., M.K. Quartey, C.L. Liebeler, and G.S. Giebink.** 1995. Timing of penicillin treatment influences the course of *Streptococcus pneumoniae*-induced middle ear inflammation. Antimicrob. Agents Chemother. **39:**1896–1898.

132. **Sato, K., M.K. Quartey, C.L. Liebeler, C.T. Le, and G.S. Giebink.** 1996. Roles of autolysin and pneumolysin in middle ear inflammation caused by a type 3 *Streptococcus pneumoniae* strain in the chinchilla otitis media model. Infect. Immun. **64:**1140–1145.

133. **Scalon, K.L., W.F. Diven, and R.H. Gelw.** 1989. Purification and properties of *Streptococcus pneumoniae* neuraminidase. Enzyme **41:**143–150.

134. **Schneerson, R., J.B. Robbins, J.C. Parke Jr., et al.** 1986. Quantitative and qualitative analysis of serum antibodies elicited in adults by *Haemophilus influenzae* type b and pneumococcus type 6A capsular polysaccharide-tetanus toxoid conjugates. Infect. Immun. **52:**519–528.

135. **Sharon, N.** 1987. Bacterial lectins, cell-cell recognition and infectious disease. FEBS Lett. **217:**145–157.

136. **Shimamura, K., H. Shigemi, Y. Kurono, and G. Mogi.** 1990. The role of bacterial adherence in otitis media with effusion. Arch. Otolaryngol. Head Neck Surg. **116:**1143–1146.

137. **Shurin, P.A., G.S. Giebink, D.L. Wegman, et al.** 1988. Prevention of pneumococcal otitis media in chinchillas with human bacterial polysaccharide immune globulin. J. Clin. Microbiol. **26:**755–759.

138. **Shyu, W.C., J. Haddad, J. Reilly, W.N. Khan, D.A. Campbell, Y. Tsai, and R.H. Barbhaiya.** 1994. Penetration of cefprozil into the middle ear fluid of patients with otitis media. Antimicrob. Agents Chemother. **39:**2210–2212.

139. **Sloyer, J.L. Jr., V.M. Howie, J.H. Ploussard, et al.** 1974. Immune response to acute otitis media in children. J. Immunol. **118:**248–250.

140. **Sloyer, J.L., V.M. Howie, J.H. Ploussard, G. Schiffman, and R.B. Johnston, Jr.** 1976. Immune response to acute otitis media: Association between middle ear fluid antibody and the clearing of clinical infection. J. Clin. Microbiol. **4:**306–308.

141. **Steinfort, C., R. Wilson, T. Mitchell, et al.** 1989. Effect of *Streptococcus pneumoniae* on human respiratory epithelium in vitro. Infect. Immun. **57:**2006–2013.

142. **Sturen, E.D., R. Essner, and J.S. Economou.** 1989. Overview of biological response modifiers. Surg. Oncol. **5:**379–384.f

143. **Takeuchi, K., K. Maesako, A. Yuta, and Y. Sakakura.** 1994. Interleukin-8 gene expression in middle ear effusions. Ann. Otol. Rhinol. Laryngol. **103:**404–407.

144. **Toews, G.B., D.A. Hart, and E.J. Hansen.** 1985. Effect of systemic immunization in pulmonary clearance of *Haemophilus influenzae* type b. Infect. Immun. **48:**343–349.

145. **Tuomanen, E., H. Liu, B. Hengstler, et al.** 1985. The induction of meningeal inflammation by components of the pneumococcal cell wall. J. Infect. Dis. **151:**859–868.

146. **Tuomanen, E., A. Tomasz, B. Hengstler, and O. Zak.** 1985. The relative role of bacterial cell wall and capsule in the induction of inflammation in pneumococcal meningitis. J. Infect. Dis. **151:**535–540.

147. **Tuomanen, E.** 1986. Piracy of adhesins: Attachment of superinfecting pathogens to respiratory cilia by secreted adhesins of Bordetella pertussis. Infect. Immun. **54:**905–908.

148. **Tuomanen, E., B. Hengstler, O. Zak, and A. Tomasz.** 1986. The role of complement in inflammation during experimental pneumococcal meningitis. Microbial. Pathogen. **1:**15–32.

149. **Tuomanen, E., R. Rich, and O. Zak O.** 1987. Induction of pulmonary inflammation by components of the pneumococcal cell surface. Am. Rev. Resp. Dis. **135:**869–874.

150. **Vance-Bryan, K., T.A. Larson, M.W. Garrison, J.P. Toscano, D.M. Canafax, and J.C. Rotschafer.** 1992. An in vitro pharmacodynamic model to stimulate acute otitis media with effusion. Pharmaceut. Res. **9:**920–924.

151. **Vogelman, B., S. Gudmundson, J. Leggett, et al.** 1988. Correlation of antimicrobial pharmacokinetic parameters with therapeutic efficacy in an animal model. J. Infect. Dis. **158:**831–847.

152. **Wissner, A., R.E. Schaub, P.E. Sum, et al.** 1986. Analogues of platelet activating factor 4. Some modifications of the phosphocholine moiety. J. Med. Chem. **29:**328–333.

153. **Yellon, R.F., G. Leonard, P.T. Marucha, et al.** 1991. Characterization of cytokines present in middle ear effusions. Laryngoscope **101:**165–169.

154. **Yellon, R.F., G. Leonard, P. Marucha, et al.** 1992. Demonstration of interleukin-6 in middle ear effusions. Arch. Otolaryngol. Head Neck Surg. **118:**745–748.

155. **Yuan, Z., H.Q. Russlie, and D.M. Canafax.** 1996. Determination of amoxicillin in human and chinchilla plasma and middle ear fluid by solid phase extraction and reversed phase HPLC. In Proceedings of the 6th International Symposium on Recent Advances in Otitis Media, June 4–8, 1995, Ft. Lauderdale, FL. (in press).

156. **Yuan, Z., H.Q. Russlie, and D.M. Canafax.** 1995. Sensitive assay for measuring amoxicillin in human plasma and middle ear fluid using solid phase extraction and reversed-phase high-performance liquid chromatography. J. Chromatogr. **674:**93–99.

157. **Zollinger, W.D., and J.W. Boslego.** 1981. A general approach to standardization of the solid-phase radioimmunoassay for quantitation of class-specific antibodies. J. Immunol Methods **46:**129–140.

Address reprint requests to:
Dr. G. Scott Giebink
Box 296 Mayo
420 Delaware Street S.E.
Minneapolis, MN 55455

Streptococcus pneumoniae
Copyright © 2000 Mary Ann Liebert, Inc., 2 Madison Avenue, Larchmont, NY 10538

Immunization and Protection in Pneumococcal Otitis Media Studied in a Rat Model

KARIN PRELLNER,[1] ANN HERMANSSON,[1] PETER WHITE,[1] ÅSA MELHUS,[1] and DAVID BRILES[2]

ABSTRACT

The recent and growing problem of bacterial resistance to common antibiotics has generated great interest in different methods for prevention of infections. The treatment of the pathogens causing upper airway infections and especially acute otitis media (AOM) is especially interesting in this context because these infections are a common cause of prescription of antibiotics all over the world. Both in AOM and recurrent AOM, *Streptococcus pneumoniae*, the most frequently occurring bacterium is isolated in 30–50% of all AOM attacks.[16] In the last decade, multiresistant *S. pneumoniae* have emerged as a major problem. Thus, it is important to explore possibilities that immunization may protect against pneumococcal OM. In a well-defined animal model using Sprague-Dawley rats, we have investigated the effects of different routes of immunization with different antigens and whole cells. Together with otomicroscopical evaluation of middle ear (ME) status, samples for bacterial cultivation as well as for studies of histopathological changes have been collected. Antibody titers have been followed during and after pneumococcal AOM by an enzyme-linked immunosorbent assay (ELISA) method.

ANIMAL MODELS IN MIDDLE EAR RESEARCH

EVEN TAKING INTO CONSIDERATION the difficulty in translating results from animal studies to human conditions, studies in animal models provide opportunities not otherwise available. In the animal model, variables can be controlled and those of special interest can be isolated from the others. Repeated observations can be made and different types of sampling is possible. Animal models of otitis media (OM) have been used for many years,[9] and have proven to be a valuable complement to *in vitro* studies and clinical studies when dealing with questions concerning etiology (anatomy, physiology, bacteriology, histology, etc.), prevention, and treatment as well as sequelae.

We are working with a rat model using Sprague-Dawley rats.[11] All common pathogens of acute otitis media (AOM) in humans, *i.e.*, *Streptococcus pneumoniae*, *Haemophilus influenzae*, *Moraxella catarrhalis*, and *Streptococcus pyogenes* cause AOM in the rat when inoculated into the middle ear (ME). Several different types of *S. pneumoniae* have been used, and all types tested have caused AOM when inoculated into the ME in a sufficient dose. When frozen inocula have been used, 10^6

colony-forming units or more might be needed to cause purulent infections. When fresh bacteria are used, the number of bacteria needed is smaller. The infections are, as in humans, usually self-limiting and the animals are not prone to develop general sepsis. There is, again as in humans, a considerable difference in the clinical course of the infection depending on what agent is inoculated into the ME of the animal.

A number of different animals have been used as models for ME research, but chinchillas, gerbils, guinea pigs, and rats are those used most frequently. The rat has been thoroughly described regarding ME anatomy and histology.[2,10] The ME mucosa of the rat resembles that of humans, as does the function of the Eustachian tube.[35] In contrast to chinchillas and gerbils,[7] rats do develop spontaneous AOM but they are not prone to develop sepsis when infected by *S. pneumoniae*. The tympanic membrane of the rat is accessible to inspection and myringotomy using an ordinary otomicroscope.

Different strategies for immunization have been tested in the rat model. Both local and the general defenses seem to be of interest in the protection against AOM.[18,31] The protection after a pneumococcal AOM[33] as well as after different routes of immunization with whole bacteria and pneumococcal polysac-

[1]Department of Otorhinolaryngology, University of Lund, Lund, Sweden.
[2]Department of Microbiology, University of Alabama at Birmingham, Birmingham, AL 35294.
Reprinted from *Microbial Drug Resistance*, Vol. 5, No. 1, 1999.

A

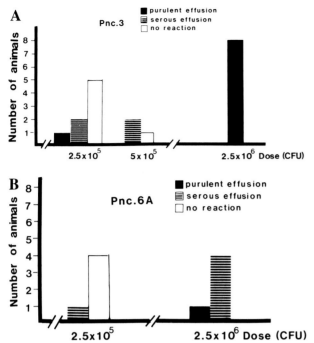

FIG. 1. **(A)** Number of animals developing OM with purulent vis-á-vis serous effusion or no reaction when challenged with *S. pneumoniae* type 3 at different doses. **(B)** Number of animals developing OM with purulent vis-á-vis serous effusion or no reaction when challenged with *S. pneumoniae* type 6A at different doses. (Reprinted from Am. J. Otolaryngol **9:**97–101, 1988, with kind permission of W.B. Saunders Company, USA.)

charides and passive immunization have been investigated. Antibody titers after immunization and after pneumococcal challenge have been followed with an enzyme-linked immunosorbent assay (ELISA) and Western blot studies.

THE RAT MODEL

Male Sprague-Dawley rats, weighing 250–300 g at the beginning of the studies, were used in most studies. The animals were kept under standard laboratory conditions and given food (pellets) and water *ad libitum*. Before undergoing operation or examination, the animals were anesthetized by intravenous injection of methohexital (Brietal®; Eli Lilly & Co., Indianapolis, IN) into a tail vein. Both operations and subsequent examinations were performed under a conventional otomicroscope. The tympanic bulla was exposed on both sides through a ventral midline incision.[11] A fine needle was used to make injections into the ME cavity through the bony wall of the bulla.

The rat ME is embedded in the temporal bone. The architecture of the tympanic cavity is similar to that of humans except that the rat lacks mastoid air cells and the floor of its tympanic cavity protrudes to form the tympanic bulla. The lateral wall of the tympanic cavity consists of the tympanic membrane, which has quite a large pars flaccida, the loose upper part of the membrane. The vascular supply for the tympanic membrane is almost identical to that of humans. On the opposite medial

wall, the orifice of the Eustachian tube can be found. The rat tube is more horizontal than that in humans and is, as in humans, usually closed. The Eustachian tube is lined with a pseudo-stratified ciliated columnar respiratory epithelium with goblet cells. This type of epithelium also extends from the tubal opening in the ME cavity as an anterior and an inferior tract along the medial wall of the cavity. The human ciliary transportation system in the ME cavity is roughly the same. The rest of the cavity is lined with squamous or cuboidal epithelium. The subepithelial tissue is composed of fibroblasts, blood vessels, nerve fibers, macrophages, and mast cells. The mast cells are confined to areas covered by ciliated epithelium, which are the floor of the tympanic bulla, the pars flaccida, and along the manubrial vessels. The uninfected ME mucosa contains very few lymphocytes and no lymphoid tissue. However, as discussed below, the rat ME mucosa undergoes extensive changes during and after AOM, as does that of the human. These changes can persist for a considerable time.

Several capsular types of *S. pneumonia* have been shown to cause AOM in the rat model. Frozen bacteria were used in early studies, but in later studies they have been exchanged for fresh bacteria. When using frozen bacteria, log-phase pneumococci

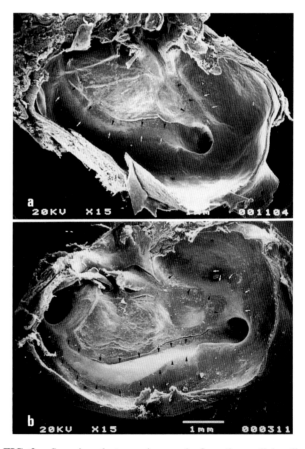

FIG. 2. Scanning electron micrographs from the medial wall of the tympanic cavity of the rat. **(a)** Normal mucosa; **(b)** 2 months after inoculation of *S. pneumoniae* type 3. Note the distribution of ciliated cells (arrows) with broadened tracts anterior and inferior to the promontory. (Reprinted from Acta Otolaryngol. **109:**421–430, 1990, with kind permission of Scandinavian University Press.)

were prepared and stored in aliquots at −80°C.[3] In most studies, types 3 and 6A *S. pneumonia* were used, but several other types have also been shown to cause AOM. All types tested are known to be associated with AOM in humans. Todd-Hewitt broth was used to dilute the bacteria to the concentration used at challenge, and the suspended bacteria were injected into the ME in a volume of approximately 0.05 ml.

The ME infections thus induced are self-limiting. The animals do not show any signs of deterioration except when doses 100 times or more of what are required to cause ME infection are given. In the otomicroscope, a bulging eardrum with pus in the ME cavity and dilated vessels over the malleus are seen after 2–3 days. After 10–12 days, all otomicroscopical signs of infection have usually disappeared. The dose of bacteria as well as the capsular type are of consequence for the outcome (Fig. 1a,b). At a sufficient dose, the animals develop AOM. If more bacteria are given, the animals will ultimately develop sepsis. If a lower dose is given, the animals either will not show any signs of ME infection or will only develop serous effusion behind the tympanic membrane.

When frozen bacteria are used, the doses needed to cause AOM vary between 10^3–10^6 CFU. Considerably lower doses

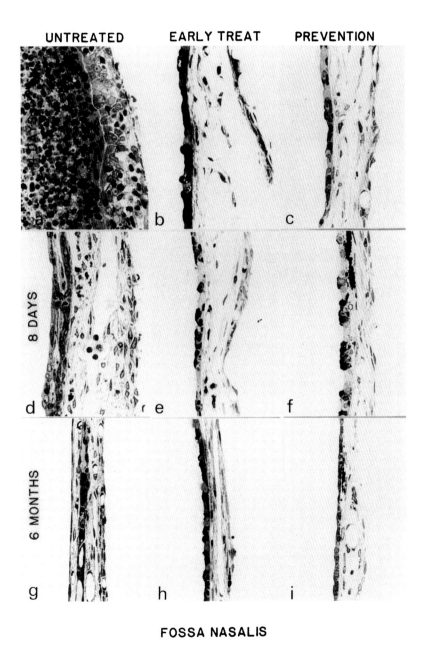

FIG. 3. Light micrographs (480×) representing the fossa nasalis on day 4, day 8, and after 6 months. Untreated animals (**a, d,** and **g**) are compared to animals given early treatment with pcV (**b, e,** and **h**) and animals given preventive treatment with pcV (**c, f,** and **i**). (Reprinted from Otolaryngol. Head Neck Surg. **105:**578–585, 1991, with kind permission of Mosby Publisher, St. Louis, MO.)

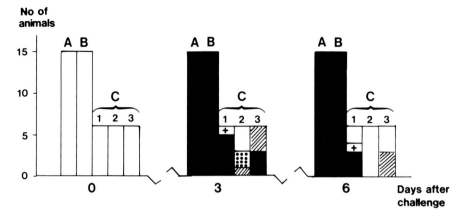

FIG. 4. Otomicroscopy findings, in the right, challenged ear, days 0, 3, and 6. A, Untreated controls; B, systemic gamma-globulin given 24 hr before (1), simultaneously with (2), and 24 hr after (3) challenge; C, intrabullar gammaglobulin given 24 hours before (1), simultaneously with (2), and 24 hr after (3) challenge. (●) Purulent OM; (◑) serous OM; (◉) clear fluid; (○) normal ME; (⊕) dead. (Reprinted from Acta Otolaryngol. **109:**300–306, 1990, with kind permission of Scandinavian University Press.)

are needed when using fresh bacteria. Blood samples for de-termination of antibodies as well as bacteriological samples from ME, blood, and nasopharynx have been currently col-lected. Using an ELISA method, a rise in specific im-munoglobulin G (IgG) antibodies has been found to reach a

peak concentration 7–10 days after pneumococcal challenge. Western blot studies have revealed the presence of antibodies to a 35-kDa protein after pneumococcal challenge.

Bacterial samples from ME effusions yielded pneumococci from all purulent effusions as well as from some serous effu-

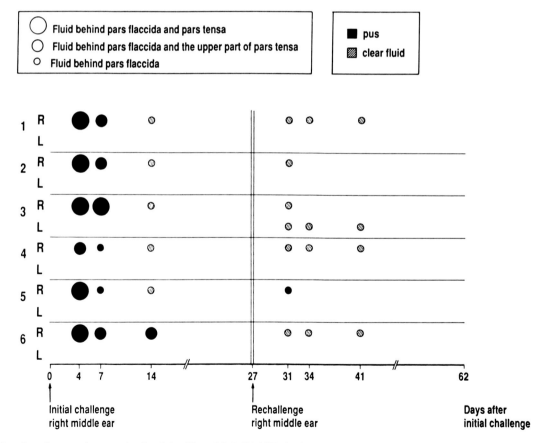

FIG. 5. Otomicroscopic status in the right (R) and left (L) MEs in 6 rats (nos. 1–6) after unilateral (R) challenge and ipsilat-eral (R) rechallenge. No indications on scheduled days means absence of fluid in the ME. (Reprinted from Acta Otolaryngol. **111:**1083–1089, 1991, with kind permission of Scandinavian University Press.)

sions. The nasopharynx is transiently colonized in most animals developing purulent ME effusion, but only for some days. Bacteremia has only been noted in septic animals.

Phenoxymethylpenicillin (pcV) has been shown not only to be effective as treatment but also, when given prior to bacterial challenge, to be effective as prevention.[14] The histopathology of the rat ME was studied after an episode of pneumococcal AOM.[12] After this transient infection, changes were recorded at all mucosal sites in the ear. The normally flat epithelium had become more cuboidal or cylindrical and numerous ciliated cells occurred in areas normally devoid of these cells (Fig. 2). Epithelial cells penetrated into the subepithelium, forming gland-like structures. These changes partly persisted for more than 6 months. The changes, in many respects, resembled those recorded in humans in conjunction with episodes of purulent OM.[1,4]

After antibiotic treatment, the changes seen in the ME mucosa at all sites were less pronounced.[14] The long-lasting mucosal changes recorded after an untreated episode of pneumococcal AOM were largely prevented (Fig. 3).

Acute purulent OM caused by *H. influenzae* and *M. catarrhalis* have also been extensively studied in the rat model and compared to each other and to pneumococcal infections. Different clinical courses as well as histopathological changes are seen after infections with the different bacteria.[19,34]

EFFECT OF IMMUNIZATION ON AOM

No differences have been found in the total serum concentrations of IgG, IgA, or IgM between rAOM children and healthy children. rAOM children have, however, been found to have lower concentrations of specific IgG antibody against certain types of pneumococci as well as aberrations in the complement system.[26] Both in humans and experimental animals, ME effusions have been shown to contain immunoglobulins.[23] That active as well as passive immunization can affect the course of OM, or even prevent it in certain cases, has been shown in both humans and animals. The number of AOM episodes has been reported to be reduced by pneumococcal vaccination in older children and in animal models[8,27] and by immunoglobulin given systemically to chinchillas.[30]

Effect of passive immunization with gammaglobulin

Gamma globulin (Sandoglobulin®) was administered to rats in conjunction with an episode of pneumococcal OM[13] (Fig. 4). The gamma globulin was either given intravenously or directly into the ME; administration was 24 hr before bacterial challenge, simultaneously with challenge, or 24 hr after challenge.

Intravenous administration of gamma globulin given 24 hr before, simultaneously with, or 24 hr after challenge failed to

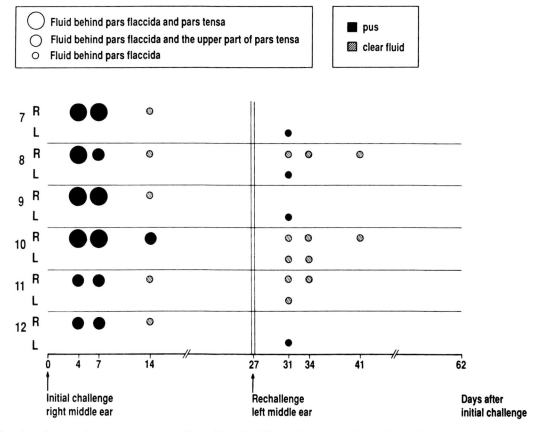

FIG. 6. Otomicroscopic status in the right (R) and left (L) MEs in 6 rats (nos. 7–12) after unilateral (R) challenge and ipsilateral (L) rechallenge. No indications on scheduled days means absence of fluid in the ME. (Reprinted from Acta Otolaryngol. **111:**1083–1089, 1991, with kind permission of Scandinavian University Press.)

affect the course of the infection. Cultures from purulent ME effusion showed growth of pneumococci. The intrabullar administration of gamma globulin 24 hr before challenge did not affect the infection while intrabullar administration of gamma globulin 24 hr after or simultaneously with challenge gave a significant reduction in the number of animals developing purulent AOM. These results indicate that the presence of IgG antibodies in the ME of the rat can modify and even prevent the establishment of AOM induced by ME challenge of pneumococci.

Effect of a previous AOM

To study the protection achieved after an episode of pneumococcal OM, animals were rechallenged after a period of 1 month. Rechallenge was performed either in the ipsilateral or the contralateral ear[31] (Fig. 5). Ipsilateral protection was almost total. After contralateral rechallenge, there was no significant reduction in the numbers of animals developing OM, but the infection was modified and thus was less severe and lasted for a shorter period (Fig. 6). When antibody concentrations were followed measuring specific serum IgG-antibodies against pneumococcal type-3-polysaccharide, the antibody level rose after the initial infection but had almost returned to baseline at the time of rechallenge (Fig. 7).

The clinical observations described are in accordance with observations made after AOM caused by *H. influenzae* in the rat.[18] In these studies, rechallenge in the ipsilateral ear with the same type of *H. influenzae* offers good protection against reinfection with the same type of *H. influenzae*, whereas there is a reduction in the intensity of the OM after rechallenge in the contralateral ear. Cross protection between different types of *H. influenzae* was also investigated. There was no cross protection between different types of nontypeable *H. influenzae* (NTHi),

but a resolved AOM caused by *H. influenzae* type b could confer cross protection against reinfection with NTHi. Although a specific response could not be ruled out, a role for nonspecific response responses had to be considered.

To explore this cross protection further, rats challenged with pneumococci were rechallenged with NTHi. A cross protection did occur and was comparable to that achieved after initial challenge with *H. influenzae* type b. No cross-reacting serum antibodies were detected. To achieve cross protection, the pneumococci had to be viable and presented locally in the ME cavity, which suggests that the protection could be due to local inflammatory reactions.

The viability of bacteria has been shown to be important for the induction of inflammation in ME infections. Because only encapsulated bacteria have shown cross protection so far, it seems probable that events in the ME associated with the capsular properties are essential. Histologically, the rat ME mucosa, after an episode of infection with an encapsulated bacterial strain, differs considerably from the mucosa seen after an infection with a nonencapsulated bacteria.[17] Encapsulated bacteria yield intense and severe inflammatory changes, but the inflammation appears to be of relatively short duration whereas unencapsulated bacteria yield a less violent course but long-lasting inflammation.[19] Thus, it seems probably that unspecific responses are important for the protection of the rat ME.

Effect of vaccination through various routes

Immunization with pneumococcal vaccine (Pneumovax®) or live pneumococci type 3 by different routes[33] was tested in the rat model. It was performed intraperitoneally or into the gastrointestinal tract, and rechallenge was performed with type 3 pneumococci either 4 days, 4 weeks, or 8 weeks later. Sera from all animals were collected and analyzed for the presence of spe-

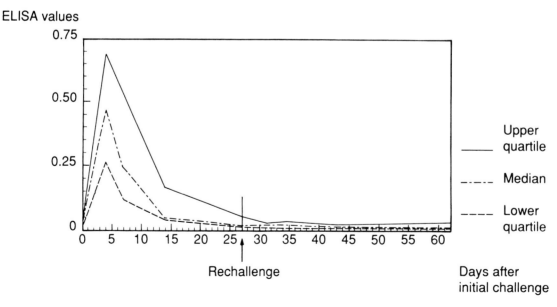

FIG. 7. Concentrations of specific serum IgG-antibodies against pneumococcal type 3 polysaccharide in rats with experimentally induced pneumococcal AOM, as measured by ELISA. The values are followed from day 0, before initial challenge, and throughout the study. (Reprinted from Acta Otolaryngol. **111:**1083–1089, 1991, with kind permission of Scandinavian University Press.)

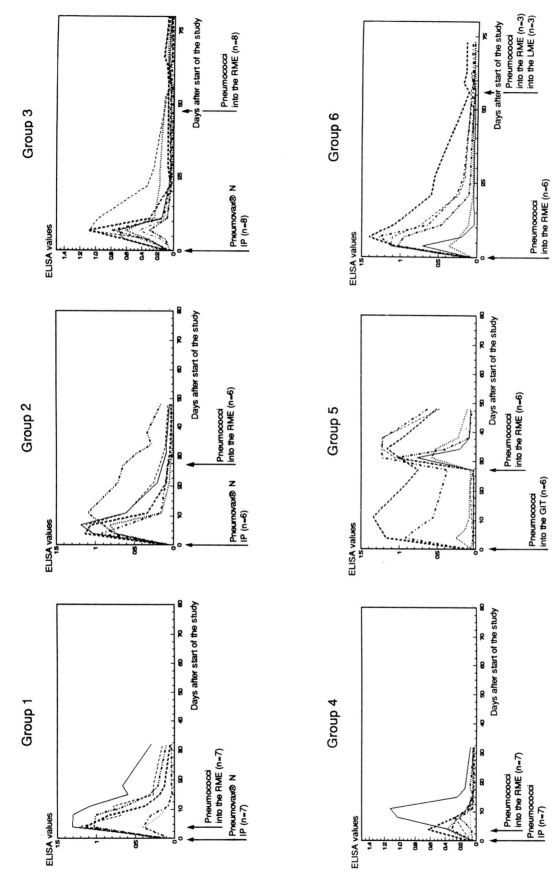

FIG. 8. The specific serum IgG antibody response in each rat in all groups (1–6) is shown in relation to the route [intraperitoneal (IP), into the right ME (RME), or into the gastrointestinal tract (GIT)] for primary immunization with pneumococci or pneumovax®N, and the subsequent pneumococcal ME challenge into the RME (groups 1–5) or rechallenge of the RME or left ME (group 6). (Reprinted from Int. J. Pediatr. Otorhinolaryngol. **25:**91–103, 1993, with kind permission of Elsevier Science NL Burgerhartstraaat 25 1055 KV Amsterdam, The Netherlands.)

cific IgG antibodies (Fig. 8). Both the rats given intraperitoneal immunization with Pneumovax® or pneumococci type 3 and 3 of the rats immunized in the gastrointestinal tract with live pneumococci exhibited a specific serum IgG response that reached a maximum within a week. With the exception of the group immunized in the gastrointestinal tract, a decrease to preimmunization level was observed within 2–4 weeks and no new antibody was produced after subsequent ME challenge. The 6 rats immunized in the gastrointestinal tract manifested two different patterns of serum IgG antibody response. In 3 rats, antibody response after immunization was present, and after ME challenge a new rise in antibody levels was recorded. In the other 3 rats, no initial response was recorded. The reaction after challenge in these 3 rats matched unimmunized controls. The only rats showing decreased incidence of AOM in this study were the 3 rats that had manifested an initial rise in serum IgG after gastrointestinal immunization. However, the resolution of pus from the ME was faster than in the controls in the other groups, with the exception of those given intraperitoneal Pneumovax® 4 days prior to challenge, where no difference from control animals was seen.

The possibility of using the gastrointestinal route for immunization has been shown by other investigators. In a study by Yoshimura and colleagues,[37] a pneumococcal immunization into the duodenum of guinea pigs induced protection against AOM induced by pneumococcal ME challenge.

It is also of interest to note that, although no absolute protection was achieved after immunization intraperitoneally with either live pneumococci or Pneumovax®, there was a faster resolution of the infection induced 4 days after immunization in the group immunized with live pneumococci. This was not the case in the group immunized by Pneumovax®. At the time of immunization, the groups showed the same level of specific serum IgG response. It might be that serum antibodies to other

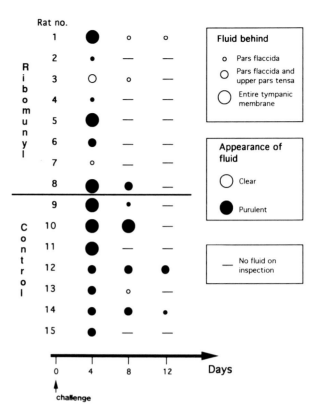

FIG. 10. Otomicroscopical results after pneumococcal challenge with (Nos. 1–8) or without (Nos. 9–15) Ribomunyl®. (Reprinted from Immunobiology in Otorhinolaryngology— Progress of a decade, pp. 115–120. Proceedings of the 4th International Academic Conference, Oita, Japan, 1994, G. Mogi, J.E. Veldman, and H. Kawauchi, eds., with kind permission of Kugler Publications, Amsterdam/New York.)

pneumococcal antigens also are of importance for the defense against AOM.

AOM IN THE RAT EVOKES ANTIBODIES TO A 35-KDA PROTEIN

In the discussion of a non-type-specific immune response, the pneumococcal proteins have attracted interest. Several proteins have been identified on the pneumococcus, of which at least three seem to influence virulence, *i.e.*, the toxin pneumolysin, the major pneumococcal autolysin, and the pneumococcal surface protein A.[24] In one study, the antibody response to proteins after an episode of AOM in rats[32] was investigated (Fig. 9). Rats were inoculated with *S. pneumoniae* type 3 in the ME, the tympanic membrane was inspected, and blood samples were collected on days 4, 7, 14, and 56. Using a Western blot method, an antibody response to a 35-kDa protein was found in the sera of 5 out of the 6 rats. In one rat, this response already was seen 4 days after inoculation and in all 5 rats it was present on day 14. Two other bands (28-kDa and 45-kDa proteins) were also observed in 5 of the 6 rats, but these bands were not persistent throughout the study.

These results indicate an activation of a systemic immune

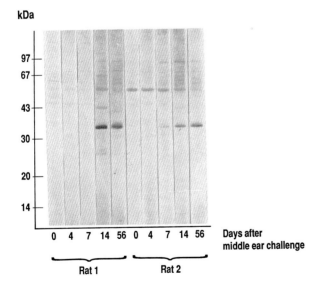

FIG. 9. SDS-PAGE for crude preparations of pneumococci types 1, 3, 6A, 18C, 19F, and 23F demonstrating the similarity in electrophoretic pattern of proteins. (Reprinted from Acta Otolaryngol. **112:**518–523, 1992, with kind permission of Scandinavian University Press.)

response to pneumococcal proteins following a pneumococcal AOM. It is known that protein antigens and their antibodies may contribute to an inflammatory reaction in the ME, *i.e.*, OM with effusion (OME) in guinea pig.[28] In humans, it has been reported that OME might be exacerbated by immune complexes.[25] The finding that proteins elicit an immune response in experimental AOM in the rat make it seem possible that proteins contribute to the inflammatory reaction as well as to protection. One might also speculate regarding the similarity in molecular weight of the protein detected in this study (approximately 35 kDa) and the 37-kDa protein homologous to the pneumococcal surface-associated protein A that is a putative member of the streptococcal adhesins.[29]

Effects of vaccination with surface protein A

The surface protein A (PspA) is present on all pneumococcal isolates examined.[6] Antibodies to PspA as well as immunization with this protein have been shown to protect mice from fatal infection.[20] Thus, PspA is not type specific and seems to be able to elicit a protective immune response. The possibility of protecting against a localized infection such as AOM was investigated in the rat model. *Streptococcus pneumoniae* type 6A was used for challenge. In the animals immunized with PspA, there was evidence of protection against purulent ME infection.

EFFECT OF NONSPECIFIC IMMUNOSTIMULATION

The possibility of triggering an immune response by oral vaccines has been widely used, *e.g.*, in poliomyelitis vaccines.[5] Knowledge of the gut-associated lymphoid tissue (GALT) indicates that oral vaccines contribute to both local and systemic immunization.[21] A preparation for oral delivery composed of bacterial ribosomes combined with a cell wall adjuvant, "Ribomunyl®", has previously been shown to increase the number of specific antibody-forming cells in human tonsil tissue, indicating an enhancement of local infectious defense in the upper respiratory tract. The Ribomunyl® preparation is a mixture of ribosomes from *Klebsiella pneumoniae*, *H. influenzae*, *S. pneumoniae*, and *S. pyogenes*, supplemented with membrane proteoglycans from a noncapsular strain of *K. pneumoniae*[22] (Pierre Fabre Médicament, Place Abel Gance 45, Boulogne, France). Previous studies of oral immunization with specific bacterial strains have shown that it can induce protection against experimental AOM.[15]

The rat OM model was used to evaluate the effect of Ribomunyl® on OM.[36] Ribomunyl® was given to 8 rats prior to challenge with *S. pneumoniae*. Seven untreated rats were challenged with the same dose of the same bacteria simultaneously. An effusion was seen in all MEs of all rats 4 days after challenge (Fig. 10). The ME effusion was purulent in 6 out of 8 MEs in the Ribomunyl®-treated group and in 7 out of 7 in the control group. On day 8, a reduced amount of ME effusion was seen in both groups with more effusion in the untreated group.

Although previous studies concerning immunostimulants have demonstrated a stimulation of specific antibody-producing cells in the upper respiratory tract after oral administration

of a ribosomal preparation, there was no AOM protection. The effects of the ribosomal preparation may have a nonspecific effect on the course of bacterial or viral infections although the possibility of preventing an infection after direct inoculation into the ME was not demonstrated.

REFERENCES

1. **Akaan-Pentitilä, E.** 1980. "Middle ear mucosa in newborn infants. A topographical and microanatomical study." Thesis. University of Helsinki.

2. **Albiin, N., S. Hellström, L.E. Stenfors, and A. Cerne.** 1986. Middle ear mucosa in rats and humans. Ann. Otol. Rhinol. Laryngol. **95** (Suppl. 126).

3. **Alwmark, A., S. Bengmark, P. Gullstrand, and C. Schalén.** 1981. Improvement of the splenectomized rat model for overwhelming pneumococcal infection. Standardisation of the inocula. Eur. Surg. Res. **13**:339–343.

4. **Bak-Pedersen, K., and M. Tos.** 1973. Mucous glands in the middle ear and osseous ET. Ann. Otol. Rhinol. Laryngol. **82**:80–88.

5. **Briles, D.E., J.D. King, M.A. Gray, L.S. McDaniel, E. Swiatlo, and K.A. Benton.** 1996. PspA, a protection-eliciting pneumococcal protein: immunogenicity of isolated native PspA in mice. Vaccine **14**:858–867.

6. **Crain, M.J., W.D. Waltman, J.S. Turner, J. Yother, D.F. Talkington, L.S. McDaniel, R.M. Gray, and D.E. Briles.** 1990. Pneumococcal surface protein A (PspA) is serologically highly variable and is expressed by all clinically important capsular serotypes of Streptococcus pneumoniae. Infect. Immun. **58**:3293–3299.

7. **Daniel, H.J., H.C. Forrest, R.A. Cook.** 1971. Otitis media in two strains of laboratory rats. J. Aud. Res. **11**:276–278.

8. **Giebink, G.S., G. Schiffman, K. Petty, and P.G. Quie.** 1978. Modification of otitis media following vaccination with the capsular polysaccharide of Streptococcus pneumoniae in chinchillas. J. Infect. Dis. **138**:480–487.

9. **Giebink, G.S.** 1987. Animal models of otitis media with effusion. *In* J. Bernstein and P. Ogra (eds.). Immunology of the Ear. Raven Press, New York.

10. **Hellström, S., B. Salén, and L.E. Stenfors.** 1982. Anatomy of the rat middle ear. A study under the dissection microscope. Acta Anat. **112**:346–352.

11. **Hermansson, A., P. Emgård, K. Prellner, S. Hellström.** 1988. A rat model for pneumococcal otitis media. Am. J. Otolaryngol. **9**:97–101.

12. **Hermansson, A., K. Prellner, S. Hellström.** 1990. Persistent structural changes in the middle ear mucosa of the rat after an experimentally induced episode of pneumococcal otitis media. Acta Otolaryngol. **109**:421–430.

13. **Hermansson, A., and K. Prellner.** 1990. Effect of gammaglobulin on pneumococcal otitis media in the rat. Acta Otolaryngol. **109**:300–306.

14. **Hermansson, A., S. Hellström, and K. Prellner.** 1991. Mucosal changes induced by experimental pneumococcal otitis media are prevented by penicillin V. Otolaryngol. Head Neck Surg. **105**:578–585.

15. **Lee, C.-J., S.D. Banks, and J.P. Li.** 1991. Virulence, immunity, and vaccine related to Streptococcus pneumoniae. Crit. Rev. Microbiol. **18**:89–114.

16. **Luotonen, J., E. Herva, P. Karma, M. Timonen, M. Leinonen, H. Mäkelä.** 1981. The bacteriology of acute otitis media in children with special reference to *Streptococcus pneumoniae* as studied by bacteriological and antigen detection methods. Scand. J. Infect. Dis. **13**:177–183.

17. **Magnuson, K., A. Hermansson, Å. Melhus, and S. Hellström.**

1999. The tympanic membrane and middle ear mucosa during nontypeable Haemophilus influenzae and Haemophilus influenzae type b acute otitis media. A study in the rat. (in press).

18. **Melhus, Å., A. Hermansson, M. Akkoyunlu, K. Prellner, and A. Forsgren.** 1995. Experimental recurrent otitis media induced by Hemophilus influenzae. Protection and serum antibodies. Am. J. Otolaryngol. **16:**383–390.

19. **Melhus, Å., A. Hermansson, and K. Prellner.** 1994. Nontypeable and encapsulated *Haemophilus Influenzae* yield different clinical courses of experimental otitis media. Acta Otolaryngol. **114:**289–294.

20. **McDaniel, E., K.A. Swiatlo, Benton.** 1996. PspA, a protection-eliciting pneumococcal protein: Immunogenicity of isolated native PspA in mice. Vaccine **14:**858–867.

21. **Michel, F.B., L. Dussourd d'Hinterland, J. Bousquet, A.M. Pinel, and G. Normier.** 1978. Immunostimulation by a ribosomal vaccine associated with a bacterial cell wall adjuvant in humans. Infec Immunity **20:**760–769.

22. **Millet, I., S. Lafont, A. De Fraissinette, M. Jeannin, J.P. Revillard, G. Normier, and L. Dussourd D'Hinterland.** 1987. Polyclonal activation of murine B cells by a membrane proteoglycan of *Klebsiella pneumoniae.* Clin. Exp. Immun. **70:**201–208.

23. **Mogi, G.** 1974. Mucosal immunity of the middle ear. Acta Otolaryngol. **Suppl. 414:**127–130.

24. **Paton, J.C.** 1993. Molecular analysis of the pathogenicity of Streptococcus pneumoniae: The role of pneumococcal proteins. Annu. Rev. Microbiol. **47:**89–115.

25. **Prellner, K.** 1987. Complement an other amplification mechanisms in otitis media, pp. 345–361. *In* J. Bernstein and P. Ogra (eds.). Immunology of the Ear. Raven Press, New York.

26. **Prellner, K., and O. Kalm.** 1988. Humoral immune response in otitis media. Acta Otolaryngol. **Suppl. 457:**133–138.

27. **Rosén, C., P. Christensen, J. Henrichsen, B. Hovelius, and K. Prellner.** 1984. Beneficial effect of pneumococcal vaccination on otitis media in children over two years old. Int. J. Pediatr. Otolaryngol. **7:**239–246.

28. **Ryan, R.F., and A. Catanzaro.** 1983. Passive transfer of immune mediated middle ear inflammation and effusion. Acta Otolaryngol. **95:**123–130.

29. **Sampson, J.S., S.P. O'Conner, A.R. Sinson, J.A. Tharpe, and H. Russel.** 1994. Cloning and nucleotide sequence analysis of a 37-kilodalton protein homologous to previously reported Streptococcus sp. antigens. Infect. Immun. **62:**319–324.

30. **Shurin, P.A., G.S. Giebink, D.L. Wegman, D. Ambrosino, J. Rholl, M. Overman, T. Bauer, and G.R. Siber.** 1988. Prevention of pneumococcal otitis media in chinchillas with human bacterial polysaccharide immune globulin. J. Clin. Microbiol. **26:**755–759.

31. **Svinhufvud, M., K. Prellner, A. Hermansson, C. Schalén.** 1991. Experimental recurrent pneumococcal otitis media: protection and serum antibodies. Acta Otolaryngol. **111:**1083–1089.

32. **Svinhufvud, M., M. Akkoyunlu, J. Rennberg, P. Christensen, and K. Prellner.** 1992. Occurrence of antibodies to pneumococcal protein antigens in experimental acute otitis media. Acta. Otolaryngol. **112:**518–523.

33. **Svinhufvud, M., A. Hermansson, K. Prellner.** 1993. Active immunisation and resistance to experimental acute pneumococcal otitis media. Int. J. Pediatr. Otorhinolaryngol. **25:**91–103.

34. **Westman, E., Å. Melhus, S. Hellström, and A. Hermansson.** Acute otitis media induced by Moraxella catarrhalis in the rat middle ear. (Accepted APMIS).

35. **White, P., A. Hermansson, and M. Svinhufvud.** 1990. Surfactant and Isoprenaline effect on Eustachian tube opening in rats with acute otitis media. Am. J. Otolaryngol. **11:**389–392.

36. **White, P., A. Hermansson, Å. Melhus, and K. Prellner.** 1994. Effect of an immunomodulating substance, Ribomunyl®, on the course of experimental otitis media in rats, pp. 115–120. *In* G. Mogi, J.E. Veldman, and H. Kawauchi (eds.). Immunobiology in Otorhinolaryngology—Progress of a decade. Proceedings of the 4th International Academic Conference, Oita, Japan. Kugler Press,

37. **Yoshimura, H., N. Watanabe, J. Bundo, M. Shinoda, and G. Mogi.** 1991. Oral vaccine therapy for pneumococcal otitis media in an animal model. Arch. Otolaryngol. Head Neck Surg. **117:** 889–894.

Address reprint requests to:
Prof. Karin Prellner
Department of Otorhinolaryngology
University Hospital
S-221 85 Lund
Sweden

Incidence of Invasive Pneumococcal Disease in Denmark

JØRGEN HENRICHSEN and SUSANNE VINTHER NIELSEN

ABSTRACT

The incidence of invasive pneumococcal disease has increased more than 10 times over the last two decades as judged by the number of isolates of *Streptococcus pneumoniae* from blood and cerebrospinal fluid. The overall incidence in 1996 was 27 cases per 100,000 inhabitants. In the elderly, that is, those aged 60 years or more, it was 80 per 100,000. Figures from 1997 are slightly lower. The 10 most common types in children account for 85% of all invasive infections, while in adults they only account for 69%. On the basis of these facts, different vaccine strategies are discussed. Only a minority of all capsular types of *Streptococcus pneumoniae* cause invasive disease in humans. The existing 23-valent polysaccharide vaccines in most places of the world thus cover around 90% of such infections. Recently, six new types were described, bringing the total number of types up to 90; in additon, the history of the nomenclature of types was reviewed.[5] This study extends recent data indicating that there has been a steady increase in the number of cases of invasive pneumococcal infections in Denmark and other countries over the past 20 years.[9–11] It also gives typing data with a view to the possibility of constructing a conjugate vaccine for the use in adults in addition to those presently subject to trials in children under 2 years of age.

INTRODUCTION

In Denmark the incidence of invasive pneumococcal disease has been followed closely for decades because all strains of pneumococci isolated from such cases in the country have been sent to Statens Serum Institut for typing.

MATERIALS AND METHODS

Almost all pneumococci isolated from blood and cerebrospinal fluid (CSF) in Denmark are sent to our institute for verification of diagnosis and typing. Typing is done by the capsular reaction test as described elsewhere.[1,4,7]

RESULTS

Table 1 shows the number of isolates of invasive pneumococci in Denmark during the years 1989–1996 as well as the incidence. Both nearly tripled. The total number of blood or CSF isolates in the 6-year period 1983–1988 was 2,294[8] compared to 5,950 in the 6-year period 1992–1996. Certainly, the present number of invasive isolates is at least ten times higher than it was 20 years ago as has also been observed in Norway.[10]

The rise in the number of invasive isolates during the 1989–1996 period was entirely due to rise in the number of blood isolates. The number of CSF isolates was just close to 100 during the whole period.

The incidence was higher in the very young and in the elderly (Fig. 1). In 1996, it had reached 80 per 100,000 in those 60 years of age and older. Tables 2 and 3 show the types of the pneumococcal isolates from blood or CSF from all age groups

TABLE 1. NUMBER OF ISOLATES OF PNEUMOCOCCI FROM BLOOD OR CSF,[a] 1989–96, IN DENMARK

Year	Number of isolates	Incidence per 100,000 inhabitants
1989	520	10
1990	642	13
1991	749	15
1992	821	16
1993	962	19
1994	926	18
1995	1,075	21
1996	1,417	27

[a]CSF, cerebrospinal fluid (<100 isolates annually).
From Nielsen and Henrichsen,[9] with permission.

Divisions of Microbiology and Diagnostics, Statens Serum Institut, Copenhagen, Denmark.

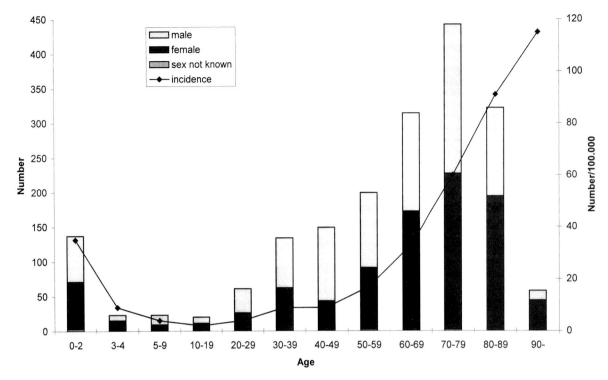

FIG. 1. Incidence, age, and sex distribution of invasive pneumococcal disease in Denmark, 1993–94. (From Nielsen and Henrichsen,[9] with permission of Cambridge University Press.)

and from children, respectively. Types 6A and 6B are looked at as one type in this context because they have been shown to be cross-protective.[12] The types in the two tables are not all the same. It is also noteworthy that, while the 10 most common types from all ages represent 69% of all invasive isolates, in children they represent 85% of all.

DISCUSSION

The pronounced increase in invasive pneumococcal disease in Denmark is very similar to what has been noticed in Nor-

way. There is no obvious explanation for this other than the well-known waxing and waning over decades of infections due to capsulated bacteria.

The incidence found by us in the elderly (80/100,000) compares with that found in a recent study from Israel.[11] Bacteremia is often associated with pneumonia, which is a common disease in the elderly.[3] Recently, outbreaks of pneumococcal pneumonia among unvaccinated residents in chronic-care facilities in three U.S. states (Massachusetts, Oklahoma, Maryland) have been described.[2]

With the high morbidity and mortality of pneumococcal pneumonia and especially with the increase in resistance against

TABLE 2. *Streptococcus pneumoniae* ISOLATED FROM BLOOD OR CSF IN DENMARK, 1989–94, ALL AGES[a]

Order of frequency	Type	No. of strains[b]
1	1	575
2	4	397
3	14	387
4	6A + B[c]	385
5	7F	340
6	9V	292
7	3	250
8	12F	218
9	8	172
10	18C	168

[a]Total no. of strains: 4,620.
[b]The 10 first types represent 69% of all.
[c]6A: 173 and 6B: 212.
From Nielsen and Henrichsen,[9] with permission.

TABLE 3. *Streptococcus pneumoniae* ISOLATED FROM BLOOD OR CSF IN DENMARK 1989–94, LESS THAN 14 YEARS OF AGE[a]

Order of frequency	Type	No. of strains[b]
1	6A + B[c]	92
2	18C	67
3	14	60
4	1	48
5	7F	44
6	19F	34
7	9V	29
8	4	16
9	23F	13
10	5	9

[a]Total no. of strains: 482.
[b]The 10 first types represent 85% of all.
[c]6A: 34 and 6B: 58.
From Nielsen and Henrichsen,[9] with permission.

penicillin and many other antibiotics,[6] vaccination becomes a high priority and may be even a necessity. Of course, the existing 23-valent polysaccharide vaccine may be used much more extensively than at present.

On the other hand, another possibility to consider could be the use of a conjugate vaccine in adults composed either of the 10 most common disease causing adult types or of the ten most common disease causing types in adults *other* than the types included in a childhood vaccine. By comparing Table 3 in this paper with Table 2 in Nielsen and Henrichsen,[9] the vaccine in the latter case should include types 3, 8, 9N, 11A, 12F, 19A, 20, 22F, 24F, and 38. Such a vaccine could be used very successfully in conjunction with the childhood vaccine and they could both be boosted by the presently available 23-valent polysaccharide vaccine.

REFERENCES

1. **Austrian, R.** 1976. The quellung reaction, a neglected microbiologic technique. Mt. Sinai J. Med. **43:**699–709.
2. **CDC.** 1997. Outbreaks of pneumococcal pneumoniae among unvaccinated residents in chronic-care facilities—Massachusetts, October 1995; Oklahoma, February 1996; and Maryland, May–June 1996. M.M.W.R. **46:**60–62.
3. **Fedson, D., J. Henrichsen, P.H. Mäkelä, and R. Austrian.** 1989. Immunization of elderly people with polyvalent pneumococcal vaccine. Infection **17:**437–441.
4. **Henrichsen, J.** 1979. The pneumococcal typing system and pneumococcal surveillance. J. Infect. **1:**31–37.
5. **Henrichsen, J.** 1995. Six newly recognized types of *Streptococcus pneumoniae.* J. Clin. Microbiol. **33:**2759–2762.
6. **Klugman, K.P.** 1990. Pneumococcal resistance to antibiotics. Clin. Microbiol. Rev. **3:**171–196.
7. **Lund, E., and J. Henrichsen.** 1978. Laboratory diagnosis, serology and epidemiologi of *Streptococcus pneumoniae. In* T. Bergan and J.R. Norris (eds.), Methods in microbiology. Academic Press, London, pp. 241–262.
8. **Nielsen, S.V., and J. Henrichsen.** 1993. Capsular types and susceptibility to penicillin of pneumococci isolated from cerebrospinal fluid or blood in Denmark, 1983–1988. Scand J. Infect. Dis. **25:**165–170.
9. **Nielsen, S.V., and J. Henrichsen.** 1996. Incidence of invasive pneumococcal disease and distribution of capsular types of pneumococci in Denmark, 1989–94. Epidemiol. Infect. **117:**411–416.
10. **Nøkleby, H., and A. Lystad.** 1996. Use of pneumococcal vaccine in Norway (in Norwegian). M.S.I.S. **24:**15.
11. **Raz, R., G. Elhanan, T. Shimoni, R. Kitzes, C. Rudinski, Y. Ygra, A. Ynnon, and the Israeli Adult Pneumococcal Bacteremic Group.** 1997. Pneumococcal bacteremia in Israeli adults: epidemiology and resistance to penicillin. Clin. Infect. Dis. **24:**1164–1168.
12. **Robbins, J.B., R. Austrian, C.-J. Lee, S.C. Rastogi, G. Schiffman, J. Henrichsen, P.H. Mäkelä, C.V. Broome, R.R. Facklam, R.H. Tiesjema, and J.C. Parke, Jr.** 1983. Considerations for formulating the second-generation pneumococcal capsular polysaccharide vaccine with emphasis on the cross-reactive types within groups. J. Infect. Dis. **148:**1136–1159.

Address reprint requests to:
Jørgen Henrichsen
Division of Microbiology
Statens Serum Institut
Artillerivej 5
DK-2300 Copenhagen S
Denmark

Part 5

Antibiotic Resistance

Streptococcus pneumoniae
Copyright © 2000 Mary Ann Liebert, Inc., 2 Madison Avenue, Larchmont, NY 10538

Serotypes and Clones of Antibiotic-Resistant Pneumococci

LESLEY McGEE,[1] KEITH P. KLUGMAN,[1] and ALEXANDER TOMASZ[2]

HISTORY

AS PART OF THE DEVELOPMENT of a pneumococcal vaccine, it was discovered that the serum of a patient who had recovered from pneumococcal pneumonia could, in some instances, agglutinate pneumococci isolated from other patients. Thus groups of strains came to be recognized in South Africa by Sir Spencer Lister[1] and by Griffith[2] in the United States. Today there are 90 pneumococcal serotypes recognized using the Quellung reaction and Danish serotype-specific antisera.[3]

In 1933 DNA was discovered to be the basis of heritable changes in living organisms, when it was found that DNA from a killed pneumococcus could transform a living strain to a new serotype.[4] Soon after the commercial production of penicillin, it was recognized that penicillin-resistance could similarly be transformed by DNA from penicillin-resistant killed pneumococci to live susceptible strains.[5] It was another 40 years before the unlinked genes encoding capsular transformation[6,7] and penicillin-resistance were discovered.[8] Wild-type pneumococci are now described that have clearly switched both their penicillin-resistance genes and capsular genes.[9,10]

CARRIAGE OF RESISTANT SEROTYPES

Although the first penicillin-resistant pneumococcus was identified in an adult,[11] the first multiply resistant strains were found in children,[12] and resistant strains have been shown to be more common in children than in adults wherever this has been studied.[13] The reason for this association is unclear, but probably reflects widespread use of antibiotics in children, who more frequently carry pneumococci than do adults. This affords a greater chance of conditions conducive to transformation occurring in the nasopharynx of children. Penicillin therapy reduces the carriage of penicillin-susceptible strains in children, but often does not eliminate them,[14,15] and, because penicillin therapy also selects for colonization of the nasopharynx of children with resistant strains,[15,16] the co-existence of resistant and susceptible strains is favored by penicillin therapy. In multiply resistant strains, exposure to one antibiotic, *e.g.,* trimethoprim-sulfamethoxazole, may select penicillin resistance, more readily than does penicillin therapy itself.[17]

SEROTYPES AND INVASIVE DISEASE

Penicillin-resistance (MIC ≥ 2.0 mg/L) and multiple resistance are restricted worldwide to a few serogroups. These same serogroups dominate the intermediately resistant strains, although a much wider range of serogroups are occasionally implicated in relative penicillin resistance.

Penicillin resistance and multiple resistance were first associated with serotypes 6A, 6B, and 19A pneumococci in hospitalized children in South Africa.[12,18] Early epidemics in the United States were also restricted to serotypes 19A[19] and 6B.[20] Serogroups 6 and 19 and serotype 14 account for 28–67% of pneumococcal bacteremias in children, but only 1–16% of pneumococcal bacteremias in adults.[13]

In Spain, fully resistant strains predominantly belong to serogroup 23, although serogroup 6, serotype 15, and nontypeable strains were found in Barcelona,[21] in the early 1980s. Multiply resistant serogroup 23 strains were reported in two outbreaks in the United Kingdom in 1987.[22,23] In the United States in 1997, 92% of pneumococcal strains with MIC > 2 μg/mL were associated with serogroups 23, 6, 19, 9, and 14.[24]

RESISTANT CLONES WITHIN AND BETWEEN SEROTYPES

An analysis of the evolution of pneumococci suggests that the global increase in the incidence of penicillin-resistant pneumococci involves at least two processes: (i) the importation and spread of a small number of resistant clones[25–27] with advantages over local strains in an environment in which antibiotics are often misused and (ii) *in vivo* selection of indigenous strains with modified penicillin binding proteins (PBPs),[28] either by replacement of part of PBP genes by interspecies or homologous recombinational events or by the acquisition of point mutations in PBP genes.[29,30]

Spanish serotype 23F[25] strains resistant to penicillin, tetracycline, chloramphenicol, and variably resistant to erythromycin, have been described as a distinct clone that has spread to numerous countries in Europe,[31–38] the United Kingdom,[9] the United States,[25,39] South Africa,[40] South America,[41–44] and some regions in the Far East.[27,45,46] The clone has been found in France without tetracycline resistance.[32] The same bacterial

[1]MRC/SAIMR/Wits Pneumococcal Diseases Research Unit, P.O. Box 1038, Johannesburg, South Africa.
[2]Rockefeller University, New York, NY 10021.

clone, but with a 19F capsule, has been found in Spain,[9] France,[32] Iceland,[47] Italy,[37] the United States,[24] the United Kingdom,[9] Taiwan,[46] and South Korea.[27,45] In 1991 Barnes et al.[48] isolated a serotype 14 organism from a child in a day-care center in the United States who had previously carried the 23F strain. PFGE and PBP typing revealed the serotype 14 to be a variant of the Spanish 23F, suggesting capsular switching. This serotype 14 variant has since been identified in Spain[49] and South Korea.[27] Nesin et al. describe serotype 9N and 3 variants of the Spanish 23F clone in two hospitals in New York City.[50] A recent study[24] conducted in the United States on 328 penicillin-resistant pneumococci from 39 states revealed that close to 40% of all highly penicillin-resistant isolates belonged to the Spanish 23F clone, suggesting that a major part of the increase in the incidence of penicillin-resistant pneumococci is due to the spread of a limited number of pneumococcal clones. The serotype 23F pneumococci resistant to extended spectrum cephalosporins, isolated in Tennessee, probably evolved locally and are distinct from the Spanish clone.[51] A penicillin-resistant 23F strain from Finland represents another distinct clone of this serotype that probably evolved in Finland.[31] Serotype 23F clones unique to certain areas have also been identified in Italy,[37] Israel,[52] Colombia,[41] Brazil,[53] and Taiwan.[46] It should be noted that strain BM4200 isolated in France in 1978 has all the phenotypic attributes of the "Spanish" clone.[54] Because the clone from Spain was only described from isolates in the 1980s, molecular analysis of this French isolate may change designation of the clone to the "French" clone!

A serotype 6B strain, also previously described in Spain, has become the dominant pneumococcus isolated from children in Iceland[26] where it accounts for 75% of multiresistant pneumococci.[47] It has also been identified in France,[32] Germany,[33] the United States,[55] the United Kingdom,[26] and Taiwan.[46] A variant of this clone with different PBP genes has been found in Finland.[31] A distinct type 6B clone, intermediately resistant to penicillin and variably resistant to trimethoprim-sulfamethoxazole and to erythromycin, has been described in Bethel, Alaska.[56] Distinct clones of serotype 6B have also been identified in Israel,[52] Bulgaria,[38] the United States,[57] Brazil,[53] Taiwan,[56] and South Africa[63] and have probably evolved locally in each country.

The widespread use of erythromycin has lead to the emergence of a type 14 clone resistant only to erythromycin in the United Kingdom.[59] The clone is widely dispersed throughout the country, and because 29% of blood or CSF isolates from children belonged to serotype 14 in that study, the clone is responsible for a considerable percentage of invasive pneumococcal disease in children in the United Kingdom at this time. Coffey et al.[49] identified a novel serotype 14 clone present in Spain that is highly resistant to penicillin and, in some cases, erythromycin. In a study on strains from Slovakia and the Czech Republic,[60] all serotype 14 isolates with a very high penicillin MIC (8–16 μg/mL) shared a common, highly abnormal PBP pattern with only two (instead of the normal four) high-molecular-size PBPs detectable, both of which showed greatly reduced penicillin affinity. Novel serotype 14 clones present solely in Bulgaria[38] and Brazil[53] have also been identified.

A penicillin-resistant serotype 9V clone present in Spain[9] and France[32] has become widely disseminated throughout the world and has been identified in Italy,[37] Sweden,[61] Germany,[33] the United States,[24] the United Kingdom,[9] and in South America[41,43] and the Far East.[27,46] The PBP genes are identical to those from the Spanish 23F clone.[9] The probable parental fully susceptible 9V clone also exists in the United Kingdom[58] and France.[32] The same bacterial clone but with a serotype 14 capsule has been found in the United States[48] and in a number of countries in South America.[41–44,54]

A clone of multiply resistant serotype 19A strains first identified in Hungary[62] has been described in the Czech Republic and Slovakia.[60] A second clone of 19A with penicillin MICs between 1 and 4 μg/mL has also been identified in these two countries. An analysis of the very wide diversity of resistant pneumococcal isolates in South Africa has identified two clones of serogroup 19A.[63] The first clone representing strains isolated from blood cultures and CSFs of children are intermediately resistant to penicillin (0.12–0.25 μg/mL). The second multiply resistant clone has high-level resistance to penicillin (MIC 4–8 μg/mL), chloramphenicol (MIC 32 μg/mL), tetracycline (MIC 64 μg/mL), erythromycin (MIC > 64 μg/mL), clindamycin (MIC > 64 μg/mL), and rifampicin (MIC 32 μg/mL). Two novel serotype 19 clones have also been described in Bulgaria[38] and Taiwan,[46] respectively. The Bulgarian serotype 19 strains are resistant to tetracycline, trimethoprim-sulfamethoxazole (SXT), and cefotaxime and show extremely high levels of penicillin and erythromycin resistance. This clone did not react with either the erm or mef DNA probes and the mechanism of macrolide resistance in this group of pneumococci remains to be elucidated. Isolates of the Taiwan-19F clone were resistant to penicillin, tetracycline, and erythromycin but were susceptible to chloramphenicol.

A clone of multiply resistant serotype 15F strains unique to Spain[49] has been described. Cluster analysis suggests that the genetic background of these isolates is similar to that of the members of the major multiresistant serotype 23F clone using multilocus enzyme electrophoresis (MLEE) and REP-PCR, but has dissimilar PBP genes to that of the Spanish 23F clone.

An analysis of the clonal structure of pneumococci suggests a freely combining population with epidemic clones, particularly amongst antibiotic-resistant strains.[59]

CONJUGATE VACCINE IMPACT ON SEROTYPES

Analysis of the leading serotypes causing invasive disease in developing and developed countries has led to the formulation of seven valent conjugate vaccines for each group of countries respectively.[64] In a study in Israel[65] where children aged 12–18 months old were immunized with a heptavalent conjugate pneumococcal vaccine, carriage of vaccine-type pneumococci was reduced. The vaccine had no effect on carriage of non-vaccine-type pneumococci. Data from studies on the impact of conjugate vaccines on nasopharyngeal carriage of pneumococci in The Gambia[66] and South Africa[67] is also available. They show that immunization significantly reduces carriage of vaccine-associated and antibiotic-resistant strains, but that non-vaccine serotypes, which are less likely to cause invasive disease, are more prevalent. Clinical trials of immunogenicity and impact on carriage of various global conjugate vaccine formulations are now ongoing. Because the vaccine-associated serotypes are the same as those associated with resistance, increasing resistance widens the potential coverage of the vaccine.[68] Studies have shown that infant immunization reduces carriage of pneumococci and this may potentially have a dramatic impact on the problem of antibiotic resistance in the pneumococcus.

IMPACT OF HUMAN IMMUNODEFICIENCY VIRUS ON PNEUMOCOCCAL SEROTYPES

The impact of the human immunodeficiency virus (HIV) epidemic on pneumococcal pneumonia and bacteremia was described as early as 1984.[69] Subsequent to this report from New York, workers in San Francisco showed that the incidence of pneumococcal bacteremia in acquired immunodeficiency syndrome (AIDS) patients was approximately 100-fold greater than in controls.[70]

An association of HIV infection with pneumococcal resistance has been found in Kenya,[71] and a similar association has been made in the United States.[72] Meynard and co-workers[73] have also documented the association of HIV infection with exposure to antimicrobial agents and infection with resistant pneumococci. The association of penicillin-resistance with HIV infection has been expanded with our observation that HIV-infected patients are infected with pediatric serotypes more often than uninfected controls.[74] This association exists even in the absence of penicillin-resistance. The observation raises the possibility that HIV infection recreates susceptibility to childhood serotypes in these immunocompromised adults.

REFERENCES

1. **Lister, F.S.** 1913. Specific serological reactions with pneumococci from different sources. South African Inst. Med. Res. **2:**103–114.
2. **Griffith, F.** 1928. The significance of pneumococcal types. J. Hyg. **27:**113–159.
3. **Henrichsen, J.** 1995. Six newly recognised types of *Streptococcus pneumoniae*. J. Clin. Microbiol. **32:**2759–2762.
4. **Avery, O., MacLeod, C., and McCarty, M.** 1944. Studies on the chemical nature of the substance inducing transformation of pneumococcal types. J. Exp. Med. **79:**137–158.
5. **Hotchkiss, R.D.** 1951. Transfer of penicillin resistance in pneumococci by the deoxyribonucleate derived from resistant cultures. Cold Spring Harb. Symp. Quant. Biol. **16:**457–461.
6. **Dillard, J.P., and Yother, J.** 1994. Genetic and molecular characterisation of capsular polysaccharide biosynthesis in *Streptococcus pneumoniae* type 3. Mol. Microbiol. **12:**959–972.
7. **Guidolin, A., Morona, J.K., Morona, R., Hansman, D., and Paton, J.C.** 1994. Nucleotide sequence analysis of genes essential for capsular polysaccharide biosynthesis in *Streptococcus pneumoniae* type 19F. Infect. Immun. **62:**5384–5396.
8. **Dowson, C.G., Hutchinson, A., Brannigan, J.A., George, R.C., Hansman, D., Linares, J., Tomasz, A., Smith, J.M., and Spratt, B.G.** 1989. Horizontal transfer of penicillin-binding protein genes in penicillin-resistant clinical isolates of *Streptococcus pneumoniae*. Proc. Natl. Acad. Sci. USA **86:**8842–8846.
9. **Coffey, T.J., Dowson, C.G., Daniels, M., Zhou, J., Martin, C., Spratt, B.G., and Musser, J.M.** 1991. Horizontal transfer of multiple penicillin-binding protein genes, and capsular biosynthetic genes, in natural populations of *Streptococcus pneumoniae*. Mol. Microbiol. **5:**2255–2260.
10. **Kell, C.M., Jordens, J.Z., Daniels, M., Coffey, T.J., Bates, J.,**

11. **Hansman, D., and Bullen, M.M.** 1967. A resistant pneumococcus. Lancet **ii:**264–265.
12. **Jacobs, M.R., Koornhof, H.J., Robins-Browne, R.M., Stevenson, C.M., Vermaak, Z.A., Freiman, I., Miller, G.B., Witcomb, M.A., Isaacson, M., Ward, J.I., and Austrian, R.** 1978. Emergence of multiply resistant pneumococci. N. Engl. J. Med. **299:**735–740.
13. **Klugman, K.P.** 1990. Pneumococcal resistance to antibiotics. Clin. Microbiol. Rev. **3:**171–196.
14. **Gray, B.M., Converse, III, G.M., and Dillon, Jr., H.C.** 1980. Epidemiologic studies of *Streptococcus pneumoniae* in infants: acquisition, carriage, and infection during the first 24 months of life. J. Infect. Dis. **142:**923–933.
15. **Koornhof, H.J., Wasas, A., and Klugman, K.P.** 1992. Antimicrobial resistance in *Streptococcus pneumoniae*: A South African perspective. Clin. Infect. Dis. **15:**84–94.
16. **Robins-Browne, R.M., Kharsany, A.B.M., and Koornhof, H.J.** 1984. Antibiotic-resistant pneumococci in children. J. Hygiene **93:**9–16.
17. **Melander, E., Molstad, S., Persson, K., Hansson, H.B., Sodestrom, M., and Ekdahl, K.** 1998. Previous antibiotic consumption and other risk factors for carriage of penicillin-resistant *Streptococcus pneumoniae* in children. Eur. J. Clin. Microbiol. Infect. Dis. **17:**834–883.
18. **Oppenheim, B., Koornhof, H.J., and Austrian, R.** 1986. Antibiotic-resistant pneumococcal disease in children at Baragwanath Hospital, Johannesburg. Pediatr. Infect. Dis. **5:**520–524.
19. **Simberkoff, M.S., Lewkaszewski, M., Cross, A., Al-Ibrahim, M., Baltch, A.L., Smith, R.P., Geiseler, P.J., Nadler, J., and Richmond, A.S.** 1986. Antibiotic-resistant isolates of *Streptococcus pneumoniae* from clinical specimens: a cluster of serotype 19A organisms in Brooklyn, New York. J. Infect. Dis. **153:**78–82.
20. **Radetsky, M.S., Istre, G.R., Johansen, T.L., Parmelee, S.W., Lauer, B.A., Wiesenthal, A.M., and Glode, M.P.** 1981. Multiply resistant pneumococcus causing meningitis: Its epidemiology within a day-care centre. Lancet **ii:**771–773.
21. **Linares, J., Garau, J., Dominguez, C., and Perez, J.L.** 1983. Antibiotic resistance and serotypes of *Streptococcus pneumoniae* from patients with community-acquired pneumococcal disease. Antimicrob. Agents Chemother. **23:**545–547.
22. **Moore, E.P., and Williams, E.W.** 1988. Hospital transmission of multiply antibiotic-resistant *Streptococcus pneumoniae*. J. Infect. **16:**199–208.
23. **Paton, J.H., and Reeves, D.S.** 1987. First multiresistant pneumococcus in Britain. Br. Med. J. **295:**810–811.
24. **Corso, A., Severina, E.P., Petruk, V.F., Mauriz, Y., and Tomasz, A.** 1998. Molecular characterization of penicillin-resistant *Streptococcus pneumoniae* isolates causing respiratory disease in the United States. Microb. Drug Resist. **4:**325–337.
25. **Munoz, R., Coffey, T.J., Daniels, M., *et al.*** 1991. Intercontinental spread of a multiresistant clone of serotype 23F *Streptococcus pneumoniae*. J. Infect. Dis. **164:**302–306.
26. **Soares, S., Kristinsson, K.G., Musser, J.M., Tomasz, A.** 1993. Evidence for the introduction of a multiresistant clone of serotype 6B *Streptococcus pneumoniae* from Spain to Iceland in the late 1980s. J. Infect. Dis. **168:**158–163.
27. **McGee, L., Klugman, K.P., Friedland, D., and Lee, H.-J.** 1997. Spread of the Spanish multi-resistant serotype 23F clone of *Streptococcus pneumoniae* to Seoul, Korea. Microb. Drug Resist. **3:**253–257.
28. **Zighelboim, S., and Tomasz, A.** 1980. Penicillin-binding proteins of multiply antibiotic resistant South African strains of *Streptococcus pneumoniae*. Antimicrob. Agents Chemother. **17:**434–442.

29. **Laible, G., Spratt, B.G., and Hakenbeck, R.** 1991. Interspecies recombinational events during the evolution of altered PBP2X genes in penicillin-resistant clinical isolates of *Streptococcus pneumoniae*. Mol. Microbiol. **5**, 1993–2202.

30. **Dowson, C.G., Coffey, T.J., and Spratt, B.G.** 1998. Origin and molecular epidemiology of penicillin protein-mediated resistance to β-lactam antibiotics. Trends Microbiol. 2:361–366.

31. **Sibold, C., Wang, J., Henrichsen, J., and Hakenbeck, R.** 1992. Genetic relationships of penicillin-susceptible and -resistant *Streptococcus pneumoniae* strains isolated on different continents. Infect. Immun. **60**:4119–4126.

32. **Lefèvre, J.C., Bertrand, M.A., and Faucon, G.** 1995. Molecular analysis by pulsed-field gel electrophoresis of penicillin-resistant *Streptococcus pneumoniae* from Toulouse, France. Eur. J. Clin. Microbiol. Infect. Dis. **14**:491–497.

33. **Reichmann, P., Varon, E., Günther, E., et al.** 1995. Penicillin-resistant *Streptococcus pneumoniae* in Germany: genetic relationship to clones from other European countries. J. Med. Microbiol. **43**:377–385.

34. **Vaz Pato, M.V., de Carvalho, C.B., and Tomasz, A.** 1995. The multicenter study group. Antibiotic susceptibility of *Streptococcus pneumoniae* isolates in Portugal. A multicenter study between 1989 and 1993. Microb. Drug Resist. **1**:59–69.

35. **Tarasi, A., Sterk-Kuzmanovic, N., Sieradzki, K., Schoenwald, S., Austrian, R., and Tomasz, A.** 1995. Penicillin-resistant and multidrug-resistant *Streptococcus pneumoniae* in a paediatric hospital in Zagreb, Croatia. Microb. Drug Resist. **1**:169–176.

36. **Sluijter, M., Faden, H., de Groot, R., et al.** 1998. Molecular characterization of pneumococcal nasopharynx isolates collected from children during their first 2 years of life. J. Clin. Microbiol. **36**:2248–2253.

37. **Marchese, A., Ramirez, M., Schito, G.C., and Tomasz, A.** 1998. Molecular epidemiology of penicillin-resistant *Streptococcus pneumoniae* isolates recovered in Italy from 1993 to 1996. J. Clin. Microbiol. **36**:2944–2949.

38. **Setchanova, L., and Tomasz, A.** 1999. Molecular characterization of penicillin-resistant *Streptococcus pneumoniae* isolates from Bulgaria. J. Clin. Microbiol. **37**:638–648.

39. **McDougal, L.K., Facklam, R., Reeves, M., et al.** 1992. Analysis of multiply antimicrobial resistant isolates of *Streptococcus pneumoniae* from the United States. Antimicrob. Agents Chemother. **36**:2176–2184.

40. **Klugman, K.P., Coffey, T.J., Smith, A., Wasas, A., Meyers, M., and Spratt, B.G.** 1994. Cluster of an erythromycin-resistant variant of the Spanish multiply resistant 23F clone of *Streptococcus pneumoniae* in South Africa. Eur. J. Clin. Microbiol. Infect. Dis. **13**:171–174.

41. **Castañeda, E., Tomasz, A., and Vela, M.C.T.** 1998. Penicillin-resistant *Streptococcus pneumoniae* in Colombia: Presence of international epidemic clones. Microb. Drug Resist. **4**:233–239.

42. **Rossi, A., Corso, A., Pace, J., Regueira, M., and Tomasz, A.** 1998. Penicillin-resistant *Streptococcus pneumoniae* in Argentina: Frequent occurrence on an internationally spread serotype 14. Microb. Drug Resist. **4**:225–231.

43. **Echániz-Aviles, M., Carnalla-Barajas, N., Velàzquez-Meza, M.E., Soto-Noguerón, A., Espinoza-de los Monteros, L.E., and Solórzano-Santos, F.** 1995. Capsular types of *Streptococcus pneumoniae* causing disease in children from Mexico City. Pediatr. Infect. Dis. J. **14**:907–909.

44. **Camou, T., Hortal, M., and Tomasz, A.** 1998. The apparent importation of penicillin-resistant capsular type 14 Spanish/French clone of *Streptococcus pneumoniae* into Uruguay in the early 1990s. Microb. Drug Resist. **4**:219–224.

45. **Tarasi, A., Chong, Y., Lee, K., and Tomasz, A.** 1997. Spread of the serotype 23F multidrug-resistant *Streptococcus pneumoniae* clone to South Korea. Microb. Drug Resist. **3**:105–109.

46. **Shi, Z.-Y., Enright, M.C., Wilkinson, P., Griffiths, D., and Spratt, B.G.** 1998. Identification of three major clones of multiply antibiotic-resistant *Streptococcus pneumoniae* in Taiwanese hospitals by multilocus sequencing typing. J. Clin. Microbiol. **36**:3514–3519.

47. **Kristinsson, K.G.** 1995. Epidemiology of penicillin-resistant pneumococci in Iceland. Microb. Drug Resist. **1**:121–125.

48. **Barnes, D.M., Whittier, S., Gilligan, P.H., Soares, S., Tomasz, A., and Henderson, F.W.** 1995. Transmission of multidrug-resistant serotype 23F *Streptococcus pneumoniae* in group day care: Evidence suggesting capsular transformation of the resistant strain in vivo. J. Infect. Dis. **171**:890–896.

49. **Coffey, T.J., Berrón, S., Daniels, M., et al.** 1996. Multiply antibiotic-resistant *Streptococcus pneumoniae* recovered from Spanish hospitals (1988–1994): novel major clones of serotypes 14, 19F and 15F. Microbiology **142**:2747–2757.

50. **Nesin, M., Ramirez, M., and Tomasz, A.** 1998. Capsular transformation of a multi-drug resistant *Streptococcus pneumoniae* in vivo. J. Infect. Dis. **177**:707–713.

51. **McDougal, L.K., Rasheed, J.K., Biddle, J.W., and Tenover, F.C.** 1995. Identification of multiple clones of extended-spectrum cephalosporin-resistant *Streptococcus pneumoniae* isolates in the United States. Antimicrob. Agents Chemother. **39**:2282–2288.

52. **Yagupsky, P., Porat, N., Fraser, D., et al.** 1998. Acquisition, carriage, and transmission of pneumococci with decreased antibiotic susceptibility in young children attending a day care facility in Southern Israel. J. Infect. Dis. **177**:1003–1012.

53. **Brandileone, M.C., Di Fabio, J.L., Dias Vierira, V.S., et al.** 1998. Geographic distribution of penicillin resistance of *Streptococcus pneumoniae* in Brazil: genetic relatedness. Microb. Drug Resist. **4**:209–217.

54. **Buu-Hoi, A., Goldstein, F.W., and Acar, J.F.** 1988. A seventeen-year epidemiological survey of antimicrobial resistance in pneumococci in two hospitals. Antimicrob. Agents Chemother. **22(Suppl. B)**:41–52.

55. **Versalovic, J., Kapur, V., Mason, E.O., et al.** 1993. Penicillin-resistant *Streptococcus pneumoniae* strains recovered in Houston: Identification and molecular characterization of multiple clones. J. Infect. Dis. **167**:850–856.

56. **Munoz, R., Musser, J.M., Crain, M.J., et al.** 1992. Geographic distribution of penicillin-resistant clones of *Streptococcus pneumoniae*: Characterization by penicillin-binding protein profile, surface protein A typing, and multilocus enzyme analysis. Clin. Infect. Dis. **15**:112–118.

57. **Harakeh, H., Bosley, G.S., Keihlbauch, J.A., and Fields, B.S.** 1994. Heterogeneity of rRNA gene restriction patterns of multiresistant serotype 6B *Streptococcus pneumoniae* strains. J. Clin. Microbiol. **32**:3046–3048.

58. **Hsueh, P-R., Teng, L-J, Lee, L-N, Yang, P-C, Ho, S-W, and Luh, K-T.** 1999. Dissemination of high-level penicillin-, extended-spectrum cephalosporin-, and erythromycin-resistant *Streptococcus pneumoniae* clones in Taiwan. J. Clin. Microbiol. **37**:221–224.

59. **Hall, L.M.C., Whiley, R.A., Duke, B., George, R.C., and Efstratiou, A.** 1996. Genetic relatedness within and between serotypes of *Streptococcus pneumoniae* from the United Kingdom: analysis of multilocus enzyme electrophoresis, pulsed-field gel electrophoresis, and antimicrobial resistance patterns. J. Clin. Microbiol. **34**:853–859.

60. **Figueiredo, A.M., Austrian, R., Urbaskova, P., Teixeira, L.A., and Tomasz, A.** 1995. Novel penicillin-resistant clones of *Streptococcus pneumoniae* in the Czech Republic and in Slovakia. Microb. Drug Resist. **1**:71–78.

61. **Melander, E., Ekdahl, K., Hansson, H.B., et al.** 1998. Introduction and clonal spread of penicillin- and trimethoprim/sulfamethoxazole-resistant *Streptococcus pneumoniae*, serotype 9V, in Southern Sweden. Microb. Drug Resist. **4**:71–78.

62. **Marton, A., Gulyas, M., Munoz, R., and Tomasz, A.** 1991. Extremely high incidence of antibiotic resistance in clinical isolates of *Streptococcus pneumoniae* in Hungary. J. Infect. Dis. **163**:542–548.

63. **Smith, A.M., and Klugman, K.P.** 1997. Three predominant clones identified within penicillin-resistant South African isolates of *Streptococcus pneumoniae*. Microb. Drug Resist. **3**:385–389.

64. **Snaidack, D.H., Schwartz, B., Lipman, H., Bogaerts, J., Butler, J.C., Dagan, R., Echániz-Aviles, G., Lloyd-Evans, N., Fenoll, A., Girgis, N.I., Henrichsen, J., Klugman, K.P., Lehmann, D., Takala, A.K., Vandepitte, J., Gove, S., and Breiman, R.F.** 1995. Potential interventions for the prevention of childhood pneumonia: Geographic and temporal differences in serogroup distribution of sterile-site pneumococcal isolates from children—implications for vaccine strategies. Paediatr. Infect. Dis. J. **14**:503–510.

65. **Dagan, R., Melamed, R., Muallem, M., Piglansky, L., Greenberg, D., Abramson, O., Mendelman, P.M., Bohidar, N., and Yagubsky, P.** 1996. Reduction of nasopharyngeal carriage of pneumococci during the second year of life by a heptavalent conjugate pneumococcal vaccine. J. Infect. Dis. **174**:1271–1278.

66. **Obaro, S.K., Adegbola, R.A., Banya, W.A.S., and Greenwood, B.M.** 1996. Carriage of pneumococci after pneumococcal vaccination. Lancet **348**:271–272.

67. **Mbelle, N., Wasas, A., Huebner, R., Kimura, A. Chang, I., and Klugman, K.P.** 1999. Immunogenicity and impact on nasopharyngeal carriage of non-valent pneumococcal conjugate vaccine J. Infect. Dis. (in press).

68. **Dagan, R., Yagupsky, P., Goldbart, A., Wasas, A., and Klugman, K.P.** 1994. Increasing prevalence of penicillin-resistant pneumococcal infections in children in southern Israel: implications for future immunization policies. Pediatr. Infect. Dis. J. **13**:782–786.

69. **Simberkoff, M.S., El Sadr, W., Schiffman, G., and Rahal, J.J. Jr.** 1984. *Streptococcus pneumoniae* infections and bacteremia in patients with acquired immune deficiency syndrome, with report of a pneumococcal vaccine failure. Am. Rev. Respir. Dis. **130**:1174–1176.

70. **Redd, S.C., Rutherford, G.W.I., Sande, M.A., Lifson, A.R., Hadley, W.K., Facklam, R.R., and Spike, J.S.** 1990. The role of human immunodeficiency virus infection in pneumococcal bacteremia in San Francisco residents. J. Infect. Dis. **162**:1012–1017.

71. **Paul, J., Kimari, J., and Gilks, C.F.** 1995. *Streptococcus pneumoniae* resistant to penicillin and tetracycline associated with HIV seropositivity. Lancet **346**:1034–1035.

72. **Mao, C., Harper, M., McIntosh, K., Reddington, C., Cohen, J., Bachur, R., Caldwell, B., and Hsu, H.W.** 1996. Invasive pneumococcal infections in human immunodeficiency virus-infected children. J. Infect. Dis. **173**:870–876.

73. **Meynard, J.L., Barbut, F., Blum, L., Guiguet, M., Chouaid, C., Meyohas, M.C., Picard, O., Petit, J.C., and Frottier, J.** 1996. Risk factors for isolation of *Streptococcus pneumoniae* with decreased susceptibility to penicillin G from patients infected with human immunodeficiency virus. Clin. Infect. Dis. **22**:437–440.

74. **Crewe-Brown, H.H., Karstaedt, A.S., Saunders, G.L., Khoosal, M., Jones, N., Wasas, A., and Klugman, K.P.** 1997. Streptococcus pneumoniae blood culture isolates from patients with and without human immunodeficiency virus infection: alterations in penicillin susceptibilities and in serogroups or serotypes. Clin. Infect. Dis. **25**:1165–1172.

Address reprint requests to:
Dr. Lesley McGee
Department of Clinical Microbiology
and Infectious Diseases
Room 103, Main Building
South African Institute for Medical Research
P.O. Box 1038
Cnr Hospital and De Korte Sts
Hillbrow
Johannesburg 2000
South Africa

Molecular Bases of Three Characteristic Phenotypes of Pneumococcus: Optochin-Sensitivity, Coumarin-Sensitivity, and Quinolone-Resistance

ADELA G. De La CAMPA,[1] ERNESTO GARCÍA,[2] ASUNCIÓN FENOLL,[3] and ROSARIO MUÑOZ[1]

ABSTRACT

Streptococcus pneumoniae is uniquely sensitive to amino alcohol antimalarials in the *erythro* configuration, such as optochin, quinine, and quinidine. The protein responsible for the optochin (quinine)-sensitive (Opt^s, Qin^s) phenotype of pneumococcus is the proteolipid *c* subunit of the F_0F_1 H^+-ATPase. Opt^R/Qin^R isolates arose by point mutations in the *atpC* gene and produce different amino acid changes in one of the two transmembrane α-helices of the *c* subunit. In addition, comparison of the sequence of the *atpCAB* genes of *S. pneumoniae* R6 (Opt^s) and M222 (an Opt^R strain produced by interspecies recombination between pneumococcus and *S. oralis*), and *S. oralis* (Opt^R) revealed that, in M222, an interchange of *atpC* and *atpA* had ocurred. We also demonstrate that optochin, quinine, and related compounds specifically inhibited the membrane-bound ATPase activity. Equivalent differences between Opt^s/Qin^s and Opt^R/Qin^R strains, both in growth inhibition and in membrane ATPase resistance, were found.

Pneumococci also show a characteristic sensitivity to coumarin drugs, and a relatively high level of resistance to most quinolones. We have cloned and sequenced the *gyrB* gene, and characterized novobiocin resistant mutants. The same amino acid substitution (Ser-127 to Leu) confers novobiocin resistance on four isolates. This residue position is equivalent to Val-120 of *Escherichia coli* ryGB, a residue that lies inside the ATP-binding domain but is not involved in novobiocin binding in *E. coli*, as revealed by crystallographic data. In addition, the genes encoding the ParC and ParE subunits of topoisomerase IV, together with the region encoding amino acids 46 to 172 (residue numbers as in *E. coli*) of the pneumococcal ryGA subunit, were characterized in respect to fluoroquinolone resistance. The *gyrA* gene maps to a physical location distant from the *gyrB* and *parEC* loci on the chromosome. Ciprofloxacin-resistant (Cp^R) clinical isolates had mutations affecting amino acid residues of the quinolone resistance-determining region of ParC (low-level Cp^R), or in both resistance-determining regions of ParC and GyrA (high-level Cp^R). Mutations were found in residue positions equivalent to Ser-83 and Asp-87 of the *E. coli* GyrA subunit. Transformation experiments demonstrated that topoisomerase IV is the primary target of ciprofloxacin, DNA gyrase being a secondary one.

S*treptococcus pneumoniae* exhibits three characteristic phenotypes of drug sensitivity with different clinical and diagnostic relevance. These are: antimalarial drugs, quinolones, and coumarins. Within the antimalarial group of drugs, pneumococcus is particularly sensitive to optochin (Opt^S [ethylhydrocupreine hydrochloride]) and quinine (Qin^S).[51] Optochin sensitivity is a test routinely used in clinical laboratories to differentiate pneumococcus from other α-haemolytic "viridans" streptococci. This feature, together with bile solubility, colony morphology on blood agar plates, and immunological reaction with type-specific antisera ("Quellung" test) allows the identification of pneumococcus.[44] It has been reported that some pneumococcal isolates show atypical responses in one or more of these tests and that viridans streptococci can give positive results in some of them.[27,36,43,64,68,87,93] Although optochin was used in the beginning of this century for the treatment of pneumococcal infections, and optochin resistance was probably the first observation of the development of resistance *in vivo* to an

[1]Centro Nacional de Biología Fundamental and [3]Centro Nacional de Microbiología, Instituto de Salud Carlos III, 28220 Majadahonda, and [2]Centro de Investigaciones Biológicas, Consejo Superior de Investigaciones Científicas, 28006, Madrid, Spain.

Reprinted from *Microbial Drug Resistance*, Vol. 3, No. 2, 1997.

antibacterial drug, both in mice[53] and man,[52] very little was known about the genetic and biochemical bases of the optochin-sensitive/resistant phenotype. Optochin inhibition to an *S. pneumoniae* diaphorase (dehydrogenase) has been reported, but a direct correlation between growth inhibition and the level of resistance of the purified enzyme could not been demonstrated.[38] We have cloned, sequenced, and characterized the gene responsible for the optochin-sensitivity/resistance trait of *S. pneumoniae* and *S. oralis*.[15,16]

Plasmodium falciparum is the etiological agent of malaria, one of the most serious infectious diseases worldwide.[56] Although chloroquine has been the mainstay of antimalarial treatment for the past 40 years, resistance in *P. falciparum* is now widespread, making more difficult to select appropriate drugs for both prophylaxis and treatment.[83] Quinine and quinidine are the only drugs available for the parenteral treatment of severe chloroquine-resistant *P. falciparum* malaria.[55,19] In spite of years of intensive research, the mechanism of action of antimalarial compounds is still controversial. The precise mechanism of action of these compounds is difficult to analyze by studying field isolates or *in vitro* selected *P. falciparum* strains, because it is impossible to control for the effect of unknown background genes. In addition, a procedure to introduce modified genes in *P. falciparum* is not currently available. For these reasons, it would be very useful to develop an alternative model system for a better understanding of the mechanism of action of antimalarials. We have selected *S. pneumoniae* for this purpose and demonstrated that optochin and quinine specifically inhibit the membrane-associated F_0F_1 H^+-ATPase of *S. pneumoniae*. Opt^R/Qin^R pneumococcal mutants have point mutations in the *atpC* gene encoding the transmembranal *c* subunit of the F_0 complex.[59] The H^+-ATPases utilize the electrochemical transmembrane proton gradient to drive ATP synthesis or, in reverse, the hydrolysis of ATP to extrude protons from the cell.[18,73] The streptococcal F_0F_1 H^+-ATPase functions as a regulator of cytoplasmic pH.[74]

The second and third phenotypes that we have analyzed are the relatively high sensitivity of pneumococci to coumarins and its relatively high resistance to quinolones. Given the emergence and widespread distribution of penicillin-resistant strains,[2,3,37] which are often multiple resistant, it is mandatory to look for new antimicrobial agents for the treatment of the infections caused by these multi-drug-resistant strains. Among the antimicrobial drugs that could be used for the treatment of pneumococcal infections are the fluoroquinolones. Unfortunately, pneumococci show a relatively high level of resistance to most quinolones,[90] and these drugs are, in general, less active against gram-positive than against gram-negative bacteria. The coumarins, in contrary to quinolones, have not yet enjoyed the same pharmaceutical success, probably due to its low activity against gram-negative bacteria, its toxicity in eukaryotes, and its poor solubility in water. However, it is not clear whether the differences in drug susceptibility between the gram-positive and the gram-negative bacteria to quinolones and coumarins are due to drug accessibility or to the structures of their DNA topoisomerase type II enzymes or both. The characterization of the genes responsible for the synthesis of these enzymes will help to resolve this issue. Studies on the mechanisms of action of quinolones and coumarins in pneumococcus would lead to develop new drugs for clinical use with increased activity against *S. pneumoniae* and, in general, against gram-positive bacteria.

The coumarins and the quinolones act on the bacterial type II DNA topoisomerases (DNA gyrase and topoisomerase IV),

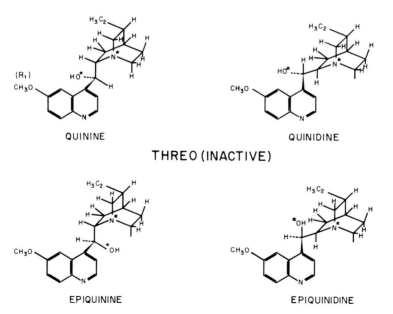

FIG. 1. Chemical structure of relevant amino alcohol antimalarial agents. Optochin is as quinine is but R1 is CH_3–CH_2–. Important N and O atoms for the reactivity of the molecules are indicated by asterisks. (Reprinted with permission from Muñoz et al.[59])

inhibiting chromosome replication and partitioning. DNA gyrase and topoisomerase IV enzymes function by passing a DNA helix through another, utilizing a double strand break (reviewed in ref. 45), and require ATP hydrolysis for the reaction. DNA gyrase is an essential bacterial enzyme that consists of two A and two B subunits, which are encoded by the gyrA and gyrB genes, respectively. It catalyzes ATP-dependent negative supercoiling of DNA and is involved in DNA replication, recombination, and transcription (reviewed in refs. 21, 85). Whereas DNA gyrase is an essential enzyme in prokaryotes, it has not been found in mammalian cells. Hence, it has been seen as a selective target for the design of antibiotics. Topoisomerase IV, recently described in Escherichia coli,[34] is encoded by two closely linked genes, parC and parE, and it is believed that this enzyme plays an essential role in partitioning replicated chromosomes. As already mentioned for DNA gyrase, topoisomerase IV consists of four subunits ($ParC_2ParE_2$), being ParC and ParE homologous to GyrA and GyrB, respectively. The ParC and GyrA subunits are involved in the breakage–rejoining process and GyrB and ParE in energy transduction via ATP hydrolysis.

Bacterial resistance to quinolones can arise through point mutations in any subunit of DNA gyrase (reviewed in ref. 70). However, in E. coli, high-level resistance mutations map primarily to the quinolone resistance-determining region (QRDR) spanning residues 67–106 of the GyrA sequence;[92] in this region the homology between GyrA and ParC is the highest. Recent studies have identified similar mutations in the equivalent region of ParC from Neisseria gonorrhoeae,[4] Staphylococcus aureus,[17] and Haemophilus influenzae.[23] In the gram-negative bacteria, N. gonorrhoeae and H. influenzae, GyrA has been identified as the primary target of ciprofloxacin. Amino acid changes in ParC were only observed with the simultaneous presence of one or more resistance mutations in gyrA. Interestingly, the opposite was observed in the gram-positive bacterium S. aureus. We have characterized the parE, parC, and gyrA genes of S. pneumoniae in relation to the formation of the fluoroquinolone resistance phenotype. Sequence analysis and transformation experiments indicated that ParC is the primary target of ciprofloxacin and that it cooperates with GyrA mutants to increase the resistance level.[58]

The coumarins, which include novobocin and coumermycin A1, are naturally occurring compounds, isolated from certain strains of Streptomyces, which inhibit the ATPase activity of GyrB.[22,49] Topoisomerase IV is also inhibited in vitro by novobiocin,[66] but parE resistance mutations have not yet been described. Mutations in gyrB that confer coumarin resistance have been described in E. coli,[10,13] Borrelia burgdorferi,[72] and Haloferax.[28] We have genetically characterized the pneumococcal gyrB gene and also identified mutations that cause novobiocin resistance.[57] This represented the first characterization of a coumarin resistance mutation in the gyrB gene of a gram-positive bacterium.[57] Recently, mutations also conferring resistance to coumarins and to the new drugs, cyclothialidines, from the gram-positive bacterium S. aureus have been identified.[75] Although coumarins are not used for the treatment of pneumococcal infections, new less toxic compounds, the cyclothialidines, that also inhibit the ATPase activity of the B subunit of the DNA gyrase,[61] would represent new drugs with a promising future for the treatment of pneumococcal infections.

MOLECULAR BASES OF THE OPTOCHIN/QUININE SENSITIVITY PHENOTYPE

Optochin, quinine, and quinidine are compounds derived from the Cinchona bark tree.[84] All three are amino alcohol antimalarials that can have an erythro- or threo- structure that is relevant for their antimalarial activity.[78] Of primary importance is the N–O distance (Fig. 1). This distance is larger in the erythro forms (intermolecular interactions are favored) than in the threo forms, in which intramolecular interactions are preferred. The sensitivity of S. pneumoniae to several cinchona alkaloids was determined (Table 1). Only those alkaloids having antimalarial properties (i.e., those in the erythro configuration) also possess antipneumococcal activity. In addition, a different susceptibility to quinine and quinidine has been found (Table 1) which agrees with that previously reported for P. falciparum.[69,88]

Construction of Opt^R and Qin^R S. pneumoniae strains

We first transformed the pneumococcal M22 strain (Opt^S),[71] using DNAs from different Opt^R streptococci (S. sanguis, S. mitis, S. gordonii, and S. oralis) taxonomically related to S. pneumoniae and found that only S. oralis DNA showed significant transformation efficiency, which is in accordance with the high genetic relationship between S. oralis and S. pneumoniae.[35] One Opt^R M22 colony obtained by transformation with S. oralis DNA was kept and designated as M222 strain. Afterwards, we isolated several spontaneous Opt^R mutants (frequency of spontaneous mutation to Opt^R being about 10^{-7}) and Qin^R mutants (MJQ1 to 7) by plating R6 cells in plates containing quinine (60 μg/ml).

Cloning and sequencing the genes conferring Opt^R to M222

Chromosomal M222 DNA was digested with several restriction endonucleases and the residual Opt^R transforming activity was assayed using strain M22 (Opt^S) as recipient. EcoRV fragments of 5–7 kb isolated from agarose gels were cloned

TABLE 1. SUSCEPTIBILITY OF S. PNEUMONIAE STRAINS TO SEVERAL CINCHONA ALKALOIDS

Strain	MIC (mM) of[a]			
	Optochin	Quinine	Quinidine	Epiquinine -epiquinidine
R6, M22	3	80	1,000	1,000
MJ11	63	100	500	1,000
MJ2	63	320	500	ND[b]
MJQ3[c]	8	200	1,000	ND
MJQ4	31	250	50	ND

[a]For the determination of MICs, cells were grown in Todd–Hewitt broth, supplemented with 0.5% yeast extract containing different concentrations of drugs.
[b]ND, not determined.
[c]As MJQ1, MJQ2, MJQ5, MJQ6, and MJQ7.
(Reprinted with permission from Muñoz et al.[59])

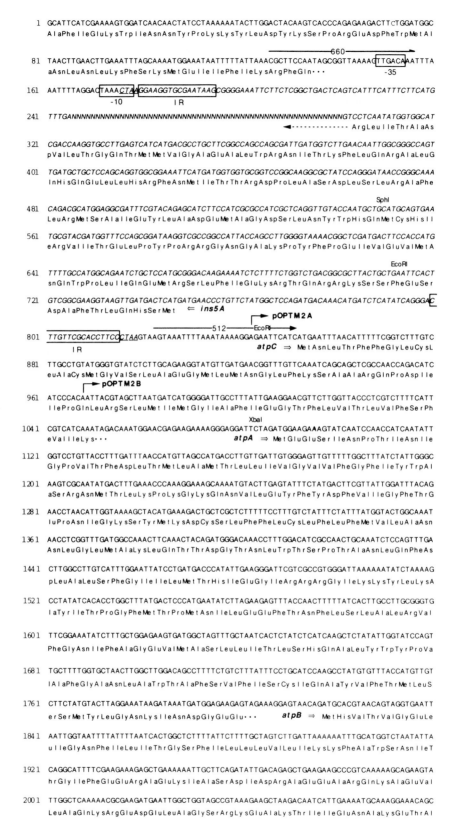

FIG. 2. Nucleotide and deduced amino acid sequences of pertinent regions of plasmid pOPTM1 and pOPTM2. Only the strand corresponding to the mRNA sequence is shown. The sequence corresponding to the IS5 element is shown in italics, the integration site is underlined, and inverted repeats (IR) are boxed. The -35 and -10 regions of the putative *atp* promoter are also boxed. Oligonucleotides used in PCR experiments are indicated by arrows. The extent of the deletions in the derivative plasmids pOPTM2A and -2B are indicated by curved arrows. *N*, not determined nucleotide sequence.

```
2081   TGAGCAAAGTAAGGCTAATATCTTAGCAGATGCTAAAGTAGAAGCAGGTCGCTTAAAAGAGAAGGCGAATCAAGAAATTG
       aGluGlnSerLysAlaAsnIleLeuAlaAspAlaLysValGluAlaGlyArgLeuLysGluLysAlaAsnGlnGluIleA
                                                     ←————594————
2161   CTCAGAATAAAGCTGAGGCTTTGCAAAGTGTTAAGGGCGAGGTGGCAGATTTGACCGTTAGTCTCGCTGGTAAAATCATC
       laGlnAsnLysAlaGluAlaLeuGlnSerValLysGlyGluValAlaAspLeuThrValSerLeuAlaGlyLysIleIle
2241   TCAAAAAACCTTGACAGTCATGCTCATAAGGAACTCATTGATCAGTATATCGATCAGCTAGGAGAAGCCTAATGGACAAG
       SerLysAsnLeuAspSerHisAlaHisLysGluLeuIleAspGlnTyrIleAspGlnLeuGlyGluAla··MetAspLys
                                                                          atpX ⇒
       SphI
2321   AAAACAGCAAAGGTAATTGAAAAATACAGCATGCCTTTTGTCCAATTAGTGATTGAAAAAGGAGAAGAGGACCGGATTTT
       LysThrAlaLysValIleGluLysTyrSerMetProPheValGlnLeuValIleGluLysGlyGluGluAspArgIlePh
2401   TTCAGACTTGGATCAAATCAAGCAAGTCGCAGAAGAAACGGGCTTACCTTCTTTTTTAGCTCAGGTGGCAGTTGATGAGT
       eSerAspLeuAspGlnIleLysGlnValAlaGluGluThrGlyLeuProSerPheLeuAlaGlnValAlaValAspGluS
2481   CTGATAAGGAAAAAACAGTTGGTTTCTTTCAAGACTCTGTCTCACCTTTAATGCAAAACTTTATTCAGGTTCTGATTTAC
       erAspLysGluLysThrValGlyPhePheGlnAspSerValSerProLeuMetGlnAsnPheIleGlnValLeuIleTyr
2561   AATCACAGAGCAAATCTTTTTTATGAT
       AsnHisArgAlaAsnLeuPheTyrAsp
```

FIG. 2. *(Continued)*

into *E. coli* using *Sma*I-cut pUC13 and the ligated products used to transform to ampicillin resistance. Alkaline lysates of these transformants were tested for the ability to transform the M22 strain to Opt^R. One clone harboring a recombinant plasmid (pOPTM1) with a 6.7 kb DNA insert was isolated from about 1,500 recombinant colonies and used for further studies. The gene responsible for the Opt^R phenotype was localized in a 1.8 kb *Sph*I fragment that was subcloned, yielding plasmid pOPTM2. The nucleotide sequence obtained from the inserts of pOPTM1 and pOPTM2 revealed four complete open reading frames (ORF) (Fig. 2). The first ORF corresponded to the Ins5A protein encoded by the IS5 element of *E. coli*.[39] Sequence in Fig. 3 shows the characteristic duplication of the site of integration (CTAA box) of the IS5 element and the inverted repeat sequences. We concluded that a complete IS5 element was present in pOPTM1. However, additional experiments using

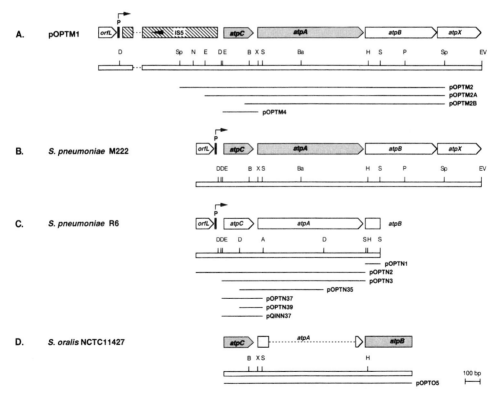

FIG. 3. Genetic structure and physical maps of the *atp* regions of plasmid pOPTM1 (A), *S. pneumoniae* M222 (B), *S. pneumoniae* R6 (C), and *S. oralis* (D) as deduced from the nucleotide sequence. The top lane shows in each case the genetic structure of the region. P indicates the putative promoter and genes are indicated by empty (*S. pneumoniae* R6) or shaded (*S. oralis*) arrows. The physical maps of the plasmid inserts of pertinent plasmids are also indicated. A, *Ase*I; B, *Bst*EII; Ba, *Bal*I; D, *Dra*I; E, *Eco*RI; EV, *Eco*RV; H, *Hph*I; N, *Nco*I; P, *Pvu*II; S, *Ssp*I; Sp, *Sph*I; X, *Xba*I. (Reprinted with permission from Fenoll et al.[16])

PCR amplification (see below) showed that IS5 was not present in either of the streptococcal genomes and, consequently, is presumed to be a cloning artifact.

The other three complete ORFs are oriented in the opposite direction for transcription to IS5. They could encode proteins of about 7 kDa, 27 kDa, and 18 kDa that were homologous to the genes coding for the c, a, and b subunits, respectively, of the F_0 portion of the H^+-ATPase. We, therefore, named these genes atpC, A, and B. The insertion of the IS5 element would interfere with the expression of the complete atp operon. A similar fact has been observed in the atp operon of E. coli, in which insertion of IS5 between the promoter and the first gene of the operon limits the expression of the a subunit, otherwise inhibitory of the cell growth.[33] These results suggest that overproduction of the a subunit of the streptococcal H^+-ATPase would also be toxic for E. coli. Moreover, deletions including the atpA gene of Enterococcus hirae (formerly S. faecalis) have been observed when cloning in E. coli.[74] It is conceivable that the insertion of the IS5 element into plasmid pOPTM1 would represent a fortuitous event that allowed the cloning of these genes in E. coli.

Two features differentiate the pneumococcal atp operon from others previously described. First, the gene order is atpCAB in contrast to the atpACB gene order found in other organisms[73] including related species as Enterococcus hirae.[74] Interestingly, as found in E. hirae, there is no ORF in S. pneumoniae homologous to the atpI gene present in other bacteria.[73] Second,

an ORF, preceded by a putative RBS, and beginning in an ATG codon that overlapped the stop codon of atpB is at the 3′ end of the atpCAB operon. As this gene seems to be part of the atp operon, we preliminary named it atpX. An additional gene has also been found in the ATPase genes of Rhodopseudomomas blastica,[82] but we have not been able to find any significant homology between the atpX genes of S. pneumoniae and R. blastica or other genes included in the EMBL data bank.

To identify which of the genes carried by pOPTM2 conferred Opt^R, plasmids with 5′ deletions were used to transform M22 to Opt^R. Plasmid pOPTM2A (Fig. 2 and Fig. 3) showed high efficiency of transformation whereas pOPTM2B did not, suggesting that the 38 N-terminal amino acids of the ATPase c subunit were responsible for the Opt^R phenotype. To confirm this hypothesis, a fragment containing the complete atpC gene was cloned to yield plasmid pOPTM4 (Fig. 3). Unexpectedly, this plasmid did not transform the pneumococcal M22 strain to Opt^R.

Genetic characterization of the atp genes of S. pneumoniae and S. oralis

As just indicated, M222 is a hybrid strain originated by transformation of S. pneumoniae with S. oralis DNA. To elucidate the recombination events that rendered strain M222, it was necessary to analyze the genetic structure of the atp genes of S. pneumoniae and S. oralis. Fragments of DNA from the atp operon of S. oralis and S. pneumoniae R6 (Opt^S), and MJ11 (Opt^R) were cloned in E. coli after PCR amplification with synthetic oligonucleotides derived from the sequence of the pOPTM1 insert. Oligonucleotides 660 and 512 are located before and after the insertion site of IS5 in pOPTM1, respectively, whereas oligonucleotide 594 is located near the 3′ end of atpB (Fig. 2). The PCR products are shown in Fig. 4. When the set 660/594 was used, all S. pneumoniae DNAs tested (including M222 DNA) showed a major band of about 1.4 kb, whereas no amplification was observed with S. oralis DNA (not shown). With this set of primers, pOPTM1 showed a band of about 2.5 kb, as expected from the insertion of an IS5 element (1,165 bp) in this plasmid. The results of PCR amplification with oligonucleotides 660/594 showed that the IS5 element was absent in the M222 strain and that the element was probably introduced into pOPTM1 during cloning in E. coli. When oligonucleotides 512/594 were used, M222, pOPTM1 and S. oralis showed a band of the expected size (1.4 kb), whereas that observed with the S. pneumoniae DNAs was of about 1.7 kb. The accuracy of the amplified products was tested by transformation of strain M22 to Opt^R using DNA fragments of 1.4 and 1.7 kb corresponding to the amplification of the MJ11 (Opt^R) DNA.

The atp genes of S. oralis and S. pneumoniae were cloned from PCR products of an amplification experiment with oligonucleotides 512/594 and the inserts of the resulting plasmids (Fig. 3) were sequenced. Comparison between the DNA sequences of strain M222 (insert of plasmid pOPTM1), S. pneumoniae R6 (inserts of plasmids pOPTN1 and 2), and S. oralis (inserts of plasmid pOPT05) (not shown) showed that the atpC and atpA genes of M222 and S. oralis were identical, whereas nucleotides coincide in M222 and R6 in the region extending from the 5′ end of the sequence to near the integration site of the IS5 element as well as in the atpB gene (Fig. 3). These find-

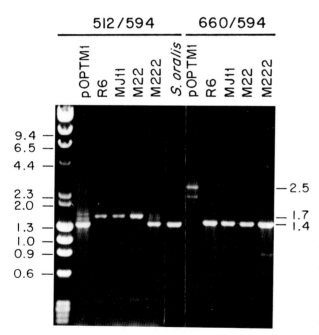

FIG. 4. Products of PCR amplification of atp genes. Plasmid pOPTM1 or chromosomal DNA from S. oralis and the indicated S. pneumoniae strains were used for PCR amplification with oligonucleotides 660/594 or 512/594. Products were subjected to agarose gel electrophoresis and stained with ethidium bromide. Left lane, HindIII-cleaved λ DNA plus HaeIII-cleaved ΦX174 RF DNA. Numbers indicate molecular sizes in kb.

TABLE 2. MUTATIONAL SUBSTITUTIONS ON SEVERAL
NATURAL AND LABORATORY OPT[R]/QIN[R] ISOLATES

Strain	Source	Capsular group	Amino acid change (codon change)
R6 derivatives			
MJ11	SM[a]	Rough[b]	[49]A→T(GCC→ACC)
MJ2,-4,-5,-6	SM[a]	Rough[b]	[48]V→L(GTT→CTT)
MJQ1,-2,-3,-5,-6,-7	SM[a]	Rough[b]	[23]M→I(ATG→ATA)
MJQ4	SM[a]	Rough[b]	[20]G→A(GGT→GCT)
Clinical isolates			
MJ959/89	Blood	19	[49]A→T(GCC→ACC)
MJ455/89	CSF[c]	6	[48]V→F(GTT→TTT)
MJ1996/89	Blood	14	[50]F→L(TTT→TTG)
MJ4133/89	Sputum	NT[d]	[48]V→F(GTT→TTT)

[a]SM, spontaneous mutant isolated in the laboratory.
[b]The progenitor of these strains was of serogroup 2.
[c]CSF, cerebrospinal fluid.
[d]NT, nontypable.

ings demonstrated the interchange of the *atpC* and *atpA* genes in M222.

Based on sequence similarities between several genes of *S. pneumoniae* and *S. oralis*, it has been suggested that interspecific transformation occurred in nature.[9,14,48] On the other hand,

TABLE 3. TRANSFORMATION OF *S. PNEUMONIAE*
STRAIN M22 WITH CHROMOSOMAL DNAS,
PCR PRODUCTS, AND CLONED *atpC* GENES

	Efficiency of transformation (10^4 transformants/ml) with[a]:			
	Optochin (μM)		Quinine (μM)	
Donor DNA	8	4	80	100
R6				
Chromosomal	<0.01	<0.01	<0.01	<0.01
PCR product	<0.05	<0.05	<0.05	<0.05
MJ11				
Chromosomal	50	ND[b]	4	<0.01
PCR product	45	ND	15	<0.05
Cloned *atpC*	10	ND	25	<0.01
MJ2				
Chromosomal	20	ND	19	24
PCR product	37	ND	50	60
MJQ3[c]				
Chromosomal	ND	1	25	1
PCR product	ND	2	40	1
MJQ4				
Chromosomal	26	ND	70	31
PCR product	20	ND	150	100
Cloned *atpC*	23	ND	100	100

[a]Transformation was performed as described elsewhere[81] and transformants were selected in C medium[81] containing 0.08% yeast extract and the indicated drug concentration.
[b]ND, not done.
[c]Identical results were obtained using either MJQ1, MJQ2, MJQ5, MJQ6, and MJQ7.
(Reprinted with permission from Muñoz et al.[59])

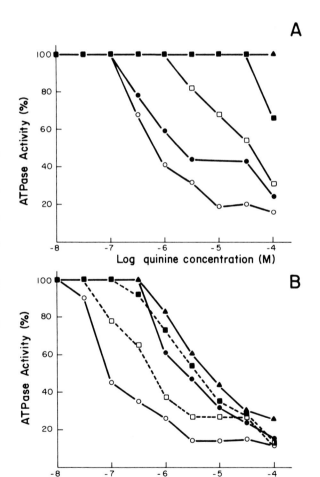

FIG. 5. Effects of quinine (A) and optochin (B) on ATPase activity in membranes from wild type (○, R6) and mutants (▲, MJ2; ●, MJ11; □, MJQ3; and ■, MJQ4). Values are the average of at least three independent determinations. (Reprinted with permission from Muñoz et al.[59])

it has been shown that *N. meningitidis* can be transformed to increased penicillin resistance using chromosomal DNA from other *Neisseria* species providing a laboratory demonstration of interspecies recombination events that mimic what is presumed to occur in nature.[6] The comparison of the nucleotide sequence of the *atpC* and *atpA* genes of *S. oralis* and *S. pneumoniae* revealed about 80% identity, a value that might account for the successful transformation of *S. pneumoniae* using *S. oralis* DNA. The absence of transformation observed when using pOPTM4 as donor DNA might be due to an incompatibility in the organization of an F_0 complex with a *c* subunit from one species and an *a* subunit from another.

Characterization of mutations responsible for the Opt^R/Qin^R phenotype

Transformation to Opt^R with plasmids derived from pOPTN3 (pOPTN35, 37, and 39) (Fig. 3) showed that the mutation responsible for the Opt^R phenotype of the MJ11 strain was a G to A transition located in the *atpC* gene. Moreover, the nucleotide sequence of the *atpC* gene from four Opt^R, seven Qin^R R6 derivatives, and several clinical isolates of *S. pneumoniae* either Opt^R (four strains), or Opt^S (three isolates), was determined in the same way. The sequence of the *atpC* gene from the Opt^S clinical isolates was identical to that of R6 whereas all the Opt^R have point mutations that produce different changes in the corresponding amino acid residues: Val-48 (four R6 derivatives and two clinical isolates), Ala-49 (one clinical isolate), and Phe-50 (one clinical isolate). The Qin^R strains had mutations altering amino acids Met-23 and Gly-20 (Table 2). Our results show that, apart from the laboratory strain M222, none of the naturally Opt^R pneumococci analyzed so far has a mosaic structure in their *atp* genes.

Direct evidence showing that *atpC* mutations are responsible for optochin and quinine resistance was obtained by genetic transformation performed with chromosomal DNAs, PCR products containing the *atpCA* genes, or cloned *atpC* genes (including the one from strain MJQ4 into plasmid pQINN37) (Fig.

3). The DNAs from the Opt^R mutants transformed with high efficiency the Opt^S M22 strain not only to Opt^R but also to Qin^R (Table 3). Furthermore, DNAs from the Qin^R mutants were also able to transform the M22 strain to both Qin^R and Opt^R. The Opt concentration used to select transformants was 8 μM (3 μg/ml), except when the donor DNA was prepared from MJQ1, 2, 3, 5, 6, or 7, where transformants were scored at 4 μM according to the MIC for optochin of these strains (8 μM). Also according to the MIC of MJ11 for quinine (Table 2), no Qin^R M22 transformants were obtained when scored at 100 μM (Table 3). These results indicated that the Opt^R and Qin^R phenotypes were determined by the same mutation.

Biochemical characterization of AtpC

ATPase activity was determined on isolated membranes of Opt^S/Qin^S (M22, R6) and both Opt^R/Qin^R *S. pneumoniae*. All strains were equally inhibited by dicyclohexylcarbodiimide (DCCD), a typical inhibitor of the F_0F_1 H^+-ATPases (not shown), whereas Opt and Qin inhibited differently the ATPase activity of the various strains in correspondence to their different MICs (compare Fig. 5 with Tables 1 and 3). Interestingly, a mixture of 9-epiquinine and 9-epiquinidine, the *threo* cinchona alkaloids, did not inhibit the ATPase activity of R6 even at the highest concentration used (1 mM). These experiments confirmed the biochemical functionality of the *atp* genes and its relation with the Opt/Qin resistant/sensitive phenotypes.

Combined genetic and chemical modification studies support a hairpin-like structure for the *c* subunit with two α-helices that transverse the membrane antiparallelly, separated by a conserved polar loop region that possibly forms the F_1-binding region.[18] Mutations that eliminate the carboxyl group of Asp-61 in the *E. coli c* subunit (equivalent to Glu-52 in *S. pneumoniae*) in helix-2 inhibit H^+ translocation.[18] Glu-52 was not altered in the Opt^R/Qin^R pneumococcal mutants, although inhibition of H^+-ATPase activity was observed. The mutations that confer both Opt^R and Qin^R phenotypes to *S. pneumoniae* would produce changes in Gly-20 or Met-23 of helix-1 (those

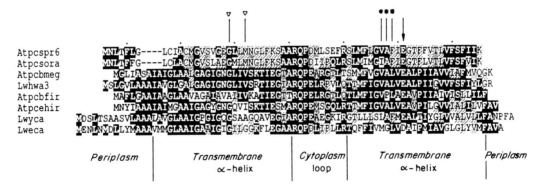

FIG. 6. Amino acid sequence comparison between different *c* subunits of the F_0F_1 H^+-ATPase. Amino acid residues conserved in at least four species are shown in black boxes whereas those present in at least two species are either shadowed or dotted. Amino acids that are mutated in laboratory strains obtained *via* quinine resistance are indicated by inverted triangles, whereas those mutated in strains obtained *via* optochin resistance and in Opt^R clinical strains are indicated by asterisks. The amino acid involved in proton translocation is indicated by an arrow. The putative localization of the different regions when the protein is folded within the membrane bilayer are also indicated.[73] Atpcspr6, *S. pneumoniae* R6; Atpcsora, *S. oralis;* Atpcbmeg, *Bacillus megaterium;*[7] Lwhwa3, thermophyllic bacterium PS 3;[30] Atpcbfir, *B. firmus*[31] Atpcehir, *E. hirae;*[74] Lwyca, *Synechococcus* sp.;[11] Lweca, *E. coli.*[20] (Reprinted with permission from Fenoll et al.[16])

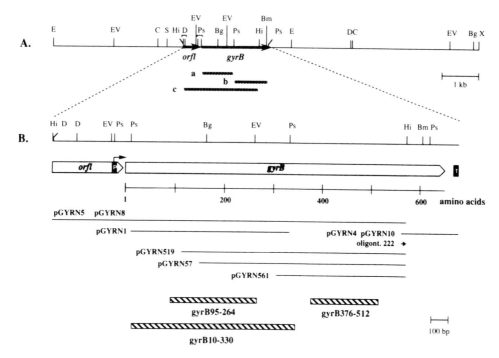

FIG. 7. Restriction map of the *gyrB* region of *S. pneumoniae* (A) and genetic structure as deduced from the nucleotide sequence (B). P indicates the putative promoter, and RBS the ribosome binding site. The physical maps of the inserts of pertinent plasmids, PCR products, and oligonucleotides are also indicated. Bm, *Bam*HI; Bg, *Bgl*II; C, *Cla*I; D, *Dra*I; E, *Eco*RI; EV, *Eco*RV; Hi, *Hind*III, Ps, *Pst*I; X, *Xba*I. The DNA probes used in Southern blot experiments are indicated as bars labeled a (insert of plasmid pGYRN1), b (insert of plasmid pGYRN7), and c (insert of plasmid pGYRN5). The location of the ORFs are indicated by arrows.

isolated via quinine resistance), and Val-48 or Ala-49 of helix-2 (those isolated *via* optochin resistance) (Fig. 6). Moreover, an Opt[R] clinical isolate has altered Phe-50 of helix-2 (Table 2). The altered amino acid residues located in helix-2 are near to Glu-52 which, in all the species studied so far, is directly involved in proton translocation). It has been shown in *E. coli* that Gly-58 (equivalent to Ala-49 in *S. pneumoniae,* Fig. 6) is also an important residue for proton conduction.[54] Moreover, in *Saccharomyces cerevisiae,* olygomicin and venturicidin resistance can be induced by an Ala to Thr change in the mitochondrial H[+]-ATPase *c* subunit in a position equivalent to the Ala-49 residue of *S. pneumoniae.*[60]

A functional ATPase from a double mutant *E. coli* strain in which the Asp-61 carboxyl group was eliminated and its function replaced by an Asp residue at position 24 in helix-1 (equivalent to Val-15 of *S. pneumoniae*) has been isolated and characterized.[50] The functioning of the double mutant suggests that both helices may interact as a unit to present the essential carboxyl group during H[+] translocation. However, the amino acids of helix-1 and helix-2 would be closely juxtaposed within the membrane bilayer when the protein is folded and associated with the *a* and *b* subunits to form the F_0 complex of the H[+]-ATPase. Therefore, the interaction of Qin and Opt with the *c* subunit would cause a conformational change in F_0 hindering the proper presentation of the essential carboxyl group of Glu-52 for H[+] translocation. These results support the idea that the interaction of the chemically similar (see Fig. 1) optochin and quinine with the *c* subunit occurs in the same region of the protein.

It is tempting to speculate that the primary target for quinine in *P. falciparum* would also be the subunit equivalent to the

bacterial *c* protein of the mitochondrial F_0F_1 H[+]-ATPase because an appropriate functioning of mitochondria is critical for survival of erythrocytic stages of malarial parasites.[5,25] However, the vacuolar H[+]-ATPase[65] could also be an alternative target because its proteolipid subunit and the eubacterial proteolipid are evolutionary related.[47,62] Antimalarials increase the vacuolar pH. This increase inhibits parasite growth, possibly because the acid proteases of the parasite could not longer degrade hemoglobin.[29] Quinine and quinidine could bind to the proteolipid subunit of the vacuolar ATPase and inhibit the proton pump which would result in an increase of the vesicle pH. In agreement with this hypothesis, it has been observed that quinine strongly inhibits a vacuolar membrane ATPase activity of *P. falciparum.*[8] Notwithstanding that further experiments with *P. falciparum* will be necessary to demonstrate that the primary target of quinine in *S. pneumoniae* is similar to that in the malarial parasite, the pneumococcal system described here is an interesting model system to test the putative antimalarial activity of new compounds, either natural or synthetic, structurally related to the *Cinchona* alkaloids.

MOLECULAR BASES OF THE COUMARIN AND QUINOLONE SENSITIVE/RESISTANT PHENOTYPES

Genetic characterization of gyrB of S. pneumoniae

We used plasmid pNOV35, which carries the *nov-1* allele[67] from the Nov[R] *S. pneumoniae* 533 strain.[41] The nucleotide se-

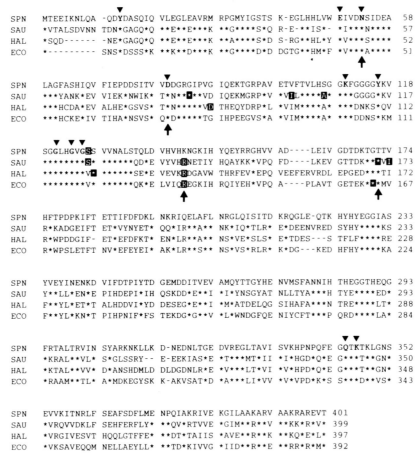

FIG. 8. Comparison of protein sequences of the N-terminus of DNA gyrase B from *S. pneumoniae* R6 (SPN), *S. aureus* (SAU),[46] *Haloferax* sp. (HAL),[28] and *E. coli* (ECO).[1] Residues of *E. coli* GyrB involved in ATP binding or hydrolysis (▼) are doubly-underlined in the *S. pneumoniae* sequence. Residues involved in novobiocin resistance are doubly-underlined and boxed. Important residues for the interaction of *E. coli* GyrB with novobiocin are indicated by black arrows. Asterisks, amino acid identity; dashes, gaps introduced to maximize similiarities.

quence of the 0.9-kb *Pst*I insert of pNOV35 was determined after subcloning, yielding plasmid pGYRN1 (Fig. 7). This sequence showed an incomplete ORF homologous to the N-terminus of the gyrase B proteins (GyrB) previously reported. A partial physical map of the *gyrB* chromosomal region of *S. pneumoniae* was constructed by Southern blotting and hybridization with the 0.9-kb *Pst*I probe from within the *gyrB* gene that showed that the probe was included in a 2.1 kb-*Hind*III fragment. Pneumococcal DNA from the 533 strain was digested with *Hind*III, and fragments showing high efficiency of transformation for novobiocin resistance (those about 2.1 kb) were cloned into *E. coli* using pUC18 as vector plasmid. Two independent plasmids (pGYRN8 and pGYRN5) containing an identical 2.1-kb *Hind*III insert, carried the 5′moiety of the pneumococcal *gyrB* gene. To clone the C-terminus of *gyrB*, PCR experiments were performed with a single primer, oligonucleotide 222 (Fig. 7), under conditions that allowed the mispriming of the oligonucleotide. A PCR product of about 400 bp was cloned into pUC18, rendering plasmids pGYRN4 and pGYRN10. The nucleotide sequences of the inserts of these plasmids were shown to be identical and corresponded to the 3′moiety of *gyrB*. The deduced product of *gyrB* is a protein of 648 amino acid residues (72.1

kDa). The TAA stop codon was followed by a putative transcription terminator. No sequence for *gyrA* is found in the cloned region suggesting that *gyrB* is transcribed independently of *gyrA*, as happens in *Bacillus subtilis*.[63]

Identification of gyrB mutations responsible for novobiocin resistance

Plasmids with deletions extending to the triplet encoding the amino acid residue 114 (taking the first GyrB residue as number 1), as plasmid pGYRN519 (Fig. 8), were able to transform a Nov[S] strain to Nov[R]. However, plasmids with deletions extending to the triplet encoding residue 149 and further, as pGYRN57 and pGYRN561 did not. This localized the mutation into the DNA region encoding residues 114 to 149. Then, the chromosomal region coding for residues 95 to 264 (gyrB95–264, Fig. 7) from the wild type strain R6, the Nov[R] 533 strain, and three independent, spontaneous Nov[R] strains (MJN10, MJN11 and MJN17), was amplified with specific oligonucleotides. The direct nucleotide sequence of the PCR products showed a point mutation, TTG (Ser-127) to TCG (Leu) in the four Nov[R] strains. The nucleotide change is a transition

T to C which is consistent with the low efficiency transformation described for the *nov-1* allele.[26,40]

The structure of the N-terminal fragment (residues 2 to 392) of *E. coli* GyrB determined by X-ray crystallography[89] identified two subdomains: an N-terminal subdomain (residues 2 to 220) containing the ATPase site and the binding site for coumarin antibiotics (24) and a C-terminal subdomain (residues 221–393) which is thought to constitute part of the DNA-binding site. The *S. pneumoniae* protein (Fig. 8) shows a 54% identity with that of *E. coli* and conserves the residues involved in ATP binding (89) and hydrolysis (Glu-42).[32]

The Ser127-Leu change increases novobiocin resistance by 100 fold in *S. pneumoniae* mutant cells (the MICs of Nov^S R6 and Nov^R strains being 1 and 128 μg/ml, respectively) but has no effect in coumermycin A1 resistance (MICs of the Nov^S and Nov^R strains being 0.125 μg/ml). Interestingly, the same differences in susceptibility to novobiocin and coumermycin A1 are found in Ser128-Leu (equivalent to Ser127-Leu of *S. pneumoniae*) in *S. aureus* mutants, that although are resistant to novobiocin, exhibit a sensitivity to coumermycin almost equal to that of the wild type.[75] The three-dimensional structure of *E. coli* GyrB shows that Val-120 (equivalent to Ser-127 of *S. pneumoniae*) lies within the ATP-binding domain. In *S. pneumoniae* the change occurred in a residue that is not conserved and that did not appear to be essential for ATP binding[89] or hydrolysis.[32] This would allow ATP-binding because the mutant cells grew normally (i.e., they have an active gyrase). Nevertheless, it has been reported that coumarin-resistant DNA gyrase B subunits from *E. coli* have a reduced ATPase activity.[10] The coumarin-binding region in the gyrase B subunit has been genetically identified in Arg-136 and Gly-164 of *E. coli*[10,13] and in Arg-133 of *B. burgdorferi* (equivalent to Arg-136 of *E. coli*).[72] These residues are conserved in all known GyrB proteins with two exceptions: at position 136, a Thr residue is present in *Streptomyces sphaeroides*,[80] the producer of novobiocin, with and a Lys residue is present in place of Arg in *S. pneumoniae* (Fig. 8). A possible explanation for our observation is

that Val-120 contributes to both ATP- and coumarin-binding sites, as suggested by the crystallographic data and the point mutations. This would be consistent with the reported competition between novobiocin and ATP for the GyrB protein.[76] Moreover, mutations in the Asp-81, Ser-121, and Arg-136 (residue numbers are as in *E. coli*)[28] GyrB residues have been reported for an *Haloferax* Nov^R strain. The combination of mutations in both the ATP- and coumarin-binding regions confers the Nov^R phenotype and agrees with the existence of overlapping binding sites for ATP and coumarins, as it has been recently demonstrated.[42]

Mutations that change Gly-164 to Val in *E. coli* GyrB confer a greater-than-10-fold increase in novobiocin and chlorobiocin resistance but only 2-fold increase in coumermycin A1 resistance.[10] On the other hand, mutations that change Arg-136 of *E. coli* GyrB conferred a 10-fold increase in novobiocin resistance and a 5- or greater-that-20-fold in coumermycin A1 resistance, depending of the amino acid change.[10,13] The differences in drug susceptibility suggest that different specific interactions are required for the different coumarins. This has been proved for the binding of novobiocin, coumermycin A1 and a cyclothialidine[42] to the *E. coli* GyrB subunit. However, in the crystallographic structure of the *E. coli* GyrB N-terminal fragment accomplished with novobiocin, Val-120 (equivalent to Ser-127 of *S. pneumoniae*) is not involved in novobiocin binding. In *E. coli* GyrB, the key amino acids implicated in novobiocin binding appear to be Asn-46, Asp-73, Arg-136, and Thr-165[42] (Fig. 8). This data is consistent with the localization of the mutations conferring Nov^R in *E. coli* and *B. burgdorferi* but not with the mutations found in *S. pneumoniae*. This might indicate that the structures of the GyrB subunits of *E. coli* and *S. pneumoniae* are different. Moreover, the location of mutations conferring resistance to different GyrB inhibitors in the ATP-binding site of the GyrB protein of *S. pneumoniae* (novobiocin) and in *S. aureus* (novobiocin, coumermycin A1, and cyclothialidine)[75] would made the assumption extensive to gram-positive bacteria. This maybe would explain the differences in

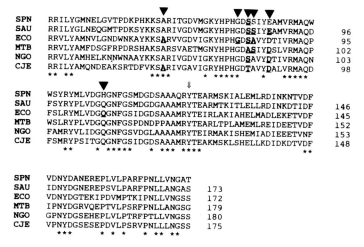

FIG. 9. Comparison of the amino acid sequences of a region of the DNA gyrase A containing the QRDR from *S. pneumoniae* (SPN), *S. aureus* (SAU),[46] *E. coli* (ECO),[77] *Mycobacterium tuberculosis* (MTB),[79] *N. gonorrhoeae* (NGO),[4] and *Campylobacter jejuni* (CJE).[86] The residues involved in quinolone resistance (▼) are set in boldface type and underlined; double-tailed arrow, active residue which links to DNA; asterisks, amino acid identity. (Reprinted with permission from Muñoz et al.[58])

TABLE 4.   AMINO ACID CHANGES OF QRDRs OF PARC AND GYRA OF *S. PNEUMONIAE* ISOLATES

Strain	Ciprofloxacin MIC (μg/ml) (increase)	Amino acid change (codon change)[a] ParC	GyrA
R6, M22	0.5	[75]PHGD**SS**IY**D**AMVR[87]	[79]PHGD**SS**IYEAMVR[91]
937	1	None	None
5145	1	None	None
13925	8 (8×)	[83]D→Y (GAT→T**A**T)	None
3429	8 (8×)	[79]S→Y (TCT→T**A**T)	None
3305	8 (8×)	[79]S→Y (TCT→T**A**T)	None
517	64 (64×)	[79]S→F (TCT→T**T**T)	[83]S→Y (TCC→T**A**C)
1244	128 (128×)	[79]S→F (TCT→T**T**T)	[83]S→F (TCC→T**T**C)
R1[13925-C]	4 (8×)	[83]D→Y (GAT→T**A**T)	None
R1[3429-C]	4 (8×)	[79]S→Y (TCT→T**A**T)	None
R2[13925-C/517-A]	16 (32×)	[83]D→Y (GAT→T**A**T)	[83]S→Y (TCC→T**A**C)
R2[3429-C/517-A]	32 (64×)	[79]S→Y (TCT→T**A**T)	[83]S→Y (TCC→T**A**C)
R2[517-C/1244-A]	32 (64×)	[79]S→F (TCT→T**T**T)	[83]S→F (TCC→T**T**C)
R2[1244 genomic]	32 (64×)	[79]S→F (TCT→T**T**T)	[83]S→F (TCC→T**T**C)

[a]The amino acid positions indicated for GyrA refer to the corresponding positions in the *E. coli* GyrA sequence.
R1[13925-C] and R1[3429-C] is the nomenclature for transformants of M22 to the first level of ciprofloxacin resistance, obtained with the parC50–152 PCR products of strains 13925 and 3429, respectively. R2[13925-C/517-A], R2[517-C/1244-A], and R2[3429-C/517-A] are transformants to the second level of ciprofloxacin resistance, obtained from R1[13925-C], and R1[3429-C] using the gyrA46–172 PCR products of strains 517 and 1244, respectively. R2[1244genomic] is a transformant obtained from M22 with chromosomal DNA from the 1244 strain.

susceptibilities exhibited by these two kinds of bacteria to the coumarin and cyclothialidines antibacterial agents.

Cloning and sequencing the gyrA QRDR of S. pneumoniae

The *gyrA* gene was identified by an approach successfully used for the isolation of *gyrA* homologues from other bacterial species.[4,17] Degenerated oligonucleotide primers were designed based on the sequence conservation found among known *gyrA* genes corresponding to regions 39–45 and 173–180 of the

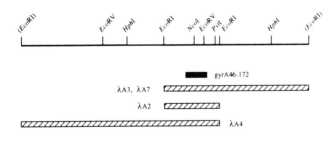

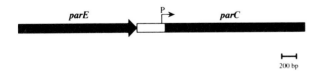

FIG. 10. Restriction map of the *S. pneumoniae* genome DNA region containing the *parE* and *parC* genes. The inserts of λA2, λA3, λA4, and λA7 (hatched bars) and the gyrA46–172 fragment used as a probe (black bars) are shown. The *Eco*RI targets in parenthesis are derived from the cloning strategy and do not necessary represent real targets in the pneumococcal DNA. P indicates the putative promoter. (Reprinted with permission from Muñoz et al.[58])

amino acid sequence of *E. coli gyrA*. Amplification using DNA from the *S. pneumoniae* wild type strain R6 resulted in the production of a PCR product that should encode 127 amino acid residues, corresponding to positions 46 to 172 of the *E. coli* GyrA subunit, which includes the QRDR region and was designated gyrA46–172 (Fig. 9). Subsequently, DNA samples from clinical isolates of *S. pneumoniae,* either ciprofloxacin-sensitive (Cp[S]) or -resistant (Cp[R]) were amplified and the nucleotide sequence of the corresponding *gyrA* region was determined directly from the PCR products. All clinical strains had a sequence identical to that of the wild type strain R6 or silent nucleotide changes, except the two strains showing high-level of resistance Cp (MICs ≥ 64 μg/ml) in which point mutations were observed (Table 4). Mutations in these two strains would result in changes affecting a Ser residue in a position equivalent to Ser-83 of *E. coli* GyrA (Fig. 9). This residue position is the most commonly associated to high-level quinolone resistance in *E. coli*[12,92] and in other bacteria (see Fig. 9).

Transformation experiments were performed using Cp[S] pneumococcal strains as recipients and both chromosomal DNAs and the gyrA46–172 PCR products from strains 517 and 1244 as donor DNAs. Only chromosomal DNAs were able to transform to Cp[R] (see below). Unexpectedly, no Cp[R] transformants were observed using the PCR products as donor DNAs when the selection was carried out at concentrations of ciprofloxacin ranging from 1 to 16 μg/ml. To discard the possibility of a very low efficiency of transformation due to the small size of the PCR fragments, these were cloned into pUC18 and, again, no transformation to Cp[R] was observed.

The region encoding the residues 376–512 of *S. pneumoniae* of the C-terminus of GyrB was amplified with specific oligonucleotides and, subsequently, the gyrB376–512 PCR products (Fig. 7) were sequenced. Only silent nucleotide changes were found. These results suggested that *gyrB* is not involved in Cp resistance in pneumococcus, in sharp contrast to what happens in other bacteria.[70]

Cloning and sequencing the parE *and* parC *genes of S. pneumoniae*

We approached the cloning of the complete *gyrA* gene by using the amplified gyrA46–172 DNA as a probe to screen a λgt11 library of *S. pneumoniae* DNA, and several recombinant phages were identified (Fig. 10) and their inserts sequenced. Amino acid sequence comparisons showed that the first ORF (*parE*) was homologous to ParE, and the second (*parC*) to ParC. The region homologous between the gyrA46–172 probe and showed a 65.5% identity at the nucleotide level that could account for the nonspecific hybridization between the *gyrA* probe and the 780 bp *Eco*RI fragment included in *parC*. On the other hand, ParE of *S. pneumoniae* showed higher identity with ParE of *S. aureus* (68.4%) than with GyrB of *S. pneumoniae* (48.9%).

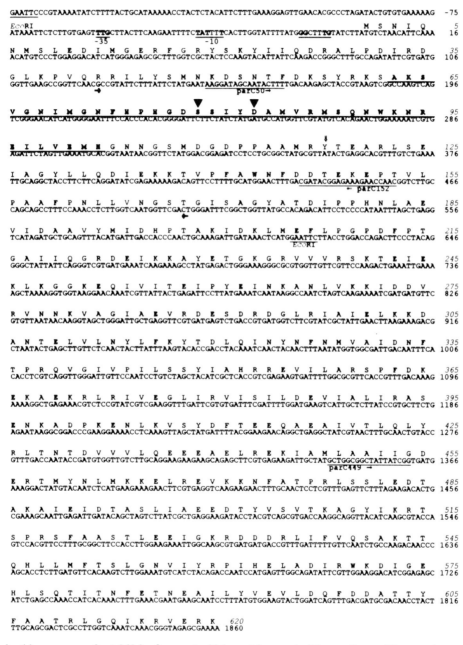

FIG. 11. Nucleotide sequence of a 1,860-bp fragment which contains most of the *parC* gene. The strand corresponding to the mRNA sequence is shown. Nucleotides and amino acids are numbered by taking the firt *parC* nucleotide as nt 1 and the first ParC residue as number 1. Putative consensus regulatory elements are underlined and set in bold face. Oligonucleotides and *Eco*RI sites are indicated and underlined. The amino acid residues that constitute the QRDR are underlined and set in boldface. The nucleotide sequence between the two black arrows corresponded to the region homologous to the gyrA46–172 probe. The residues involved in ciprofloxacin resistance (▼), and the active Y-118 site which links DNA (double-tailed arrow) are indicated. (Reprinted with permission from Muñoz et al.[58])

Location of gyrA, gyrB, and parC genes in the S. pneumoniae genome

Chromosomal DNA prepared from strain R6 was digested with different restriction endonucleases, subjected to pulsed-field gel electrophoresis and the resulting fragments blotted and hybridized with probes specific for parC (parC449–620) (Fig. 11), gyrA, (gyrA46–172) (Fig. 9) and gyrB (gyrB10–330) (Fig. 7). Both gyrB and parC probes detected a SmaI fragment of 380 kb, an ApaI fragment of 330 kb and a SacII fragment of 160 kb (not shown), corresponding to fragment numbers 1/2, 1, and 5, respectively, of the S. pneumoniae genome.[19] The hybridization of the gyrB probe confirmed the previous localization of the nov-1 allele by chromosomal transformation. However, when gyrA was used as a probe, the detected fragments were a 340-kb SmaI, a 330-kb ApaI and a 310-kb SacII, corresponding to fragment numbers 2, 1, and 1, respectively. These results clearly showed that the gyrA gene maps far (at least 90 kb apart) from the gyrB and parC loci on the R6 chromosome. The parC and parE genes are located contiguously in the chromosome as in S. aureus.[17]

Genetic basis of the mechanism of ciprofloxacin resistance in S. pneumoniae

To learn if the Cp[R] pneumococcal isolates had mutations in the parC gene as it has been described in other bacteria, PCR fragments spanning amino acids 50–152 of ParC (designated as parC50–152) were obtained after amplification with specific oligonucleotides (Fig. 11) and sequenced. Analysis of the nucleotide sequences showed that all Cp[R] strains (MIC $\geq$ 8 μg/ml) had mutations altering amino acids Ser-79 or Asp-83 (Table 4), whereas sensitive strains (MIC = 1 μg/ml) did not. Three strains had single mutations in parC (Table 4). Direct evidence showing that the parC mutations are responsible for Cp resistance was obtained by genetic transformation. Both chromosomal DNAs and the parC50–152 PCR products were used as donor DNAs to transform the competent S. pneumoniae strain M22 (Cp[S], MIC = 0.50 μg/ml). The frequencies of transformation to Cp[R] achieved with both DNAs (1–5 $\times$ 10[5] transformants/ml) were similar when the selection was done at 0.55 μg/ml. However, when selection was performed at 8 μg/ml, only chromosomal DNAs were able to transform although at frequencies 100 times lower. This latter frequency is consistent with transformation by two unlinked markers. One of these transformants, R[1244-genomic] (Table 4) was shown to have all the nucleotide changes detected in parC and gyrA of the donor strain 1244. Transformants obtained with parC50–152 from Cp[R] isolates 13925 and 3429 increased the MICs of the recipient M22 strain (MIC = 0.5 μg/ml) to Cp to 4 μg/ml, an 8-fold increase. The same 8-fold increase of resistance is observed in the Cp[R] isolates as compared with sensitive clinical isolates (usually with a MIC = 1 μg/ml). The sequences of the parC and gyrA regions of two of these transformants, R1[13925-C] and R1[3429-C], showed some of the parC nucleotide changes present in the donor strains. Transformant R1[13925-C] had the G-to-T transversion that produces the Asp-83-Tyr change but no other two nucleotide changes present in the donor strain. This result identified the Asp-83-Tyr change as the responsible for Cp[R] in strain 13925. Moreover, Ser-79 is a residue involved in Cp susceptibility as deduced from the parC sequence of the transformant R1[3429-C] (Table 4).

Most Cp[R] strains have alterations at Ser-79, a position analogous to Ser-83 of GyrA. We found no substitution in the QRDR of GyrA of low-level Cp[R] pneumococcal clinical isolates (MIC = 8 μg/ml); however, a change of Ser-79 of ParC (equivalent to Ser-83 of GyrA) did occur. The nature of the changes affecting these two Ser residues were equivalent: Ser to Tyr or Ser to Phe amino acid changes. Mutations in the S. pneumoniae gyrA were only observed in high-level Cp[R] isolates, and in these cases, the amino acid substitutions observed were Ser-83 to Tyr or Phe. These same substitutions have been associated with gyrA mutation in Cp[R] strains of N. gonorrhoeae (Ser to Phe).[4] The absence of substitutions in the QRDR of GyrA in low-level Cp[R] isolates suggests that ParC is the primary target for fluoroquinolones in S. pneumoniae and that mutation in parC is a prerequisite before mutations in gyrA occur. Once the cells have acquired low-level resistance to Cp by gaining mutations in parC, it was possible to transform to a higher level of resistance using the gyrA46–172 DNAs from the high-level Cp[R] strains. Sequencing of the pertinent regions of parC and gyrA confirmed that the second-level transformants, R2[13925-C/517-A], R2[517-C/1244-A] and R2[3429-C/517-A] contained mutations both in parC and gyrA that are present in the donor DNAs. The new transformants had MICs of 16 μg/ml (32-fold increase) if the Ser-83-Tyr or Phe changes of GyrA are combined with the Asp-83-Tyr change of ParC, or 32 μg/ml (64-fold increase) if the GyrA changes are combined with mutations in equivalent positions of ParC (Ser-79-Tyr or Phe). The combination of the two mutations (Ser-83-Tyr in GyrA and Ser-79-Phe in ParC) in strain 517 (Table 4) resulted in a MIC of 64 μg/ml (a 64-fold increase); likewise, in M22 strain, with a MIC = 0.5 μg/ml, the simultaneous occurrence of these two mutations raised the MIC to 32 μg/ml. However, with strain 1244, the differences in increase of the MICs values between the clinical isolate (128 μg/ml, Table 1) and the transformants possessing the same mutations (R2[517-C/1244-A] and R[1244-genome] with MICs of 32 μg/ml; Table 2), were twice higher. The difference between the MICs of the clinical isolate and that of the transformants could be attributed to alterations in drug permeability or to other mutations in regions not sequenced in this study of the genes encoding the subunits of the type II topoisomerases of S. pneumoniae.

Table 4 illustrates how both the type and number of mutations are important to the overall level of Cp resistance. High-level resistance is due to mutations causing a Ser to Phe or Tyr changes in both of the two equivalent Ser residues of ParC and GyrA. Although a detailed three-dimensional structure of the GyrA and ParC proteins is not available, these observations provide evidence that Ser-83 of GyrA and Ser-79 of ParC are essential amino acids for interactions with DNA and the fluoroquinolones.

Amino acid sequence comparison between the QRDRs (corresponding to positions 67–106 of the E. coli GyrA) of the pneumococcal ParC and GyrA subunits with that of the gram-negative bacteria (E. coli and N. gonorrhoeae) and the gram-positive S. aureus were performed. In the gram-negatives, the primary target for fluoroquinolones is GyrA whereas in S. aureus the primary target for these drugs is ParC. The highest identities among ParC and GyrA sequences were found between S. pneumoniae and S. aureus (65% and 87.5%, respectively), being the identities between the other ParC and GyrA lower than 53% and 70%, respectively. This high amino acid sequence similarity is consistent with the intrinsic resistances of *S. pneumoniae* and *S. aureus* (ca., 1 μg/ml) to Cp, and with ParC being more sensitive to Cp than GyrA in these species. These comparisons support the idea that amino acid sequences of the QRDRs of ParC and GyrA are mainly responsible for the different susceptibilities of topoisomerase IV and DNA gyrase to fluoroquinolones. It is tempting to speculate that, given the evolutionary relationship between gram-positive and gram-negative bacteria, the primary target for fluoroquinolones in the former would be ParC (as in *S. aureus* and *S. pneumoniae*), whereas GyrA would be the primary target in gram-negative bacteria.

REFERENCES

1. **Adachi, T., M. Mizuuchi, E.A. Robinson, E. Appella, M.H. O'Dea, M. Gellert, and K. Mizuuchi.** 1987. DNA sequence of *E. coli gyrB* gene: Application of a new sequencing strategy. Nucleic Acids Res. **15:**771–784.

2. **Appelbaum, P.C.** 1992. Antimicrobial resistance in *Streptococcus pneumoniae*: An overview. Clin. Infect. Dis. **15:**77–83.

3. **Baquero, F.** 1995. Pneumococcal resistance to β-lactam antibiotics: A global overview. Microb. Drug Resist. **1:**115–120.

4. **Belland, R., S. Morrison, C. Ison, and W. Huang.** 1994. *Neisseria gonorrhoeae* acquires mutations in analogous regions of *gyrA* and *parC* in fluoroquinolone-resistant isolates. Mol. Microbiol. **14:**371–380.

5. **Blum, J.J., A. Yayon, S. Friedman, and H. Ginsburg.** 1984. Effects of mitochondrial protein synthesis inhibitors on the incorporation of isoleucine into *Plasmodium falciparum*. J. Protozool. **31:**475–479.

6. **Bowler, L.C., Q.-Y. Zhang, J.-Y. Riou, and B.G. Spratt.** 1994. Interspecies recombination between the *penA* genes of *Neisseria meningitidis* and comensal *Neisseria* species during the emergence of penicillin resistance in *N. meningitidis:* Natural events and laboratory simulation. J. Bacteriol. **176:**333–337.

7. **Brusilow, W.S., M.A. Scarpetta, C.A. Hawthorne, and W.P. Clark.** 1989. Organization and sequence of the genes coding for the proton-translocating ATPase of *Bacillus megaterium*. J. Biol. Chem. **264:**1528–1533.

8. **Choi, I., and J.L. Mego.** 1988. Purification of *Plasmodium falciparum* digestive vacuoles and partial characterization of the vacuolar membrane ATPase. Mol. Biochem. Parasitol. **31:**71–78.

9. **Coffey, T.J., C.G. Dowson, M. Daniells, and B.G. Spratt.** 1993. Horizontal spread of an altered penicillin-binding protein 2B gene between *Streptococcus pneumoniae* and *Streptococcus oralis*. FEMS Microbiol. Lett. **110:**335–340.

10. **Contreras, A., and A. Maxwell.** 1992. *gyrB* mutations which confer coumarin resistance also affect DNA supercoiling and ATP hydrolysis by *Escherichia coli* DNA gyrase. Mol. Microbiol. **6:**1617–1624.

11. **Cozens, A.L., and J.E. Walker.** 1987. The organization and sequence of the genes of the ATP synthase in the cyanobacterium *Synechococcus* 6301: Support for an endosymbiotic origin of chloroplasts. J. Mol. Biol. **194:**359–383.

12. **Cullen, M., A. Wyke, R. Kuroda, and L. Fisher.** 1989. Cloning and characterization of a DNA gyrase gene from *Escherichia coli* that confers clinical resistance to 4-quinolones. Antimicrob. Agents. Chemother. **33:**886–894.

13. **del Castillo, I., J.L. Vizán, M.C. Rodriguez-Sáinz, and F. Moreno.** 1991. An unusual mechanism for resistance to the antibiotic coumermycin A1. Proc. Natl. Acad. Sci. USA **88:**8860–8864.

14. **Dowson, C.G., A. Hutchison, N. Woodford, A.P. Johnson, R.C. George, and B.G. Spratt.** 1990. Penicillin-resistant viridans streptococci have obtained altered penicillin-binding protein genes from penicillin-resistant strains of *Streptococcus pneumoniae*. Proc. Natl. Acad. Sci. USA **87:**5858–5862.

15. **Fenoll, A., R. Muñoz, E. García, and A.G. de la Campa.** 1994. Molecular basis of the optochin-sensitive phenotype of pneumococcus: Characterization of the genes encoding the F_0 complex of the *Streptococcus pneumoniae* and *Streptococcus oralis* H$^+$-ATPases. Mol. Microbiol. **12:**587–598.

16. **Fenoll, A., R. Muñoz, E. García, and A.G. de la Campa.** 1995. Optochin sensitivity is encoded by the *atpC* gene of the *Streptococcus pneumoniae* F_0F_1 H$^+$-ATPases. Dev. Biol. Stand. **85:**287–291.

17. **Ferrero, L., B. Cameron, B. Manse, D. Lagneaux, J. Crouzet, A. Famechon, and F. Blanche.** 1994. Cloning and primary structure or *Staphylococcus aureus* DNA topoisomerase IV: A primary target of fluoroquinolones. Mol. Microbiol. **13:**641–653.

18. **Futai, M., T. Noumi, and M. Maeda.** 1989. ATP synthase (H$^+$-ATPase): Results by combined biochemical and molecular biological approaches. Annu. Rev. Biochem. **58:**111–136.

19. **Gasc, A.-M., L. Kauc, P. Barraillé, M. Sicard, and S. Goodgal.** 1991. Gene localization, size, and physical map of the chromosome of *Streptococcus pneumoniae*. J. Bacteriol. **173:**7361–7367.

20. **Gay, N.J., and J.E. Walker.** 1981. The *atp* operon: Nucleotide sequence of the promoter and the genes for the membrane proteins, and the δ subunit of *Escherichia coli* ATP-synthase. Nucleic Acids. Res. **9:**3919–3926.

21. **Gellert, M.** 1981. DNA topoisomerases. Annu. Rev. Biochem. **50:**879–910.

22. **Gellert, M., M.H. O'Dea, T. Itoh, and J.-I. Tomizawa.** 1976. Novobiocin and coumermycin inhibit DNA supercoiling catalyzed by DNA gyrase. Proc. Natl. Acad. Sci. USA **73:**4474–4478.

23. **Georgiou, M., R. Muñoz, F. Román, R. Cantón, R. Gómez-Lus, J. Campos, and A.G. de la Campa.** 1996. Ciprofloxacin-resistant *Haemophilus influenzae* possess mutations in analogous positions of GyrA and ParC. Antimicrob. Agents Chemother. **40:**1741–1744.

24. **Gilbert, E.J., and A. Maxwell.** 1994. The 24 kDa N-terminal subdomain of the gyrase B protein binds coumarin drugs. Mol. Microbiol. **12:**365–373.

25. **Ginsburg, A., A.A. Divo, T.G. Geary, M.T. Borland, and J.B. Jensen.** 1986. Effects of mitochondrial inhibitors on intraerythrocytic *Plasmodium falciparum in vitro* cultures. J. Protozool. **33:**121–125.

26. **Guild, W.R., and N.B. Shoemaker.** 1976. Mismatch correction in pneumococcal transformation: Donor length and *hex*-dependent marker efficiency. J. Bacteriol. **125:**125–135.

27. **Holmberg, H., D. Danielsson, J. Hardie, A. Krook, and R. Whiley.** 1985. Cross-reactions between alpha-streptococci and omniserum, a polyvalent pneumococcal serum, demonstrated by direct immunofluorescence, immunoelectrophoresis and latex agglutination. J. Clin. Microbiol. **21:**745–748.

28. **Holmes, M.L., and M.L. Dyall-Smith.** 1991. Mutations in DNA gyrase result in novobiocin resistance in halophyilic archaebacteria. J. Bacteriol. **173:**642–648.

29. **Homewood, C.A., D.C. Warhust, W. Peters, and V.C. Baggaley.** 1972. Lysosomes, pH, and the antimalarial action of chloroquine. Nature **235:**50–52.

30. **Hoope, J., and W. Sebald.** 1980. Amino acid sequence of the proteolipid subunit of the proton-translocating ATPase complex from the thermophilic bacterium PS-3. Eur. J. Biochem. **107:**57–65.

31. **Ivey, D.M., and T.A. Krulwich.** 1991. Organization and nucleotide sequence of the *atp* genes encoding the ATP synthase from alkaliphilic *Bacillus firmus* OF4. Mol. Gen. Genet. **229:**292–300.

32. **Jackson, A.P., and A. Maxwell.** 1993. Identifying the catalytic residue of the ATPase reaction of DNA gyrase. Proc. Natl. Acad. Sci. USA **90:**11232–11236.

33. **Kanazawa, H., T. Kitasu, T. Noumi, and M. Futai.** 1984. Overproduction of the *a* subunit of the F$_0$ component of proton-translocating ATPase inhibits growth of *Escherichia coli.* J. Bacteriol. **158:**300–306.

34. **Kato, J., Y. Nishima, R. Imamura, H. Niki, S. Higara, and H. Suzuki.** 1990. New topoisomerase essential for chromosome segregation in *E. coli.* Cell **63:**393–404.

35. **Kilpper-Bälz, R., P. Wenzig, and K.H. Schleiffer.** 1985. Molecular relationships and classification of some viridans streptococci as *S. oralis* and emended description of *Streptococcus oralis* (Bridge and Sneath 1982). Int. J. Syst. Bacteriol. **35:**482–488.

36. **Kontiainen, S., and A. Sivonen.** 1987. Optochin resistance in *Streptococcus pneumoniae* strains isolated from blood and ear fluid. Eur. J. Clin. Microbiol. **6:**422–424.

37. **Klugman, K.P.** 1990. Pneumococcal resistance to antibiotics. Clin. Microbiol. Rev. **2:**171–196.

38. **Kreger, A.S., and R.H. Olsen.** 1986. Purification and properties of mutants and wild-type diaphorases from *Diplococcus pneumoniae.* J. Bacteriol. **96:**1029–1036.

39. **Kröger, M., and G. Hobom.** 1982. Structural analysis of insertion sequence IS5. Nature **97:**159–162.

40. **Lacks, S.A., J.J. Dunn, and B. Greenberg.** 1982. Identification of base mismatches recognized by the heteroduplex-DNA-repair system of *Streptococcus pneumoniae.* Cell **31:**327–336.

41. **Lacks, S.A., and B. Greenberg.** 1975. A deoxyribonuclease of *Diplococcus pneumoniae* specific for methylated DNA. J. Biol. Chem. **250:**4060–4066.

42. **Lewis, R.J., O.M.P. Singh, C.V. Smith, T. Skarzynski, A. Maxwell, A.J. Wonacott, and D.B. Wigley.** 1996. The nature of inhibition of DNA gyrase by the coumarins and the cyclothialidines revealed by X-ray crystallography. EMBO J. **15:**1412–1420.

43. **Lund, E.** 1950. Antigenic relationships between pneumococci and nonhaemolytic streptococci. Acta Pathol. Microbiol. Scand. **27:**110–118.

44. **Lund, E., and J. Henrichsen.** 1978. Laboratory diagnosis, serology and epidemiology of *Streptococcus pneumoniae.* Methods Microbiol. **12:**241–262.

45. **Luttinger, A.** 1995. The twisted life of DNA in the cell: Bacterial topoisomerases. Mol. Microbiol. **15:**601–606.

46. **Magerrison, E.E.C., R. Hopewell, and L.M. Fisher.** 1992. Nucleotide sequence of the *Staphylococcus aureus gyrB-gyrA* locus encoding the DNA gyrase A and B proteins. J. Bacteriol. **174:**1596–1603.

47. **Mandel, M., Y. Moriyama, J.D. Hulmes, Y.-C.E. Pan, H. Nelson, and N. Nelson.** 1988. cDNA sequence encoding the 16-kDa proteolipid of chromaffin granules implies gene duplication in the evolution of H$^+$-ATPases. Proc. Natl. Acad. Sci. USA **85:**5521–5524.

48. **Martin, C., T. Briese, and R. Hakenbeck.** 1992. Nucleotide sequences of genes encoding penicillin-binding proteins from *Streptococcus pneumoniae* and *Streptococcus oralis* with high homology to *Escherichia coli* penicillin-binding proteins 1A and 1B. J. Bacteriol. **174:**4517–4523.

49. **Maxwell, A.** 1993. The interaction between coumarin drugs and DNA gyrase. Mol. Microbiol. **9:**681–686.

50. **Miller, M.J., M. Oldenburg, and R.H. Fillingame.** 1990. The essential carboxyl group in subunit *c* of the F$_1$F$_0$ ATP synthase can be moved and H$^+$-translocating function retained. Proc. Natl. Acad. Sci. USA **87:**4900–4904.

51. **Moore, H.F.** 1915. The action of ethylhydrocuprein (optochin) on type strains of pneumococci *in vitro* and *in vivo,* and on some other microorganisms *in vitro.* J. Exp. Med. **22:**269–285.

52. **Moore, H.F., and A.M. Chesney.** 1917. A study of ethylhydrocuprein (optochin) in the treatment of acute lobar pneumonia. Arch. Intern. Med. **19:**611–682.

53. **Morgenroth, J., and M. Kaufmann.** 1912. Arzneifestigkeit bei bakterien (pneumokokken). Z. Immunitätsforsch. Exp. Ther. **15:**610–624.

54. **Mosher, M.E., L.K. Peters, and R.H. Fillingame.** 1983. Use of lambda *unc* transducing bacteriophages in genetic and biochemical characterization of H$^+$-ATPase mutants of *Escherichia coli.* J. Bacteriol. **156:**1078–1092.

55. **Most, H.** 1984. Treatment of parasitic infections of travelers and immigrants. N. Engl. J. Med. **310:**298–304.

56. **Muller, R., and J.R. Baker.** 1990. Medical parasitology. Gower Medical Publishing, London.

57. **Muñoz, R., M. Bustamante, and A.G. de la Campa.** 1995. Ser-127-to Leu substitution in the DNA gyrase B subunit of *Streptococcus pneumoniae* is implicated in novobiocin resistance. J. Bacteriol **177:**4166–4170.

58. **Muñoz, R., and A.G. de la Campa.** 1996. ParC subunit of the DNA topoisomerase IV of *Streptococcus pneumoniae* is a primary target of fluoroquinolones and cooperates with the DNA gyrase A subunit in forming resistance phenotype. Antimicrob. Agents Chemother. **40** (in press).

59. **Muñoz, R., E. García, and A.G. de la Campa.** 1996. Quinine specifically inhibits the proteolipid subunit of the F$_0$F$_1$ H$^+$-ATPase of *Streptococcus pneumoniae.* J. Bacteriol. **178:**2455–2458.

60. **Nagley, P., R.M. Hall, and B.G. Ooi.** 1086. Amino acid substitutions in mitochondrial ATPase subunit 9 of *Saccharomyces cerevisiae* leading to oligomycin or venturicidin resistance. FEBS Lett. **195:**159–163.

61. **Nakada, N., H. Gmünder, T. Hirata, and M. Arisawa.** 1994. Characterization of the binding site for cyclothialidine on the B subunit of DNA gyrase. J. Biol. Chem. **24:**14286–14291.

62. **Nelson, H., and N. Nelson.** 1989. The progenitor of ATP synthases was closely related to the current vacuolar H$^+$-ATPase. FEBS Lett. **247:**147–153.

63. **Ogasawara, N., S. Moriya, and H. Yoshikawa.** 1985. Structure and function of the region of the replication origin of the *Bacillus subtilis* chromosome. IV. Transcription of the *oriC* region and expression of DNA gyrase genes and other open reading frames. Nucleic Acids Res. **7:**2267–2279.

64. **Pease, A.A., C.W.I. Douglas, and R.C. Spencer.** 1986. Identifying noncapsulate strains of *Streptococcus pneumoniae* isolated from eyes. J. Clin. Pathol. **39:**871–875.

65. **Pedersen, P.L., and E. Carafoli.** 1987. Ion motive ATPases. I. Ubiquity, properties, and significance to cell function. Trends Biochem. Sci. **12:**146–150.

66. **Peng H., and J. Marians.** 1993. *Escherichia coli* topoisomerase IV. Purification, characterization, subunit structure, and subunit interactions. J. Biol. Chem. **268:**24481–24490.

67. **Pérez-Ureña, M.T., M.E. Pons, A. Salgado, G. del Solar, S. Ballester, P. López, A. Puyet, and M. Espinosa.** 1987. Enrichment of genes and location of mutations in cloned DNA fragments of *Streptococcus pneumoniae.* FEMS Microbiol. Lett. **42:**153–158.

68. **Phillips, G., R. Barker, and O. Brogan.** 1988. Optochin resistant *Streptococcus pneumoniae.* Lancet **ii:**281.

69. **Phillips, R.E., D.A. Warrel, N.J. White, S. Looareesuwan, and J. Karbwang.** 1985. Intravenous quinidine for the treatment of severe falciparum malaria: Clinical and pharmacokinetic studies. N. Engl. J. Med. **312:**1273–1278.

70. **Reece, R., and A. Maxwell.** 1991. DNA gyrase: Structure and function. Crit. Rev. Biochem. Mol. Biol. **26:**335–375.

71. **Ronda, C., J.L. García, and R. López.** 1988. Characterization of genetic transformation in *Streptococcus oralis* NCTC 11427: Expression of the pneumococcal amidase in *S. oralis* using a new shuttle vector. Mol. Gen. Genet. **215:**53–57.

72. **Samuels, D.S., R.T. Marconi, W.M. Huang, and C.F. Garon.** 1994. *gyrB* mutations in coumermycin A1-resistant *Borrelia burgdorferi.* J. Bacteriol. **176:**3072–3075.

73. **Senior, A.E.** 1990. The proton-translocating ATPase of *Escherichia coli.* Annu. Rev. Biophys. Biophys. Chem. **19**:7–41.

74. **Shibata, C., T. Ehara, K. Tomura, K. Igarashi, and H. Kobayashi.** 1992. Gene structure of *Enterococcus faecalis* F_1F_0-ATPase which functions as a regulator of cytoplasmic pH. J. Bacteriol. **174**:6117–6124.

75. **Stieger, M., P. Angehrn, B. Wohlgensiger, and H. Gmünder.** 1996. GyrB mutations in *Staphylococcus aureus* strains resistant to cyclothialidine, coumermycin, and novobiocin. Antimicrob. Agents Chemother. **40**:1060–1062.

76. **Sugino, A., N.P. Higgins, P.O. Brown, C.L. Peebles, and N.R. Cozzarelli.** 1978. Energy coupling in DNA gyrase and the mechanism of action of novobiocin. Proc. Natl. Acad. Sci. USA **75**:4838–4842.

77. **Swanberg, S.L., and J.C. Wang.** 1986. Cloning and sequencing of the *Escherichia coli gyrA* gene coding for the A subunit of the DNA gyrase. J. Mol. Biol. **197**:729–736.

78. **Sweeney, T.R., and R.E. Strube.** 1979. Antimalarials. *In* M.E. Wolf (ed.), Burger's medicinal chemistry, 4th ed. John Wiley & Sons, Inc., New York, pp. 333–413.

79. **Takiff, H.E., L. Salazar, C. Guerrero, W. Philipp, W.H. Huang, B. Kreiwirth, S.T. Cole, W. R. Jr. Jacobs, and A. Telenti.** 1994. Cloning and nucleotide sequence of *Mycobacterium tuberculosis gyrA* and *gyrB* genes and detection of quinolone resistant mutations. Antimicrob. Agents Chemother. **38**:773–780.

80. **Thiara, A.S., and E. Cundliffe.** 1993. Expression and analysis of two *gyrB* genes from the novobiocin producer, *Streptomyces sphaeroides.* Mol. Microbiol. **8**:495–506.

81. **Tomasz, A.** 1970. Cellular metabolism in genetic transformation of pneumococci: Requirement for protein synthesis during induction of competence. J. Bacteriol. **101**:860–871.

82. **Tybulewicz, V.L.J., G. Falk, and J.E. Walker.** 1984. *Rhodopseudomonas blastica atp* operon: Nucleotide sequence and transcription. J. Mol. Biol. **179**:185–214.

83. **van Es, H.H. G., E. Skamene, and E. Schurr.** 1993. Chemotherapy of malaria, a battle against all odds? Clin. Invest. Med. **16**:285–293.

84. **Verpoorte, R., J. Schripsema, and T. van der Leer.** 1988. *Cinchona* alkaloids. *In* A. Brossi (ed.), The alkaloids, chemistry and pharmacology, vol. 34. Academic Press, Inc., San Diego, CA, pp. 331–398.

85. **Wang, J. C.** 1985. DNA topoisomerases. Annu. Rev. Biochem. **54**:665–697.

86. **Wang, Y., W. M. Huang, and D. E. Taylor.** 1993. Cloning and nucleotide sequence of the *Campylobacter jejuni gyrA* gene and characterization of quinolone resistance mutations. Antimicrob. Agents Chemother. **37**:457–463.

87. **Wasilauskas, B. I., and K. D. Hampton.** 1984. An analysis of *Streptococcus pneumoniae* identification using biochemical and serological procedures. Diagn. Microbiol. Infect. Dis. **2**:301–307.

88. **White, N. J., S. Looareesuwan, D. A. Warrell, T. Chongsuphajaisiddhi, D. Bunnag, and T. Harinasuta.** 1981. Quinidine in falciparum malaria. Lancet **ii**:1069–1071.

89. **Wigley, D. B., G. J. Davies, E. J., Dodson, A. Maxwell, and G. Dodson.** 1991. Crystal structure of an N-terminal fragment of the DNA gyrase B protein. Nature **351**:624–629.

90. **Wolfson, J. S., and D. C. Hooper.** 1989. Fluoroquinolone antimicrobial agents. Clin. Microbiol. Rev. **2**:378–424.

91. **Wyler, D. J.** 1983. Malaria: Resurgence, resistance and research. N. Engl. J. Med. **308**:875–878; 934–940.

92. **Yoshida, H., M. Bogaki, M. Nakamura, and S. Nakamura.** 1990. Quinolone resistance determining region in the DNA gyrase *gyrA* gene of *Escherichia coli.* Antimicrob. Agents Chemother. **34**:1271–1272.

93. **Yurchah, A., and R. Austrian.** 1966. Serologic and genetic relationship between pneumococci and other respiratory streptococci. Trans. Assoc. Amer. Phys. **79**:368–37523.

Address reprint requests to:
Adela G. De La Campa
Centro Nacional de Biología Fundamental
Instituto de Salud Carlos III
28220 Majadahonda, Madrid, Spain

Antibiotic Resistance in *Streptococcus pneumoniae* in Spain: An Overview of the 1990s

JOSEFINA LIÑARES, FE TUBAU, and M. ANGELES DOMÍNGUEZ

ABSTRACT

Antibiotic-resistant *Streptococcus pneumoniae* have been increasingly isolated in Spain over the past two decades. In the 1980s, there was a gradual increase in the resistance of *S. pneumoniae* to penicillin and other antibiotics. In the 1990s, the prevalence of penicillin resistance has remained stable ($\approx$40%) among invasive strains isolated from adult patients, but has increased among invasive and noninvasive pediatric isolates, with rates of approximately 50% and 60%, respectively. In Spain, the rates of resistance to macrolides, lincosamides and streptogramin B of *S. pneumoniae* have increased dramatically from <5% in 1986 to 30% in 1998. Of great concern in the 1990s is the increase in strains with decreased susceptibility to third generation cephalosporins ($\approx$20%), such as cefotaxime or ceftriaxone, which are antibiotics of choice for penicillin resistant pneumococcal meningitis. Resistance to co-trimoxazole is 40–50%, to tetracycline is 30–40%, and to chloramphenicol is 20–30%. Currently, resistance to three or more antimicrobial groups is found in 30–40% of pneumococcal strains, and this limits the antibiotic options for treatment of pneumococcal infections. The majority of these isolates are of serogroups/types 6, 14, 23, 19, and 15. The molecular characterization of these strains suggests that the increase in the incidence of these resistant pneumococci is due to the spread of a limited number of clones.

INTRODUCTION

*S*TREPTOCOCCUS PNEUMONIAE remains a major cause of morbidity and mortality in humans as a common etiological agent in community-acquired pneumonia and meningitis, particularly in adults, and in acute otitis media in children. In the past, treatment of these infections was straightforward due to the high penicillin susceptibility of *S. pneumoniae*. However, antibiotic resistant pneumococci are being isolated at an increasing rate, and they have become a serious worldwide problem.[1–2,24]

Clinical resistance to penicillin in *S. pneumoniae* was first reported by investigators in Boston in 1965, but they failed to recognize the significance of that resistance. Subsequently this phenomenon was reported from Australia in 1967 and especially in South Africa in 1977 where strains with both a high level of penicillin resistance and multiple antibiotic resistance were reported.[23] Penicillin resistance spread rapidly throughout the world in the 1980s, mainly in South Africa, Spain, Hungary, and France.[5–7,11–21,26–44,49–56] The principal mechanism of penicillin resistance is the production of altered penicillin-binding proteins, which leads to cross-resistance to other beta-lactam antibiotics, including even third generation cephalosporins and carbapenems.[22,36,60] In Spain, penicillin-resistant *S. pneumoniae* was first detected in 1979,[6,34] and since then an increasing incidence of strains with resistance to penicillin and other antibiotics has been reported.[11,12,16,37] The aim of this paper is to review the trends in pneumococcal antibiotic resistance in Spain in the 1990s.

TRENDS IN ANTIBIOTIC RESISTANCE IN *Streptococcus pneumoniae*

During the past two decades in Spain, we have witnessed a gradual increase in the resistance of *S. pneumoniae* to beta-lactam antibiotics and to other nonrelated antimicrobials.[11,12,37] Recently updated data from the Spanish Pneumococcal Reference Laboratory in Madrid, reports a statistically significant increase in antibiotic resistance among 6,817 invasive pneumococcal strains studied. Intermediate resistance to penicillin (IRP, MIC 0.1–1 μg/ml) increased from 6.0% in 1979 to 30.3% in 1996, high resistance to penicillin (HRP, MIC $\geq$ 2 μg/ml) from 0% to 11.7% in 1996 and resistance to erythromycin from 0.9%

Microbiology Department, Ciutat Sanitària i Universitària de Bellvitge, Barcelona, Spain.

to 23% in 1996. At the same time, resistance to chloramphenicol decreased from 55.2% in 1979 to 23% in 1996, and resistance to tetracycline from 76.7% in 1979 to 31.3% in 1996.[11,12] Similar trends in antimicrobial resistance were observed at the Hospital de Bellvitge in Barcelona among 1,494 invasive pneumococci isolated from adult patients (Fig. 1).[37] These changes could be related, at least in part, to trends in antibiotic use in Spain.[3] Data obtained from the Spanish Ministry of Health showed that community use of macrolides has increased significantly from 3.48 million prescriptions in 1985 to 8.68 million in 1995; cephalosporins from 4.26 million prescriptions in 1985 to 9.11 million in 1995. The use of aminopenicillins by outpatients was approximately 30 million prescriptions/year during the past decade. In contrast, the use of tetracycline decreased from 1.99 million prescriptions in 1985 to 0.94 million in 1995, and chloramphenicol from 0.09 to 0.004 million prescriptions.[3,42]

From January 1990 to December 1996, a total of 9,243 invasive and noninvasive isolates were studied at the Pneumococcal Reference Laboratory in Madrid, revealing an overall rate of penicillin-resistant pneumococci (PRP) of 49% (IRP 39% and HRP 10%). In this study, the frequency of antibiotic resistance among noninvasive pneumococci ($n = 3,892$) was significantly higher than among invasive pneumococci ($n = 4,720$): resistance to penicillin 59.4% versus 39.4% (IRP 31% and HRP 8.4%), resistance to cefotaxime 25.1% versus 18.6%, resistance to erythromycin 28.8% versus 16.7%, resistance to tetracycline 51.6% versus 36%, and resistance to chloramphenicol 36.5% versus 25.7%.[12]

The rates of PRP reported at several Spanish National Congresses of Infectious Disease and Clinical Microbiology from different regions in Spain were as follows: Catalonia (43–64%), Asturias (47–61%), Aragon (65–70%), Basque Country (30–45%), Galicia (33–50%), Castilla (32–89%), Madrid (49–64%), Valencia (26–69%), Murcia (40–68%), Andalucia (47–71%), and Canary Islands (52%). Although there is considerable regional and local variation in these figures, the differences in PRP rates among regions could be due to age of patients, previous use of antibiotics, previous hospitalization, HIV infection, type of specimen studied and serogroup/type distribution in the population studied.

When only invasive isolates from adult patients were considered, similar rates of penicillin resistance (25.7–32.9%) were found among different cities, but the proportion of PRP isolated from blood in children was 42.1–58%, higher than in adults (Table 1).

Studies at Hospital de Bellvitge in Barcelona, analyzing the frequency of antibiotic resistance among 2,593 consecutive clinical strains from adult patients isolated between 1991 and 1997 showed penicillin resistance 45.4% (IRP 25.0%, HRP 20.4%), cefotaxime resistance 21.7% (16.0% with MIC of 1 μg/ml and 5% with MIC of 2 μg/ml), erythromycin resistance 19.6%, clindamycin resistance 18.9%, chloramphenicol resistance 26.5%, tetracycline resistance 34.2%, co-trimoxazole resistance 47.3%, and ciprofloxacin resistance 1.9%. Rates of antibiotic resistance were related to the clinical origin of the pneumococcal strains: blood isolates were less resistant to penicillin and other antimicrobials than were sputum isolates. In

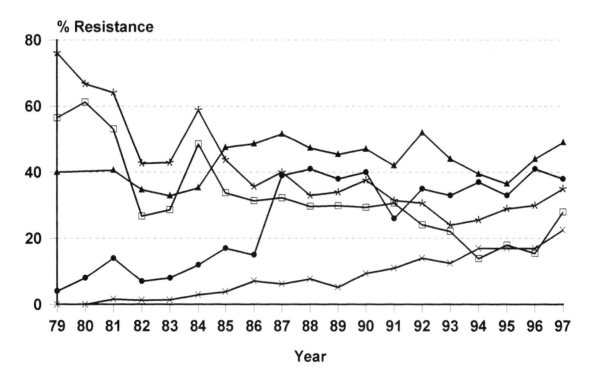

FIG. 1. Trends in antibiotic resistance of 1,494 invasive pneumococci isolated from adult patients from 1979 to 1997 in Hospital de Bellvitge, Barcelona.

TABLE 1. FREQUENCY OF PENICILLIN RESISTANCE AMONG BLOOD *S. pneumoniae* ISOLATES

Geographical area	No. of strains	% Resistance	Age	Period	References
Spain[a]	2,160	31.5%	Adults	1990–96	Fenoll et al.[12]
Barcelona	403	30.5%	Adults	1991–97	Liñares et al.[c]
San Sebastián	323	25.7%	Adults	1990–98	Perez-Trallero et al.[c]
La Coruña	184	31.0%	Adults	1991–97	Moure et al.[46]
Murcia	71	32.9%	Adults	1989–93	Gomez et al.[21]
Oviedo	183[b]	31.1%	Adults	1990–93	Fleites et al.[13]
Madrid	402	33.0%	Adults + Children	1992–96	Torres et al.[62]
Barcelona	236[b]	35.1%	Adults + Children	1996	Latorre et al.[29]
Spain[a]	424	50.9%	Children	1990–96	Fenoll et al.[12]
Barcelona	87[b]	43.7%	Children	1989–97	Latorre et al.[31]
San Sebastián	57	42.1%	Children	1990–98	Perez-Trallero et al.[c]
La Coruña	26	50%	Children	1991–97	Moure et al.[46]
Madrid	87	58%	Children	1989–93	Ramos et al.[54]

[a]Data from Pneumococcal Reference Laboratory, Madrid, Spain.
[b]The majority of strains were blood isolates, but CSF and pleural fluid isolates were also included.
[c]Unpublished data.

Table 2, percentages of resistance to seven antimicrobial agents among blood and sputum pneumococcal strains isolated between 1985 and 1990 are compared with those isolated between 1991 and 1997 at Hospital de Bellvitge. In the 1990s, we observed an increase in resistance to cefotaxime, macrolides, clindamycin, and resistance to three or more antibiotics.

The evolution of antimicrobial resistance in 1,165 pneumococci isolated between 1992 and 1996 was analyzed at Hospital Gregorio Marañón in Madrid. Overall resistance to penicillin, cefotaxime, and erythromycin was 51%, 22%, and 23%, respectively. Isolates from ear and eye were more resistant to penicillin (68%) than were blood isolates (33%) and CSF isolates (38%).[62]

In an analysis of 236 consecutive invasive pneumococcal strains collected during 1996 in 16 hospitals in Catalonia, resistance to penicillin was found in 83 (35.1%) pneumococci, (IRP 27.1% and HRP 8%); resistance to cefotaxime was observed in 29 strains (12.3%: 10.1% had MIC of 1 μg/ml and 2.1% had MIC of 2 μg/ml); resistance to erythromycin was found in 42 (17.8%) strains.[29]

The prevalence of resistance to penicillin and other antimicrobials was higher in pediatric isolates than in adult isolates, regardless of the source of specimen. The Pneumococcal Reference Laboratory reported a rate of penicillin resistance of 54.5% among 580 invasive pneumococci isolated from children and 62.9% among 1,686 noninvasive isolates from children.[12] In a study of 210 consecutive blood pneumococcal strains from 184 adults and 26 children isolated between 1991 and 1997 at

TABLE 2. COMPARISON OF ANTIBIOTIC RESISTANCE OF PNEUMOCOCCAL STRAINS FROM DIFFERENT SOURCES AND PERIODS ISOLATED FROM ADULT PATIENTS AT HOSPITAL DE BELLVITGE, BARCELONA

Antimicrobial agents	Blood (% R)		Sputum (% R)	
	1985–90 n = 253	1991–97 n = 403	1985–90 n = 627	1991–97 n = 1,855
Penicillin	23.3	30.5	47.2	49.4
MIC 0.1–1 μg/mL	14.6	12.1	26.6	28.3
MIC $\geq$ 2 μg/mL	8.7	18.4	20.6	21.1
Cefotaxime	2.4	19.1	ND	22.5
MIC = 1 μg/mL	1.9	14.9	ND	16.6
MIC $\geq$ 2 μg/mL	0.5	4.2	ND	5.9
Erythromycin	7.9	13.2	12.1	21.0
Clindamycin	7.9	12.9	12.1	20.3
Tetracycline	30.0	24.8	47.5	39.6
Chloramphenicol	28.0	18.6	35.8	28.3
Co-trimoxazole	42.3	36.1	59.5	50.5
Resistance to 3 or more antibiotics	21.7	26.5	39.0	42.3

ND, not done.

a hospital in La Coruña, Galicia, rates of antibiotic resistance were higher ($p < 0.05$) in pediatric isolates than in adult isolates: penicillin 50% versus 31%, cefotaxime 38% versus 16%, co-trimoxazole 65% versus 45%, and multiple resistance 38% versus 20%.[46] The antibiotic susceptibility of 100 pneumococcal pediatric strains isolated between 1984 and 1985 was compared with 100 pneumococci isolated between 1994 and 1995 at a children's hospital in Barcelona. Increases had occurred in penicillin resistance, MIC > 0.1 μg/ml (51% versus 61%), erythromycin resistance (6% versus 36%), and intermediate cefotaxime resistance (10% versus 16%), whereas the percentages of strains with MIC of cefotaxime of 2 μg/ml remained stable (2% versus 2%).[30]

Healthy children are an important reservoir of multiple resistance in the community in Spain.[18,50,51] In an analysis of pneumococcal carriage in 306 healthy school children performed in 1991 in Seville, the carriage rate was 67.6%. The percentages of antibiotic resistance in 207 pediatric carriers were: penicillin resistance 53.5% (IRP 39.1% and HRP 14.4%), erythromycin resistance 28.5% and chloramphenicol resistance 16.4%.[50] These rates were higher than those found by our team in 1983 in Barcelona among 159 carrier children: penicillin resistance 35.9% (IRP 32.7% and HRP 3.2%), and erythromycin resistance 5.7%.[51] However, the percentage of penicillin resistance (30%) reported in pediatric carriers in Valencia in 1995 was lower than those found in Barcelona and in Seville, although rates of erythromycin resistance (22.6%) and co-trimoxazole resistance (83%) were similar to those reported in Seville.[18] In a study performed in Cádiz, Andalucia, 71% of 385 pneumococci isolated between 1991 and 1995 showed resistance to penicillin, but the incidence of penicillin resistance in nasopharyngeal carrier children (75.8%) was more marked than in invasive strains (30.2%).[19]

Resistance to non–beta-lactam antibiotics was observed more frequently in strains with resistance to penicillin than in susceptible strains.[37] In a selected sample of 175 S. pneumoniae strains susceptible to penicillin and 317 strains with decreased susceptibility to penicillin, PRP exhibited a significantly higher percentage of resistance ($p < 0.1$) to erythromycin (31.2 versus 5.2), tetracycline (61.5 versus 18.9), chloramphenicol (54.5 versus 15.4), and co-trimoxazole (83.9 versus 24.1) than did penicillin susceptible pneumococci isolated during the same period of time. Although the percentages of resistance to ciprofloxacin (3.1 versus 0.6) were greater in the PRP group, differences were not statistically significant.[40]

Of great concern is the rise in resistance to third generation cephalosporins such as cefotaxime or ceftriaxone, which are antibiotics of choice for penicillin resistant pneumococcal meningitis. In our hospital, a statistically significant increase in penicillin and cefotaxime resistance among meningeal isolates was observed when comparing the periods 1979–86 ($n = 74$) and 1987–94 ($n = 59$). Penicillin resistance rose from 19% during the first period to 40% during the second period; intermediate cefotaxime resistance (MIC $= 1$ μg/ml) increased from 1% to 10%, and cefotaxime resistance (MIC $= 2$ μg/ml) from 0% to 7%.[38]

The distribution of MICs of cefotaxime of 9,243 pneumococci studied between 1990 and 1996 by the Spanish Pneumococcal Reference Laboratory was: MIC ≤ 0.5 μg/ml in 7,235

(78.3%) strains; MIC $= 1$ μg/ml in 1,776 (19.2%) strains; MIC $= 2$ μg/ml in 196 (2.1%) strains; MIC $= 4$ μg/ml in 28 (0.3%) strains; and MIC $= 8$ μg/ml in eight (0.08%) strains. It is important to note that eight strains with MICs of cefotaxime of 8 μg/ml were isolated from respiratory tract, and six of them were atypical pneumococci (noncapsulated, optoquine resistant and/or bile negative).[12]

Although there have been several reports in the literature regarding a high incidence of erythromycin resistance in S. pneumoniae in Hungary[44] and France,[20] until 1985, macrolide resistance remained at a low level ($<3\%$) in Spain.[11,37] However, in the past 12 years, a progressive increase in macrolide resistance in S. pneumoniae has been observed throughout the country. This evolution may be due to the epidemic spread of serogroup/type strains 6, 14, 15, 19, and 23 under selective pressure of increased macrolide use. At Hospital de Bellvitge, Barcelona, the macrolide resistance increased from 7.1% in 1986 to 29% in 1997.[37,41] This increase is consistent with those recently reported by different Spanish authors.[7,12,15,17,35,50,52,56,58,62] In a recent study where 1,220 respiratory pneumococcal isolates from outpatients were collected in 14 different medical centers throughout Spain from May 1996 to April 1997, 422 (34.6%) of them showed resistance to erythromycin. Rates of erythromycin resistance differed greatly between noninvasive strains isolated in children (36–60%) and invasive strains (13–16%).[17] The majority of erythromycin-resistant strains showed multiple resistance.[18] A total of 501 erythromycin-resistant isolates were collected in our hospital from 1991 to 1997 and 96.8% of them were resistant to clindamycin, 89.6% to penicillin, 44.3% to cefotaxime, 92.4% to tetracycline, 61.6% to chloramphenicol, and 74.6% to co-trimoxazole.

There are two recognized mechanisms of macrolide resistance to S. pneumoniae: target modification and efflux. Target modification occurs at the level of the ribosomes via an *erm* gene encoding a 23S rRNA methylase and renders the strains resistant to macrolides, lincosamides, and streptogramin B compounds (MLS$_B$ phenotype). A novel mechanism of resistance due to an efflux system has been described in S. pneumoniae and S. pyogenes.[59] This mechanism confers resistance to 14- and 15-membered macrolides, but susceptibility to lincosamides and streptogramin B antibiotics (M phenotype). Table 3 shows that the majority ($>97\%$) of macrolide-resistant pneumococci isolated in Spain have MLS$_B$ phenotype (resistance to clindamycin, and streptogramin$_B$ compounds), and that the M phenotype is rare (0.5–3%). In the United States, however, the M phenotype is found in $>40\%$ of erythromycin-resistant pneumococci.[59]

Regarding resistance to 4-fluoroquinolones (4-FQ) in S. pneumoniae, it has been found to be low in Spain ($<3\%$).[39] Although, the in vitro activity of old 4-FQ, ciprofloxacin, and ofloxacin, against S. pneumoniae strains is low, and clinical failures have been described. In the past years new compounds with higher activity against S. pneumoniae, such as sparfloxacin, grepafloxacin, moxifloxacin, clinafloxacin, and trovafloxacin have been developed and may be considered alternatives for the treatment of respiratory infections.[39,40] In a study conducted at our hospital, the frequency of resistance (%) and in vitro activities of 4-FQ against 337 clinical isolates of S. pneumoniae obtained during 1997 from 336 consecutive

TABLE 3. PHENOTYPES OF MACROLIDE-RESISTANT PNEUMOCOCCI IN SPAIN

Period	City	No. of strains	Phenotype MLS_B[a]	ermB[b]	Phenotype M[c]	mefE[b]	References
1994–97	San Sebastián	76	93.4%	+	6.6%	+	Perez-Trallero et al.[53]
1996–97	Logroño	70	98.5%	+	1.5%	+	Landero et al.[26]
1996–97	Madrid	124	98.4%	ND	1.6%	ND	Cercenado et al.[7]
1990–97	Barcelona	501	96.8%	+[d]	3.2%	+	Liñares et al.[e]

[a]Resistance to macrolides, lincosamides, and streptogramin$_B$.
[b]Presence of ermB or mefE determinants by PCR.
[c]Resistance to 14- and 15-membered macrolides.
[d]Only 35 strains studied by PCR.
[e]Unpublished data.

adult patients were as follows: trovafloxacin MIC_{90} 0.12 μg/ml (0.9%); sparfloxacin MIC_{90} 0.25 μg/ml (2.6%); ofloxacin MIC_{90} 2 μg/ml (2.6%); and ciprofloxacin MIC_{90} 2 μg/ml (3.5%). No differences in activity against penicillin-susceptible or -resistant strains were noted for any of the 4-FQs tested. Eight strains (2.3%) with MICs of ciprofloxacin and ofloxacin of >32 μg/ml were inhibited by 1–4 μg/ml of trovafloxacin and 8–32 μg/ml of sparfloxacin. These strains with high level resistance to ciprofloxacin had changes in the quinolone resistance determining regions of ParC (S^{79} → F or Y) and GyrA (S^{80} → F or Y). Four strains (1.2% with low level resistance to ciprofloxacin (MIC 4–8 μg/ml) had only ParC mutations (S^{79} → F or Y), and were inhibited by 0.12–0.25 μg/ml of trovafloxacin. Transformation experiments suggest that ParC is the primary target of

ciprofloxacin is S. pneumoniae strains and that DNA gyrase is a secondary target.[41,48]

RESISTANCE PATTERNS AND SEROGROUPS

Table 4 summarizes the antibiotic resistance patterns found between 1991 and 1997 and compares those found between 1979 and 1990 in Hospital de Bellvitge. In the 1990s, we observed a statistically significant increase in the penicillin and co-trimoxazole resistance pattern (P, SxT) from 6.4% to 10.5%, and in two of the multiresistance patterns (P, E, CI, T, C, SxT; and P, E, CI, T, SxT), which rose from 4.9% to 12.8%. The rates of strains susceptible to all antibiotics tested increased

TABLE 4. COMPARISON OF RESISTANCE PATTERNS OF 3,738 PNEUMOCOCCAL STRAINS STUDIED DURING TWO PERIODS AT HOSPITAL DE BELLVITGE, BARCELONA (SPAIN)

Resistance pattern[a]	1991–96 no. (%) of strains	1979–90 no. (%) of strains
P, SxT	236 (10.5)	95 (6.4)
P, T, C, SxT	197 (8.8)	203 (13.6)
P, E, CI, T, C, SxT	190 (8.4)	54 (3.6)
SxT	124 (5.5)	134 (9.0)
P, E, CI, T, SxT	98 (4.4)	20 (1.3)
P	77 (3.4)	20 (1.3)
P, T, SxT	48 (2.1)	39 (2.6)
T, C	40 (1.8)	84 (5.6)
T	35 (1.6)	60 (4.0)
T, C, SxT	31 (1.4)	82 (5.5)
T, SxT	29 (1.3)	58 (3.9)
Other different patterns	195 (8.7)	196 (13.1)
Susceptible[b]	946 (40.8)	447 (29.9)
Total	2,246 (100.0)	1,492 (100.0)

[a]P, resistant to penicillin; T, resistant to tetracycline; C, resistant to chloramphenicol; E, resistant to erythromycin; Cl, resistant to clindamycin; SxT, resistant to co-trimoxazole.
[b]Susceptible to all antibiotics tested.

from 29.9% in 1979–90 to 40.8% in 1990–97. This observation might be explained by the fact that the patterns with resistance to tetracycline and chloramphenicol have decreased throughout the 1990s period. The most frequent resistance pattern in the 1980s (P, T, C, SxT, 13.6%) represented only 8.8% of isolates during the 1990s. Similar trends in the evolution of pneumococcal resistance patterns were reported by the Spanish Pneumococcal Reference Laboratory.[12]

The six serogroups or serotypes (SGTs) found most frequently in Spain in the 1990s were SGT 19 (12%), 6 (11.8%), 23 (10.5%), 3 (9.7%), 14 (9.6%), and 9 (7.4%) representing 61% of the 9,243 pneumococci studied. The prevalence of SGTs 9, 14, and 19 increased from 2 to 7%, 6 to 14% and 5 to 7.5%, respectively. Serogroup 6 remained between 8% and 12% during the whole period. Serogroup 23, which was increasing at the beginning of the 1980s, decreased during the 1990s representing 10% by 1996. When blood isolates from adult patients were analyzed, the most prevalent SGTs, in order of frequency, were 3, 9, 14, 8, 4, 19, 6, 23, 1, and 18, whereas the order of frequency in blood isolates from children was 19, 6, 14, 18, 23, 1, 5, 6, 12, and 3.[12] The SGTs most frequently found in respiratory pneumococcal isolates in a recent study of 1,102 strains collected throughout Spain were 6 (14.0%), 19 (10.3%), 23 (9.1%), 9 (5.9%), and 14 (4.5%).[17] At our hospital, the ten most frequent SGTs found among 274 pneumococci isolated from blood during the 1990–97 period were as follows: 3 (11.2%), 14 (10.6%), 9 (8.0%), 4 (7.7%), 19 (6.6%), 6 (6.2%), 8 (5.8%), 1 (4.4%), 18 (4.4%), and 23 (4.4%). The significant increase in blood isolates of SGT 14 during the 1990s (10.6%) is noteworthy, since it represented only 2% of strains isolated from blood in adult patients admitted to our hospital in the 1980s. Approximately 50% of strains of SGT 14 had the characteristic resistant pattern (P, SxT) of serotype 9V.

The distribution of the most frequent SGTs among penicillin-resistant isolates is shown in Table 5 adapted from Fenoll et al.[12] SGTs 6, 14, 23, 19, and 9 accounted for 92.2% of penicillin resistant isolates. Multiresistance associated with macrolide resistance (PTCE and PTE) was observed in 73% of SGT 6, 63% of SGT 15, 35% of SGT 14, 29% of SGT 23, 27% of SGT 19, and 2% of SGT 9.[12]

In Spain, ≈90% of penicillin resistant pneumococci are resistant to SxT, and although resistance to SxT was not studied at the Pneumococcal Reference Laboratory, the majority of pneumococci with penicillin resistance (pattern P) were probably also resistant to SxT. It is interesting to note that 87% of strains SGT 9 and 53% of SGT 14 have this resistant pattern. In our experience, the genotypes (determined by pulsed field gel electrophoresis–PFGE–) of 26/28 serotype 9V strains and 16/37 serotype 14 strains were identical to French/Spanish epidemic clone 9V. This finding could suggest that one of the most frequent clones in Spain among adult patients is now the French/Spanish international clone 9V, as has been occurred in other American and European countries.[32,45,61]

Coffey et al.[8,9] suggested that serogroup 19 multiresistant strains, 19F and 19A, are a serotype variant of the Spanish multiresistant serotype 23F clone, which presumably has arisen by recombination at the capsular locus. As shown in Table 5, the majority of these multiresistant strains share the multiple resistance pattern PTC (60% of SGT 23 and 47% of SGT 19). The two most common Spanish clones, 23 F and 6B serotypes, have been studied in detail by several groups. The Spanish serotype 23F clone has been identified in at least six other countries across three continents.[47] The second major clone 6B has been found in the U.K. and Iceland.[57]

CONCLUSION

In Spain, the antibiotic resistance rates for *S. pneumoniae* are among the highest in Europe, coinciding with high antibiotic consumption by outpatients and widespread use of antibiotics as growth promoters in farm animals.[3] This review confirms that the prevalence of macrolide and third generation cephalosporin resistance in clinical isolates of *S. pneumoniae* has increased dramatically in Spain in the 1990s. There is a clear trend towards acquiring resistance to multiple antibiotics and these strains are now major components of the nasopharygeal flora in children. The selective pressure resulting from injudicious use of antimicrobials favors the geographical

TABLE 5. PENICILLIN-RESISTANT *S. pneumoniae*: MOST FREQUENT RESISTANCE PATTERNS AND SEROGROUPS (1990–96)

	PTCE	PTE	PTC	P	Other penicillin-resistant patterns
Serogroup 6 n = 896	55%	18%	19%	2%	6%
Serotype 14 n = 846	28%	7%	8%	53%	4%
Serogroup 23 n = 816	26%	3%	60%	5%	6%
Serogroup 19 n = 781	22%	5%	47%	12%	14%
Serogroup 9 n = 559	0.3%	1.6%	0.7%	87%	10.4%

P, resistant to penicillin; T, resistant to tetracycline; C, resistant to chloramphenicol; E, resistant to erythromycin; Co-trimoxazole was not tested.
Adapted from Fenoll et al.[12]

spread of multiresistant epidemic clones of *S. pneumoniae*[25] and could explain the high rates of antimicrobial resistance found in Spain.[3] Since most of these resistant strains belong to only a limited number of SGTs, which are also among the most common causes of pediatric and adult infections, conjugate pneumococcal vaccine aimed at these antigens may be able to reduce the carriage rate of resistant pneumococci among toddlers[10] and is an important future tool for the control of resistant pneumococcal disease.

REFERENCES

1. **Appelbaum, P.C.** 1992. Antimicrobial resistance in *Streptococcus pneumoniae*: an overview. Clin. Infect. Dis. **15**:77–83.

2. **Baquero, F.** 1995. Pneumococcal resistance to β-lactam antibiotics: a global geographic overview. Microb. Drug Resist. **1**:115–120.

3. **Baquero, F., and the Task Force of the General Direction for Health Planning of the Spanish Ministry of Health.** 1996. Antibiotic resistance in Spain: what can be done? Clin. Infect. Dis. **23**:819–823.

4. **Baquero, F.** 1996. Epidemiology and management of penicillin-resistant pneumococci. Curr. Opin. Infect. Dis. **9**:372–379.

5. **Bouza, E., and P. Muñoz.** 1995. Penicillin-resistant pneumococci in adult disease with especial reference to AIDS patients. Microb. Drug Resist. **1**:9–28.

6. **Casal, J.** 1982. Antimicrobial susceptibility of *Streptococcus pneumoniae*: serotype distribution of penicillin-resistant strains in Spain. Antimicrob. Agents Chemother. **22**:222–225.

7. **Cercenado, E., C. Sanchez-Carrillo, C. Garcia-Rey, and E. Bouza.** 1997. Erythromycin resistance in *Streptococcus pyogenes* and *Streptococcus pneumoniae*: high incidence of M phenotype among clinical isolates [Abstract E-110]. Presented at the 37th Annual Meeting of the Interscience Conference on Antimicrobial Agents and Chemotherapy, American Society for Microbiology, Toronto.

8. **Coffey, T.J., M.C. Enright, M. Daniels, P. Wilkinson, S. Berrón, A. Fenoll, and B. Spratt.** 1998. Serotype 19A variants of the Spanish serotype 23F multiresistant clone of *Streptococcus pneumoniae*. Microb. Drug Resist. **4**:51–55.

9. **Coffey, T.J., S. Berrón, M. Daniels, M.E. Garcia-Leoni, E. Cercenado, E. Bouza, A. Fenoll, and B. Spratt.** 1996. Multiply antibiotic-resistant *Streptococcus pneumoniae* recovered from spanish hospitals (1988–1994): novel major clones of serotypes 14, 19F and 15F. Microbiology **142**:2747–2757.

10. **Dagan, R., R. Melamed, M. Muallen, L. Piglansky, D. Greenberg, O. Abramson, P.M. Mendelman, N. Bohidar, and P. Yagupsky.** 1996. Reduction of nasopharyngeal carriage of pneumococci during the second year of life by a heptavalent conjugate pneumococcal vaccine. J. Infect. Dis. **174**:1271–1278.

11. **Fenoll, A., C. Martín-Bourgon, R. Muñoz, D. Vicioso, and J. Casal.** 1991. Serotype distribution and antimicrobial resistance in *Streptococcus pneumoniae* isolates producing systemic infections in Spain 1979–1989. Rev. Infect. Dis. **13**:56–60.

12. **Fenoll, A., I. Jado, D. Vicioso, A. Pérez and J. Casal.** 1998. Evolution of *Streptococcus pneumoniae*: serotypes and antibiotic resistance in Spain. Update 1990–1996. J. Clin. Microbiol. **36**:3447–3454.

13. **Fleites, A., M.J. Santos, and F.J. Mendez.** Penicillin-resistant *S. pneumoniae*: clinical and microbiological aspects. 1994 [Abstract E-21]. Presented at the 34th Annual Meeting of the Interscience Conference on Antimicrobial Agents and Chemotherapy. American Society for Microbiology, Orlando, Florida.

14. **Florez, C., J.M. Pérez, R. Aretio, P. Parras, and E. Martin.** 1992. Susceptibility of *Streptococcus pneumoniae* to five antibiotics. J. Antimicrob. Chemother. **30**:727–728.

15. **Garcia-Arenzana, J.M., M. Montes, N. Gómez, and E. Pérez-Trallero.** 1991. Resistencia a eritromicina en *Streptococcus pneumoniae*. Enf. Inf. Microbiol. Clin. **9**:613–618.

16. **García-Leoni, M.E., E. Cercenado, P. Rodeño, J.C.L. Bernaldo de Quirós, E. Martínez-Hernández, and E. Bouza.** 1992. Susceptibility of *Streptococcus pneumoniae* to penicillin: a prospective microbiological and clinical study. Clin. Infect. Dis. **14**:427–435.

17. **García de Lomas, J., and grupo Español para la Vigilancia de Patógenos Respiratorios.** 1998. Situación epidemiológica actual y resistencia de los patógenos respiratorios en España. Med. Clin. **110**:44–52.

18. **García de Lomas, J., C. Gimeno, E. Millas, M. Bermejo, M.A. Lázaro, D. Navarro, L. Garcia Ponte, and B. Garijo.** 1997. Antimicrobial susceptibility of *Streptococcus pneumoniae* isolated from pediatric carriers in Spain. Eur. J. Clin. Microbiol. Infect. Dis. **16**:11–13.

19. **García-Martos, P., F. Galan, P. Marín, and J. Mira.** 1997. Increase in high resistance to penicillin of clinical isolates of *Streptococcus pneumoniae* in Cádiz, Spain. Chemotherapy **43**:179–181.

20. **Geslin, P., A. Buu-Hoï, A. Frémaux, and J.F. Acar.** 1992. Antimicrobial resistance in *Streptococcus pneumoniae*: an epidemiological survey in France, 1970–1990. Clin. Infect. Dis. **15**:95–98.

21. **Gomez, J., V. Baños, J. Ruiz Gomez, F. Herrero, M.L. Núñez, M. Canteras, and M. Valdés.** 1995. Clinical significance of pneumococcal bacteremias in a general hospital: a prospective study 1989–1993. J. Antimicrob. Chemother. **36**:1021–1030.

22. **Hackenbeck, R., M. Tarpay, and A. Tomasz.** 1980. Multiple changes of penicillin-binding proteins in penicillin-resistant clinical isolates of *Streptococcus pneumoniae*. Antimicrob. Agents Chemother. **17**:364–371.

23. **Jacobs, M.R., H.J. Koornhof, R.M. Robins-Browne, C.M. Stevenson, Z.A. Vermaak, I. Freiman, G.B. Miller, M.A. Witcomb, M. Isaacson, J.I. Ward, and R. Austrian.** 1978. Emergence of multiply resistant pneumococci. N. Engl. J. Med. **299**:735–740.

24. **Klugman, K.P.** 1990. Pneumococcal resistance to antibiotics. Clin. Microbiol. Rev. **3**:171–196.

25. **Kristinsson, K.G.** 1997. Effect of antimicrobial use and other risk factors on antimicrobial resistance in pneumococci. Microb. Drug Resist. **3**:117–122.

26. **Landero, M., A. Portillo, M.J. Gastañares, F. Ruiz-Larrea, M. Zarazaga, I. Olarte, and C. Torres.** 1998. MLS resistance phenotypes and mechanisms in *S. pneumoniae* [Abstract 3.10]. Presented at the Fourth International Conference on the Macrolides, Azalides, Streptogramins and Ketolides, Barcelona.

27. **Latorre, C., T. Juncosa, and I. Sanfeliu.** 1982. Antibiotic susceptibility of *Streptococcus pneumoniae* from pediatric patients. J. Antimicrob. Chemother. **22**:659–665.

28. **Latorre, C., C. Muñoz, G. Trujillo, T. Juncosa, and P. Clarós.** 1994. Susceptibility of pneumococci isolated from middle ear effusions to antimicrobial agents commonly used in otitis media. J. Antimicrob. Chemother. **33**:186–187.

29. **Latorre, C., and Grupo de Microbiólogos de Hospitales Comarcales de Cataluña.** 1997. Estudio prospectivo de las cepas invasivas de *Streptococcus pneumoniae* aisladas en 16 hospitales de Cataluña [Abstract 119]. Presented at the VII Reunión de la Sociedad Española de Enfermedades Infecciosas y Microbiología Clínica, Madrid.

30. **Latorre, C.** 1998. *Streptococcus pneumoniae* isolated from a pediatric population: changes in ten years. 1998. Acta Paediatr. **87**:940–944.

31. **Latorre, C., A. Gene, T. Juncosa, C. Muñonz, and A. González.**

1999. Invasive pneumococci in a paediatric hospital [Abstract]. Presented at the 9th European Congress of Clinical Microbiology and Infectious Diseases, Berlin.

32. **Lefevre, J.C., M.A. Bertrand and G. Faucon.** 1995. Molecular analysis by pulsed-field gel electrophoresis of penicillin-resistant *Streptococcus pneumoniae* from Toulouse, France. Eur. J. Microbiol. Infect. Dis. **14:**491–497.

33. **Liñares, J., J.L. Pérez, J. Garau, and R. Martin.** 1983. Co-trimoxazole resistance in pneumococci. Eur. J. Clin. Microbiol. **2:**473–474.

34. **Liñares, J., J. Garau, C. Domínguez, and J.L. Pérez.** 1983. Antibiotic resistance and serotypes of *Streptococcus pneumoniae* from patients with community acquired pneumococcal disease. Antimicrob. Agents Chemother. **23:**545–547.

35. **Liñares, J., D. Mariscal, S. Gomez-Lus, T. Alonso, J.L. Perez, and R. Martin.** 1992. Increase of erythromycin resistence among clinical isolates of *Streptococcus pneumoniae* [Abstract 1027]. Presented at the 32nd Annual Meeting of the Interscience Conference on Antimicrobial Agents and Chemotherapy, American Society for Microbiology, Anaheim, California.

36. **Liñares, J., T. Alonso, J.L. Pérez, J. Ayats, M.A. Dominguez, R. Pallares, and R. Martin.** 1992. Decreased susceptibility of penicillin-resistant pneumococci to twenty-four beta-lactam antibiotics. J. Antimicrob. Chemother. **30:**279–288.

37. **Liñares, J., R. Pallarés, T. Alonso, J.L. Pérez, J. Ayats, F. Gudiol. P. Fernández-Viladrich, and R. Martín.** 1992. Trends in antimicrobial resistance of clinical isolates of *Streptococcus pneumoniae* in Bellvitge Hospital, Barcelona, Spain 1979–1990. Clin. Infect. Dis. **15:**99–105.

38. **Liñares, J., F. Tubau, C. Cabellos, P.F. Viladrich, F. Gudiol, R. Hakenbeck, and R. Martin.** 1995. Increase of penicillin and third generation cephalosporins resistance in meningeal isolates of *Streptococcus pneumoniae* in adult patients (1979–1994) [Abstract E24]. Presented at the 35th Annual Meeting of the Interscience Conference on Antimicrobial Agents and Chemotherapy, American Society for Microbiology, San Francisco.

39. **Liñares, J., F. Tubau, R. Pallares, C. Ardanuy, and R. Martin.** 1996. *Streptococcus pneumoniae*: susceptibility to fluoroquinolones [Abstract C3]. Presented at the 36th Annual Meeting of the Interscience Conference on Antimicrobial Agents and Chemotherapy, American Society for Microbiology, New Orleans.

40. **Liñares, J., F. Tubau, F. Alcaide, C. Ardanuy, A. Garcia, and R. Martín.** 1996. Antimicrobial resistance of *Streptococcus pneumoniae*: comparison of the *in vitro* activity of 16 antibiotics. Curr. Ther. Res. **57:**57–64.

41. **Liñares, J., C. Ardanuy, F. Tubau, M.A. Benitez, A.G. De la Campa, and R. Martin.** 1998. Comparative in vitro activities of trovafloxacin and 12 antimicrobials against *S. pneumoniae* [Abstract 13.018]. Presented at the 8th International Congress on Infectious Diseases, Boston.

42. **Liñares, J.** 1998. Community-acquired antimicrobial resistance: is it controllable? Int. J. Clin. Pract. **95:**23–26.

43. **Nava, J.M., F. Bella, J. Garau, J. Lite, M.A. Morera, C. Marti, D. Fontanals, B. Font, V. Pineda, S. Uriz, *et al.*** 1994. Predictive factors for invasive disease due to penicillin-resistant *Streptococcus pneumoniae*: a population-based study. Clin. Infect. Dis. **19:**884–890.

44. **Marton, A., M. Gulyas, and R. Muñoz.** 1991. Extremely high incidence of antibiotic resistance in clinical isolates of *Streptococcus pneumoniae* in Hungary. J. Infect. Dis. **163:**542–548.

45. **Melander, E., K. Ekdahl, H.B. Hansson, C. Kammem, M. Laurell, P. Nilsson, K. Persson, M. Söderström and S. Mölstad.** 1998. Introduction and clonal spread of penicillin- and trimethoprim/sulfamethoxazole-resistant *Streptococcus pneumoniae*, serotype 9V in southern Sweden. Microb. Drug Resist. **4:**71–78.

46. **Moure, R., M. Abalde, L.A. Rocha, E. Miguez, F. Peña, A. Echaniz, and P. Llinares.** 1997. Resistencia en *Streptococcus pneumoniae* aislados en hemocultivos [Abstract 118]. Presented at the VII Reunión de la Sociedad Española de Enfermedades Infecciosas y Microbiología Clínica, Madrid.

47. **Muñoz, R., T.J. Coffey, M. Daniels, C.G. Dowson, G. Laible, J. Casal, R. Hakenbeck, M. Jacob, J.M. Musser, B.G. Spratt, and A. Tomasz.** 1991. Intercontinental spread of a multiresistant clone of serotype 23F *Streptococcus pneumoniae*. J. Infect. Dis. **164:**302–306.

48. **Muñoz, R., and A.G. de la Campa.** 1996. Par C subunit of DNA topoisomerase IV of *Streptococcus pneumoniae* is a primary target of fluoroquinolones and cooperates with DNA gyrase A subunit in forming resistant phenotype. Antimicrob. Agents Chemother. **40:**2252–2257.

49. **Pallares, R., J. Liñares, M. Vadillo, C. Cabellos, F. Manresa, P. Fernández-Viladrich, R. Martín, and F. Gudiol.** 1995. Resistance to penicillin and cephalosporin and mortality from severe pneumococcal pneumonia in Barcelona, Spain. N. Engl. J. Med. **333:**474–480.

50. **Palomino-Nicas, J., J. Pachon, A. Garcia-Curiel, C. Toledo, A. Martin, E. Alfaro, and D. Prados.** 1992. Nasopharyngeal carriage and antimicrobial resistance of *Streptococcus pneumoniae* in healthy school children [Abstract 1536]. Presented at the 32nd Annual Meeting of the Interscience Conference on Antimicrobial Agents and Chemotherapy, American Society for Microbiology, Anaheim, California.

51. **Pérez, J.L., J. Liñares, J. Bosch, M.J. López de Goicoechea, and R. Martin.** 1987. Antibiotic resistance of *Streptococcus pneumoniae* in childhood carriers. J. Antimicrob. Chemother. **19:**278–280.

52. **Pérez-Trallero, E., J.M. Garcia-Arenzana, and M. Urbieta.** 1988. Erythromycin resistance in streptococci. Lancet **2:**444–445.

53. **Pérez Trallero, E., M. Montes, J.M., García Arenzana, J.M. Marimón and D. Vicente.** 1998. Presencia de los genes *ermB* y *mefE* en *Streptococcus pneumoniae* en Gipuzkoa [Abstract 30-10]. Presented at the VIII Congreso Sociedad Española de Enfermedades Infecciosas y Microbiología Clínica, Palma de Mallorca, Spain.

54. **Ramos Amador, J.T., J. Saavedra, E. Ruiz-Chercoles, C. Garrido, F. Sanz, J. Ruiz Contreras, and A. Rodriguez Noriega.** 1995. Invasive antibiotic-resistant *Streptococcus pneumoniae* in children: risk factors for penicillin resistance [Abstract C8]. Presented at the 35th Annual Meeting of the Interscience Conference on Antimicrobial Agents and Chemotherapy, American Society for Microbiology, San Francisco.

55. **Rodriguez-Tudela, J.L., F. López de Felipe, J.V. Martinez-Suárez, and A. Fenoll.** 1992. Comparative in-vitro activity of four peptide antibiotics against penicillin-resistant *Streptococcus pneumoniae* isolated from cerebrospinal fluid (CSF). J. Antimicrob. Chemother. **29:**299–302.

56. **Sempere, M.A., J. Gomez, and J. Ruiz.** 1992. Resistance of *Streptococcus pneumoniae* to erythromycin in adults and children. J. Antimicrob. Chemother. **29:**348–349.

57. **Soares, S., K.G. Kristinsson, J.M. Musser, and A. Tomasz.** 1993. Evidence for the introduction of a multiresistant clone of serotype 6B *Streptococcus pneumoniae* from Spain to Iceland in the late 1980s. J. Infect. Dis. **168:**158–163.

58. **Soriano, F., and R. Fernández-Roblas.** 1993. High rates of erythromycin-resistant *Streptococcus pneumoniae* among penicillin-resistant strains. J. Antimicrob. Chemother. **31:**440.

59. **Sutcliffe, J., A. Tait-Kamradt, and L. Wondrack.** 1996. *Streptococcus pneumoniae* and *Streptococcus pyogenes* resistant to macrolides but sensitive to clindamycin: a common resistance pattern mediated by an efflux system. Antimicrob. Agents Chemother. **40:**1817–1824.

60. **Tomasz, A.** 1995. The pneumococcus at the gates. N. Engl. J. Med. **333:**514–515.

61. **Tomasz, A. A. Corso, E.P. Severina, G. Echániz-Aviles, M.C. De Cunto Brandileone, T. Camou, E. Castañeda, O., Figueroa, A. Rossi, and J.L. Di Fabio.** 1998. Molecular epidemiologic characterization of penicillin-resistant *Streptococcus pneumoniae* invasive pediatric isolates recovered in six Latin-American countries: an overview. Microb. Drug Resist. **4:**195–207.

62. **Torres, L., T. Pelaez, F.J. Vasallo, L. Martinez-Sanchez, P. Muñoz, M. Rodriguez-Creixems, and E. Bouza.** 1997. Evolution of antibiotic resistance of *Streptococcus pneumoniae*: increase of penicillin resistance in blood and cerebrospinal fluid (CSF) isolates [Abstract C-168]. Presented at the 37th Annual Meeting of the Interscience Conference on Antimicrobial Agents and Chemotherapy, American Society for Microbiology, Toronto.

Address reprint requests to:
Josefina Liñares
Microbiology Department
Ciutat Sanitària i Universitària Bellvitge
Feixa Llarga s.n. 08907–L'Hospitalet
Barcelona
Spain

Impact of Antibiotic Resistance on Chemotherapy for Pneumococcal Infections

ROMAN PALLARES, PEDRO F. VILADRICH, JOSEFINA LIÑARES, CARMEN CABELLOS,
and FRANCESC GUDIOL

ABSTRACT

Over the past three decades, penicillin-resistant pneumococci have emerged worldwide. In addition, penicillin-resistant strains have also decreased susceptibility to other β-lactams (including cephalosporins) and these strains are often resistant to other antibiotic groups, making the treatment options much more difficult. Nevertheless, the present *in vitro* definitions of resistance to penicillin and cephalosporins in pneumococci could not be appropriated for all types of pneumococcal infections. Thus, current levels of resistance to penicillin and cephalosporin seem to have little, if any, clinical relevance in nonmeningeal infections (*e.g.*, pneumonia or bacteremia). On the contrary, numerous clinical failures have been reported in patients with pneumococcal meningitis caused by strains with MICs ≥ 0.12 μg/ml, and penicillin should never be used in pneumococcal meningitis except when the strain is known to be fully susceptible to this drug. Today, therapy for pneumococcal meningitis should mainly be selected on the basis of susceptibility to cephalosporins, and most patients may currently be treated with high-dose cefotaxime ($\pm$) vancomycin, depending on the levels of resistance in the patient's geographic area. In this review, we present a practical approach, based on current levels of antibiotic resistance, for treating the most prevalent pneumococcal infections. However, it should be emphasized that the most appropriate antibiotic therapy for infections caused by resistant pneumococci remains controversial, and comparative, randomized studies are urgently needed to clarify the best antibiotic therapy for these infections.

INTRODUCTION

PNEUMOCOCCAL INFECTIONS are very prevalent worldwide, and *Streptococcus pneumoniae* is a major cause of pneumonia, meningitis, acute otitis media, and acute sinusitis.[10,70] During the past 30 years, pneumococci have developed resistance to several antimicrobial agents, including tetracycline, penicillin, trimethoprim-sulfamethoxazole, chloramphenicol, erythromycin, cephalosporins, and other drugs.[5,12,17,29,54,61] But, in terms of therapy, the real problem has been the development of resistance to penicillin. This is because penicillin was the time-honored treatment for pneumococcal infections for decades, and alternative drugs were only necessary in penicillin-allergic patients.

An interesting issue is that, shortly after the introduction of penicillin in 1940, the first strain of *S. pneumoniae* with decreased susceptibility to penicillin was produced in the laboratory,[28] but the first clinical isolate did not appear until more than 20 years later in Boston.[52] In the late 1960s, pneumococcal strains with moderate penicillin resistance were isolated in Australia and New Guinea.[41,42] In the 1970s, an epidemic of high-level penicillin- and multidrug-resistant pneumococci was detected in pediatric wards in South Africa.[6,50] Subsequently, resistant strains were identified in Europe, particularly in Spain.[30,57,60] Finally, in the 1980s, penicillin-resistant pneumococci emerged in many countries. Today, the prevalence of pneumococci resistant to penicillin and other antibiotics is increasing worldwide.[14,20,21,37,39,45,65,66]

As shown in several studies, resistance rates varied with the geographic area and age of the patient, the highest being the rate of resistance among isolates from otitis media in children.[21,54,60,61] It is important to emphasize that antimicrobial consumption is a major factor contributing to penicillin resistance and other antibiotic resistance in pneumococci.[7,13]

Although antibiotic resistance is a complex phenomenon that we do not know very well, it is important to note that resistant

Infectious Diseases and Microbiology Services, Hospital Bellvitge and University of Barcelona, Barcelona, Spain.
Reprinted from *Microbial Drug Resistance*, Vol. 4, No. 4, 1998.

pneumococcal strains have the ability to spread rapidly throughout the world. For example, the Spanish clone 23F and 6B have been disseminated to other countries in Europe and to other continents.[69,82]

The mechanism of resistance of pneumococci to penicillin is due to alterations of the penicillin binding proteins (PBPs) that have reduced their affinity for penicillin and related β-lactams.[48,64,85,86] Therefore, susceptibility to other β-lactams is also affected and the minimal inhibitory concentrations (MICs) of these drugs rise in parallel with those of penicillin G, although with different degrees depending on the drug[59,67,76,83] (Table 1). Cefotaxime, ceftriaxone, cefpirome, and cefepime are the parenteral cephalosporins that yield the lowest MICs against penicillin-resistant strains. The MICs of carbapenems are smaller than those of cephalosporins. Thus, imipenem is highly active against penicillin-resistant strains, but meropenem is slightly less active in vitro than imipenem. Amongst oral β-lactams, amoxicillin yields the lowest MICs against penicillin-resistant pneumococci, and cefuroxime and cefpodoxime are the oral cephalosporins that yield the lowest MICs, although these are several times higher than those of amoxicillin. In addition, penicillin-resistant strains are more likely to be resistant to other antibiotic groups such as erythromycin, tetracycline, chloramphenicol, and trimethoprim-sulfamethoxazole.[17,54,61] However, the newest quinolones (e.g., trovafloxacin, sparfloxacin, grepafloxacin) seem to be very active compounds against penicillin-resistant and -susceptible strains.

The current in vitro definition of penicillin resistance by S. pneumoniae (National Committee for Clinical Laboratory Standards, NCCLS 1995) is as follows: susceptible strains (MIC ≤ 0.06 μg/ml of penicillin G), intermediate resistance (MIC 0.12–1.0 μg/ml of penicillin G), and high-level resistance (MIC ≥ 2.0 μg/ml of penicillin G). However, the laboratory definition of resistance to penicillin was established before the clinical relevance of this level of resistance had been deter-

mined. In other words, the current in vitro definitions of penicillin resistance are open to question, particularly for those pneumococcal strains causing nonmeningeal infections.

Although no prospective, randomized studies on the therapy of resistant pneumococcal infections have been carried out, the published data suggest that moderate penicillin-resistant pneumococci causing nonmeningeal infections such as pneumonia or bacteremia have no therapeutic significance.[11,31,33,55,74,75,80,84,91] This is because the serum concentrations achieved with penicillin or related β-lactams are several times higher than the MICs of the strains.[4] On the other hand, however, pneumococcal meningitis poses a special therapeutic problem because of the levels of penicillin achieved in the cerebrospinal fluid (CSF) are inadequate to kill penicillin-resistant pneumococci including those with intermediate resistance,[43] and several clinical failures have been reported.[19,34,36,78]

The management of pneumococcal infections caused by resistant strains has been debated in recent reviews,[19,34,36,61,78] but several important questions remain to be answered. The most important considerations in selecting empirical antibiotic therapy in patients with a suspected pneumococcal infection are the following: prevalence and patterns of resistance in the patient's geographic area; site of infection (e.g., meningitis); risk factors for penicillin-resistant strains (e.g., prior antibiotic use, young age, day-care attendance, prior hospitalization, nosocomial infection)[16,63,73,74]; severity of illness and probability of death; route of drug administration; and potential toxicity and costs.

In this review, we will discuss the treatment of the most prevalent pneumococcal infections, focusing principally on adult patients. The regimens proposed herein are based on the current levels of resistance, but these recommendations may change in the near future.

THERAPY FOR PNEUMONIA

There are several reports dealing with the response to β-lactam antibiotic therapy in penicillin-resistant pneumococcal pneumonia or bacteremia.[11,31,33,55,74,75,80,84,91]

Friedland and Klugman[33] carried out a prospective study of community-acquired pneumococcal infections in 207 South African children, most of them were treated with penicillin or ampicillin at a standard dosage. They found that the mortality rate was 14% in children with penicillin-resistant pneumococcal infections and 11% in children with penicillin-susceptible infection.

Tan and colleagues[84] reported their experience during a 3-year period in Houston. All but 1 of 19 children with systemic infections caused by intermediate penicillin-resistant pneumococci responded adequately to initial β-lactam therapy (mostly amoxicillin or cefuroxime).

Friedland[31] reported a series of 108 children with bacteremic pneumococcal infections, excluding meningitis. In children with pneumonia who were treated with ampicillin or an equivalent β-lactam agent, 88% with penicillin-resistant infections and 93% with penicillin-susceptible infections had improved by day 7 of therapy.

Recently, we conducted a prospective nonintervention study with 504 adult patients with severe pneumococcal pneumonia; 29% of them were infected with penicillin-resistant strains.[75] Although the mortality rate was significantly higher in peni-

TABLE 1. IN VITRO ACTIVITY OF SEVERAL ANTIBIOTICS IN 952 PENICILLIN-RESISTANT STREPTOCOCCUS PNEUMONIAE[a]

Antibiotic	MIC range	MIC-50/MIC-90
Penicillin	0.12–4	1/2
Amoxicillin	0.06–4	0.5/1
Cefuroxime	1–16	2/8
Cefaclor	0.5–64	32/64
Cefixime	2–64	8/32
Cefotaxime	0.03–4	0.5/1
Ceftriaxone	0.03–4	0.5/1
Cefpirome	0.03–2	0.25/0.5
Ceftazidime	1–64	16/64
Imipenem	0.03–1	0.06/0.25
Meropenem	0.03–2	0.12/0.5
Erythromycin	0.03–>128	0.12/128
Tetracycline	0.03–>128	16/64
Cotrimoxazole[b]	0.12–16	4/8
Chloramphenicol	0.25–64	4/16
Vancomycin	0.12–1	0.25/0.5

[a]Data from the Microbiology Laboratory (1990–1995), Bellvitge Hospital, Barcelona.

[b]The ratio of trimethoprim-sulfamethoxazole is 1/19.

cillin-resistant than in penicillin-susceptible cases (38% vs. 24%), after adjustment for other variables, the odds ratio for mortality in patients with penicillin-resistant strains was not statistically significant. Moreover, when we compared the mortality rate in patients treated with penicillin or ampicillin, there were no statistically significant differences between patients infected with penicillin-resistant and those infected with penicillin-susceptible strains. Likewise, among patients treated with cefotaxime or ceftriaxone, the mortality rate was not significantly different in those infected with cephalosporin-resistant strains when compared with those infected with cephalosporin-susceptible strains. Our conclusion was that current levels of resistance to penicillin and cephalosporins are not associated with increased mortality in patients with severe pneumococcal pneumonia. Thus, these antibiotics can still be used as the therapy of choice for this disease.[75]

We suggest the following antibiotic therapy for community-acquired pneumococcal pneumonia (Table 2).

Initial empirical therapy

This refers to the treatment for a patient with a clinical picture and radiologic findings highly suggestive of pneumococcal pneumonia before the culture results are known. It should be emphasized that in patients with clinical suspicion of pneumococcal pneumonia, the diagnosis may be strongly reinforced by demonstrating polymorphonuclear leukocytes (PMNs) and Gram-positive cocci in pairs in the sputum.[71] However, sometimes the clinical picture is not clear enough and the infection may be caused by other pathogens. This possibility should be taken into account in selecting empirical therapy, particularly when the patient has severe pneumonia. Empirical therapy for pneumococcal pneumonia should be classified according to the severity of the infection (Table 2).

Mild-to-moderate pneumonia. Mild-to-moderate pneumonia should be considered in a patient who is less than 65 years old and has no co-morbid conditions; in these cases, an outpatient treatment can be prescribed.

Amoxicillin may be the therapy of choice for patients with mild/moderate pneumonia in whom a characteristic clinical picture of pneumococcal pneumonia is present. However, amoxicillin-clavulanate may be preferred in some patients such as those with chronic obstructive pulmonary disease (COPD) in whom the causative organisms may be *S. pneumoniae* or other common pathogens such as *Haemophilus influenzae* (often β-lactamase positive).

Alternative drugs such as cefuroxime, erythromycin, or penicillin procaine should be selected according to the history of allergy or when the oral route is not well tolerated.

In patients in whom, after a careful clinical evaluation, his/her physician has doubts about the diagnosis of pneumococcal pneumonia versus atypical pneumonia, a macrolide (*e.g.*, erythromycin) should be given. However, it is important to know that if the causative organisms is a pneumococcus resistant to erythromycin the patient may not respond to this therapy.[68]

Severe pneumonia. Patients with severe community-acquired pneumonia should be hospitalized, and the criteria for severe pneumonia includes (one or more): age ≥ 65 years; serious underlying conditions (*e.g.*, COPD, diabetes, malignancies, heart

TABLE 2. SUGGESTED ANTIBIOTIC REGIMENS
FOR *PNEUMOCOCCAL PNEUMONIA*

1. Initial empirical therapy
   Mild/moderate pneumonia
       Primary   Oral amoxicillin 1 g/8 hour or oral
                 amoxicillin-clauvulanate 1 g/8 hr
       Alternative   Oral cefuroxime 750 mg/8–12 hour or oral
                 erythromycin 500 mg/6 hr or i.m.
                 penicillin procaine 1.2 mU/12 hr

   Severe pneumonia
       Primary   i.v. ceftriaxone 1–2 g/24 hr or i.v. cefotaxime
                 1–2 g/8 hr or i.v. amoxicillin-clavulanate
                 2 g/8 hr (+/−) i.v. erythromycin 1 g/6 hr
       Alternative   i.v. cefpirome 1–2 g/12 hr or i.v. cefepime
                 1–2 g/8–12 hr or i.v. imipenem 500 mg/
                 6 hr or i.v. meropenem 1 g/8 hr or i.v.
                 vancomycin 1 g/12 hr (+/−) i.v.
                 erythromycin 1 g/6 hr or a new quinoline

2. Therapy when *in vitro* studies are known (severe pneumonia)
   Susceptible strains to penicillin (MICs ≤0.06 μg/ml)
       Primary   i.v. penicillin G 1 mU/4 hr or i.v. ampicillin
                 1 g/6 hr
       Alternative   i.v. cefuroxime 1.5 g/8 hr or i.v.
                 ceftriaxone 1 g/24 hr or i.v. cefotaxime
                 1 g/8 hr or i.v. erythromycin 1 g/6 hr

   Strains with decreased susceptibility to penicillin
                 penicillin MICs 0.12 to 2.0 μg/ml
       Primary   i.v. penicillin G 2 mU/4 hr or i.v. ampicillin
                 2 g/6 hr
       Alternative   i.v. ceftriaxone 1–2 g/24 hr or i.v.
                 cefotaxime 1–2 g/8 hr or i.v. erythromycin
                 1 g/6 hr

                 Penicillin MICs ≥4.0 μg/ml
       Primary   Continue with the initial empirical therapy if
                 the clinical response is satisfactory
       Alternative   i.v. imipenem 500 mg/6 hr or i.v.
                 meropenem 1 g/8 hr or i.v. erythromycin
                 1 g/6 hr or i.v. vancomycin 1 g/12 hr or a
                 new quinoline

i.m., Intramuscular; i.v., intravenous; MICs, minimal inhibitory concentrations.

Dosage recommendations are approximate values for an adult patient of 60–70 kg.

Dosage and intervals can be different in infants and children and should be calculated according to their age and specific conditions. In addition, pediatric patients may have pathogens causing pneumonia different than those in adults and thus it should be considered in selecting empirical antibiotic therapy.

Primary therapy is the treatment of choice suggested.

Alternative therapy should be selected according to (i) the patterns of antibiotic resistance in the patient's geographic area or when the culture results are known should be based on the *in vitro* susceptibility studies; (ii) history of allergy; (iii) toxicity; and (iv) costs.

failure, chronic renal failure, splenectomy, cirrhosis, or chronic alcoholism); previous pneumonia <1 year ago; altered mental status; respiration rate > 30/min; blood pressure <90/60; temperature >101°F; WBC <4000 or >30,000/mm^3; PaO$_2$ <60 mmHg (<90% O$_2$ saturation); PaCO$_2$ >50; needs mechanical ventilation; chest X-ray >1 lobe; pleural effusion; Hct <30; sepsis; and extrapulmonary disease (*e.g.*, meningitis). One important clinical consideration is that in a patient with severe pneumococcal pneumonia, the possibility of having associated meningitis should be evaluated carefully because the treatment options are substantially different (see treatment of meningitis).

To treat pneumococci and other common bacteria (*e.g.*, *H. influenzae* or other Gram-negative bacilli), the initial empirical therapy for severe pneumonia should include an appropriate cephalosporin or amoxicillin-clavulanate (Table 2). Additionally, erythromycin should be added in cases in which *Legionella* or another atypical pathogen cannot reasonably be ruled out.

In patients with severe underlying diseases (*e.g.*, neutropenic patients) in whom some fastidious organisms such as *Pseudomonas* also needs to be treated, the combination of cefpirome or cefepime or imipenem or meropenem with erythromycin should be considered. It is important to know that ceftazidime has little activity against penicillin-resistant pneumococci (Table 1).

There is little experience in treating patients with pneumococcal pneumonia with vancomycin alone and this drug has no activity against other pathogens such as Gram-negative bacilli. Thus, when vancomycin is selected for empirical therapy of severe pneumonia (*e.g.*, allergy to β-lactams or in places in which a very high level cephalosporin resistance has been detected) a combination with other drugs (*e.g.*, aztreonam or ciprofloxacin) should be considered. Serum vancomycin levels should be monitored in these patients. In our opinion, and based on the current levels of antibiotic-resistant pneumococci, vancomycin should not be widely used for treating pneumonia.

The newest quinolones (e.g., trovafloxacin, sparfloxacin, grepafloxacin) may play an important role in the empirical treatment of severe pneumonia cases in the near future.

Therapy for known pneumococcal pneumonia

When culture results (*e.g.*, positive cultures from blood, pleural fluid, or a lower respiratory tract specimen) and *in vitro* studies are known, any change in antibiotic therapy should be based on the results of susceptibility tests and on the light of clinical evolution of the patient.

Penicillin or ampicillin (at standard dosage) remains the therapy of choice for susceptible strains. Alternative drugs (see Table 2) may be necessary in penicillin-allergic patients.

Patients infected with strains having penicillin MICs of 0.12–2.0 μg/ml may respond to penicillin or ampicillin therapy, although the administration of high dose (for example, 150,000–200,000 U/kg per day of penicillin G) would be prudent to achieve higher serum and pulmonary levels of the drug.

It is not well known whether patients infected with strains for which penicillin MIC ≥ 4 μg/ml could respond to intravenous (i.v.) penicillin therapy. In these patients, consecutive therapy should be based on the response to the initial empirical therapy and the results of the *in vitro* studies. In the case that the patient is doing well with a cephalosporin or amoxicillin-clavulanate, this therapy should be continued. On the contrary, if the clinical response is not satisfactory, other drugs such as imipenem, meropenem, erythromycin, vancomycin, or a new quinoline should be considered according to the results of the *in vitro* studies.

THERAPY FOR MENINGITIS

Response to therapy in penicillin-resistant and cephalosporin-resistant pneumococcal meningitis is different to that in nonmeningeal infections. We believe that clinicians should have in mind some important considerations when selecting antibiotic therapy for pneumococcal meningitis:

(i) There have been numerous case reports of failure of penicillin therapy in patients with pneumococcal meningitis caused by intermediate or high-level penicillin-resistant strains.[1,6,22,24,27,38,46,47,62,72,77,79,92] Thus, because penicillin-resistant strains are spread worldwide, the initial therapy for pneumococcal meningitis should not be penicillin or ampicillin.

(ii) Several patients with pneumococcal meningitis infected with strains showing decreased susceptibility to cephalosporins failed cefotaxime or ceftriaxone treatment.[3,8,9,18,23,51,53,58,81] In most of them, cefotaxime or ceftriaxone were administered at the standard dosage for meningitis. However, some experience in adults suggests that the administration of a higher dosage of cefotaxime may be effective for treating patients with cephalosporin-resistant pneumococcal meningitis, at least for those with intermediate resistance.[2,88,90]

(iii) Vancomycin could be a good alternative for pneumococcal meningitis caused by penicillin- and cephalosporin-resistant strains. Nevertheless, the administration of vancomycin at 30 mg/kg per day (the dosage recommended for adult patients) was associated with several failures in adult pneumococcal meningitis.[89] These failures could be due to the highly variable concentrations of vancomycin achieved in the CSF, especially when dexamethasone was given concomitantly. However, we are unaware of any reported vancomycin failure in pneumococcal meningitis in pediatric patients in whom vancomycin is administered at higher dosages (60 mg/kg per day).[56]

(iv) In penicillin-resistant pneumococcal meningitis, chloramphenicol treatment may not be appropriated. Several penicillin-resistant pneumococci are also resistant to chloramphenicol. In addition, unsatisfactory results with chloramphenicol (despite the strains that were susceptible to this drug based on the MICs) in penicillin-resistant pneumococcal meningitis have been reported.[32] These failures could be due to a poor bactericidal activity of chloramphenicol in such strains.[32]

We suggest the following antibiotic therapy for pneumococcal meningitis (Table 3).

Initial empirical therapy

This terminology refers to the initial treatment for a patient with pneumococcal meningitis (a purulent meningitis and a CSF Gram stain showing typical Gram-positive diplococci). However, in cases with purulent meningitis and a CSF Gram stain showing no microorganisms, several possible pathogens should be considered in selecting the initial therapy, depending on the clinical suspicion in each case.

In our opinion, the initial empirical therapy for pneumococcal meningitis should be a cephalosporin such as cefotaxime. However, because some strains may have decreased susceptibility to these drugs, it may be prudent to suggest high-dose cefotaxime for the initial therapy. Other cephalosporins such as cefpirome appear to be promising for resistant pneumococcal meningitis.

TABLE 3. SUGGESTED ANTIBIOTIC REGIMENS
FOR *PNEUMOCOCCAL MENINGITIS*

1. Initial empirical therapy

   Primary   i.v. cefotaxime 300–400 mg/kg per day (5–6 g/ 6 hr) (maximum 24 g/day) (+/−) i.v. vancomycin 30 mg/kg per day (1 g/12 hr) (in children 60 mg/kg per day)

   Alternative   i.v. vancomycin (+/−) i.v. rifampin 900 mg/24 hr or i.v. cefotaxime (+) i.v. rifampin

2. Therapy when *in vitro* studies are known

   Strains susceptible to penicillin (MICs ≤0.06 μg/ml)

   Primary   i.v. penicillin G 3–4 mU/4 hr

   Alternative   i.v. cefotaxime 3–4 g/6 hr or i.v. ceftriaxone 4 g/24 hr or i.v. vancomycin (+/−) i.v. rifampin or i.v. chloramphenicol 1 g/6 hr

   Strains with decreased susceptibility to penicillin
   penicillin MICs ≥0.12 μg/ml
   Cefotaxime MICs ≤0.25 μg/ml

   Primary   i.v. cefotaxime 3–4 g/6 hr or i.v. ceftriaxone 4 g/24 hr

   Alternative   i.v. vancomycin (+/−) i.v. rifampin

   Cefotaxime MICs 0.5 to 1.0 μg/ml

   Primary   i.v. cefotaxime 300–400 mg/kg per day (5–6 g/6 hr) (maximum 24 g/day)

   Alternative   i.v. vancomycin (+/−) i.v. rifampin

   Cefotaxime MICs ≥2.0 μg/ml

   Primary   i.v. cefotaxime 300–400 mg/kg per day (5–6 g/6 hr) (+/−) i.v. vancomycin 30 mg/kg per day (1 g/12 hr) (in children 60 mg/kg per day)

   Alternative   i.v. vancomycin (+/−) i.v. rifampin (or intrathecal vancomycin 5–20 mg/24–48 hr) or i.v. meropenem 2 g/8 hr or i.v. imipenem 1 g/6 hr or i.v. chloramphenicol 1 g/6 hr

i.v., intravenous; MICs, minimal inhibitory concentrations; MBCs, minimal bactericidal concentrations.

These suggested antibiotic regimens are for treating patients with pneumococcal meningitis in regions in which penicillin-resistant pneumococci are reported.

Dosage recommendations are approximate values for an adult patient of 60–70 kg.

Dosage and intervals can be different in infants and children, and should be calculated according to their age and specific conditions. In addition, pediatric patients may have pathogens causing meningitis different from those in adults and thus it should be considered in selecting empirical antibiotic therapy, particularly in cases of purulent meningitis with no microorganisms in the CSF Gram stain.

Primary therapy is the treatment of choice suggested.

Alternative therapy should be selected according to (i) the patterns of antibiotic resistance in the patient's geographic area or when the culture results are known should be based on the *in vitro* susceptibility studies; (ii) the pharmacokinetics of the drugs; (iii) history of allergy; (iv) toxicity; and (v) costs.

In places where high-level cephalosporin resistance (MICs of cefotaxime ≥2 μg/ml) has been detected, cefotaxime may be administered in combination with vancomycin. However, it is important to have in mind some considerations regarding this

combination: (i) some studies of animals with cephalosporin-resistant meningitis have suggested that the combination of cephalosporin and vancomycin is more effective than either drug alone,[35] however, to our knowledge little clinical experience with this combination has been published[56]; (ii) even if the combination is given, in adult patients cefotaxime should be administered at a high-dosage regimen because vancomycin (at the recommended dosage) may achieve insufficient CSF levels[89]; (iii) by contrast, in children in whom vancomycin may be administered at higher dose and this drug alone may be effective for pneumococcal meningitis, the concomitant administration of high-dose cefotaxime might be less important than in adults, and the standard dose of cefotaxime or ceftriaxone might be enough; (iv) vancomycin should be discontinued when *in vitro* studies are known and the pneumococcus is susceptible to penicillin or cephalosporins.

An alternative regimen for the empirical therapy may be vancomycin with or without rifampin. Vancomycin alone may be appropriate for pediatric patients. However, in adults the combination of vancomycin and rifampin may be more appropriate (see comments on vancomycin dosage and levels above).

The combination of cefotaxime or ceftriaxone and rifampin appeared to be promising. However, some *in vitro* studies in the laboratory have shown an antagonistic effect between rifampin and β-lactams, although this has not been confirmed in animal studies.[87] To date, the relevance of this phenomenon in clinical practice is not well known, although some data in children with meningitis have suggested that this combination may enhance CSF bactericidal activity compared with that of ceftriaxone alone.[56] Rifampin cannot be used as monotherapy because of the rapid development of resistance.

Therapy for known pneumococcal meningitis

When culture results (positive CSF and/or blood cultures) and *in vitro* studies are known, any change in antibiotic ther-

TABLE 4. SUGGESTED ANTIBIOTIC REGIMENS
FOR *OTITIS MEDIA* AND *SINUSITIS*

Primary	Oral amoxicillin 50–80 mg/kg per day (1 g/6—8 hr) or oral amoxicillin-clavulanate 1 g/8 hr
Alternative	Oral cefuroxime 750 mg/8–12 hr or i.m. ceftriaxone 1 g/24 hr or oral erythromycin 500 mg/6 hr or oral clarithromycin 500 mg/12 hr or oral azithromycin 1 g/24 hr or oral TMP-SMZ 160/800 mg/12 hr

i.m., Intramuscular; TMP-SMZ, trimethoprim-sulfamethoxazole.

Dosage recommendations are approximate values for adult patients. Doses/intervals in parenthesis are those recommended for an adult patient of 60–70 kg.

Dosage and intervals can be different in infants and children, and should be calculated according to their age and specific conditions.

Primary therapy is the treatment of choice suggested.

Alternative therapy should be selected according to (i) the patterns of antibiotic resistance in the patient's geographic area or if the culture results are known should be based on the *in vitro* susceptibility studies; (ii) history of allergy; (iii) toxicity; and (iv) costs.

apy should be based on the results of susceptibility tests and on the light of clinical evolution of the patient. A control lumbar puncture should be performed 24–36 hr after the start of antibiotic therapy in all patients with resistant pneumococcal meningitis.

Penicillin remains the therapy of choice for susceptible strains, and alternative drugs are only necessary in penicillin allergic patients.

Patients infected with strains with decreased susceptibility to penicillin (MICs ≥ 0.12 μg/ml) should not be treated with penicillin. In such cases, cefotaxime or ceftriaxone, using the standard dose for meningitis, may be the therapy of choice for those with MICs of cefotaxime ≤ 0.25 μg/ml.

Based on the concept that to kill a pathogen the antibiotic concentration in CSF should exceed by 8- to 10-fold the minimal bactericidal concentration (MBC) of the drug, it may be prudent to suggest high-dose cefotaxime for those cases with MICs of cefotaxime 0.5–1.0 μg/ml. This is because the cefotaxime MBC may be one dilution higher than the cefotaxime MIC, and clinical failures have been reported in patients infected with strains having cefotaxime MICs as small as 0.5 μg/ml who were treated with standard dose of cefotaxime or ceftriaxone.[3,8,9,18,23,51,53,58,81] Ceftriaxone administered at a dose higher than 4 g/day is not recommended because of potential side effects (e.g., biliary stones). To date, there is no experience with other drugs such as cefpirome or cefepime.

Up to now, several failures have been reported in cephalosporin-resistant pneumococcal meningitis (MICs of cefotaxime ≥ 2 μg/ml) using standard dose of cefotaxime or ceftriaxone.[88] However, there are some reported cases with MICs of cefotaxime of 2 μg/ml that were cured with high-dose cefotaxime.[2,88,90] In cases in which the pneumococcus has an MIC of cefotaxime ≥ 2 μg/ml and the patient is doing well with the initial empirical therapy (e.g., high-dose cefotaxime with or without vancomycin), this therapy should be continued. On the other hand, if the patient has no good clinical response, an alternative therapy should be considered in the light of the results of a second lumbar puncture. These regimens may include vancomycin with or without rifampin (or intrathecal vancomycin) or alternatively meropenem or imipenem or chloramphenicol (based on in vitro studies), or perhaps new compounds (e.g., clinafloxacin).

The MICs of meropenem may be smaller than those of cefotaxime in cephalosporin-resistant strains, but the doses recommended and the CSF levels achieved appear not to be very promising.[25] Although imipenem may have MICs smaller than those of meropenem and some patients with meningitis have been cured with this drug, the potential risk of seizures should be taken into account. In addition, meropenem and imipenem may produce hypersensitivity reactions in β-lactam-allergic patients. In the case that chloramphenicol is selected as an alternative therapy, MBCs determinations should be performed.[32]

THERAPY FOR OTITIS MEDIA AND SINUSITIS

Acute otitis media and acute sinusitis are most commonly caused by S. pneumoniae, H. influenzae, or Moraxella catarrhalis.[15,26,40,44,49] In acute otitis media, response to antibiotic therapy is often difficult to interpret due to a high rate of spontaneous resolution.[15,34]

Some case reports of "standard dose" amoxicillin treatment, failure have been reported in pneumococcal otitis media, particularly in cases with high-level penicillin resistance.[19,34,49] However, it has been suggested that the administration of high doses of amoxicillin might be effective at least in those cases with intermediate penicillin resistance.[19]

Because in most cases microbiological cultures are not available, empirical antibiotic therapy should be selected to treat the most important microorganisms. It is important to know the prevalence of pneumococci resistant to penicillin and other antibiotics, as well as the prevalence of strains of H. influenzae and M. catarrhalis producing β-lactamase in the patient's geographic area.

As shown in Table 4, the treatment of choice for acute otitis media and acute sinusitis may be amoxicillin. In regions in which penicillin-resistant pneumococci is prevalent, the administration of high-dose amoxicillin may be prudent. In places with a high percentage of H. influenzaea and M. catarrhalis producing β-lactamase, amoxicillin-clavulanate or cefuroxime may be preferred.

Because of the low penetration of the antibiotics in the middle ear, otitis media caused by high-level penicillin-resistant pneumococci may not respond to standard doses of amoxicillin or amoxicilli-clavulanate.[34] If a patient with acute otitis media has a clinical failure after 48 hr of amoxicillin-clavulanate, amoxicillin at 30–40 mg/kg per day may be added to obtain higher amoxicillin dose (total 80 mg/kg per day) while not increasing the total clavulanate dose.[19] Other alternative drugs (e.g., ceftriaxone, macrolide, or TMP-SMZ) may also be considered. Tympanocentesis may be required in patients who do not respond to therapy and this technique would allow the identification of the causative organism and susceptibility studies.

ACKNOWLEDGMENT

This paper was supported by a grant FIS 97-0716 from the National Health Service, Madrid.

REFERENCES

1. **Abronheim, G.A., B. Reich, and M.I. Marks.** 1979. Penicillin-insensitive pneumococci. Am. J. Dis. Child. **133:**187–191.
2. **Almirante, B., E. Cortes, C. Pigrau, O. del Valle, I. Gasser, and A. Pahissa.** 1995. Personal communication.
3. **Alonso, J., V. Madrigal, and M. Garcia-Fuentes.** 1991. Recurrent meningitis from a multiply resistant Streptococcus pneumoniae strain treated with erythromycin. Pediatr. Infect. Dis. J. **10:**256.
4. **Amsden, G.W., and J.J. Schentag.** 1995. Tables of antimicrobial agent pharmacology, pp. 492–528. In G.L. Mandell, J.E. Bennet, and R. Dolin (ed.). Principles and Practice of Infectious Diseases, Fourth edition. Churchill Livingstone, New York.
5. **Appelbaum, P.C.** 1996. Epidemiology and in vitro susceptibility of drug-resistant Streptococcus pneumoniae. Pediatr. Infect. Dis. J. **15:**932–939.
6. **Appelbaum, P.C., A. Bhamjee, J.N. Scragg, A.J. Hallett, A.F. Bowen, and R.C. Cooper.** 1977. Streptococcus pneumoniae resistant to penicillin and chloramphenicol. Lancet **ii:**995–997.
7. **Arason, V.A., K.G. Kristinsson, J.A. Sigurdsson, G. Stefans-**

dottir, S. Mölstad, and S. Gudmundsson. 1996. Do antimicrobials increase the carriage rate of penicillin-resistant pneumococci in children? Cross sectional prevalence study. Br. Med. J. **313:** 387–391.

8. **Asensi, F., M.C. Otero, D. Perez-Tamarit, I. Rodriguez-Escribano, J.L. Cabedo, S. Gresa, and E. Canton.** 1993. Risk/benefit in the treatment of children with imipenem-cilastatin for meningitis caused by penicillin-resistant pneumococcus. J. Chemother. **5:**133–134.

9. **Asensi, F., D. Perez-Tamarit, M.C. Otero, M. Gallego, S. Llanes, C. Abadia, and E. Canton.** 1989. Imipenem-cilastatin therapy in a child with meningitis caused by a multiply resistant pneumococcus. Pediatr. Infect. Dis. J. **8:**895.

10. **Austrian, R.** 1994. Pneumococcal infections, pp. 607–611. *In* K.J. Isselbacher, E. Braunwald, J.D. Wilson, J.B. Martin, A.S. Fauci, and D.L. Kasper (ed.). Harrison's Principles of Internal Medicine, Thirteenth Edition. McGraw-Hill, Inc., New York.

11. **Austrian, R.** 1994. Confronting drug-resistant pneumolocci. Ann. Intern. Med. **121:**807–809.

12. **Baquero, F.** 1995. Pneumococcal resistance to beta-lactam antibiotics: A global geographic overview. Microb. Drug Resist. **1:**115–120.

13. **Baquero, F.** 1996. Trends in antibiotic resistance of respiratory pathogens: An analysis and commentary on a collaborative surveillance study. J. Antimicrob. Chemother. **38(Suppl. A):**117–132.

14. **Baquero, F., J. Martinez-Beltran, and E. Loza.** 1991. A review of antibiotic resistance patterns of *Streptococcus pneumoniae* in Europe. J. Antimicrob. Chemother. **28(Suppl. C):**31–38.

15. **Berman, S.** 1995. Otitis media in children. N. Engl. J. Med. **332:**1560–1565.

16. **Boken, D.J., S.A. Chartrand, R.V. Goering, R. Kruger, and C.H. Harrison.** 1995. Colonization with penicillin-resistant Streptococcus pneumoniae in a child-care center. Pediatr. Infect. Dis. J. **14:**879–884.

17. **Bouza, E., and P. Muñoz.** 1995. Penicillin-resistant pneumococci in adult disease with special reference to AIDS patients. Microb. Drug Resist. **1:**9–28.

18. **Bradley, J.S., and J.D. Connor.** 1991. Ceftriaxone failure in meningitis caused by Streptococcus pneumoniae with reduced susceptibility to betalactam antibiotics. Pediatr. Infect. Dis. J. **10:** 871–873.

19. **Bradley, J.S., S.L. Kaplan, K.P. Klugman, and R.J. Leggiadro.** 1995. Consensus: Management of infections in children caused by Streptococcus pneumoniae with decreased susceptibility to penicillin. Pediatr. Infect. Dis. J. **14:**1037–1041.

20. **Breiman, R.F., J.C. Butler, F.C. Tenover, J.A. Elliott, and R.R. Facklam.** 1994. Emergence of drug-resistant pneumococcal infections in the United States. J. Am. Med. Assn. **271:**1831–1835.

21. **Caputo, G.M., P.C. Appelbaum, and H.H. Liu.** 1993. Infections due to penicillin-resistant pneumococci: clinical, epidemiologic, and microbiologic features. Arch. Intern. Med. **153:**1301–1310.

22. **Caputo, G.M., F.R. Sattler, M.R. Jacobs, and P.C. Appelbaum.** 1983. Penicillin-resistant pneumococcus and meningitis. Ann. Intern. Med. **98:**416–417.

23. **Catalan, M.J., J.M. Fernandez, A. Vazquez, E. Varela de Seijas, A. Suarez, and J.C.L. Bernaldo de Quiros.** 1994. Failure of cefotaxime in the treatment of meningitis due to relatively resistant Streptococcus pneumoniae. Clin. Infect. Dis. **18:**766–769.

24. **Collignon, P.J., J. Bell, I.W. Hufton, and D. Mitchell.** 1988. Meningitis caused by a penicillin- and chloramphenicol-resistant Streptococcus pneumoniae. Med. J. Aust. **149:**497–498.

25. **Dagan, R., L. Velghe, J.L. Rodda, and K.P. Klugman.** 1994. Penetration of meropenem into the cerebrospinal fluid of patients with inflamed meninges. J. Antimicrob. Chemother. **34:**175–179.

26. **Del Castillo, F., A. Garcia-Perea, and F. Baquero-Artigao.** 1996. Bacteriology of acute otitis media in Spain: A prospective study based on tympanocentesis. *Pediatr. Infect. Dis. J.* **15:** 541–543.

27. **Devitt, L., I. Riley, and D. Hansman.** 1977. Human infection caused by penicillin-insensitive pneumococci. Med. J. Aust. **1:**586–588.

28. **Eriksen, K.R.** 1945. Studies on induced resistance to penicillin in a pneumococcus type 1. Acta Pathol. Microbiol. Scand. **22:** 398–405.

29. **Felmingham, D., R.N. Grüneberg, and the Alexander Project Group.** 1996. A multicentre collaborative study of the antimicrobial susceptibility of community-acquired, lower respiratory tract pathogens 1992–1993: The Alexander Project. J. Antimicrob. Chemother. **38(Suppl. A):**1–57.

30. **Fenoll, A., C. Martin Bourgon, R. Muñoz, D. Vicioso, and J. Casal.** 1991. Serotype distribution and antimicrobial resistance of *Streptococcus pneumoniae* isolates causing systemic infections in Spain, 1979–1989. Rev. Infect. Dis. **13:**56–60.

31. **Friedland, I.R.** 1995. Comparison of the response to antimicrobial therapy of penicillin-resistant and penicillin-susceptible pneumococcal disease. Pediatr. Infect. Dis. J. **14:**885–890.

32. **Friedland, I.R., and Klugman, K.P.** 1992. Failure of chloramphenicol therapy in penicillin-resistant pneumococcal meningitis. Lancet **339:**405–408.

33. **Friedland, I.R., and K.P. Klugman.** 1992. Antibiotic-resistant pneumococci disease in South African children. Am. J. Dis. Child. **146:**920–923.

34. **Friedland, I.R., and G.H. McCracken, Jr.** 1994. Management of infections caused by antibiotic-resistant *Streptococcus pneumoniae*. N. Engl. J. Med. **331:**377–382.

35. **Friedland, I.R., M. Paris, S. Ehrett, S. Hickey, K. Olsen, and G.H. McCracken, Jr.** 1993. Evaluation of antimicrobial regimens for treatment of experimental penicillin- and cephalosporin-resistant pneumococcal meningitis. Antimicrob. Agents Chemother. **37:**1630–1636.

36. **Friedland, I.R., S. Shelton, M. Paris, S. Rinderknecht, S. Ehrett, K. Krisher, and G.H. McCracken, Jr.** 1993. Dilemmas in diagnosis and management of cephalosporin-resistant Streptococcus pneumoniae meningitis. Pediatr. Infect. Dis. J. **12:**196–200.

37. **Garcia-Leoni, M.E., E. Cercenado, P. Rodeño, J.C.L. Bernaldo de Quiros, D. Martinez-Hernandez, and E. Bouza.** 1992; Susceptibility of *Streptococcus pneumoniae* to penicillin: a prospective microbiological and clinical study. Clin. Infect. Dis. **14:**427–435.

38. **Gartner, J.C., and R.H. Michaels.** 1979. Meningitis from a pneumococcus moderately resistant to penicillin. J. Am. Med. Assn. **241:**1707–1709.

39. **Gold, H.S., and R.C. Moellering, Jr.** 1996. Antimicrobial-drug resistance. N. Engl. J. Med. **335:**1445–1453.

40. **Gwaltney, J.M. Jr.** 1995. Sinusitis, pp. 585–90. In G.L. Mandell, J.E. Bennett, and R. Dolin (ed.). Principles and Practice of Infectious Diseases, 4th Edition. Churchill Livingstone, New York.

41. **Hansman, D., L. Devitt, H. Miles, and I. Riley.** 1974. Pneumococci relatively insensitive to penicillin in Australia and New Guinea. Med. J. Australia **2:**353–356.

42. **Hansman, D., H. Glasgow, J. Surt, H.L. Devitt, and R. Douglas.** 1971. Increased resistance to penicillin of pneumococci isolated from man. N. Engl. J. Med. **284:**175–177.

43. **Hieber, J.P., and J.D. Nelson.** 1977. A pharmacologic evaluation of penicillin in children with purulent meningitis. N. Engl. J. Med. **297:**410–413.

44. **Hoberman, A. J.L. Paradise, S. Block, D.J. Burch, M.R. Jacobs, and M.I. Balanescu.** 1996. Efficacy of amoxicillin/clavulanate for acute otitis media: relation to Streptococcus pneumoniae susceptibility. Pediatr. Infect. Dis. J. **15:**955–962.

45. **Hofmann, J., M.S. Cetron, M.M. Farley, W.S. Baughman, R.R. Facklan, J.A. Elliott, K.A. Deaver, and R.F. Breiman.** 1995. The prevalence of drug-resistant Streptococcus pneumoniae in Atlanta. N. Engl. J. Med. **333**:481–486.

46. **Howes, V.J., and R.G. Mitchell.** 1976. Meningitis due to relatively penicillin-resistant pneumococcus. Br. Med. J. **1**:996.

47. **Iyer, P.V., J.H. Kahler, and N.M. Jacobs.** 1978. Penicillin-resistant pneumococcal meningitis. Pediatrics **61**:157–158.

48. **Jabes, D., S. Nachman, and A. Tomasz.** 1989. Penicillin-binding protein families: evidence for the clonal nature of penicillin resistance in clinical isolates of pneumococci. J. Infect. Dis. **159**:16–25.

49. **Jacobs, M.R.** 1996. Increasing importance of antibiotic-resistant *Streptococcus pneumoniae* in acute otitis media. Pediatr. Infect. Dis. J. **15**:940–943.

50. **Jacobs, M.R., H.J. Koornhof, R.M. Robins-Browne, R.M. Stevenson, Z.A. Vermaak, I. Freiman, G.B. Miller, M.A. Whitcomb, M. Isaacson, J.I. Ward, and R. Austrian.** 1978. Emergence of multiply-resistant pneumococci. N. Engl. J. Med. **299:** 735–740.

51. **John, C.C.** 1994. Treatment failure with use of a third-generation cephalosporin for penicillin-resistant pneumococcal meningitis: Case report and review. Clin. Infect. Dis. **18**:188–193.

52. **Kislak, J.W., L.M.B. Razavi, A.K. Daly, and M. Finland.** 1965. Susceptibility of pneumococci to nine antibiotics. Am. J. Med. Sci. **250**:262–268.

53. **Kleiman, M.B., G.A. Weinberg, J.K. Reynolds, and S.D. Allen.** 1993. Meningitis with beta-lactam-resistant Streptococcus pneumoniae: The need for early repeat lumbar puncture. Pediatr. Infect. Dis. J. **12**:782–783.

54. **Klugman, K.P.** 1990. Pneumococcal resistance to antibiotics. Clin. Microbiol. Rev. **3**:171–196.

55. **Klugman, K.P.** 1996. The clinical relevance of in-vitro resistance to penicillin, ampicillin, amoxycillin and alternative agents, for the treatment of community-acquired pneumonia caused by Streptococcus pneumoniae, Haemophilus influenzae and Moraxella catarrhalis. J. Antimicrob. Chemother. **38(Suppl. A):**133–140.

56. **Klugman, K.P., I.R. Friedland, and J.S. Bradley.** 1995. Bactericidal activity against cephalosporin-resistant Streptococcus pneumoniae in cerebrospinal fluid of children with acute bacterial meningitis. Antimicrob. Agents Chemother. **39**:1988–1992.

57. **Latorre, C., T. Juncosa, and I. Santfeliu.** 1985. Antibiotic resistance and serotypes of 100 Streptococcus pneumoniae strains isolated in a children's hospital in Barcelona, Spain. Antimicrob. Agents Chemother. **28**:357–359.

58. **Leggiadro, R.J., F.F. Barrett, P.J. Chesney, I. Davis, and F.C. Tenover.** 1994. Invasive pneumococci with high level penicillin and cephalosporin resistance at a mid-south children's hospital. Pediatr. Infect. Dis. J. **13**:320–322.

59. **Liñares, J., T. Alonso, J.L. Perez, J. Ayats, M.A. Dominguez, R. Pallares, and R. Martin.** 1992. Decreased susceptibility of penicillin-resistant pneumococci to twenty-four beta-lactam antibiotics. J. Antimicrob. Chemother. **30**:279–288.

60. **Liñares, J., R. Pallares, T. Alonso, J.L. Perez, J. Ayats, F. Gudiol, P.F. Viladrich, and R. Martin.** 1992. Trends in antimicrobial resistance of clinical isolates of *Streptococcus pneumoniae* in Bellvitge Hospital, Barcelona, Spain (1979–1990). Clin. Infect. Dis. **15**:99–105.

61. **Lister, P.D.** 1995. Multiply-resistant pneumococcus: Therapeutic problems in the management of serious infections. Eur. J. Clin. Microbiol. Infect. Dis. **14(Suppl. 1):**18–25.

62. **Mace, J.W., D.S. Janik, R.L. Sauer, and J.J. Quilligan, Jr.** 1977. Penicillin-resistant pneumococcal meningitis in an immunocompromised infant. J. Pediatr. **91**:506–507.

63. **Mannheimer, S.B., L.W. Riley, and R.B. Roberts.** 1996. Association of penicillin-resistant pneumococci with residence in a pediatric chronic care facility. J. Infect. Dis. **174**:513–519.

64. **Markiewicz, Z., and A. Thomasz.** 1989. Variation in penicillin-binding protein patterns of penicillin-resistant clinical isolates of pneumococci. J. Clin. Microbiol. **27**:405–410.

65. **Marton, A., M. Gulyas, R. Muñoz, and A. Tomasz.** 1991. Extremely high incidence of antibiotic resistance in clinical isolates of *Streptococcus pneumoniae* in Hungary. J. Infect. Dis. **163:** 542–548.

66. **Mason, E.O., S.L. Kaplan, L.B. Lamberth, and J. Tillman.** 1992. Increased rate of isolation of penicillin-resistant Streptococcus pneumoniae in a children's hospital and in vitro susceptibilities to antibiotics of potential therapeutic use. Antimicrob. Agents Chemother. **36**:1703–1707.

67. **Mason, E.O., L. Lamberth, R. Lichenstein, and S.L. Kaplan.** 1995. Distribution of Streptococcus pneumoniae resistant to penicillin in the USA and in-vitro susceptibility to selected oral antibiotics. J. Antimicrob. Chemother. **36**:1043–1048.

68. **Moreno, S., M.E. Garcia-Leoni, E. Cercenado, M.D. Diaz, J.C. Bernaldo de Quiros, and E. Bouza.** 1995. Infections caused by erythromycin-resistant Streptococcus pneumoniae: Incidence, risk factors, and response to therapy in a prospective study. Clin. Infect. Dis. **20**:1195–1200.

69. **Muñoz, R., T.J. Coffey, M. Daniels, C.G. Dowson, G. Laible, J. Casal, R. Hakenbeck, M. Jacobs, J.M. Musser, B.G. Spratt, and A. Tomasz.** 1991. Intercontinental spread of a multiresistant clone of serotype 23F Streptococcus pneumoniae. J. Infect. Dis. **164**:302–306.

70. **Musher, D.M.** 1995. *Streptococcus pneumoniae*, pp. 1811–1826. *In* G.L. Mandell, J.E. Bennett, and R. Dolin (ed.). Principles and Practice of Infectious Diseases, 4th Edition. Churchill Livingstone, New York.

71. **Musher, D.M., and S.J. Spindel.** 1996. Community-acquired pneumonia, pp. 102–124. *In* J.S. Remington, and M.N. Swartz (ed.). Current Clinical Topics in Infectious Diseases. McGraw-Hill Book Co., New York.

72. **Naraqi, S., G.P. Kirkpatrick, and S. Kabins.** 1974. Relapsing pneumococcal meningitis: isolation of an organism with decreased susceptibility to penicillin G. J. Pediatr. **85**:671–672.

73. **Nava, J.M., F. Bella, J. Garau, J. Lite, M.A. Morena, C. Marti, D. Fontanals, B. Font, V. Pineda, S. Uriz, F. Deulofeu, A. Calderon, P. Duran, M. Grau, and A. Agudo.** 1994. Predictive factors for invasive disease due to penicillin-resistant *Streptococcus pneumoniae*: A population-based study. Clin. Infect. Dis. **19**:884–890.

74. **Pallares, R., F. Gudiol, J. Liñares, J. Ariza, G. Rufi, L. Murgui, J. Dorca, and P.F. Viladrich.** 1987. Rick factors and response to antibiotic therapy in adults with bacteremic pneumonia caused by penicillin-resistant pneumococci. N. Engl. J. Med. **317**:18–22.

75. **Pallares, R., J. Liñares, M. Vadillo, C. Cabellos, F. Manresa, P.F. Viladrich, R. Martin, and F. Gudiol.** 1995. Resistance to penicillin and cephalosporin and mortality from severe pneumococcal pneumonia in Barcelona, Spain. N. Engl. J. Med. **333:** 474–480.

76. **Pankuch, G.A., M.A. Visalli, M.R. Jacobs, and P.C. Appelbaum.** 1995. Activities of oral and parenteral agents against penicillin-susceptible and -resistant pneumococci. Antimicrob. Agents Chemother. **39**:1499–1504.

77. **Paredes, A., L.H. Taber, M.D. Yow, D. Clark, and W. Nathan.** 1976. Prolonged pneumococcal meningitis due to an organism with increased resistance to penicillin. Pediatrics **58**:378–381.

78. **Paris, M.M., O. Ramilo, and G.H. McCracken, Jr.** 1995. Management of meningitis caused by penicillin-resistant Streptococcus pneumoniae. Antimicrob. Agents Chemother. **39**:2171–2175.

79. **Ridgway, E.J., K.D. Allen, T.J. Neal, M. Lombard, and A. Rigby.** 1992. Penicillin-resistant pneumococcal meningitis. Lancet **339**:931.

80. **Sanchez, C., R. Armengol, J. Lite, I. Mir, and J. Garau.** 1992.

Penicillin-resistant pneumococci and community-acquired pneumonia. Lancet **339**:988.

81. **Sloas, M.M., F.F. Barrett, P.J. Chesney, B.K. English, B.C. Hill, F.C. Tenover, and R.J. Leggiadro.** 1992. Cephalosporin treatment failure in penicillin- and cephalosporin-resistant Streptococcus pneumoniae meningitis. Pediatr. Infect. Dis. J. **11**:662–666.

82. **Soares, S., K.G. Kristinsson, J.M. Musser, and A. Tomasz.** 1993. Evidence for the introduction of a multiresistant clone of 6B Streptococcus pneumoniae from Spain to Iceland in the late 1980s. J. Infect. Dis. **168**:158–163.

83. **Spangler, S.K., M.R. Jacobs, and P.C. Appelbaum.** 1994. Susceptibilities of 177 penicillin-susceptible and -resistant pneumococci to FK 037, cefpirome, cefepime, ceftriaxone, cefotaxime, ceftazidime, imipenem, biapenem, meropenem and vancomycin. Antimicrob. Agents Chemother. **38**:898–900.

84. **Tan, T.Q., E.O. Mason, Jr., and S.L. Kaplan.** 1992. Systemic infections due to *Streptococcus pneumoniae* relatively resistant to penicillin in a children's hospital: Clinical management and outcome. Pediatrics **90**:928–933.

85. **Tomasz, A.** 1995. The pneumococcus at the gates. N. Engl. J. Med. **333**:514–515.

86. **Tomasz, A., and R. Munoz.** 1995. Beta-lactam antibiotic resistance in gram-positive bacterial pathogens of the upper respiratory tract: A brief overview of mechanisms. Microb. Drug Resist. **1**:103–109.

87. **Tubau, F., C. Cabellos, and J. Liñares.** 1996. Lack of correlation between in vitro and in vivo studies of combinations of rifampin plus vancomycin or beta-lactam antibiotics against Streptococcus pneumoniae. Antimicrob. Agents Chemother. **40**:1573–1574.

88. **Viladrich, P.F., C. Cabellos, R. Pallares, F. Tubau, J. Martinez-Lacasa, J. Liñares, and F. Gudiol.** 1996. High doses of cefotaxime in treatment of adult meningitis due to Streptococcus pneumoniae with decreased susceptibilities to broad-spectrum cephalosporins. Antimicrob. Agents Chemother. **40**:218–220.

89. **Viladrich, P.F., F. Gudiol, J. Liñares, R. Pallares, I. Sabate, G. Rufi, and J. Ariza.** 1991. Evaluation of vancomycin for therapy of adult pneumococcal meningitis. Antimicrob. Agents Chemother. **35**:2467–2472.

90. **Viladrich, P.F., F. Gudiol, J. Liñares, G. Rufi, J. Ariza, and R. Pallares.** 1988. Characteristics and antibiotic therapy of adult meningitis due to penicillin-resistant pneumococci. Am. J. Med. **84**:839–846.

91. **Ward, J.** 1981. Antibiotic-resistant Streptococcus pneumoniae: clinical and epidemiologic aspects. Rev. Infect. Dis. **3**:254–266.

92. **Willett, L.D., H.C. Dillon, Jr., and B.M. Gray.** 1985. Penicillin-intermediate pneumococci in a children's hospital. Am. J. Dis. Child. **139**:1054–1057.

Address reprint requests to:
Roman Pallares
Infectious Diseases Service
Hospital Bellvitge
08907 L'Hospitalet
Barcelona, Spain

Effect of Antimicrobial Use and Other Risk Factors on Antimicrobial Resistance in Pneumococci

KARL G. KRISTINSSON

INTRODUCTION

PENICILLIN-RESISTANT PNEUMOCOCCI have spread globally, and their prevalence has increased rapidly during the past decade. The high prevalence rates were initially only in countries with high and relatively uncontrolled antimicrobial use, but this has changed. High prevalence rates are now being reported from countries with relatively restricted antimicrobial use.[51,60] The penicillin-resistant pneumococci are often multiresistant, which may create problems in the outpatient treatment of pneumococcal infections,[24,63] and penicillin- and cephalosporin-resistant strains causing meningitis are difficult to treat.[72] If the same trend continues unabated, pneumococcal infections may become a major threat in the not so distant future.[81]

Antimicrobial use is generally considered one of the major driving forces for resistance, and this has been clearly demonstrated in the hospital setting.[64] The effect of antimicrobial use in the community has not been as well documented, and more information is needed. The rapid spread of penicillin-resistant pneumococci in Iceland, as opposed to the scarcity of such strains in the other Nordic countries, indicates that there may be other important factors that are important for the successful spread of these strains. In order to be able to slow down or reverse the trend of increasing resistance, it is important to study carefully the epidemiology of penicillin resistance among pneumococci. Only with a clear view of the major risk factors for the spread of resistance will it be possible to introduce effective control measures.

The habitat of the pneumococcus is the upper respiratory tract of humans, mainly the nasopharynx. It is a member of the normal upper respiratory tract of all individuals at some stage, and carriage rates are highest in children. In order to be able to study the risk factors, it is useful to review important aspects in the behavior of this organism.

CARRIAGE

The pneumococcal carrier state has been described in an excellent review by Austrian.[10] The main habitat of the pneumococcus is the nasopharynx of children. Carriage increases from birth, and is maximal at preschool age. It is stressed that no single method detects carriage in all individuals, and different methods have different sensitivities. Injecting samples intraperitoneally into mice may be the most sensitive method, but is not suitable for large epidemiological studies. Using selective blood agar plates containing gentamicin (5 μg/ml) increases the yield of direct inoculation onto agar.[49]

Pneumococci may be acquired as early as the first day of life, and then probably from the mother,[42] but the mean age of acquisition of the first type has been shown to be about at 6 months.[38] The duration of carriage decreases with successive types and acquisition of new types peaks in the winter.[38] At any given time, as many as 60% can be shown to carry pneumococci if examined appropriately[40] and simultaneous carriage of multiple types is not uncommon.[41] Duration of carriage ranges from 1 to 17 months, and longer carriage is associated with acquisition at younger ages.

Pneumococcal carriage is strongly age related, and increases steadily with age during the first year and is highest in 1–2-year-old children. Thereafter, carriage rates decrease slowly and adults have much lower carriage rates than children.[38] Children with siblings and children associated with day care acquire pneumococci earlier, and have more pneumococcal types and higher carriage rates than other children.[3,4,38] In addition, adults having close and frequent contact with children have higher carriage rates than others.[49]

Adherence and subsequent colonisation appears to be due to binding of the pneumococci to the disaccharide *N*-acetyl-glucosamine β1-3 galactose on pharyngeal epithelial cells.[2,25] This ability is more pronounced in pneumococci producing transparent colonies, as opposed to pneumococci producing opaque or semitransparent colonies.[26] The reason is not clear, and the bacterial adhesin is not a part of the capsule, although certain capsular types appear to be better colonisers than others. The recent description of six new capsular types brings the number of pneumococcal serotypes to 90.[50] Only a few of these serotypes are common in healthy children. The most common serogroups are groups 6, 19, and 23, which together are found in about 60% of carriers.[38,45,49] These serogroups together with another common group (group 14) are also the groups carried for significantly longer periods than other groups (mean 4.2 months, as opposed to 2.7 months).[38] Infections usually occur within 1 month of acquiring a new strain.[38]

Department of Microbiology, National University Hospital, Reykjavik, Iceland.

INFECTIONS

The pneumococcus is the commonest cause of important respiratory tract infections such as pneumonia, otitis media, and sinusitis. It is also one of the commonest causes of meningitis.[67] To be in a better position to define the major risk factors for infection, the pathogenesis of pneumococcal infections must be kept in mind. Otitis media and sinusitis normally begin by local spread of the bacteria from the nasopharynx into the sinuses or via the eustachian tube into the middle ear cavity. Local spread and/or aerosol spread is also involved in the early stages of pneumonia. The pneumococci may travel to these sites without causing infections, but certain individuals appear to be more susceptible to pneumococcal infections than others. The risk factors for pneumococcal disease differ depending on the localization of the infection.

Otitis media is extremely common in children and responsible for most of their visits to health centers[80] and for most of the use of antimicrobial agents.[8] In a prospective study of 698 children, 84% of the children had experienced one or more episodes of acute otitis media and 46% three or more episodes at 3 years of age.[79] Factors significantly associated with an increased risk of developing otitis media were: male gender, sibling history of recurrent acute otitis media, early occurrence of acute otitis media, and not being breast fed. Being looked after or being associated with day care centers, has also been shown to increase the risk of acute otitis media.[3,52,84] The increased risk of day-care attendance may be related to higher carriage rates for pneumococci and an increased risk of all kinds of upper respiratory tract infections.[83] Recent infection with respiratory viruses increases the risk of otitis media.[48,55]

The risk factors for pneumococcal pneumonia and invasive pneumococcal disease are different from those of pneumococcal upper respiratory tract infections. They include chronic obstructive airways disease and cigarette smoking (compromising the pulmonary clearance mechanisms), conditions associated with decreased humoral immune response, alcoholic cirrhosis, diabetes mellitus, and asplenia.[37,67] Recently an association has been demonstrated between invasive pneumococcal disease and season, air pollution, and isolation of respiratory viruses.[55]

The serotypes causing otitis media were mainly 14, 19F, 23F, 6B, 3, and 19A (in that order) in a study of pneumococcal infections in 314 middle ear isolates from preschool children in the United States.[20] Not surprisingly, these are virtually the same as the serotypes most frequently colonising the nasopharynx in healthy children. The serotypes causing invasive infections differ slightly, although this depends on the time and place of the study. Serotypes 14, 1, 7F, 3, 6B, 4, and 23F were most common in a study of strains mainly from Europe and the Middle East (23% children),[69] serotypes 14, 6B, 19F, 18C, 23F, and 4 in preschool children in the United States[20] and 14, 7F, 9V, 3, 6B, and 23F in Sweden (only 6% children).[47] In a comparison between the invasive serotypes in children and adults, only a slight difference was observed, with children having group 6 and type 18C more often than adults, and adults having types 3 and 8 more often than children.[69] All the above studies were done in the developing countries, but in a review of published data from six continents, a difference in the most common types was observed.[77] Also, there can be important temporal differences, as was clearly observed in a study from Boston.[36]

PROBLEMS

Antimicrobial resistance in pneumococci has become a major public health concern. In order to prevent further spread, better understanding of the underlying molecular events and the forces that drive them is essential. Epidemiological studies aimed at identifying the main risk factors for spread of resistance are needed to be able to minimise risk and monitor the effects of control measures.

EPIDEMIOLOGY OF ANTIMICROBIAL USE AND RESISTANCE

Soon after the introduction of penicillin, resistance developed in Staphylococci. Resistance could also be provoked in pneumococcal strains under controlled laboratory conditions, but was not seen in clinical isolates.[34,65] Since nasopharyngeal colonisation usually precedes pneumococcal infections and some of the more common serotypes are often carried for extended periods, it is surprising that resistance was first described in the clinical setting as late as during the 1970s.[43,44,56] This was not even taken seriously and global spread of penicillin resistant pneumococci was considered a remote possibility. Resistance in pneumococci was subsequently described in several countries, but, in the late 1980s, resistance spread fast in some places, mainly South Africa and Spain.[7,21,53,62] This was followed by the development of high-level penicillin resistance and multiresistance.[53,58]

The spread of resistance in pneumococci has been extensively reviewed,[1,5,6,11,13,58] but it is interesting to view the situation in 1990. At that time, >10% of pneumococcal strains had been reported resistant to penicillin in Mexico, Chile, Spain, Hungary, Poland, South Africa, Kenya, Israel, New Guinea, and foci in certain areas of the United States (Alaska, Colorado, Massachusetts, New Mexico, and Oklahoma). At the same time, less than 5% of strains were reported as being resistant in Western Europe (except Spain).[58] There was a clear relationship between the annual aminopenicillin consumption and the rate of penicillin resistance in pneumococci in Spain, and the spread of those strains appeared to closely parallel the use of β-lactam drugs.[13] That the highest prevalence of penicillin-resistant pneumococci was reported in Spain and Eastern European countries, where antimicrobial use was relatively unrestricted, and self-administration common, further supported the association with antimicrobial use. Antimicrobial use was much higher in Spain than in the United Kingdom and Scandinavia, where resistance rates were much lower.[13,70]

Iceland is one of the Nordic countries and has had a relatively restricted antimicrobial policy, similar to the Scandinavian countries (although it has the highest antimicrobial use of those countries).[70] Therefore, it was surprising that, after the introduction of a multiresistant strain in 1989, it spread fast and had reached about 20% incidence (in pneumococcal infections) in 1993.[59,60] That the epidemic spread on an island with excellent health service offered an ideal opportunity to study the main risk factors for carriage and spread of penicillin-resistant pneumococci.

MAIN RISK FACTORS

Several recent studies have described risk factors for infections or carriage by penicillin-resistant as opposed to penicillin-sensitive pneumococci.

Infections

In a retrospective case control study of 24 adults with bacteremic pneumonia (and 48 controls), Pallares *et al.*[71] found the following four significant risk factors (using univariate analysis) for infection with resistant pneumococci: β-lactam antibiotic therapy in the past 3 months, nosocomial pneumonia, hospitalization in the past 3 months, and pneumonia in the past year. Invasive pneumococcal infections in Atlanta in 1994 caused by drug-resistant pneumococci were more likely to be in whites than blacks and in children under 6 years of age,[51] and, in children in Ohio, such strains were much more likely ($p < 0.00001$) if they had received antibiotics in the month prior to the systemic illness.[31] In a study of acute otitis media in children in Kentucky, multivariate analysis found number of antibiotic courses and otitis-prone condition to be independently predictive of penicillin resistant as opposed to penicillin-sensitive pneumococci.[17] Additional factors associated with penicillin resistant pneumococci, by univariate analysis were young age, day-care center attendance, recent antimicrobial use, number of prior antibiotic courses, and antibiotic prophylaxis. In a study of children from Slovakia with otitis media, bacteremia, or meningitis, frequent antibiotic use, prior hospitalisation, and length of hospital stay were significantly associated with infection with resistant strains.[76] A large national survey in France looked at the epidemiological features and risk factors for infection by pneumococci with diminished susceptibility to penicillin. The study was retrospective and based on microbiological and clinical data on 10,350 pneumococci isolated from infected patients.[16] A logistic regression model identified the following factors as being associated with insensitive pneumococci: age of less than 15 years, isolation from the upper respiratory tract, HIV infection, β-lactam antimicrobial therapy in the previous 6 months, and nosocomial acquisition. A smaller prospective study (112 isolates and 95 patients) identified previous use of β-lactam antibiotics, alcoholism, and noninvasive disease as significant risk factors for infection due to penicillin-resistant strains and the extremes of age (<5 or >65 years) and previous use of β-lactam antibiotics as risk factors for multiresistant strains (multivariate analysis).[22] In patients infected with HIV, treatment with antibacterial agents, particularly trimethoprim-sulphamethoxazole in the previous 3 months, was associated with an increased risk for isolation of pneumococci with decreased susceptibility to penicillin.[66]

Carriage

Child-to-child transmission of pneumococci occurs readily in the day-care setting, and day-care centers have been shown to facilitate the spread of resistant pneumococci.[15,73,74] Risk factors for carriage of penicillin-resistant pneumococci have been studied in areas of high prevalence of such strains. In Kentucky, nasopharyngeal cultures were performed on 240 healthy children, and their parents asked about history of otitis media and antimicrobial drug use.[32] Current acute otitis media, child day-care center attendance, antimicrobial use in the preceding 6 months and younger age were associated with pneumococcal drug resistance by univariate and multivariate analysis. In a large cross-sectional and analytical prevalence study conducted in five different communities in Iceland, 919 children were studied for the possible correlation of antimicrobial consumption and carriage of penicillin-resistant and multiresistant pneumococci.[8] The study population included 15–38% of the peer population groups in the different areas. By multivariate analysis, age (<2 years), area (highest antimicrobial consumption), and individual use of antimicrobials significantly influenced the odds of carrying penicillin-resistant pneumococci. By univariate analysis, recent antimicrobial use (2–7 weeks) and use of co-trimoxazole were also significantly associated with carriage of penicillin resistant pneumococci. Within a day-care center, children that had received prophylactic antibiotics or frequent courses of antibiotics were significantly more likely to carry penicillin-resistant than penicillin-sensitive pneumococci.[74] In hospitalized children in Slovakia, frequent antimicrobial drug use, prior hospitalization and length of hospital stay were associated with infection with a particular penicillin-resistant strain.[75] More recent studies have confirmed antimicrobial use and white race,[9] young age (but not antibiotic use),[82] and antimicrobial prophylaxis[18] as risk factors for carrying nonsusceptible pneumococci. Antimicrobial treatment of otitis media in children has been shown to adversely affect the nasopharyngeal flora by increasing the proportion of penicillin nonsusceptible strains.[23,27,30]

A summary of the risk factors that have been associated with carriage and/or infection by penicillin-resistant or multiresistant pneumococci can be seen in Table 1. The association with prior antimicrobial use has been clearly demonstrated. Day-care centers have also been shown to facilitate the spread of resistant pneumococci, and some studies have shown an increased risk associated with hospitalisation. Antimicrobial use is therefore a driving force for resistance, which can be facilitated by day-care centers and hospitals.

The risk factors associated with pneumococcal infections are related to risk factors for pneumococcal resistance. This relationship is demonstrated in Fig. 1. The interaction of risk factors is clearly demonstrated by the epidemiology of penicillin-resistant pneumococci in Iceland. Multiresistant pneumococci were introduced into the country in 1989 and spread fast to reach almost 20% yearly incidence in 1992.[60,78] This was a much higher incidence than was known in other Northern European countries, despite the fact that antimicrobials are only available by prescription in Iceland and the total use is similar to the use in Sweden and Finland. Although antimicrobial use was considered important, day-care centers (most of the Icelandic children attend and then spend a large time inside during the long winters), large families, and relatively high use of co-trimoxazole were also considered important.[59] On the other hand, hospitals were not considered a risk factor in Iceland. The

TABLE 1. RISK FACTORS THAT HAVE BEEN SHOWN TO BE SIGNIFICANTLY
ASSOCIATED WITH CARRIAGE (C) OR INFECTION (I) WITH A RESISTANT
PNEUMOCOCCUS AS OPPOSED TO A SENSITIVE PNEUMOCOCCUS

Risk factor	C/I	References
Recent antimicrobial use	C, I	8,9,16,17,22,30–32,66,71,73
Young age	C, I	8,16,17,22,32,35,51,82
Repeated antimicrobial courses	C, I	8,17,31,35,74
DCC attendance	C, I	17,32,35
Otitis prone condition	C, I	17,32,74
Prior hospitalisation	C, I	16,17,71
Antimicrobial prophylaxis	C, I	17,18,74
Recent β-lactam use	C, I	16,23,27,71
Recent trim-sulpha use	C, I	8,66
Isolation from URT	I	16,22
White race	C, I	9,51
Living in a high prevalence area	C	8
HIV infection	I	16
Otitis media not responsive to AM	C	74
Nosocomial pneumonia	I	71
Old age	I	22

interplay of risk factors considered important in Iceland can be seen in Fig. 2.

Studies *in vitro* have indicated that certain antimicrobial classes[68] and certain pharmacokinetic parameters may be more likely to encourage resistance than others.[14] There is a lack of clinical studies investigating these aspects, although β-lactam antibiotics have been identified as risk factors in some of the studies[13,16,23,27,71] and trimethoprim-sulpha in a few.[8,66] A recent French study investigating the risk factors for carriage of penicillin nonsusceptible pneumococci in 941 healthy school children, found that low daily dose and long treatment duration with an oral β-lactam increased the risk of carrying nonsus-

ceptible strains ($p = 0.002$ and 0.02, respectively).[39] This suggests that pharmacokinetic and pharmacodynamic parameters may have a significant role in selecting resistant strains.

POSSIBLE SOLUTIONS

Five of the 16 risk factors listed in Table 1 relate to antimicrobial therapy. Other prominent risk factors are young age, day-care center attendance, otitis-prone condition, and prior hospitalization. All those risk factors are centered around children, which is not surprising as children are the main reservoir for pneumococci. In addition, of all age groups, antimicrobials are most frequently prescribed for children, and antimicrobial use is likely to have an influence on pneumococci just as on other commensal flora. Measures to reduce the prevalence of penicillin-resistant pneumococci must therefore be centered on

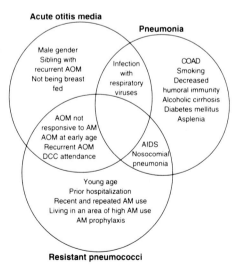

FIG. 1.   Relationship between risk factors of pneumococcal infections and antimicrobial resistance in pneumococci. AM, antimicrobials; AOM, acute otitis media; COAD, chronic obstructive airways disease.

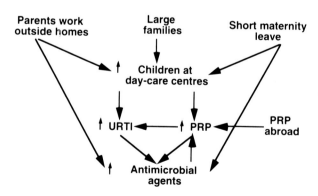

FIG. 2.   Summary of factors promoting increased prevalence of penicillin resistant pneumococci in Iceland, and how they can create a vicious cycle in day-care centers. URTI, upper respiratory tract infection; PRP, penicillin resistant pneumococci. (From Kristinsson,[59] with permission.)

reduction of antimicrobial use in children and on good infection control in day-care centers and hospitals.

The rapid increase in the incidence of penicillin-resistant pneumococci in Iceland from 1989 to 1993 triggered much publicity. It was considered that the problem was due to high use of antimicrobials in children together with the fact that most Icelandic children attend day-care centers. This created the vicious circle seen in Fig. 2.[59] In order to break this cycle, a campaign against the overuse of antimicrobials, aimed at both the public and physicians, was started. In addition, children receiving antimicrobials or carriers of penicillin-insensitive pneumococci with cold or coughing were discouraged from going to day-care centers. This led to reduced antimicrobial use and subsequently reduced incidence of penicillin-insensitive pneumococci.[61] By using active infection control measures (denying preschool children carrying resistant pneumococci attendance at group day care) and measures to reduce antimicrobial use, epidemiological data suggest that the intervention may have limited the dissemination of penicillin-resistant strains in Malmohus County, Southern Sweden.[33] These examples indicate that it may be possible to influence the prescribing habits of whole communities and, by doing so, reduce resistance.

Health authorities in many other countries have recognized the potential public health problems associated with increasing resistance in pneumococci. In 1994, a working group, sponsored by the Centers for Disease Control and Prevention, was set up. The group has developed strategies for surveillance investigation, prevention, and control of infections due to drug-resistant pneumococci.[54] Also in 1994 a task force was formed in Spain, under the auspices of the Spanish Ministry of Health. This task force produced a unique document "Antibiotic Resistance in Spain: What can be done?," where the problem of antimicrobial resistance in the community is recognized and described, and general recommendations given to limit the emergence, evolution, and spread of resistant microorganisms.[12] Since then many other National Governments, the World Health Organization, and the European Union have officially recognized the problem and set up strategies for the surveillance of resistance and interventions. The Institute of Medicine recently issued a report on antimicrobial resistance following a Forum on Emerging Infections workshop.[46]

The currently available vaccines are polyvalent polysaccharides, containing 23 different serotypes.[19] They are not immunogenic in young children, especially not for the most commonly resistant serotypes, and are therefore not likely to reduce the reservoir of resistant pneumococci. Experimental vaccines with protein-conjugated capsular polysaccharides have been shown to be immunogenic in children and safe.[57] A study from Israel indicates that such vaccines may also reduce the carriage of resistant serotypes in children.[28,29] If this is confirmed in larger studies, then vaccination may be a useful method in reducing the reservoir of resistant pneumococci.

Antimicrobial use has continued to rise in most countries and so does resistance in most bacteria. Health authorities around the world must combine their efforts, not only in monitoring the emergency of resistance, but also, the main driving force for resistance, antimicrobial use. Monitoring antimicrobial use is important for programs aimed at reducing antimicrobial resistance, and concerted action is needed to maintain the efficacy of antimicrobials.

REFERENCES

1. **Allen, K.D.** 1991. Penicillin-resistant pneumococci [Review]. J. Hosp. Infect. **17:**3–13.

2. **Andersson, B., E.H. Beachey, A. Tomasz, E. Tuomanen, and C. Svanborg-Eden.** 1988. A sandwich adhesion on *Streptococcus pneumoniae* attaching to human oropharyngeal epithelial cells *in vitro*. Microb. Pathog. **4:**267–278.

3. **Aniansson, G., B. Alm, B. Andersson, A. Håkansson, P. Larsson, O. Nylén, H. Peterson, P. Rignér, M. Svanborg, H. Sabharwal, and C. Svanborg.** 1994. A prospective cohort study on breast-feeding and otitis media in Swedish infants. Pediatr. Infect. Dis. J. **12:**183–188.

4. **Aniansson, G., B. Alm, B. Andersson, P. Larsson, O. Nylén, H. Peterson, P. Rignér, M. Svanborg, and C. Svanborg.** 1992. Nasopharyngeal colonization during the first year of life. J. Infect. Dis. **165:**S38–S42.

5. **Appelbaum, P.C.** 1992. Antimicrobial resistance in *Streptococcus pneumoniae*: an overview [Review]. Clin. Infect. Dis. **15:**77–83.

6. **Appelbaum, P.C.** 1987. World-wide development of antibiotic resistance in pneumococci [Review]. Eur. J. Clin. Microbiol. **6:**367–377.

7. **Appelbaum, P.C., A. Bhamjee, J.N. Scragg, A.F. Hallett, A.J. Bowen, and R.C. Cooper.** 1977. *Streptococcus pneumoniae* resistant to penicillin and chloramphenicol. Lancet **2:**995–997.

8. **Arason, V.A., K.G. Kristinsson, J.A. Sigurdsson, G. Stefansdottir, S. Mölstad, and S. Gudmundsson.** 1996. Do antimicrobials increase the carriage rate of penicillin resistant pneumococci in children? B.M.J. **313:**387–391.

9. **Arnold, K.E., R.J. Leggiadro, R.F. Breiman, H.B. Lipman, B. Schwartz, M.A. Appleton, K.O. Cleveland, H.C. Szeto, B.C. Hill, F.C. Tenover, J.A. Elliott, and R.R. Facklam.** 1996. Risk factors for carriage of drug-resistant *Streptococcus pneumoniae* among children in Memphis, Tennessee. J. Pediatr. **128:**757–764.

10. **Austrian, R.** 1986. Some aspects of the pneumococcal carrier state. J. Antimicrob. Chemother. **18:**35–45.

11. **Baquero, F.** 1995. Pneumococcal resistance to β-lactam antibiotics: a global geographic overview. Microb. Drug Resist. **1:**115–120.

12. **Baquero, F., and the Task Force of the General Direction for Health Planning of the Spanish Ministry of Health.** 1996. Antibiotic resistance in Spain: what can be done? Clin. Infect. Dis. **1996:**819–823.

13. **Baquero, F., J. Martinez-Beltran, and E. Loza.** 1991. A review of antibiotic resistance patterns of *Streptococcus pneumoniae* in Europe [Review]. J. Antimicrob. Chemother. **28:**31–38.

14. **Baquero, F., and M.C. Negri.** 1997. Strategies to minimize the development of antibiotic resistance. J. Chemother. **9:**29–37.

15. **Barnes, D.M., S. Whittier, P.H. Gilligan, S. Soares, A. Tomasz, and F.W. Henderson.** 1995. Transmission of multidrug-resistant serotype 23F *Streptococcus pneumoniae* in group day care: evidence suggesting capsular transformation of the resistant strain *in vivo*. J. Infect. Dis. **171:**890–896.

16. **Bédos, J.-P., S. Chevret, C. Chastang, P. Geslin, B. Régnier, and a.t.F.C.P.S. Group.** 1996. Epidemiological features of and risk factors for infection by *Streptococcus pneumoniae* strains with diminished susceptibility to penicillin: findings of a French Survey. Clin. Infect. Dis. **22:**63–72.

17. **Block, S.L., C.J. Harrison, J.A. Hedrick, R.D. Tyler, R.A. Smith, E. Keegan, and S.A. Chartrand.** 1995. Penicillin-resistant *Streptococcus pneumoniae* in acute otitis media: risk factors, susceptibility patterns and antimicrobial management. Pediatr. Infect. Dis. J. **14:**751–759.

18. **Brook, I., and A.E. Gober.** 1996. Prophylaxis with amoxicillin or sulfisoxazole for otitis media: effect on the recovery of penicillin-resistant bacteria from children. Clin. Infect. Dis. **22:**143–145.

19. Broome, C.V., and R.F. Breiman. 1991. Pneumococcal vaccine—past, present, and future [Editorial]. N. Engl. J. Med. 325:1506–1508.

20. Butler, J.C., R.F. Breiman, H.B. Lipman, J. Hofmann, and R.R. Facklam. 1995. Serotype distribution of *Streptococcus pneumoniae* infections among preschool children in the United States, 1978–1994: implications for development of a conjugate vaccine. J. Infect. Dis. 171:885–889.

21. Casal, J. 1982. Antimicrobial susceptibility of *Streptococcus pneumoniae*: serotype distribution of penicillin-resistant strains in Spain. Antimicrob. Agents Chemother. 22:222–225.

22. Clavo-Sanchez, A.J., J.A. Giron-Gonzalez, D. Lopez-Prieto, J. Canueto-Quintero, A. Sanchez-Porto, A. Vergara-Campos, P. Marin-Casanova, and J.A. Cordoba-Dona. 1997. Multivariate analysis of risk factors for infection due to penicillin-resistant and multidrug-resistant *Streptococcus pneumoniae*: a multicenter study. Clin. Infect. Dis. 24:1052–1059.

23. Cohen, R., E. Bingen, E. Varon, F. de La Rocque, N. Brahimi, C. Levy, M. Boucherat, J. Langue, and P. Geslin. 1997. Change in nasopharyngeal carriage of *Streptococcus pneumoniae* resulting from antibiotic therapy for acute otitis media in children. Pediatr. Infect. Dis. J. 16:555–560.

24. Cohen, R., F. de la Rocque, M. Boucherat, C. Dolt, E. Bingen, and P. Geslin. 1994. Treatment failure in otitis media: an analysis. J. Chemother. 4:17–22.

25. Cundell, D., H.P. Masure, and E.I. Tuomanen. 1996. The molecular basis of pneumococcal infection: a hypothesis. Clin. Infect. Dis. 21:S204–S212.

26. Cundell, D.R., J.N. Weiser, J. Shen, A. Young, and E. Tuomanen. 1995. Relationship between colonial morphology and adherence of *Streptococcus pneumoniae*. Infect. Immunol. 63:757–761.

27. Dabernat, H., P. Geslin, F. Megraud, P. Bégué, J. Boulesteix, C. Dubreuil, F. de La Roque, A. Trinh, and A. Scheimberg. 1998. Effects of cefixime or co-amoxiclav treatment on nasopharyngeal carriage of *Streptococcus pneumoniae* and *Haemophilus influenze* in children with acute otitis media. J. Antimicrob. Chemother. 41:253–258.

28. Dagan, R., R. Melamed, O. Zamir, and O. Leroy. 1997. Safety and immunogenicity of tetravalent pneumococcal vaccines containing 6B, 14, 19F and 23F polysaccharides conjugated to either tetanus toxoid or diphtheria toxoid in young infants and their boosterability by native polysaccharide antigens. Pediatr. Infect. Dis. J. 16:1053–1059.

29. Dagan, R., M. Muallem, R. Melamed, O. Leroy, and P. Yagupsky. 1997. Reduction of pneumococcal nasopharyngeal carriage in early infancy after immunization with tetravalent pneumococcal vaccines conjugated to either tetanus toxoid or diphtheria toxoid. Pediatr. Infect. Dis. J. 16:1060–1064.

30. del Castillo, F., F. Baquero-Artigao, and A. Garcia-Perea. 1998. Influence of recent antibiotic therapy on antimicrobial resistance of *Streptococcus pneumoniae* in children with acute otitis media in Spain. Pediatr. Infect. Dis. J. 17:94–97.

31. Doone, J.L., S.L. Klespies, and C. Sabella. 1997. Risk factors for penicillin-resistant systemic pneumococcal infections in children. Clin. Pediatr. 36:187–191.

32. Duchin, J.S., R.F. Breiman, A. Diamond, H.B. Lipman, S.L. Block, J.A. Hedrick, R. Finger, and J.A. Elliott. 1995. High prevalence of multidrug-resistant *Streptococcus pneumoniae* among children in a rural Kentucky community. Pediatr. Infect. Dis. J. 19:745–750.

33. Ekdahl, K., H.B. Hansson, S. Mölstad, S. Söderström, M. Walder, and K. Persson. 1998. Limiting the spread of penicillin-resistant *Streptococcus pneumoniae*: experiences from the South Swedish pneumococcal intervention project. Microb. Drug Resist. 4:99–105.

34. Eriksen, K.R. 1945. Studies on induced resistance to penicillin in

35. Fairchok, M.P., W.S. Ashton, and G.W. Fischer. 1996. Carriage of penicillin-resistant pneumococci in a military population in Washington, DC: risk factors and correlation with clinical isolates. Clin. Infect. Dis. 22:966–972.

36. Finland, M., and M.W. Barnes. 1977. Changes in occurrence of capsular serotypes of *Streptococcus pneumoniae* at Boston City Hospital during selected years between 1935 and 1974. J. Clin. Microbiol. 5:154–166.

37. Gillespie, S.H. 1989. Aspects of pneumococcal infection including bacterial virulence, host response and vaccination. J. Med. Microbiol. 28:237–248.

38. Gray, B.M., G.M. Converse III, and H.C. Dillon Jr. 1980. Epidemiologic studies of *Streptococcus pneumoniae* in infants: acquisition, carriage, and infection during the first 24 months of life. J. Infect. Dis. 142:923–933.

39. Guillemot, D., C. Carbon, B. Balkau, P. Geslin, H. Lecoeur, F. Vauzelle-Kervroedan, G. Bouvenot, and E. Eschwége. 1998. Low dosage and long treatment duration of β-lactam. Risk factors for carriage of penicillin-resistant *Streptococcus pneumoniae*. J.A.M.A. 279:365–370.

40. Gundel, M. 1933. Bakteriologische und epidemiologische Untersuchungen über die Besiedlung der oberen Atmungswege Gesunder mit Pneumokokken. Z. Hyg. Infektionskrankheit 114:923–933.

41. Gundel, M., and G. Okura. 1933. Untersuchungen über das gleichzeitige Vorkommen mehrer Pneumokokkentypen bei Gesunden und ihre Bedeutung für die Epidemiologie. Z. Hyg. Infektionskrankheit 114:678–704.

42. Gundel, M., and F.K.T. Schwartz. 1932. Studien über die Bakterienflora der obern Atmungswege Neugeborner (im vergleich mit der Mundhöhlenflora der Mutter und des Pflegepersonals) unter besonderer Berucksichtigung ihrer Bedeutung für das Pneumonieproblem. Z. Hyg. Infektionskrankheit 113:411–436.

43. Hansman, D., and M.M. Bullen. 1967. A resistant pneumococcus. Lancet 2:264–265.

44. Hansman, D., H. Glasgow, J. Sturt, L. Devitt, and R. Douglas. 1971. Increased resistance to penicillin of pneumococci isolated from man. N. Engl. J. Med. 284:175–177.

45. Hansman, D., and S. Morris. 1988. Pneumococcal carriage amongst children in Adelaide, South Australia. Epidemiol. Infect. Dis. 101:411–417.

46. Harrison, P.F., and J. Lederberg (ed.). 1998. Antimicrobial resistance: issues and options. Workshop report. Institute of Medicine, National Academy Press, Washington, DC.

47. Hedlund, J., S.B. Svenson, M. Kalin, J. Henrichsen, B. Olsson-Liljequist, G. Möllerberg, and G. Källenius. 1995. Incidence, capsular types and antibiotic susceptibility of invasive *Streptococcus pneumoniae* in Sweden. Clin. Infect. Dis. 21:948–953.

48. Henderson, F.W., A.M. Collier, M.A. Sanyal, J.M. Watkins, D.L. Fairclough, W.A. Clyde, and F.W. Denny. 1982. A longitudinal study of respiratory viruses and bacteria in the etiology of acute otitis media with effusion. N. Engl. J. Med. 306:1377–1383.

49. Hendley, J.O. 1975. Spread of *Streptococcus pneumoniae* in families. I. Carriage rates and distribution of types. J. Infect. Dis. 132:55–61.

50. Henrichsen, J. 1995. Six newly recognized types of *Streptococcus pneumoniae*. J. Clin. Microbiol. 33:2759–2762.

51. Hofmann, J., M.S. Cetron, M.M. Farley, W.S. Baughman, R.R. Facklam, J.A. Elliott, K.A. Deaver, and R.F. Breiman. 1995. The prevalence of drug-resistant *Streptococcus pneumoniae* in Atlanta. N. Engl. J. Med. 333:481–486.

52. Hurwitz, E.S., W.J. Gunn, P.F. Pinsky, and L.B. Schonberger. 1991. Risk of respiratory illness associated with day-care attendance: a nationwide study. Pediatrics 87:62–69.

53. Jacobs, M.R., H.J. Koornhof, R.M. Robins-Browne, C.M.

a pneumococcus type 1. Acta Pathol. Microbiol. Scand. 22:398–401.

Stevenson, Z.A. Vermaak, I. Freiman, G.B. Miller, M.A. Witcomb, M. Isaacson, J.I. Ward, and R. Austrian. 1978. Emergence of multiply resistant pneumococci. N. Engl. J. Med. **299:**735–740.

54. **Jernigan, D.B., M.S. Cetron, and R.F. Breiman.** 1996. Minimizing the impact of drug-resistant *Streptococcus pneumoniae* (DRSP). A strategy from the DRSP Working Group. J.A.M.A. **275:**206–209.

55. **Kim, P.E., D.M. Musher, W.P. Glezen, M.C. Rodriguez-Barradas, W.K. Nahn, and C.E. Wright.** 1996. Association of invasive pneumococcal disease with season, atmospheric conditions, air pollution, and the isolation of respiratory viruses. Clin. Infect. Dis. **22:**100–106.

56. **Kislak, J.W., L.M.B. Razavi, A.K. Daly, and M. Finland.** 1965. Susceptibility of pneumococci to nine antibiotics. Am. J. Med. Sci. **250:**261–268.

57. **Klein, D.L.** 1995. Pneumococcal conjugate vaccines: review and update. Microb. Drug Resist. **1:**49–58.

58. **Klugman, K.P.** 1990. Pneumococcal resistance to antibiotics [Review]. Clin. Microbiol. Rev. **3:**171–196.

59. **Kristinsson, K.G.** 1995. Epidemiology of penicillin-resistant pneumococci in Iceland. Microb. Drug Resist. **1:**121–125.

60. **Kristinsson, K.G., M.A. Hjalmarsdottir, and O. Steingrimsson.** 1992. Increasing penicillin resistance in pneumococci in Iceland [Letter]. Lancet **339:**1606–1607.

61. **Kristinsson, K.G., M.Á. Hjalmarsdottir, and T. Gudnason.** 1998. Continued decline in the incidence of penicillin non-susceptible pneumococci in Iceland [Abstract C022]. Presented at the 38th. Interscience Conference on Antimicrobial Agents and Chemotherapy, American Society for Microbiology, San Diego.

62. **Linares, J., J. Garau, D. Domínguez, and J.L. Pérez.** 1983. Antibiotic resistance and serotypes of *Streptococcus pneumoniae* from patients with community-acquired pneumococcal disease. Antimicrob. Agents Chemother. 23:545–547.

63. **McCracken, G.H., Jr.** 1995. Emergence of resistant *Streptococcus pneumoniae*: a problem in pediatrics. Pediatr. Infect. Dis. J. **14:**424–428.

64. **McGowan, J.E.J.** 1983. Antimicrobial resistance in hospital organisms and its relation to antibiotic use. Rev. Infect. Dis. **5:**1033–1039.

65. **McKee, C.M., and C.L. Houck.** 1943. Induced resistance to penicillin of cultures of staphylococci, pneumococci and streptococci. Proc. Soc. Exp. Biol. Med. **53:**33–34.

66. **Meynard, J.L., F. Barbut, L. Blum, M. Guiguet, C. Chouaid, M.C. Meyohas, O. Picard, J.C. Petit, and J. Frottier.** 1996. Risk factors for isolation of *Streptococcus pneumoniae* with decreased susceptibility to penicillin G from patients infected with human immunodeficiency virus. Clin. Infect. Dis. **22:**437–440.

67. **Musher, D.M.** 1992. Infections caused by *Streptococcus pneumoniae*: clinical spectrum, pathogenesis, immunity, and treatment [Review]. Clin. Infect. Dis. 14:801–807.

68. **Negri, M.C., M.I. Morosini, E. Loza, and F. Baquero.** 1994. *In vitro* selective antibiotic concentrations of beta-lactams for penicillin-resistant *Streptococcus pneumoniae* populations. Antimicrob. Agents Chemother. **38:**122–125.

69. **Nielsen, S.V., and J. Henricksen.** 1992. Capsular types of *Streptococcus pneumoniae* isolated from blood and CSF during 1982–1987. Clin Infect Dis. **15:**794–798.

70. **Nordiska-läkamedelsnämnden.** 1993. Nordic statistics on medicines 1990–1992. Vol. 34. NLN, Uppsala.

71. **Pallares, R., F. Gudiol, J. Linares, J. Ariza, G. Rufi, L. Murgui, J. Dorca, and P.F. Viladrich.** 1987. Risk factors and response to antibiotic therapy in adults with bacteremic pneumonia caused by penicillin-resistant pneumococci. N. Engl. J. Med. **317:**18–22.

72. **París, M.M., O. Ramilo, and G.H. McCracken.** 1995. Management of meningitis caused by penicillin-resistant *Streptococcus pneumoniae* [Review]. Antimicrob. Agents Chemother. **39:**2171–2175.

73. **Radetsky, M.S., G.R. Istre, T.L. Johansen, S.W. Parmelee, B.A. Lauer, A.M. Wiesenthal, and M.P. Glode.** 1981. Multiply resistant pneumococcus causing meningitis: its epidemiology within a day-care centre. Lancet. **2:**771–773.

74. **Reichler, M.R., A.A. Allphin, R.F. Breiman, J.R. Schreiber, J.E. Arnold, L.K. McDougal, R.R. Facklam, B. Boxerbaum, D. May, R.O. Walton, et al.** 1992. The spread of multiply resistant *Streptococcus pneumoniae* at a day care center in Ohio. J. Infect. Dis. **166:**1346–1353.

75. **Reichler, M.R., J. Rakovsky, M. Sláciková, B. Hlavácová, L. Krajcíková, T. Tarina, A. Sobotová, F.R.R., and B.R.F.** 1996. Spread of multidrug-resistant *Streptococcus pneumoniae* among hospitalized children in Slovakia. J. Infect. Dis. **173:**374–379.

76. **Reichler, M.R., J. Rakovsky, A. Sobotova, M. Slacikova, B. Hlavacova, B. Hill, L. Krajcikova, P. Tarina, R.R. Facklam, and R.F. Breiman.** 1995. Multiple antimicrobial resistance of pneumococci in children with otitis media, bacteremia, and meningitis in Slovakia. J. Infect. Dis. **171:**1491–1496.

77. **Sniadack, D.H., B. Schwartz, H. Lipman, J. Bogaerts, J.C. Butler, R. Dagan, G. Echaniz-Aviles, N. Lloyd-Evans, A. Fenoll, N.I. Girgis, J. Henrichsen, K. Klugman, D. Lehmann, A.K. Takala, J. Vandepitte, S. Gove, and R. Breiman.** 1995. Potential interventions for the prevention of childhood pneumonia: geographic and temporal differences in serotype and serogroup distribution of sterile site pneumococcal isolates from children—implications for vaccine strategies. Pediatr. Infect. Dis. J. **14:**503–510.

78. **Soares, S., K.G. Kristinsson, J.M. Musser, and A. Tomasz.** 1993. Evidence for the introduction of a multiresistant clone of serotype 6B *Streptococcus pneumoniae* from Spain to Iceland in the late 1980s. J. Infect. Dis. **168:**158–163.

79. **Teele, D.W., J.O. Klein, B. Rosner, and a.t.G.B.O.M.S. Group.** 1989. Epidemiology of otitis media during the first seven years of life in children in Greater Boston: a prospective cohort study. J. Infect. Dis. **160:**83–94.

80. **Teele, D.W., J.O. Klein, B. Rosner, and t.G.B.O.M.S. Group.** 1983. Middle ear disease and the practice of pediatrics: burden during the first five years of life. J.A.M.A. **249:**1026–1029.

81. **Tomasz, A.** 1994. Multiple-antibiotic-resistant pathogenic bacteria. A report on the Rockefeller University Workshop. N. Engl. J. Med. **330:**1247–1251.

82. **Ussery, X.T., B.D. Gessner, H. Lipman, J.A. Elliott, M.J. Crain, P.C. Tien, A.J. Parkinson, M. Davidson, R.R. Facklam, and R.F. Breiman.** 1996. Risk factors for nasopharyngeal carriage of resistant *Streptococcus pneumoniae* and detection of a multiply resistant clone among children living in the Yukon-Kuskokwim delta region of Alaska. Pediatr. Infect. Dis. J. **15:**986–992.

83. **Wald, E.R.** 1991. Frequency and severity of infections in day care: three-year follow-up. J. Pediatr. **118:**509–514.

84. **Wald, E.R., N. Guerra, and C. Byers.** 1991. Upper respiratory tract infections in young children: duration of and frequency of complications. Pediatrics **87:**129–133.

Address reprint requests to:
Karl G. Kristinsson
Department of Microbiology
National University Hospital
P.O. Box 1465
121 Reykjavik
Iceland

Molecular Evolution of Rifampicin Resistance in *Streptococcus pneumoniae*

MARK ENRIGHT,[1] PIOTR ZAWADSKI,[1] PAUL PICKERILL,[2] and CHRISTOPHER G. DOWSON[2]

ABSTRACT

Rifampicin resistance has arisen in several different species of bacteria because of alterations to one or more regions in the target of the antibiotic, the β-subunit of RNA polymerase encoded by *rpoB*. Nucleotide sequence analysis of a 270 bp fragment of *rpoB* from 16 clinical rifampicin-susceptible isolates of *Streptococcus pneumoniae*, 8 clinical rifampicin-resistant isolates, and 3 spontaneous rifampicin-resistant mutants, has revealed that, as with previously examined species, point mutations within the cluster I region of *rpoB*, at sites encoding Asp_{516} and His_{526}, also confer resistance to rifampicin in this important human pathogen. Moreover, the residues within cluster I, that were altered within the rifampicin-resistant mutants of *S. pneumoniae*, were in the same position as those previously found to alter in resistant isolates of *Escherichia coli* and *Mycobacterium tuberculosis*. Sequence analysis of *rpoB*, both from these isolates of *S. pneumoniae* and from two strains of *S. mitis*, reveals that, among a number of clinical isolates, resistance to rifampicin in *S. pneumoniae* has arisen by point mutation. However, the nucleotide sequence of *rpoB* from one isolate examined suggests that interspecies gene transfer may also have played a role in the evolution of rifampicin-resistance in *S. pneumoniae*.

INTRODUCTION

THE EMERGENCE OF ISOLATES OF *STREPTOCOCCUS PNEUMONIAE* with resistance to antimicrobial agents has been observed in most countries. Many studies have focused on the increased isolation rates for strains that are resistant to β-lactam antibiotics but resistance to other agents, such as chloramphenicol, erythromycin, clindamycin, tetracycline, and rifampicin, have also been reported, as are strains that are multiply resistant.[1,15,21] Resistance usually arises because of the acquisition of novel determinants that either inactivate, or reduce the accumulation of, an antibiotic by an organism. However, there are a number of instances where resistance occurs because of alteration of the target of an antibiotic. The evolution of target-mediated resistance to β-lactams—penicillin-binding-protein (PBP) mediated resistance—has occurred in a number of naturally transformable bacterial species, including *S. pneumoniae*, by horizontal gene transfer and homologous recombination, but has not yet arisen by this means in non-transformable organisms. Alternatively, target-mediated resistance to rifampicin—RNA polymerase subunit B (*rpoB*) mediated resistance—has

been shown to evolve by point mutation in a number of non-transformable species.

β-lactam resistance in *S. pneumoniae* has been well studied in both clinical isolates and laboratory mutants,[13] and involves alterations of three targets, PBPs 1A, 2B, and 2X, that lead to forms with a decreased affinity for the antibiotic.[2] Among clinical isolates, PBP genes from strains resistant to β-lactams show a mosaic structure with regions very similar to sensitive strains (DNA sequence divergence <1%) but with blocks of sequence varying by up to 23% compared to sensitive strains. These resistant blocks have been shown to emerge by recombination with related species of streptococci, such as *Streptococcus mitis*,[11] and the subsequent spread of these low affinity PBPs has occurred by both intra- and inter-species recombination.[6,5,10] Mosaic PBPs have also been found to evolve by point mutation, presumably in response to selection by the therapeutic use of different classes of β-lactam antibiotics.[4] The PBPs of pathogenic *Neisseria spp.* also show a characteristic mosaic structure in strains resistant to β-lactams.[27]

The rarity of rifampicin-resistant pneumococci isolated in hospitals indicates that there is currently little selective pres-

[1]Department of Biochemistry, University of Sussex, Brighton BN1 9QG, UK.
[2]Department of Biological Sciences, University of Warwick, Coventry CV4 7AL, UK.
Reprinted from *Microbial Drug Resistance*, Vol. 4, No. 1, 1998.

sure for resistance. In the few studies where rifampicin-resistant *S. pneumoniae* isolates have been found, the isolation rates were much lower than were those for isolates resistant to other agents. For example, a study in a Spanish hospital from 1979–1990,[22] found that, whereas 21.8% of strains were resistant to penicillin, only 0.1% were rifampicin-resistant. In the same study, 36.6% of isolates were resistant to chloramphenicol, 45.6% to tetracycline, and 42.2% to co-trimoxazole. Similar low isolation rates of rifampicin resistance are found in the USA (0.5%)[9] and in Brasil (3.1%).[25] Rifampicin is not used routinely in the treatment of pneumococcal infections although it is sometimes used in combination with vancomycin or cefataxime/ceftriaxone against multiply-resistant pneumococci.[18,20] *Mycobacterium tuberculosis* infections are usually treated with rifampicin, often in combination with other drugs, and rifampicin is used prophylactically to reduce carriage of *Neisseria meningitidis* in contacts of patients with meningococcal meningitis.[8] Nevertheless, rifampicin resistance in these two organisms is still infrequent: a recent review of the literature[7] estimated that fewer than 3% of *M. tuberculosis* isolates were rifampicin-resistant and two Spanish studies of resistant meningococci found no rifampicin-resistant strains.[12,24]

Rifampicin acts by binding to the β-subunit of RNA polymerase, causing premature termination during DNA transcription in *E. coli*[17] and point mutations, most of which map to two regions in the centre of the *rpoB* gene, clusters I and II, which have been described and which lead to rifampicin resistance.[16] DNA studies on the sequence of *rpoB* from *Neisseria meningitidis*,[3] *Mycobacterium tuberculosis*,[19,29,30] and *Mycobacterium leprae*[14] show that clusters I and II are largely conserved in these organisms and that many of the mutations described in *E. coli* are present in rifampicin-resistant strains of these species, especially in cluster I mutations.

In this study, we have examined the molecular basis of rifampicin resistance in *S. pneumoniae* to determine the relative importance of point mutation or horizontal gene transfer in the evolution of the *rpoB* locus. To this end, we also have looked at the nucleotide sequence of *rpoB* from two strains of *S. mitis*, as this species previously has been found to donate PBP2B genes to *S. pneumoniae* in the evolution of penicillin resistance.

MATERIALS AND METHODS

Strains and culture conditions

All isolates were from our collection: the details are shown in Table 1. Isolates were stored at −70°C in brain heart infu-

TABLE 1. DETAILS OF STRAINS USED IN THIS STUDY

Strain	Country of origin	MIC (ug ml)	Serogroup	Year of isolation	Mutation
R6	United States	<0.064	NC	1930	
R6r	United States	>20	NC	—	70 H ⇒ D
VA1	United States	<0.064	19	1983	
7	United Kingdom	<0.064	NT	1993	
29044	Czech republic	<0.064	14	1987	
36	South Africa	6	19	1989	70 H ⇒ N
3307	United Kingdom		3	1995	
630	Spain	<0.064	16	1987	
ATCC 6323	United States		23	1944	
GM169	Spain	<0.064	19	1989	
KD18	Kenya	<0.064	23	1991	
KD5	Kenya	<0.064	14	1991	
KD6	Kenya	<0.064	19	1991	
110K/70	Papua New Guinea	<0.064	42	1970	
4865	Papua New Guinea	<0.064	15	Unknown	
Sp1	Spain	<0.064	23	1988	
233	Poland	64	23	1994	
234	Poland	64	23	1994	
13 (*S. mitis*)	United Kingdom	<0.064	NT	1993	
1 (*S. mitis*)	United Kingdom	<0.064	NT	1993	
3026	Spain	8	Unknown	1994	60 D ⇒ N
3051	Spain	8	Unknown	1994	60 D ⇒ N
3275	Spain	>256	Unknown	1994	70 H ⇒ Y
2349	Spain	<0.064	Unknown	Unknown	
2349r	Spain	12	Unknown	Unknown	70 H ⇒ N
S3	Spain	<0.064	3	Unknown	
S3r	Spain	16	3	Unknown	70 H ⇒ Y
3331	Spain	>256	23	1995	70 H ⇒ N
3443	Spain	>128	23	1995	70 H ⇒ N

NC, non-capsulate; NT, non-typable; Mutation, amino-acid alteration; r, spontaneous mutant from susceptible isolate.

sion (BHI) broth (Oxoid, Basingstoke, Hants, United Kingdom) with 15% glycerol. *S. pneumoniae* and *S. mitis* isolates were plated on blood agar (Todd-Hewitt agar containing 5% sheep blood) and incubated overnight at 37°C in air with 5% CO_2.

Rifampicin MICs and generation of rifampicin resistant mutants

Rifampicin MICs were determined using E-test strips (AB Biodisk, Solna, Sweden) on brain heart infusion (BHI) blood agar plates. Spontaneous rifampicin-resistant mutants were obtained by spreading a single colony from an overnight culture on blood agar containing (10 μg ml^{-1}) rifampicin (Sigma chemicals, Poole, Dorset, United Kingdom). One of the resulting colonies was then spread on blood agar and incubated overnight. Spontaneous mutants were also obtained for strains S3 and 2349, although these were in vivo mutants recovered from a rat treated with rifampicin.

Polymerase chain reaction

To enable amplification of the pneumococcal *rpoB*, two degenerate primers were designed based on conserved regions of the *rpoB* amino-acid sequence of *E. coli* (PIR database accession number A00688) and *B. subtilis* (SWISS-PROT database accession number P37870). The positions of these oligonucleotides correspond to amino-acids 399–406 and 518–525 in the *B. subtilis* protein sequence. The primer sequences are

399up 5' GAY GAY ATN GAY CAY YTN GGN AA 3'

525dn 5' DAT RTT NGG NCC YTC NGG NGY YTC 3'

where Y = C or T, R = A or G, D = A, G or T and N = inosine.

one μg of each primer was added to a buffer containing 0.2M KCl, 0.2M Tris, pH8.5, 0.2M $MgCl_2$, 2 mg ml^{-1} gelatin, and 25 mM of each of the four nucleotide trisphosphates. Chromosomal DNA (5 ng ul^{-1}) and 0.050 units ul^{-1} *Taq* polymerase (Perkin-Elmer, Foster City, CA) were added before thermal cycling in a PTC-100 thermal controller from MJ Research Inc. (Massachusetts). Samples were heated to 95°C for 5 min before 27 cycles of denaturation (95°C, 1 min), annealing (55°C, 2 min), and extension (72°C, 2 min). Products were visualized on 0.8% agarose gels stained with 0.03% ethidium bromide.

DNA sequencing

PCR products were purified using Qiaquick PCR purification columns (Qiagen, Dorking, Surrey, United Kingdom) to remove unincorporated nucleotides and primers. Sequencing was performed directly using an ABI Prism 377 DNA sequencer (ABI, Warrington, United Kingdom). Purified templates were sequenced using AmpliTaq© DNA Polymerase FS (ABI) and 12 ng of each PCR primer.

Transformation

PCR fragments using primers 399up and 525dn were purified using quiquick columns and then cloned into TA vector

and used to transform *E. coli* strain DH5αF' (Invitrogen, San Diego, California). Mini-prep DNA (Wizard miniprep, Promega, Madison, Wisconsin) was then used to transform *S. pneumoniae* strain R6.[2]

RESULTS

Sequences of 270bp fragments of the *rpoB* gene were obtained from 29 different isolates using primers 399up and 525dn. The region sequenced is homologous to part of the *rpoB* gene from *E. coli*, which includes *rpoB* cluster I.[16] These 29 isolates comprised two clinical susceptible *S. mitis* isolates (1 and 13), one susceptible serotype 3 *S. pneumoniae* strain isolated from a racehorse (3307), the laboratory strain R6, and three spontaneous rifampicin mutants generated from sensitive pneumococcal strains (R6, S3 and 2349), as well as 22 clinical *S. pneumoniae* isolates (see Table 1). Of the 22 clinical pneumococcal isolates, 8 were resistant to rifampicin (MIC 6 to >265ug ml-1).

These 26 sequences (discounting the 3 spontaneous mutants) were aligned to each other without the need for gaps and the level of DNA divergence was calculated (see Table 2). Fig. 1 shows the DNA differences (polymorphisms) present in all the strains studied compared to the *rpoB* sequence from a susceptible pneumococcal strain R6. Many pneumococcal isolates had identical DNA sequence in this region, for example, strains 630, GM169, KD5, 110K/70, and KD6, Sp1, 233, 234, 2349. The 270bp nucleotide sequence of all pneumococcal strains, both susceptible and resistant, differed by $\geq$ 3.0% when compared to each other. The DNA sequences from *S. mitis* isolates 1 and 13 differed by 5.2% and 4.1% from *S. pneumoniae* strain R6.

No relationship between serogroup/serotype and DNA sequence appears to be present among the isolates and the sequences of the eight naturally rifampicin-resistant strains are not markedly distinct from sensitive isolates. Indeed, two resistant strains from Poland (233 and 234, isolated from different patients) have identical DNA sequences to the sensitive strains Sp1 and KD6. The spontaneous mutants created from susceptible strains R6, S3, and 2349 differ by only one base compared to the sensitive strains leading to a single amino-acid alteration His_{70} within this sequence (see Table 1). To ensure that the mutants generated from sensitive strains were responsible for rifampicin resistance, the 270bp *rpoB* PCR product from strain R6[r] was cloned and used to transform a sensitive strain 110K/70 to rifampicin resistance. The resulting transformants had a rifampicin MIC of >20 ug ml-1 (the same as the donor strain R6[r]) compared to <0.064 ug ml-1 for the recipient 110K/70. Transformation frequencies were ~ 4 × 10^{-5}.

The deduced amino-acid polymorphisms present only in rifampicin-resistant strains are shown in Fig. 2. The resistant strains all have one of two amino-acid alterations compared to sensitive strains, with the most common mutation being a replacement of the His residue at position 70 (equivalent to residue His_{526} in *E. coli*) with one of three others (Asp, Asn, or Tyr). Two Spanish strains, 3026 and 3051, had a replacement of the Asp_{60} residue by Asn. None of these substitutions are present in sensitive strains, although there are numerous synonymous (silent) nucleotide alterations.

The 270 bp fragment of *rpoB* from strain 3331 was found to

TABLE 2.   PERCENTAGE NUCLEOTIDE DIVERGENCE WITHIN A 270BP FRAGMENT OF *rpoB*
FROM RIFAMPICIN-RESISTANT AND -SUSCEPTIBLE ISOLATES OF *S. PNEUMONIAE*, AND *S. MITIS*

Strain	2	3	4	5	6	7	8	9	10	11	12	13
1. R6/VA1/7/KD18/4865/S3	5.2	4.1	0.4	0.4	0.7	0.4	0.4	0.7	0.7	2.2	1.1	0.7
2. 1 (*S. mitis*)		3.3	4.8	5.6	5.2	4.8	5.6	5.9	5.2	4.4	5.6	6.0
3. 13 (*S. mitis*)			3.7	4.4	4.1	3.7	4.4	4.8	4.1	4.1	4.4	4.8
4. 29044				0.7	1.1	0.7	0.7	1.1	1.1	1.9	1.5	1.1
5. 630/KD5/GM169/110K70					0.4	0.7	0.7	0.4	1.1	2.6	1.5	3.7
6. 6323						0.4	1.1	0.7	0.7	2.2	1.1	0.7
7. KD6/SP1/**233/234**/2349							0.7	1.1	0.4	1.9	0.7	1.1
8. **36**								1.1	0.7	1.9	0.7	1.1
9. **3026/3051**									1.5	3.0	1.9	0.7
10. **3275**										1.9	0.7	1.5
11. **3331**											1.9	3.0
12. **3443**												1.9
13. 3307												

Strains in bold are resistant clinical isolates.

be the most divergent when compared against other pneumococci. The six nucleotide alterations shown in Fig. 1 are located between nucleotides 135–267 and flank the sites known to confer resistance to rifampicin. The nucleotide divergence over this region is 4.5%, including the alteration at 208 that confers resistance to rifampicin. Without this alteration, the divergence is reduced to 3.8% over this region of 132 nucleotides. Apart from the alteration at position 208 (see Fig. 1) the other five nucleotide alterations are synonymous and, therefore, not involved in resistance. This level of divergence between *rpoB* from strain 3331 and the other isolates of *S. pneumoniae* is similar to that between *S. mitis* and *S. pneumoniae*. Moreover, the polymorphisms involved suggest that they may have been introduced by recombination.

DISCUSSION

Rifampicin resistance in *S. pneumoniae*, as found previously for *E. coli*, *M. tuberculosis*, *N. meningitidis,* and *M. leprae,* involves amino-acid alterations to the β-subunit of RNA polymerase, with mutations responsible for resistance typically being found in the conserved cluster I region. All but two Polish strains used in this study have cluster I alterations. The two rifampicin-resistant Polish isolates that have cluster I amino-acid sequences identical to susceptible pneumococci may, however, possess cluster II mutations, as found in some rifampicin-resistant *E. coli*.[26] However, this was not investigated further. Using the *E. coli* numbering, cluster I amino acid alterations within rifampicin-resistant pneumococci occurred at two sites, Asp_{516} and His_{526}, which are known to confer rifampicin resistance in *E. coli*: Asp_{516} to Asn and His_{526} to Tyr, being found in both *E. coli* and *S. pneumoniae*. Although His_{526} to Asn or Asp has not been reported previously as occurring in *E. coli*,[16,17] His_{526} to Asp has been found in rifampicin-resistant isolates of *Mycobacterium tuberculosis*.[29]

The DNA sequence of *rpoB* from most of the *S. pneumoniae* isolates studied were very similar, although the variation found between some isolates (up to 3% over the whole 270 bp

```
                                                     1111111111111111111111111111111122222222222222222222
                                     111122223333455556777788889999900012223333455556677888899999000001112223444566666
                                     392345124804682347323681346013459268768935684456928184569235681457803605846895145 67
R6/VA1/7/KD18/4865/S3    TGTGCCAGATGCTAAATCATGCGCATACTGACAAATCACAGAGTATCAAGAGGCACCGCTTTGGTTCCACTACAGCTCCATAT
R6r                      ...................................................................G................
1                       ........GCT.......AT........G..C.....G.G...........T.A................AA.T....
13                      ........CT..G.......AT.C.............G................T.................AA.T....
29044                   .................................G................................................
630/KD5/GM169/110K70    .................................T................................................
6323                    ...............................T.........................................T....
KD6/Sp1/233/234/2349    ...............................T.........................................T....
36                      ......................................................................A.........
3026/3051               .................................T...............A................................
3275                    ........................................................................T.......T....
2349                    ........................................................................T........T....
2349r                   ........................................................................A........T....
3331                    .......................G............A.......A..............A.T...C
3443                    ..........................................................AA.............T....
S3r                     ......................................................................T.........
3307                    ......T......................T....................................
```

FIG. 1.   Polymorphic sites present in the 270 bp sequenced region of *rpoB*. Only those nucleotides that differ from those of strain R6 are shown. The positions of the polymorphic sites are shown in vertical format above the sequence. Numbering: nucleotide 3 corresponds to position 1372 of the *E. coli rpoB* gene. Isolates in bold are rifampicin resistant. r represents spontaneous mutants of susceptible isolates in this study. Bold underlined polymorphisms are those identified as confering rifampicin resistance in this and in previous studies.[16,17,28,29]

```
         41                                                                          N
S.p      P    V    T    A    A    V    K    E    F    F    G    S    S    Q    L    S    Q    F    M    D
S.p      CCT  GTA  ACA  GCT  GCA  GTT  AAA  GAA  TTC  TTT  GGT  TCA  TCA  CAG  TTG  TCA  CAG  TTC  ATG  GAC
E.c           I    S    A    A    V    K    E    F    F    G    S    S    Q    L    S    Q    F    M    D
         497                                                                       F    L         F    M    V
                                                                                   P    P                   N
                                                                                   R                   Y
M.t                                                                                L    L                   A
                                                                                                            V

                                                                    _____
                                                                              E.coli CLUSTER I


                                          D
                                          Y
         61                               N
S.p      Q    H    N    P    L    S    E    L    S    H    K    R    R    L    S    A    L    G    P    G
S.p      CAA  CAC  AAC  CCG  CTT  TCT  GAG  TTG  TCT  CAC  AAA  CGC  CGT  TTG  TCA  GCC  TTA  GGA  CCT  GGT
E.c      Q    N    N    P    L    S    E    I    T    H    K    R    R    I    S    A    L    G    P    G
         517                     F                        Y              S         Y    E    P    D
                                                          P              C         F    V
                                                          R              L
                                                          Q              H
M.t                         P                             D                        L         P
                                                          Y
                                                          P

      _____
                              E.coli CLUSTER I

         81
S.p      G    L    T    R    D    R    A    G    Y    E
S.p      GGT  TTG  ACT  CGT  GAC  CGT  GCC  GGA  TAT  GAA
E.c      G    L    T    R    E    R    A    G    F    E
         537
```

FIG. 2. Derived amino-acid substitutions in *rpoB* responsible for rifampicin resistance in *S. pneumoniae* and *E. coli*. Amino-acid residues are numbered according to their position in the sequenced fragment and also according to the *E. coli* numbering system.[16–17]

fragment) was greater than that found at other housekeeping gene loci, such as glucose-6-phosphate dehydrogenase, alcohol dehydrogenase, adenylate kinase, and glutamine synthase, typically <1.0% (unpublished results). The divergence of 130 bp region *rpoB* from strain 3331 was found to be as high as 4.5%. However, the number of polymorphic sites in our data set was not sufficient to prove statistically the presence of recombination at the *rpoB* locus of this strain, even though there appears to be some visual evidence for recombination and for the possibility that this may have been responsible for the introduction of the His_{526} to Asn polymorphism that confers resistance.

Recently we have obtained unpublished *rpoB* sequences from 26 *Neisseria meningitidis* strains from a study of *rpoB* mutations leading to rifampicin resistance.[3] A region homologous to that sequenced in this work varies by 0–2% between all strains of *N. meningitidis* belonging to one of five serogroups, although the six naturally rifampicin-resistant meningococci in the study had identical DNA sequences, suggesting a clonal origin. This level of DNA sequence variation at *rpoB* (0–2%) is similar to that found in meningococcal housekeeping loci such as *adk, fbp* and *recA*,[31] suggesting that, generally, in susceptible isolates there is an absence of recombination (in the isolates examined) at this locus in meningococci. However, meningococcal loci such as *argF*[31] clearly have evolved by recombination and the results from Carter et al.[3] do not rule out the possibility that *rpoB*-mediated rifampicin resistance in *N. meningitidis* could also evolve by horizontal gene transfer.

Sulphonamide resistance in *S. pneumoniae* can arise by alterations to the chromosomally encoded dihydropterate synthase (*sulA*). Maskell et al.[23] have shown that 3-6-bp duplications within *sulA* can lead to resistance in clinical isolates. However, it is also clear that members of a serotype 9V clone possess a divergent *sulA* and that horizontal gene transfer has been involved in the acquisition (or loss) of resistance within this clone. Unlike rifampicin, sulphonamides in combination with trimethoprim, as co-trimoxazole, have been used frequently in the treatment of pneumococcal infections.

The increasing prevalence of multi-drug-resistant *S. pneumoniae* has prompted the suggestion that rifampicin be used in combination with other agents in treating resistant infections. From our results, and a general knowledge of the evolution of pneumococcal targets for several different antibiotics,[11,23] we surmise that an increase in the use of rifampicin will lead inevitably to increased isolation rates of rifampicin-resistant pneumococci due to mutation and, perhaps, recombination between strains which may lead to to both the spread and increased levels of rifampicin resistance among pneumococci.

ACKNOWLEDGMENTS

This work was funded by the Wellcome Trust.

REFERENCES

1. **Applebaum, P.C., A. Bhamjee, J.N. Scragg, A.F. Hallet, A.J. Bowen, and R.C. Cooper.** 1977. *Streptococcus pneumoniae* resistant to penicillin and chlorampheticol. Lancet **2**:995–997.

2. **Barcus, V.A., K. Ghanekar, M. Yeo, T.J. Coffey, and C.G. Dowson.** 1995. Genetics of high level penicillin resistance in clinical isolates of *Streptococcus pneumoniae*. FEMS Micro. Lett. **126**:299–304.

3. **Carter, P.E., F.J.R. Abadi, D.E. Yakubu, and T.H. Pennington.** 1994. Molecular characterization of rifampicin-resistant *Neisseria meningitidis*. Antimicrob. Agents. Chemother. **38**:1256–1261.

4. **Coffey, T.J., M. Daniels, L.K. McDougal, C.G. Dowson, F.C. Tenover, and B.G. Spratt.** 1995. Genetics analysis of clinical isolates of *Streptococcus pneumoniae* with high-level resistance to expanded-spectrum cephalosporins. Antimicrob. Agents Chemother. **39**:1306–1313.

5. **Coffey, T.J., C.G. Dowson, M. Daniels, and B.G. Spratt.** 1993. Horizontal spread of an altered penicillin-binding-protein 2B gene between *Streptococcus pneumoniae* and *Streptococcus oralis* FEMA Micro. Lett. **110**:335–340.

6. **Coffey, T.J., C.G. Dowson, M. Daniels, J. Zhou, C. Martin, B.G. Spratt, and J.M. Musser.** 1991. Horizontal transfer of multiple penicillin-binding protein genes, and capsular biosynthetic genes, in natural populations of *Streptococcus pneumoniae*. Mol. Microbiol. **5**:2255–2260.

7. **Cohn, D.L., F. Bustreo, and M.C. Raviglione.** 1997. Drug-resistant tuberculosis: Review of the worldwide situation and the WHO/IUATLD global surveillance project. Clin. Infect. Dis. **24**:S1(suppl.) S121–S130.

8. **Deal, W.B., and E. Saunders.** 1969. Efficacy of rifampicin in treatment of meningococcal carriers. N. Engl. J. Med. **281**:641–645.

9. **Doern, G.V., A. Brueggemann, H.P. Holley, and A.M. Rauch.** 1996. Antimicrobial resistance of *Streptococcus pneumoniae* recovered from outpatients in the United States during the winter months of 1994 to 1995—results of a 30-center national surveillance study. Antimicrob. Agents. Chemother. **40**:1208–1213.

10. **Dowson, C.G., A. Hutchison, N. Woodford, A.P. Johnson, R.C. George, and B.G. Spratt.** 1990. Penicilli-resistant viridans streptococci have obtained altered penicillin-binding protein genes from penicillin-resistant strains of *Streptococcus pneumoniae*. Proc. Natl. Acad. Sci. **87**:5858–5862.

11. **Dowson, C.G., T.J. Coffey, C. Kell, and R.A. Whiley.** 1993. Evolution f penicillin resistance in *Streptococcus pneumoniae*: the role of *Streptococcus mitis* in the formation of a low affinity PBP2B in *S. pneumoniae*. Mol. Microbiol. **9**:635–643.

12. **Florez, C., J.L. Garcia-Lopez, and E. Martin Mazuelos.** 1997. Susceptibilities of 55 strains of *Neisseria meningitidis* isolated in Spain in 1993 and 1994. Chemotherapy **43**:168–170.

13. **Hakenbeck, R., C. Martin, C.G. Dowson, and T. Grebe.** 1994. Penicillin-binding Protein 2b of *Streptococcus pneumoniae* in piperacillin-resistant laboratory mutants. J. Bacteriol. **177**:5574–5577.

14. **Honoré, N., and S.T. Cole.** 1993. Molecular basis of rifampicin resistance in *Mycobacterium leprae*. Antimicrob. Agents Chemother. **37**:414–418.

15. **Jacobs, M.R., H.J. Koornhof, R.M. Robins-Browne, C.M. Stevenson, Z.A. Vermaak, I. Freiman, G.B. Miller, M.A. Witcomb, M. Isaacson, J.I. Ward, and R. Austrian.** 1978. Emergence of multiply resistant pneumococci. N. Engl. J. Med. **299**:735–740.

16. **Jin, D.J., and C.A. Gross.** 1988. Mapping and sequencing of mutations in the *Escherichia coli rpoB* gene that lead to rifampicin resistance. J. Mol. Biol. **202**:45–58.

17. **Jin, D.J., M. Cashel, D.I. Friedman, Y. Nakamura, W.A. Walter, and C.A. Gross.** 1988. Effects of rifampicin resistant *rpoB* mutations on antitermination and interaction with *nusA* in *Escherichia coli*. J. Mol. Biol. **204**:247–261.

18. **John, C.C.** 1994. Treatment failure with use of a 3rd-generation cephalosporin for penicillin-resistant pneumococcal meningitis—case report and review. Clin. Infect. Dis. **18**:188–193.

19. **Kapur, V., L.L. Li, S. Iordanescu, M.R. Hamrick, A. Wanger, B.N. Kreiswirth, and J.M. Musser.** 1994. Characterization by automated DNA-sequencing of mutations in the gene (*rpoB*) encoding the RNA-polymerase Beta-subunit in rifampicin-resistant *Mycobacterium tuberculosis* strains from New York City and Texas. J. Clin. Micro. **32**:1095–1098.

20. **Klugman, K.P., I.R. Friedland, and J.S. Bradley.** 1995. Bactericidal activity against cephalosporin-resistant *Streptococcus pneumoniae* in cerebrospinal fluid of children with acute bacterial-meningitis. Antimicrob. Agents. Chemother. **39**:1988–1992.

21. **Klugman, K.P., T. Kapper, and A. Bryskier.** 1996. *In-vitro* susceptibility of penicillin-resistant *Streptococcus pneumoniae* to levofloxacin, selection of resistant mutants, and time-kill synergy studies of levofloxacin combined with vancomycin, tecoplanin, fusidic acid, and rifampicin. Antimicrob. Agents Chemother. **40**:2802–2804.

22. **Liñares, J., R. Pallares, T. Alonso, J.L. Pérez, J. Ayats, F. Gudiol, P.F. Viladrich, and R. Martin.** 1992. Trends in antimicrobial resistance of clinical isolates of *Streptococcus pneumoniae* in Bellvitge Hospital, Barcelona, Spain (1979–1990). Clin. Infect. Dis. **15**:99–105.

23. **Maskell, J.P., A. Sefton, and L.M.C. Hall.** 1997. Mechanism of sulphonamide resistance in clinical isolates of *Streptococcus pneumoniae*. Anti. Microb. Agents. Chemother. **41**:2121–2126.

24. **Pascual, A., P. Joyanes, L. Martinez Martinez, A.I. Suarez, and E.J. Perea.** 1996. Comparison of broth microdilution and E-test for susceptibility testing of *Neisseria meningitidis*. J. Clin. Micro. **34**:588–591.

25. **Sessegolo, J.F., A.S.S. Levin, C.E. Levy, M. Asensi, R.R. Facklam, and L.M. Teixeira.** 1994. Distribution of serotypes and antimicrobial resistance of *Streptococcus pneumoniae* strains isolated in Brasil from 1988 to 1992. J. Clin. Micro. **32**:906–911.

26. **Severinov, K., M. Soushko, A. Goldfarb, and V. Nikiforov.** 1993. New rifampicin-resistant and streptolydigin-resistant mutants in the b subunit of *Escherichia coli* RNA polymerase. J. Biological Chem. **268**:14820–14825.

27. **Spratt, B.G.** 1988. Hybrid penicillin-binding proteins in penicillin-resistant strains of *Neisseria gonorrhoeae*. Nature **332**:173–176.

28. **Spratt, B.G.** 1994. Resistance to antibiotics mediated by target alterations. Science **264**:388–393.

29. **Taniguchi, H., H. Aramaki, Y. Nikaido, Y. Mizuguchi, M. Nakamura, T. Koga, and S. Yoshida.** 1996. Rifampicin resistance and mutation of the *rpoB* gene in *Mycobacterium tuberculosis*. FEMS Micro. Lett. **144**:103–108.

30. **Telenti, A., P. Imboden, F. Marchesi, T. Schmidheini, and T. Bodmer.** 1993. Direct automated detection of rifampicin-resistant *Mycobacterium tuberculosis* by polymerase chain-reaction and single-strand conformation polymorphism analysis. Antimicrob. Agents. Chemother. **37**:2054–2058.

31. **Zhou, J., and B.G. Spratt.** 1992. Sequence diversity within *argF*, *fbp* and *recA* genes of natural isolates of *Neiseria meningitidis*: Interspecies recombination within the *argF* gene. Mol. Microbiol. **6**:135–2146.

Address reprint requests to:
Dr. Chris Dowson
Department of Biological Sciences
University of Warwick
Coventry CV4 7AL, UK

Penicillin-Binding Proteins in β-Lactam-Resistant *Streptococcus pneumoniae*

REGINE HAKENBECK,[1] KRISTINA KAMINSKI,[2] ANDREA KÖNIG,[2] MARK VAN DER LINDEN,[1] JOHANNA PAIK,[2] PETER REICHMANN,[1] and DOROTHEA ZÄHNER[1]

INTRODUCTION

NON-β-LACTAMASE–MEDIATED PENICILLIN RESISTANCE in *Streptococcus pneumoniae* has been the subject of investigations in the laboratory since the early 40s. As a phenomenon in clinical isolates, however, penicillin resistance appeared only several decades later. Using the penicillin-binding protein 2x (PBP2x) as an example, we investigated the evolution of a penicillin target protein into a resistance determinant that can be transferred not only between different clones of *S. pneumoniae* but also across species barrier thereby contributing substantially to the rapid increase in resistant isolates. The problems of identifying PBP alterations relevant for penicillin resistance in clinical isolates will become evident by this scenario, which implies an important role of natural transformation for the evolution of a species.

The dissection of the mutational pathway of penicillin resistance in laboratory mutants has provided insights into PBP mutations that confer an increase in resistance. Unexpectedly, it has also revealed mechanisms that provide protection from β-lactam action at a level distinct from that of the target-PBP mediated resistance. Resistance development in this setting is accompanied by loss of the ability to develop genetic competence, and the identification of two proteins involved in both phenotypes—the histidine-protein kinase CiaH and a putative glycosyltransferase CpoA—has revealed an unknown complexity in the mechanism of β-lactam action.

PBPs AS PENICILLIN RESISTANCE DETERMINANTS IN *S. pneumoniae*

Penicillin resistance is mediated by the alteration of penicillin target enzymes, the penicillin-binding proteins (PBPs). PBPs catalyze important steps in the assembly of peptidoglycan, with the transpeptidation between two peptide side chains of the murein subunits representing the crucial penicillin-sensitive reaction. PBPs interact with β-lactams enzymatically by forming a covalent complex via the active site serine. Alterations in PBPs of resistant strains result in decreased affinity to the antibiotic so that higher penicillin concentrations are required for binding and inhibition of the enzyme.

S. pneumoniae contains six PBPs: the high molecular weight (hmw) class A PBPs 1a (79.7 kDa according to the deduced peptide sequence), PBP1b (89.6 kDa), PBP2a (80.8 kDa), the class B hmw PBP2x (82.3 kDa), and PBP2b (82.3 kDa), and the low molecular weight (lmw) PBP3 (45.2 kDa)[12] (Fig. 1). All six PBPs can occur as low-affinity variants. Whereas selection of β-lactam–resistant mutants in the laboratory reveals point mutations in PBP genes,[13,18,20,23,39,44] resistance in clinical isolates of *S. pneumoniae* appears to be a property acquired via genetic transformation. Resistant clinical isolates of *S. pneumoniae* contain mosaic PBP genes that result from gene transfer events from related species, followed by homologous recombination of resistance determinants.[4,25,27] This process results in replacement of sequences that diverge approximately 20% compared to the gene sequences of penicillin-susceptible strains, generally leading to approximately 10% amino acid substitutions.

Low-affinity forms of PBPs 2b and 2x confer low level resistance when transformed into a penicillin susceptible recipient strain,[6,24] and are prerequisites for high level β-lactam resistance. This indicates that both of these proteins are essential, and indeed, attempts to delete either one of these PBPs were unsuccessful.[16,22] PBP1a confers high level resistance only in recipients where at least PBP2x or both class B hmw PBPs are low-affinity variants. The role of PBP2a as a resistance determinant, again requiring at least an altered PBP2x in order to be able to contribute to resistance, has clearly been established, whereas the role of PBP1b in resistance development is not yet clear.[12] PBP1a is a secondary resistance determinant and dispensable,[11,16] and mutants with interrupted *pbp2a* and *pbp1b* genes can also be obtained.[30] The lmw PBP3 can also be deleted, but mutant cells exhibit gross morphological changes and, similar to all class A hmw PBP mutants, grow slower than the wild type.[35] PBP3 has been described as a resistance determinant so far only in a cefotaxime-resistant laboratory mutant.[18]

A remarkable feature of PBP2b is that it does not interact with third generation cephalosporins such as cefotaxime, so that alterations in PBP2b are not required for cefotaxime resistance.

[1]Department of Microbiology, University of Kaiserslautern, Kaiserslautern, Germany.
[2]Max Planck Institut für Molekulare Genetik, Berlin, Germany.
Reprinted from *Microbial Drug Resistance*, Vol. 5, No. 2, 1999.

This class of β-lactams does not induce a lytic response in *S. pneumoniae*, indicating that inhibition of PBP2b is crucial for lysis induction.[14] In agreement with this notion, lysis is almost completely suppressed in strains harboring a low-affinity PBP2b.[6] Thus, although a low-affinity PBP2b variant confers only a twofold resistance increase, the biological consequences are much more dramatic and may contribute substantially to survival during antibiotic treatment *in vivo*. Several reports document indeed that the tolerant phenotype is important for survival of the pathogen in the host.[26,42,43]

The use of third generation cephalosporins has been encouraged in areas with a high prevalence of penicillin-resistant isolates. In view of the results described above, however, one should realize that since cefotaxime has one target less compared to other β-lactam antibiotics, cefotaxime resistance may develop relatively easy. The appearance of isolates in the United States preferentially resisting third generation cephalosporins, one of which contains a single point mutation in PBP2x known to be selectable by cefotaxime in the laboratory, is completely consistent with this notion.[1,28]

MOSAIC GENES IN *Streptococcus sp.*

What is the origin of the divergent sequence blocks in the mosaic PBP genes? Since no naturally resistant streptococci exist, we searched for homologous PBP genes in penicillin-susceptible streptococci that are part of the human oral flora.[36] Genes homologous to the *S. pneumoniae* PBP2x were found in

S. mitis NCTC10712 (isolated in Britain) and *S. oralis* M3 (a South African isolate) with MIC values for β-lactam antibiotics almost identical to penicillin-sensitive *S. pneumoniae* strains (e.g., 0.02–0.03 μg/ml for cefotaxime).[36,37] Surprisingly, when the *S. oralis* and the *S. mitis* *pbp2x* were compared to each other, a central sequence block of the *pbp2x* genes differed by approximately 20%, whereas 3' and 5' sequences were less than 5% divergent. A similar situation was found for the *pbp2b* gene of sensitive streptococci.[3] Thus, in case of *Streptococcus* sp., mosaicism is not confined to PBP genes of resistant isolates but clearly occurs in penicillin-sensitive strains as well.

Most intriguingly, it was possible to transform the penicillin-sensitive *S. pneumoniae* R6 strain with *pbp2x* genes of *S. mitis* 10712 or *S. oralis* M3 to confer a minor but selectable 1.5- to 2-fold increase in MIC.[37] This and similar experiments showed that genetic exchange of PBP genes can occur already at the level of "penicillin-sensitive" genes, giving rise to new mosaic gene variants and a change of β-lactam susceptibility of the recipient (Fig. 2).

Sequences highly related to those of the *S. mitis* 10712 or the *S. oralis* M3 *pbp2x* were found in a variety of penicillin-resistant *S. pneumoniae*.[17,37] In transformation experiments, the *pbp2x* genes of β-lactam–resistant pneumococci conferred a resistance level of at least 0.2 μg/ml cefotaxime, much higher than that of the sensitive streptococci mentioned above. The critical difference that relates to the potential to clearly function as a resistance determinant appears to reside in only a few amino acids (aa) of the PBP. It is likely that β-lactam resistance first arose in commensal streptococci via the introduction

S. pneumoniae PBP

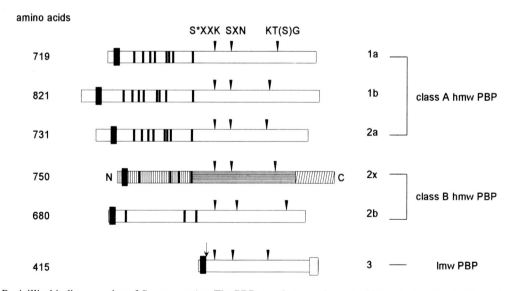

FIG. 1. Penicillin-binding proteins of *S. pneumoniae*. The PBPs are drawn as bars. An N-terminal hydrophobic region is shown as a black box. The conserved sequence motifs within the N-terminal domain are shown as black bars (there are eight conserved regions in class A hmw PBPs, and four motifs described in class B hmw PBPs[5,12]); the three conserved peptide motifs of the central penicillin-binding domain are marked by arrows. Different shading of PBP2x indicates N-terminal, penicillin-binding/transpeptidase, and C-terminal domain according to the three-dimensional structure.[31] In PBP3, a putative processing site is indicated by an arrow, and a C-terminal amphiphilic helix is shown in gray.[18]

of point mutations in the target PBPs before being transferred into the pneumococcus as outlined in Fig. 3. Not only contain all resistant *S. pneumoniae* low-affinity PBPs, which are encoded by mosaic PBP genes, but resistance levels of commensal streptococci often exceed those of *S. pneumoniae* isolates. In fact, we were able to transfer very high levels of β-lactam resistance (cefotaxime MIC of 50 μg/ml and oxacillin MIC of 100 g/ml) using DNA of a resistant *S. mitis* into *S. pneumoniae*. The *S. pneumoniae* transformants contained low-affinity PBP2x, 2b, 2a, 1a, and 1b encoded by altered PBP genes, demonstrating that sequences of all hmw PBPs can be exchanged.[12] In other words, the appearance of penicillin-resistant pneumococci may well be a secondary event, with the genetic potential for penicillin resistance first evolving in commensal bacteria.

VARIATION OF PBPs IN CLONES OF PENICILLIN-RESISTANT *S. pneumoniae*

The pneumococcal clones that have been characterized in our laboratory and served as the basis for investigating the evolution and spread of PBP genes are shown in Fig. 4.[34,38] They include the first three main clones found in Spain of serotype 23F, 6B, and 9V, at least another three genetically distinct serotype 23F clones from other European countries, and the Hungarian

serotype 19A clonal group previously described.[29] Serotype 6B isolates occur in different countries and appear to be all members of a closely related clonal group that includes the Spanish serotype 6B clone. Most β-lactam–resistant as well as sensitive *S. pneumoniae* clones as defined by MLEE and capsular type contained an almost uniform set of PBPs as judged by electrophoretic mobility, biochemical properties, epitope mapping, and MIC values for β-lactam antibiotics.[10,15,38]

Sequence analyses confirmed that the uniform PBP pattern of the multiresistant "Spanish" serotype 23F clone is a reflection of almost identical PBP genes: e.g., the *pbp1a* gene of two strains isolated in Spain in 1984 and South Africa in 1987 differed by only one nucleotide over the 2-kb sequenced region,[27] and the *pbp2x* gene of two strains isolated 12 years apart in Spain and Germany differed by only four nucleotides.[17] There are, however, also clones that harbor a variety of PBP alleles, with the most pronounced example being one Hungarian 19A clone where different PBP1a and PBP2b variants were recognized on the basis of epitope mapping,[34] and there were four *pbp2x* variants that contained distinct mosaic sequence blocks.[33] A clonal group of serotype 6B isolates was found throughout Europe,[34] with isolates from Finland, France, Spain, and Hungary containing mosaic *pbp2x* genes with related mosaic blocks but distinct borders, showing that they must have arisen by independent recombination events[17] (Fig. 4).

Sequence comparisons of more than 30 *pbp2x* genes from

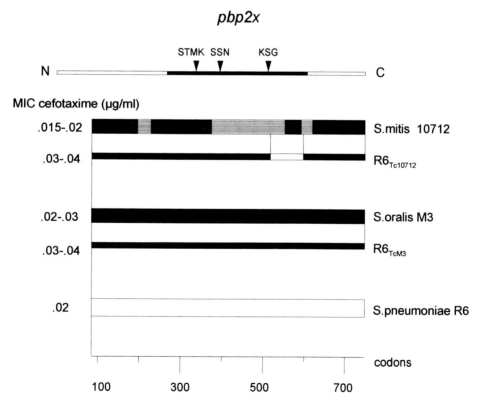

FIG. 2. Homologous *pbp2x* genes in penicillin-susceptible *Streptococcus mitis, S. oralis,* and *S. pneumoniae*. White, gray, and black bars indicate sequences that are 16–25% different from each other. R6$_{Tc10712}$/R6$_{TcM3}$:*pbp2x* in transformants of the *S. pneumoniae* R6 strain obtained with chromosomal DNA of the indicated strains and selection with cefotaxime. The black bars indicate sequence blocks in *pbp2x* of the transformants that were identical to those of the donor DNA.[37] The dimensions of the *pbp2x* gene and the three homology boxes in the penicillin-binding domain of PBP2x are indicated on top.

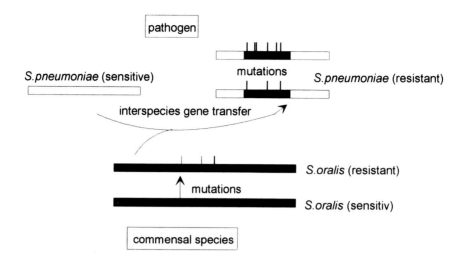

FIG. 3. Hypothetical evolution of a *pbp2x* allele into a penicillin-resistance determinant. A penicillin susceptible *S. oralis* is arbitrarily chosen as potential ancestor of a *pbp2x* gene. *pbp2x* functions as a resistance determinant after acquisition of point mutations (indicated as vertical bars) in *S. oralis* and also in *S. pneumoniae* (or other related streptococci) after gene transfer, presumably via transformation. More mutations can then occur, resulting in a PBP with improved properties relating to resistance or other functions.

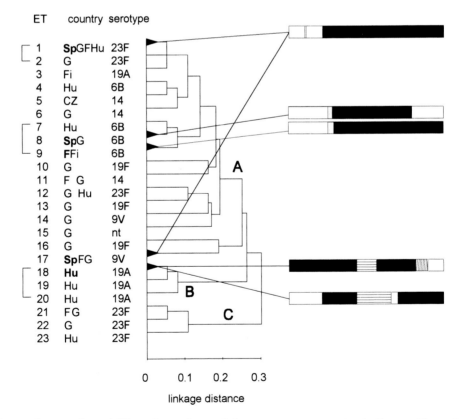

FIG. 4. *pbp2x* mosaic genes in penicillin-resistant clones of *Streptococcus pneumoniae* in Europe. Shown is a dendrogram based on a cluster analysis of a collection of *S. pneumoniae* isolates from Europe.[34] The mosaic structures of *pbp2x* of three clones from Spain (23F, 6B, and 9V), a member of the serotype 6B clonal group from France, and of two members of the same Hungarian serotype 19A clone are shown. Same shading refers to highly related sequences: white, penicillin-sensitive *S. pneumoniae* isolates; black, *S. oralis* M3; horizontal striped, *S. mitis* 10712. CZ, Czech Republic; F, France; G, Germany; Fi, Finland; Hu, Hungary; Sp, Spain; ET, electrophoretic type as determined by MLEE analysis.

different clones isolated from different parts of the world revealed that at least five different alleles with approximately 20% divergence to each other must have contributed to the various mosaic structures. Moreover, at least ten distinct combinations of mosaic blocks were recognized.[17]

A major class of closely related mosaic *pbp2x* genes contains one divergent sequence block with variable length up to almost 600 of the 750 codon *pbp2x* gene. The divergent block is very similar (<5% divergence) to the *pbp2x* gene of the susceptible *S. oralis* M3. This class is found in a variety of distinct *S. pneumoniae* clones as well as in *S. mitis* and *S. oralis* isolates distributed in Eastern and Western Europe and even in different continents (Fig. 5). Their susceptibilities vary from sensitive to high-level cephalosporin resistance. This confirms the existence of a global gene pool that is shared by a wide range of streptococcal species.[32]

The *pbp2x* gene of the multiple resistant "Spanish" serotype 23F clone belongs to this mosaic gene class. The restriction enzyme cleavage pattern of *pbp2x*, *pbp2b*, and *pbp1a* genes, and even the entire *pbp2x* sequence are completely identical to that of the penicillin-resistant serotype 9V clone. These findings further establish gene transfer events between distinct clones of one species.[2,9] The mosaic structure of the *pbp2x* gene of the serotype 6B clone, although it also contains sequences identical to the 23F clone, suggests a different source,[37] and analysis of their *pbp1a* genes confirmed this.[27] Highly cephalosporin-resistant *S. mitis* from Spain contained essentially the same divergent *pbp2x* block that was present in the *S. pneumoniae* 23F clone, except for a few amino acid alterations that may be crucial for high level cephalosporin resistance.[32] In addition, the *S. mitis* genes contain distinct sequences at the 5'-end of the gene, illustrating further allelic variation.

The history of a mosaic gene can only be deduced if both donor and recipient are known, and, of course, this information is not available for clinical isolates. Other factors, such as multiple recombinations during transformation, add to the complexity of the situation and the deduced mosaic structures therefore reflect only a best guess of the genetic structure of a particular sequence.[9]

POINT MUTATIONS IN PBP2x

Single amino acid alterations in PBP2x can confer only a slight increase in resistance, and the high resistance levels observed in clinical isolates or in laboratory mutants are the result of multiple mutations in several genes. Analysis of *pbp2x* in laboratory mutants selected with cefotaxime revealed that an amazing variety of distinct mutational pathways lead to low-affinity PBP2x variants.[20,23] Fourteen different point mutations in PBP2x were identified after four to six selection steps, with combinations of up to four occurring in individual mutants. All of these were located within the penicillin-binding/transpeptidase domain. Single mutations located between positions 596 and 601 conferred an MIC for cefotaxime of 0.04–0.08 μg/ml. A potent cefotaxime-specific mutation is a Thr550 to Ala change directly adjacent to the K547SG motif. A Gly550 (the result of two mutations in the same codon) confers cefotaxime MIC of 03. μg/ml.[20] Most mosaic genes from resistant strep-

tococci confer cefotaxime MICs of approximately 0.15–0.2 μg/ml, and higher values appear exceptional[32] (Fig. 6).

Some mutations confer low level resistance to a wide variety to β-lactams, such as the mutations at the C-terminal end of the penicillin-binding domain between Gly597 and Gly 601. Others are specific for cefotaxime only, and a most dramatic example is the change Thr550 to Ala that at the same time confers hypersensitivity to oxacillin.[1,20] The oxacillin hypersensitivity is not expressed in the Gly550 mutant, although cefotaxime resistance is further increased.[6] Mutations that confer resistance in a temperature-dependent manner have also been found.[20]

The identification of specific amino acid alterations that produce resistance of resistant clinical isolates is more problematic. The mosaic sequences in *pbp2x* that can span the entire 750-codon gene result in approximately 10% aa alterations. These changes are not evenly distributed: in the C-terminal domain of PBP2x, there are up to 23% aa changes versus up to 13% changes in the central penicillin-binding/transpeptidase domain. Out of over 30 PBP2x sequences, the smallest number of alterations in the transpeptidase domain, 11 aa changes, was found in the PBP2x from a New Guinea isolate, followed by the PBP2x of an isolate from England with 22 aa.[25] If one subtracts those changes that occur in the related *pbp2x* genes of the sensitive *S. mitis* 10712 and *S. oralis* M3, the number of aa changes potentially relevant for resistance is reduced to six and eight, respectively.

All mosaic PBP2x genes from resistant streptococci analyzed so far contain alterations in one of two aa: at position 338 within the S337TMK motif, the Thr is substituted by Ala, or in rare cases by Gly or Pro, and at position 552 close to the K547TG box the Gln is substituted by Glu. Site directed mutagenesis at position 338 showed that all three substitutions confer increased resistance,[19] and, similarly, the Glu552 mutations could be selected as cephalosporin resistant laboratory mutants.[39] In addition, single cases with identified mutations include the Thr550 to Ala change that conferred high-level cephalosporin resistance in a clinical *S. pneumoniae* isolate from the United States,[1] probably an example of a mutation acquired recently in areas where the use of third generation cephalosporins is encouraged; and a serotype 23F isolate contains the same His394 to Tyr mutation described in a particular cefotaxime-resistant laboratory mutant.[17,20] Whether substitutions in the region between residues 597 and 601 that occur in a few *pbp2x* genes from clinical isolates contribute to resistance, similar to the situation in laboratory mutants, remains to be seen (Fig. 6).

The three-dimensional structure of a PBP2x derivative in which the hydrophobic N-terminal membrane spanning domain was deleted has contributed significantly to our understanding of the interaction between antibiotic inhibitors and their target proteins.[31] Similar to the related structures of β-lactamases, the three conserved motifs of the central penicillin binding domain in PBP2x form the active site cavity. In addition to the mutations that are closely linked to these motifs, sequences at the end of the penicillin-binding/transpeptidase domain between amino acid 596 and 601 also appear to affect the active site. Interestingly, the two mutations at positions 422 and 426 are located close to the interface between the transpeptidase domain and the C-terminal domain, but their relationship to the interaction with β-lactam antibiotics is not obvious. Clearly, the res-

pbp2x

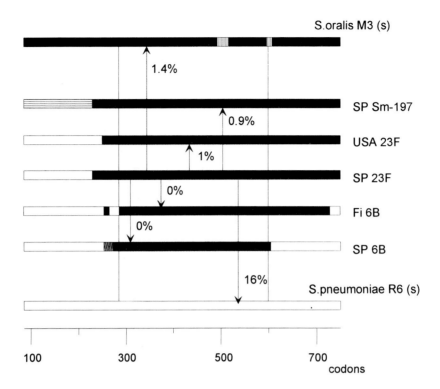

FIG. 5. A common class of mosiac *pbp2x* genes in penicillin-resistant streptococci. Black regions represent sequences that are highly related to each other (<1% divergence); they are closely related to *pbp2x* of *S. oralis* M3. The difference in nucleotide sequence (%) is indicated for the shaded area. Shown are mosaic *pbp2x* genes of the penicillin-resistant serotype 23F *S. pneumoniae* from Spain (SP 23F), of high-level cephalosporin resistant isolates from the US (USA 23F); serotype 6B clones from Finland (Fi 6B) and Spain (SP 6B), and a Spanish *S. mitis* isolate 197 (SP Sm-197).[1,17,32]

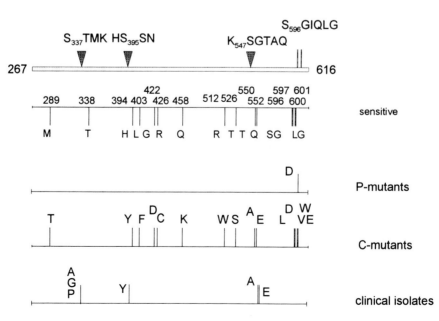

FIG. 6. Point mutations in PBP2x of laboratory mutants and clinical isolates involved in β-lactam resistance. Single mutations within the PBP2x penicillin-binding domain occur in laboratory mutants isolated with cefotaxime (C-mutants) or piperacillin (P); each mutation occurs in a different mutant at different selection steps. The mutations in the clinical isolates are discussed in the text.

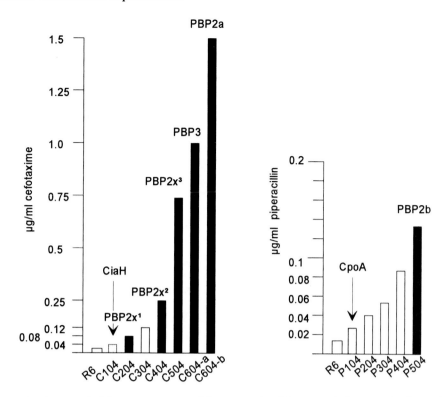

FIG. 7. Resistance development in laboratory mutants of *S. pneumoniae*. Mutants resisting stepwise increasing concentrations of cefotaxime or piperacillin were isolated from the laboratory strain R6. Cefotaxime and piperacillin MICs of one cefotaxime resistant (C) and one piperacillin resistant (P) mutant family are indicated as bars. Genes that play a role as resistance determinants are marked at the step where mutations were selected in the resistant mutants. Black bars show mutations in PBP genes.

olution of the structure of a low-affinity PBP2x variant, preferably one with only a few mutations rather than a highly altered mosaic PBP2x of a clinical isolate, will provide more insight into the structural impact of such alterations.

Sites homologous to those of PBP2x mutations are found in other *S. pneumoniae* PBPs. Mutations within the S370TMK box, Thr371 to Ala or Ser, are frequent in PBP1a of clinical isolates[17,40]; the mutation Thr446 to Ala directly adjacent to the S443SN box is crucial in low-affinity PBP2b[6,41]; the mutation Gly617 to Ala, which is part of the K615SG box occurs in PBP2b of a laboratory mutant,[13] and the lmw PBP3 mutant Thr246 to Ile, close to K239TG, confers cefotaxime resistance.[18] Mutations at the end of the penicillin-binding domain have been described in *S. pneumoniae* PBP2b.[12] The position equivalent to the Thr550 to Ala mutation in PBP2x has been investigated on the atomic level in the *Streptomyces* R61 enzyme, revealing why this particular mutation affects specifically the interaction with cefotaxime.[21] Thus, the emerging structure-function information from PBP2x appears to be generally relevant to the analysis of resistance determinants in other PBPs as well.

PBP AND NON-PBP GENES AS RESISTANCE DETERMINANTS IN LABORATORY MUTANTS

A series of mutants resistant to cefotaxime, a nonlytic β-lactam that does not interact with PBP2b, or to piperacillin, a typ-

ical lytic β-lactam, were selected stepwise on increasing concentrations of the antibiotic.[23] Characterization of the PBP profiles of the mutants already suggested that not all steps of resistance increase were mediated by mutations of PBP genes, and this was confirmed by genetic analysis. In the cefotaxime-resistant mutants (C-mutants), mutations occurred primarily in PBP2x, but only two to four mutations were found in mutants selected with five or six selection steps. In addition, PBP2a was affected in three cases and could not be visualized by fluorography due to alterations in the *pbp2a* gene,[44] and in one mutant, the lmw PBP3 was affected.[18] In the piperacillin-resistant mutants (P-mutants), PBP2b was the first PBP affected, followed by a PBP2x mutation in two of the three mutant families. In none of the mutant families, however, did the number of point mutations that were found in PBP genes match the number of selection steps, and sometimes even in the mutant isolated at the first selection step, no PBP alteration was apparent. In other words, resistance was not necessarily associated with a PBP mutation. Figure 7 summarizes the results obtained with one C- and one P-mutant lineage. Most remarkably, selection of either one of the β-lactams was inevitably coupled with loss of transformability of the mutants, although the step at which this phenotype appeared varied in different mutant lineages.[7,8,45]

In all C-mutant lineages, mutations in a histidine protein kinase CiaH contributed to cefotaxime resistance either at the first or at a later selection step.[8,44,45] In two of the three P-mutant lineages, a mutation in a putative glycosyltransferase, CpoA, occurred in the first step.[7] In both, *ciaH* and *cpoA*, different mutations occurred in different mutant families similar to the situations concerning PBP2x, PBP2a, and PBP2b. Some *ciaH* alleles, and both *cpoA* alleles conferred defects in transformability when introduced into the parental R6 strain. The *cpoA* alleles resulted in a third phenotype, an apparent reduction in the amount of PBP1a. The results confirmed that the two classes of β-lactams—lytic and nonlytic—act via different primary mechanisms.

The resistance mediated by the mutations in the non-PBP genes in the parental R6 strain is comparable to those mediated by single point mutations of the PBPs: the *cpoA* alleles conferred an increase in piperacillin MIC from 0.04 μg/ml in the parent strain to 0.06 μg/ml compared to 0.06–0.08 μg/ml conferred by PBP2b mutations, and the *ciaH* mutants had a twofold increase in cefotaxime MIC compared to the 2- to 10-fold increase conferred by PBP2x mutations.[6,7,45]

The *ciaH* gene is part of an operon and overlaps by eight nucleotides with the *ciaR* gene encoding a cognate response regulator. Homology searches with the sensor domain of the kinase did not reveal relatedness to any other protein, and the signal sensed by CiaH is not known. Moreover, the genes controlled by the *cia* system remain to be identified. The function of CpoA, a member of a superfamily of glycosyltransferases that act on essential cellular components, is still unclear. The fact that mutations in non-PBP genes are selected by β-lactam treatment suggests that they counteract the β-lactam induced changes of the bacterial cell wall, which may occur below MIC levels. They have not been found in resistant clinical isolates, indicating that they may not be tolerated outside the laboratory.

Other resistance determinants in the laboratory mutants remain to be identified. By further unraveling the complex resistance pathway exhibited by the laboratory mutants we hope to learn new aspects of the mechanism of action of β-lactam antibiotics. We will also learn more about the regulation of genetic competence, which is clearly an important route for the acquisition of penicillin resistance determinants in clinical isolates.

ACKNOWLEDGMENTS

This work was supported by DFG Ha 1011/7-1 and BMBF FKZ 01K19703/1. We thank Jeff Stock for helpful discussions.

REFERENCES

1. **Coffey, T.J., M. Daniels, L.K. McDougal, C.G. Dowson, F.C. Tenover, and B.G. Spratt.** 1995. Genetic analysis of clinical isolates of *Streptococcus pneumoniae* with high-level resistance to expanded-spectrum cephalosporins. Antimicrob. Agents Chemother. **39:**1306–1313.
2. **Coffey, T.J., C.G. Dowson, M. Daniels, J. Zhou, C. Martin, B.G. Spratt, and J.M. Musser.** 1991. Horizontal transfer of multiple penicillin-binding protein genes, and capsular biosynthetic genes, in natural populations of *Streptococcus pneumoniae.* Mol. Microbiol. **5:**2255–2260.
3. **Dowson, C.G., T.J. Coffey, C. Kell, and R.A. Whiley.** 1993. Evolution of penicillin resistance in *Streptococcus pneumoniae*; the role of *Streptococcus mitis* in the formation of a low-affinity PBP2B in *S. pneumoniae.* Mol. Microbiol. **9:**635–643.
4. **Dowson, C.G., A. Hutchison, J.A. Brannigan, R.C. George, D. Hansman, J. Liñares, A. Tomasz, J.M. Smith, and B.G. Spratt.** 1989. Horizontal transfer of penicillin-binding protein genes in penicillin-resistant clinical isolates of *Streptococcus pneumoniae.* Proc. Natl. Acad. Sci. U.S.A. **86:**8842–8846.
5. **Ghuysen, J.-M. and G. Dive.** 1994. Biochemistry of the penicilloyl-serine transferases. *In* J.-M. Ghuysen and R. Hakenbeck (eds.), Bacterial cell wall. Elsevier Sciences BV, Amsterdam, pp. 103–129.
6. **Grebe, T., and R. Hakenbeck.** 1996. Penicillin-binding proteins 2b and 2x of *Streptococcus pneumoniae* are primary resistance determinants for different classes of β-lactam antibiotics. Antimicrob. Agents Chemother. **40:**829–834.
7. **Grebe, T., J. Paik, and R. Hakenbeck.** 1997. A novel resistance mechanism for β-lactams in *Streptococcus pneumoniae* involves CpoA, a putative glycosyltransferases. J Bacteriol. **179:**3342–3349.
8. **Guenzi, E., A.M. Gasc, M.A. Sicard, and R. Hakenbeck.** 1994. A two-component signal-transducing system is involved in competence and penicillin susceptibility in laboratory mutants of *Streptococcus pneumoniae.* Mol. Microbiol. **12:**505–515.
9. **Hakenbeck, R.** 1997. Evolution of penicillin-binding protein genes in sensitive streptococci into resistance determinants of *Streptococcus pneumoniae. In* B.A.M. van der Zeijst, W.P.M. Hoekstra, J.D.A. van Embden, and A.J.W. van Alphen (eds.), Ecology of pathogenic bacteria: molecular and evolutionary aspects. Royal Netherlands Academy of Arts and Sciences, Amsterdam, pp. 225–235.
10. **Hakenbeck, R., T. Briese, L. Chalkley, H. Ellerbrok, R. Kalliokoski, C. Latorre, M. Leinonen, and C. Martin.** 1991. Antigenic variation of penicillin-binding proteins from penicillin resistant clinical strains of *Streptococcus pneumoniae.* J. Infect. Dis. **164:**313–319.
11. **Hakenbeck, R., H. Ellerbrok, C. Martin, G. Morelli, G. Schuster, A. Severin and A. Tomasz.** 1993. Penicillin-binding protein 1a and 3 in *Streptococcus pneumoniae*: what are essential PBP's. *In* M.A. De Pedro, J.-V. Höltje, and W. Löffelhardt (eds.), Bacterial growth and lysis metabolism and structure of the bacterial sacculus. Plenum Press, New York, pp. 335–340.
12. **Hakenbeck, R., A. König, I. Kern, M. van der Linden, W. Keck, D. Billot-Klein, R. Legrand, B. Schoot, and L. Gutmann.** 1998. Acquisition of five high-M_r penicillin-binding protein variants during transfer of high-level β-lactam resistance from *Streptococcus mitis* to *Streptococcus pneumoniae.* J. Bacteriol. **180:**1831–1840.
13. **Hakenbeck, R., C. Martin, C. Dowson, and T. Grebe.** 1994. Penicillin-binding protein 2b of *Streptococcus pneumoniae* in piperacillin-resistant laboratory mutants. J. Bacteriol. **176:**5574–5577.
14. **Hakenbeck, R., S. Tornette, and N.F. Adkinson.** 1987. Interaction of non-lytic β-lactams with penicillin-binding proteins in *Streptococcus pneumoniae.* J. Gen. Microbiol. **133:**755–760.
15. **Jabes, D., S. Nachman, and A. Tomasz.** 1989. Penicillin-binding protein families: evidence for the clonal nature of penicillin resistance in clinical isolates of pneumococci. J. Infect. Dis. **159:**16–25.
16. **Kell, C.M., U.K. Sharma, C.G. Dowson, C. Town, T.S. Balganesh, and B.G. Spratt.** 1993. Deletion analysis of the essentiality of penicillin-binding proteins 1A, 2B and 2X of *Streptococcus pneumoniae.* F.E.M.S. Microbiol. Lett. **106:**171–175.
17. **König, A., J. Paik, R. Reinhardt, and R. Hakenbeck.** Unpublished data.
18. **Krauβ, J., and R. Hakenbeck.** 1997. Mutations in PBP3 of a cefotaxime resistant laboratory mutant C604 and penicillin resistant clinical isolates of *Streptococcus pneumoniae.* Antimicrob. Agents Chemother. **41:**936–942.
19. **Krauβ, J., A. König, and R. Hakenbeck.** Unpublished data.

20. Krauβ, J., M. van der Linden, T. Grebe, and R. Hakenbeck. 1996. Penicillin-binding proteins 2x and 2b as primary PBP-targets in *Streptococcus pneumoniae*. Microbial Drug Resist. 2:183–186.

21. Kuzin, A.P., J. Liu, J.A. Kelly, and J.R. Knox. 1995. Binding of cephalothin and cefotaxime to D-ala-D-ala-peptidase reveals a functional basis of a natural mutation in a low-affinity penicillin-binding protein and in extended-spectrum β-lactamases. Biochemistry 34:9532–9540.

22. Laible, G., and R. Hakenbeck. Unpublished data.

23. Laible, G., and R. Hakenbeck. 1991. Five independent combinations of mutations can result in low-affinity penicillin-binding protein 2x of *Streptococcus pneumoniae*. J. Bacteriol. 173:6986–6990.

24. Laible, G., R. Hakenbeck, M.A. Sicard, B. Joris, and J.-M. Ghuysen. 1989. Nucleotide sequences of the *pbpX* genes encoding the penicillin-binding protein 2x from *Streptococcus pneumoniae* R6 and a cefotaxime-resistant mutant, C506. Mol. Microbiol. 3:1337–1348.

25. Laible, G., B.G. Spratt, and R. Hakenbeck. 1991. Inter-species recombinational events during the evolution of altered PBP 2x genes in penicillin-resistant clinical isolates of *Streptococcus pneumoniae*. Mol. Microbiol. 5:1993–2002.

26. Liu, H.H., and A. Tomasz. 1985. Penicillin tolerance in multiply drug-resistant natural isolates of *Streptococcus pneumoniae*. J. Infect. Dis. 152:365–372.

27. Martin, C., C. Sibold, and R. Hakenbeck. 1992. Relatedness of penicillin-binding protein 1a genes from different clones of penicillin-resistant *Streptococcus pneumoniae* isolated in South Africa and Spain. E.M.B.O. J. 11:3831–3836.

28. McDougal, L.K., J.K. Rasheed, J.W. Biddle, and F.C. Tenover. 1995. Identification of multiple clones of extended-spectrum cephalosporin-resistant *Streptococcus pneumoniae* isolates in the United States. Antimicrob. Agents Chemother. 39:2282–2288.

29. Muñóz, R., J.M. Musser, M. Crain, D.E. Briles, A. Marton, A.J. Parkinson, U. Sorensen, and A. Tomasz. 1992. Geographic distribution of penicillin-resistant clones of *Streptococcus pneumoniae*: characterization by penicillin-binding protein profile, surface protein A typing, and multilocus enzyme analysis. Clin. Infect. Dis. 15:112–118.

30. Paik, J., I. Kern, R. Lurz, and R. Hakenbeck. 1999. Mutational analysis of the *Streptococcus pneumoniae* bimodular class A penicillin-binding proteins. J. Bacteriol., in press.

31. Pares, S., N. Mouz, Y. Pétillot, R. Hakenbeck, and O. Dideberg. 1996. X-ray structure of *Streptococcus pneumoniae*. PBP2x, a primary penicillin target enzyme. Nat. Struct. Biol. 3:284–289.

32. Reichmann, P., A. König, J. Liñares, F. Alcaide, F.C. Tenover, L. McDougal, S. Swidsinski, and R. Hakenbeck. 1997. A global gene pool for high-level cephalosporin resistance in commensal *Streptococcus spp.* and *Streptococcus pneumoniae*. J. Infect. Dis. 176:1001–1012.

33. Reichmann, P., A. König, A. Marton, and R. Hakenbeck. 1996. Penicillin-binding proteins as resistance determinants in clinical isolates of *Streptococcus pneumoniae*. Microbial Drug Resist. 2:177–181.

34. Reichmann, P., E. Varon, E. Günther, R.R. Reinert, P. Lütticken, A. Marton, P. Geslin, J. Wagner, and R. Hakenbeck.

35. Schuster, C., B. Dobrinski, and R. Hakenbeck. 1990. Unusual septum formation in *Streptococcus pneumoniae* mutants with an alteration in the D,D-carboxypeptidase penicillin-binding protein 3. J. Bacteriol. 172:6499–6505.

36. Sibold, C. 1993. Epidemiologie von Penicillin-Resistenz in *Streptococcus pneumoniae*: Verwandtschaftsanalyse klinischer Isolate und Verbreitung homologer Penicillin-bindender Proteine. Dissertation. Freie Universität, Berlin.

37. Sibold, C., J. Henrichsen, A. König, C. Martin, L. Chalkley, and R. Hakenbeck. 1994. Mosaic *pbpX* genes of major clones of penicillin-resistant *Streptococcus pneumoniae* have evolved from *pbpX* genes of a penicillin-sensitive *Streptococcus oralis*. Mol. Microbiol. 12:1013–1023.

38. Sibold, C., J. Wang, J. Henrichsen, and R. Hakenbeck. 1992. Genetic relationship of penicillin-susceptible and -resistant *Streptococcus pneumoniae* strains isolated on different continents. Infect. Immunol. 60:4119–4126.

39. Sifaoul, F., M.-D. Kitzis, and L. Gutmann. 1996. *In vitro* selection of one-step mutants of *Streptococcus pneumoniae* resistant to different oral β-lactam antibiotics is associated with alterations of PBP2x. Antimicrob. Agents Chemother. 40:152–156.

40. Smith, A.M., and K.P. Klugman. 1998. Alterations in PBP1A essential for high-level penicillin resistance in *Streptococcus pneumoniae*. Antimicrob. Agents Chemother. 42:1329–1333.

41. Spratt, B.G. 1994. Resistance to β-lactam antibiotics. *In* J.-M. Ghuysen and R. Hakenbeck (eds.), Bacterial cell wall. Elsevier Science B.V., Amsterdam, pp. 517–534.

42. Tomasz, A. 1988. Resistance and tolerance to β-lactam antibiotics in pneumococci and in *Staphylococcus aureus*. *In* P. Actor, L. Daneo-Moore, M.L. Higgins, M.R.J. Salton, and G.D. Shockman (eds.), Antibiotic inhibition of bacterial cell surface assembly and function. American Society for Microbiology, Washington, D.C., pp. 616–627.

43. Tuomanen, E., and A. Tomasz. 1991. Mechanism of phenotypic tolerance of nongrowing pneumococci to beta-lactam antibiotics. Scand. J. Infect. Dis. 23(Suppl 74):S102–S112.

44. van der Linden, M., and R. Hakenbeck. Unpublished data.

45. Zähner, D., T. Grebe, E. Guenzi, J. Krauβ, M. van der Linden, K. Terhune, J.B. Stock, and R. Hakenbeck. 1996. Resistance determinants for β-lactam antibiotics in laboratory mutants of *Streptococcus pneumoniae* that are involved in genetic competence. Microbial Drug Resis. 2:187–191.

1995. Penicillin-resistant *Streptococcus pneumoniae* in Germany: genetic relationship to clones from other European countries. J. Med. Microbiol. 43:377–385.

Address reprint requests to:
Regine Hakenbeck
University of Kaiserslautern
Department of Microbiology
Paul-Ehrlichstrasse 23
D-67663 Kaiserslautern
Germany

The Molecular Mechanisms of Tetracycline Resistance in the Pneumococcus

CAROL A. WIDDOWSON and KEITH P. KLUGMAN

ABSTRACT

Tetracycline resistance in the pneumococcus is a result of the acquisition of one of two resistance determinants, *tet*(M) or *tet*(O). These genes encode ribosomal protection proteins that have homology to the elongation factors G and Tu. Tet(M) and Tet(O) both have GTPase activity that appears to be important in the displacement of tetracycline from the ribosome. Modification of tRNA may also be important for tetracycline resistance. Transcription of *tet*(M) is thought to be regulated by transcriptional attenuation. Transcription of *tet*(O) is constitutive, however, upstream of the gene are sequences that also appear to be involved in transcriptional attenuation. *tet*(M) is transferred on the conjugative transposons, Tn*1545* and Tn*5151*. It is not yet known whether *tet*(O) is transported on transposons or plasmids, or whether it is chromosomally integrated, in pneumococci.

INTRODUCTION

TETRACYCLINE IS A BROAD-SPECTRUM ANTIBIOTIC used in the treatment of both Gram-positive and Gram-negative infections.[14] The wide activity range of this antibiotic and the fact that it can be administered orally, is relatively inexpensive, and has few side effects for older children and adults, has made it a popular choice to prescribe for bacterial infections.[55] Such widespread use, however, has resulted in resistance developing in many bacteria, including pneumococci. Tetracycline resistance in the pneumococcus was first reported in 1963. This strain was isolated from a 10-month-old child in New South Wales, Australia, suffering from pneumococcal meningitis.[21] Since 1963, tetracycline resistance has been found in pneumococci globally. The spread of this resistance can, to a large extent, be attributed to the presence of tetracycline resistance genes on mobile, conjugative transposons.

TETRACYCLINE: STRUCTURE AND MODE OF ACTION

All clinically useful tetracyclines have a four-ring basic structure, with substituent variations at carbons 5, 6 or 7 (see Reference 13). These variations do not usually affect the activity of the antibiotic in bacteria.[14] Tetracyclines cause bacteristasis by binding to a high affinity site, the acceptor site (A site), on the 30S ribosomal subunit of the bacteria.[20] Where aminoacetyl-tRNA binding is at a high level, the tetracycline also binds to the peptidyl-donor site (P site) on the ribosome.[22] The antibiotic reduces the affinity of the A site for aminoacyl-tRNA by 80%[20] and the affinity of the P site for aminoacyl-tRNA by 50%.[20,22] Such binding disrupts the interactions between the aminoacyl-tRNA and the mRNA, thus preventing translation.

There are a few tetracycline analogues, such as chleocardin and 6-thiatetracycline, that are bactericidal in all susceptible bacteria and are thought to disrupt the cellular membrane of the bacteria.[44] However, these tetracyclines are not used clinically because they are thought to disrupt mammalian cellular membranes also (see Reference 13).

THE GENETIC BASIS OF TETRACYCLINE RESISTANCE IN PNEUMOCOCCI

The most commonly found tetracycline resistance gene in pneumococci, is *tet(M)*. This gene was first described in *Streptococcal* species by Burdett, Inamine, and Rajagopalan.[9] It has since been described in diverse species such as *Clostridium*,[50] *Listeria*,[42] *Mycoplasma*,[49] *Ureaplasma*,[48] *Gardnerella*,[47] *Neisseria*,[39] *Eikenella*,[28] *Kingella*,[28] and *Haemophilis*.[45]

Pneumococcal Diseases Research Unit of the Medical Research Council, the South African Institute for Medical Research and the University of Witwatersrand, Department of Clinical Microbiology and Infectious Diseases, South African Institute for Medical Research, P.O. Box 1038, Johannesburg 2000, South Africa.
Reprinted from *Microbial Drug Resistance*, Vol. 4, No. 1, 1998.

Recently *tet(O)* has also been described in South African pneumococci,[64] tet(O) is more commonly a resistance determinant in *Campylobacter* species[54] but has been described in streptococcal species, such as *S. mutans,*[30] *S. milleri,* and group B streptococci.[67]

The *tet(O)* and *tet(M)* genes are closely related, sharing ~76% nucleotide sequence homology and 77% amino acid homology.[54] Both genes have open reading frames of 1917 bases which encode 72,5 kDa proteins in pneumococci.[35,64]

MECHANISMS OF TETRACYCLINE RESISTANCE

Three different mechanisms have been described in bacteria for resistance to tetracycline. Active efflux of tetracycline from the cell is a method used by both Gram-positive and Gram-negative bacteria, for protection against tetracycline. This is brought about through membrane-bound efflux proteins that exchange one proton for a tetracycline-cation complex.[32] The genes *tet(A–E), (G), (H), (K), (L),* and *(P)* encode proteins involved in active efflux.[25,26,31,37,38,41,53] Ribosomal protection is another mechanism of resistance to tetracycline. The genes *tet(M), (O), (S), B*(P), and *(Q),* and Otr A encode proteins involved in ribosomal protection.[4,12,19,40,46,53,54] Enzymatic alteration of tetracycline has also been reported,[41] however, this form of resistance appears to only have developed in *Bacteroides.* Ribosomal protection is the only mechanism of tetracycline resistance in pneumococci described thus far. In vitro protein synthesising systems have shown that protein synthesis is not prevented by tetracycline when cell extracts are prepared from cells carrying *tet(M)*[4] or *tet(O).*[34] In addition, tetracycline accumulates in susceptible cells at the same rate as it does in resistant cells, indicating that active efflux does not occur,[4] and the tetracycline extracted from resistant cells retains its biologic activity and is unmodified.[4]

Numerous models have been proposed for the mechanism of tetracycline resistance through ribosomal protection. However, most of these models have been disputed. While various, important observations have been made, a feasible model has only been proposed very recently, with new findings by Burdett.[8]

HOMOLOGY OF RIBOSOMAL PROTECTION PROTEINS TO ELONGATION FACTORS

Both *tet(O)* and *tet(M)* encode proteins of approximately 72kDa, as do all ribosomal protection proteins involved in tetracycline resistance (see Reference 58). The N-terminal regions of these proteins show homology to 5 different translational elongation factors, particularly to elongation factors Tu and G (Ef-Tu and Ef-G).[51] The N-terminal region of the elongation factors consists of five conserved motifs, designated G1 to G5, which are involved in GTP-GDP binding (see Reference 58). It has been suggested that Tet(M) could act as a tetracycline-resistant elongation factor.[51]

Of the two elongation factors, Ef-G and Ef-Tu, ribosomal protection proteins resemble Ef-G more closely.[34] Ef-Tu is abundant in the cell, whereas Ef-G is only produced in small amounts (1 molecule per ribosome). Ef-G has a higher degree of homology with the ribosomal protection proteins than Ef-Tu, and these factors share similar molecular masses (80kDa and ~72kDa respectively) (see Reference 34). A specific Gly residue that is critical for Ef-Tu function[27] is replaced by Ala in both Ef-G and the ribosomal protection proteins.[34]

Ef-G is a catalyst for the translocation step of protein synthesis, in which the mRNA, together with the associated tRNAs, moves relative to the ribosome, placing the next codon of the mRNA in position to be translated.[1] Ef-G is a GTPase that functions as a molecular switch where Ef-G is active in the GTP conformation, and inactive in the GDP conformation.[1] Translocation can occur when Ef-G is absent[23]; however, translocation occurs faster and more efficiently with Ef-G as a catalyst.[52]

Tet(M) has been purified and shown to have GTPase activity that appears to be catalytic.[6] Substitutions in the GTP-binding domain of *tet(O)* cause a loss of tetracycline resistance conferred by Tet(O).[24] Very small quantities of ribosomal protection proteins are required for resistance, as revealed by protein analysis of S-100 fractions used to convert sensitive ribosomes to resistance.[34] Both RP-HPLC and SDS are unable to detect ribosomal protection proteins in active tetracycline resistant 100-S fractions. Manavathu and co-workers[34] were also unable to overproduce Tet(O) using three different expression vectors (*tac, λ*PL and T7) into which *tet(O)* had been cloned. Tet(O) was undetectable by coomassie blue staining despite the resistance phenotype. These observations suggest a catalytic function for both *tet(M)* and *tet(O).*

Despite the similarities between ribosomal protection proteins and Ef-G, however, Tet(M) is unable to replace Ef-G in *Escherichia coli* mutants (and Ef-Tu in *Bacillus subtilis*) that are temperature sensitive for Ef-G (or Ef-Tu).[6] In addition, translocation and ribosome-dependent hydrolysis of GTP, the functions of Ef-G, are not inhibited by tetracycline.[7]

TETRACYCLINE RELEASE FROM THE RIBOSOME

Previously, it was shown that Tet(O) does not interfere with the binding of tetracycline to the ribosome.[24,34] This has now been disputed by Burdett.[8] In a recently published paper, Burdett showed that in the absence of GTP, tetracycline binding to the ribosome occurs at the same rate in the presence or absence of Tet(M). However, with the addition of GTP, Tet(M) promotes the release of tetracycline from ribosomes. This release is limited when 5′ guanylylimidodiphosphate, a nonhydrolyzable analogue of GTP, is substituted for GTP. Hydrolysis of GTP therefore appears to be necessary for full release of tetracycline from the ribosomes.[8] This is a particularly significant finding because, previously, all models have discounted the ability of ribosomal protection proteins to dislodge tetracycline from the ribosome. The necessary hydrolysis of GTP may account for the similarities between Tet(M) and the elongation factors.

tRNA MODIFICATION

E. coli strains containing mutations in the *miaA* locus, show reduced levels of tetracycline resistance in the presence of

Tet(M).[7] The *miaA* gene is responsible for encoding an activity that modifies position A37 immediately 3' of the anticodon of tRNA that reads codons beginning with U, such as tRNAs for phenylalanine, tryptophan, tyrosine, cysteine, leucine, and serine.[56] Aberrant translation results from undermodification of these tRNAs.[3,66] It therefore appears that modification of tRNA is important for efficient translation. Burdett[7] suggested that tRNA modification may be important in the mechanism of tetracycline inhibition of protein synthesis. Tet(M) may be involved in modifying the tRNA appropriately, thus preventing tetracycline inhibition. When a mutation is present in the *miaA* locus, Tet(M) may not be able to stabilize the tRNA interactions sufficiently for protein synthesis to occur normally.

REGULATION OF TET(*M*) TRANSCRIPTION

Transcription of *tet(M)* is controlled by a simple regulatory system, transcriptional attenuation, encoded upstream from the structural gene. Resistant bacteria, growing under drug-free conditions, are able to restrict the amount of Tet(M) produced to a low basal level. With exposure to tetracycline, exaggerated amounts of Tet(M) are synthesized.

Transcriptional attenuation is made possible by the presence of a short open reading frame upstream of the structural gene that encodes GC rich RNA that easily forms secondary hairpin structures because of the presence of inverted repeat sequences and that are followed by a run of U residues.[29] These hairpins and U residues act as transcription terminators in the following way (see Reference 65). The regulatory region is transcribed by polymerase, producing RNA that naturally forms hairpin structures. These structures are formed within the transcription bubble that occurs when the DNA uncoils during transcription. The presence of the hairpin structure may cause the polymerase to pause. If the RNA/DNA hybrid downstream of the hairpin is weakly stabilized, the RNA will be released, the DNA bubble will close and the polymerase will dissociate from the DNA. This weak stabilization of the RNA/DNA hybrid can be a result of a run of U residues, since oligo(dU).oligo(dA), formed by RNA/DNA interactions, is particularly unstable in comparison to oligo(dT).oligo(dA), formed by DNA/DNA interactions.

Su and co-workers[57] described a short open reading frame upstream from *tet(M)*, encoding a 28 amino-acid peptide. This open reading frame is preceded by a potential ribosomal binding site and a putative promoter. There is also a stop codon for this open reading frame very close to the ribosome binding site of *tet(M)*. There are 4 methionines present within the first 8 amino acid residues and 4 pairs of inverted repeats. The 3rd pair of inverted repeats is followed by a run of U residues. Su and co-workers[57] suggested that this is involved in transcriptional attenuation. The following mechanism for transcriptional attenuation has been proposed[57] for *tet(M)*: Under drug-free conditions, translation continues normally for the first peptide bond of the leader peptide upstream from *tet(M)*. Translation is then retarded because 5 out of the next 7 codons require rare aminoacyl-tRNAs. Transcription continues until it reaches the termination site, created by the secondary RNA structure and the 5 U residues. Either termination of transcription occurs, or read through may occur and transcription is then either terminated at the weaker termination site, created by the fourth in-

verted repeat sequence, which is also followed by a series of U residues, or read through continues through to *tet(M)*. Read-through to *tet(M)* is possible particularly if the ribosome translating the RNA is close to the transcription bubble. This may be the reason for a low-level basal production of Tet(M) prior to exposure to tetracycline. When tetracycline is present in the bacteria, all transcription and translation is delayed because of tetracycline occupying the A and P sites on the ribosomes. This increases the availability of all aminoacyl-tRNAs, including the rare ones. Increased availability of these aminoacyl-tRNAs speeds up translation of the leader peptide. When translation occurs shortly behind transcription, the ribosome destabilises the secondary structure of the developing mRNA, allowing transcription to continue through to *tet(M)*. This is possible because the leader peptide stop site, the Shine and Dalgarno site, and the translation initiation site are optimal for Tet(M) synthesis.

Thus, translation of *tet(M)* is highly regulated. It has been suggested with respect to translational attenuation,[33] that one of the reasons for attenuation as opposed to the usual regulation involving regulatory proteins, is that a low level of the resistance proteins can be maintained in the cell before exposure to the drug. This may have be advantageous when the bacterium is first exposed to the drug, allowing time for high levels of the resistance proteins to be produced. This may also be a reason for transcriptional regulation as a means of genetic control. As previously stated, read through of the termination sites can occur, particularly if translation occurs immediately after transcription, resulting in low levels of Tet(M) in resistant bacteria prior to exposure to tetracycline. Although Su and coworkers[57] were working on *tet(M)* from Tn*916*, there also appears to be a similar regulatory system for *tet(M)* on Tn*1545*, in which there is a stemloop structure extending from positions 51–99 upstream of the structural gene start codon consisting of 2 perfect inverted repeat sequences separated by 6bp.[35]

Although, leader peptides have not been described in *tet(O)*, the DNA sequences flanking *tet(M)* and *tet(O)* share a higher degree of homology than the actual protein-coding sequences.[35] There are two palimdromic sequences followed by 5 T residues 41 nucleotides upstream of *tet(O)*, which resembles a transcription terminator.[63] These upstream sequences appear to be important to full expression of tetracycline resistance.[63] This suggests a control sequence. However, expression of tetracycline resistance in *Campylobacter C. jejuni* is constitutive.[59] It is not yet known whether expression is constitutive or inducible in pneumococci.

TRANSFER OF TETRACYCLINE RESISTANCE DETERMINANTS IN PNEUMOCOCCI

The *tet*(M) gene is situated on two transposons in pneumococci. Tn*1545* is a 25,3kb conjugative transposon containing the resistance determinants *aph*A-3, for resistance to kanamycin and other structurally related aminoglycosides, *erm*Am, for resistance to macrolide, lincosamide and streptogramin-B type antibiotics, and *tet(M)*, for resistance to tetracycline.[11,17] Tn*1545* shares a high degree of homology, having identical termini, to another transposon, Tn*916*, first isolated in *E. faecalis*.[10,16] Tn*1545* is able to conjugate and transpose to a variety of organisms such as *E. faecalis*,[17] *S. lactis*,[17] *S.*

diacetylactis,[17] *S. cremoris,*[17] *S. sanguis,*[17] *S. aureus,*[17] *B. subtilis*[18] and *Lysteria monocytogenes.*[17]

The *tet*(M) gene was also found to be part of a 65,5kb conjugative transposon, originally called Ω(cat-tet),[62] and now called Tn*5253*.[2] It has since been found that Tn*5253* comprises two independent transposons, Tn*5251,* carrying tet*(M),* inserted into Tn*5252,* carrying a chloramphenicol resistance gene.[2] Tn*5251* resembles the Tn*1545*/Tn*916* class of elements.[2,43] In a 4419 base pair segment containing *tet(M),* only 73 nucleotides differ in Tn*5251* and Tn*916*.[4] Most of these differences occur in the *tet(M)* regions, which are 90% homologous.[5,43] The tet genes from Tn*5251* and Tn*1545* are identical.[43] It is not clear whether Tn*5251* is able to conjugate independently of Tn5253.[43,2]

tet(O) in streptococci can be conjugatively transferred to other Gram-positive bacteria on plasmids.[67] Plasmids are not common in pneumococci, however. It is possible that pneumococci received the *tet(O)* gene via a streptococcal plasmid through conjugation. The gene may have integrated into the chromosome by homologous recombination, losing the rest of the plasmid. This may account for the relative scarcity of *tet(O)* in pneumococci. Alternatively, pneumococci are naturally transformable and could have acquired the *tet(O)* gene through transformation.

It is thought that *tet(M)* and *tet(O)* diverged from a common Gram-positive ancestor. While *tet(M)* became common in other streptococci and enterococci, *tet(O),* became rare in these Gram-positive bacteria, and more common in the Gram-negative *Campylobacter* species. There are several reasons for believing that *tet(O)* originated in Streptococci and not *Campylobacter* species. First, the G-C content of *tet(O)* is significantly higher than that from *C. jejuni,* and *C. coli* (40% compared to 31% and 33%, respectively).[54] Second, the codon usage in *tet(O)* is close to the codon usage of streptococcal genes.[54] Third, there is complimentarity between the tet*(O)* ribosomal binding site and the 3′ terminus of the 16S rRNA of *B. subtilis.*[54] The ribosomal binding site is a feature which is able to distinguish Gram-positive from Gram negative bacteria.[36] And fourth, the kanamycin resistance gene *aph*A3, which is common in Gram-positive cocci, is present with *tet(O)* on the plasmid pIP1433, a plasmid in *Campylobacter.*[60,61] The acquisition of *aph*A3 by *C. coli* is thought to be recent and to have occurred by in vivo transfer from Gram-positive to Gram-negative bacteria.[60]

The significance of the location of *tet(M)* and *tet(O)* on conjugative transposons and plasmids is enormous. Tn*916*/Tn*1545* class of transposons have been either introduced into or occur naturally in at least 52 different Gram-positive and Gram-negative bacterial species (see Reference 15). Such spread of antibiotic resistance genes and obvious positive selection for bacteria containing these genes, has resulted in tetracycline ceasing to be a feasible treatment for many infections.

REFERENCES

1. AEvarsson, A., E. Brazhnikov, M. Garber, J. Zheltonosova, Y. Chirgadze, S. Al-Karadaghi, L.A. Svensson, and A. Liljas. 1994. Three dimensional structure of the ribosomal translocase: elongation factor G from *Thermus thermophilus.* EMBO J. **13**:3669–3677.

2. Ayoubi, P., A.O. Kilic, and M.N. Vijayakumar. 1991. Tn*5253,* the pneumococcal Ω(*cat tet*) BM6001 element, is a composite structure of two conjugative transposons, Tn*5251* and Tn*5252.* J Bacteriol. **173**:1617–1622.

3. Bouadloun, F., T. Srichaiyo, L.A. Isaksson, and G.R. Bjork. 1986. Influence of modification next to the anticodon in tRNA on codon sensitivity of translational suppression and accuracy. J Bacteriol. **166**:1022–1027.

4. Burdett, V. 1986. Streptococcal tetracycline resistance mediated at the level of protein biosynthesis. J Bacteriol. **165**:564–569.

5. Burdett, V. 1990. Nucleotide sequence of the *tet*(M) gene of Tn*916.* Nucleic Acids Res. **18**:6137.

6. Burdett, V. 1991. Purification and characterisation of Tet(M), a protein that renders ribosomes resistant to tetracycline. J. Biol. Chem. **266**:2872–2877.

7. Burdett, V. 1993. tRNA Modification actvity is necessary for Tet(M)-mediated tetracycline resistance. J. Bacteriol. **175**:7209–7215.

8. Burdett, V. 1996. Tet(M)-promoted release of tetracycline from ribosomes is GTP dependent. J. Bacteriol. **178**:3246–3251.

9. Burdett, V., J. Inamine, and S. Rajagopalan. 1982. Heterogeneity of tetracycline resistance determinants in *Streptococcus.* J. Bacteriol. **149**:995–1004.

10. Caillaud, F. and P. Courvalin. 1987. Nucleotide sequence of the ends of the conjugative shuttle transposon Tn*1545.* Mol. Gen. Genet. **209**:110–115.

11. Caillaud, F., C. Carlier, and P. Courvalin. 1987. Physical analysis of the conjugative shuttle transposon Tn*1545.* Plasmid **17**:58–60.

12. Charpentier, E., G. Gerbaud, and P. Courvalin. 1993. Characterization of a new class of tetracycline-resistance gene *tet*(S) in *Listeria monocytogenes* BM4210. Gene **131**:27–34.

13. Chopra, I., P.M. Hawkey, and M. Hinton. 1992. Tetracyclines, molecular and clinical aspects. J. Antimicrob. Chemother. **29**:245–277.

14. Chopra, I., T.G.B. Howe, A.H. Linton, K.B. Linton, M.H. Richmond, and D.C.E. Speller. 1981. The tetracyclines: prospects at the beginning of the 1980s. J. Antimicrob. Chemother. **8**:5–21.

15. Clewell, D.B., S.E. Flannagan, and D.D. Jaworski. 1995. Unconstrained bacterial promiscuity: the Tn*916*-Tn*1545* family of conjugative transposons. Trends in Microbiol. **3**:229–236.

16. Clewell, D.B., S.E. Flannagan, Y. Ike, J.M. Jones, and C. Gawron-Burke. 1988. Sequence analysis of the termini of conjugative transposon Tn*916.* J. Bacteriol. **170**:3046–3052.

17. Courvalin, P. and Carlier, C. 1986. Transposable multiple antibiotic resistance in *Streptococcus pneumoniae.* Mol. Gen. Genet. **205**:291–297.

18. Courvalin, P., and C. Carlier. 1987. Tn*1545:* A conjugative shuttle transposon. Mol. Gen. Genet. **206**:259–264.

19. Dittrich, W., and H. Schrempf. 1992. The unstable tetracycline resistance gene of *Streptomyces lividans* 1326 encodes a putative protein with similarities to translational elongation factors and Tet(M) and Tet(O) proteins. Antimicrob. Agents Chemother. **36**:1119–1124.

20. Epe, B., P. Woolley, and H. Hornig. 1987. Competition between tetracycline and tRNA at both P and A sites of the ribosome of *Escherichia coli.* FEB **213**:443–447.

21. Evans, W., and D. Hansman. 1963. Tetracycline-resistant pneumococcus. Lancet **1**:451.

22. Geigenmuller, U., and K.H. Nierhaus. 1986. Tetracycline can inhibit tRNA binding to the ribosomal P site as well as to the A site. Eur. J. Biochem. **161**:723–726.

23. Gravrilova, L.P., O.E. Kostiashkina, V.E. Koteliansky, N.M. Rutkevitch, and A.S. Spirin. 1976. Factor-free ("non-enzymatic") and factor-dependent systems of translation of polyurdylic acid by *Escherichia coli* ribosomes. J. Mol. Biol. **101**:537–552.

24. Grewal, J., E.K. Manavathu, and D.E. Taylor. 1993. Effect of

mutational alteration of Asn-128 in the putative GTP-binding domain of tetracycline resistance determinant Tet(O) from *Campylobacter jejuni*. Antimicrob. Agents Chemother. **37**:2645–2649.

25. **Guay, G.G., S.A. Khan, and D.M. Rothstein.** 1993. The *tet*(K) gene of plasmid pT181 of *Staphylococcus aureus* encodes an efflux protein that contains 14 transmembrane helices. Plasmid **30**:163–166.

26. **Hansen, L.M., L.M. McMurry, S.B. Levy, and D.C. Hirsh.** 1993. A new teracycline resistance determinant, Tet H, from *Pasteurella multocida* specifying active efflux of tetracycline. Antimicrob. Agents Chemother. **37**:2699–2705.

27. **Jacquet, E., and A. Parmeggiani.** 1988. Structure–function relationships in the GTP binding domain of Ef-Tu: mutation of Val20, the residue homologous to position 12 in p21. EMBO J. **7**:2861–2867.

28. **Knapp, J.S., S.R. Johnson, J.M. Zenilman, M.C. Roberts, and S.A. Morse.** 1988. High-level tetracycline resistance resulting from Tet M in strains of *Neisseria* species, *Kingella denitrificans,* and *Eikenella corrodens*. Antimicrob. Agents Chemother. **32**:765–767.

29. **Landick, R. and C. Yanofsky.** 1987. Transcription attenuation, pp1276–1301. *In* F.C. Neidhardt, J.L. Ingraham, K.B. Low, B. Magasanik, M. Schaechter, and H.E. Umbarger (eds.), Escherichia coli and Salmonella Typhimurium: Cellular and Molecular Biology, vol. 2, American Society for Microbiology, Washington D.C.

30. **LeBlanc, D.J., L.N. Lee, B.M. Titmas, C.J. Smith, and F.C. Tenover.** 1988. Nucleotide sequence analysis of tetracycline resistance gene *tetO* from *Streptococcus mutans* DL5. J. Bacteriol. **170**:3618–3626.

31. **Levy, S.B.** 1989. Evolution and spread of tetracycline resistance determinants. J. Antimicrob. Chemother. **24**:1–3.

32. **Levy, S.B.** 1992. Active efflux mechanisms for antimicrobial resistance. Antimicrob. Agents Chemother. **36**:695–703.

33. **Lovett, P.S.** 1990. Translational attenuation as the regulator of inducible *cat* genes. J. Bacteriol. **172**:1–6.

34. **Manavathu, E.K., C.L. Fernandez, B.S. Cooperman, and D.E. Taylor.** 1990. Molecular studies on the mechanism of tetracycline resistance mediated by Tet(O). Antimicrob. Agents Chemother. **34**:71–77.

35. **Martin, P., P. Trieu-Cuot, and P. Courvalin.** 1986. Nucleotide sequence of the *tetM* tetracycline resistance determinant of the streptococcal conjugative transposon Tn*1545*. Nucleic Acids Res. **14**:7047–7058.

36. **McLaughlin, J.R., C.L. Murray, and J.C. Rabinowitz.** 1981. Unique features in the binding site sequence of the Gram-positive *Staphylococcus aureus* β-lactamase gene. J. Biol. Chem. **256**:11283–11291.

37. **McMurry, L., R.E. Petrucci, Jr., and S. Levy.** 1980. Active efflux of tetracycline encoded by four genetically different tetracycline resistance determinants in *Escherichia coli*. Proc. Natl. Acad. Sci. USA **77**:3974–3977.

38. **McMurry, L., B.H. Park, V. Burdett, and S.B. Levy.** 1987. Energy-dependent efflux mediated by class L (TetL) tetracycline resistance determinant from streptococci. Antimicrob. Agents Chemother. **31**:1648–1650.

39. **Morse, S.A., S.R. Johnson, J.W. Biddle, and M.C. Roberts.** 1986. High-level tetracycline resistance in *Neisseria gonorrhoeae* is a result of acquisition of streptococcal *tetM* determinant. Antimicrob. Agents Chemother. **30**:664–670.

40. **Nikolich, M.P., N.B. Shoemaker, and A.A. Salyers.** 1992. A *Bacteroides* tetracycline resistance gene represents a new class of ribosome protection tetracycline resistance. Antimicrob. Agents Chemother. **36**:1005–1012.

41. **Park, B.H., and S.B. Levy.** 1988. The cryptic tetracycline resistance determinant on Tn*4400* mediates tetracycline degradation as well as tetracycline efflux. Antimicrob. Agents Chemother. **32**:1797–1800.

42. **Poyart-Salmeron, C., P. Trieu-Cuot, C. Carlier, A. MacGowan, J. McLauchlin, and P. Courvalin.** 1992. Genetic basis of tetracycline resistance in clinical isolates of Listeria monocytogenes. Antimicrob. Agents Chemother. **36**:463–466.

43. **Proveddi, R., R. Manganelli, and G. Pozzi.** 1996. Characterization of conjugative transposon Tn*5251* of *Streptococcus pneumoniae*. FEMS Microb. Letts. **135**:231–236.

44. **Rasmussen, B., H.F. Noller, G. Daubresse, B. Oliva, Z. Misulovin, D.M. Rothstein, G.A. Ellestad, Y. Gluzman, F.P. Tally, and I. Chopra.** 1991. Molecular basis of tetracycline action: identification of analogs whose primary target is not the bacterial ribosome. Antimicrob. Agents Chemother. **35**:2306–2311.

45. **Roberts, M.C.** 1989. Plasmid-mediated Tet M in *Haemophilus ducreyi*. Antimicrob. Agents Chemother. **33**:1611–1613.

46. **Roberts, M.C.** 1994. Epidemiology of tetracycline-resistance determinants. Trends in Microbiology **2**:353–357.

47. **Roberts, M.C., S.L. Hillier, J. Hale, K.K. Holmes, and G.E. Kenny.** 1986. Tetracycline resistance and *tetM* in pathogenic urogenital bacteria. Antimicrob. Agents Chemother. **30**:810–812.

48. **Roberts, M.C., and G.E. Kenny.** 1986. Dissemination of the *tetM* tetracycline resistance determinant to *Ureaplasma urealyticum*. Antimicrob. Agents Chemother. **29**:350–352.

49. **Roberts, M.C., L.A. Koutsky, K.K. Holmes, D.L. LeBlanc, and G.E. Kenny.** 1985. Tetracycline-resistant *Mycoplasma hominis* strains contain streptococcal *tetM* sequences. Antimicrob. Agents Chemother. **28**:141–143.

50. **Roberts, M.C., L.V. McFarland, P. Mullany, and M.E. Mulligan.** 1994. Characterization of the genetic basis of antibiotic resistance in *Clostridium difficile*. J. Antimicrob. Chemother. **33**: 419–429.

51. **Sanchez-Pescador, R., J.T. Brown, M. Roberts, and M.S. Urdea.** 1988. Homology of the TetM with translational elongation factors: implications for potential modes of tetM conferred tetracycline resistance. Nucleic Acid Res. **16**:1218.

52. **Schilling-Bartetzko, S., A. Bartetzko, and K.H. Nierhaus.** 1992. Kinetic and thermodynamic parameters for tRNA binding to the ribosome and for the translocation reaction. J. Biol. Chem. **267**:4703–4712.

53. **Sloan, J., L.M. McMurry, D. Lyras, S.B. Levy, and J.I. Rood.** 1994. The *Clostridium perfringens* Tet P determinant comprises two overlapping genes: *tetA*(P), which mediates active tetracycline efflux, and *tetB*(P), which is related to the ribosomal protection family of tetracycline-resistance determinants. Mol. Microbiol. **11**:403–415.

54. **Sougakoff, W., B. Papadopoulou, P. Nordmann, and P. Courvalin.** 1987. Nucleotide sequence and distribution of gene *tetO* encoding tetracycline resistance in *Campylobacter coli*. FEMS Microbiol. Lett **44**:153–159.

55. **Speer, B.S., N.B. Shoemaker, and A.A. Salyers.** 1992. Bacterial resistance to tetracycline: mechanisms, transfer, and clinical significance. Clin. Microbiol. Rev. **5**:387–399.

56. **Sprinzl, M., T. Hartmann, F. Meissner, J. Moll, and T. Vorderwulbecke.** 1987. Compilation of tRNA sequences and sequences of tRNA genes. Nucleic Acids Res. **15 Suppl**:r53–r188.

57. **Su, Y.A., P. He, and D.B. Clewell.** 1992. Characterization of the *tet*(M) determinant of Tn*916*: evidence for regulation by transcriptional attenuation. Antimicrob. Agents Chemother. **36**:769–778.

58. **Taylor, D.E., and A. Chau.** 1996. Tetracycline resistance mediated by ribosomal protection. Antimicrob. Agents Chemother. **40**: 1–5.

59. **Taylor, D.E., K. Hiratsuka, H. Ray, and E.K. Manavathu.** 1987. Characterization and expression of a cloned tetracycline resistance determinant from *Campylobacter jejuni* plasmid pUA466. J Bacteriol. **169**:2984–2989.

60. **Trieu-Cuot, P., and P. Courvalin.** 1986. Evolution and transfer

of aminoglycoside resistance genes under natural conditions. J. Antimicrob. Chemother. **18 Suppl. C:** 93–103.

61. **Trieu-Cuot, P., G. Gerbaud, T. Lambert, and Courvalin, P.** 1985. In vivo transfer of genetic information between Gram-positive and Gram-negative bacteria. EMBO J. **4:**3583–3587.

62. **Vijayakumar, M.N., S.D. Priebe, and W.R. Guild.** 1986. Structure of a conjugative element in *Streptococcus pneumoniae.* J. Bacteriol. **166:**978–984.

63. **Wang, Y., and D.E. Taylor.** 1991. A DNA sequence upstream of the *tet*(O) gene is required for full expression of tetracycline resistance. Antimicrob. Agents Chemother. **35:**2020–2025.

64. **Widdowson, C.A., K.P. Klugman, and D. Hanslo.** 1996. Identification of the tetracycline resistance gene, tet(O), in *Streptococcus pneumoniae.* Antimicrob. Agents Chemother. **40:**2891–2893.

65. **Yagar, T.D. and P.H. van Hippel.** 1987. Transcription elongation and termination in *Escherichia* coli, pp1241–1275. *In* F.C. Neidhardt, J.L. Ingraham, K.B. Low, B. Magasanik, M. Schaechter, and H.E. Umbarger (eds.), *Escherichia coli* and *Salmonella typhimurium:* Cellular and Molecular Biology, vol. 2, American Society for Microbiology, Washington D.C.

66. **Yanofsky, C. and L. Soll.** 1977. Mutations affecting tRNA-Trp and its charging and their effect on regulation of transcription at the attenuator of the tryptophan operon. J. Mol. Biol. **111:**663–677.

67. **Zilhao, R., B. Papadopoulou, and P. Courvalin.** 1988. Occurrence of the *Campylobacter* resistance gene *tetO* in *Enterococcus* and *Streptococcus* spp. Antimicrob. Agents Chemother. **32:**1793–1796.

Address reprint requests to:
Keith P. Klugman
South African Institute for Medical Research
Department of Medical Microbiology
P.O. Box 1038
Johannesburg 2000, South Africa

Part 6

Surveillance and Intervention

Streptococcus pneumoniae
Copyright © 2000 Mary Ann Liebert, Inc., 2 Madison Avenue, Larchmont, NY 10538

CEM/NET: Clinical Microbiology and Molecular Biology in Alliance

HERMINIA DE LENCASTRE,[1,2] ILDA SANTOS SANCHES,[3] and ALEXANDER TOMASZ[1]

BACKGROUND

ONE OF THE MOST IMPORTANT COMPONENTS of the emerging diseases in our era is the emergence and worldwide spread of antibiotic-resistant bacterial pathogens. That this process does not recognize national boundaries was most strikingly demonstrated by the intercontinental spread of multidrug-resistant epidemic clones of methicillin-resistant *Staphylococcus aureus* (MRSA) and multidrug-resistant *Streptococcus pneumoniae* clones. Clearly there is urgent need for operating international surveillance systems. The creation of such an international surveillance network is most naturally the mission of international and national public health agencies such as the World Health Organization (WHO) and the Centers for Disease Control (CDC), which private initiatives may supplement but cannot replace. However, it is conceivable that the resources of at least some of the currently burgeoning private, national, and regional surveillance efforts may gradually become integrated into an international surveillance system with harmonized methodologies and electronic communication link-ups to WHO.

The CEM/NET initiative to be described below has neither the capacity nor the intention to replace such a longitudinal surveillance system. Nevertheless, CEM/NET has already made, and can continue to make in the future, significant contributions to the international effort to control the emergence and spread of resistant bacteria through its unique and flexible organization, its heavily science-based operations, and its primarily prospective and problem-oriented undertakings.

The basic philosophy of CEM/NET recognizes the mutual dependence of clinical microbiologists and molecular microbiologists in understanding and contributing to the control of antibiotic-resistant pathogens. The interest of clinical microbiologists in collaborating with basic scientists is based on the fact that conventional methods for the typing of multidrug-resistant nosocomial and community-acquired pathogens are rapidly becoming obsolete. This is particularly true for multidrug-resistant Gram-positive pathogens such as *S. aureus*, coagulase-negative staphylococci, enterococci, *S. pneumoniae,* as well as *Mycobacterium.* Clinical microbiologists in search for new typing tools depend on the skills of molecular biologists to develop and streamline molecular fingerprinting methods to replace conventional typing techniques for tracking bacterial pathogens and other types of epidemiological problem solving.

The interest of molecular biologists

The introduction of massive quantities of antibacterial agents into the clinical environment during the past 50 years has created an evolutionary-scale force selecting for the emergence and worldwide spread of antibiotic-resistant pathogens that carry intriguing and novel genetic and biochemical mechanisms. This process is taking place entirely in the "real world" environment of microbes: in hospitals, day care centers, *etc., i.e.,* outside the walls of basic science microbiology laboratories. Yet this phenomenon is full of fascinating scientific novelty and it offers the basic scientist precious insights into the forces that shape this accelerated evolution, involving the movement of genes across species boundaries, processes by which new genotypes assemble, acquisition of regulatory mechanisms by the bacteria that allow optimal expression of a "foreign-born" resistance gene, properties essential for the virulence and epidemic spread of bacterial pathogens. Understanding these mechanisms is both a challenge and a unique opportunity for molecular biologists. The molecular biologist depends on the skills of clinical microbiologists for identifying the resistant isolates and for providing access to them for mechanistic analysis.

A disturbing aspect of the phenomenon of the resurgence of infectious diseases in our era is that the overwhelming majority of fatalities occur in the developing parts of the world due to a variety of factors, including the lack of availability of conventional antibacterial agents and the appearance of strains with drug resistance.

Building two kinds of bridges

The above scenario suggests the importance of building two kinds of bridges: one between the clinical environment in which the resistant pathogens emerge and the world of the microbiology science laboratory where these microbes can be taken apart

---

[1]Laboratory of Microbiology, The Rockefeller University, New York, NY 10021.
[2]Unidade de Genética Molecular, Instituto de Tecnologia Química e Biológica da Universidade Nova de Lisboa (ITQB/UNL), Oeiras, Portugal.
[3]Faculdade de Ciências e Tecnologia, Universidade Nova de Lisboa (FCT/UNL), Monte da Caparica, Portugal.

and their properties analyzed and understood. A second bridge is between science in developed countries and appropriate centers in developing countries, which receive an unusually large burden of the resurgent infectious diseases in our era. The first kind of "bridge" should be a mechanism by which microbial samples collected in epidemiologically meaningful projects are transferred into the basic science laboratories for analysis. Projects involve surveillance-type operations and basic science studies on the mechanisms of resistance. The second kind of "bridge" would involve exporting modern technology. For this reason, a major current activity of CEM/NET is educational: training clinical microbiologist colleagues in molecular fingerprinting techniques.

THE CEM/NET INITIATIVE:
UNIQUE STRUCTURE

It was the recognition of this need to build bridges of the two types that in 1994 led to the formation of CEM/NET (Center for Molecular Epidemiology and Network for Epidemiological Tracking of Antibiotic-Resistant Pathogens). Unlike most other surveillance systems, the core of CEM/NET initiative is two basic science microbiology laboratories, each with a considerable track record in the basic microbiology (genetics, biochemistry, and physiology) of antibiotic resistance and virulence: Laboratory of Microbiology at The Rockefeller University (headed by Alexander Tomasz), and the Molecular Genetics Unit at the Instituto de Tecnologia Química e Biológica (ITQB) affiliated with the Universidade Nova de Lisboa in Portugal (headed by Herminia de Lencastre) (Fig. 1).

CEM/NET may be defined as a loosely structured grass-roots initiative for collaborative projects between the core laboratories and clinical microbiologists and infectious diseases colleagues. For the clinical microbiologist, CEM/NET provides the high-powered tools of molecular fingerprinting for the analysis of epidemiological problems and surveillance. For the molecular biologist in the core laboratories, CEM/NET provides access to antibiotic resistant clinical isolates with their interesting and novel genetic and biochemical mechanisms. Membership in CEM/NET is voluntary, built on personal ties and collaboration, and may vary from project to project. This is an informal, grass-roots initiative, with minimal or no bureaucracy at all.

Virtually all surveillance-type operations of CEM/NET involve prospective studies, the exceptions being outbreak investigations in Portuguese hospitals and hospitals in New York City, the aim of which is tracking transmission routes and identifying in-hospital reservoirs of nosocomial pathogens. Many of the surveillance-type operations of CEM/NET are integrated with the major activity of the initiative, which is teaching molecular fingerprinting techniques. This is done through personalized training of clinical microbiologist colleagues in molecular fingerprinting techniques through working visits to The Rockefeller University and/or to the CEM Laboratory in Oeiras, Portugal. Because of the complexity of these techniques, such hands-on tutorial kind of teaching is essential. The international training at Rockefeller University is supported by National Institutes of Health (NIH), the Scandinavian Society for Microbiology, and several private foundations. A special international training program at the Portuguese laboratory (1996–present) is supported by the Calouste Gulbenkian Foundation and the Portuguese grant

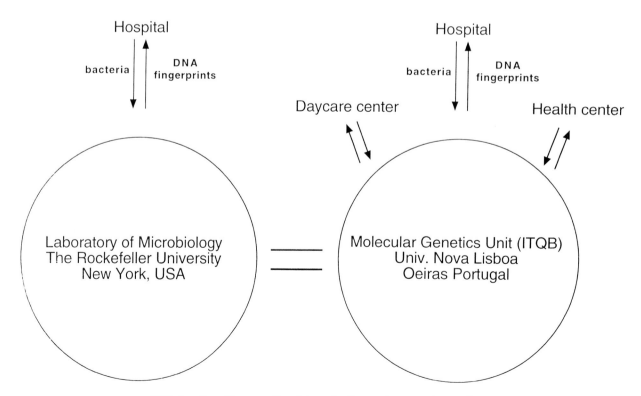

FIG. 1. Surveillance, outbreak investigation, and prospective studies.

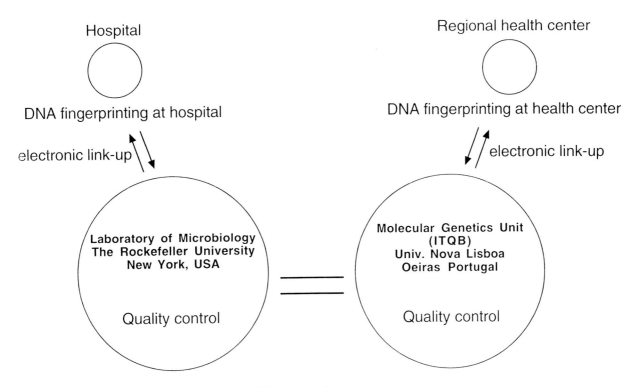

FIG. 2. Aim for the future.

agency PRAXIS XXI from the Ministry of Science and Technology. The format of the Gulbenkian-supported program is as follows: two to three clinical microbiologist colleagues arrive at the same time to join the staff of the CEM laboratory in Portugal for 3-month periods of learning molecular fingerprinting techniques using collections of their own isolates. After characterization of the isolates, the intention is to make the data available through manuscripts submitted to well-referred international journals for publication. Since mid-1995 to 1999, 30 colleagues from 18 different countries (Latin America, Europe, Japan, and Africa) have taken part in these programs. The productivity of the collaborative surveillance-type projects is documented by the 52 co-authored publications that have appeared in print between 1994 and 1999. Findings of considerable importance documented in these molecular epidemiology papers include the identification of multiresistant epidemic clones of MRSA: the "Iberian" epidemic clone (spread to Spain, Portugal, Italy, Scotland, Belgium, Germany, and, most recently, to New York City); the "Brazilian" epidemic clone (spread over 5,000 kilometers between Porto Alegre, Rio de Janeiro, Manaus, and, most recently, to Portugal and the Czech Republic), the "Hungarian" epidemic clone (spread over several hundred kilometers in eight provincial cities in Hungary); the "Pediatric Clone" (characteristic of pediatric MRSA isolates and found in several countries); intercontinental spread of the multidrug-resistant serotype 23F clone of *S. pneumoniae* (the "Spanish/USA epidemic clone") between Spain and the United States; the abrupt appearance and massive spread of a multidrug-resistant serotype 6B clone of *S. pneumoniae* (the "Spanish/Icelandic epidemic clone") in Iceland; multiplicity of genetic backgrounds among vancomycin resistant *Enterococcus faecium* (VRE) in hospitals in New York City; characterization of one of the first

MRSA isolates with decreased vancomycin susceptibility; and detection of spontaneous capsular switch among multidrug-resistant strains of penumococci.

Other type of educational activities of CEM/NET included the International Workshop on the Epidemiology of Antibiotic-Resistant Gram-Positive Pathogens, May 1995, in Oeiras, Portugal; international meeting entitled "*Streptococcus pneumoniae: Molecular Biology and Mechanism of Disease—Update for the 1990s*" held at ITQB in Oeiras, Portugal in September, 1996 (will appear in book form in 1999); Harmonization Workshop in Eastern Europe for clinical microbiologists, Warsaw, Poland, December, 1996 (co-sponsored by European Society for Microbiology); molecular characterization of penicillin-resistant *S. pneumoniae* collected in a trans-European study (Rockefeller University, October–December, 1996); molecular characterization of *S. pneumoniae* collected in six South American countries through the Pan American Health Organization (PAHO) study (Rockefeller University, January–May, 1997).

The ultimate aim of CEM/NET is to build an international network of independent and high-quality centers in specific parts of the world, with emphasis on countries from the developing world selected on the basis of prior collaboration (Fig. 2).

PUBLICATIONS IN MOLECULAR EPIDEMIOLOGY (MRSA, MRCNS, VRE, AND *STREPTOCOCCUS PNEUMONIAE*)

1. **Soares, S., K.G. Kristinsson, J.M. Musser, and A. Tomasz.** 1993. Evidence for the introduction of a multiresistant clone of serotype 6B *Streptococcus pneumoniae* from Spain to Iceland in the late 1980s. J. Infect. Dis. **168:**158–163.

2. De Lencastre, H., I. Couto, I. Santos, J. Melo-Cristino, A. Torres-Pereira, and A. Tomasz. 1994. Methicillin-resistant *Staphylococcus aureus* disease in a Portuguese hospital: characterization of clonal types by a combination of DNA typing methods. Eur. J. Clin. Microbiol. Infect. Dis. **13**:64–73.

3. Dominguez, M.A., H. de Lencastre, J. Liñares, and A. Tomasz. 1994. Spread and maintenance of a dominant methicillin-resistant *Staphylococcus aureus* (MRSA) clone during an outbreak of MRSA disease in a Spanish hospital. J. Clin. Microbiol. **32**:2081–2087.

4. Barnes, D.M., S. Whittier, P.H. Gilligan, S. Soares, A. Tomasz, and F.W. Henderson. 1995. Transmission of multidrug-resistant serotype 23F *Streptococcus pneumoniae* in group day care: evidence suggesting capsular transformation of the resistant strain *in vivo*. J. Infect. Dis. **171**:890–896.

5. Vaz Pato, M.V., C.B. de Carvalho, A. Tomasz, and The Multicenter Study Group. 1995. Antibiotic susceptibility of *Streptococcus pneumoniae* isolates in Portugal. A multicenter study between 1989 and 1993. Microb. Drug Resist. **1**:59–69.

6. Figueiredo, A.M.S., R. Austrian, P. Urbaskova, L.A. Teixeira, and A. Tomasz. 1995. Novel penicillin-resistant clones of *Streptococcus pneumoniae* in the Czech Republic and in Slovakia. Microb. Drug Resist. **1**:71–78.

7. Santos Sanches, I., M. Ramirez, H. Troni, M. Abecassis, M. Padua, A. Tomasz, and H. de Lencastre. 1995. Evidence for the geographic spread of a methicillin-resistant *Staphylococcus aureus* clone between Portugal and Spain. J. Clin. Microbiol. **33**:1243–1246.

8. Teixeira, L.A., C.A. Resende, L.R. Ormonde, R. Rosenbaum, A.M.S. Figueiredo, H. de Lencastre, and A. Tomasz. 1995. Geographic spread of epidemic multiresistant *Staphylococcus aureus* clone in Brazil. J. Clin. Microbiol. **33**:2400–2404.

9. Tarasi, A., N. Sterk-Kuzmanovic, K. Sieradzki, S. Schoenwald, R. Austrian, and A. Tomasz. 1995. Penicillin-resistant and multidrug-resistant *Streptococcus pneumoniae* in a pediatric hospital in Zagreb, Croatia. Microb. Drug Resist. **1**:169–176.

10. Couto, I., J. Melo-Cristino, M.L. Fernandes, T. Garcia, N. Serrano, M.J. Salgado, A. Torres-Pereira, I. Santos Sanches, and H. de Lencastre. 1995. Unusually large number of methicillin-resistant *Staphylococcus aureus* clones in a Portuguese hospital. J. Clin. Microbiol. **33**:2032–2035.

11. Montecalvo, M.A., H. de Lencastre, M. Carraher, C. Gedris, M. Chung, K. van Horn, and G.P. Wormser. 1995. Natural history of colonization with vancomycin-resistant *Enterococcus faecium*. Infect. Control Hosp. Epidemiol. **16**:680–685.

12. Santos Sanches, I., M. Aires de Sousa, L. Sobral, I. Calheiros, L. Felicio, I. Pedra, and H. de Lencastre. 1995. Multidrug-resistant Iberian epidemic clone of methicillin-resistant *Staphylococcus aureus* endemic in a hospital in northern Portugal. Microb. Drug Resist. **1**:299–306.

13. Mato, R., H. de Lencastre, R.B. Roberts, and A. Tomasz. 1996. Multiplicity of genetic backgrounds among vancomycin-resistant *Enterococcus faecium* isolates recovered from an outbreak in a New York City hospital. Microb. Drug Resist. **2**:309–317.

14. De Lencastre, H., E.P. Severina, R.B. Roberts, B.N. Kreiswirth, A. Tomasz, and the BARG Initiative Pilot Study Group. 1996. Testing the efficacy of a molecular surveillance network: methicillin-resistant *Staphylococcus aureus* (MRSA) and vancomycin-resistant *Enterococcus faecium* (VREF) genotypes in six hospitals in the metropolitan New York City area. Microb. Drug Resist. **2**:343–351.

15. De Lencastre, H., A. de Lencastre, and A. Tomasz. 1996. Methicillin resistant *Staphylococcus aureus* isolates recovered from a New York City hospital: analysis by molecular fingerprinting techniques. J. Clin. Microbiol. **34**:2121–2124.

16. Aires de Sousa, M., I. Santos Sanches, A. van Belkum, W. van Leeuwen, H. Verbrugh, and H. de Lencastre. 1996. Characterization of methicillin-resistant *Staphylococcus aureus* isolates from Portuguese hospitals by multiple genotyping techniques. Microb. Drug Resist. **2**:331–341.

17. Santos Sanches, I., M. Aires de Sousa, L. Cleto, M. Baeta de Campos, and H. de Lencastre. 1996. Tracing the origin of an outbreak of methicillin-resistant *Staphylococcus aureus* infections in a Portuguese hospital by molecular fingerprinting methods. Microb. Drug Resist. **2**:319–329.

18. Dominguez, M.A., J. Linares, A. Pulido, J.L. Perez, and H. de Lencastre. 1996. Molecular tracking of coagulase-negative staphylococcal isolates from catheter-related infections. Microb. Drug Resist. **2**:423–427.

19. Ramirez, M., D.A. Morrison, and A. Tomasz. 1997. Ubiquitous distribution of the competence related genes *comA* and *comC* among isolates of *Streptococcus pneumoniae*. Microb. Drug Resist. **3**:39–52.

20. Tarasi, A., Y. Chong, K. Lee, and A. Tomasz. 1997. Spread of the serotype 23F multidrug-resistant *Streptococcus pneumoniae* clone to South Korea. Microb. Drug Resist. **3**:105–109.

21. De Lencastre, H., E.P. Severina, H. Milch, M. Konkoly Thege, and A. Tomasz. 1997. Wide geographic distribution of a unique methicillin-resistant *Staphylococcus aureus* clone in Hungarian hospitals. Clin. Microbiol. Infect. **3**: 289–296.

22. Kloos, W.E., D.N. Ballard, J.A. Webster, R.J. Hubner, A. Tomasz, I. Couto, G.L. Sloan, H.P. Dehart, F. Fiedler, K. Schubert, H. de Lencastre, I.S. Sanches, H.E. Heath, P.A. Leblanc, and A. Ljungh. 1997. Ribotype delineation and description of *Staphylococcus sciuri* subspecies and their potential as reservoirs of methicillin resistance and staphylolytic enzyme genes. Intl. J. Systematic Bacteriol. **47**:313–323.

23. Tarasi, A., Y. Chong, K. Lee, and A. Tomasz. 1997. Spread of the serotype 23F multidrug-resistant *Streptococcus pneumoniae* clone to South Korea. Microb. Drug Resist. **3**:105–109.

24. McNeeley, D.F., A.E. Brown, G.J. Noel, M. Chung, and H. de Lencastre. 1998. An investigation of vancomycin-resistant *Enterococcus faecium* within the pediatric service of a large urban medical center. Pediatr. Infect. Dis. **17**:184–188.

25. Nesin, M., A. Severin, and A. Tomasz. 1997. Stability of clonally related DNA fingerprints and cell wall peptide patterns in geographic isolates of multiresistant epidemic clones of *Streptococcus pneumoniae*. Int. J. Infect. Dis. **2**:1–8.

26. Sieradzki, K., P. Villari, and A. Tomasz. 1998. Decreased susceptibilities to teicoplanin and vancomycin among coagulase-negative methicillin-resistant clinical isolates of staphylococci. Antimicrob. Agents Chemother. **42**:100–107.

27. Mato, R., I. Santos Sanches, M. Venditti, D.J. Platt, A. Brown, and H. de Lencastre. 1998. Spread of the multiresistant Iberian clone of methicillin-resistant *Staphylococcus aureus* (MRSA) to Italy and Scotland. Microb. Drug Resist. **4**:107–112.

28. Oliveira, D., I. Santos-Sanches, R. Mato, M. Tamayo, G. Ribeiro, D. Costa, and H. de Lencastre. 1998. Virtually all methicillin-resistant *Staphylococcus aureus* (MRSA) infections in the largest Portuguese teaching hospital are caused by two internationally spread multiresistant strains: the "Iberian" and the "Brazilian" clones of MRSA. Clin. Microbiol. Infect. **4**:373–384.

29. Santos Sanches, I., Z. Saraiva, T. Tendeiro, J. Serra, D. Dias, and H. de Lencastre. 1998. Extensive intra-hospital spread of a multiresistant staphylococcal clone. Int. J. Infect. Dis. **3**:26–31.

30. Aires de Sousa, M., I. Santos-Sanches, M.L. Ferro, M.J. Vaz, Z. Saraiva, T. Tendeiro, J. Serra, and H. de Lencastre. 1998. Intercontinental spread of a multidrug resistant methicillin-resistant *Staphylococcus aureus* clone. J. Clin. Microbiol. **36**:2590–2596.

31. Leski, T., D. Oliveira, K. Trzcinski, I. Santos Sanches, M. Aires de Sousa, W. Hryniewicz, and H. de Lencastre. 1998. Clonal

distribution of methicillin-resistant *Staphylococcus aureus* in Poland. J. Clin. Microbiol. **36**:3532–3539.

32. **Corso, A., I. Santos Sanches, M. Aires de Sousa, A. Rossi, and H. de Lencastre.** 1998. Spread of a methicillin-resistant and multiresistant epidemic clone of *Staphylococcus aureus* in Argentina. Microb. Drug Resist. **4**:277–288.

33. **Sieradzki, K., R.B. Roberts, D. Serur, J. Hargrave, and A. Tomasz.** 1998. Recurrent peritonitis in a patient on dialysis and prophylactic vancomycin. The Lancet (Research Letters) **351**:880–881.

34. **Roberts, R.B., A. de Lencastre, W. Eisner, E.P. Severina, B. Shopsin, B.N. Kreiswirth, A. Tomasz, and the MRSA Collaborative Study Group.** 1998. Molecular epidemiology of methicillin-resistant *Staphylococcus aureus* in twelve New York hospitals. J. Infect. Dis. **178**:164–171.

35. **Tomasz, A., A. Corso, and Members of the PAHO/Rockefeller University Workshop: E.P. Severina, G. Echániz-Aviles, M.C. de Brandileone, T. Camou, E. Castañeda, O. Figueroa, A. Rossi, and J.L. di Fabio.** 1998. Molecular epidemiologic characterization of penicillin-resistant *Streptococcus pneumoniae* invasive pediatric isolates recovered in six Latin-American countries: an overview. Microb. Drug Resist. **4**:195–207.

36. **Brandileon, M.C. de C., J.L. di Fabio, V.S.D. Vieira, R.C. Zanella, S.T. Casagrande, M.L.L.S. Guerra, S. Bokermann, A.C. Pignatary, and A. Tomasz.** 1998. Geographic distribution of penicillin resistance of *Streptococcus pneumoniae* in Brazil: genetic relatedness. Microb. Drug Resist. **4**:209–217.

37. **Camou, T., M. Hortal, and A. Tomasz.** 1998. The apparent importation of penicillin-resistant capsular type 14 Spanish/French clone of *Streptococcus pneumoniae* into Uruguay in the early 1990s. Microb. Drug Resist. **4**:219–224.

38. **Rossi, A., A. Corso, J. Pace, M. Regueira, and A. Tomasz.** 1998. Penicillin resistant *Streptococcus pneumoniae* in Argentina: frequent occurrence of an internationally spread serotype 14 clone. Microb. Drug Resist. **4**:225–231.

39. **Castañeda, E., I. Peñuela, M.C. Vela, The Colombian Pneumococcal Study Group, and A. Tomasz.** 1998. Penicillin-resistant *Streptococcus pneumoniae* in Colombia: Presence of international epidemic clones. Microb. Drug Resist. **4**:233–239.

40. **Echániz-Aviles, G., M.E. Velázquez-Meza, M.N. Carnalla-Barajas, A. Soto-Noguerón, J.L. di Fabio, F. Solórzano-Santos, Y. Jiménez-Tapia, and A. Tomasz.** 1998. Predominance of the multiresistant 23F international clone of *Streptococcus pneumoniae* among isolates from Mexico. Microb. Drug Resist. **4**:241–246.

41. **Marchese, A., M. Ramirez, G.C. Schito, and A. Tomasz.** 1998. Molecular epidemiology of penicillin-resistant *Streptococcus pneumoniae* isolates recovered in Italy from 1993 to 1996. J. Clin. Microbiol. **36**:2944–2949.

42. **Corso, A., E.P. Severina, V.F. Petruk, Y.R. Mauriz, and A. Tomasz.** 1998. Molecular characterization of penicillin resistant *Streptococcus pneumoniae* isolates causing respiratory disease in the United States. Microb. Drug Resist. **4**:325–337.

43. **Nesin, M., M. Ramirez, and A. Tomasz.** 1998. Capsular transformation of a multidrug-resistant *Streptococcus pneumoniae* in vivo. J. Infect. Dis. **177**:707–713.

44. **Sieradzki, K., R.B. Roberts, D. Serur, J. Hargrave, and A. Tomasz.** 1999. Heterogeneously vancomycin-resistant *Staphylococcus epidermidis* strain causing recurrent peritonitis in a dialysis patient during vancomycin therapy. J. Clin. Microbiol. **37**:39–44.

45. **Setchanova, L., and A. Tomasz.** 1999. Molecular characterization of penicillin-resistant *Streptococcus pneumoniae* isolates from Bulgaria. J. Clin. Microbiol. **37**:638–648.

46. **Sieradzki, K., R.B. Roberts, S.W. Haber, and A. Tomasz.** 1999. The development of vancomycin resistance in a patient with methicillin-resistant *Staphylococcus aureus* infection. N. Engl. J. Med. **340**:517–523.

47. **De Lencastre, H., K. Kristinsson, A. Brito-Avô, I. Santos Sanches, R. Sá-Leão, J. Saldanha, E. Sigvaldadottir, S. Karlsson, D. Oliveira, R. Mato, M.A. de Sousa, and A. Tomasz.** 1999. Carriage of respiratory tract pathogens and molecular epidemiology of *Streptococcus pneumoniae* colonization in healthy children attending day care centers in Lisbon, Portugal. Microb. Drug Resist. **5**:19–29.

48. **Sá-Leão, R., I. Santos Sanches, D. Dias, I. Peres, R.M. Barros, and H. de Lencastre.** 1999. Detection of an archaic clone of *Staphylococcus aureus* with low level resistance to methicillin in a pediatric hospital in Portugal and in international samples: relics of a formerly widely disseminated strain? J. Clin. Microbiol. **37**:1913–1920.

49. **Tamayo, M., R. Sá-Leão, I.S. Sanches, E. Castañeda, and H. de Lencastre.** 1999. Dissemination of a chloramphenicol- and tetracycline-resistant but penicillin-susceptible invasive clone of serotype 5 *Streptococcus pneumoniae* in Colombia. J. Clin. Microbiol. **37**:2337–2342.

50. **De Lencastre, H., A.E. Brown, D. Armstrong, M. Chung, and A. Tomasz.** 1999. Role of transposon Tn5482 in the epidemiology of vancomycin-resistant *Enterococcus faecium* in the Pediatric Oncology Unit of a New York City hospital. Microb. Drug Resist. **5**:113–129.

51. **De Lencastre, H, I. Santos Sanches, A. Brito-Avô, R. Sá-Leão, J. Saldanha, K.G. Kristinsson, and A. Tomasz.** 1999. Carriage and antibiotic resistance of respiratory pathogens and molecular epidemiology of antibiotic resistant *Streptococcus pneumoniae* colonizing children in day care centers in Lisbon: The Portuguese Day Care Center Initiative. Clin. Microbiol. Infect. **5**(Suppl. 4): 55–63.

52. **Melter, O., I. Santos Sanches, J. Schindler, M. Aires de Sousa, R. Mato, V. Kovárova, H. Zemlickova, and H. de Lencastre.** 1999. Methicillin-resistant *Staphylococcus aureus* (MRSA) clonal types in the Czech Republic. J. Clin. Microbiol. **37**(9):September issue, in press.

Address reprint requests to:
Herminia de Lencastre
Laboratory of Microbiology
The Rockefeller University
New York, NY 10021

Penicillin-Resistant *Streptococcus pneumoniae*: An International Molecular Epidemiological Study

PETER W.M. HERMANS, KARIN OVERWEG, MARCEL SLUIJTER, and RONALD DE GROOT

ABSTRACT

An international study was undertaken to investigate the epidemiological dynamics of penicillin-resistant pneumococci. We compared the molecular epidemiological characteristics of 316 penicillin-resistant isolates, originating from The Netherlands, Thailand, the United States, Spain, Greece, Poland, Cuba, Germany, Finland, U.K., Iceland, South Africa, Hungary, Portugal, Croatia, and the Czech Republic. A total of 131 distinct restriction fragment end labeling (RFEL) types were observed. Thirty-six genetic types were shared by two or more strains (clusters). Seven RFEL clusters consisted of strains originating from different countries, demonstrating international dissemination of penicillin-resistant pneumococci. The two most predominant RFEL types corresponded with the pandemic clones 23F and 9V, and were found in 10 and six different countries, respectively. This clearly demonstrates the pandemic behavior of these two clones. Fifteen out of the 36 RFEL clusters contained two or more serotypes. This finding indicates frequent horizontal transfer of capsular genes. Within distinct RFEL types identical penicillin-binding protein (PBP) genotypes were often observed, demonstrating a high frequency of horizontal DNA transfer of penicillin resistance genes. The most predominant PBP type comprised 40% of the entire collection. This PBP type was found in 20 distinct RFEL types and was observed in 11 countries. The vast majority of the strains belonging to the pandemic clones 23F and 9V shared this predominant PBP type. We hypothesize that the clones 23F and 9V are responsible for the worldwide increase of penicillin-resistance, since they serve as an important genetic reservoir for susceptible pneumococci to acquire penicillin resistance.

INTRODUCTION

STREPTOCOCCUS PNEUMONIAE (pneumococcus) continues to be a common cause of serious and life-threatening infections such as pneumonia, bacteremia, and meningitis, and of noninvasive infections such as otitis media and sinusitis. In the late 1970s and 1980s, the incidence of penicillin-resistant pneumococci has increased in Western countries, particularly in Spain, reaching levels up to 50%.[6,12,14,22] An epidemiological study in the United States in 1995 has demonstrated that 25% of invasive pneumococci were intermediate level or high-level resistant to penicillin.[11] The emergence of high-level resistance to penicillin, particularly in combination with other resistance determinants, poses serious problems for the institution of adequate antimicrobial therapy.

The high incidence of infections caused by pneumococci and the emergence of drug-resistant isolates form major objectives for molecular epidemiological surveillance. In order to obtain meaningful epidemiological information, genetic markers are needed that reflect an adequate rate of genetic rearrangements over time. Various pheno- and genotypical methods have been developed to assist in epidemiological investigations. These methods include serotyping, multilocus enzyme electrophoresis, pneumococcal surface protein A typing and penicillin-binding protein (PBP) typing, and DNA fingerprint methods such as pulsed-field gel electrophoresis, ribotyping and DNA fingerprinting of the PBP genes. We have recently investigated the usefulness of various DNA fingerprint methods to study the molecular epidemiology of pneumococcal infections. The potentials of (i) ribotyping, (ii) BOX fingerprinting using the BOX repetitive sequence of *S. pneumoniae* as a DNA probe, (iii) polymerase chain reaction fingerprinting using a primer homologous to the enterobacterial repetitive intergenic consequence sequence or homologous to the pneumococcal BOX repetitive sequence, (iv) pulsed-field gel electrophoresis of large-size DNA fragments, and (v) restriction fragment end la-

Department of Pediatrics, Sophia Children's Hospital, Erasmus University Rotterdam, Rotterdam, The Netherlands.

beling (RFEL) to detect restriction fragment length polymorphism of small-size DNA fragments have been compared.[10,30] Although the discriminatory power of the DNA fingerprint techniques differs significantly, the deduced genetic clustering of the pneumococcal strains is comparable. The ease to perform computerized analysis and the potential to create reliable fingerprint libraries also differs significantly. Ribotyping, BOX fingerprinting and RFEL analysis are very suitable for computerized analysis of the fingerprints. RFEL analysis, a technique which has also proved to be relatively stable over time,[24] is currently routinely used in our laboratory to generate a data library of pneumococcal DNA fingerprints.[10]

Several examples of international spread of resistant pneumococcal clones have been reported: (i) Soares et al.[28] have documented the spread of a multiresistant clone of serotype 6B from Spain to Iceland in the late 1980s. This has resulted in an epidemic of this clone, which was isolated with a frequency up to 12% already in 1992.[13] (ii) In 1991, Munoz and colleagues have reported evidence for the intercontinental spread of a multiresistant clone of S. pneumoniae serotype 23F from Spain to the United States.[16] This clone has subsequently disseminated through the United States.[15] (iii) Gasc et al.[5] have reported in 1995 the spread of a penicillin-resistant pneumococcal clone of serogroup 9 from Spain to France. The latter clone has also recently been observed in Germany.[19] Besides the international spread of the clones 6B, 23F and 9V, novel penicillin-resistant and multiresistant clones have been reported in former Czechoslovakia, Spain, Japan, and South Africa that tend to spread in an epidemic manner within these countries.[2,21,26,32]

In the present study, we investigated the international epidemiological dynamics of penicillin-resistant pneumococci. For this purpose, we compared the molecular epidemiological characteristics of 316 penicillin-resistant isolates, originating from 16 distinct countries including The Netherlands, Thailand, the United States, Spain, Greece, Poland, Cuba, Germany, Finland, U.K., Iceland, South Africa, Hungary, Portugal, Croatia, and the Czech Republic.

MATERIALS AND METHODS

Bacterial isolates

Penicillin-resistant pneumococcal isolates ($n = 316$) were collected in 16 different countries. A total of 188 penicillin-resistant isolates [minimum inhibitory concentration (MIC) ≥ 0.1 mg/L] were collected in The Netherlands. Thirty-nine Dutch medical microbiology laboratories participated in this study, and sent all penicillin-resistant pneumococci isolated between March 1995 and March 1997 to our laboratory. These 39 laboratories offer microbiological services to the majority of the Dutch hospitals. The participating hospitals provide medium-, high- and intensive care facilities, and are distributed all over The Netherlands. The laboratories performed susceptibility testing on all pneumococcal isolates, and all penicillin-resistant pneumococci were included in the study. Duplicate isolates from patients were excluded. The clinical origin of the Dutch isolates was sputum ($n = 126$), nasopharynx ($n = 21$), nose ($n = 19$), blood ($n = 7$), cerebrospinal fluid ($n = 3$), pus ($n =$

3), bronchial secretion fluid ($n = 3$), ear ($n = 2$), vagina ($n = 1$), hypopharynx ($n = 1$), and conjunctiva ($n = 1$). One pneumococcal isolate was of unknown clinical origin.

Fifty-three penicillin-resistant isolates from Thailand were collected between February 1993 and May 1994 in six hospitals located in five distinct regions of the country. The isolates all originated from the nasopharynx of single individuals under the age of five with acute respiratory infections.

Nine penicillin-resistant isolates were collected between February 1994 and September 1995 in Kyriakou Children's Hospital in Athens, Greece. These strains originated from patients under the age of 14 years (mean age 2.75 years), suffering from otitis media ($n = 5$), rhinitis ($n = 2$), bronchiolitis ($n = 1$), or bacteremia ($n = 1$).

Five penicillin-resistant isolates were collected in Cuba. The isolates all originated from the nasopharynx of single individuals under the age of 5 with respiratory infections.

We further received five penicillin-resistant pneumococci from Poland, which were isolated in three distinct hospitals from children suffering from otitis media ($n = 1$), sinusitis ($n = 1$), or pharyngitis ($n = 3$).

In order to expand our pneumococcal collection with DNA fingerprints from penicillin-resistant strains, we asked various colleagues to provide us with clinical isolates. These strains originated from the United States ($n = 10$, Facklam[8]; $n = 9$, Faden[25]; $n = 4$, Tomasz; $n = 1$, Tenover), Spain ($n = 3$, Hakenbeck[19]; $n = 10$, Casal), Germany ($n = 4$, Hakenbeck[19]), Finland ($n = 3$, Hakenbeck[23]), U.K. ($n = 3$, Hall[7]), Iceland ($n = 3$, Kristinsson), South Africa ($n = 2$, Hakenbeck[23]), Hungary ($n = 1$, Hakenbeck[19]), Portugal ($n = 1$, Tomasz), Croatia ($n = 1$, Tomasz), and the Czech Republic ($n = 1$, Hakenbeck[19]).

Biochemical characterization, serotyping and susceptibility testing

Species identification of the S. pneumoniae isolates was performed using optochine susceptibility and bile solubility testing.[17] Pneumococci were serotyped on the basis of capsular swelling (Quellung reaction) observed microscopically after suspension in antisera prepared at Statens Seruminstitut, Copenhagen, Denmark,[4]

The MICs of the pneumococcal strains were determined by agar dilution. The MIC was defined as the lowest concentration of the antimicrobial agent preventing visible growth. For this purpose, serial ^{2}log concentrations of antibiotics were prepared in IsoSensitest agar (Oxoid, Unipath Ltd., Basingstoke, U.K.), supplemented with 5% horse blood. The pneumococcal isolates were removed from storage at $-70°C$, and sub-cultured at $37°C$ on Columbia agar (Oxoid) supplemented with 5% sheep blood using 5% CO_2. Bacterial suspensions were prepared in 0.9% NaCl from 24-h agar cultures, and adjusted to a McFarland turbidity of 0.5. Suspensions were further diluted (1:10) in saline. The inocula were applied on the test plates using a multipoint inoculator, resulting in about 10^4 colony forming units per spot. MIC values were read after 24 h of incubation at $37°C$ using 5% CO_2.

The antimicrobial agents tested were penicillin G (Sigma Chemical Co., St. Louis, MO), erythromycin (Abbott Lab. Ltd, Queenborough, Kent, U.K.), doxycycline (Pfizer S.A., Brussels, Belgium), vancomycin (Eli Lilly, Indianapolis, IN), rifampicin (Sigma), cotrimoxazole, i.e., the combination (1:19) of trimethoprim (Sigma) and sulphamethoxazole (Sigma), and ciprofloxacin (Bayer, Wuppertal, Germany). Breakpoints of the antibiotics to discriminate between susceptible and nonsusceptible strains were used according to the NCCLS guidelines for susceptibility testing.[18]

RFEL analysis

Typing of pneumococcal strains by RFEL was performed as described by Van Steenbergen et al.,[31] and adapted by Hermans et al.[10] Briefly, purified pneumococcal DNA was digested by the restriction enzyme EcoRI. The DNA restriction fragments were end-labeled at 72°C with [α-^{32}P]dATP using Taq DNA polymerase (Goldstar, Eurogentec, Seraing, Belgium). The radiolabeled fragments were denatured, and separated electrophoretically on a 6% polyacrylamide sequencing gel containing 8M urea. Subsequently, the gel was transferred onto filter paper, vacuum-dried (HBI, Saddlebrook, NY), and exposed for variable periods at room temperature to ECL Hyperfilms (Amersham, Bucks, U.K.).

PBP genotyping

Genetic polymorphism of the PBP genes pbp1a, pbp2b, and pbp2x was investigated by RFLP analysis. For this purpose, we amplified the genes by PCR, and analyzed the digested DNA products by agarose gel electrophoresis. PCR amplification of the PBP genes was performed in a 50-μl PCR buffer system containing 75 mM Tris-HCl pH 9.0, 20 mM (NH$_4$)$_2$SO$_4$, 0.01% (w/v) of Tween 20, 1.5 mM MgCl$_2$, 0.2 mM dNTP, 10 pmol of the individual primers, 0.5 units of DNA polymerase (Eurogentec), and 10 ng/μl of purified chromosomal DNA. Cycling was performed in a PTC-100 Programmable Thermal Controller (MJ Research, Watertown, MA, USA), and consisted of the following steps: pre-denaturation at 94°C for 1 min, 30 cycles of 1 min 94°C, 1 min 52°C, 2 min 72°C, and final extension at 72°C for 3 min. The primers used to amplify the PBP 1a, 2b, and 2x genes were described previously.[1,3,16] The amplification products (5 μl) were digested by restriction endonuclease HinfI, and separated by electrophoresis in 2.5% agarose gels containing 0.5 × TBE and 0.1 μg/ml of ethidium bromide (5 mm thick; Agarose MP, Boehringer Mannheim, Almere, The Netherlands). Gels were run in 0.5 × TBE containing 0.1 μg/ml of ethidium bromide at a constant current of 20 mA for 4 h. Prior to electrophoresis, samples were mixed with a 5× concentrated layer mix consisting of 50% glycerol in water and 0.8 mg bromo phenol blue per ml. Gels were photographed with a Polaroid MP4 Landcamera and Polaroid 667 films. The different PBP genotypes are represented by a three-number code (i.e., 06-05-19), referring to the RFLP patterns of the PBP genes 1a (06), 2b (05), and 2x (19), respectively.

Computer-assisted analysis of the DNA fingerprints

The RFEL types were analyzed using the Windows version of the Gelcompar software version 4 (Applied Maths, Kortrijk, Belgium) after scanning the RFEL autoradiograms using the Image Master DTS (Pharmacia Biotech, Uppsala, Sweden). For this purpose, the DNA fragments in the molecular weight range of 160–400 base pairs were explored. The fingerprints were normalized using pneumococcus-specific bands present in the RFEL banding patterns of all strains. Comparison of the fingerprints was performed by unweighted pair group method using arithmetic averages (UPGMA),[20] and using the Jaccard similarity coefficient applied to peaks.[27] Computer-assisted analysis, and methods and algorithms used in this study were carried out according to the instructions of the manufacturer of Gelcompar. A tolerance of 1.5% in band positions was applied during comparison of the fingerprint patterns. Identical DNA types were arbitrarily defined as RFEL homologies higher than 95%. A genetic cluster was defined being a genotype (RFEL or PBP type) that was shared by two or more pneumococcal strains. The degree of genetic clustering was defined as the percentage of strains displaying genotypes (RFEL or PBP types) that were observed twice or more.

RESULTS AND DISCUSSION

All 316 penicillin-resistant pneumococcal strains were analyzed by serotyping, RFEL and PBP genotyping, and the resistance patterns were determined. The results are summarized in Fig. 1. One hundred and thirty-one distinct RFEL types were observed, representing 36 genetic clusters (RFEL types shared by two or more strains) and 96 unique RFEL types. The largest collections of strains originated from The Netherlands (n = 188) and Thailand (n = 53), and demonstrated 76% and 68% of genetic clustering, respectively. The degree of clustering was much higher among the penicillin-resistant strains from both countries compared with a group of 153 penicillin-susceptible strains isolated in The Netherlands in 1994, which displayed only 33% of genetic clustering.[9] These data clearly demonstrate that the transmission behaviour of these strains is comparable in both countries. We have recently investigated in a one-year survey the epidemiological characteristics of penicillin-resistant pneumococci in The Netherlands. The data obtained from this study have demonstrated that multiple clones of penicillin-resistant pneumococci are frequently introduced in this low-prevalence country. Some of these isolates are able to spread among the population in and outside hospitals, in particular in sub-populations with a high risk for pneumococcal infections and a high consumption of antibiotics.[9]

Among the 316 penicillin-resistant pneumococci, 236 strains (75%) were intermediately resistant to penicillin and 77 (24%) displayed high-level resistance. Forty-seven percent of the penicillin-resistant strains were co-resistant to erythromycin, 56% to doxycycline and 87% to cotrimoxazole. All isolates were in vitro susceptible to vancomycin and ciprofloxacin. The resistance patterns of the penicillin-resistant pneumococci originating from The Netherlands are summarized in Table 1. Comparison of the pneumococci with penicillin MIC values of <1 mg/L and those with MIC values of ≥1 mg/L clearly demonstrated that the penicillin-resistant pneumococci with MIC values of ≥1 mg/L were more frequently multiply resistant to four antibiotics (resistance pattern PCDE). In addition, the degree of genetic clustering using both RFEL typing and PBP typing is also higher among the penicillin-resistant isolates displaying

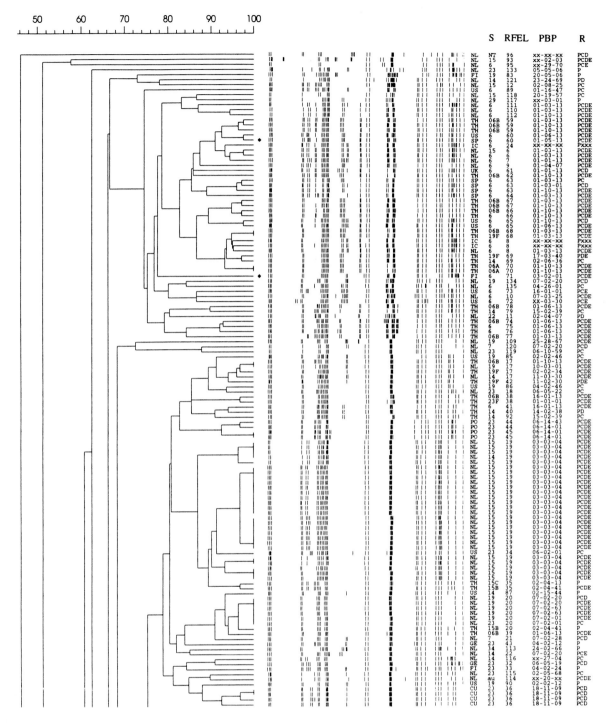

FIG. 1. Dendrogram of the RFEL banding patterns of 316 penicillin-resistant pneumococci originating from The Netherlands (NL, $n = 188$), Thailand (TH, $n = 53$), USA ($n = 24$), Spain (SP, $n = 13$), Greece (GR, $n = 9$), Poland (PO, $n = 5$), Cuba (CU, $n = 5$), Germany (GE, $n = 4$), Finland (FI, $n = 3$), UK (UK, $n = 3$), Iceland (IC, $n = 3$), South Africa (SA, $n = 2$), Hungary (HU, $n = 1$), Portugal (PT, $n = 1$), Croatia (CR, $n = 1$) and the Czech Republic (CZ, $n = 1$). Characters in brackets indicate serogroup (S), RFEL type (RFEL), PBP type (PBP), and resistance pattern (R). The arbitrary cut-off value for an identical RFEL type is 95%, except for RFEL type 19.[9] The previously described pandemic clones 23F (■[29]), 9V (●[19]) and 6B (◆[19]) are also depicted. P, penicillin G; C, cotrimoxazole; D, doxycycline; E, erythromycin; R, rifampicin.; xx, unknown PBP type; NT, non-typable.

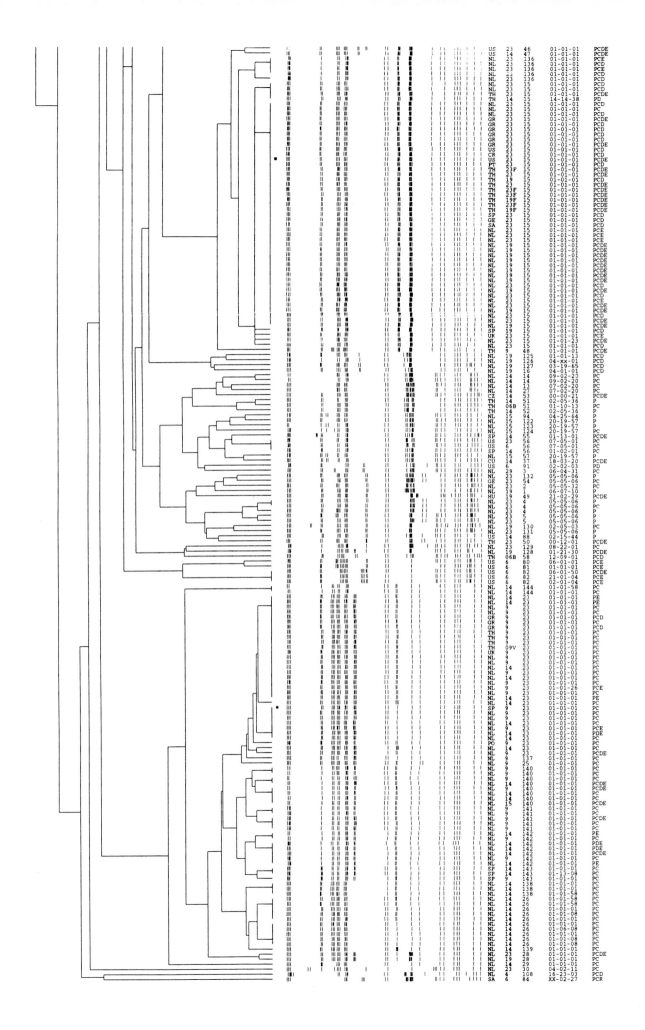

TABLE 1. RESISTANCE PATTERNS OF PENICILLIN-RESISTANT PNEUMOCOCCI IN THE NETHERLANDS ($n = 188$)

	MIC for penicillin (mg/L)					
	0.1–1			≥1		
		Genetic clustering (%)			Genetic clustering (%)	
Resistance pattern	Number of strains	RFEL	PBP	Number of strains	RFEL	PBP
P	16	25	56	1		
PC	18	0	39	45	87	91
PD	2	0	0	0		
PE	0			6	100	100
PCD	10	0	30	11	91	91
PCE	0			6	83	83
PDE	1			1		
PCDE	10	30	20	61	87	87

P, penicillin G; C, cotrimoxazole; D, doxycycline; E, erythromycin; R, rifampicin.

TABLE 2. GENOTYPIC AND PHENOTYPIC PROPERTIES OF PENICILLIN-RESISTANT PNEUMOCOCCI SHARING IDENTICAL RFEL TYPES

RFEL type[a]	Number of strains	Number of countries	Serogroup (number of strains)	RFEL type[a]	Number of strains	Number of countries	Serogroup (number of strains)
15[b]	53	10	23 (37) 19 (15) 14 (1)	63	3	1	06 (3)
				82	3	1	06 (3)
23[c]	32	6	09 (22) 14 (10)	138	3	1	14 (3)
				6	2	1	06 (1) 15 (1)
19	27	1	15 (26) 14 (1)	28	2	1	19 (1) 23 (1)
26	10	1	14 (10)				
140	8	1	09 (4) 14 (4)	38	2	1	06 (1) 23 (1)
20	7	2	19 (5) 15 (1) 23 (1)	51	2	1	06 (1) 14 (1)
142	7	1	14 (5) 09 (2)	68	2	1	06 (1) 19 (1)
136	5	1	23 (5)	69	2	1	14 (1) 19 (1)
141	5	1	09 (5)	60	2	2	06 (2)
17	4	2	19 (2) 14 (1) 06 (1)	5	2	1	23 (2)
				14	2	1	14 (2)
				35	2	1	15 (2)
36	4	1	23 (4)	44	2	1	23 (2)
56	3	2	06 (1) 14 (1) 23 (1)	45	2	1	23 (2)
				65	2	1	06 (2)
143	3	1	14 (2) 09 (1)	66	2	1	06 (2)
				67	2	1	06 (2)
8	3	2	06 (3)	70	2	1	06 (2)
4	3	1	23 (3)	144	2	1	14 (2)
59	3	1	06 (3)				

[a]RFEL types displayed by two or more strains (RFEL clusters) were exclusively included.
[b]RFEL type 15 represents pandemic clone 23F.[16]
[c]RFEL type 23 represents pandemic clone 9V.[5]

TABLE 3. GENOTYPIC AND PHENOTYPIC PROPERTIES OF PENICILLIN-RESISTANT PNEUMOCOCCI SHARING IDENTICAL PBP TYPES

PBP type[a] (1a-2b-2x)	Number of strains	Number of countries	RFEL type (number of strains)	Serogroup (number of strains)
01-01-01[b]	127	11	15 (51)	23 (37)
			23 (31)	09 (21)
			140 (8)	19 (16)
			142 (7)	14 (16)
			136 (5)	06 (1)
			141 (5)	
			26 (4)	
			28 (2)	
			138 (2)	
			143 (2)	
			25 (1)	
			29 (1)	
			38 (1)	
			46 (1)	
			47 (1)	
			48 (1)	
			81 (1)	
			137 (1)	
			139 (1)	
			144 (1)	
03-03-04	27	1	19 (27)	15 (26)
				14 (1)
01-10-13	13	4	59 (2)	06 (13)
			66 (2)	
			70 (2)	
			17 (1)	
			51 (1)	
			62 (1)	
			63 (1)	
			65 (1)	
			67 (1)	
			70 (1)	
			112 (1)	
01-03-13	12	3	06 (2)	06 (10)
			68 (2)	15 (1)
			08 (1)	19 (1)
			59 (1)	
			63 (1)	
			64 (1)	
			67 (1)	
			77 (1)	
			110 (1)	
			111 (1)	
05-05-06	9	2	04 (3)	23 (9)
			05 (2)	
			54 (1)	
			131 (1)	
			132 (1)	
			133 (1)	
01-06-13	7	2	39 (1)	06 (7)
			60 (1)	
			65 (1)	
			74 (1)	
			75 (1)	
			76 (1)	
			78 (1)	
07-02-20	7	1	20 (2)	14 (3)
			13 (1)	19 (3)
			22 (1)	07 (1)

(cont.)

TABLE 3. GENOTYPIC AND PHENOTYPIC PROPERTIES OF PENICILLIN-RESISTANT PNEUMOCOCCI SHARING IDENTICAL PBP TYPES (CONT'D)

PBP type[a] (1a-2b-2x)	Number of strains	Number of countries	RFEL type (number of strains)	Serogroup (number of strains)
20-19-57	5	1	27 (1) 120 (1) 134 (1) 57 (1) 118 (1) 122 (1) 123 (1) 124 (1)	15 (5)
01-01-58	4	1	26 (2) 138 (1) 144 (1)	14 (4)
18-11-09	4	1	36 (3) 37 (1)	23 (4)
01-01-13	3	2	07 (1) 61 (1) 125 (1)	06 (2) 09 (1)
06-14-01	3	1	44 (1) 45 (2)	23 (3)
01-01-08	3	1	26 (3)	14 (3)
02-04-41	2	1	20 (1) 35 (1)	15 (2)
02-15-14	2	1	87 (1) 88 (1)	14 (2)
07-02-01	2	1	20 (2) 23 (1)	19 (1)
07-05-01	2	1	56 (2) 23 (1)	06 (1)
15-02-39	2	1	40 (1) 79 (1)	14 (2)
16-01-13	2	1	51 (1) 52 (1)	06 (2)
02-05-36	2	1	51 (2)	14 (2)
07-02-63	2	1	20 (2)	19 (2)
09-02-20	2	1	14 (2)	14 (2)

[a]RFEL types displayed by two or more strains (RFEL clusters) were exclusively included.
[b]Includes the vast majority of the strains belonging to the pandemic clones 23F[16] and 9V.[5]

MICs of ≥ 1 mg/L. These data suggest that the epidemic behaviour of the penicillin-resistant strains is enhanced by increasing levels of penicillin resistance. Moreover, we hypothesize that horizontal co-transfer of antibiotic resistance genes other than PBP genes occurs frequently among pneumococci with a high level of resistance to penicillin.

Seven out of the 36 RFEL clusters often consisted of strains originating from different countries (Table 2). The strains displaying the two predominant RFEL types 15 and 23 were found in 10 and six different countries, respectively. These data demonstrate the pandemic spread of these two genotypes.

Fifteen out of the 36 RFEL clusters harbored two or more serogroups (Table 2). This indicates frequent horizontal transfer of capsular genes among pneumococci. The high frequency of capsular transfer may have consequences with regard to the outcome of current vaccine strategies, which focus entirely on the use of capsular polysaccharides representing a restricted number of capsular types. The use of multivalent conjugate vaccines may shift the capsular distribution towards capsular types that are not present in these vaccines. Such a shift might be enhanced by the frequent horizontal exchange of capsular genes.

All 316 penicillin-resistant pneumococci were analyzed by PBP genotyping. Ninety-two distinct PBP types were observed, representing 22 PBP clusters (PBP genotypes shared by two or more strains) and 70 unique PBP types (Fig. 1, Table 3). No overlap was seen between the PBP types of the penicillin-resistant pneumococci and more than 200 susceptible isolates (data not shown). Within distinct RFEL types identical PBP types were often observed. Forty percent of the collection of 316 penicillin-resistant pneumococci displayed PBP type 01-01-01. This predominant PBP type was observed in 11 countries and displayed by 20 distinct RFEL types (Table 3). This observation suggests frequent horizontal exchange of PBP genes, which has resulted in the spread of PBP type 01-01-01 among various pneumococcal RFEL types.

Within the group of 316 penicillin-resistant strains, the previously described pandemic clones 23F (16), 9V (5), and 6B (28) were also included (Fig. 1). The predominant RFEL type 15, observed in 10 countries, was identical with the RFEL type of the pandemic clone 23F, whereas RFEL type 23, observed in six countries, was displayed by the pandemic clone 9V, respectively. Interestingly, all isolates from Greece ($n = 9$) matched either with clone 23F ($n = 6$) or with clone 9V ($n = 3$), indicating the significance of both clones in this country (Fig. 1). In addition, the vast majority of the strains belonging to the pandemic clones 23F and 9V shared the predominant PBP type 01-01-01 (Table 3). We hypothesize that the predominant pandemic clones 23F and 9V are primarily responsible for the increase of penicillin resistance worldwide, because they are an important penicillin resistance reservoir for susceptible pneumococci.

The previously identified pandemic 6B-type strains, which displayed genetically related multilocus enzyme electrophoresis patterns,[19] only shared 79% of the RFEL DNA bands. Interestingly, the two RFEL types belonged to a genetic family which branched at 75% genetic relatedness (Fig. 1). Within this genetic family, serogroup 6 was displayed by 82% of the members. Only 27% of the serogroup 6 strains did not match within this family. These data indicate that most of the serogroup 6 strains are clonally related, and linked within a single genetic family. Genetic polymorphism observed by PBP typing was also restricted within this family, and *pbp*2x type 13 was predominantly (68%) and almost exclusively present among the family members (Fig. 1).

This study aimed to identify the clones of penicillin-resistant pneumococci that are currently displaying pandemic behaviour. Our data clearly show the importance of the pandemic clones 23F and 9V, as they were detected in 10 and six out of the 16 countries, respectively. In addition, serogroup 6 strains were also frequently observed. However, the genetic homogeneity of these strains is reduced. This finding is consistent with the observations of Harakeh *et al.*[8] who have demonstrated genetic heterogeneity within serotype-6B pneumococci isolated in the United States. Using a genetic relatedness ≥75%, serogroup 6 strains were observed in seven countries. These observations suggest that the introduction and subsequent pandemic spread of clone 6B has occurred earlier in the antibiotic era compared with the international clones 23F and 9V. The contribution of clone 6B to the global increasing prevalence of penicillin-resistant pneumococci is at present overruled by the rapidly spreading clones 23F and 9V.

Detection and reduction of transmission of alarming drug-resistant pneumococci that are currently spreading all over the world is an important goal in the battle against pneumococcal disease. Obviously, restrictive use of antibiotics remains the major defence against the epidemic dissemination of such strains. In addition, the emergence of multidrug resistant pneumococci increases the need for vaccination of patients at risk for pneu-

mococcal disease such as the elderly, and the importance to improve conjugate vaccines to efficiently protect young children. Detailed studies on the epidemiology and epidemic behaviour of (multi)resistant pneumococci will assist to identify emerging clones. To this respect, close collaboration between the laboratories sharing interests in pneumococcal molecular epidemiology is of utmost importance. Extensive collaboration can be facilitated by the establishment of a freely accessible electronic network. Such a network can be used to exchange information on technical aspects of DNA fingerprinting, aimed to standardize the methodological procedures. In addition, the network can be used to construct and distribute an international data library containing DNA fingerprints of (multi)resistant pneumococcal strains. Such approach will facilitate adequate worldwide monitoring of the epidemiology of emerging (multi)resistant pneumococcal strains.

ACKNOWLEDGMENTS

We would like to thank all our colleagues who were willing to provide us with strains from The Netherlands (A.T. Bernards, R.W. Brimicombe, A.G.M. Buiting, J. Dankert, B.I. Davies, J. de Jong, B.M. de Jongh, R.J.A. Diepersloot, S.I.S. Dirks-Go, A. Fleer, H.M.E. Frénay, J. Goudswaard, W.D.H. Hendriks, B. Hendrikx, M.G.R. Hendrix, C. Hol, A.R. Jansz, E.E.J. Ligtvoet, Y.J. Kraat, B.T. Lim, J.G. Mulder, H.L.J. Nieste, B.P. Overbeek, P.G.H. Peerbooms, H. Schreuder, F.W. Sebens, C.P. Timmerman, G.J. van Asselt, C. Vandenbroucke-Grauls, B.J. van Dijke, J.M. van Duin, A.J.A. van Griethuysen, M. van Weyenberg-Blaauw, J. Verhoef, F. Vlaspolder, R.W. Vreede, and G. Weers-Pothoff), Thailand (S. Dejsirilert), Greece (V. Deliyianni), Cuba (I. Tamargo), Poland (W. Hryniewicz), USA (H. Faden, R.R. Facklam, F. Tenover, A. Tomasz), Spain (J. Casal), UK (L.M.C. Hall), Iceland (K. Kristinsson), Portugal and Croatia (A. Tomasz), and Germany, Finland, Hungary, South Africa, and the Czech Republic (R. Hakenbeck). N. Lemmens, K. Elzenaar, A. van Veen, A.J. de Neeling, W.J. van Leeuwen, and W.H.F. Goessens are greatly acknowledged for their technical support.

REFERENCES

1. **Coffey, T.J., C.G. Dowson, M. Daniels, J. Zhou, C. Martin, B.G. Spratt, and J.M. Musser.** 1991. Horizontal transfer of multiple penicillin-binding protein genes, and capsular biosynthetic genes, in natural populations of *Streptococcus pneumoniae.* Mol. Microbiol. **5:**2255–2260.

2. **Coffey, T.J., S. Berron, M. Daniels, E. Garcia-Leoni, E. Cercenado, E. Bouza, A. Fenoll, and B.G. Spratt.** 1996. Multiply antibiotic-resistant *Streptococcus pneumoniae* recovered from Spanish hospitals (1988–1994): Novel major clones of serotypes 14, 19F and 15F. Microbiology **142:**2747–2757.

3. **Dowson, C.G., A. Hutchison, and B.G. Spratt.** 1989. Extensive re-modelling of the transpeptidase domain of penicillin-binding protein 2B of a penicillin-resistant South African isolate *Streptococcus pneumoniae.* Mol. Microbiol. **3:**95–102.

4. **Facklam, R.R., and J.A. Washington.** 1991. II. Streptococcus and related catalase-negative gram positive cocci In: Balows, A., W.J. Hausler, R.L. Hermann, H.D. Isenberg, H.J. Shadomy, eds. Man-

ual of clinical microbiology, 5th ed. American Society for Microbiology, Washington, DC, pp. 238–257.

5. **Gasc, A.M., P. Geslin, and M. Sicard.** 1995. Relatedness of penicillin-resistant *Streptococcus pneumoniae* serogroup 9 strains from France and Spain. Microbiology **141:**623–627.

6. **Gómez, J., J. Ruiz-Gómez, Hernández-Cardona, Núñez, M. Canteras, and M. Valdés.** 1994. Antibiotic resistance patterns of *Streptococcus pneumoniae, Haemophilus influenzae* and *Moraxella catarrhalis*: A prospective study in Murcia, Spain, 1983–1992. Chemotherapy **40:**299–303.

7. **Hall, L.M.C., R.A. Whiley, B. Duke, R.C. George, and A. Efstratiou.** 1996. Genetic relatedness within and between serogroups of *Streptococcus pneumoniae* from the United Kingdom: analysis of multilocus enzyme electrophoresis, pulsed-field gel electrophoresis, and antimicrobial resistance patterns. J. Clin. Microbiol. **34:**853–859.

8. **Harakeh, H., G.S. Bosley, J.A. Keihlbauch, and B.S. Fields.** 1994. Heterogeneity of rRNA gene restriction patterns of multiresistant serotype 6B *Streptococcus pneumoniae* strains. J. Clin. Microbiol. **32:**3046–3048.

9. **Hermans, P.W.M., M. Sluijter, K. Elzenaar, A. van Veen, J.J.M. Schonkeren, F.M. Nooren, W.J. van Leeuwen, A.J. de Neeling, B. van Klingeren, H.A. Verbrugh, and R. de Groot.** 1996. Penicillin-resistant *Streptococcus pneumoniae* in The Netherlands: results of a 1-year molecular epidemiologic survey. J. Infect. Dis. **175:**1413–1422.

10. **Hermans, P.W.M., M. Sluijter, T. Hoogenboezem, H. Heersma, A. van Belkum, and R. de Groot.** 1995. Comparative study of five different DNA fingerprint techniques for molecular typing of *Streptococcus pneumoniae* strains. J. Clin. Microbiol. **33:**1606–1612.

11. **Hofmann, J., M.S. Cetron, M.M. Farley, W.S. Baughman, R.R. Facklam, J.A. Elliott, K.A. Deaver, and R.F. Breiman.** 1995. The prevalence of drug resistant *Streptococcus pneumoniae* in Atlanta. N. Engl. J. Med. **333:**481–486.

12. **Klugman, K.** 1990. Pneumococcal resistance to antibiotics. Clin. Microbiol. Rev. **3:**171–196.

13. **Kristinsson, K.G., M.A. Hjalmarsdottir, and O. Steingrimsson.** 1992. Increasing penicillin resistance in pneumococci in Iceland. Lancet **339:**1606–1607.

14. **Lister, P.D.** 1995. Multiply-resistant pneumococcus: therapeutic problems in the management of serious infection. Eur. J. Clin. Microbiol. Infect. Dis. **4:**18–25.

15. **McDougal, L.K., R. Facklam, M. Reeves, S. Hunter, J.M. Swenson, B.C. Hill, and F.C. Tenover.** 1992. Analysis of multiply antimicrobial-resistant isolates of *Streptococcus pneumoniae* from the United States. Antimicrob. Agents Chemother. **36:**2176–2184.

16. **Munoz, R., T.R. Coffey, M. Daniels, C.G. Dowson, G. Laible, J. Casal, R. Hakenbeck, M. Jacobs, J.M. Musser, B.G. Spratt, and A. Tomasz.** 1991. Intercontinental spread of a multiresistant clone of serotype of 23F *Streptococcus pneumoniae*. J. Infect. Dis. **164:**302–306.

17. **Murray, P.R., E.J. Baron, M.A. Pfaller, F.C. Tenover, and R.H. Yolken (eds.).** 1995. Manual of clinical microbiology. Washington, DC, American Society for Microbiology Press.

18. **National Committee for Clinical Laboratory Standards.** 1995. Performance standards for antimicrobial susceptibility testing.

Sixth informational supplement. NCCLS document M100-S6. Wayne, PA, NCCLS.

19. **Reichmann, P., E. Varon, E. Günther, R.R. Reinert, R. Lüttiken, A. Marton, P. Geslin, J. Wagner, and R. Hakenbeck.** 1995. Penicillin-resistant *Streptococcus pneumoniae* in Germany: genetic relationship to clones from other European countries. J. Med. Microbiol. **43:**377–385.

20. **Romesburg, H.C.** 1990. Cluster analysis for researchers. Krieger, Malabar, Florida.

21. **Sa Figueiredo, A.M., R. Austrian, P. Urbaskova, L.A. Teixeira, and A. Tomasz.** 1995. Novel penicillin-resistant clones of *Streptococcus pneumoniae* in the Czech Republic and in Slovakia. Microb. Drug Resist. **1:**71–78.

22. **Schreiber, J., and M. Jacobs.** 1995. Antibiotic-resistant pneumococci. Pediatr. Clin. North Am. **42:**519–537.

23. **Sibold, C., J. Wang, J. Henrichsen, and R. Hakenbeck.** 1992. Genetic relationships of penicillin-susceptible and -resistant *Streptococcus pneumoniae* strains isolated on different continents. Infect. Immunol. **60:**4119–4126.

24. **Sluijter, M.** Personal communication.

25. **Sluijter, M., H. Faden, R. de Groot, N. Lemmens, W.H.F. Goessens, A. van Belkum, and P.W.M. Hermans.** 1998. Molecular characterization of pneumococcal nasopharynx isolates collected from children during their first 2 years of life. J. Clin. Microbiol. **36:**2248–2253.

26. **Smith, A.M., and K.P. Klugman.** 1997. Three predominant clones identified within penicillin-resistant South-African isolates of *Streptococcus pneumoniae*. Microb. Drug Resist. **3:**385–389.

27. **Sneath, P.H.A., and R.R. Sokal.** 1973. Numerical taxonomy. Freeman, San Francisco.

28. **Soares, S., K.G. Kristinsson, J.M. Musser, and A. Tomasz.** 1993. Evidence for the introduction of a multiresistant clone of serotype 6B *Streptococcus pneumoniae* from Spain to Iceland in the late 1980s. J. Infect. Dis. **168:**158–163.

29. **Tenover, F.** Personal communication.

30. **Van Belkum, A., M. Sluijter, R. de Groot, H.A. Verbrugh, and P.W.M. Hermans.** 1996. A novel BOX-repeat PCR assay for high resolution typing of *Streptococcus pneumoniae* strains. J. Clin. Microbiol. **34:**1176–1179.

31. **Van Steenbergen, T.J.M., S.D. Colloms, P.W.M. Hermans, J. de Graaff, and R.H.A. Plasterk.** 1995. Genomic DNA fingerprinting by restriction fragment end labeling (RFEL). Proc. Natl. Acad. Sci. U.S.A. **92:**5572–5576.

32. **Yoshida, R., Y. Hirakata, M. Kaku, H. Takemura, H. Tanaka, K. Tomono, H. Koga, S. Kohno, and S. Kamahira.** 1997. Genetic relationship of penicillin resistant *Streptococcus pneumoniae* serotype 19B strains in Japan. Epidemiol. Infect. **118:**105–110.

Address reprint requests to:
Peter W.M. Hermans
Department of Pediatrics
Sophia Children's Hospital
Erasmus University Rotterdam
P.O. Box 1738
3000 DR Rotterdam
The Netherlands

Pneumococcal Disease and the Role
of Conjugate Vaccines

DAVID L. KLEIN

THE PROBLEM FROM AN
EPIDEMIOLOGICAL VIEWPOINT

*S*TREPTOCOCCUS *PNEUMONIAE* (pneumococcus) in the postantibiotic era, remains a major cause of morbidity and mortality both in the United States and throughout the developing world (Table 1). With the elimination of *Haemophilus influenzae* type b as a major invasive pathogen for children in well-immunized populations,[7] *S. pneumoniae* has become the most important bacterial pathogen in infants and children. It is the leading cause of bacterial pneumonia, bacteremia, and otitis media, and one of the three most common causes of bacterial meningitis in children <5 years of age.[34,36,61] In the United States, infections due to *S. pneumoniae* remain among the top ten causes of death and display a mortality rate twice that of the two other leading causes of meningitis.[44] Worldwide, approximately 4 million children die each year from pneumonia, of which 1 million have been attributed to *S. pneumoniae.* Most of these deaths occur in children living in developing countries who are <1 year of age.[56] Surveys have shown that 5–70% of healthy adults carry *S. pneumoniae* in their upper respiratory tract.[22,24,37] Thus, the many diseases of *S. pneumoniae* may be considered endemic throughout the world.

Current concerns about the epidemiology and pathogenesis of pneumococci include changing patterns of virulence and antimicrobial susceptibility and the increased opportunity for spread in communal settings such as day care centers. The global perspective of communicable diseases has been reflected in the spread of antibiotic resistant pneumococci across borders and into all continents. The widespread, indiscriminate overuse of antibiotics such as penicillin, amoxicillin, chloramphenicol, and cephalosporins has created a situation which has led to the emergence of *S. pneumoniae* strains that harbor resistance to multiple antibiotics.[25] Other factors contributing to the evolution of resistance include prescribing practices, increasing human morbidity, inappropriate usage of antibiotics, availability of relatively inexpensive drugs, and the creation of ideal settings such as hospitals and day care facilities which enhance the transmission of infectious agents. The mechanism of transferring fragments of genes or entire plasmids directly among different strains of bacteria and even between different species of bacteria, has successfully allowed for a common means of

acquiring resistance to antibiotics.[46] The problem of multidrug-resistant bacteria is most serious in many developing countries where reliable supplies of alternate forms of antimicrobial therapy are generally not available. Under these conditions, antibiotic treatment now becomes less effective and more expensive.[1] Despite the continuing development of new antibiotics, the ability to effectively treat pneumococcal disease is impaired by the rapid worldwide spread of antibiotic-resistant forms of pneumococci.[45] Major research efforts are now focused on the molecular mechanisms responsible for drug resistance, as well as research to develop and evaluate new or improved therapeutic and prophylactic approaches for disease intervention and prevention.

THE PROBLEM FROM AN
IMMUNOLOGICAL VIEWPOINT

The concerns about changing patterns of pneumococcal infection may be balanced by the recent introduction of conjugate vaccine technology. The development of conjugate vaccines against *S. pneumoniae* represents a significant strategy to offset drug resistance and protect against the spread of uncontrolled invasive strains of this pathogen. This effort has been a high priority among vaccine manufacturers to help prevent dramatic increases in morbidity and mortality due to *S. pneumoniae.*

It is generally accepted that immunity to *S. pneumoniae* results from the development of specific antibodies against the type-specific capsular polysaccharides of the pneumococcus. These capsular polysaccharides, therefore, represent important virulence factors. Although there are at least 90 distinct types of pneumococcal capsular polysaccharides, most human infections are caused by only 23 serotypes, each having a different polysaccharide capsule. Thus, a vaccine composed of a mixture of purified polysaccharides from these 23 serotypes is now used to immunize adults over the age of 65, children >2 years of age who are at risk for pneumococcal infections, and other high-risk groups such as diabetics and patients with renal or cardiovascular disease.[27]

Unfortunately, the current available 23-valent pneumococcal vaccine does not provide adequate protection to children <2

Bacterial Respiratory Disease Program Officer, Respiratory Diseases Branch, DMID/NIAID, National Institutes of Health, Bethesda, Maryland.

Reprinted from *Microbial Drug Resistance,* Vol. 5, No. 2, 1999.

TABLE 1. INCIDENCE OF PNEUMOCOCCAL DISEASE

I. Worldwide
  A. Pneumonia
    1. Estimated number of cases: 20,000,000
    2. Estimated number of deaths: 1,050,000
  B. Meningitis
    1. Estimated number of deaths: 75,000
  C. Total pneumococcal deaths: 1,125,000
    (9% of all childhood deaths)
II. United States
  A. Pneumonia—estimated number of cases: 500,000
  B. Meningitis—estimated number of cases: 3,000
  C. Bacteremia—estimated number of cases: 50,000
  D. Otitis media—estimated number of cases: 7,000,000

Case fatality rates: >40% for bacteremia and 55% for meningitis.

years, who are at greatest risk of disease, in addition to immunocompromised patients and the extreme elderly.[26,54] This lack of responsiveness among various high-risk groups is due to their inability to promote a T-cell–dependent immune response to free polysaccharide antigens.[41] Even in healthy adults, free polysaccharide vaccines are often poor immunogens. One year after a single immunization with the licensed pneumococcal vaccine, a gradual decline in antibody titer can be detected.[43] Five years after immunization of healthy young adults, antibody titers are about three fourths of their peak value. Ten years after immunization, anticapsular antibodies remained high only for two of six capsule types tested.[42]

Several case-control studies and serotype prevalence evaluations have suggested an overall efficacy for the 23-valent polysaccharide vaccine of 50–70% for vaccine type strains in adults with bacteremia disease (Table 2).[53] Efficacy for young children, immunocompromised patients, including individuals carrying HIV, and the elderly who are medically compromised was less, especially for the pediatric serotypes (i.e., 6B, 14, 19F, 23F) that are less immunogenic. Table 2 further shows that with increasing age and increasing years following vaccination, efficacy of the licensed polysaccharide vaccine declines.

CONJUGATE VACCINES AND THE IMMUNE SYSTEM

Like most polysaccharide vaccines, immune responses to purified pneumococcal polysaccharides are T-independent and variable, again being most limited in immunocompromised patients and young infants. Other interesting properties associated with T-independent immune responses include (1) the production of disproportionate amounts of IgM antibody; (2) the inability to induce a booster response (i.e., lack of immunological memory) upon repeated immunizations; (3) an immune response which is short-lived (i.e., rapidly waning antibody); and (4) the failure to produce high affinity antibody.[51,58]

Several different approaches have been used to overcome the poor immunogenicity of pneumococcal polysaccharide vaccines. In addition to the polysaccharide capsule, other virulence factors, generally protein in nature, have been examined as potential vaccine candidates when used alone or as a conjugate carrier. These virulence determinants are generally protein in nature and consist of excreted or released toxins and enzymes in addition to various surface proteins such as pneumolysin, autolysin, neuraminidase, pneumococcal surface protein A (PspA), and pneumococcal surface adhesin A, a 37-kD outer membrane protein.[38,52] For each of these candidate vaccines, protective antibodies have been identified in animal studies; only PspA has undergone phase I/II clinical trials.

The most current approach to immunizing infants against infections caused by encapsulated bacteria is to present the capsular antigens to the immune system in a form that is more immunogenic such as a protein-polysaccharide conjugate vaccine.[51] Using this approach, weakly immunogenic or non-immunogenic antigens can be made immunogenic by covalently coupling them to an immunogenic carrier protein. In this way, the antigen acquires the immunogenic character of its carrier and now becomes recognized by the immune system as T-dependent. Proteins are broken down into peptides that associate with class II major histocompatibility complex molecules on the cell surface and then are presented to T-cells to stimulate antibody production by B-cells.[18] This defines proteins as T-dependent antigens. Such complexes can stimulate a T-helper cell response, which in turn generates stronger booster responses on restimulation.

This approach is similar to that used for Hib conjugate vaccines, which has proved to be successful in controlling invasive Hib disease in vaccinated infants, especially meningitis. In the United States, between 1989 and 1997, the incidence of invasive Hib diseases in children less than 5 years of age declined by >99%. Of the 74 Hib cases identified in 1995 for whom information about age and vaccine status was available, 33 (45%) were unvaccinated.[2,9] Given the lack of an apparent animal reservoir, it is conceivable that universal vaccination with Hib conjugate vaccines could eradicate invasive Hib diseases. This

TABLE 2. EFFICACY OF POLYVALENT PNEUMOCOCCAL VACCINE IN IMMUNOCOMPETENT PATIENTS, ACCORDING TO AGE GROUP AND TIME SINCE VACCINATION

Age (years)	No. of case-control pairs	Time since vaccination, percent protective efficacy (95% confidence interval)		
		<3 years	3–5 years	>5 years
<55	125	93 (82 to 97)	89 (74 to 96)	85 (62 to 94)
55–64	149	88 (70 to 95)	82 (57 to 93)	75 (38 to 90)
65–74	213	80 (51 to 92)	71 (30 to 88)	58 (−2 to 83)
75–84	188	67 (20 to 87)	53 (−15 to 81)	32 (−67 to 72)
>85	133	46 (−31 to 78)	22 (−90 to 68)	−13 (−174 to 54)

dramatic reduction in Hib disease underscores the potential for pneumococcal polysaccharide conjugate vaccines and serves as the technical and medical basis for its use in infants.

DEVELOPMENT OF CONJUGATE VACCINES

Fortunately, not all serotypes are equally prevalent so that an effective conjugate pneumococcal vaccine needs to contain only those serotypes most commonly associated with pneumococcal disease.[8] In addition, the number of vaccine serotypes are generally limited because of the need to conjugate each serotype individually and the concerns about limiting the total dose of carrier protein to control carrier-induced tolerance.[5] The most frequently occurring pneumococcal serotypes in the United States (i.e., 3, 4, 6B, 9V, 14, 18C, 19F, and 23F) have, thus far, been included in most of the candidate vaccines (Table 3).[48] Currently, conjugate vaccines containing seven to 11 serotypes are undergoing clinical evaluation in various populations using the same chemical parameters and constructs as used for the Hib conjugate vaccines. Several different protein carriers and conjugation techniques have been employed and include (1) reductive amination that employs a CRM 197 carrier (Wyeth-Lederle Vaccines and Pediatrics); (2) cyanogen bromide activated linkage to a 6 carbon adipic dihydride spacer using either tetanus toxoid or diphtheria toxoid as a carrier (Pasteur/Merieux/Connaught); (3) a bivalent linker model (i.e., thioether) using a meningococcal outer membrane protein complex (OMPC) as the carrier (Merck Research Laboratories [MRL]); and (4) a nontypeable *H. influenzae* OMP carrier produced by SmithKline Beecham (SB) (Table 3).[14,60] It should be noted that other proteins have been considered and tested as potential carriers including bovine serum albumin, human immunoglobulin G, flagellar protein of *Salmonella typhi*, pneumolysin, PspA, and pertussis toxoids.

Conditions for the development of conjugates to different capsular serotypes differ for each of the above methodologies. The biochemical issues involved in constructing optimal pneumococcal polysaccharide conjugate vaccines have been shown to vary by serotype. Thus, specific formulations have been necessary for certain serotypes to maximize the immune response and account for its variability following exposure to different pneumococcal polysaccharides.[54] Other important factors which may influence the immunogenicity of conjugate vaccines include (1) the selection of a protein carrier and avoidance of carrier-mediated suppression of the antibody response; (2) the physical nature of the saccharide such as the amount of crosslinking and the number of repeat units; (3) the saccharide:protein ratio; (4) the method used to covalently couple molecules; (5) the frequency of immunization; (6) the use of adjuvants; and (7) the age and immunocompetency of the host.[15,16]

CLINICAL USE OF CONJUGATE PNEUMOCOCCAL VACCINES

Many phase I, II, and III clinical trials have been conducted during the past 8 years with several different pneumococcal conjugate vaccines. Although older children and adults, particularly immunocompromised individuals and those at high disease risk, will be candidates for vaccines, the primary target population for immunization will be young infants, who are expected to be immunized with three doses of the vaccine during the first six months of life. This is appropriate to prevent occult bacteremia, most common in children during the first two years of life, and to prevent pneumococcal meningitis. It is also appropriate to prevent severe bacterial pneumonias that are a major cause of death in young infants in developing countries as well as to prevent otitis media in developed countries. Based on preliminary studies and safety, covalent coupling of polysaccharides to protein carriers appears to be an excellent method for improving the immunogenicity of pneumococcal vaccines and offers an efficient way to protect infants and young children from disease.[16]

Early clinical studies first examined mono- and bivalent conjugate vaccines; over the years, these vaccines progressed rapidly into multivalent products containing various formulations, dosages, and combinations of serotypes. These vaccines have all been evaluated for safety and immunogenicity to assess optimal dose, ratio of serotype components, maximal number of serotypes, and amount of carrier that can be combined. Without exception, current multivalent vaccines now in clinical trials in infants contain, at a minimum, serotypes 4, 6B, 9V, 14, 18C, 19F, and 23F, which account for approximately 78% of all invasive disease in U.S. children.[6] Interestingly, the same seven serotypes in U.S. adults would cover only 50% of the pneumococcal isolates due to the low prevalence of serotypes 14 and 6B in this population. Thus, pneumococcal conjugate vaccines have now been developed which contain additional serotypes to accommodate different populations, age groups, and geographical needs. For example, serotypes 1 and 5 are known to be important in preventing disease in developing countries while in adults worldwide, serotypes 3, 8, and 19A cause a preponderance of disease.[6,11]

Some of the most promising and interesting results with the pneumococcal conjugate vaccines have been observed in infant populations. Clinical studies revealed few mild or transient reactions with the pneumococcal conjugate vaccines in addition to markedly improved immunogenicity to each of the various serotypes included in the vaccine. Several serotypes such as 3, 4, 18C, 19F are more immunogenic than others and provide a better and more consistent immune response following the administration of just one or two doses of vaccine between 2 and 6 months of age compared to types 6B and 23F, which consistently elicits some of the weakest immune responses of all serotypes. These latter types generally require a minimum of three doses to generate a good anti-6B or anti-23F IgG response. This pattern of serotype immunogenicity is observed regardless of the chemistry and conjugate vaccine formulation used.

The main target population for pneumococcal conjugate vaccine studies up to now has been infants and children. Primary objectives of phase I and II studies in infants have been to evaluate the safety and immunogenicity of the conjugate vaccines and to define various parameters associated with dose, time of administration, interaction with other vaccines, and impact on colonization. One such study examined the difference between administering two versus three doses of conjugate vaccine. A more rigorous antibody response was generally observed in toddlers who received two doses of a quadrivalent conjugate vaccine spaced 2 months apart compared to those who received only one dose. Similarly, a greater antibody response was observed in infants receiving three doses of a similar vaccine at

TABLE 3. SELECTED CHARACTERISTICS OF GLYCOPROTEIN CONJUGATE PNEUMOCOCCAL VACCINES

Manufacturer	Protein carrier	Linker	Saccharide length	Vaccine serotypes	Clinical studies
Pasteur/Merieux/Connaught	Tetanus toxoid + diphtheria toxoid	Short linker	—	1, 3, 4, 5, 6B, 7F, 9V, 14, 18C, 19F, 23F (D carrier—3, 6B, 14, 18C) (T carrier—1, 4, 5, 7F, 9V, 19F, 23F)	Phase I/II
Wyeth/Lederle Vaccines and Pediatrics	CRM 197	Reductive amination (amine)	Long	7-valent: 4, 6B, 9V, 14, 18C, 19F, 23F 9-valent: 1, 4, 5, 6B, 9V, 14, 18C, 19F, 23F 11-valent: 1, 3, 4, 5, 6B, 7F, 9V, 14, 18C, 19F, 23F	Phase III Phase III Preclinical
Merck Research Laboratories	OMP-meningococcus B	Bivalent linker (thioether)	Long	4, 6B, 9V, 14, 18C, 19F, 23F	Phase II/III
SmithKline Beecham	Nontypeable H. influenzae OMP	—	Long	4-valent: 6B, 14, 19F, 23F 11-valent: 1, 3, 4, 5, 6B, 7F, 9V, 14, 18C, 19F, 23F	Phase I Phase I

2, 4, and 6 months of age compared with those who received only two doses starting at a later age of 4 and 6 months.[28]

In general, most of the multivalent pneumococcal conjugate vaccines tested in infants provide a good antibody response following three doses for all included serotypes with 70–100% of vaccinees achieving an antibody response >1.0 μg IgG antipneumococcal polysaccharide/ml. Because many of the serotypes elicit poor to minimal antibody responses following one or two doses of vaccine, vaccine manufacturers have found it necessary to reformulate their products by increasing the antigen concentrations of the weaker immunogens. Thus, some conjugate vaccines contain up to four different concentrations of individual polysaccharide antigens, based on the ability of each to induce an effective immune response.

The promise of an effective conjugate pneumococcal vaccine capable of reducing the burden of local and invasive disease must be tempered by the recognition that the vaccine will cover only about three-quarters of the serotypes causing disease and that the vaccine serotypes may differ according to geographical need. Even if these penumococcal conjugate vaccines prove to be highly immunogenic, they still may not offer enough protection against all pneumococcal infections. Based on the example of Hib conjugate vaccines, it is very likely that pneumococcal conjugates, which induce a satisfactory production of high-affinity IgG antibodies, will protect against bacteremic pneumococcal infections. The real problem, however, is that the majority of pneumococcal morbidity is associated with mucosal infections such as pneumonia and otitis media. At this time, we do not know how effective the pneumococcal conjugates will be in protecting against diseases associated with mucosal surfaces following parenteral immunization. Nor do we know what impact they will have on colonization and herd immunity. To answer these questions, investigators have been conducting clinical trials in several different populations, which are at increased risk of pneumococcal infections.[17]

PHASE I/II STUDIES IN DIFFERENT POPULATIONS

Only recently was a consensus reached on the quantitation and standardization of serum antibody to pneumococci as measured by ELISA. This fact makes it very difficult to provide generalized statements regarding clinical trial outcomes or to compare the results among different study vaccines and different laboratories. There are also inherent dangers when discussing data not based on equivalent reference sera. Therefore, it is not the intent of the following review to compare immunogenicity data generated by any of the conjugate vaccines, but to provide the results of many studies done over the past several years under various settings.

The early clinical studies with the pneumococcal conjugate vaccines were first done in adults and toddlers for safety reasons. One such study, using an MRL heptavalent conjugate vaccine, demonstrated that a 1.0-μg dose of each vaccine serotype given to adults induced a relatively weak antibody response and a low rate of seroconversion to certain serotypes such as 6B and 19F probably due to the high pre-vaccination levels of serotype specific antibody (Table 4).[30] These findings contrast with earlier adult studies with the Haemophilus PRP-OMPC vaccine, which induced high anti-PRP responses. The reason for this difference is unknown. Table 4 further indicates that although an increase was observed for all anti-pneumococcal polysaccharide IgG responses in both children and adults following a single dose of vaccine, toddlers showed a consistently greater fold-increase for GMTs to each serotype (i.e., 1.3- to 2.2-fold for adults versus 3.0- to 13.2-fold for toddlers). Interestingly, priming of infants with three doses of a similar heptavalent-OMPC vaccine generates a more vigorous immune response to serotype 6B (i.e., 2.6-fold increase), one of the weakest of all pneumococcal serotypes, than that observed in many adults (Table 5).[40] Furthermore, toddlers immunized with a single dose of heptavalent-OMPC vaccine often produce as much if not more antibody to all the vaccine serotypes than infants immunized with three doses of the same vaccine.

Another study was performed with a Wyeth-Lederle five-valent oligosaccharide conjugate vaccine to examine the phenomenon of immunologic memory. Children 17–20 months of age were given a primary dose of the conjugate vaccine and boosted two months later with either the pneumococcal polysaccharide vaccine (group 1) or the same conjugate vaccine (group 2). The antibody response in both groups was compared to a control group which received a pneumococcal polysaccharide vaccine followed by a meningococcal polysaccharide vaccine (group 3). Other than drowsiness, which was increased in the conjugate group after dose two compared with the other two groups, the data did not demonstrate significant differences for other adverse events, which were minor for all groups. Ex-

TABLE 4. IMMUNOGENICITY OF A MRL HEPTAVALENT PNEUMOCOCCAL CONJUGATE VACCINE IN ADULTS AND CHILDREN

	Serotype		GMT of antibody (μg/ml)						
			6B	14	19F	23F	9V	18C	4
(A)	N		20	21	20	21	21	19	21
	Day	0	6.0	4.8	7.3	4.8	5.8	7.8	12.2
	Day	30	9.2	9.1	9.5	10.5	11.8	15.0	26.3
(C)	N		16	16	16	16	16	16	15
	Day	0	0.9	0.5	0.8	0.4	0.8	1.1	2.0
	Day	30	2.7	4.6	5.4	3.4	9.1	5.8	26.4

(A), adults.
(C), children.

TABLE 5. HEPTAVALENT PNEUMOCOCCAL-OMP COMPLEX:
SERUM IgG ANTIBODY CONCENTRATIONS PREVACCINATION
AND POST THREE DOSES (GIVEN AT 2, 4, AND 6 MONTHS)

Serotypes	EIA GMT mg/ml			
	Pre	Post dose 1	Post dose 2	Post dose 3
4	1.18	3.86	6.39	16.56
6B	0.74	0.59	0.69	1.95
9V	0.73	1.52	2.26	5.81
14	0.51	1.04	3.03	5.23
18C	0.73	0.65	0.86	2.31
19F	0.63	2.22	2.50	4.45
23F	0.56	0.48	0.62	1.46

cept for type 6B, the children in groups 1 and 2 demonstrated equivalent antibody responses to the remaining serotypes following the booster dose, with the anti-18C IgG response being the most vigorous (Table 6).[10] Furthermore, children in groups 1 and 2, who had received at least a single dose of conjugate vaccine, had higher antibody responses to all serotypes than children in group 3, who were primed initially with a plain pneumococcal vaccine, and subsequently boosted with a meningococcal vaccine. Thus, a single dose of the pneumococcal polysaccharide vaccine administered 2 months before priming with the conjugate vaccine (i.e., group 2) was capable of eliciting a good booster response indicative of immunologic memory.

The ability to establish a priming event is clearly one of the strong features associated with pneumococcal conjugate vaccines. This is reflected by an increase in the percent of individuals demonstrating antibody responses of ≥ 1.0 μg/ml, a level considered to be biologically significant, but not proven clinically to be a surrogate for protection. The presence of functional antibody is also becoming recognized as an important indicator of immune responsiveness following immunization with pneumococcal vaccines. This was exemplified in a study in which toddlers received two doses of a MRL tetravalent pneumococcal conjugate vaccine. Opsonophagocytic antibody activity was measured consistently (94%) in children whose ELISA titers for each serotype were ≥ 2 μg/ml IgG, suggesting a strong correlation between functional antibody and positive ELISA responses ≥ 2 μg/ml IgG.[20]

In another study using a Pasteur-Merieux-Connaught (PMC)

quadrivalent pneumococcal vaccine conjugated to a tetanus carrier (i.e., Pn-T), young adults received either two doses of one of three different concentrations of a Pn-T vaccine spaced one month apart or one dose of a plain pneumococcal polysaccharide vaccine. All three concentrations of Pn-T were equally immunogenic and safe. There were no significant differences among the conjugate vaccines and the pneumococcal polysaccharide vaccine with regard to safety and immunogenicity. Serologically, a single dose of pneumococcal polysaccharide vaccine was almost as immunogenic as two doses of the conjugate vaccine for all serotypes and antigen concentrations.[49] Furthermore, there was no evidence of a booster effect following a second dose of conjugate Pn-T vaccine given four weeks later. However, this same vaccine when given to infants as a three dose series was very immunogenic and demonstrated immunological memory to a subsequent challenge with a plain pneumococcal polysaccharide vaccine.

As previously indicated, pneumococcal resistance to multiple antibiotics is a growing problem in many countries worldwide.[35] Several studies recently demonstrated that nasopharyngeal carriage plays a significant role in the transmission of resistant forms of pneumococci.[11] The majority of multiple-resistant pneumococci belong to a small number of childhood serotypes including groups 6B, 9V, 14, 19F, and 23F. Fortunately, most of the multivalent conjugate vaccines now undergoing clinical evaluation contain these important serotypes. With this in mind, a study was performed in Israel to assess the ability of a MRL heptavalent conjugate vaccine to provide protection against resistant forms, and reduce the frequency and prevalence of nasopharyngeal cultures of penicillin-resistant pneumococcal organisms. Two doses of the vaccine were given to 12–18-month-old children. The data in Table 7 show that the carriage rates for penicillin-resistant and nonresistant pneumococci were significantly reduced for vaccine-type organisms.[12] A 50% reduction was seen in the penicillin-resistant vaccine types after both the first and second doses of vaccine. Although not shown in the table, increases in the GMTs for IgG were also observed following each dose of vaccine for all serotypes. These results suggest that conjugate vaccines are able to significantly reduce the carriage of the vaccine-related pneumococcal serotypes in children as well as decrease the burden of antibiotic-resistant strains.

More recent data from the Gambia demonstrated that infants immunized with a pneumococcal conjugate vaccine had a similar reduction in the carriage rates of serotypes associated with

TABLE 6. IMMUNOGENICITY OF A QUINQUEVALENT PNEUMOCOCCAL-CRM$_{197}$ CONJUGATE VACCINE IN HEALTHY TODDLERS

	Geometric mean antibody levels (EIA μg/ml) and foldrise over prevaccination levels ( )				
	6B	14	18C	19	23F
Grp 1	2.82 (67X)	4.23 (29X)	7.36 (194X)	1.77 (6X)	1.59 (19X)
Grp 2	1.06 (16X)	2.64 (14X)	6.26 (163X)	3.86 (9X)	2.10 (14X)
Grp 3	0.26 (1X)	0.24 (1X)	0.50 (9X)	0.71 (2X)	0.34 (2X)

Grp 1: two doses of conjugate vaccine 2 months apart.
Grp 2: one dose of conjugate vaccine followed 2 months later with a dose of pneumococcal capsular polysaccharide vaccine.
Grp 3: one dose of pneumococcal polysaccharide vaccine followed 2 months later by a quadrivalent meningococcal polysaccharide conjugate vaccine.

TABLE 7. REDUCTION OF NASOPHARYNGEAL CARRIAGE OF PENICILLIN-RESISTANT
PNEUMOCOCCI BY PNEUMOCOCCAL-OMP COMPLEX CONJUGATE VACCINE IN TODDLERS

	Predose 1		3-month postdose 1		1-month postdose 2	
Nonvacc. type—pneumococci	21/91	(23%)	14/78	(18%)	11/64	(17%)
Vacc. type—pneumococci	22/91	(24%)	8/78	(10%)	5/64	(8%)
Vacc. type—penicillin resis. pneumococci	12/91	(13.1%)	5/78	(6.4%)	2/64	(3%)

the vaccine. However, an increase in the carriage of other non-vaccine pneumococcal serotypes was observed suggesting that serotype replacement may have occurred after vaccination against *S. pneumoniae*.[47]

Compared to infants and toddlers, very few studies have been conducted in the elderly with conjugate pneumococcal vaccines. Two of the more recent studies, using a five-valent oligosaccharide conjugate vaccine produced by Wyeth-Lederle, demonstrated equivocal results. Immunogenicity levels for some serotypes were better following the use of the conjugate vaccine whereas other serotypes responded better to a dose of polysaccharide vaccine.[50,55] These results were disappointing and suggest that the induction of an antibody response in the elderly, following the use of a certain conjugate vaccine, overall, is no better or worse than the conventional 23-valent polysaccharide vaccine.

Additional studies in the elderly indicate that aging has no consistent effect on antipneumococcal polysaccharide IgG levels following immunization with a plain capsular polysaccharide vaccine.[21] Therefore, the increased susceptibility of elderly individuals to pneumococcal invasive disease does not appear to be due to age in general, or to lower IgG antibody production in response to pneumococcal polysaccharide antigens specifically, but rather to conditions associated with poor health, which compromises the immune response.[23] The use of newer and more advanced conjugate vaccines (i.e., additional serotypes and different formulations), in addition to the use of more aggressive immunization schedules and adjuvants, are now being examined to determine whether elderly individuals will benefit in any way following an exposure to a conjugate pneumococcal vaccine.

Limited studies have been conducted in infants with pneumococcal conjugate vaccines to examine the way they interact immunologically when given simultaneously with licensed pediatric vaccines. A monovalent pneumococcal-OMPC vaccine was administered at 2, 4, and 6 months of age concomitantly with an Hib conjugate vaccine, using either HbOC or PRP-OMPC. In this study, the anti-6B GMTs were significantly lower after dose three in a group receiving concurrent Hib conjugate vaccine (regardless of type) compared to a group receiving just the monovalent 6B-OMPC nonconcurrently with one of the Hib conjugate vaccines; the anti-PRP GMTs were unaffected.[62] However, it should be noted that other studies with the same and different pneumococcal conjugate vaccines have demonstrated that infants respond adequately to each of the vaccine related pneumococcal polysaccharides following the concurrent administration of pneumococcal and Hib conjugate vaccines and that Hib vaccine provides no significant degree of interference. Obviously, additional studies will be nec-

essary to closely examine the effects of combining different childhood vaccines with pneumococcal conjugate products.

Another important study examined immunologic memory in infants who had been primed with a heptavalent conjugate vaccine at 2, 4, and 6 months and boosted with a plain pneumococcal polysaccharide vaccine at 15 months of age compared to an unprimed control group immunized with a single dose of polysaccharide at 15 months of age. The antipneumococcal polysaccharide IgG response measured 7 days postbooster dose was significantly higher in the primed recipients than in the unprimed control group. Nearly all primed vaccinees achieved antibody responses of ≥ 1.0 μg antipneumococcal polysaccharide/ml to all seven serotypes.[39] These data provide good evidence that the conjugate vaccine is conferring properties of T-dependent antigens to the various polysaccharides and is capable of eliciting immunologic memory in infants subsequently exposed to pneumococcal antigens.

Several clinical trials in infants have been performed with the Wyeth-Lederle pneumococcal-CRM$_{197}$ vaccine containing multiple serotypes at different concentrations and different formulations (i.e., oligosaccharide-Os versus polysaccharide-Ps). The trials were designed to examine the response of infants to three different antigen concentrations of multivalent pneumococcal Os and Ps vaccines containing up to five different serotypes. Overall, the Ps formulation provided a higher antipneumococcal polysaccharide response than a corresponding Os formulation following three doses of vaccine.[13] No significant differences were noted for any of the local reactions (i.e., no measured adverse events were associated with the two prototype vaccines). It has been hypothesized that the Ps formulation is more immunogenic than a comparable Os design due to

TABLE 8. IMMUNE RESPONSE IN INFANTS TO FOUR
DIFFERENT QUADRIVALENT PNEUMOCOCCAL CONJUGATE
VACCINES ADMINISTERED AT 2, 4, AND 6 MONTHS OF AGE

Vaccine	Antibody concentrations (μg/ml) at 7 months of age			
	6B	14	19F	23F
Pn-CRM	0.40	2.50	0.79	1.10
Pn-OMP	1.30	8.27	9.85	1.90
Pn-D	0.88	2.30	529	0.88
Pn-T	0.77	3.06	3.20	0.67

Pn-CRM, Wyeth/Lederle; Pn-OMPC, Merck Research Laboratories; Pn-D, Pasteur/Merieux/Connaught; Pn-T, Pasteur/Merieux/Connaught.

TABLE 9. IMMUNOGENICITY OF A QUINQUEVALENT PNEUMOCOCCAL-CRM$_{197}$
CONJUGATE VACCINE IN HIV$^+$ AND NON–HIV-INFECTED CHILDREN

Group[a]	Vaccine	Total ≥threefold rises (%)	Fold-rise in type-specific antibody (ng/ml) pre- to postvaccine				
			6B	23F	24	18C	19F
1. HIV$^+$	Conjugate[b]	36/56 (64%)[d]	66[e]	229	40[e]	2512[d]	19
2. HIV$^+$	Ps[c]	26/64 (41%)[e]	22[e]	23	5[e]	42[e]	35
3. HIV$^-$	Conjugate[b]	21/25 (84%)[e]	2818[e]	1318	2399[e]	479[e]	427
4. HIV$^-$	Ps[c]	30/46 (65%)[e]	955	42[e]	295[e]	1122[e]	224

[a]30 HIV$^+$ and 30 HIV$^-$ children, having a mean age of 4.4 years, received either the Os conjugate vaccine containing 10 μg of each Ps or the 23-valent licensed vaccine containing 25 μg of each Ps.
[b]Conjugate pneumococcal vaccine.
[c]Plain polysaccharide vaccine.
[d]$p < 0.05$ between groups 1 and 2.
[e]$p < 0.05$ between groups 2 and 4.

the Ps having more epitopes than the Os.[3,17] These results, as well as additional phase II and III studies, have emphasized the use of the Ps formulation for all serotypes (except 18C) in current Wyeth-Lederle multivalent pneumococcal conjugate vaccines.

A recent phase I/II double-blind, placebo-controlled trial was conducted in Finnish infants using two different quadrivalent vaccines (Pn-T and a pneumococcal conjugate diphtheria [Pn-D]) manufactured by PMC. Each vaccine contained serotypes 6B, 14, 19F, 23F at concentrations of 1, 3, or 10 μg for each capsular polysaccharide. The incidence of local adverse events for both vaccines was very low when administered at 2, 4, and 6 months of age. Compared to DTP and PRP-T control vaccines given simultaneously, fewer and less serious adverse events were noted for both conjugate vaccines. Both pneumococcal conjugate vaccines were similarly immunogenic postdose-3 at concentrations of 1 and 3 μg.[3] Pn-D vaccine induced a slightly higher anti-6B and 23F response than did Pn-T, as well as a consistently higher antibody response for all serotypes at the 10-μg level. Although not statistically significant, it appeared that there was a dose-dependent immune response for Pn-D, which was not evident with Pn-T. Additional studies using a combination of Pn-T and Pn-D conjugates, are now undergoing clinical evaluation.

Studies in Finland have tested most of the available multivalent pneumococcal conjugate vaccines in different age groups. The protocols for these trials were similar and involved administering vaccine at 2, 4, and 6 months of age and measuring serum IgG antipneumococcal polysaccharide in both unimmunized controls and immunized infants pre- and postvaccination. The results presented in Table 8 describe post third-dose antibody levels elicited by quadrivalent vaccines from the four vaccine developers.[29] All four vaccines induced antibody to each of the serotypes in infants; certain serotypes such as 19F induced more antibody than others. This is the only study which has compared antibody levels elicited by different conjugate vaccines and measured in a single laboratory using a standardized ELISA technique. However, these studies were not done comparatively, nor did they use final optimized formulations currently employed in phase III efficacy and licensure studies. Under these circumstances, the ability to make fair, unbiased comparisons for each of the different vaccines are limited.

Studies have also been conducted in high-risk groups including AIDS patients. The safety and immunogenicity of a five-valent pneumococcal-CRM$_{197}$ vaccine produced by Wyeth-Lederle was compared to pneumococcal polysaccharide vaccine in HIV($^+$) and HIV($^-$) children. The pattern and intensity of adverse events were similarly low and transient for both groups, although up to 40% of vaccine recipients did complain of local pain. The results in Table 9 reveal that the HIV($^+$) patients responded with lower antibody levels to both the polysaccharide and conjugate vaccines than HIV($^-$) patients.[32] However, the percentage of HIV($^+$) children showing a ≥threefold increase in antipneumococcal polysaccharide levels was

TABLE 10. DIFFERENT TYPES OF EFFICACY TRIALS

Protection against invasive, bacteremic pneumococcal infections
Protection against common mucosal infections, e.g., pneumonia and otitis media
Protection against mortality
Impact on pneumococcal carriage

TABLE 11. PROBLEMS ASSOCIATED WITH PNEUMOCOCCAL CONJUGATE VACCINES

Cost of producing vaccine and limited potential in developing countries
Need for multivalent products made up of individual vaccines
Need for different formulations, dosages, and combinations or serotypes to accommodate different population, age groups, and geographical needs
Problem with carrier-induced tolerance due to large total dose of carrier protein
Currently, vaccine covers, at best, only three-quarters of types causing disease which may vary over time
Majority of pneumococcal morbidity is associated with mucosal infections
All conjugate vaccine antigens are not created equally; each conjugated antigen is a unique, separate vaccine with different immunological properties

significantly greater in those receiving conjugate vaccine than those receiving the pneumococcal polysaccharide vaccine regardless of $CD4^+$ lymphocyte counts. The use of a similar five-valent pneumococcal-CRM_{197} vaccine in adult $HIV(^+)$ patients produced results closely resembling those observed in $HIV(^+)$ children.[4] Thus, $HIV(^+)$ individuals, who suffer from low levels of T-helper cells, but still maintain functional B-cell activity, may benefit from the use of Pn conjugate vaccines, especially when provided during the early phase of the disease.

CURRENT STATUS OF CONJUGATE VACCINES

Several previous studies provided indirect evidence that pneumococcal conjugate vaccines can protect against disease; this included the following: (1) promising immunogenicity of pneumococcal conjugates and the presence of functional antibody[20,31]; (2) passive immunization studies with pneumococcal immune globulin preparations demonstrating protection against invasive pneumococcal infections and pneumococcal otitis media[57]; (3) the prevention or attenuation of experimental otitis media in chinchillas following pneumococcal conjugate vaccination[19]; and (4) good experience and background information with Hib conjugate vaccines demonstrating both efficacy and a reduction in nasopharyngeal carriage rates against invasive Hib infections.[11,47] Recent published data from a trial in Northern California revealed for the first time protective efficacy of a pneumococcal conjugate vaccine produced by Wyeth-Lederle. The trial was conducted in infants using invasive disease, based on vaccine serotypes, as the primary clinical end point. These results are very encouraging and hopefully will be a harbinger of things to come.

Several different sets of efficacy trials are in progress worldwide, each examining different clinical end points (Tables 3 and 10). These trials are all designed as randomized, double-blind, and placebo-controlled. Many examined not only the efficacy of multivalent pneumococcal conjugate vaccines, but the safety and impact on carriage as well. At this time, only vaccines produced by MRL and Wyeth-Lederle Vaccines and Pediatrics have undergone phase III studies. All these studies involve vaccines containing seven or more serotypes. Two trials, one in progress (Finland) and one recently completed (United States), have evaluated the impact these vaccines have on otitis media. In addition to the above-mentioned study in Northern California, two other efficacy studies, now in progress, are also examining invasive disease as a primary endpoint. These studies involve infant populations in South Africa, and a Navajo/Apache population in the Southwest United States. A fourth efficacy trial is scheduled to begin in 1999 in the Gambia following an on-going phase II study and will look at both morbidity and mortality end points. Other efficacy trials are expected to begin in the near future and will incorporate PMC conjugate vaccines containing anywhere from nine to 11 serotypes. These trials will be done, most likely, in settings where the incidence of disease is sufficiently high to demonstrate the effect of a conjugate vaccine on invasive pneumococcal disease and carriage.

Pneumococcal conjugate vaccines have evolved considerably over the past several years from simple monovalent vaccines to products containing multiples of up to 11 serotypes. Further changes are likely as new carriers are tested, new adjuvant systems are introduced, epidemiological shifts occur among disease-producing serotypes, and geographical needs prevail.

The interest in developing and promoting pneumococcal conjugate vaccines are many and are based on several needs such as (1) providing protection to various high-risk groups; (2) offsetting drug resistance; (3) protecting against the spread of uncontrolled invasive strains; and (4) the potential for reducing the transmission of pneumococci in community and specialized settings. However, as good as these conjugate vaccines sound, they must be tempered by several limiting factors (Table 11). Overall, the conjugate pneumococcal vaccines appear to be relatively safe and produce increased immunological responses for various high-risk groups compared to the licensed polysaccharide vaccines. The immunogenicity has been shown to vary significantly among serotypes in terms of magnitude and kinetics of response. Furthermore, there are no antibody data that show what levels of antibody concentrations are needed for protection. Nevertheless, the routine use of pneumococcal conjugate vaccines may represent the most successful means for decreasing the burden of antibiotic-resistant strains of pneumococci.

REFERENCES

1. **Acute Respiratory Infections.** 1998. The forgotten pandemic. Int. J. Tuberc. Lung. Dis. **2**:2–4.

2. **Adams, W.G., K.A. Deaver, and S.L. Cochi.** 1993. Decline of childhood *Haemophilus influenzae* type b (Hib) disease in the Hib vaccine era. J.A.M.A. **269**:221–226.

3. **Ahman, H., H. Kayhty, O. Leroy, J. Froeschle, and J. Eskola.** 1995. Immunogenicity of tetravalent pneumococcal conjugate vaccines (PncD, PncT) in Finnish infants [Abstract G69]. *In* 35th Interscience Conference on Antimicrobial Agents and Chemotherapy (ICAAC), San Francisco, p. 170.

4. **Ahmed, F., M.C. Steinhoff, M.C. Rodriguez-Barradas, R.G. Hamilton, D.M. Muscher, and K.E. Nelson.** 1996. Effect of human immunodeficiency virus type 1 infection on the antibody response to glycoprotein conjugate pneumococcal vaccine: results from a randomized trial. J. Infect. Dis. **173**:83–90.

5. **Baltimore, R.** 1992. New challenges in the development of a conjugate pneumococcal vaccine. J.A.M.A. **268**:3366–3367.

6. **Berman, S.** 1991. Epidemiology of acute respiratory infections in children of developing countries. Rev. Infect. Dis. **13**:5454–5462.

7. **Bisgard, K.M., A. Kao, J. Leake, P.M. Strebel, B.A. Perkins, and M. Wharton.** 1998. *Haemophilus influenzae* invasive disease in the United States, 1994–1995: Near disappearance of a vaccine-preventable childhood disease. Emerg. Infect. Dis. **4**:229–237.

8. **Butler, J.C., R.F. Breiman, H.B. Lipman, J. Hofmann, and R.R. Facklam.** 1995. Serotype distribution of *Streptococcus pneumoniae* infections among preschool children in the United States, 1978–1994: implications for development of a conjugate vaccine. J. Infect. Dis. **171**:885–889.

9. **Centers for Disease Control.** 1996. Progress toward elimination of *Haemophilus influenzae* type b diseases among infants and children—United States, 1987–1995. M.M.W.R. **45**:901–906.

10. **Chiu, S.S., D.P. Grenberg, S. Partridge, S.J. Chang, C.Y. Chiu, S.M. Marcy, and J.I. Ward.** 1995. Safety and immunogenicity of a pentavalent pneumococcal conjugate vaccine in healthy toddlers [Abstract G71]. *In* 35th Interscience Conference on Antimicrobial Agents and Chemotherapy (ICAAC), San Francisco, p. 171.

11. **Dagan, R., R. Melamed, M. Muallem, L. Piglansky, D. Greenberg, O. Abramson, P.M. Mendelman, and P. Yagupsky.** 1996. Reduction of nasopharyngeal carriage of antibiotic-resistant pneumococci during second year of life by a heptavalent pneumococcal conjugate vaccine. J. Infect. Dis. **174:**1271–1278.

12. **Dagan, R., R. Muallem, and P. Yagupsky.** 1995. Reduction of nasopharyngeal carriage of penicillin-resistant pneumococci by pneumococcal-OMPC conjugate vaccine during second year of life [Abstract G2]. *In* 35th Interscience Conference on Antimicrobial Agents and Chemotherapy (ICAAC), San Francisco, p. 158.

13. **Daum, R.S., M. Steinhoff, M. Rennels, E. Rothstein, K. Resinger, H. Keyserling, S. Black, K. Bewley, and F. Malinoski.** 1995. Immunogenicity of *S. pneumoniae* oligo- and polysaccharide-CRM197 conjugate vaccines in healthy U.S. infants [Abstract GG5]. *In* 35th Interscience Conference on Antimicrobial Agents and Chemotherapy (ICAAC), San Francisco, p. 170.

14. **Dick, W.E., Jr., and M. Beurret.** 1989. Glyconjugates of bacterial carbohydrate antigens. A survey and consideration of design and preparation factors. Contrib. Microbiol. Immunol. **10:**48–114.

15. **Dintzis, R.Z.** 1992. Rational design of conjugate vaccines. Pediatr. Res. **32:**376–385.

16. **Eby, R., M. Koster, D. Hogerman, F. Malinoski, IBS Department, and Scale-up and Development Department.** 1994. Pneumococcal conjugate vaccines. *In* E. Norrby, F. Buren, R.M. Charock, and H.S. Ginsberg (eds.), Vaccines 1994: modern approaches to new vaccines including prevention of AIDS. Cold Spring Harbor Press, Cold Spring Harbor, NY, pp. 119–124.

17. **Eby, R.** 1995. Pneumococcal conjugate vaccines. *In* M.F. Powell and M.J. Newman (eds.), Vaccine design: the subunit and adjuvant approach. Plenum Press, New York, pp. 695–718.

18. **Germain, R.N., and L.R. Hendrix.** 1991. MHC class II structure, occupancy and surface expression determined by post-endoplasmic reticulum antigen binding. Nature **353:**134–139.

19. **Giebink, G.S., M. Koskela, P.P. Vella, M. Harris, and C.T. Le.** 1993. Pneumococcal capsular polysaccharide-meningococcal outer membrane protein complex conjugate vaccines: immunogenicity and efficacy in experimental pneumococcal otitis media. J. Infect. Dis. **167:**347–355.

20. **Gray, B.M., and E.L. Anderson.** 1995. Quantitative and functional antibody responses in children given a tetravalent pneumococcal conjugate vaccine [Abstract 393]. *In* Infectious Diseases Society of America, Annual Meeting, San Francisco, p. 115.

21. **Groover, J.E., D.M. Musher, E.A. Graviss, and R.E. Baughn.** 1995. Does antibody response to pneumococcal capsular polysaccharides decrease with aging? [Abstract 390]. Infectious Diseases Society of America, Annual Meeting, San Francisco, p. 114.

22. **Hansman, D., S. Morris, M. Gregory, and B. McDonald.** 1985. Pneumococcal carriage amongst Australian aborigines in Alice Springs, Northern Territory. J. Hyg. (Lond.) **95:**677–684.

23. **Hedlund, J., M. Kalin, A. Ortqvist, and J. Henrichsen.** 1994. Antibody response to pneumococcal vaccine in middle-aged and elderly patients recently treated for pneumonia. Arch. Intern. Med. **154:**1961–1965.

24. **Hendley, J.O., M.A. Sande, P.M. Stewart, and J.M. Gwaltney, Jr.** 1975. Spread of *Streptococcus pneumoniae* in families. I. Carriage rates and distribution of types. J. Infect. Dis. **132:**55–61.

25. **Hofmann, J., M.S. Cetron, M.M. Farley, W.S. Baughman, R.R. Facklam, J.A. Elliott, K.A. Deaver, and R.F. Breiman.** 1995. The prevalence of drug-resistant streptococcus pneumoniae in Atlanta. N. Engl. J. Med. **333:**481–486.

26. **Immunization Practices Advisory Committee.** 1989. Pneumococcal polysaccharide vaccine. M.M.W.R. **38:**64–76.

27. **Janoff, E.N., and J.B. Rubins.** 1997. Invasive pneumococcal disease in the immunocompromised host. Microb. Drug Resist. **3:**215–232.

28. **Kayhty, H., H. Ahman, P.-R. Ronnberg, R. Tillikainen, and J. Eskola.** 1995. Pneumococcal polysaccharide-meningococcal outer membrane protein complex conjugate vaccine is immunogenic in infants and children. J. Infect. Dis. **172:**1273–1278.

29. **Käyhty, H., and J. Eskola.** 1996. New vaccines for the prevention of pneumococcal infections. Emerg. Infect. Dis. **2:**289–298.

30. **Keyserling, H., C. Bosley, S. Starr, B. Watson, D. Laufer, E. Anderson, E. Shapiro, P. Mendelman, C. Rusk, J. Donnelly, D. Loy, C. Shadle, L. Feeley, and H. Matthews.** 1994. Immunogenicity of pneumococcal type 14 conjugate vaccine in infants [Abstract 1087]. *In* Annual Meeting of the American Pediatric Society/Society for Pediatric Research, Seattle, p. 184A.

31. **Keyserling, H.L., S. Romero-Steiner, L.B. Pais, J. Dykes, and G.M. Carlone.** 1995. Opsonophagocytic titers correlate with IgG ELISA antibody levels in infants immunized with a streptococcus pneumoniae protein oligosaccharide conjugate vaccine [Abstract 1060]. *In* Annual Meeting of the American Pediatric Society/Society of Pediatric Research, San Diego, p. 179A.

32. **King, J.C., P. Vink, M. Smilie, M. Parks, D. Madore, and F. Malinoski.** 1995. Safety and immunogenicity of a 5-valent conjugate pneumococcal vaccine in HIV[+] and non–HIV-infected children [Abstract 1064]. *In* Annual Meeting of the American Pediatric Society/Society for Pediatric Research, San Diego, p. 180A.

33. **Klein, J.O.** 1981. The epidemiology of pneumococcal disease in infants and children. Rev. Infect. Dis. **3:**246–253.

34. **Klein, J.O.** 1994. Otitis media. Clin. Infect. Dis. J. **19:**823–833.

35. **Klugman, K.P.** 1990. Pneumococcal resistance to antibiotics. Clin. Microbiol. Rev. **3:**171–196.

36. **Leowski, J.** 1986. Mortality from acute respiratory infections in children under 5 years of age: global estimates. World Health Stat. Q. **39:**138–144.

37. **Lloyd-Evans, N., T.J. O'Dempsey, I. Baldeh, O. Secka, E. Demba, J.E. Todd, T.F. Mcardle, W.S. Banya, and B.M. Greenwood.** 1996. Nasopharyngeal carriage of pneumococci in Gambian children and in their families. Pediatr. Infect. Dis. J. **10:**866–871.

38. **McDaniel, L.S., J.S. Sheffield, P. Delucchi, and D. Briles.** 1991. PspA, a surface protein of *Streptococcus pneumoniae*, is capable of eliciting protection against pneumococci of more than one capsular type. Infect. Immunol. **59:**222–228.

39. **Mendelman, P.M., E.L. Anderson, and J. Donnelly.** 1995. Immunologic memory in young infants induced by a pneumococcal conjugate vaccine. Presented at the Immune Workshop in Sickle Cell Disease, Bethesda, MD, September 27–28.

40. **Mendelman, P.M., S. Block, J. Hedrick, E. Anderson, H. Keyserling, R. Yogev, D. Greenberg, C. Rusk, C. Shadle, D. Lov, M. Chung, M. Stallworth, G. Calandra, H. Matthews, J. Ward, L. Feeley, J. Donnelly, M. Liu, R. Ellis, and J.L. Ryan.** 1994. Immunogenicity of a 7-valent pneumococcal conjugate vaccine in 2-month-old infants [Abstract 1109]. *In* Annual Meeting of the American Pediatric Society/Society for Pediatric Research, Seattle, p. 187A.

41. **Mosier, D.E., and B. Subbarao.** 1982. Thymus independent antigens: complexity of B lymphocyte activation revealed. Immunol. Today **3:**217–225.

42. **Mufson, M., H. Krause, G. Schiffman, and D.F. Hughey.** 1987. Pneumococcal antibody levels one decade after immunization of healthy adults. Am. J. Med. Sci. **293:**279–284.

43. **Mufson, M.** 1990. *Streptococcus pneumoniae*. *In* G.L. Mandell, R.G. Douglas, and J.E. Bennett (eds.), Principles and practices of infectious diseases. Churchill Livingstone, New York, pp. 1539–1550.

44. **Mufson, M.A.** 1981. Pneumococcal infections. J.A.M.A. **246:**1942–1948.

45. **Munoz, R., J.M. Musser, M. Crain, D.E. Briles, A. Marton, A.J. Parkinson, U. Sorensen, and A. Tomasz.** 1991. Geographic distribution of penicillin-resistant clones of *Streptococcus pneumoniae*: characterization by penicillin-binding protein (PBP) profile,

surface protein A typing and multilocus enzyme analysis. Clin. Infect. Dis. **15**:112–118.

46. **Nesin, M., M. Ramirez, and A. Tomasz.** 1998. Capsular transformation of a multidrug-resistant *Streptococcus pneumoniae in vivo.* J. Infect. Dis. **177**:707–713.

47. **Obaro, S.K., R.A. Adegbola, W.A.S. Banya, and B.M. Greenwood.** 1996. Carriage of pneumococci after pneumococcal vaccination. Lancet **348**:271–272.

48. **Orange, M., and B.M. Gray.** 1993. Pneumococcal serotypes causing disease in children in Alabama. Pediatr. Infect. Dis. J. **12**:244–246.

49. **Portier, H., P. Choutet, M. Duong, M. Moreau, B. Danve, and M. Cadoz.** 1994. Serum antibody response to a tetravalent pneumococcal-tetanus toxoid conjugate vaccine in adult volunteers [Abstract G91]. *In* 34th Interscience Conference on Antimicrobial Agents and Chemotherapy (ICAAC), Orlando, FL p. 237.

50. **Powers, D.C., E.L. Anderson, and C.M. Mink.** 1996. Reactogenicity and immunogenicity of a protein-conjugated pneumococcal polysaccharide vaccine in older adults. J. Infect. Dis. **173**:1014–1018.

51. **Robbins, J.B., and R. Schneerson.** 1990. Polysaccharide-protein conjugates: a new generation of vaccines. Rev. Infect. Dis. **161**:821–832.

52. **Rubins, J.B., D. Charboneau, C. Fasching, A.M. Berry, J.C. Paton, J.E. Alexander, P.W. Andrew, T.J. Mitchell, and E.N. Janoff.** 1996. District roles for pneumolysin's cytotaxic and complement activities in the pathogenesis of pneumococcal pneumonia. Am. J. Respir. Crit. Care Med. **153**:1339–1346.

53. **Shapiro, E.D., A.T. Berg, R. Austrian, D. Schroeder, V. Parcells, A. Margolis, R.K. Adair, and J.D. Clemens.** 1991. The protective efficacy of polyvalent pneumococcal polysaccharide vaccine. N. Engl. J. Med. **325**:1453–1460.

54. **Shapiro, E.D.** 1991. Pneumococcal vaccines. Semin. Pediatr. Infect. Dis. **2**:147–152.

55. **Shelly, M.A., B. Graves, G.J. Riley, and J.J. Treanor.** 1994. Comparison of pneumococcal polysaccharide (PS) and CRM-197 conjugated pneumococcal polysaccharide (CRM-PS) vaccines in young and older adults [Abstract 393]. *In* Infectious Diseases Society of America, Annual Meeting, Orlando, FL, p. 115.

56. **Sniadack, D.H., B. Schwartz, H. Lipman, J. Bogaerts, J.C. Butler, R. Dagan, G. Echaniz-Aviles, N. Lloyd-Evans, A. Fenoll, and N.I. Girgis.** 1995. Potential interventions for the prevention of childhood pneumonia: geographic and temporal differences in serotype and serogroup distribution of sterile site pneumococcal isolates from children—implications for vaccine strategies. Pediatr. Infect. Dis. J. **14**:503–510.

57. **Shurin, P.A., G.S. Giebink, D.L. Wegman, D. Ambrosino, J. Rholl, M. Overman, T. Bauer, and G. Siber.** 1988. Prevention of pneumococcal otitis media in chinchillas with human bacterial polysaccharide immune globulin. J. Clin. Microbiol. **26**:755–759.

58. **Stein, K.E.** 1985. Network regulation of the immune response to bacterial polysaccharide antigens. Curr. Top. Microbiol. Immunol. **119**:57–74.

59. **Steinhoff, M.C., K. Edward, H. Keyserling, M.L. Thoms, C. Johnson, D. Madore, and D. Hogerman.** 1994. A randomized comparison of three bivalent *Streptococcus pneumoniae* glycoprotein conjugate vaccines in young children: effect of polysaccharide size and linkage characteristics. Pediatr. Infect. Dis. J. **13**:368–372.

60. **Vella, P.P., S. Marburg, J.M. Staub, P.J. Kniskern, W. Miller, A. Hagopian, C. Ip, R.L. Tolman, C.M. Rusk, L.S. Chupak, and R.W. Ellis.** 1992. Immunogenicity of conjugate vaccines consisting of pneumococcal capsular polysaccharide types 6B, 14, 19F, and 23F and a meningococcal outer membrane protein complex. Infect. Immun. **60**:4977–4983.

61. **WHO Technical Advisory Group on ARI.** 1984. A program for controlling acute respiratory infections in children: memorandum from a WHO meeting. Bull. W.H.O. **64**:47–58.

62. **Yogev, R., S. Gupta, B. Emanuel, K. William, and J. Adams.** 1993. Safety, tolerability and immunogenicity of tetravalent (6B, 14, 19F, 23F) pneumococcal (Pn) conjugate vaccine in infants given concurrently with routine immunizations [Abstract 170]. *In* 33rd Interscience Conference on Antimicrobial Agents and Chemotherapy (ICAAC), New Orleans, p. 150.

Address reprint requests to:
David L. Klein
Bacterial Respiratory Disease Program Officer
Respiratory Diseases Branch
DMID/NIAID
National Institutes of Health
6700-B Rockledge Dr., Room 3130
Bethesda, MD 20892

Streptococcus pneumoniae
Copyright © 2000 Mary Ann Liebert, Inc., 2 Madison Avenue, Larchmont, NY 10538

Epidemiology of Pneumococcal Serotypes and Conjugate Vaccine Formulations

JAY C. BUTLER

ABSTRACT

The incidence of bacteremia and meningitis due to *Streptococcus pneumoniae* is highest among preschool age children, particularly those <2 years of age. Clinical trials of capsular polysaccharide vaccines among young children have been disappointing. Conjugation of bacterial polysaccharides to proteins can increase antibody responses following vaccination of young children. Conjugate vaccines under evaluation in clinical trials contain a limited number (seven to 11) of serotypes. To identify serotypes most commonly associated with infection in young children, we serotyped pneumococcal isolates submitted to the CDC through national surveillance from 3,884 children <6 years old with pneumococcal bacteremia ($n = 3169$), meningitis ($n = 401$), or otitis media ($n = 314$) from 1978 to 1994. Seven serotypes (14, 6B, 19F, 18C, 23F, 4, and 9V) accounted for 3045 (78%) isolates. A conjugate pneumococcal vaccine protecting against these seven serotypes and serologically cross-reactive serotypes could potentially prevent 86% of bacteremia, 83% of meningitis, and 65% of otitis media cases. The proportion of isolates covered by such a vaccine increased from 78% to 87% from 1978 to 1994. Of 70 isolates submitted during 1992–94 that were nonsusceptible to penicillin (minimal inhibitory concentration [MIC] > 0.1 μg/mL, 56 (80%) were among the seven most prevalent serotypes. All 21 isolates resistant to penicillin (MIC $\geq$ 2.0 μg/mL) were among these seven serotypes.

INTRODUCTION

Streptococcus pneumoniae is a leading cause of bacteremia, meningitis, pneumonia, and upper respiratory tract infection worldwide.[4] In community-based studies in the United States, annual incidence rates of pneumococcal bacteremia are 15–30 cases/100,000 population for all persons, 45–90 cases/100,000 population for persons $\geq$65 years of age, and >150 cases/100,000 population for children $\leq$2 years of age.[6,9,26,27,41] Although the incidence of invasive pneumococcal disease is highest among young children, effective vaccines are not yet available for persons younger than 2 years old. T-cell–independent antigens such as polysaccharides produce limited antibody responses in children under age 2 years, and clinical trials of the pneumococcal capsular polysaccharide vaccines among young children have demonstrated limited or no evidence of efficacy.[17,30,32] Conjugation of bacterial polysaccharides to proteins can result in T-cell dependent immune responses, increasing antibody levels following primary vaccination of young children and booster responses to subsequent doses.[29,37,47] This strategy has led to the development of *Haemophilus influenzae*, type b (Hib) vaccines that are safe and

efficacious in children younger than 2 years of age.[7,18] The use of conjugated Hib vaccines has been accompanied by a dramatic reduction in the incidence of invasive Hib infections.[1]

Conjugation of pneumococcal polysaccharide antigens to a carrier protein may provide the means for preventing invasive *S. pneumoniae* infections during early childhood. An obstacle to this approach is that there are 90 serotypes of *S. pneumoniae*,[25] and currently, it does not appear possible to include more than a limited number of antigens in a conjugated formulation.[23,47] Most conjugate pneumococcal vaccines proposed to date have been seven-, nine- or 11-valent.[2,14,16,47] The choice of antigens to include in a pneumococcal polysaccharide conjugate vaccine should be based primarily on the predominant serotypes causing disease in the population targeted for vaccination. For example, a vaccine designed to prevent invasive infection in the United States may be inadequate in other parts of the world because of differences in serotype prevalence in various locales. A vaccine based on the serotypes most commonly causing bacteremia among adults may not be well suited for prevention of otitis media in children. Moreover, shifts in serotype distribution over time may eventually make a given vaccine formulation obsolete. The goal of this review is to pro-

---

Arctic Investigations Program, Centers for Disease Control and Prevention, Anchorage, Alaska.

vide an overview of epidemiology of pneumococcal serotypes among patients reported to the Centers for Diseases Control and Prevention's (CDC) National Pneumococcal Sentinel Surveillance,[10] to compare the data on serotype distribution from the United States with that from other countries, and to discuss factors other than serotype prevalence which may be considered in conjugate vaccine formulation.

From 1978 to 1994, pneumococcal isolates were submitted from 3,884 children <6 years old; of these patients, 3,007 (77.4%) were <2 years old.[11] Isolates were from the blood (n = 3,169), cerebrospinal fluid (n = 401), or middle ear fluid (n = 314). Differences in serotype prevalence by body site were greatest for serotype 3, which accounted for 9% of middle ear fluid isolates but ≤1% of blood or CSF isolates (Fig. 1). A similar association between serotype 3 and otitis media was observed by Gray among children in Birmingham, Alabama during the late 1970s.[24] Serotypes 18C and 4 were somewhat more common among patients with bacteremia or meningitis compared to patients with otitis.

Overall, seven serotypes (14, 6B, 19F, 18C, 23F, 4, and 9V, in decreasing order of frequency) accounted for 3,045 (78.4%) isolates. These seven most common serotypes are included in a heptavalent vaccine that has been evaluated for safety and immunogenicity in young children[2,16,43] and that has been shown to prevent invasive pneumococcal infection in a double blind

randomized trial among 37,000 children enrolled in a northern California health maintenance organization.[8] The most common serotypes not included in the vaccine were 19A (3.7% of all isolates), 6A (3.5%), 3 (1.5%), 7F (1.3%), and 1 (1.2%); all other serotypes each accounted for <1%.[11] This heptavalent vaccine would potentially provide protection against additional serotypes (primarily 6A, but also 9A, 9L, 18B, 18F) involved in 206 (5.3%) infections because of serologic cross-reactivity.[31,45,50] Heterologous immune responses between 19A and 19F are limited[40]; therefore, a vaccine containing 19F was not considered potentially protective against 19A. Thus, 83.7% of these infections among preschool aged children in the United States could potentially be prevented by an efficacious heptavalent conjugated pneumococcal vaccine, including 2,719 (86%) of those associated with an isolate from blood, 331 (85%) with meningitis, but only 203 (65%) with an isolate from middle ear fluid.

The seven most common serotypes accounted for 80% of 3,570 isolates from the blood of CSF of children <6 years old. By comparison, of blood and CSF isolates from 2,322 unvaccinated persons ≥6 years old reported by the same surveillance during 1978–92 (of whom 93.0% were ≥18 years old and 33.5% were ≥65), 1,171 (50%) isolates were one of these seven serotypes.[12] Serotype 4 was the most prevalent serotype among older children and adults, accounting for 13.4% of cases (Fig. 2). The most common serotype isolated from older patients which was not among the seven most prevalent serotypes among young children was 12F—this serotype caused 6.2% of invasive infections in older children and adults but only 0.6% of those among children <6 years old.

The proportion of isolates from children <6 years old which would be covered by the heptavalent vaccine described above increased from 78% in 1978 to 87% in 1994, primarily due to the increasing prevalence of serotype 14.[11] While only modest changes in serotype prevalence were observed during the 16 years of CDC surveillance, more substantial shifts may occur over longer periods. At Boston City Hospital, serotypes 1, 2, and 3 accounted for roughly one-half of isolates from all sites prior to 1950, but by 1979–1982 they accounted for <5%.[3,20,51] Of 3,644 isolates from blood of patients at 10 U.S. hospitals submitted to and serotyped by Austrian and colleagues between 1967 and 1975, serotypes 1, 2, and 3 accounted for 8.5%, 0.3%, and 7.1%, respectively.[3] Among the blood and CSF isolates submitted to CDC, serotype 1 and 3 together accounted for only 2.7% from children <6 years old during 1978–94 and 8.2% from unvaccinated persons ≥6 years old during 1978–92. Only one of over 7,000 blood isolates serotyped at CDC from 1978 though 1995 was serotype 2.

Antimicrobial susceptibility testing was performed on all blood and CSF isolates submitted during 1992 through 1994 (Table 1). Of 508 isolates tested, 438 (86.2%) were susceptible to penicillin (minimal inhibitory concentration [MIC] <0.1 μg/mL), 49 (9.6%) were penicillin-intermediate (MIC 0.1–1.0 μg/mL), and 21 (4.1%) were penicillin-resistant (MIC ≥ 2.0 μg/mL). The majority of penicillin-resistant isolates were serotype 6B. Among the 10 most prevalent serotypes, two—18C and 4—were uniformly susceptible to penicillin. Of 14 serogroup 19A isolates, only 5 (35.7%) were penicillin-susceptible. A heptavalent vaccine based on the seven most prevalent serotypes would cover 88% of penicillin-susceptible, 73%

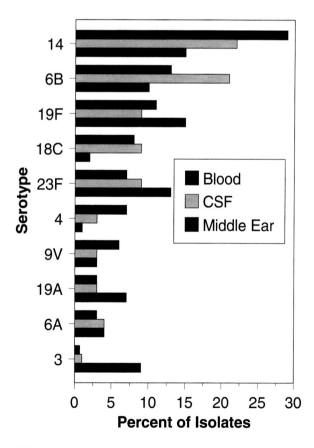

FIG. 1. Serotype prevalence by recovery site for isolates from patients <6 years old in the United States, 1978–94, including 3,169 from the blood, 401 from the CSF, and 314 from middle ear fluid.

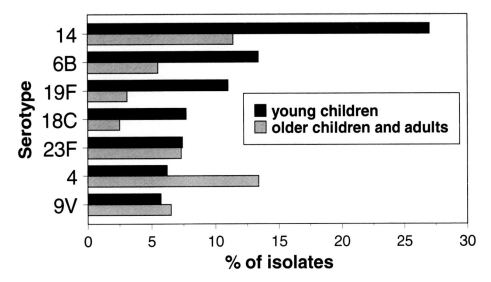

FIG. 2. Prevalence of selected pneumococcal serotypes among isolates from 3,884 young children (<6 years old) and 2,322 unvaccinated older children and adults (≥6 years old).

of penicillin intermediate, and 100% of penicillin-resistant isolates.

The proportion of isolates that would be covered by the proposed heptavalent conjugate vaccine did not differ substantially among regions of the United States.[11] However, when the serotype distribution from the United States is compared to similar surveillance data from other parts of the world, substantial differences are noted,[49] and it is apparent that a vaccine that is based on the most prevalent serotypes among children in one country may not be appropriate for children in a different region of the world. The seven most common serogroups in the United States accounted for 84% of isolated from Finland and 78% from Australia but only 33% of isolates from Rwanda and 31% from Papua New Guinea. In Rwanda and Papua New Guinea, as well as several other countries (South Africa, Israel, and a number of South American nations), >10% of isolated are either serotype 1 or serotype 5, yet in the United States, these two serotypes together accounted for only 1.3% of inva-

sive pneumococcal infections.[28,49] Based on comparisons of serogroup distribution among 16 countries, Sniadack et al.[49] recommended that a nonavalent vaccine ("global-9") incorporating serotypes 1, 5, 6B, 7F, 9V, 14, 18C, 19F, and 23F would be optimal for global use to prevent invasive pneumococcal pneumonia among children. A similar conjugate vaccine which differs from the "global-9" by inclusion of serotype 4 instead of 7F is currently being evaluated in clinical trials.[14]

The inclusion of >9 antigens in a conjugate vaccine for global use would result in limited increases in coverage against serotypes causing bacteremia and meningitis among young children in most areas for which surveillance data are available, but additional serotypes could substantially improve protection against otitis media (serotype 3 and 19A) or against invasive infections in adults (serotypes 4 and 12F). Trials evaluating the efficacy of pneumococcal conjugate vaccine for the prevention of acute otitis media are ongoing, but preliminary data suggest that the heptavalent conjugate vaccine may reduce nasopha-

TABLE 1. PNEUMOCOCCAL SEROTYPE PREVALENCE BY PENICILLIN SUSCEPTIBILITY FOR ISOLATES SUBMITTED TO THE CENTERS FOR DISEASE CONTROL AND PREVENTION FROM BLOOD OR CEREBROSPINAL FLUID OF 508 PATIENTS <6 YEARS OLD, 1992–94

	Susceptibility to penicillin (minimal inhibitory concentration)			
Serotype	<0.1 μg/mL, no. (% of serotype)	0.1–1.0 μg/mL, no. (% of serotype)	≥2.0 μg/mL, no. (% of serotype)	Total, no. (% of all isolates)
14	147 (32.0)	10 (20.4)	1 (4.8)	158 (32.0)
6B	58 (13.2)	10 (20.4)	11 (52.4)	79 (15.6)
19F	50 (11.4)	6 (12.2)	0	56 (11.0)
9V	31 (7.1)	6 (12.2)	4 (19.0)	41 (8.1)
23F	21 (4.8)	3 (6.1)	5 (23.8)	29 (5.7)
18C	28 (6.4)	0	0	28 (5.5)
4	18 (4.1)	0	0	18 (3.5)
19A	5 (1.1)	9 (18.4)	0	14 (2.8)
6A	13 (3.0)	1 (2.0)	0	14 (2.8)
Other	67 (15.3)	4 (8.2)	0	71 (14.0)

ryngeal colonization with vaccine-type strains among young children[16] and thus may have a role in prevention of otitis media and the development of "herd immunity" by reducing transmission from colonized children. The role of conjugate vaccine for prevention of pneumococcal disease in adults has not been defined.[35,42] Nevertheless, immunologic priming with conjugate vaccine followed with a booster dose of 23-valent polysaccharide vaccine may be a method to improve immunogenicity among adults.[15] Therefore, inclusion of serotypes that are prevalent among adults may be an important consideration in a conjugate vaccine with >9 serotypes. A proposed 11-valent vaccine incorporating serotypes 1, 3, 4, 5, 6B, 7F, 9V, 14, 18C, 19F, and 23F[14] would cover (assuming cross-protection between 6B and 6A) 86% of isolates submitted from children to CDC, including 87% of those from blood, 85% from CSF, and 76% from middle ear fluid, and 64% of blood and CSF isolates from unvaccinated older children and adults.

Factors other than serotype prevalence among populations targeted for immunization may need to be considered in vaccine formulation. Serotypes possibly associated with higher mortality, such as serotype 3,[36] may deserve special emphasis for inclusion in pneumococcal vaccines. Certain pneumococcal serotypes are more immunogenic than others. It two serotypes are equally prevalent in the target population, preference for the more immunogenic serotype is justified. Unfortunately, there are limited data available to define the quantity of anticapsular antibody which is protective, and the protective antibody level may not be the same for all serotypes. There is considerable cross-reactivity among certain of the 90 recognized serotypes, and a single antigen may provide protection against several types within a given serogroup.[12,44] For example, adult volunteers given nonconjugated vaccine containing either 50 μg of 6A polysaccharide or 50 μg of both 6A and 6B polysaccharides showed no difference in antibody responses to serotype 6A or 6B.[45] However, cross-immunogenicity is more limited among other types within the same groups, as is the case with 19A and 19F.[40]

Antigen stability under field conditions is another important consideration for pneumococcal vaccine formulation. Serotype 6A, a component of the 14-valent polysaccharide vaccine, was found to be subject to degradation,[52] and 6A was replaced by the more stable 6B antigen in the 23-valent vaccine. Epidemiologic observations suggest that persons immunized with the 23-valent vaccine (containing 6B) had greater protection against invasive 6A infection than did persons receiving the 14-valent vaccine (containing 6A).[12]

Finally, the clinical impact of emerging drug-resistant pneumococcal strains may need to be considered in future vaccine formulations. Anecdotal reports of treatment failures and mortality in children and adults with pneumococcal meningitis suggest that outcome may be worse for patients infected with resistant strains.[13,21,48] However, studies among adults and children with bacteremic pneumonia have not demonstrated increased mortality among those infected with penicillin-nonsusceptible pneumococci, even among patients treated with penicillin or ampicillin.[22,39] However, it is important to note that the vast majority of patients in these studies were infected with pneumococci intermediate to penicillin (MIC 0.1–1.0 μg/mL). Additional studies are needed to comprehensively assess the clinical impact of resistance to penicillin (MIC $\geq$ 2 μg/mL) and

the morbidity and economic costs associated with penicillin-resistant infections. Preliminary data from CDC surveillance suggest that increased mortality is associated with invasive pneumococcal infections with penicillin-resistant but not penicillin-intermediate strains.[19]

A promising complementary or alternative approach for prevention of all pneumococcal infections is to develop vaccines directed against an antigenic moiety common to all pneumococcal serotypes.[33,34,38,46] However, such species-wide vaccines are unlikeky to be available in the near future. In the meantime, widened and intensified national and international surveillance is needed to track the epidemiology of pneumococcal serotypes and the emergence of drug-resistant pneumococcal strains. These data will be needed to assess the impact of pneumococcal vaccines on the rates of disease caused by serotypes included in the vaccines, to determine whether the incidence of disease caused by nonvaccine serotypes is influenced by the introduction of conjugate vaccines, and to assure that components of pneumococcal polysaccharide and conjugate vaccines are based on the serotypes actually causing disease.

REFERENCES

1. **Adams, W.G., K.A. Deaver, S.L. Cochi, B.D. Plikaytis, E.R. Zell, C.V. Broome, J.D. Wenger, for the *Haemophilus influenzae* Study Group.** 1993. Decline of childhood *Haemophilus influenzae* type b (Hib) disease in the Hib vaccine era. J.A.M.A. **269:**221–226.

2. **Anderson, E.L., D.J. Kennedy, K.M. Geldmacher, J. Donnelly, and P.M. Mendelman.** 1996. Immunogenicity of heptavalent pnuemococcal conjugate vaccine in infants. J. Pediatr. **128:**649–653.

3. **Austrian, R., R.M. Douglas, G. Schiffman, A.M. Coetzee, H.J. Koornhof, S. Hayden-Smith, and R.D.W. Reid.** 1976. Prevention of pneumococcal pneumonia by vaccination. Trans. Assoc. Am. Physicians **89:**184–194.

4. **Baltimore, R.S., and E.D. Shapiro.** 1991. Pneumococcal infections. *In* A.S. Evans and P.S. Brachman (eds.), Bacterial infections of humans: epidemiology and control. Plenum, New York, pp. 525–546.

5. **Barry, M.A., D.E. Craven, and M. Finland.** 1984. Serotypes of *Streptococcus pneumoniae* isolated from blood cultures at Boston City Hospital between 1979 and 1982. J. Infect. Dis. **149:**449–452.

6. **Bennett, N.M., J. Buffington, and F.M. LaForce.** 1992. Pneumococcal bacteremia in Monroe County, New York. Am. J. Public Health **82:**1513–1516.

7. **Black, S.B., H.R. Shinefield, D. Lampert, B. Fireman, R.A. Hiatt, M. Polen, E. Vittinghoff, and the Northern California Kaiser Permanente Vaccine Study Center Pediatrics Group.** 1991. Safety and immunogenicity of oligosaccharide conjugate *Haemophilus influenzae* type b (HbOC) vaccine in infancy. Pediatr. Infect. Dis. J. **10:**92–96.

8. **Black, S.B., H. Shinefield, P. Ray, E. Lewis, B. Fireman, the Kaiser Permanente Vaccine Study Group, R. Austrian, G. Siber, J. Hackell, R. Kohberger, and I.H. Chang.** 1998. Efficacy of heptavalent conjugate pneumococcal vaccine (Wyeth Lederle) in 37,000 infants and children: results of The Northern California Kaiser Permanente Efficacy Trial [Abstract LB-9]. *In* Final Program, Abstract, and Exhibits Addendum of the 38th Interscience Conference on Antimicrobial Agents and Chemotherapy, San Diego, California, September 24–27, 1998, p. 23.

9. **Breiman, R.F., J.S. Spika, V.J. Navarro, P.M. Darden, and C.P.**

Darby. 1990. Pneumococcal bacteremia in Charleston County, South Carolina. Arch. Intern. Med. 150:1401–1405.

10. Broome, C.V., and R.R. Facklam. 1981. Epidemiology of clinically significant isolates of Streptococcus pneumoniae in the United States. Rev. Infect. Dis. 3:277–280.

11. Butler, J.C., R.F. Breiman, H.B. Lipman, J. Hofmann, and R.R. Facklam. 1995. Serotype distribution of Streptococcus pneumoniae infections among preschool children in the United States, 1978–1994: implications for development of a conjugate vaccine. J. Infect. Dis. 171:885–889.

12. Butler, J.C., R.F. Breiman, J.F. Campbell, H.B. Lipman, C.V. Broome, and R.R. Facklam. 1993. Pneumococcal polysaccharide vaccine efficacy: an evaluation of current recommendation. J.A.M.A. 270:1826–1831.

13. Catalán, M.J., J.M. Fernández, A. Vazquea, E. Varela de Seijas, A. Suárez, and J.C.L. Bernaldo de Quirós. 1994. Failure of cefotaxime in the treatment of meningitis due to relatively resistant Streptococcus pneumoniae. Clin. Infect. Dis. 18:766–769.

14. Children's Vaccine Initiative. 1996. A pneumococcal vaccine to save children of all ages nears final testing. C.V.I. Forum 13:3–11.

15. Chan, C.Y., D.C. Molrine, S. George, N.J. Tarbell, P. Mauch, L. Diller, R.C. Shamberger, N.R. Phillips, A. Goorin, and D.M. Ambrosino. 1996. Pneumococcal conjugate vaccine primes for antibody responses to polysaccharide pneumococcal vaccine after treatment of Hodgkin's disease. J. Infect. Dis. 173:256–258.

16. Dagan, R., R. Melamed, M. Muallem, L. Piglansky, D. Greenberg, O. Abramson, P.M. Mendelman, N. Bohidar, and P. Yagupsky. 1996. Reduction of nasopharyngeal carriage of pneumococci during the second year of life by a heptavalent conjugate pneumococcal vaccine. J. Infect. Dis. 174:1271–1278.

17. Douglas, R.M., J.C. Paton, S.J. Duncan, and D.J. Hansman. 1984. Antibody response to pneumococcal vaccination in children younger than five years of age. J. Infect. Dis. 149:861–869.

18. Eskola, J., H. Käyhty, A.K. Takala, H. Peltola, P.R. Rönnberg, E. Kela, E. Pekkanen, P.H. McVerry, and P.H. Mäkelä. 1990. A randomized, prospective field trial of a conjugate vaccine in the protection of infants and young children against invasive Haemophilus influenzae type b disease. N. Engl. J. Med. 323:1381–1387.

19. Feikin, D., M. Cetron, A. Schuchat, R. Facklam, J. Jorgenson, M. Kolczak, and the Active Surveillance Team. 1997. Multistate population-based assessment of drug resistant S. pneumoniae mortality [Abstract 48]. In Program and Abstracts of the 35th Annual Meeting of the Infectious Diseases Society of America, September 13–16, 1997, San Francisco, California, p. 80.

20. Finland, M., and M.W. Barnes. 1977. Changes in occurrence of capsular serotypes of Streptococcus pneumoniae at Boston City Hospital during selected years between 1935 and 1974. J. Clin. Microbiol. 5:154–166.

21. Friedland, I.R., and K.P. Klugman. 1992. Failure of chloramphenicol therapy in penicillin-resistant pneumococcal meningitis. Lancet 339:405–408.

22. Friedland, I.R. 1995. Comparison of the response to antimicrobial therapy of penicillin-resistant and penicillin-susceptible pneumococcal disease. Pediatr. Infect. Dis. J. 14:885–890.

23. Giebink, G.S. 1994. Immunology: promise of new vaccines. Pediatr. Infect. Dis. J. 13:1064–1068.

24. Gray, B.M., G.M. Converse III, and H.C. Dillon, Jr. 1979. Serotypes of Streptococcus pneumoniae causing disease. J. Infect. Dis. 140:979–983.

25. Henrichsen, J. 1995. Six newly recognized types of Streptococcus pneumoniae. J. Clin. Microbiol. 33:2759–2762.

26. Hofmann, J., M.S. Cetron, M.M. Farley, W.S. Baughman, R.R. Facklam, J.A. Elliot, K.A. Deaver, and R.F. Breiman. 1995. The prevalence of drug-resistant Streptococcus pneumoniae in Atlanta. N. Engl. J. Med. 333:481–486.

27. Istre, G.R., M. Tarpay, M. Anderson, A. Pryor, D. Welch, and the Pneumococcus Study Group. 1987. Invasive disease due to Streptococcus pneumoniae in an area with a high rate of relative penicillin resistance. J. Infect. Dis. 156:732–735.

28. Kertez, D.A., J.L. Di Fabio, M.C.C. Brandileone, E. Castañeda, G. Echániz-Aviles, I. Heitmann, A. Homma, M. Hortal, M. Lovgren, R.O. Ruvinsky, J.A. Talbot, J. Weekes, J.S. Spika, and the PAHO Pneumococcal Surveillance Study Group. 1998. Invasive Streptococcus pneumoniae infection in Latin American children: results of the Pan American Health Organization surveillance study. Clin. Infect. Dis. 26:1355–1361.

29. Klein, D.L. 1995. Pneumococcal conjugate vaccines: review and update. Microb. Drug Resist. 1:49–58.

30. Koskela, M., M. Leinonen, V.M. Häivä, M. Timonen, and P.H. Mäkelä. 1986. First and second dose antibody responses to pneumococcal polysaccharide vaccine in infants. Pediatr. Infect. Dis. 5:45–50.

31. Krishnamurthy, T., C.J. Lee, J. Henrichsen, D.J. Carlo, T.M. Stoudt, and J.B. Robbins. 1978. Characterization of the cross-reaction between type 19F(19) and 19A(57) pneumococcal polysaccharides. I. compositional analysis and immunologic relation determined with rabbit typing antisera. Infect. Immunol. 22:727–735.

32. Leinonen, M., A. Säkkinen, R. Kalliokoski, J. Luotonen, M. Timonen, and P.H. Mäkelä. 1986. Antibody response to 14-valent pneumococcal capsular polysaccharide vaccine in pre-school age children. Pediatr. Infect. Dis. 5:39–44.

33. Lock, R.A., J.C. Paton, and D. Hansman. 1988. Comparative efficacy of pneumococcal neuraminidase and pneumolysin as immunogens protective against Streptococcus pneumoniae. Microb. Pathol. 5:461–467.

34. McDaniel, L.S., J.S. Sheffield, P. Delucchi, and D.E. Briles. 1991. PspA, a surface protein of Streptococcus pneumoniae, is capable of eliciting protection against pneumococci of more than one capsular serotype. Infect. Immunol. 59:222–228.

35. Molrine, D.C., S. George, N. Tarbell, P. Mauch, L. Diller, D. Neuberg, R.C. Shamberger, E.L. Anderson, N.R. Phillips, K. Kinsella, and D.M. Ambrosino. 1995. Antibody responses to polysaccharide and polysaccharide-conjugate vaccines after treatment of Hodgkin disease. Ann. Intern. Med. 123:828–834.

36. Mufson, M.A., D.M. Kruss, R.E. Wasil, and W.I. Metzger. 1974. Capsular types and outcome of bacteremic pneumococcal disease in the antibiotic era. Arch. Intern. Med. 134:505–510.

37. Obaro, S.K., Z. Huo, W.A.S. Banya, D.C. Henderson, M.A. Monteil, A. Leach, and B.M. Greenwood. 1997. A glycoprotein pneumococcal conjugate vaccine primes for antibody responses to a pneumococcal polysaccharide vaccine in Gambian children. Pediatr. Infect. Dis. J. 16:1135–1140.

38. Paton, J.C., R.A. Lock, C.J. Lee, J.P. Li, A.M. Berry, T.J. Mitchell, P.W. Andrew, D. Hansman, and G.J. Boulnois. 1991. Purification and immunogenicity of genetically obtained pneumolysin toxoids and their conjugation to Streptococcus pneumoniae type 19F polysaccharide. Infect. Immunol. 59:2297–2304.

39. Pallares, R., J. Liñares, M. Vadillo, C. Cabellos, F. Manresa, P.F. Viladrich, R. Martin, and F. Gudiol. 1995. Resistance to penicillin and cephalosporins and mortality from severe pneumococcal pneumonia in Barcelona, Spain. N. Engl. J. Med. 333:474–480.

40. Penn, R.L., E.B. Lewin, R.G. Douglas Jr., G. Schiffman, C.J. Lee, and J.B. Robbins. 1982. Antibody responses in adult volunteers to penumococcal polysaccharide types 19F and 19A administered singly and in combination. Infect. Immunol. 36:1261–1262.

41. Plouffe, J.F., R.F. Breiman, R.R. Facklam, for the Franklin County Pneumonia Study Group. 1996. Bacteremia with Streptococcus pneumoniae in adults: implications for therapy and prevention. J.A.M.A. 275:194–198.

42. Powers, D.C., E.L. Anderson, K. Lottenbach, and C.M. Mink. 1996. Reactogenicity and immunogenicity of a protein-conjugate

pneumococcal oligosaccharide vaccine in older adults. J. Infect. Dis. **173:**1014–1018.

43. **Rennels, M.B., K.M. Edwards, H.L. Keyserling, K.S. Reisinger, D.A. Hogerman, D.V. Madore, I. Chang, P.R. Paradiso, F.J. Malinoski, and A. Kimura.** 1998. Safety and immunogenicity of heptavalent pneumococcal vaccine conjugated to CRM_{197} in United States infants. Pediatrics **101:**604–611.

44. **Robbins, J.B., R. Austrian, C.J. Lee, S.C. Rastogi, G. Schiffman, J. Henrichsen, P.H. Mäkelä, C.V. Broome, R.R. Facklam, R.H. Tiesjema, and J.C. Parke, Jr.** 1983. Considerations for formulating the second-generation pneumococcal capsular polysaccharide vaccine with emphasis on the cross-reactive types within groups. J. Infect. Dis. **148:**1136–1159.

45. **Robbins, J.B., C.J. Lee, S.C. Rastogi, G. Schiffman, and J. Henrichsen.** 1979. Comparative immunogenicity of group 6 pneumococcal type 6A(6) and type 6B(26) capsular polysaccharides. Infect. Immunol. **26:**1116–1122.

46. **Russell, H., J.A. Tharpe, D.E. Wells, E.H. White, and J.E. Johnson.** 1990. Monoclonal antibody recognizing a species-specific protein from *Streptococcus pneumonia.* J. Clin. Microbiol. **28:**2191–2195.

47. **Siber, G.R.** 1994. Pneumococcal disease: prospects for a new generation of vaccines. Science **265:**1385–1387.

48. **Sloas, M.M., F.F. Barrett, P.J. Chesney, B.K. English, B.C. Hill, F.C. Tenover, and R.J. Leggiadro.** 1992. Cephalosporin treatment failure in penicillin- and cephalosporin-resistant *Streptococcus pneumoniae* meningitis. Pediatr. Infect. Dis. J. **11:**662–666.

49. **Sniadack, D.H., B. Schwartz, H. Lipman, J. Bogarts, J.C. Butler, R. Dagan, G. Echiniz-Aviles, N. Lloyd-Evans, A. Fenoll, N.I. Girgis, J. Henrichsen, K. Klugman, D. Lehmann, A.K. Takala, J. Vandepitte, S. Gove, and R.F. Breiman.** 1995. Potential interventions for the prevention of childhood pneumonia: geographic and temporal differences in serotype and serogroup distribution of sterile site pneumococcal isolates from children—implications for vaccine strategies. Pediatr. Infect. Dis. J. **14:**503–510.

50. **Szu, S.C., C.J. Lee, J.C. Parke, Jr., G. Schiffman, J. Henrichsen, R. Austrian, S.C. Rastogi, and J.B. Robbins.** 1982. Cross-immunogenicity of pneumococcal group 9 capsular polysaccharides in adult volunteers. Infect. Immunol. **35:**777–782.

51. **Tilghman, F.C., and M. Finland.** 1937. Clinical significance of bacteremia in pneumococcal pneumonia. Arch. Intern. Med. **59:**602–619.

52. **Zon, G., S.C. Szu, W. Egan, J.D. Robbins, and J.B. Robbins.** 1979. Hydrolytic stability of pneumococcal group 6 (type 6A and 6B) capsular polysaccharides. Infect. Immunol. **37:**89–103.

Address reprint requests to:
Jay C. Butler
Arctic Investigations Program
Centers for Disease Control and Prevention
4055 Tudor Centre Dr.
Anchorage, AK 99508

Streptococcus pneumoniae:
At the Threshold of the 21st Century

DANIEL M. MUSHER,[1] ROBERT F. BREIMAN,[2] and ALEXANDER TOMASZ[3]

INTRODUCTION

As it has been since it was first identified more than 100 years ago, *Streptococcus pneumoniae* remains a major pathogen for humans. The pneumococcus is the most commonly identified etiologic agent in acute otitis media, sinusitis, pneumonia requiring hospitalization of adults, and meningitis—infections that continue to cause substantial morbidity and mortality in developed countries. Among children in poorer nations, it is the most frequent cause of severe pneumonia, which is now the leading cause of death in most developing countries. After the Second World War, probably because of the remarkable efficacy of penicillin, interest in pneumococcal infection appeared to wane. In the 1990s, however, concern over the important role of this pathogenic bacterium as a cause of mortality in the developing world, a high incidence of infection in HIV-infected persons, and, especially, worldwide emergence of antimicrobial resistance have contributed to a remarkable resurgence of interest in the pneumococcus. The purpose of this volume is to bring together many of those investigators who have contributed to the explosion of knowledge about pneumococcus in order to exchange questions and ideas.

S. pneumoniae is able to cause disease because it readily colonizes the nasopharynx and then, in a small proportion of persons, migrates to spaces from which it is not cleared, such as the alveoli, the blood and meninges, and the paranasal sinuses or the middle ear. It escapes ingestion and killing by phagocytic cells, a capacity largely determined by the polysaccharide capsule but, perhaps, with some contribution by surface proteins such as pneumococcal surface protein A (PspA). The disease state, itself, generally reflects the presence of intense inflammation that is triggered by cell wall substances, with some contribution by capsule and intracellular products, together with damage to tissues by intracellular products that are released by autolysins. Much of the genome of *S. pneumoniae* has been mapped. The cell wall has been studied by modern techniques, as has the vaccine potential of capsule and noncapsular constituents. Vaccines made up of several serotypes of capsular polysaccharide conjugated to carrier proteins are now being evaluated for efficacy in prevention of pneumococcal illness in infants and children. Finally, a wealth of information is now available about the mechanisms and risk factors for antimicrobial resistance.

THE GENOME PROJECT

By use of sampling methods, at least partial sequencing of 90% of genes of *S. pneumoniae* has been achieved. This method enables a rapid and efficient overview of the genome. All individual genes have not been identified, and some sequences will inevitably be subject to revision. Also, no attempt to focus attention on genes of special clinical significance has been made, but this can soon follow. Attempting to attain a completely annotated genomic sequence by means of multiple redundancies may have been preferable but would have required vastly more resources. Even when such an effort was made, as in the case of *Haemophilus influenzae* type b, subsequent revisions to a greater or lesser extent have been required. Information from this project will facilitate cloning of individual gene products such as capsular constituents or pneumolysin, which could have diagnostic use. Further, such products may be targeted by novel therapeutic agents, a factor that might become increasingly important with progressive antimicrobial resistance.

NASOPHARYNGEAL COLONIZATION

Pneumococcal infection usually does not occur without prior colonization of the nasopharynx. Nasopharyngeal colonization varies with age and exposure (including living and school/working conditions), the season, and the presence of coexisting viral respiratory illness. Such colonization, in turn, depends upon the interaction between the pneumococcal cell surface and nasopharyngeal epithelial cells. The bacterial surface is actually far more complex and subsists in a vastly more dynamic state than was previously recognized. In addition to peptidoglycan, the unique phosphocholine moiety, and polysaccharide capsule, a number of other substances are expressed. Lipoteichoic and teichoic acid structures that protrude from the surface have identical chain structures, a characteristic that suggests common biosynthetic steps and may be unique to pneumococci. These

---

[1]Veterans Affairs Medical Center and the Baylor College of Medicine, Houston, Texas.
[2]Centers for Disease Control and Prevention, Atlanta, Georgia.
[3]Rockefeller University, New York, New York.

substances mediate adherence to mammalian epithelial cell glycoconjugates containing GalNacβ1-4Gal. Pneumococcal surface adhesin is homologous with lipoprotein adhesin molecules
of certain other oral streptococci. Mutants that lack this adhesin
are less likely to colonize and cause disease after intranasal
challenge but, less understandably, also after intraperitoneal
challenge.

Pneumococci replicate *in vitro* in colonies that are either
transparent or opaque. Transparent colony forms contain up to
eightfold greater choline than opaque ones and show far greater
attachment to tissue-cultured epithelial cells *in vitro* or to mouse
epithelial cells *in vivo;* nonetheless, the opaque phenotype
seems to be associated with greater virulence, at least in animal models. Larger amounts of capsular polysaccharides may
render opaque colonies less adherent, but more directly invasive. The importance of these observations in the ability of wild
strains to cause disease remains to be determined.

It is, as yet, unknown, whether transmission of contagion occurs primarily via contact, aerosol or droplet, and it is unclear
why some persons become colonized when others do not, although upregulation of receptors on epithelial cell surfaces, for
example during viral infection, is likely to play a role. The relative importance of IgG and sIgA in terminating colonization
is not established. In any case, the pneumococcus has the potential to become invasive when it migrates out of the nasopharynx, either being carried into spaces from which clearance is impaired, such as the middle ear, the paranasal sinuses,
or the bronchial tree, or directly invading epithelium and penetrating into the blood streams as is seen with *H. influenzae* and
Neisseria meningitidis. Direct invasion by pneumococci has
not, in fact, been documented. However, choline-containing cell
wall constituents activate platelet adhesion factor in endothelial cells, a reaction that increases adherence and stimulates the
appearance of intracellular translocation vesicles which may be
responsible for transporting pneumococci across endothelial
cells. It is unclear why colonization is innocuous for the vast
majority who are infected with *S. pneumoniae* (*i.e.,* why invasion is a relatively rare phenomenon); the rapid emergence of
capsular type-specific systemic antibodies after colonization,
and (perhaps prior to the production of type-specific antibodies) the presence of antibodies to other surface constituents, as
well as structural integrity of local mechanisms of clearance are
thought to play important roles.

RESISTANCE TO INGESTION

If the body's normal clearance mechanisms fail to remove
pneumococci that have been carried beyond the nasopharynx,
it becomes the job of the secondary defense system—in this
case, consisting largely of professional phagocytes—to clear
them. The polysaccharide capsule plays the predominant role
in preventing ingestion and killing by phagocytic cells, mainly
because it hides the Fc of IgG (ubiquitous in humans) that reacts with cell wall and the C3b that is fixed during that reaction or by the alternative complement pathway. Surface protein
A (PspA) may also contribute to resistance to uptake.

The antigenic nature of capsular polysaccharide has been
used historically to identify pneumococci. With the recent addition of seven new serotypes, a total of 90 are now recognized.

Close relatedness of certain types has led to the concept of
serogroups of which there are now 21. Within each group, the
initial type identified is called F (for first), and subsequent ones
are A, B, etc.; thus, group 7 includes types 7F, 7A, 7B, etc. Exceptions to this nomenclature include group 6 (consisting of
types 6A and 6B) and group 9 (consisting of types 9A, 9L, 9N
and 9V).

Although laboratories have traditionally identified pneumococci by the capsular polysaccharide phenotype, there appear
to be variants, both natural and laboratory-induced, that contain the genetic characteristics of one type, yet with the capsule
of another type. Capsular "switching" has been observed between serotypes 23F and 6B and 23F and 19F. For example,
certain clinical isolates are typed as 19F or 6B, but have the genetic fingerprint of the multidrug resistant type 23 clone first
recognized in Europe. This suggests the occurrence in nature
of transfer of genetic material among pneumococci. Still unex-
plained is the interesting observation that the virulence of certain laboratory mutants has been determined by the transformed
organism, not by the capsule; perhaps the interaction between
complement and surface proteins is responsible.

Differences in the interactions with complement help to explain biologic differences among different pneumococcal
serotypes. Even in the absence of antibody, the C3 component
of complement deposits on capsule; a 10-kD segment of the alpha chain of C3 is cleaved, exposing a thioester site that is essential for covalent binding. Pneumococci make proteins that
rapidly degrade C3b. Proteins of *S. pneumoniae* types 3 and 4
degrade C3b to iC3d, which is well recognized by CR2 on B
cells but not by polymorphonuclear leukocytes, whereas types
6A and 14 cleave C3b to iC3b, which readily interacts with the
complement receptor CR3 on PMN but not with CR2. Thus,
capsules of *S. pneumoniae* types 3 and 4 are potent immunogens although in the absence of antibody to capsule, these organisms are poorly ingested, whereas types 6A and 14 are readily ingested but are poor immunogens. These observations help
explain differences in the susceptibility of various serotypes to
phagocytosis by PMN or macrophages and perhaps differences
in virulence, as well.

PspA, which extends through the cell wall from attachments
to choline residues of lipoteichoic acid within cell membranes,
also appears to contribute to resistance to ingestion. Antibodies to PspA confer some degree of protection in mice. In fact,
despite a fair amount of molecular diversity (which can be used
as a marker for pneumococcal clones), antibodies to one PspA
seem to be widely cross-protective within the species.

OTHER VIRULENCE FACTORS

The virulence potential of a number of pneumococcal substances have been studied extensively. For example, pneumolysin contributes to the inflammatory response and also damages mammalian cells. This protein stimulates release of tumor
necrosis factor (TNF) and interleukins by macrophages, binds
IgG nonspecifically to active the complement cascade and activates phospholipase A_2 in endothelial cells, thus stimulating
inflammation. At the same time, pneumolysin damages cells
and, in doing so, inhibits an effective host response. Related
properties include the capacities to lyse cell membranes by

punching large holes at cholesterol-containing sites; inhibit random or directed migration, respiratory burst and bactericidal capacity of PMN and monocytes; and reduce IgG synthesis by B-lymphocytes. In the lungs, pneumolysin inhibits ciliary action (a similar effect on hair cells might help to explain deafness in pneumococcal meningitis) and increases vascular permeability by damaging vascular endothelium. Higher levels of antibody to pneumolysin at the time of hospitalization for pneumococcal pneumonia are inversely associated with the severity of the infection.

Autolysin contributes to tissue damage by lysing pneumococci and releasing damaging substances. Mutants that lack pneumolysin or autolysin have reduced virulence, and antibody to either of these substances is partially protective. The observation that antibodies to autolysin do not reduce disease in experimental animals infected by pneumolysin-deficient mutants suggests that the principal virulence effect of autolysin is to release pneumolysin from pneumococci. The neuraminidase of *S. pneumoniae* may also contribute to pathogenicity as shown by reduction of virulence with anti-neuraminidase antibody. Although a gene knockout of neuraminidase A does not alter virulence, it is thought that a compensatory increase in neuraminidase B is responsible. Finally, while the mechanism is not clear, pneumococcal hyaluronidase may contribute to the process of mucosal invasion.

Pneumococci grow in chains, dividing at an equatorial zone, a site for numerous events in the life-cycle of pneumococcus. The presence of choline in this zone is crucial for autolysin-mediated remodeling that leads to cell division and PspA release. Growth in the absence of choline (e.g., with ethanolamine as a substitute) leads to long chains that are not susceptible to autolysin and do not release PspA or divide normally. Substances make their way into or are extruded from the pneumococcus, and enzymes, either autolytic or bacteriophage-produced, act at these sites. In fact, phages in the Cp and Dp series act only at choline-containing sites in the equatorial zone; the genes encoding their autolytic enzymes closely resemble the genes of pneumococcus that control autolysin.

The lytic enzymes of pneumococcus have a modular design that evolved, presumably to enable pneumococcus to survive in its own ecological niche. It remains unclear what proportion of clinical pneumococcal isolates carry bacteriophages; there is a possibility that the capacity of bacteriophages to attach pneumococcus may eventually be clinically useful by identifying a surface point for attack by a novel antibacterial substance.

SUSCEPTIBILITY TO INFECTION

For reasons that remain unclear, the incidence of pneumococcal disease may be increasing in developed countries and remain high in developing ones. HIV infection has recently been added to the traditional list of susceptible persons, which includes people who are malnourished, alcoholics, diabetics, and those with hepatic or renal insufficiency, myeloma, and lymphoma. The incidence of pneumococcal pneumonia is >100-fold increased in men with AIDS when compared with non–HIV-infected persons of similar age; in certain communities, the proportion of young adult males with pneumococcal pneumonia who have HIV infection is so high (perhaps 40%)

that such infection should prompt an HIV antibody test. The mechanism for the susceptibility is thought principally to be diminished IgG responses.

Certain groups such as Native Americans (including Eskimos) and African-Americans have a higher incidence of pneumococcal disease. Bacteremic pneumococcal infection is highly associated with the R131 allele of FcγRIIa, a surface receptor on PMN that recognizes Fc of IgG2 but binds poorly when compared to the H131 form. The capacity to respond to capsular polysaccharide vaccine is inherited as a codominant trait. Although the racial and ethnic associations remain to be elucidated, similarly deficient responses to the PRP capsule of *H. influenzae* are thought to be associated with Ig allotype.

The frequency with which certain serotypes cause disease varies dramatically from one era and one country to another, precluding grand generalizations about the relation between serotype and, for example, socioeconomic factors. For example, studies in Israel have suggested that *S. pneumoniae* serotype 1 affects groups that live in primitive conditions rather than urban dwellers; in the United States, this type has not been implicated in more than 2% of cases of pneumococcal disease in decades. Nevertheless, type 1 is a very important cause of invasive disease among children in developing countries and, surprisingly, it has recently re-emerged as the most common cause of adult pneumococcal disease in Denmark, accounting for 15% of bacteremic cases. Some serotypes, such as 2, that were major causes of disease 50 years ago have nearly disappeared. Reasons for these fluctuations are unknown.

PNEUMOCOCCAL SEPSIS

S. pneumoniae is the most common gram positive organism to cause community-acquired septicemia and death. The incidence of serious pneumococcal infection has risen in locations where its prevalence has been carefully studied during the past few decades. The death rate is age-related, increasing from <2% among bacteremic children to 40–50% in older adults, and has not changed since the early antibiotic era.

Lethality in pneumococcal sepsis results from stimulation of interleukin 1, 6, and 8 and TNF, and activation of a number of cascades, including (but not limited to) coagulation and complement pathways, together with vessel injury pathways. Peptidoglycan is largely responsible for stimulating these pathways. The conical conformation of this molecule is thought to be important, since similarly constituted, but cylindrical molecules have no such effects.

Like lipopolysaccharide, soluble peptidoglycan seems to interact wtih macrophages at the CD14 receptor; not surprisingly, muramyl dipeptide, a well-known activator of macrophages, is central to this reaction, although other macrophage receptors may play a lesser role. When interleukin production is stimulated (for example by viral infection), internalization of peptidoglycan constituents may increase, potentiating this series of events. *In vitro*, it requires 1,000 times more peptidoglycan than lipopolysaccharide to activate macrophages; this finding may be an artifact of the experimental model, since smaller fragments as they occur in nature may be both more numerous and more active. Antibodies that have sufficient affinity to peptidoglycan to block this effect have not been identified, and substances that interact with CD-14 have not prevented death from advanced pneumococcal infection. The belief remains, however, that administration of some substances such as antagonists of platelet-activating factor, CD14, antibody to interleukins, TNF, cyclooxygenase inhibitors, or glucocorticosteroids will eventually be shown to inhibit the progression of the cascade with its lethal consequences.

The interaction of phosphocholine and the receptor for platelet-activating factor may also contribute to the physiologic alterations of sepsis. Sugars, such as lacto-*N*-neotetraose, that block the interaction with the receptor for platelet-activating factor seem to modify the evolution of experimental pneumococcal infection of any serotype even after infection has been initiated.

By disrupting bacteria, antimicrobial therapy may initially increase the ill effects of the bacteria on the host. Based on theoretical considerations outlined above and experiments in rabbits, some experts recommend administration of glucocorticoids 30 min prior to antibiotics, especially when treating meningitis, though studies done to date have been inconclusive.

SOME USES OF ANIMAL MODELS

Investigations into both the pathogenesis and the treatment of otitis media and meningitis have benefited greatly from the availability of animal models. Local and systemic immune responses are seen after direct inoculation of the middle ear of rats with pneumococci, enabling local and humoral responses to be compared. In infant rats or in mice, it is possible to titrate the precise amount of IgG to a pneumococcal capsular polysaccharide that needs to be given systemically to protect against a known challenge dose of *S. pneumoniae*. Such experiments have helped to validate ELISAs currently in use to measure antibodies to pneumococcal capsular polysaccharides Protection against colonization has also been shown by passive administration of immune globulin, an observation consistent with observed effects of vaccination against pneumococcal or *Haemophilus* infection. Use of the rabbit model of meningitis has given direct evidence for participation by C5A, TNF, IL-1, and IL-6 in the inflammatory process and has helped to identify cell wall components as the principal mediators of the process. Interferon, IL-1, and IL-6 all contribute to increased permeability of the blood-brain barrier, but it is unclear whether this is a direct mechanism or a result of the inflammation. Nitrous oxide production may also play a role.

Administration of penicillin to chinchillas with pneumococcal otitis media initially causes a great increase in the number of white blood cells in middle ear fluid. This increase is blunted in pneumolysin-deficient mutants and is absent in autolysin-deficient ones, thus supporting other studies that evaluate the contribution to pathogenesis of these virulence factors.

ANTIBIOTIC RESISTANCE

Certainly, the biggest news in pneumococcal infection in the 1980s and 1990s was the emergence, selection, and global spread of antibiotic-resistant strains of *S. pneumoniae*. Early recognition of a major problem was in countries, such as Spain and Hungary, where antibiotics are readily available without prescription. Certain clones seem to have had a special capacity to spread thanks to world travel. However, overuse of antibiotics worldwide has selected for antibiotic resistance.

PENICILLIN-BINDING PROTEINS

The cell membrane of *S. pneumoniae* contains enzymes (transpeptidases) that create ala-ala cross linking of peptidoglycan. Beta-lactam compounds bind these enzymes at their active sites, thereby preventing them from fulfilling their contribution to cell wall formation. Because these enzymes are identifiable by their interaction with radiolabeled penicillin, they have been called penicillin-binding proteins (PBPs). Five have been well described: 1A, 1B, 2A, 2B, 2X. In strains from the 1940s, these PBPs are saturable with very low concentrations of penicillin (≤ 0.002 μg/mL). Alterations in these enzymes occur in the laboratory as a result of exposure to stepwise increases in penicillin; pneumococci that are bred in this fashion end up with enzymes that have greatly reduced affinity for penicillin and, therefore, appear to be penicillin resistant. This same sequence may occur in nature although, as shall be discussed below, acquisition of an entire package ("cassette") of DNA that confers broad resistance to a number of antimicrobial agents seems to be more commonly responsible. An increasing number of pneumococcal strains cultured from ill patients have acquired varying degrees of resistance to penicillin. Current isolates that are not inhibited by 0.002 μg/mL, but are inhibited by 0.06 μg/mL penicillin have probably already undergone some alteration in the PBPs.

Changes in PBP 1A and 2A probably explain low-level (intermediate) penicillin decreased susceptibility; higher levels of resistance to penicillin requires alterations of PBPs 1A, 2X, and 2B. In contrast, higher level resistance to third generation cephalosporins (cefotaxime and ceftriaxone) probably result from altered PBPs 1A and 2X alone. Examination of antibiotic saturation and other chemico-physical properties enable similarities to be sought among pneumococcal isolates. Crystallographic analysis of PBP 2x reveals unique properties of the three domains where penicillin is bound and shows changes in these domains that are associated with resistance. Mutations in other genes (such as ciaH and ciaR) may also lead to resistance by mechanisms that do not involve PBPs.

Laboratory-induced penicillin-resistant pneumococci have altered peptidoglycan composition. The proportion of monomer peptides relative to cross-linked dipeptides is greatly elevated. Also alanine-serine bridging replaces alanine-alanine bridging at some sites. It is uncertain whether these changes merely occur as a result of the changes in PBPs—whether they are part of the price paid by the bacteria for acquiring resistance—or whether they actually contribute to the penicillin resistance. The physiologic significance of these changes, and the extent to which they occur in naturally emerging penicillin-resistant strains remains to be fully elucidated. It has been hypothesized that acquisition of altered PBP genes, while enabling pneumococci to thrive in environments where penicillin and other antimicrobials are ever-present, might have a "cost" to the resistant organism that would diminish its capacity to compete if the selective pressure was removed; however, thus far no substantial costs of acquiring resistance has been shown for *S. pneumoniae.*

Resistance to tetracycline generally reflects the acquisition of the tet M gene on a transposon, for example Tn*916*-Tn*1545.* The precise mechanism by which the resistance is expressed is still not fully known. There appears to be substantial variability among strains in the tet M allele, in contrast to a single allele for chloramphenicol acetyl transferase and two alleles for the gene that encodes erythromycin resistance.

"Competence" is the term used to describe the capacity to take up DNA from the environment. The notable competence of pneumococci is due to a 41-kD protein called competence-stimulating peptide (CSP) that acts as a pheromone; when a certain population density is reached, the gene *comC* or the closely related *comA* (others use different terminology, calling these genes *comC1* and *comC2*, respectively) is upregulated leading to increased production of competence stimulating protein. All pneumococci have *comA* and/or *comC* genes. Upregulation is demonstrable in about two-thirds of isolates studied to date, with no apparent relation between serotype and competence. Once DNA is taken into the pneumococcus, assimilation of the donor strand is mediated by the *recA* gene.

Antimicrobial resistance may first have been selected among other streptococcal species such as *Streptococcus mitis* and *S. oralis,* organisms that acquired (from an unknown source) genetic material that encodes resistance to a broad array of antibiotics including penicillin, trimethoprim/sulfamethoxazole and erythromycin, as well as heavy metals and other substances. The remarkable competence of pneumococci enabled them to incorporate an entire "cassette" of this genetic information. The result is that antimicrobial-resistant pneumococci contain DNA sequences that closely resemble those in other streptococci and that resistance to a similarly broad array of antimicrobial substances.

EPIDEMIOLOGY OF ANTIBIOTIC RESISTANCE AMONG PNEUMOCOCCI

The emergence of antibiotic resistance has been studied in many countries. In Spain, the proportion of pneumococci intermediate to penicillin (MIC, 0.1–1.0 μg/mL) or with resistance (MIC $\geq$ 2 μg/mL) rose from 6% to 38% and 0% to 6%, respectively, since 1979. Certain adult populations, especially persons with AIDS who are on nearly constant treatment with trimethoprim/sulfamethoxazole have a particular high likelihood of carrying resistant strains, as has been shown in Houston, Texas. In Atlanta, Georgia, a network for examining every invasive isolate of *S. pneumoniae* has documented that nearly one-half of isolates are intermediate or resistant to penicillin, including 15% that are resistant. High-level cefotaxime resistance was detected in 8% of isolates recently among the Atlanta isolates. These numbers have increased substantially since 1994. It is hoped that efforts of the Centers for Disease Control, organized into surveillance, epidemiologic investigation, prevention, and control components, will help to contain the further spread of drug resistance in *S. pneumoniae.*

Antimicrobial-resistant pneumococci emanate from day-care centers or their equivalents, where close physical contact of young children, facilitated by intercurrent viral infection that causes rhinitis, and excessive—in some cases, constant—antibiotic use by a remarkably high proportion of attendees create perfect conditions for breeding, selecting, and spreading resistant mutants. Thus, the rapid increase in antibiotic-resistant *S. pneumoniae* is multifactorial, related to the introduction of resistant strains into the community and the spontaneous emergence of newly resistant strains, together with conditions that enhance spread and selection.

Educating physicians and the public in Iceland as to the need for more conservative antibiotic use may have begun to limit the spread and reduce the incidence of resistant strains in that country. An extremely low incidence of antibiotic resistance in the Netherlands may be due to societal norms that include much less use of day care and more limited (or better directed) antibiotic therapy for otitis media. In Sweden, where the proportion of pneumococci that are resistant is low, children who are pneumococcal carriers are sent home if they are sneezing and coughing, thereby reducing the likelihood of spread. Thus, lessons can be learned from those countries that have had lower rates of antibiotic resistance among pneumococci.

Parallel experience with the spread of methicillin-resistant *Staphylococcus aureus* teaches us that these experiences are not unique to *S. pneumoniae.* With both of these organisms, we are dealing with bacteria that are carried in the nares or nasopharynx by healthy persons and are spread by close personal contact among human beings. Persons may be colonized for weeks, months, or years, and accessibility of rapid worldwide travel suggests that spread will eventually occur. The preeminence of methicillin-resistant *S. aureus* in hospitals shows the importance of spread by close contact and selection by antibiotic use.

IMPLICATIONS FOR THERAPY

Pulmonary infection

Pneumonia in adults or children caused by intermediately resistant strains is still successfully treated with "ordinary" (post-1980) doses of penicillin such as 2–3 million units every 4–6 h or ampicillin/amoxicillin 1 g every 6 h. Reasonable alternatives in adults include cefotaxime 1 g every 6 h or ceftriaxone 1 g every 24 h. Pneumonia due to organisms that are resistant to penicillin may still respond to high dose penicillin (3–4 million units every 4 h), although it seems more reasonable to use cefotaxime or ceftriaxone as noted above. When pneumococci are resistant to these cephalosporins as well as to penicillin, it is still possible that the disease will be cured by higher doses (*e.g.,* 2 g cefotaxime every 6 h or 1 g ceftriaxone every 12 h). Because pneumonia due to organisms inhibited by 1–2 μg/mL penicillin has responded as well as more susceptible strains, there may be a redefinition of susceptibility based on the site infected and pharmacokinetic considerations. Thus when *S. pneumoniae* causes meningitis, present definitions would apply but, in cases of pneumonia, sensitive organisms would have MIC $\leq$ 1 μg/mL intermediate = 2 μg/mL, and resistant $\geq$ 4 μg/mL for penicillin, cefotaxime or ceftriaxone. Amoxicillin is probably somewhat more active than penicillin, although a similar definition will probably be adopted. A quinolone or vancomycin could be used for patients who are allergic to beta-lactams. Vancomycin is the only one of these drugs that is uniformly effective against pneumococci at the time of this writing.

The problem is, of course, that the susceptibility is not known when treatment is begun. Empiric therapy can be selected based on the resistance patterns in the community and the severity of disease. However, the use of vancomycin is discouraged unless organisms are proven to be resistant to other antibiotics. In the United States, the attempt to limit the emergence of vancomycin resistance has restricted the use of this drug to situations in which infection is caused by an organism that will not respond to other treatments. The progressive spread of antimicrobial resistance among pneumococci will certainly strain infection control efforts to limit use of vancomycin.

Otitis media

Therapy for pneumonia due to intermediately or even highly resistant strains remains successful because the respiratory tract is an open system in which intimate contact with serum constituents allows instant access for high concentrations of antibiotic and drainage via the bronchial tree allow for constant clearance. Otitis media is more of a problem for several reasons: (a) it occurs in a closed space and therefore is more dependent upon achieving bactericidal concentrations; (b) the accumulation of antibiotics may be altered by pressure; (c) pneumococci are more likely to be intermediately or highly resistant; and (d) the treating physician usually does not know the causative organism because tympanic membrane puncture is not routinely done. Most authorities have continued to recommend amoxicillin at 80 mg/kg/day in 2–3 divided doses, although others feels that the prevalence of beta-lactamase production among *Haemophilus* and *Moraxella* mandates addition of clavulanic acid or alternate therapy. Giving one-half of the amoxicillin in a form that includes a beta-lactamase inhibitor will reduce the side-effects and the expense without reducing efficacy. If this fails, ceftriaxone can be given parenterally 1 g daily. If there is not a rapid response, health-care providers should give immediate consideration to collecting middle ear fluid (by myringotomy) to document the etiologic pathogen and determine drug susceptibility.

Meningitis

Meningitis due to *S. pneumoniae* should be treated from the start with cefotaxime 2 g q 6 h or ceftriaxone 2 g q 12 h. Many experts support the addition of vancomycin, pending antimicrobial susceptibility testing. Pneumococcal meningitis is sufficiently dangerous and rare that empiric use of vancomycin pending susceptibility results will not adversely affect antibiotic susceptibility patterns. Also controversial in treating meningitis is the addition of rifampin which *in vitro* appears to inhibits the bactericidal effect of penicillins, but which in limited studies of rabbits and infected humans may have appeared to offer some benefit.

PREVENTION

Concern over emerging resistance has stimulated research into prevention of infection. Pneumococcal capsular polysaccharides stimulate antibody responses in healthy adults of all ages, and a number of studies have shown efficacy of pneumococcal polysaccharide vaccine particularly for preventing pneumococcal bacteremia among immunocompetent patients at risk for disease (particularly the elderly). Some authorities continue, however, to question its efficacy in populations that are at highest risk, such as immunosuppressed patients. If such persons are not protected, it is unclear whether (a) their antibody levels are not high enough; (b) antibody declines at a much faster rate; (c) antibody of poor avidity for the pneumococcus is responsible; or (d) other factors relating to their health are more important determinants of outcome than the level of anticapsular antibody in their bloodstream. Not surprisingly, persons who have defects in IgG production, such as those infected with HIV (particularly late in the course of HIV infection), or persons with lymphoma or myeloma have diminished responses to pneumococcal vaccination although it still seems reasonable to vaccinate them and to repeat vaccination (at least once) after an interval of 5 years.

Polysaccharide vaccines are well recognized to be poorly antigenic in children under the age of 2 years because bacterial polysaccharides produce T-cell–independent responses. Conjugation of *H. influenzae* type b capsule (PRP) to one of several proteins has generated a spectacularly successful immunogen; serious disease due to this organism has been nearly eradicated in countries with good vaccine programs.

Conjugate pneumococcal vaccines have been developed using at least three different carrier proteins and doses of capsular polysaccharide ranging from 1 to 10 μg/ml. Thus far, it has been possible to include only a limited number (seven to nine) of serotype-specific capsular polysaccharides in conjugate vaccines currently being evaluated. One problem is that the serotype distribution varies geographically and temporally; as noted above, the serotype distribution for children in developing countries tends to be somewhat different than for those in developed countries: serotypes 1 and 5 are important types in developing countries and less so in developed settings (except as noted recently in Denmark). Some serotypes (6B, 14, 19F, 23F), however, are common causes of invasive diseases in all settings and these types are also most frequently associated with drug resistance. Thus, an ideal vaccine would include types prevalent globally (covering 60–80% of invasive pneumococcal disease), avoiding the complication of developing and licensing multiple vaccines for different settings (which would likely have severely adverse effects on costs of the vaccine).

A series of three vaccinations successfully induces antibody production in children under the age of 2 and is expected to reduce the incidence of pneumococcal otitis, pneumonia, and meningitis. Some studies in toddlers have shown a reduction in pneumococcal carriage. The use of conjugate vaccines in adults has not been so promising. Whereas protein-conjugated PRP leads to vastly higher antibody levels in adults when compared with PRP alone, conjugated pneumococcal polysaccharides have often induced antibody levels that are not as high as those that follow nonconjugate vaccine. This could be due to the fact that the total amount of polysaccharide administered is lower for conjugate vaccines (1–5 μg) than it is for nonconjugated vaccines (25 μg). Evaluations of conjugate vaccines are now underway in several settings for their efficacy in preventing a variety of conditions, including pneumococcal otitis media, pneumonia, and invasive pneumococcal disease.

There is some suggestion that a single (priming) dose of conjugate vaccine followed by a (boosting) dose of polysaccharide vaccine will stimulate higher antibody levels than polysaccharide vaccine alone. This was shown in one study of persons with Hodgkins' disease but not confirmed in elderly subjects or those with HIV infection. Even if this kind of schedule of administration were to be successful, knowing how difficult it has been to get adults vaccinated, it is probably impractical to develop vaccines for adults that require administration of two or more doses.

Because the number of serotypes that can be included in a conjugate vaccine will always be limited and account for only a proportion of pneumococci that could potentially cause disease, there is great interest in studying species wide antigens that could potentially induce protective immunity against all pneumococci. PspA, pneumolysin, and the 37-kD (PsaA) are being evaluated in animal models as vaccine candidates. Potential problems include whether enough cell wall antigens are exposed (due to presence of capsular material) to allow antibodies against them to protect against disease. Additional consideration is whether these immunogenic proteins could be combined into a multicomponent vaccine or whether they could be used as carrier proteins in a capsular polysaccharide-conjugate vaccine.

The theoretical benefits of mucosal immunization, for example by intranasal insufflation of pneumococcal polysaccharides deserve more intensive study. A vigorous local immune response might provide the best protection in all regards against pneumococcal infection. Even the development of temperature-sensitive mutants might eventually be possible.

REMAINING QUESTIONS

So many questions remain to be answered; many have not yet even been addressed. In addition to all those cited above in the text summarizing this colloquium, other areas that warrant investigation include the nature of acquisition of colonization (droplet spread versus direct contact) and the kind of separation that might reduce spread of pneumococci; whether some strains have a special advantage to spread globally and what that advantage might involve; changes that occur at a molecular level when a passaged pneumococcus becomes increasingly virulent; the importance of g proteins in activating cell receptors (such as platelet activating factor), thereby contributing to increased disease; mechanisms by which tight cellular junctions of the normal blood-brain barrier become attenuated during meningitis and the possible further role of pinocytosis; the mechanism for the antibacterial action of tetracycline; and whether antibiotic resistant pneumococci have diminished virulence.

A critically important area that is not addressed in this volume is the development of diagnostic tests for pneumococcal disease. It is the absence of rapid, sensitive, and specific diagnostic tests that is responsible for the widespread use of empiric antimicrobial drugs that is driving the spread of antimicrobial resistance. Having useful diagnostic tests available would target antimicrobial therapy, reducing costs, and would add substantial precision to epidemiologic studies of pneumococcal disease, particularly those designed to evaluate prevention modalities such as vaccine use. It is hoped that the increasing understanding of the molecular biology of *S. pneumoniae* will lead to development of useful methods for better documenting its clinical impact.

In light of the global importance of *S. pneumoniae* as a cause of illness, sequelae, and death, and the emergence of drug resistance that is making these infections more difficult to treat successfully, it is time for a concerted effort to apply scientific advances to overcoming obstacles of critical clinical and public health importance. As a beginning toward this goal, it is hoped that this volume will be of value. It blends observations arising out of scientific exploration and intellectual curiosity with issues of intense public health significance. Because of space limitations, only a fraction of those contributing to the science of *S. pneumoniae* are included; nonetheless, the depth of research to better define its molecular biology, pathophysiology, and epidemiology is impressive. Sharing of information will undoubtedly spark additional investigations and achievements until we have effective solutions to the urgent emerging problems of pneumococcal disease.

Address reprints requests to:
Daniel M. Musher
Room 4B-370
Veterans Affairs Medical Center
2002 Holcombe Blvd.
Houton, TX 77030-4211

Index

Page numbers in *italics* indicate figures. Page numbers followed by "t" indicate tables.